Practical Manual of
Physical Medicine
and Rehabilitation

Diagnostics, Therapeutics, and Basic Problems

Practical Manual of
Physical Medicine and Rehabilitation

Diagnostics, Therapeutics, and Basic Problems

Jackson C. Tan, M.D., P.T., Ph.D.
Adjunct Assistant Clinical Professor
Rusk Institute of Rehabilitation Medicine
New York University Medical Center
New York, NY and
Medical Director
Occupational and Rehabilitation Center
Jacksonville, Florida

EDITORIAL CONSULTANT:
Sheila E. Horn, D.O.
Assistant Clinical Professor
Rusk Institute of Rehabilitation Medicine
New York University Medical Center
New York, NY and
Associate Medical Director
The New York Times
New York, NY

ILLUSTRATORS:
Jackson C. Tan, M.D., P.T., Ph.D.
and Cristina Burwell

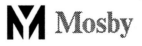 Mosby

St. Louis Baltimore Boston Carlsbad Chicago Minneapolis New York Philadelphia Portland
London Milan Sydney Tokyo Toronto

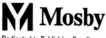

Mosby
Dedicated to Publishing Excellence

A Times Mirror Company

Vice President and Publisher: Anne S. Patterson
Executive Editor: Robert Hurley
Associate Developmental Editor: Marla Sussman
Project Manager: Chris Baumle
Production Editor: Eric Van Gorden
Designer: Carolyn O'Brien
Manufacturing Manager: William A. Winneberger, Jr.

Printed in the United States of America
Composition by Maryland Composition
Printing/binding by R. R. Donnelley

Mosby-Year Book, Inc.
11830 Westline Industrial Drive
St. Louis, Missouri 63146

Library of Congress Cataloging in Publication Data

Tan, Jackson C.
    Practical manual of physical medicine & rehabilitation :
diagnostics, therapeutics, and basic problems / by Jackson C. Tan ;
editor, Sheila E. Horn: illustrators, Jackson C. Tan and Cristina
Burwell.
        p. cm.
    Includes bibliographical references and index.
    ISBN 0-8151-8708-4
    1. Physical therapy—Handbooks, manuals, etc.   2. Medical
rehabilitation—Handbooks, manuals, etc.   I. Horn, Sheila E.
II. Title.   III. Title: Practical manual of physical medicine and
rehabilitation.
    [DNLM: 1. Physical Medicine—handbooks.   2. Rehabilitation—
handbooks. WB 39 T161p 1998]
    RM701.T36   1998
    615.8'2—DC21
    DNLM/DLC
    for Library of Congress   97-22255
                                                                    CIP

98 99 00 01 02/9 8 7 6 5 4 3 2 1

This book is dedicated to the late *Howard A. Rusk, M.D.,* who started a wonderful legacy for the care of the disabled, and to all physiatrists, who together with other members of the rehabilitation team, continue to enrich and ennoble this legacy.

I dedicate this book, with love and gratitude, to
Un Beng Tan and *Ah Wan Chio,* my parents, who gave me the spark of life,
Margareta Nordin, P.T., Dr.Sci., who ignited in me the spark of writing,
Sheila Horn, D.O., whose encouragement and invaluable insight nurtured my spark
    of writing,
Rev. Cynthia Heller, whose spiritual wisdom gave soul to my spark of writing,
Nancy Kress, whose imagination gave the wings of flight to my spark of writing,
and my niece, *Merry June Grace Tan,* and nephew, *Fred Gerald Tan,* who are the
    sparks of the future.

FOREWORD

Over the past fifty years the speciality of physical medicine and rehabilitation (PM&R) has grown exponentially. We have seen an increased interest in alternative medicine and a more informed public. With the graying of America, increases in managed care, sicker patients, and shorter hospitalizations, it is imperative that physiatrists keep abreast with the current milieu of practice and its changing views. In these rapidly-changing times, physiatrists must adapt and serve as the primary guardians of the disabled.

The genesis of this book commenced when Dr. Tan was in residency training. Dr. Tan is certainly qualified to write this book because of his unique background in clinical medicine as well as in research and teaching. Aside from being a physiatrist, he is also a physical therapist and has a Ph.D. in physical therapy.

Although this book is not meant to replace other major comprehensive textbooks, it is a handy, concise, and practical resource for residents, practicing clinicians, and allied health practitioners who have to juggle the patient's clinical, social, and financial issues in their fast-paced practices.

This book deals not only with diagnostic tools but primarily with practical therapeutic tools, including physical modalities, pharmacotherapeutics, and injection therapies. It also deals with the diagnosis and management of basic clinical problems commonly encountered in PM&R. Knowledge of these basic problems can be applied to the management of most adult and geriatric PM&R cases in both in- and outpatient settings.

Each of the book's chapters are classified and outlined for easy reading and for easy referencing. At the end of the book is a useful mini-atlas of normal radiographic and MRI films. Also included is a compilation of useful PM&R resources.

It is auspicious that this book's publication coincides with the 50th anniversary of the Rusk Institute of Rehabilitation Medicine. Thousands of physicians and therapists have received their training here at the Rusk Institute and we are proud of their contributions to the medical literature and the clinical care they have rendered throughout the world.

One of the first major comprehensive textbooks of PM&R was from the Rusk Institute (Rusk HA, editor: *Rehabilitation Medicine*, St. Louis, 1958, C.V. Mosby) and I had the privilege of having contributed to its subsequent editions. At present, I am proud to have the privilege of contributing the foreword for this practical manual of PM&R written by a Rusk-trained physician. Dr. Tan represents the next generation of physiatrists who will continue Dr. Rusk's legacy of excellence and achievement and carry the torch into the next millennium.

Mathew H.M. Lee, M.D., M.P.H., F.A.C.P.
Professor and Director
Rusk Institute of Rehabilitation Medicine
New York University Medical Center

PREFACE

*"Knowledge is of two kinds. We know a subject ourselves, or we know where
we can find information upon it."*
—*Samuel Johnson*

In the past few decades, the field of physical medicine and rehabilitation (PM&R) has grown so drastically that it seems impossible for one practitioner to reasonably tackle each subject matter with cutting-edge quality. However, the knowledge explosion in PM&R has been coupled with the advancement of computer technology and the increased accessibility of excellent textbooks, journals, videotapes, and conferences in PM&R and related fields. Thus, given these circumstances, it has become possible for one person with a unique background in physiatry, physical therapy, research, teaching, and computer technology to write a medical textbook with the desired cutting-edge quality.

The concept of a single-authorship is an illusion. The material contained in this book is based on published and unpublished knowledge that I learned from other authorities in the field. Moreover, each chapter has been reviewed and critiqued by different experts and I incorporated their suggestions, which improved the chapters they reviewed. Indeed, as shown in the acknowledgments, it took a global community to write this book.

Instead of "single-author," a more accurate description of this textbook would be "single-style." One of the main advantages of a single-style book is that the author can ensure a consistent quality and style throughout the book. The individual chapters can also be easily integrated and cross-referenced so that the whole book becomes greater than the sum of its parts.

This manual is designed to be portable, concise, practical, and user-friendly with the intention of supplementing (not replacing) other major, comprehensive textbooks of PM&R. It is written for the ever-busy, modern practitioner of PM&R whose reading time may be severely limited and who needs a quick reference source in the clinics. Although the primary target audience of this book is physiatrists, nevertheless physicians in other medical specialities (e.g., gerontology, family practice, internal medicine, rheumatology, neurology, orthopedics, and neurosurgery) as well as allied health practitioners (e.g., physical and occupational therapists, speech-language pathologists, prosthetists, orthotists, nurses, nutritionists, psychologists, social workers, and vocational counselors) will benefit from these pages, especially in facilitating communication with physiatrists.

Although other portable PM&R books have been published recently, this book has the following features, which distinguish it from other books:

- Tight, strict, and practical classification of subject matters, with each chapter written in an outline format for easy understanding, easy cross-referencing, and easy retention;
- In-depth concise coverage of basic clinical problems in PM&R with emphasis on practical and conservative diagnostic and therapeutic measures, the knowledge of which are essential in managing most of the cases seen in PM&R;

- A section on treatment modalities, which includes not only the traditional PM&R modalities but also pharmacologic and injection therapies;
- Extensive use of composite illustrations and tables to clarify the text;
- Appendices that include commonly-used reference values, normal anatomy, and a mini-atlas of normal skeletal radiographs and MRIs of the brain and spine; and
- Updated addresses and phone numbers of information resources for the disabled and for medical and nonmedical professionals taking care of the disabled.

This volume primarily deals with the PM&R care of adult and geriatric patients and does not include pediatric patients. Conceptually, it is divided into five sections. The first part deals with physiatric evaluation, the second part with diagnostic test, the third part with differential diagnoses, the fourth part with therapeutic modalities, pharmacology, and injection therapies, and the fifth part with basic clinical problems in PM&R. By learning how to manage these basic clinical problems, one can practically apply them to any disease encountered in a regular PM&R practice.

The recommendations presented in this manual (some of which may be controversial) are meant to be used as guidelines, not dogmas. These guidelines are certainly not "recipes" of treatment but should be considered "menus" or "tools" from which one can judiciously choose in designing the overall management plan for the patient. In writing this book, every effort has been made to ensure that the recommendations are based upon current standards of practice of PM&R and of medicine.

Although most sections can be read "from beginning to end," other sections (e.g., part 1 on clinical evaluation and part 3 on differential diagnoses) consist of listings intended to be used as a quick reference. To maintain the portable size of the book, the bibliography is kept light-to-moderate and generally cites other major textbooks or review articles, from which a more detailed bibliography can be obtained. Moreover, less emphasis has been placed on pathophysiology and epidemiology, in order to pack in more detail on practical clinical management. Likewise, certain chapters, such as the one on electrodiagnostic tests, were intentionally limited since they are well-covered in other reference manuals. Basic medical knowledge is also presumed to have been learned by the reader during medical school (e.g. how to elicit deep tendon reflexes or test cranial nerves). Emphasis is placed on physiatric procedures, such as how to perform motor point blocks, rather than surgical interventions for the treatment of spasticity.

In this type of book, there is always the difficulty of balancing portability or conciseness with depth of content, in addition to the risk of oversimplification and omission of important details. In writing this book, my dictum has always been to present the most relevant clinical information in a clear, concise, and easy-to-read manner with as much depth as is needed to maintain practicality. Comments from readers are welcomed, as these suggestions will be used to improve subsequent editions.

Perfection is a constantly changing goal,
an unattainable state of mind.
It is the journey that counts.

Jackson C. Tan, M.D., P.T., Ph.D.
New York, NY

ACKNOWLEDGMENTS

"If I have seen further, it is by standing upon the shoulders of Giants."
—*Sir Isaac Newton*

Throughout my life, I have been blessed with the support and grace of my family, friends, and colleagues. They have all given meaning to and enriched my life's journey and work. Without them, this book would have remained unwritten. I am particularly indebted to the following individuals for their help in my arduous writing journey:

- Sheila Horn, D.O., editor extraordinaire and kindred spirit, who read, critiqued, and improved every single chapter from the initial to the final drafts;
- Jung Ahn, M.D. and Horatio Pineda, M.D. (both excellent teachers), and Michelle Stern, M.D. and Conway Chin, D.O. (both friends and former co-residents), who each reviewed and critiqued multiple chapters;
- Arthur Jimenez, M.D., Normal Berger, M.S., Fred Frieden, M.D., Martha Taylor-Sarno, M.A., M.D., Edwin Richter, M.D., Hossein Firooznia, M.D., Joseph DeVito, M.D., Edward Allcock, D.O., Eric Lippman, M.D., David Rodriguez, D.O., Nancy Whyte, O.T.R., and all my other mentors, colleagues, and friends at the New York University Medical Center, as well as Carlos Oteyza, M.D. and Cynthia Eng, M.D. (both friends and colleagues), who each reviewed and critiqued early drafts;
- Ben Willems, M.S., Ali Sheikhzadeh, Ph.D., Nihat Ozkaya, Ph.D., and Dawn Leger, Ph.D., for computer assistance and for writing advice;
- Lourdes Willems, B.A., and Rev. Cynthia Heller, for manuscript preparation;
- Cristina Burwell, for assistance with the illustrations;
- Ronald Cahn, P.T. and Xiang-Bin Kong, M.D., for assistance in acquiring medical literature;
- The staff of the Frederick L. Ehrman Medical Library of the New York University Medical Center (in particular, Arthur Strange) and the Herman Robbins Medical Library of the Hospital for Joint Diseases-Orthopedic Institute (in particular, Claudia Lascar), for courteous and generous services;
- Robert Hurley, Executive Editor of Mosby-Year Book, who believed in my dream and guided it through the reality of the medical publishing world;
- The wonderful staff of Mosby-Year Book, in particular Eric Van Gorden and Marla Sussman, for editorial assistance;
- Mathew Lee, M.D., M.P.H., Bruce Grynbaum, M.D., Howard Thistle, M.D., Lori Garjian, M.D., Laura Dunlop, O.T.R., Charng-Shen Wang, M.S., P.T., Aris Oteyza, R.N., Nelia Jimenez, R.N., the excellent and friendly staff of Occupational and Rehabilitation Center (Jacksonville, FL), and my parents, brothers (Freddie, Stevenson, and Dennis), sister (Marianne), sisters-in-law (Emerald and Jereny), relatives, and other friends and colleagues (both in America and in the Philippines), for moral and emotional support;
- Writers of imaginative literature, for nourishment of the creative soul, and compeers at the S.A.M. (Parent Assembly no. 1) and I.B.M. (Ring no. 26), for moments of true magic and friendship;
- and, last but not least, all my patients who have taught me so much about the art of medicine.

CONTENTS

PART I   **PM&R Clinical Examination**
          1.1   Clinical Evaluation and Documentation, 3

PART II   **PM&R Diagnostic Tests**
          2.1   Laboratory Tests, 23
          2.2   Noninvasive Imaging Studies, 30
          2.3   Invasive Imaging Studies, 38
          2.4   Electrodiagnostic Tests, 44
          2.5   Musculoskeletal and Work-Related Tests, 51
          2.6   Pulmonary Function Tests, 68
          2.7   Exercise Tolerance Testing, 79
          2.8   Functional Assessment Instruments, 95
          2.9   Psychologic Tests, 99

PART III   **PM&R Differential Diagnoses**
          3.1   Differential Diagnoses of Pain, 105
          3.2   Differential Diagnoses of Nonpain Problems, 124

PART IV   **PM&R Management Tools**
          4.1   Physical Modalities, 133
          4.2   Therapeutic Exercises, 156
          4.3   Orthoses, 178
          4.4   Prostheses, 229
          4.5   Adaptations for Activities of Daily Living, 260
          4.6   Gait Aids and Gait Patterns, 283
          4.7   Manual- and Powered-Mobility Systems, 293
          4.8   Pharmacologic Agents, 321
          4.9   Joint and Soft Tissue Injections, 386
          4.10   Nerve Blocks, 401
          4.11   Trigger Point Therapy, 411

PART V   **Basic PM&R Problems**
          5.1   Deconditioning, 425
          5.2   Pressure Ulcers, 431
          5.3   Venous Thromboembolism, 445
          5.4   Spasticity, 460
          5.5   Neurogenic Communication Disorders, 482
          5.6   Dysphagia, 514

5.7   Voiding Dysfunctions, 538
5.8   Bowel Dysfunction, 553
5.9   Problems in Human Sexuality, 580
5.10   Acute and Chronic Pain, 607
5.11   Work-Related Musculoskeletal Problems, 645
5.12   Chronic Pulmonary Problems, 665
5.13   Cardiac Problems, 708

Appendices and Resources

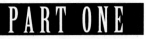

PART ONE

PM&R Clinical Examination

CHAPTER 1.1

CLINICAL EVALUATION AND DOCUMENTATION

Physical medicine and rehabilitation (PM&R) encompasses the diagnosis and treatment of physical and functional disorders involving the neuromuscular, musculoskeletal, and cardiopulmonary systems. PM&R as a specialty was officially sanctioned by the American Board of Medical Specialties in 1947. The shortened name of the specialty is physiatry (from the Greek *physio*, or nature), and its practitioner is called a physiatrist.

Unlike other fields of medicine, the primary concern of PM&R is not the identification and cure of disease. Rather, its primary goal is the patient attaining the fullest physical, psychological, social, vocational, avocational, and educational potential consistent with physiologic or anatomic impairment and environmental limitations. This is achieved by an interdisciplinary team approach consisting of the patient and his or her support system (family or significant others), physiatrist, physical therapist (PT), occupational therapist (OT), psychologist, speech-language pathologist (SLP), rehabilitation nurse, social worker, vocational counselor, recreational therapist (RT), prosthetist-orthotist, nutritionist, and other health professionals involved in the rehabilitation of the patient (e.g., psychiatrist, respiratory therapist, kinesiotherapist or corrective therapist, chaplain, maxillofacial prosthetist, dentist, podiatrist, audiologist, bioengineer, hospital-based or special education teacher, pharmacist, durable medical equipment vendor, child life specialist, horticultural therapist, music therapist, dance therapist, animal-assisted therapy specialist).

To be proficient in functional assessments, the physiatrist must understand the distinctions between impairment, disability, and handicap (as defined by the World Health Organization).

- **Impairment** refers to "any loss or abnormality of psychological, physiological, or anatomical structure or function." It represents the problem at the tissue and organ level. Examples include muscular weakness, limited joint range of motion, pain, and confusion.
- **Disability** refers to "any restriction or lack resulting from an impairment of the ability to perform an activity in the manner or within the range considered normal for a human being." It represents the problem at the whole-person level. Examples include the inability to walk, run, or ski after suffering a stroke.
- **Handicap** refers to "a disadvantage for a given individual, resulting from an impairment or a disability, that limits or prevents the fulfillment of a role that is normal (depending on the age, sex, and social and cultural factors) for that individual." It represents the problem at the societal level. Examples include difficulties with social integration, economic self-sufficiency, and negotiation of architectural barriers (e.g., wheelchair inaccessibility).

The basic elements of a physiatric evaluation are the same as with other medical specialties. Although the emphasis is on the assessment of functions and activities of daily living (ADL), a thorough history taking and physical examination is important for a comprehensive evaluation.

I. History

A. Chief complaint (CC), i.e., reason for seeking physiatric attention. If possible, record in the patient's own words to assess patient's intellect, perception, and concerns about existing illness and dysfunction.

B. Source of information. As much as possible, try to obtain information from the patient. If necessary, the patient's primary caregiver or medical records may corroborate. In patients with communication disorders, such as in a stroke or traumatic brain injury patient, assistance from a family member is needed (if available, a speech therapist would be helpful).

C. History of present illness (HPI), i.e., chronological narrative of the patient's chief complaint. Describe each symptom using the "**O-PP-Q-RR-S-TTT** or **OP²QR²ST³**" mnemonic:

- **O**ther associated manifestations
- **P**rovocative (aggravating) factors
- **P**alliative (relieving) factors
- **Q**uality (character)
- **R**egion (location and extension)
- **R**adiation to a distant site (if present)
- **S**everity (intensity)
- **T**iming (onset, duration, frequency, pattern of involvement, progression)
- **T**ests results
- **T**reatments effects

   In the HPI, record the hand dominance and the functional history (compare current with premorbid functioning). The functional history describes how the chief complaint affects the patient's physical and functional independence at home, at work, or at school. The key functions include self-care (feeding, grooming, bathing, dressing, and toileting), sphincter control (bladder and bowel), mobility/transfers (bed, chair, toilet, and shower), locomotion (ambulation on level-ground and stairs, with or without gait aids; use of mobility devices such as wheelchair; operation of motor vehicles), social cognition (social interaction, problem solving, and memory), and communication. The degree of independence (or dependence) can be briefly described as full independence, modified independence (i.e., with an assistive device or modification of the environment), requiring close or distant supervision by another person, requiring assistance (minimal, moderate, or maximal assistance), or fully dependent.

D. Past history. General state of health, prior hospitalizations (medical, surgical, psychiatric, and rehabilitation), past traumas and accidents, past surgeries, blood transfusions and reactions, vaccinations (flu and pneumococcal), recent travels, past minor and major psychiatric illnesses, and past illnesses (diabetes, hypertension, coronary artery disease, pneumonia, bronchitis, chronic obstructive pulmonary disease, hepatitis, rheumatic fever, cancer). For pediatric patients, include birth history, growth and developmental milestones, significant childhood illnesses, and immunizations.

E. Allergies. Type of allergic reaction to any food, drug, chemicals, or pets.

F. Current medications. All current prescription and nonprescription drugs; record their dose, frequency, and duration.

G. Personal history provides the clinician with opportunity to modify the patient's unhealthy behavior through counseling. Knowing the patient's current and premorbid lifestyle or personality can help in setting realistic rehabilitation goals.

Table 1.1-1.   CAGE questionnaire for screening of alcohol abuse or alcohol dependency

C:	Have you ever felt you ought to **C**ut down on drinking?
A:	Have people **A**nnoyed you by criticizing your drinking?
G:	Have you ever felt bad or **G**uilty about your drinking?
E:	Have you ever had a drink first thing in the morning to steady your nerves or get rid of a hangover (**E**ye-opener)?

Tabulated from Ewing JA: Detecting alcoholism: The CAGE questionnaire; *JAMA* 252: 1905-1907, 1984, copyright © 1984, American Medical Association, with permission.

1. **Life style and habits**
    a. **Avocational (recreational or leisure) interests.** Indoor and outdoor sports (note frequency, duration, and intensity to estimate fitness level), intellectual pursuits, social interactions, organizations, and group functions.
    b. **Diet.** Usual dietary habits, special diets, caffeine use, ability to prepare meals and snacks.
    c. **Cigarette smoking.** Quantity in pack years.
    d. **Recreational drug use.** Depressants, stimulants, opiates, cannabis derivatives, and hallucinogens.
    e. **Sexual history.** Sexual preference, sexual promiscuity, most recent sexual experience.
    f. **Alcohol use.** A "yes" response on the CAGE questionnaire (see Table 1.1-1) is suspicious of alcohol abuse and, therefore, warrants further investigation.
2. **Religious beliefs** relevant to health and rehabilitation.
3. **Premorbid personality** and emotional response to previous illnesses and family troubles.

H. **Social history.** Knowing the patient's home situation and available support systems can help in discharge planning.
    1. **Home situation and architectural barriers.** Owns or rents home, location of home (urban, suburban, or rural), distance between home and rehabilitation facilities, number of outside and inside steps, accessibility to elevator or ramps, availability of space for entry ramps, and accessibility of the kitchen, bath, bedroom, living room, and laundry room. Also ask patient's specific expectations regarding household chores, such as meal preparation, shopping, home maintenance, cleaning, and child-rearing.
    2. **Marriage history and status**
    3. **Family, significant others, support system**

I. **Vocational (and economic) history** helps in retraining patients for possible return to the workforce or in assisting patient in securing alternative employment or gainful activities.
    1. **Educational and training history.** Educational level, abilities, special skills, licenses, and certifications.
    2. **Work and/or military history.** Type and place of work, work environment (include physical barriers at work and use of any special supports or adaptive aids), military service, return-to-work history after previous injury.
    3. **Financial situation, insurance, and litigation.** Sources of income, investments, insurance resources, disability classifications, debts, and litigation status.

J. Family history helps in understanding patient's support structure and in genetic counseling of inheritable disease. Record the age and health status of each immediate family member. If deceased, indicate the age and probable cause of death. Ask for family history of diabetes, heart disease, hypertension, cancer, rheumatic disease (rheumatoid arthritis, osteoarthritis, seronegative spondyloarthropathies, e.g., ankylosing spondylitis), gout, stroke, kidney stones, psychiatric disorders, neuromuscular disorders, or any hereditary conditions.

K. Review of systems (ROS). Carefully screen all the systems for clues to disease (not previously identified in history taking) that may adversely affect the rehabilitation outcome.

1. **General.** Overall state of health, usual weight, recent weight change, sleeping habits, appetite, fever, chills, night sweats, fatigue.

2. **Skin.** Pressure ulcer, rash (with or without sun sensitivity), pruritus, color (or ischemic) changes, pigmentation, nodules.

3. **Lymphatic.** "Swollen glands" or masses in the neck, axilla, groin; lymphedema.

4. **HEENT**
   a. **Head.** Headache, trauma.
   b. **Eyes.** Pain, dryness, conjunctivitis, scotoma.
   c. **Ears.** Earache, ear discharge.
   d. **Nose and sinuses.** Epistaxis, nasal stuffiness or congestion, drainage, sinusitis.
   e. **Mouth and throat.** Condition of teeth, gums, and tongue; last dental examination; mouth disorders (sores, masses, dryness, tightness); sore throat; change in voice.

5. **Breasts.** Pain, history of lumps, bleeding, symmetry, nipple discharge. In female patients, ask if she performs self-examination and note her last mammogram date.

6. **Respiratory.** Cough, sputum (quantity, color), hemoptysis, wheezing, shortness of breath, pain associated with breathing.

7. **Cardiac.** Chest pain, palpitations, dyspnea, orthopnea, paroxysmal nocturnal dyspnea, edema, heart murmurs, history of high blood pressure, syncope, exercise tolerance.

8. **Peripheral vascular.** Varicose veins, thrombophlebitis, claudication, Raynaud's phenomenon.

9. **Gastrointestinal.** Swallowing problems, reflux symptoms, abdominal pain, nausea, vomiting, increased girth, jaundice, blood from mouth or rectum, change in bowel habits (constipation, diarrhea, incontinence), use of laxatives.

10. **Genitourinary.** Dysuria, frequency, urgency, hesitation, nocturia, pyuria, flank pain, hematuria, renal stones, discharge, venereal disease, bleeding. In patients with neurogenic bladder, ask about fluid intake, voiding schedules, bladder emptying techniques, incontinence, retention, and incomplete emptying.
    a. **Male sexuality.** Libido, erection, ejaculation, fertility, dyspareunia.
    b. **Female sexuality:** Libido, vaginal and clitoral sensation, orgasm, fertility, dyspareunia.
    c. **Gynecologic/reproductive:** Age at menarche, last menstrual period, frequency and duration of periods, number and complications of pregnancies, live births, miscarriages, age at menopause, contraception.

11. **Musculoskeletal.** Pain, swelling, stiffness, limitation of range of motion,

arthritis, gout, cramps, myalgia, fasciculation, atrophy, hypertrophy, fracture, deformity.

12. Neurologic

   a. Consciousness level. Change in level of consciousness, convulsions.

   b. Cognitive. Change in memory or thinking.

   c. Speech and language. Change in reading, speaking, and writing ability.

   d. Cranial nerves

     • **I.** Altered sense of smell

     • **II, III, IV, VI.** Diplopia, blurred vision, field cuts, glasses

     • **V.** Weakness of muscles of mastication

     • **VII.** Facial weakness, dysarthria, loss of taste

     • **VIII.** Deafness, imbalance, dizziness, vertigo, tinnitus

     • **IX, X, XII.** Difficulties in swallowing and speaking

     • **XI.** Difficulties in turning head or in shrugging

   e. Sensory. Loss or change of sensation (touch, pain, temperature), dysesthesia, hyperpathia.

   f. Motor. Weakness, paralysis, tremors, involuntary movements.

   g. Gait. Stability, use of assistive or mobility devices, falls, endurance.

13. Psychiatric. Personality changes, extreme mood change, insomnia, anxiety, depression, obsessive and phobic ideas, past major and minor psychiatric care, history of psychotherapy or psychotropic pharmacological intervention, suicidal ideation or prior suicidal attempts.

14. Endocrine. Heat or cold intolerance, polydypsia, polyuria, polyphagia

15. Hematologic. Easy bruising, transfusion reactions, excessive bleeding, history of anemia.

II. Physical Examination. The basic techniques of physiatric physical examination (i.e., inspection, palpation, percussion, and auscultation) are the same as with other medical specialties (see supplemental references). Emphasis is placed on musculoskeletal, neurological, and functional examinations.

  A. Vital signs (VS). Blood pressure (indicate which arm; measure in supine, sitting, and standing to rule out orthostasis), pulse (rate and regularity), respiration (rate and rhythm), temperature, weight, height.

  B. General description. State of health, general appearance, apparent age, nutritional status, body development, personal hygiene, cooperativeness, hostile or threatening behavior, signs of anxiety or distress.

  C. Integument.

    1. Skin. Color, temperature, turgor, atrophy, lesions.

    2. Pressure ulcers. Location (usually over bony prominence), diameter (cm), depth, wound type (e.g., abrasion, scab, blister, ulcer with eschar or slough), appearance, color, drainage (character, volume, or odor), and presence of epithelization and/or granulation tissue, edema, and tunneling or sinus tracts. The periwound area (e.g., erythema, induration, maceration) should also be described. For clinical grading or staging of pressure ulcers, refer to Table 5.2-1 in Chapter 5.2.

    3. Hair. Distribution, amount, texture, hair loss spots, facial hairs.

    4. Nail. Infection, hygiene, long toenails, ingrown toenails.

  D. Lymph nodes. Posterior auricular, cervical, supraclavicular, axillary, inguinal areas (if with lymphadenopathy, note size, consistency, mobility, tenderness).

  E. HEENT

    1. Head. Size, shape, symmetry, lesions, craniofacial anomalies, neurosurgical procedures, shunt sites, shunt bulb compressibility.

2. **Eyes.** Eye dryness, conjunctival and scleral color, corneal lesions, eyelid nodules, adequacy of lid closure, fundi.

3. **Ears.** Drainage, tympanic membrane.

4. **Nose and sinuses.** Polyps, lesions, drainage, sinus tenderness (frontal and maxillary).

5. **Mouth and throat.** Lesions, ulcers, teeth loss, dentures, hygiene.

6. **Temporomandibular joint.** Crepitation, tenderness, swelling, mouth opening size.

F. **Neck.** Nuchal rigidity, carotid pulsations and bruits, jugular venous distention, thyroid gland, trachea, skin around tracheostomy site (type and size of tracheostomy tube).

G. **Thorax and diaphragm.** Chest wall shape, tenderness, deformity, breathing pattern, chest expansion (normal is >6 cm at nipple line), use of accessory muscles, cough force and efficiency, hiccups.

H. **Lungs.** Quality and intensity of breath sounds, "e" to "a" change, whispered pectoriloquy ("ninety-nine"), wheezes, crackles (rales), rhonchi, or rubs.

I. **Heart.** Thrills, point of maximal impulse, S_1 and S_2 intensity and splitting, murmurs (timing, intensity, pitch, location, radiation, quality), abnormal heart sounds (S_3, S_4, clicks, rubs, snaps, gallops).

J. **Breasts and nipples.** Masses, tenderness, rashes, ulceration, discharge.

K. **Abdomen.** Obesity, scars, rigidity, distention, ascites, venous pattern, masses (pulsatile and nonpulsatile), tenderness, guarding, bowel sounds, abdominal bruits, hepatosplenomegaly.

L. **Rectal.** Lesions, inflammation, masses, hemorrhoids, perineal sensation, sphincter tone, fecal occult blood, prostate (size, shape, and consistency), bulbocavernosus reflex.

M. **Genitourinary.** Costovertebral angle tenderness, hernia.

   1. **Male genitalia.** Circumcision, ulcers, nodules, masses, scars, inflammation, tenderness, discharge, fistulas, hypospadia, testicular descension and symmetry.

   2. **Female genitalia.** Nodules, masses, discharge, swelling.

N. **Peripheral vascular system.** Peripheral arteries (describe symmetry and grade intensity of brachial, radial, popliteal, femoral, dorsalis pedis, and posterior tibialis pulses), femoral bruits, edema (severity and presence of pitting), distal clubbing, and cyanosis.

O. **Musculoskeletal system.** Note any pain behavior (e.g., marked grimacing, groans, limping) during examination. Refer to Table 1.1-2 for sequence of musculoskeletal examination (for more details, see Hoppenfeld's *Physical Examination of the Spine and Extremities* and Magee's *Orthopedic Physical Assessment* [both listed under supplemental references]).

   1. **Spine.** Surgical scars, spinal posture (cervical lordosis, scoliosis, dorsal kyphosis, lumbar lordosis), shoulder height, pelvic level, trunk tilt (neck range of motion [ROM], back ROM [e.g., Schober's test], neck and trunk strength, spinal and paraspinal tenderness, muscle tightness and spasm, compression tests (Spurling's test), traction maneuvers (e.g., straight leg raising [SLR] and Gaenslen's test).

   2. **Limbs.** Alignment (e.g., genu varum or valgum), contractures, deformities, limb length discrepancy, limb girth asymmetry, winging (scapular), erythema, hematoma, scar, callous, lesions, swelling, masses, crepitation, fasciculation, atrophy, hypertrophy, tenderness, trigger point, tender point, spasm, spasticity, rigidity, tests that provoke symptoms (e.g., Tinel's test, Phalen's wrist flexion test), amputation (note residual limb

Table 1.1-2. **Sequence of physiatric examination with emphasis on musculoskeletal system. Testing position and sequence may be modified in patients who cannot assume all positions**

POSITION	TESTS
A. Standing	1. Posture and gait analyses, functional lower limb strength (heel-walk, toe-walk, squatting, transfer in and out of bed or chair) 2. Lower limb alignment and deformities, position of ankles and feet (e.g., flatfeet, inversion or eversion) 3. Back motion (flexion, extension, lateral bending, Schober's test)

B. Seated	1. Head and neck motion in all planes (include Spurling's test)
	2. TMJ examination
	3. Thoracolumbar rotation with pelvis fixed
	4. Routine medical (VS, skin, HEENT, neck, thorax, breasts, lungs, heart, flank) and neurologic exam (mental status, cranial nerves, reflexes, sensory, coordination)
	5. Upper limb: inspect, palpate, measure girth, screen strength (see Table 1.1-4), and functional ROM:
	  a. Shoulder complex (arm elevation from side to 180° above head; internal rotate by reaching dorsum of hand to highest level of spinous process; external rotate by putting hand behind the neck or head)
	  b. Glenohumeral joint (fix scapula, abduct arm, and do internal and external rotations)
	  c. Elbow: flexion and extension
	  d. Wrist and hands (wrist motion, fist, grip and pinch, pronation and supination, thumb distal phalange flexion and extension, opposition)
	6. Lower limb: inspect, palpate, screen strength (see Table 1.1-4), and ROM
	  a. Hip flexion
	  b. Knee extension and flexion
	  c. Ankle dorsiflexion, plantar flexion, inversion, eversion

C. Supine	1. Routine medical exam (skin, abdomen, genitalia, peripheral vascular systems) and neurologic exams 2. Low back (abdominal strength, traction maneuvers, e.g., SLR, Gaenslen) 3. Hips: rolling, abduction, adduction, flexion (knee to chest), internal and external rotation with hips flexed to 90°; maneuvers (Thomas', Ober's). 4. Leg length measurement; girth 5. Knees: patella (patellar click sign, bulge sign), popliteal area (synovial cyst), knee stability (Drawer's, Lachman's, Apley's, medial and lateral stress tests) 6. Ankle and feet: malleoli, dorsiflexion and plantarflexion, subtalar motion inversion and eversion 7. Toes: alignment and deformity
D. Sidelying	1. Hip abduction and adduction 2. Rectal and perineal exam
E. Prone	1. Inspect and palpate cervical, thoracic, lumbosacral, sacroiliac, gluteal areas 2. Hip extension (knee straight and bent) 3. Head, neck, and trunk extension

shape, length, scar, skin integrity, sensation, ROM, strength). See Table 1.1-3 for screening tests of upper and lower limbs used to grossly assess the musculoskeletal system (ROM and strength) as well as the central and peripheral nervous system. The screening tests are used to determine which specific muscle or joint needs further testing. For muscle strength, the numerical or word/letter grading system may be used (see Table 1.1-4).

a. **Range-of-motion (ROM).** Measure active and passive ROM; use the 0° to 180° system (i.e., anatomic position is the zero starting point, except for rotation that uses a point midway between normal rotation range as the zero starting point); record the patient's position and starting joint position during testing; note the stabilization, alignment, and goniometer type used, as well as the factors affecting the ROM such as pain, swelling, spasm, spasticity, motivation, cooperation, fear, obesity, and contractures. For functional ROM testing, refer to Tables 1.1-2 and 1.1-3. ROM limitations can be estimated by using the percentage system, i.e., 0 limitation = full ROM; minimal limitation = lacks 1% to 33% to full ROM; moderate limitation = lacks 33% to 66% to full ROM; maximal limitation = lacks 66% to 100% to full ROM. Average ROMs for the spine and limbs are summarized in Appendices A-1 and A-2. Further details on ROM testing can be found in Norkin and White's *Measurement of joint motion: A guide to goniometry* (see supplemental references) as well as Chapter 2.5, section I.

b. **Joint stability.** Determine ankylosis, hypo- or hypermobility, instability, subluxation, and dislocation. Perform maneuvers such as Drawer's test, Lachman's test, and pivot-shift test.

c. **Muscle strength.** Manual muscle testing (MMT) and dynamometry (see Chapter 2.5, section II) are tests of voluntary movement used to assess weakness due to disorders primarily involving the contractile muscle elements, the myoneural junction, and the lower motor neurons. They are inaccurate for disorders of the upper motor neurons (UMN) or the brain (e.g., cerebral palsy, stroke) because of alteration in reflex activity, which brings about abnormal muscle tone and synergy patterns. Screening tests of muscle strength are presented in Table 1.1-3.

  1) **Manual muscle testing (MMT).** Note distribution of muscle weakness (proximal vs. distal, upper vs. lower limbs); document patient's position and stabilization as well as co-contractions and substitution patterns used during testing; and record factors affecting MMT such as pain, swelling, spasm, spasticity, motivation, cooperation, effort, fear, fatigue, contractures, size, physical condition, and conversion reaction of patient. For grading manual muscle strength, see Table 1.1-4. If possible, MMT must be compared with uninvolved side. Further details about MMT procedures can be found in Hislop and Montgomery's *Daniels and Worthingham's muscle testing* and Kendall, McCreary, and Provance's *Muscles testing and function* (see supplemental references).

  2) **Dynamometry.** Hand-held, isometric, isokinetic, isoinertial dynamometers (for specific dynamometers, see Chapter 2.5, section II).

P. **Neurologic**
  1. **Mental status.**
    a. **Level of consciousness.** Classify level of consciousness using the Glasglow "coma" or responsiveness scale (see Table 1.1-5).

Table 1.1-3.   Screening tests of upper and lower limbs used to grossly assess the musculoskeletal system (ROM and MMT) as well as the central and peripheral nervous system

MUSCLE	SPINAL ROOTS*	PERIPHERAL NERVE	TEST
UPPER LIMB†:			
Upper trapezius	Cranial nerve XI, C3, C4	Spinal accessory; Cervical roots	Shrugging
Deltoid	**C5**, C6	Axillary	Shoulder abduction
Biceps brachii	C5, C6	Musculocutaneous	Elbow flexion of supinated arm
Brachioradialis	C5, **C6**	Radial	Elbow flexion of neutral arm
Triceps brachii	C6, **C7**, C8	Radial	Elbow extension
Extensor pollicis longus	**C7**, C8	Radial	Thumb distal phalange extension
Extensor carpi ulnaris	**C7**, C8	Ulnar	Wrist extension
Flexor pollicis longus	C7, **C8**	Median	Thumb distal phalange flexion
Opponens pollicis	C8, **T1**	Median	Thumb opposition
Opponens digiti minimi	C8, **T1**	Ulnar	5th digit opposition
LOWER LIMB‡:			
Iliopsoas	**L1, L2**, L3	Lumbar plexus	Hip flexion
Adductor longus	**L2, L3**, L4	Obturator	Hip adduction
Quadriceps femoris	L2, **L3, L4**	Femoral	Knee extension
Gluteus medius	**L4, L5**, S1	Superior gluteal	Hip abduction
Gluteus maximus	**L5, S1**, S2	Inferior gluteal	Hip extension
Hamstrings	L5, **S1**, S2	Sciatic	Knee flexion
Tibialis anterior	**L4**, L5	Deep peroneal	Ankle dorsiflexion and inversion
Extensor hallucis longus	**L5**, S1	Deep peroneal	Big toe extensor
Peroneus longus	L5, S1	Superficial peroneal	Ankle eversion
Gastrocnemius	S1, S2	Tibial	Ankle plantarflexion

* A **bold** designation indicates the predominant root supply.
† Pronator drift can be used to screen proximal shoulder and arm weakness.
‡ Heel tapping can be used to screen proximal lower extremity muscle weakness whereas forefoot tapping screens for distal lower limb muscle weakness.

Table 1.1-4. Grading of manual muscle testing using number, word, and letter system

NUMBER GRADE[1]	WORD GRADE[2]	LETTER GRADE[2]	DEFINITION
0	Zero	0	No observable or palpable muscle contraction
1	Trace	T	Visible or palpable muscle contraction but no joint motion
2−	Poor minus	P−	Joint moves through incomplete ROM in gravity-decreased position
2	Poor	P	Joint moves through complete ROM in gravity-decreased position
2+	Poor plus	P+	Joint moves through incomplete ROM (<50%) against gravity or through complete ROM against slight resistance in gravity-decreased position
3−	Fair minus	F−	Joint moves through incomplete ROM (>50%) against gravity
3	Fair	F	Joint moves through complete ROM against gravity
3+	Fair plus	F+	Joint moves through complete ROM against gravity and slight resistance*
4	Good	G	Joint moves through complete ROM against gravity and moderate resistance†
5	Normal	N	Joint moves through complete ROM against gravity and full resistance†

Adapted from: [1] Guarantors of Brain: *Aids to the examination of the peripheral nervous system,* London, 1986, Balliere Tindall; [2] Daniels L, Worthingham C: *Muscle testing,* ed 5, Philadelphia, 1986, WB Saunders.
* Resistance for grades 3+ and above are given at the end range of motion (i.e., break test).
† Grades 4 and 5 have poor interrater reliability and do not need plus or minus designation.

    b. Cognition. Alertness, orientation (to time, place, and person), attention (digit repetition), recent and immediate memory recall (recall three named objects or numbers within 5, 10, and 15 minutes), general information (appropriate for age and educational/cultural background), calculations (count by sevens), proverbs explanation, describing similarities (e.g., between apple and orange), and judgment (e.g., how to find a friend in an unfamiliar city). The level of cognitive function or recovery can be classified by using the Rancho Los Amigos descriptive scale (Table 1.1-6).

    c. Perception. Agnosia (identification of common objects or body parts), unilateral environmental neglect, right-left disorientation, safety awareness (i.e., is patient aware of his or her deficit and the environment? does patient take adequate safety precautions?).

  2. Speech and language. Communicative skills (residual and premorbid), hearing function, aphasia, apraxia, dysarthria.

    a. Listening. Ability to follow verbal commands (single- and multisteps).

    b. Reading. Ability to follow written commands (single- and multisteps).

Table 1.1-5.   Glasgow "coma" or responsiveness scale (GCS) classifies and scores the patient's eye, motor, and verbal responses to verbal and physical stimuli

PARAMETER	PATIENT'S RESPONSE	SCORE*
Eye opening (**E**)	Spontaneous eye opening	E 4
	Opens eyes in response to speech	E 3
	Opens eyes in response to pain	E 2
	No eye opening	E 1
Best motor response (**M**)	Obeys verbal commands	M 6
	Localizes painful stimulus	M 5
	Flexion withdrawal from painful stimulus	M 4
	Abnormal flexion response to painful stimulus	M 3
	Extensor response to painful stimulus	M 2
	No motor response	M 1
Best verbal response (**V**)	Oriented; able to converse	V 5
	Disoriented; confused conversation	V 4
	Inappropriate words	V 3
	Incomprehensible sounds	V 2
	No verbal response	V 1

Tabulated with permission from Jennett B, Teasdale G: Aspects of coma after severe head injury. *Lancet* 1:878-881, 1977. Copyright © 1977 The Lancet Ltd.
* The GCS score is calculated by adding the E, M, and V scores (lowest possible score is 3 and highest is 15). GCS scores can be used to classify head injury (8 or less = severe; 9-12 = moderate; 13-15 = mild).

c. **Speaking.** Naming of at least three objects or pictures indicated by the examiner; ability to state his or her own name, address, and phone; ability to read aloud short paragraphs; ability to say a prolonged "aaah" (test for phonation and resonance deficits), "pa-pa-pa" (lip closure test), "ta-ta-ta" (test of tongue function), "ka-ka-ka" (test of speed, regulatory, and posterior pharyngeal function).

d. **Writing:** Ability to write his or her own name, address, phone, and a brief paragraph.

3. **Cranial nerves (CN)**
   - **I.** Sense of smell
   - **II.** Visual acuity (near and far, with and without eyewear), visual fields, color
   - **III.** Eye adduction (medial rectus muscle), eye depression (inferior rectus muscle), eye elevation (superior rectus and inferior oblique muscles), pupillary constriction (with CN II), upper lid elevation
   - **IV.** Eye intortion with depression and adduction (superior oblique muscle)
   - **V.** Mastication (masseter, pterygoids), sensory of forehead, face, and jaw
   - **VI.** Eye abduction (lateral rectus muscle)
   - **VII.** Facial expression, blink or corneal reflex (with CN V), taste in anterior two thirds of tongue, "ba-ba-ba"
   - **VIII.** Hearing (whisper or use ticking watch), Weber, Rinne, nystagmus
   - **IX, X.** Sensory and motor functions of pharynx and larynx (gag reflex, position of uvula, swallowing), "ka-ka-ka"

Table 1.1-6.   Rancho Los Amigos Levels of Cognitive Functioning or Recovery*

COGNITIVE LEVEL	DESCRIPTION OF PATIENT
I. No response	Unresponsive to any stimuli
II. Generalized response	Nonspecific, inconsistent, and nonpurposeful response to any stimuli; response may be physiologic changes, gross body movement, and/or vocalization
III. Localized response	Specific but inconsistent response to stimulus; may follow simple commands (e.g., closing eyes, squeezing hands) but in an inconsistent, delayed manner
IV. Confused, agitated	Heightened state of activity; bizarre, incoherent, and nonpurposeful behavior relative to immediate environment; gross attention to environment is brief; no selective attention; lacks short- and long-term recall; unable to cooperate directly with treatment; may confabulate; may be hostile; needs maximum assistance for self-care
V. Confused, inappropriate	Appears alert; consistent response to simple commands, but when command is complex or lack any external structure, responses are nonpurposeful or fragmented; gross attention to the environment but highly distractible; unable to focus on specific task; with structure, may be able to converse on a social automatic level for short period; often confabulatory; memory is severely impaired; unable to learn new information; needs assistance for self-care and supervision for feeding; may wander off either randomly or with vague intention of "going home"
VI. Confused, appropriate	Shows goal-directed behavior but is dependent on external input or direction; responses may be incorrect due to memory problems, but they are appropriate to the situation; follows simple commands consistently with carryover for relearned tasks such as self-care; needs at least supervision for old learning and maximal supervision for new learning with little or no carryover; past memories show more depth and detail than recent memory; no longer wanders and is oriented (inconsistently) to time and space
VII. Automatic, appropriate	Appears appropriate and oriented within the hospital and home setting; goes through daily routine automatically but robotlike; if with structure, able to initiate social or recreational activities; judgment is impaired; independent in self-care but needs supervision in home and community skills for safety; prevocational evaluation and counseling may be indicated
VIII. Purposeful, appropriate	Alert and oriented; able to recall and integrate past and recent events and is aware of and responsive to environment; shows carryover for new learning and needs no supervision once activities are learned; may continue to have decreased abilities relative to premorbid abilities; decreased level of social, emotional, and intellectual capacities but still functional within society; independent in home and community skills (within patient's physical abilities); vocational rehabilitation is indicated

Condensed from: Professional Staff Association: *Rehabilitation of the head injured adult: Comprehensive physical management,* Downey, CA 1979, Rancho Los Amigos Hospital, pp. 87-88, with permission from the Adult Brain Unit Service, Rancho Los Amigos Medical Center, Downey, CA.
* Does not address specific cognitive deficits; No reliability data is available; Useful for communicating general cognitive and/or behavioral status particularly in patients with traumatic brain, injury, where this scale is commonly used.

- **XI.** Shrugging of shoulders (trapezius), movement of head (sternocleidomastoid)
- **XII.** Tongue movement, "la-la-la"
4. **Sensory.** (see Appendices B-1 and B-2 for dermatomes).
    a. **Superficial sensation.** Pinprick (use disposable safety pin), light touch (use wisp of cotton), temperature (use hot and cold test tubes).

b. Deep sensation. Joint position or proprioception, deep pain (for upper limb hyperextend small finger; for lower limb, firmly compress calf muscle or Achilles tendon), vibration.

c. Cortical sensation. Two-point discrimination, graphesthesia, stereognosis, double simultaneous stimulation (cortical extinction).

5. Reflexes.

a. Muscle-stretch or deep tendon reflexes (DTR). Commonly tested DTRs include (the main segment is **bolded**): biceps brachii (**C5**, 6), brachioradialis (C5, **6**), triceps brachii (**C7**, C8), quadriceps (L2, **L3**), gastrocnemius-soleus (**S1**, S2). Less frequently tested DTRs include: jaw jerk (cranial nerve V), internal hamstring (L4, L5, S1, S2), and external hamstring (L5, S1, S2). DTRs on both sides must be compared and graded as: 0 = absent, 1+ = hypoactive, 2+ = normal, 3+ = brisker than average, 4+ = hyperactive, with clonus and pathologic reflexes.

b. Superficial (segmental) reflexes. Corneal (cranial nerves V and VII), gag (cranial nerves IX and X), epigastric (T6-9), hypogastric (T11-L1), cremasteric (L1-L2), bulbocavernosus (S2-4), and anal (S3-5) reflexes.

c. Pathologic reflexes. Babinski (Chaddock or Oppenheim), Hoffman, Kernig, bite, tongue thrust, chewing, and suck-swallow reflexes.

d. Developmental or primitive reflexes and reactions. Asymmetric tonic neck reflex (ATNR), symmetric tonic neck reflex (STNR), tonic labyrinthine reflex (TLR), positive supporting reaction, crossed extension reflex, associated reactions, grasp reflex, righting reactions, equilibrium reactions, protective extension (parachute), sucking, and rooting reflexes.

6. Motor control.

a. Muscle tone. Spasticity (for clinical grading, see Table 5.4-1 in Chapter 5.4), flaccidity (e.g., pendulum and drop arm test), rigidity, dystonia.

b. Coordination. Tests for upper limbs include finger-to-nose and knee-pat tests; tests for lower limbs include toe-to-finger and heel-to-shin tests.

c. Alternate motion rate. Rapid alternating hand movements, tongue wiggling, finger wiggling, foot-patting.

d. Involuntary movements. Tremors, chorea, athetosis, ballismus, dystonia, myoclonus, asterixis, tics.

e. Motor planning ability. Dressing apraxia (inability to put on a coat), constructional apraxia (inability to draw the face of a clock).

f. Balance/postural reactions. Romberg test, sway excursion, verticality (perception of body position in space), balance responses to external displacement and during volitional displacements, adaptability to repeated displacements (see Table 1.1-7 for functional grading of balance).

g. Flexibility (or ROM; see section II.O.2.a under musculoskeletal examination).

h. Movement patterns. Flexion or extension synergy patterns (see Table 1.1-8 for differentiation and Table 1.1-9 for grading of movement patterns), primitive reflexes (see section II.P.5.d).

i. Strength (see section II.O.2.c under musculoskeletal examination).

7. Gait. Document any gait aids used (note hand used, appropriate sequencing, condition of device; see chapter 4.6). Observe the gait parameters

Table 1.1-7. Functional grading of balance

BALANCE GRADE	DEFINITION
Zero	Patient needs maximal assistance to maintain balance
Poor	Patient needs support to maintain balance
Fair	Patient is able to maintain balance without support; cannot tolerate challenge; cannot maintain balance while shifting weight
Good	Patient is able to maintain balance without support; accepts moderate challenge and can shift weight, although limitations are evident
Normal	Patient is able to maintain balance without support; accepts maximal challenge and can shift weight in all directions

From Leahy P: Motor control assessment. In Montgomery P, Connolly B, eds: *Motor control and physical therapy: Theoretical framework and practical applications.* Hixson, TN, 1991, Chattanooga Group, p. 75, with permission.

(described in Table 1.1-10) from front, side, and rear, and note type of pathologic gait (e.g., antalgic, short-leg, coxalgic, metatarsalgic gait). Refer to Chapter 2.5, section VI for details about gait analyses.

- **Q. Functional neuromuscular assessment** for screening of disabilities (see Table 1.1-11).
- **R. Functional (ADL) scales.** The most widely used general (global) scale of function is the *Functional Independence Measure* (FIM) (see Chapter 2.8, section I). The FIM assesses 18 activities of self-care, mobility, locomotion, communication, and social cognition on a seven-point scale from fully independent to fully dependent. Other ADL scales that are more task specific include *Barthel Index, PULSES profile, Klein-Bell ADL Scale, Katz index of independence in ADL,* and *Kenny self-care evaluation* (see Chapter 2.8).

Table 1.1-8. Synergy patterns of the limbs

LIMBS	FLEXION SYNERGY COMPONENTS	EXTENSION SYNERGY COMPONENTS
Upper	Scapular retraction/elevation or hyperextension	Scapular protraction
	Shoulder abduction, external rotation	Shoulder adduction,* internal rotation
	Elbow flexion*	Elbow extension
	Forearm supination	Forearm pronation*
	Wrist and finger flexion	Wrist and finger flexion
Lower	Hip flexion,* abduction, external rotation	Hip extension, adduction,* internal rotation
	Knee flexion	Knee extension*
	Ankle dorsiflexion, inversion	Ankle plantarflexion,* inversion
	Toe dorsiflexion	Toe plantarflexion

From O'Sullivan SB: Stroke. In O'Sullivan SB, Schmitz TJ, eds: *Physical rehabilitation: Assessment and treatment.* ed 3, Philadelphia, 1994, F A Davis, p. 334, with permission.
* The components which are generally the strongest or most prominent.

Table 1.1-9.   Grading system of movement patterns in patients with upper motor neuron disease

GRADE	DEFINITION
0	Unable to initiate movement
1	Initiates movement through 25% of range of motion (ROM)
2	Carries movement through 50% of ROM
3	Carries movement through 75% of ROM
4	Carries movement through full range

Adapted from: Sawner K, Lavigne J: Brunnstrom's movement therapy in hemiplegia: A neurophysiological approach, ed 2, Philadelphia, 1992, JB Lippincott, p. 207, with permission.

Table 1.1-10.   Clinical gait analysis

PARAMETERS	OBSERVATION
A. Standing balance	Steadiness of position; Patient's attempt to regain balance as examiner pushes patient off balance
B. Body part movements during walking	
1. Posture	Fixed or abnormal postures; Inadequate, excessive, or asymmetrical movements of body parts
2. Head and trunk	Listing or tilting
3. Shoulder	Dipping, elevation, depression, protraction and retraction
4. Arm swing	Protective positioning or posturing
5. Pelvis and hip	Hip hiking, dropping (Trendelenburg), or lateral thrust
6. Knee	Genu varum, valgum, or recurvatum
7. Ankle and foot	Excessive inversion or eversion
C. Gait cycle factors	
1. Cadence	Rate, symmetry, fluidity and consistency
2. Stride width	Narrow or broad base; Knee and ankle clearance
3. Stride length	Shortened, lengthened, or asymmetrical
4. Stance phase	Normal heel-strike, foot flat, push off; Knee stability during all components of stance; Coordination of knee and ankle movements
5. Swing phase	Adequate and synchronized knee and ankle dorsiflexion during swing; Abduction or circumduction

From: Erickson RP, McPhee MC: Clinical evaluation. In DeLisa JA, Gans BM, eds: *Rehabilitation medicine: Principles and practice.,* ed 2, Philadelphia, 1993, JB Lippincott, p. 92, with permission.

Table 1.1-11.   Functional neuromuscular assessment for screening of disabilities

ACTIVITY	PATIENT TASKS
A. Bed mobility	
1. Rolling to side	Turn from side to side
2. Supine to sit	Sit at edge of bed
B. Sitting	
1. Static balance	Sit at edge of bed unsupported
2. Dynamic balance reactions	Put on shoes or slippers while seated
C. Transfers	
1. Sit to stand	Stand up from seated position
2. Bed to other surface	Transfer from bed to chair or other surface (note standing pivot ability and equipment used, e.g., sliding board)
D. Standing	
1. Static balance	Stand unsupported
2. Dynamic balance reactions	Put on robe or coat while standing
E. Gait	
1. Level surface	Walk on level surface
2. Stairs	Ascend and descend a flight of stairs
F. Wheelchair mobility	
1. Level surface	Propel wheelchair on level surface
2. Ramp	Propel wheelchair up and down ramp

III. **Summary and problem list** include a summary of the history and physical findings and a separate listing of medical and PM&R problems. The problem list must include diagnoses, secondary abnormalities, specific losses in self-care functions, social functions, vocational functions, and psychological functions. Record date of onset and date of resolution of problems.

IV. **Physiatric orders/referrals** include primary and secondary diagnoses with onset; whether evaluation and/or treatment is requested; goals of treatment with expected duration of treatment or hospital stay; intensity, frequency, and initial duration of treatment desired; precautions (weight-bearing status, assistive devices needed, current medications, associated medical diagnosis); and follow-up date.

V. **Admission orders.** Use the "**ADC-VAAN-DISML**" mnemonic.
- **A**dmit to: Ward or room; attending and resident physicians responsible for the patient
- **D**iagnosis: Admitting diagnosis, secondary diagnosis pertinent to nursing care
- **C**ondition: Patient's general condition (stable, fair, poor, critical)
- **V**ital signs: Type, frequency, and parameters for notifying physician
- **A**llergies: Medications and food products (describe past reactions)
- **A**ctivity limitations: Bed rest, out of bed to wheelchair (specify type of assistance, precautions)
- **N**ursing orders: Wound care, input and output monitoring, weighing of patient, catheter care
- **D**iet: Regular diet, restricted diet (e.g., 2 gm sodium, 2 gm potassium, 300 mg/day cholesterol), diabetic diet (e.g., 1800 cal), dysphagia diet (see Chapter 5.6, section V.A.2.b.1)

- Intravenous fluids: IV solutions and rate of infusion
- Sedatives, analgesics, and other prn medications (GI medications, bowel routine medications, antipyretics)
- Medications: Specify dose, route, frequency, duration, and special restrictions
- Laboratory and other diagnostic tests (see Chapter 2.1): Routine labs (CBC, SMAG, PT/aPTT, LFT, UA), chest radiographs, ECG, special tests

VI. Progress notes. Use the "**SOAP**" mnemonic.
- Subjective: Patient complaints/symptoms and personal impressions
- Objective: Physical signs, test data (lab, radiograph, ECG), and quantified progress.
- Assessment: Analysis of subjective and objective data with tentative diagnosis or impression
- Plan: Diagnostic studies, therapeutic regimen, additional consults, patient education required

VII. Discharge summary. Use the "**ROTC-DIC**" mnemonic.
- Reason for admission: Chief complaint, admission diagnosis, and brief history of the present illness
- Objective findings: Physical examinations, laboratory, radiograph, special tests (include pertinent negative findings too)
- Treatment given (medical, surgical, PM&R, PT, OT, psychology, etc.) and patient's response to it
- Complications and Consultations
- Diagnosis: Final diagnosis and final secondary diagnoses
- Instructions on continuing care: Medications (specify dose, route, frequency, and duration), diet, physical activity limitations, home exercises, home equipment, referrals (PT, OT, SLP, nursing, home health attendant), and follow-up appointments
- Condition upon discharge: ambulation status, self-care, ability to work

BIBLIOGRAPHY

Cifu DX, Markowski J: Physical medicine and rehabilitation: Philosophy, patient care issues and physiatric evaluation. In Garrison SJ, editor: *Handbook of physical medicine and rehabilitation basics*, Philadelphia, 1995, JB Lippincott, pp. 1-12.

Erickson RP, McPhee MC: Clinical evaluation. In DeLisa JA and Gans BM, editors: *Rehabilitation medicine: Principles and practice*, ed 2, Philadelphia, 1993, JB Lippincott, pp. 51-95.

Ferri FF: *Practical guide to the care of the medical patient*, ed 3, St. Louis, 1995, Mosby.

Grynbaum BB, Sury R: Evaluation. In Goodgold J, editor: *Rehabilitation medicine*, St. Louis, 1988, Mosby, pp. 3-23.

Sinaki M, editor: *Basic clinical rehabilitation medicine*, St. Louis, 1994, Mosby.

McPeak LA: Physiatric history and examination. In Braddom RL, editor: *Physical medicine and rehabilitation*, Philadelphia, 1996, WB Saunders, pp. 3-42.

Stolov WC, Hays RM: Evaluation of the patient. In Kottke FJ, Lehmann JF, editors: *Krusen's handbook of physical medicine and rehabilitation*, ed 4., Philadelphia, 1990, WB Saunders, pp. 1-19.

Wood PHN: Appreciating the consequences of disease: The International Classification of Impairments, Disabilities and Handicaps (ICIDH). *WHO Chronicle* 34:376-380, 1980.

Supplemental References

Adams V: *Principles of neurology*, ed 5, New York, 1993, McGraw-Hill.

Bates B: *A guide to physical examination and history taking*, ed 6, Philadelphia, 1995, JB Lippincott.

DeGowin EL, DeGowin RL: *Bedside diagnostic examination*, ed 6, New York, 1994, Macmillan.

Hislop HJ, Montgomery J: *Daniels and Worthingham's Muscle testing: Techniques of manual examination*, ed 6, Philadelphia, 1995, WB Saunders.

Hoppenfeld S: *Physical examination of the spine and extremities*, New York, 1976, Appleton-Century.

Jenkins DB: *Hollingshead's Functional anatomy of the limbs and back*, ed. 6, Philadelphia, 1991, WB Saunders.

Kendall F, McCreary EK, Provance P: *Muscles testing and function*, ed 4, Baltimore, 1993, Williams & Wilkins.

Magee DJ: *Orthopedic physical assessment*, ed 2, Philadelphia, 1992, WB Saunders.

Norkin CC, White DJ: *Measurement of joint motion: A guide to goniometry*, ed 2, Philadelphia, 1995, FA Davis.

O'Sullivan SB, Schmitz TJ, editors: *Physical rehabilitation: Assessment and treatment*, ed 3, Philadelphia, 1994, FA Davis.

Seidel HM, Ball JW, Dains JE, et al.: *Mosby's guide to physical examination*, ed 3, St. Louis, 1995, Mosby.

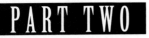

PART TWO

PM&R Diagnostic Tests

CHAPTER 2.1

LABORATORY TESTS

Understanding the rationale of any test is important in proper patient care. This chapter covers some of the common laboratory tests used in PM&R. Although some of the tests are clearly in the realm of other specialties (e.g., rheumatology), they are commonly ordered for patients undergoing rehabilitation. All laboratory tests must be interpreted in the context of a careful history, thorough physical examination, and other related tests and measures. For normal values of common laboratory tests, refer to Appendix A-3.

I. Routine tests commonly ordered upon hospital admission include:
   A. Laboratory. Complete blood count (CBC) with differential count, erythrocyte sedimentation rate (ESR), serum electrolytes with glucose (SMAG), liver function tests (LFT or FLEX), coagulation profile (prothrombin time or PT and activated partial thromboplastin time or aPTT), urinalysis.
   B. Plain Radiograph. Chest radiograph (described in Chapter 5.13, section III. C.1) to rule out cardiac and pulmonary pathology; postoperative skeletal radiograph.
   C. Electrocardiogram (ECG; described in Chapter 5.13, section III. C.2.a): Baseline ECG especially in patients with cardiac history.

II. Special laboratory studies
   A. Serum protein electrophoresis (SPEP) detects monoclonal and polyclonal patterns of serum proteins. The presence of monoclonal proteins in patients with back pain is suggestive of multiple myeloma. Polyclonal proteins are seen in connective tissue (autoimmune) disorders, chronic infection, chronic active hepatitis, lymphoproliferative disease, and sometimes are found in normal individuals.
   B. Acid phosphatase is used to provide clues of prostatic malignancy in men with metastatic bone tumor.
   C. Muscle enzymes are increased in myopathies, muscle trauma, strenuous physical exertion (marathon running), and after intramuscular injections. Muscle enzymes commonly measured are creatinine kinase (CK), aldolase, lactic dehydrogenase (LDH), and aspartate aminotransferase (AST). CK, specifically the MM isoform of CK (CK-MM), is probably the most reliable indicator of skeletal muscle damage.
   D. Thyroid function tests
      1. Serum thyroid-stimulating hormone (TSH) is the least expensive and most sensitive marker for primary hypothyroidism. TSH is elevated in primary hypothyroidism (even before the T_4 level falls to an abnormal level); while in secondary hypothyroidism (caused by pituitary or hypothalamic failure), it is decreased.
      2. Serum total T_4 is increased in hyperthyroidism, and decreased in hypothyroidism; however, it is also greatly affected by the level of serum binding protein (most commonly thyroglobulin binding globulin [TBG]) because over 99% of T_4 are bound to TBG. An increase in TBG (e.g., pregnancy, use of oral contraceptives, acute hepatitis or chronic active liver disease, use of marijuana or heroin or methadone, fluorouracil use, and acute inter-

mittent porphyria) will decrease total T_4; while decreased TBGs (e.g., androgen or glucocorticoid excess; nephrotic syndrome; severe illness; cirrhosis; intake of such drugs as phenytoin, furosemide, and salicylate) will increase total T_4.

3. **T_3 resin uptake (T_3RU)** is used to circumvent the problem of changes in serum TBG; however, it must be used only in conjunction with simultaneous measures of total T_4. The T_3 RU reflects the unsaturated thyroid binding sites on TBG and is not a measure of circulating T_3. The T_3RU is high in hyperthyroidism and low in hypothyroidism and pregnancy.

4. **Free T_4 and free T_3** are theoretically the ideal tests of thyroid function, but serum concentrations are so low they are difficult to measure.

E. **Cerebrospinal fluid (CSF) analysis** is used to identify subarachnoid hemorrhage, meningeal inflammation (meningitis) and neoplasia, presence of various abnormal antigens, antibodies, and other abnormal proteins (e.g., syphilis, multiple sclerosis [MS]). It is obtained by lumbar puncture (LP), which is a relatively simple procedure. LP contraindications include clinical evidence of increased intracranial pressure, local infection at the puncture site, or poor patient cooperation.

F. **Dystropin** is a cytoskeletal protein normally found in equal quantities in skeletal and cardiac muscle. Deficiency in dystrophin is seen in Duchenne and Becker's muscular dystrophy.

III. **Rheumatologic laboratory tests**

A. **Acute-phase reactants**

1. **Erythrocyte sedimentation rate (ESR)** is the rate of fall in millimeters per hour of red blood cells (RBCs) in a standard tube (Westergren method). Normal Westergren ESR values are 0-15 mm/hour for males and 0-20 mm/hour for females. Rates in the range of 30 mm/h are considered normal in persons 60 years old or older. Elevated ESR indicates nonspecific tissue inflammation (e.g., in the presence of infection, anemia, chronic disease, allergic reaction, malignancy, or in patients taking heparin). However, normal ESR tends to exclude active inflammatory disorders such as acute rheumatic fever, systemic lupus erythematosus (SLE), rheumatoid arthritis (RA), temporal arteritis–polymyalgia rheumatica (TA-PMR). ESR can be used to follow the course (including therapeutic responses) of chronic inflammatory disorders. Falsely low ESRs are found in polycythemia, anisocytosis, spherocytosis, sickle cell disease, or heart failure. Falsely high ESR may be seen in prolonged storage of blood to be tested or tilting of the calibrated tube.

2. **C-reactive protein (CRP)** is an acute-phase reactant serum protein that is present in low concentration in normal serum. Because of its ability to give a precipitin reaction with pneumococcal C-polysaccharide, it can be measured by a latex agglutination test or rocket electrophoresis. CRP levels rise rapidly in the presence of inflammation, then fall as the inflammation subsides. Thus, it is usually used to monitor the progress of osteomyelitis during antibiotic treatment. The major advantage of CRP testing over ESR testing is that it can be performed on freeze-stored serum. However, both are nonspecific tests of inflammation. In the absence of infection in patients with SLE or scleroderma, CRP levels are inappropriately low.

B. **Rheumatoid factors (RF)** are autoantibodies against the Fc (i.e., heavy-chain constant fragment) portion of IgGs, which are primarily associated with RA but are also found in other rheumatic diseases, such as Sjogren's syndrome, SLE, scleroderma, and mixed connective disease. They have also been associated with acute viral infections (e.g., mononucleosis, hepatitis, influenza, postvaccination), parasitic infections (e.g., malaria, schistosomiasis, filariasis), chronic inflammatory disease (e.g., TB, leprosy, syphilis, subacute bacterial endocarditis, salmonellosis), and other hyperglobulinemic states (e.g., cryoglobulinemia, sarcoid, chronic liver disease, other chronic pulmonary disease).

C. **Antinuclear antibodies (ANAs)** react to a variety of nuclear and cytoplasmic cellular antigens found in systemic rheumatic disease, such as SLE, progressive systemic sclerosis (PSS), mixed connective tissue disease (MCTD), and rheumatoid arthritis (RA). ANA studies are usually reported by pattern, intensity of fluorescence (1+ to 4+), or titer. Values of 2+ to 4+ or titers greater than 1:40 are usually considered significant. By determining reactivity of ANA-positive sera with nuclear constituents (e.g., double stranded DNA [dsDNA], single-stranded DNA [ssDNA], histones, etc.), greater diagnostic specificity is attained. For example, antibody to dsDNA is highly specific for SLE and particularly corresponds to active renal disease (dsDNA disappears with remission after immunosuppressive or steroid therapy). Although steroid or immunosuppressive therapy may affect the ANA titer, most clinicians do not rely on serial changes in ANA to monitor disease activity. Instead, ANA studies are done as an initial screening test for autoantibodies.

1. **Antineutrophil cytoplasmic antibody (ANCA)** is a special case of ANA, which binds relatively selectively to cytoplasmic proteins within neutrophils. A granular cytoplasmic staining pattern (C-ANCA) is highly specific for Wegener's granulomatosis (present in approximately 80% of cases), while a perinuclear pattern (P-ANCA) is seen in polyarteritis nodosa and in other forms of glomerulonephritis. ANCA is also useful in confirming the diagnosis of vasculitis in the presence of histopathological diagnosis.

2. **Anticardiolipin antibody** is another form of ANA found in up to 50% of patients with SLE but also occurs in individuals without SLE. It is associated with recurrent fetal loss, recurrent venous and arterial thrombosis, thrombocytopenia, and labile hypertension. It has also been reported (but unconfirmed) in patients with stroke and early myocardial infarct.

D. **Immune complexes**

1. **Cryoglobulins** are special types of immunoglobulins that precipitate from serum in the cold (0-5°C). Testing for cryoglobins is the simplest way of detecting immune complexes.

   a. **Mixed cryoglobulins** consist usually of IgM-IgG immunoglobulins and constitute two-thirds of the cryoglobulins seen in the Western world. They are used in identifying the immune complex syndrome called mixed, or essential, cryoglobulinemia. Other diseases associated with mixed cryoglobulin are autoimmune diseases (e.g., SLE, RA, polyarteritis nodosa [PN], Sjogren's syndrome, scleroderma), lymphoproliferative diseases (e.g., chronic lymphocytic leukemia, macroglobulinemia), renal diseases (e.g., proliferative glomerulonephritis), and liver diseases (Laennec's cirrhosis, biliary cirrhosis, chronic hepatitis). It can also be seen (often transiently) in viral, bacterial, or parasitic infections. Mixed cryoglobulin may be difficult to detect because it tends to be present in small amounts (50-500 mg/dl).

   b. **Monoclonal cryoglobulins** occur in large amounts (1-5 g/dl) and are easily detected as monoclonal components on electrophoresis of whole serum or the isolated cryoprecipitate. It is generally associated with multiple myeloma, macroglobulinemia, angioimmunoblastic lymphadenopathy, chronic lymphocytic leukemia, and other rarer neoplastic proliferations of plasma cells and lymphocytes.

2. **Complement assay** is one method of detecting immune complexes. The complement system consists of at least 20 different plasma and membrane proteins that play a major role in host defense against microbes by either modifying the membranes of the infectious agents (e.g., opsonization for ingestion by phagocytes, membrane damage), or by promoting the host inflammatory response (e.g., chemotaxis of neutrophils and monocytes, anaphylatoxic activity). It can be activated in an enzymatic cascade system (similar to the clotting system cascade) through the classical pathway (activated by the presence of antigen-antibody immune complexes) or through the alternative pathway (activated by the complex polysaccharides found in microbes). Both pathways eventually cleave C3 which subsequently lead to the activation of the membrane attack complex (MAC) with involvement of the terminal complement proteins C5-C9. The activated MAC proteins can insert into the membrane of cells and form a transmembrane channel that leads to cell lysis. They can also remove the lipid from viral envelops, thus rendering the virus noninfectious.

The irreversible proteolytic reactions in the complement cascade system result in cleaved proteins or complements that are rapidly cleared from the circulation. If there is an ongoing immunologic event that is activating the complement system in vivo (e.g., SLE or cryoglobulinemia), the plasma levels of these complements may be decreased, especially if the body is in a catabolic state (i.e., with low protein synthesis). Thus, low plasma complement (hypocomplementemia) suggests that there is a high level of circulating immune complexes.

Complements can be measured by functional immunoassays of individual components or by determining the total hemolytic complement (THC) or CH_{50} assay, which measures the ability of the test serum to lyse 50% of a standardized suspension of sheep RBCs coated with rabbit antibody. Because complement proteins are heat-labile, the collected specimen must be adequately frozen (at $-20°C$) and assayed within 2 weeks, otherwise, the results become inaccurate. Interpretation of an isolated static value is often difficult, hence serial testing is generally recommended for monitoring the disease activity (e.g., in patients with SLE or RA). While low values may suggest ongoing disease, normal or high values are less helpful because complement proteins, which are acute phase reactants, tend to be increased even with minor intercurrent illnesses. Deficiencies of complements C1 to C4 (i.e., complements during the early classical pathway) are associated with SLE-like syndromes and an increased incidence of infection; while deficiencies of complements C5 to C9 are associated with rheumatic syndromes and in increased incidence of infection, particularly Neisseria. A low CH_{50} is often seen in SLE, cryoglobulinemia, and RA vasculitis.

E. **Human leukocyte antigen (HLA) typing** is used as marker to identify certain rheumatic diseases.

1. **HLA-B27** is a major histocompatibility antigen and is positive in patients with ankylosing spondylitis (95%), Reiter syndrome (80%), psoriatic spondylitis (50% to 70%), and inflammatory bowel disease (75%). It has been shown that 20% of HLA-B27-positive persons experience ankylosing spondylitis or Reiter's disease after an infectious episode.

2. **SSA antigen** is associated with Sjogren's syndrome and SLE while **SSB antigen** is associated with Sjogren's syndrome only.
F. **Lyme serologic testing** detects antibodies or T-cell response to *Borrelia burgdorferi*. It is used to confirm clinical suspicion of Lyme disease but is not definitive because false negative results (e.g., during first week of infection before antibodies develop) and false positive results (e.g., because of cross reactivity to other spirochetes such as *Treponema pallidum,* in patients with rheumatoid factor or ANA) can occur.
  1. **Immunofluorescent assay (IFA)** detects antibodies to whole *B. burgdorferi* seen within weeks of the onset of the Lyme disease.
  2. **Enzyme-linked immunosorbent assay (ELISA)** has better specificity, sensitivity, and reproducibility than those of IFA. It detects IgM antibodies, which occurs 2-4 weeks after the erythema chronicum migrans (ECM) rash, then peaks after 8 weeks and normalizes by 4-6 months.
  3. **Western blotting** is used to confirm a positive IFA or ELISA especially late in the course of Lyme disease. It is used only when clinical and serologic tests are doubtful.
  4. **Cellular immunity testing** detects T-cell response to *B. burgdorferi* early in the course of Lyme disease, before the production of antibodies. It is difficult, however, to perform and interpret; therefore, it is not routinely used.
G. **Uric acid (serum)** is increased in gout and is primarily used to confirm gout. However, it is also increased in asymptomatic hyperuricemia, renal failure, rapidly proliferating neoplasms, postchemotherapy or irradiation, hemolytic anemias, toxemia of pregnancy, excessive dietary intake (e.g., kidney or liver food products), lead poisoning, parathyroid disorders, sarcoidosis, and in the intake of certain drugs (e.g., thiazides, loop diuretics, low-dose aspirin).
H. **Synovial fluid** obtained via arthrocentesis (see Chapter 4.9 for arthrocentesis techniques) can be classified into normal, noninflammatory (group I), inflammatory (group II), septic (group III), or hemorrhagic (group IV). The problems with such classifications include: (a) lack of uniform criteria for inclusion into any one group; (b) limited usefulness for diagnosis because a single disease may fall into any group (e.g., SLE and scleroderma can either be inflammatory [group I] or noninflammatory [group II]; gout, which is classified as inflammatory [group II] may look purulent [group III] during an acute attack; infected fluids [group III] may show inflammatory [group II] fluid during early infection or when partially treated). In general, the only two conditions that can be diagnosed using synovial fluid analysis alone are crystal–induced synovitis (group II or inflammatory) and septic arthritis (group III or purulent). As long as the clinician is aware of its limitations, the arbitrary classification of synovial fluids (see Table 2.1-1) may be used to distinguish inflammatory from ''noninflammatory'' arthritis and to alert the clinician about infectious arthritis when the WBC is high or when the fluid looks purulent. The following are some of the possible rheumatologic conditions that may be associated with each group of synovial fluid analysis (note that some conditions, e.g., SLE, may be associated with more than one group):
  1. **''Noninflammatory'' (group I):** Osteoarthritis, aseptic necrosis, trauma, osteochondritis dessicans, osteochondromatosis, neuropathic arthropathy, pigmented villonodular synovitis, SLE, scleroderma, and subsiding or early inflammation.
  2. **Inflammatory (group II):** Connective tissue diseases (RA, juvenile rheumatoid arthritis [JRA], SLE, acute rheumatic fever, scleroderma, arthritis accompanying ulcerative colitis and regional enteritis), infectious arthritis (e.g.,

Table 2.1-1.   Classification of synovial fluids*

SYNOVIAL FLUID	NORMAL	I	II	III	IV
Viscosity	High	High	Low	Variable	High
Color	Colorless to straw-colored	Straw-colored to yellow	Yellow	Variable	Red
Clarity	Transparent	Transparent	Cloudy	Opaque	Opaque
WBC/mm³	<200	200-2000	2000-75,000	often >100,000	May be <200
% PMN WBC	<25	<25	often >50	often >75	May be <25
Mucin clot	Firm	Firm	Friable	Friable	Firm
FBG	Nearly equal (± 10%) to blood	Nearly equal (± 10%) to blood	<25 mg/dl lower than in blood	>25 mg/dl lower than in blood	Nearly equal (± 10%) to blood

Adapted from: Zvaiffler NJ: Synovial fluid analysis. In Stein J, editor: *Internal Medicine*, ed 4, St. Louis, 1994, Mosby, p. 2358.
* Group I = "non-inflammatory"; group II = inflammatory; group III = septic; group IV = hemorrhagic.
WBC = white blood cell; PMN WBC = polymorphonuclear WBC; FBG = fasting blood glucose

viral), seronegative spondyloarthropathies (Reiter's syndrome, AS, psoriatic arthritis), crystal-induced synovitis (gout, pseudogout), leukemia, lymphoma.

3. **Purulent (group III):** Tuberculosis, acute bacterial infections, fungal infections, and sometimes gout and RA.

4. **Hemorrhagic (group IV):** Coagulation disorders (e.g., hemophilia, von Willebrand's disease, anticoagulation therapy, thrombocytopenia), trauma with or without fracture, postsurgical, pigmented (hypertrophic) villonodular synovitis, benign or malignant joint or synovial neoplasm, hemangioma, scurvy, neuropathic arthropathy, Ehlers-Danlos syndrome, pseudoxanthoma elasticum, sickle cell disease.

IV. Biopsy

A. **Muscle biopsy**, usually taken from the deltoid or quadriceps, is done to distinguish myopathic from neurogenic disease. In primary myopathies, the muscle is characterized by fiber size variation and evidence of degeneration (fiber necrosis and phagocytosis, possibly inflammation) and regeneration (basophilia, fiber splitting). In chronic myopathies, there may be extensive connective tissue proliferation and fatty infiltration. In denervating disease there may be evidence of active (small, angulated fibers), and chronic (fiber typed grouping and grouped atrophy) denervation. Muscle biopsy is of major diagnostic value in inflammatory muscle disease, steroid myopathy, muscular dystrophy, and infectious myositis. It is also valuable in the diagnosis of myopathy associated with various connective tissue diseases, including vasculitis.

B. **Synovial biopsy** is obtained via open arthrotomy or under direct vision with arthroscopy or blindly through closed needle biopsy. However, a closed needle biopsy should not be done unless there is excessive synovial fluid. It is performed when the diagnosis is unclear despite a thorough clinical examination in patients with chronic nontraumatic synovitis limited to a single or few joints. Its greatest value is in providing a more specific diagnosis in patients with monoarticular or oligoarticular arthritis whose diagnosis is not clear. It also has diagnostic values in acute infection (i.e., showing clusters and sheets of neutrophils and bacteria); chronic infection such as TB, fungal infections (i.e., showing large numbers of lymphocytes, plasma cells, granulomas, and tubercle bacilli or fungi); and infiltrative or deposition disease such as primary and secondary amyloidosis (i.e., showing amyloid infiltrates), ochronosis (i.e., showing brown pigment sheets), hemochromatosis (i.e., showing hemosiderin deposits), tumors (e.g., pigmented villonodular synovitis, benign and malignant tumors), and multicentric disease (e.g., reticular histiocytosis). It may also be helpful in chronic sarcoidosis, multiple synovial chondromatosus, polymyositis, and scleroderma.

C. **Sural nerve biopsy** is used to confirm vasculitis especially if there are symptoms of intermittent numbness or weakness or if nerve conduction studies shows delayed sural nerve conduction.

BIBLIOGRAPHY

Hicks JE, Sutin J: Rehabilitation in joint and connective tissue diseases. 2. Approach to the diagnosis of rheumatic diseases. *Arch Phys Med Rehabil* Suppl 69:S-78-S-83, 1988.

Paget S, Pellicci, Beary III, JF, editors: *Manual of rheumatology and outpatient orthopedic disorders*, ed 3, Boston, 1993, Little, Brown.

Stein J, editor: *Internal medicine*, ed 4, St. Louis, 1994, Mosby.

Schumacher, Jr., HR, Klipper JH, Koopman WJ, editors: *Primer on the rheumatic disease*, ed 10, Atlanta, 1993, Arthritis Foundation.

Surks MI, et al.: American Thyroid Association guidelines for the use of laboratory tests in thyroid disorders. *JAMA* 263:1529-1532, 1990.

CHAPTER 2.2

NONINVASIVE IMAGING STUDIES

Chapters 2.2 and 2.3 cover some of the widely used imaging studies in the PM& R setting. They are by no means complete. The classification of invasive versus noninvasive procedures is at best arbitrary. In this book, noninvasive imaging studies refer to those that do not involve skin puncture. Hence, imaging studies that involve swallowing of ultrasound probes (e.g., transesophageal echocardiography or TEE) or of barium (e.g., videofluoroscopic swallowing studies) are discussed under this chapter even though they can be argued as "invasive." Interpretation of any imaging studies must be closely correlated with clinical findings (as abnormal findings can possibly be found in asymptomatic individuals).

I. **Radiographic imaging**
   A. **Conventional radiography or plain radiography (plain x-ray)** is usually the initial diagnostic imaging method in the evaluation of bone and joint pain because it is readily available and has relatively low cost. For a systematic way of interpreting radiographs of the musculoskeletal system, use the "ABCs" mnemonic. First check the **A**lignment of the bone, then the **B**one itself, followed by **C**artilage and **S**oft tissue.
      1. **Limb radiograph** views commonly used are anteroposterior, lateral, oblique, patellar views of the knee, and standing views of the foot, knee, and hip. Plain radiographs are specific for the diagnosis of bony lesions such as fractures, neoplasms, and osteomyelitis but are not as sensitive as radionuclide bone scanning and magnetic resonance imaging (MRI) for early detection of these abnormalities. Radiograph evaluation of nonbony structures (e.g., cartilage, muscle, ligaments, tendons, and synovial fluid) is difficult unless fat or calcification is present. Joint space narrowing may indicate cartilage destruction. Displacement of adjacent fat pads in the knee, elbow, and ankle may be due to synovitis (this cannot be reliably detected in the hip and shoulder).
      2. **Spine radiograph** views commonly used are anteroposterior, lateral, oblique, odontoid, flexion-extension views, and tomography. Spine radiographs are useful in patients with suspected spinal trauma, scoliosis, congenital anomalies of the spine, back pain (e.g., spondylolisthesis, spondylolysis, ankylosing spondylitis), point tenderness, osteoporosis, and after spinal surgery (e.g., flexion and extension views of the spine can be used to diagnose instability and evaluate adequacy of spinal fusion). However, studies have shown there is practically no correlation between clinical findings and the osteophytes and/or neural foraminal stenosis (especially in cervical region) seen in conventional radiographs. Detection of multilevel degenerative disease is also a poor indicator of the specific source of the pain. Fractures of the pedicles or the neural arch are difficult to identify in conventional radiographs (CT scan is recommended instead).
      3. **Skull radiographs** have low diagnostic yield and should not be used routinely to screen headache, seizure, and transient or fixed neurologic deficits. In severe intracranial injury, immediate computer-assisted tomography (CT) is indicated. Most skull radiographs are currently used in the emergency

room on patients with relatively mild head trauma and without neurologic findings to detect fractures, to screen patients for CT examination, and on patients with facial injury, lacerations to the head, or penetrating missile injury. Skull radiographs can also be used in assessing congenital craniofacial abnormalities, palpable lesions in the scalp, and inflammatory conditions of the paranasal sinuses and mastoids.

B. Fluoroscopy is used to determine the position during surgical procedures (e.g., internal fixation of fractures and osteotomies) and during invasive radiologic procedures (e.g., myelography, percutaneous needle biopsy, diskography, arthrography, and facet joint injection). Fluoroscopy may be used for the evaluation of motion and to determine spinal stability. Its main disadvantage is excessive radiation exposure, which can be reduced by videotape recording, e.g., **videofluoroscopic swallowing studies** (see Chapter 5.6, section III.C.1.b) and **video-urodynamics** (see Chapter 5.7, section II.C.2.e).

C. Computer-assisted tomography (CT) is a cross-sectional imaging technique that uses a narrowly collimated x-ray beam of predetermined slice thickness to provide better soft tissue contrast than with plain radiographs. It is useful in evaluating the extent of bony and soft tissue tumors. In a CT scan, air is black, and fat, cerebrospinal fluid (CSF), white matter, gray matter, blood and bone are progressively whiter. Its disadvantage is that it exposes the patient to radiation.

1. **Head CT** without contrast is indicated in acute trauma, hydrocephalus (monitoring ventricular size in shunted patients), intracranial hemorrhage, stroke (distinguishing hemorrhagic from bland infarcts), skull base diseases, and complex craniofacial anomalies. Contrast-enhanced head CT has an intravascular component that enhances normal vessels and abnormal vascular structures, such as aneurysms and vascular malformations, and an extravascular component in which contrast material leaks out of vessels into areas of blood brain barrier disruptions such as brain tumors, cerebral infarction, and a variety of inflammatory processes. With the advent of MRI, the need for contrast head CT has diminished.

2. **Spine and pelvic CT scans** can be used to diagnose intervertebral disk herniation, spinal stenosis (assessment of the extent of hypertrophic bony changes, calcified ligaments, and bony spurs), degenerative disk and vertebral disease, vertebral and paraspinal tumors and inflammatory lesions, vertebral fractures (e.g., fractures through the pedicles or the neural arch, which are difficult to assess on plain radiographs), pelvic and sacral fractures, and congenital abnormalities. Although CT and MRI are equally helpful in diagnosing lumbar disk disease, CT is not as good as MRI in detecting cervical and thoracic disk herniation. In most patients with back pain and sciatica, CT has eliminated the need for myelography. In the diagnosis of intraspinal lesions, however, CT scan may be combined with myelography to enhance its sensitivity. Although sagittal and coronal CT images can be obtained by reformatting the obtained data, their resolutions are not as good as with the axial images. If after a CT scan, the diagnosis is not established, then MRI should be considered.

II. Magnetic resonance imaging (MRI) involves the imaging of protons (the positively charged spinning nucleus of hydrogen atoms) abundant in water, proteins, lipids, and other macromolecules. When placed in a magnetic field, protons align themselves either with or against the direction of the field. Their alignment direction is reversed when radiofrequency (RF) pulses are applied. As the RF pulse is stopped, the protons then return to their original magnetic alignment (relaxation phase). In the process of relaxation, the protons release the energy acquired during RF pulse, thus producing a voltage that is measured as the magnetic resonance (MR) signal. The relative brightness or darkness of the MR signal depends on the RF pulse sequence, the proton density of the tissue, and other factors such as blood flow and chemical shift.

MRI can be used to evaluate internal derangement of the knee (e.g., meniscal tears, cruciate tears, collateral ligament tears, quadriceps mechanism tears, and bone contusion); osteonecrosis; rotator cuff tears and glenohumeral instability; tendon, ligament, and muscle tears of the ankle, wrist, and elbow; diskovertebral instability and disk herniation; brain disorders (especially white matter diseases); spinal cord disorders (syringomyelia, intrinsic lesions such as cysts and tumors, myelopathy, conus medullaris lesions); bone and soft tissue tumors and metastases; occult fractures; vascular malformations; and hemangiomas. It is superior to the CT scan in detecting cervical and thoracic disk herniation. For the diagnosis of lumbar disk disease, however, MRI and CT are equally helpful. When extensive calcification or hypertrophic changes are present (e.g., calcification of the posterior longitudinal ligament or osteophytes), MRI is inferior to CT scan. In patients with sciatica, MRI (instead of myelography) is recommended to detect lesions of the conus medullaris and other intraspinal lesions (e.g., neoplasms), which may mimic sciatica.

MRI has the following advantages over CT scan:

- MRI does not use ionizing radiation and has no apparent adverse biologic effects;
- MRI is not subject to bone or dental artifact;
- MRI allows coronal and sagittal imaging with ease and with excellent resolution;
- MRI requires contrast enhancement less often than CT; and
- MRI uses contrasts agents, which are generally safer than the agents used for CT.

The disadvantages of MRI are:

- It is more expensive than CT;
- It has limited use in acutely ill patients on life support because of interactions between the magnetic field and life support equipment;
- It is often unacceptable to claustrophobic patients;
- It cannot be used in patients with ferromagnetic intracranial aneurysm clips, metallic objects anatomically close to a vital vascular or neural structures or in or around the eyes, pacemakers, cochlear implants, neurostimulator devices, or some bullet fragments;
- It has limited use when the area of clinical interest is close to ferromagnetic surgical hardware; and
- It is inferior to CT in detecting acute subarachnoid hemorrhage and in evaluating calcified lesions.

Most prosthetic heart valves as well as most orthopedic materials and devices (including stainless steel screws and wires) are considered safe for MRI. However, ferromagnetic metallic implants cause image artifact (''flare'' response), which may interfere with MRI interpretation. Pregnancy (especially in the first trimester) is considered a relative contraindication of MRI although there is no convincing evidence to suggest a risk to the fetus. Children as well as anxious patients may need to be sedated during MRI.

A. **Spin-echo MRI technique** uses two RF pulses to achieve soft tissue contrast by differential tissue relaxation times. Spin-echo MR images can be weighted depending on the RF pulse sequence, repetition time (TR is the interval between repetitions of the pulse sequence), and echo time (TE is the interval between RF excitation and the measurement of the MR signal). T_1-weighted MR images (short TR of <600 msec and short TE of <32 msec) are obtained quickly to show anatomical detail. T_2-weighted MR images (long TR of 2000-3000 msec; long TE of 60-120 msec) have improved contrast but less spatial resolution and take longer to obtain than T_1-weighted images. An intermediate-density-weighted MR image (or proton-density-weighted or spin-density-weighted image) uses TR of 1500-2500 msec and TE of 15-50 msec.

Table 2.2-1 shows the different signal intensities of different tissues on T_1- and T_2-weighted MR images. In general, fatty tissue (e.g., normal fatty bone marrow) exhibits a bright signal intensity on T_1-weighted sequences, with slightly less bright signal on T_2-weighted sequences. Conversely, pathologic processes (infiltrative disease, infection, bone marrow edema) appear as low signal on T_1-weighted sequences. Both cortical bone and fibrous tissue (including normal ligaments and tendons) maintain low signal intensity on all pulse sequences. Fluids (synovial fluid, edema, cysts) exhibit low signal intensity on T_1-weighted sequences, with markedly bright signal intensity with T_2-weighted.

B. **Gradient-echo MRI techniques** provides rapid image acquisition by using a single radiofrequency pulse to achieve soft tissue contrast through variation in pulse sequences. Unlike spin-echo MRI technique, there is no loss of signal associated with the outflow of blood during the interval between RF pulses. Hence, in gradient-echo MR images laminar blood flow appears bright while turbulent flow and thrombus appear dark. In contrast to spin-echo MR images in which rapid blood flow appears dark, slow blood flow appears intermediate, and thrombus appears intermediate or bright. Gradient-echo MRI is extremely useful in the evaluation of articular cartilage and in diagnosing subtle cervical disk disease. In general, bone is black and soft tissues (e.g., disk) are white on gradient-echo MRI.

C. **Gadolinium-enhanced MRI** is technically an invasive procedure but is discussed here for convenience. It uses an MRI contrast agent (gadolinium diethylenetriamine pentaacetic acid or GD-DTPA) that shortens T_1 relaxation times. Gadolinium-enhanced images appear bright on T_1-weighted images. It is used in spine and brain imaging especially for tumor diagnosis and detection of multiple sclerosis plaques. It is superior to CT in the detection of tumor-associated features such as edema, cysts, vascularity, hemorrhage, and necrosis. It can distinguish early postoperative scars (which are enhanced because of its rich vascularity) from recurrent disk herniation (which is avascular and is not enhanced). However, long after surgery the scar tissue may become progressively fibrotic with less discernible contrast enhancement. Relative contraindications to GD-DTPA administration include patients with hemolytic anemias (may promote extravascular hemolysis) and impaired renal function (GD-DTPA is cleared through glomerular filtration). The most common adverse reaction is mild headache which is reported in less than 10% of patients.

D. **Magnetic resonance angiography (MRA)** (see Chapter 2.3, section II.A.2.d).

III. **Diagnostic ultrasonography** transmits high-frequency (ultrasound) waves to the tissue and measures the amplitude of the reflected waves and the time it has

Table 2.2-1.   Summary of signal intensities on magnetic resonance imaging (MRI)

TISSUE	T₁-WEIGHTED IMAGE*	T₂-WEIGHTED IMAGE†
Fat	Very bright	Intermediate to dark
Cyst		
Simple	Very dark	Very bright
Proteinaceous	Intermediate to bright	Very bright
Brain		
White matter	Bright	Moderately dark
Gray matter	Moderately dark	Moderately bright
Cerebrospinal fluid	Very dark	Very bright
Multiple sclerosis plaque	Intermediate to dark	Bright
Bland infarct	Dark	Bright
Tumor	Dark	Bright
Meningioma	Intermediate	Intermediate
Abscess	Dark	Bright
Edema	Dark	Bright
Calcification	Variable: poorly seen, dark or bright	Variable: poorly seen or dark
Bone marrow		
Yellow	Very bright	Intermediate to dark
Red	Intermediate	Moderately dark
Bone metastasis		
Lytic	Dark	Intermediate to bright
Sclerotic	Dark	Dark
Cortical bone	Very dark	Very dark
Cartilage		
Fibrous	Very dark	Very dark
Hyaline	Intermediate	Intermediate
Intervertebral disk		
Normal	Intermediate	Bright
Degenerated	Intermediate to dark	Dark
Tendons and ligaments	Very dark	Very dark
Inflamed tendons	Intermediate	Intermediate
Torn tendons	Intermediate	Bright
Muscle	Dark	Dark
Gadolinium-enhanced tissue		
Low concentration	Very bright	Bright
High concentration	Intermediate to dark	Very dark
Hematoma		
Acute	Intermediate to dark	Dark
Subacute	Bright rim	Bright
Chronic	Dark rim (± bright center)	Dark rim (± bright center)

* T₁-weighted image = short TR (repetition time) of <600 msec and short TE (echo time) of <32 msec.
† T₂-weighted image = long TR of 2000-3000 msec; long TE of 60-120 msec.
Data adapted from: Edelman RR, Warach S: Magnetic resonance imaging, part I. *New Engl J Med* 328 (10):710, 1993, copyright © 1993 Massachusetts Medical Society. All rights reserved, used with permission.

taken the waves to travel from the transmitter to the receiving crystal. It measures tissue density at known depths and so builds a two-dimensional picture of the tissues, which can be presented in tones of gray. This is known as grayscale or B-mode imaging and is the mode commonly used for imaging solid structures. In this mode, the whiteness is inversely proportional to the density.

A. **Musculoskeletal ultrasonography** can be used to evaluate soft tissue masses and characterize them as either cystic or solid. Ultrasound waves are reflected by bone and cannot be used to evaluate the internal bony structures. Tendons are more echogenic than muscle and can be evaluated in some cases for continuity and inflammation. Ultrasonography of joints has been used in the shoulder for evaluation of the rotator cuff tendons but has not been as accurate as MRI or arthrography. Ultrasound may be used for evaluation of congenital dislocation of the hip in infants to determine the position of the nonossified femoral head with respect to the acetabulum. In contrast to both CT scan and MRI, ultrasonographs can display structures in motion. Its use in delineating musculoskeletal motion (e.g., motion of the spine and the facet joints), however, is still experimental.

B. **Echocardiography** uses ultrasound to image cardiac structures and function and to determine flow direction and velocities within cardiac chambers and vessels. It can either be performed via transthoracic or transesophageal ultrasound probes. Transesophageal echocardiography (TEE) can be classified as an invasive procedure as it entails swallowing of the probe. (The diagnostic uses of echocardiography are described in Chapter 5.13, section III.C.2.b).

C. **Thyroid US** is used to evaluate the size of the thyroid and the number, composition, and dimension of the thyroid nodule. Although both solid and cystic nodules can be malignant, solid nodules have higher incidence of malignancy.

D. **Renal US** is used to assess kidney anatomy for detecting hydronephrosis and kidney stones.

E. **Vascular doppler** is commonly used in PM&R to determine severity or location of peripheral vascular disease or carotid stenosis and to rule out deep venous thrombosis (DVT). Vascular spectral doppler is used to determine flow velocity. It may be combined with the basic B-mode imaging.

1. **Continuous-wave doppler** modality emits and receives ultrasound continuously. It can infer the speed that a target (e.g., red blood cell) is traveling, but it cannot determine from what distance the signal returns (i.e., it cannot state the location of the target). Although it is rapid, easy, inexpensive, and reproducible, it cannot localize occlusions nor provide adequate hemodynamic evaluation.

a. **Arterial continuous-wave doppler** is used for the evaluation of peripheral artery occlusive disease via the ankle/brachial ratio (ABI), which is determined by measuring arterial dopplers from the arm and ankle. The normal ABI should be about 1.1 (± 0.2). ABI of patients with intermittent claudication is 0.6 (± 0.2), ischemic rest pain is 0.3 (± 0.1), and impending tissue necrosis or loss is 0.1 (± 0.1). A change of ABI between examinations of more than 0.15 is considered significant. Obviously, these figures need clinical correlation before deciding on treatment. Also, in diabetic patients, false results may be obtained due to medial calcinosis of the artery. If ABI is greater than 0.6, tissue healing will likely occur spontaneously, thus, vascular reconstruction (e.g., vascular bypass or graft surgery) is usually not recommended because 30% of reconstructed vessels can become impatent within 5 years. Vascular reconstruction is only indicated for limb threatening ischemia (i.e., ischemic rest pain or tissue necrosis or loss).

    b. Venous continuous-wave doppler may be used to detect DVT. However, its inability to localize the occlusion makes it less useful than duplex scanning using pulsed-wave doppler.

  2. Pulsed-wave doppler modality emits a burst of ultrasound, waits for a period of time, then opens a "window" to catch the returning signal. Its advantage over continuous-wave doppler is its range resolution, which allows it to localize the source of occlusion. It is used in **duplex scanning** in combination with a high-resolution real-time B-mode imaging. In duplex scanning, the pulsed-wave doppler is used to locate the source of the abnormal flow and the B-mode ultrasound is used to provide morphologic image of the blood vessel. A color doppler flow mapping **(color-flow duplex scanning** or **CFDS)** is commonly used to facilitate duplex examination of the peripheral vessels, as it allows two-dimensional colored "images" of blood flow to be superimposed on the B-mode imaging. Duplex scanning is inexpensive and can be performed quickly; however, test interpretation is technician-dependent.

    a. Carotid duplex scanning is used to determine stenosis primarily at the carotid bifurcation (e.g., atherosclerotic plaques). For clinical purposes, a stenotic lesion that is identified using **CFDS** is classified as low grade (40%–60%); medium grade (61%–80%), or high grade (81%–90%). It is of limited use for disease above the region of the carotid bifurcations and is subject to errors of interpretation in cases of high-grade stenosis or complete occlusions.

    b. Venous duplex scanning is used to locate and quantify the severity of deep or superficial venous thrombosis, assess venous incompetence, and map the superficial veins before surgical harvest for bypass operations. In the detection of infrainguinal DVT (see Chapter 5.3, section III.B.1.a), the compressive technique is commonly used, i.e., a doppler sensor is placed on the proximal part of the vein as the ultrasound probe compresses the vein distally. An obstruction (e.g., thrombus) is detected if the doppler wave is not augmented upon distal vein compression or if the doppler wave does not fluctuate significantly during respiration or if the vein is noncompressible (i.e., the vein does not collapse under a force sufficient to distort the artery). For morphological identification of the thrombus, either a real-time B-mode grayscale imaging or a color imaging **(CFDS)** may be used.

IV. Plethysmography assesses limb volume by detecting changes in the electrical impedance between two electrodes wrapped around the calf.

  A. Arterial plethysmography measures multiple volume changes (pulse volume recording) in segmental cuffs inflated at a preset pressure. Unlike arterial dopplers, it is not affected by medial calcinosis in diabetic patients. However, it is inappropriate for patients who are obese, edematous, or with muscle tremors. Qualitative gradings of the pulse volume recording are normal if the wave has a sharp systolic peak followed by a dicrotic notch (caused by relaxation of arterial wall prior to diastole), mildly abnormal if the dicrotic notch is absent with slow downslope, moderately abnormal if the wave shows flattening of the systolic peak, and severely abnormal if the systolic peak is almost as flat as the baseline.

  B. Venous plethysmography (see also Chapter 5.3, section III.B.1.b)

    1. Impedance venous plethysmography (IPG) is used to diagnose proximal venous thrombosis. It involves inflation of a proximal thigh cuff to obstruct venous outflow. After allowing distal filling of the venous system, the cuff is deflated. In the normal limb, plethysmography shows that the leg swells during cuff inflation then rapidly (within 3 to 4 sec) returns to its normal size upon cuff deflation (because of rapid venous outflow). In the presence of proximal obstruction (most likely because of venous thrombosis), response is "blunted" (i.e., the return to baseline is delayed when the cuff is deflated).

2. **Exercise venous plethysmography** documents or screens for lower limb venous incompetence and quantifies its severity before, during, and after exercise. Normally, plethysmography shows a progressive decrease in leg volume during exercise followed by a period when the volume slowly returns to normal. In venous insufficiency, the exercise-induced decrease in venous volume is less than expected. Moreover, the postexercise return in volume is more rapid than expected when venous incompetence is present.

3. **Phleborheography (PRG)** uses multiple pneumatic cuffs to monitor changes in leg volume at various sites in the leg and thigh during respiration and leg compression. It is time-consuming and interpretation is subjective.

V. **Thermography** is the use of electronic screening devices to detect infrared rays emitted from the skin, which is directly equivalent to the body surface temperature. A pictorial heat map is then constructed, which shows areas of increased vasodilatation ("hot spots") or vasoconstriction ("cold spots") as a result of autonomic responses to disease or trauma in nerve root or peripheral nerves. It is considered a physiological instead of an anatomical test and is used in the diagnosis of neuromuscular pain or inflammation (e.g., radiculopathy, carpal tunnel syndrome, reflex sympathetic dystrophy, "trigger point"). Its usefulness as a diagnostic tool remains controversial.

BIBLIOGRAPHY

Edelman RR, Warach S: Magnetic resonance imaging, part I. *New Engl J Med* 328 (10):708-716, 1993.

Edelman RR, Warach S: Magnetic resonance imaging, part II. *New Engl J Med* 328 (11):785-791, 1993.

Firooznia HF, Golimbu C, Rafii M, et al: *MRI and CT of the musculoskeletal system*, St. Louis, 1992, Mosby.

Lanzer P, Rosch J, editors: *Vascular diagnostics*, New York, 1994, Springer-Verlag.

Merritt JL, Anderson JM, Fisher SV, et al: Rehabilitation of musculoskeletal and soft tissue disorders. Part 6: Diagnostic tests and examination. *Arch Phys Med Rehabil* Suppl 69:S-146-S-149, 1988.

Paget S, Pellicci P, Beary JF, III, editors: *Manual of rheumatology and outpatient orthopedic disorders*, ed 3, Boston, 1993, Little, Brown.

Ramsey RG: *Neuroradiology*, ed 3, Philadelphia, 1994, WB Saunders.

Stein J, editor: *Internal Medicine*, ed 4, St. Louis, 1994, Mosby.

CHAPTER 2.3

INVASIVE IMAGING STUDIES

As stated in Chapter 2.2, any imaging study is useless without close clinical correlation (because abnormal findings can possibly be found even in asymptomatic individuals). The following include some of the commonly used invasive imaging studies in the PM&R setting. The invasive imaging studies discussed in this chapter include only those that involve skin puncture (e.g., for introduction of contrast dye or radionuclide compounds).

I. Nuclear medicine

A. Bone mineral analyses are used to diagnose osteoporosis and determine fracture risk. Single- and dual-beam photon absorptiometries use radioisotopes and are considered invasive. Dual-energy x-ray absorptiometry and quantitative computed-tomography (QCT) scans are noninvasive nonnuclear medicine studies but are included here for convenience. In the diagnosis of osteoporosis, bone trabecular measurements (which can be determined more accurately by QCT scan) are more important because the trabecular bone turnover is 8 to 9 times that of cortical bone.

    1. Single-beam photon absorptiometry uses iodine-125 to measure the cortical bones in the forearm, primarily the distal radius. Although it can delineate bone density accurately (with a precision of 2%–3%), it does not distinguish trabecular from cortical bone. It has limited usefulness because the cortical density of forearm bones does not necessarily correlate with that of weight-bearing bones.

    2. Dual-beam photon absorptiometry (DPA) uses multienergy isotope (gradolinium-135) to analyze the density of both trabecular and cortical weight-bearing bones (i.e., lumbar vertebral body and femoral neck) with a precision of 2% to 3%. The scanning, however, is time consuming.

    3. Dual energy x-ray absorptiometry (DEXA) scan uses a dual x-ray source to replace the isotope source used in DPA. It measures the same bones as in DPA but has lower radiation exposure and greater precision than DPA and can be performed much more rapidly. The newer DEXA-scanner, which scans the vertebral body from the lateral side (instead of posteriorly to anteriorly), is preferred because it eliminates the inclusion of the cortical bone of the posterior varterbral elements in its measurement of bone density (hence a more accurate measurement of the trabecular density of the vertebral body can be made).

    4. Quantitative CT scan detects trabecular bone loss, independent of cortical bone loss, and is the only modality that can detect vertebral trabecular bone loss in early phases when treatment is most effective. It can also measure the amount of vertebral body collapse. Although QCT is more expensive than DEXA-scan, the information provided is more accurate. The QCT measurement of hip bone density is not done because the major determinant of hip fracture is believed to be the frequency of falls, not density of the femur.

B. Radionuclide bone scanning uses technetium 99m phosphate complexes (fluorine 18 or strontium 88m were used in the past) to detect physiologic changes in the bone as compared with anatomic changes seen on radiography. Increased uptake of the radionuclide reflects increased bone blood flow and increased osteoblastic activity due to new bone formation. However, this is nonspecific and can be caused by infection, tumor, fractures, or synovitis. A **three-phase bone scan,** which includes blood flow and blood pool scans, as well as static images 2 to 4 hours or more after injection, can be used to evaluate localized bone or joint pain (the early phases may be helpful in diagnosing infection and soft tissue abnormalities). The radiation exposure from a bone scan is similar to that from a radiograph series of the lumbar spine. Bone scan has similar sensitivity but less specificity than MRI in the early diagnosis of many bone and joint problems. It is less expensive than MRI and can survey the entire skeleton during one examination.

Bone scan is the procedure of choice in the evaluation of skeletal and spinal metastases and has largely replaced radiography for this purpose. It is more sensitive than plain radiographs in revealing metastatic tumors that are only a few millimeters in diameter, as only metastases larger than 1.5 cm in size and with more than 50% demineralization can generally be detected with plain radiographs. Bone scan is indicated in patients with bone or joint pain whose radiographs are negative or inconclusive. It is useful in diagnosing subtle nondisplaced traumatic fractures (e.g., navicular stress fracture), prosthetic loosening of total joint arthroplasty (especially of the femoral components), joint infections such as early osteomyelitis and disk space infections (increased sensitivity when triple phase bone scan is done, or in conjunction with gallium or indium scan), avascular necrosis (in early stage, there is no focal uptake, but in reparative stage, there is increased uptake; however, MRI is the current procedure of choice), metastatic disease as a cause of undiagnosed pain, and reflex sympathetic dystrophy (RSD) (may require 3 or 4 phase studies).

C. **Radionuclide infection scans** are not very specific because increased uptake may also occur in noninfectious conditions.

1. **Gallium 67 citrate scans** have high sensitivity for infection in the bones or soft tissues but is nonspecific because increased uptake may be seen in noninfectious conditions such fractures, tumors, or noninfectious inflammatory conditions (e.g. inflammatory arthritis). When used in conjunction with a bone scan, its specificity for infection may be increased. Infection is likely if the gallium scan shows more intense uptake than the bone scan at the affected site or if the uptake of gallium is not congruent with the uptake on the bone scan. Unfortunately, only one-third or less of bone infections meet these criteria. There are reports of false-negative gallium scans in chronic infections and in patients treated with antibiotics prior to the scan.

2. **Indium 111 or technetium 99m–labeled leukocyte scans** do not collect in areas of neoplasia and are more specific than bone scans or gallium scans in detecting bone or joint infection. However, increased uptake may also be seen in noninfectious conditions. It is useful in the evaluation of acute osteomyelitis, and possibly total joint arthroplasty infections. Unlike gallium, it is also useful in the presence of pseudoarthrosis. When used in conjunction with a bone scan or radiolabeled colloid scans, its specificity for infection may be increased.

D. **Radionuclide ventilation-perfusion lung scan (V/Q scan)** is commonly used to rule out pulmonary embolism. It consists of a perfusion scan and a ventilation scan. The perfusion scan is obtained by gamma camera imaging of the distribution of intravenously injected radionuclide (technetium 99m–labeled macroaggregates of albumin or iodine-labeled fibrinogen), which are trapped in the pulmonary capillary bed and which accumulate in clots. Normal perfusion scans show homogenous distribution of radioactivity throughout both lungs and thus rule out pulmonary embolism. An abnormal perfusion lung scan, however, is not specific for pulmonary embolism because any process that destroys or constricts pulmonary arterial vessels (e.g., pneumonia, emphysema) can cause perfusion defects. Hence a ventilation lung scan is performed by having the patient breathe a radioactive gas such as xenon 133, which distributes evenly throughout the lungs. In the presence of airway obstruction, the xenon 133 may be trapped in the proximal airway thus making interpretation difficult. If the ventilation scan is normal or if it does not match the perfusion defect (which is greater than or equal to one pulmonary segment), then there is a high probability of pulmonary embolism. Based on the relative size of perfusion and ventilation defects and radiographic abnormalities, a low, intermediate, or indeterminate probability may be designated.

E. Radionuclide venography for the detection of thrombi in the proximal vein of the lower limbs is still in the developmental stage.

F. Quantitative radionuclide renal scan is used to monitor renal function and drainage.

    1. Technetium 99m (^{99m}Tc) scan. ^{99m}Tc-dimercaptosuccinic acid (DMSA) is used for both differential function and evaluation of the functioning areas of the renal cortex. ^{99m}Tc-mercaptoacetyltriglycine (MAG3) is used to also assess urinary tract drainage as well as differential function.

    2. I 131 hippuran scan is used to monitor renal perfusion and determine glomerular filtration rate (GFR) and excretory renal plasma flow (ERPF).

G. Thyroid radioisotope scintiscanning uses Iodine 123 for evaluation of thyroid function and the noninvasive assessment of thyroid anatomy. It is used to assess thyroid nodules to define whether they are functional (hot or warm nodules, which are usually benign) or nonfunctional (cold nodules, which are usually malignant), to permit localization of the thyroid, localization of metastatic deposits of differentiated thyroid cancer or of residual normal thyroid tissue after surgery, to evaluate thyroid anatomy, and to distinguish multinodular goiter from other goitrous enlargements of the thyroid.

H. Single photon emission computed tomography (SPECT) uses scintigraphy and CT to evaluate overlapping structures in femoral head osteonecrosis, patellofemoral syndrome, and healing spondylotic defects. It may provide increased detail and may be helpful in diagnosing acute traumatic spondylosis or pars stress fracture, determining acute or preexisting fracture, and detecting photopenic areas in avascular necrosis.

II. Contrast imaging

  A. Contrast vascular imaging

    1. Venography (phlebography) of the lower limbs involves the injection of diluted contrast medium into a superficial vein of the foot followed by spot radiographs taken at different intervals of contrast injection. Demonstration of an intraluminal filling defect in all films and views is accepted as the final diagnostic test for determining deep vein thrombosis. MRI may be used to image the vein **(magnetic resonance venography [MRV])** with high sensitivity and specificity. However, MRV is expensive and has limited availability.

    2. Angiography

      a. Conventional or catheter cerebral angiography uses x-rays to image iodinated contrast material injected intraarterially via the femoral artery. The image may be made on a radiograph directly or the radiographic data may be digitized and electronically subtracted from another exposure obtained during contrast injection (called digital subtraction angiography). It is used in the assessment of aneurysms, vascular malformations and fistulas, arterial stenosis, occlusions, and collateral circulation in vascular occlusive diseases including atherosclerosis, trauma, and vasculitis, and in evaluation of vascular intracranial and skull base tumors.

b. Spinal angiography is used for the diagnosis of and for preembolization or presurgical mapping of spinal arteriovenous malformation and occasionally for vascular tumors such as hemangioblastomas.

c. Pulmonary angiography is the best available method of visualizing the pulmonary vasculature and in the diagnosis of pulmonary embolism. Current techniques, however, cannot show obstruction in small subsegmental arterial branches.

d. Magnetic resonance angiography (MRA) combines MRI with angiography. It uses the flow effects inherent to MRI to image vascular anatomy. Vascular images are generated either by simultaneously suppressing signal from static tissue while maximizing signal in inflowing blood **(time-of-flight angiography)** or by modifying magnetic field gradients to use information present in radiofrequency phase changes in flowing blood **(phase-contrast angiography)**. MRA is used for screening intracranial cerebrovascular disease (e.g., aneurysms) and extracranial vasculature pathology (e.g., for evaluation of carotid stenosis and suspected vessel thrombosis). It has less spatial resolution than conventional angiography and is limited by its high cost and sensitivity to patient motion (producing various artifacts).

B. Intravenous pyelography (IVP) or excretory urography is used to visualize the size, shape, and function of the whole urinary tract (kidney, ureters, and bladder) and to detect hydronephrosis, pyelonephritis, calculi, tumor, and renovascular hypertension. A radiopaque subtance is injected intravenously, and a series of radiographs are taken 3, 5, 10, 15, and 20 minutes after dye injection. At the end of the test, the patient voids and another radiograph is taken to visualize the residual dye in the bladder. The major disadvantage of IVP is patient's potential allergic reactions to the dye, radiation exposure, and patient inconvenience (patient needs to be NPO and to take laxatives). It could cause contrast nephropathy in patients with insulin-dependent diabetes mellitus [IDDM] or serum creatinine of 1.5 mg/dL.

C. Myelography is the radiographic examination of the spinal canal and spinal cord by means of contrast media, which is injected into the subarachnoid space by lumbar (and occasionally cervical) puncture. Low-osmolar, iodinated, nonionic water-soluble contrast agents are used because they are absorbed into the blood stream and excreted through the kidneys. Myelography is used to detect extradural or intradural abnormalities (herniation of the intervertebral disks, spinal stenosis, nerve root compression from bony spurs, spinal cord tumors), nerve root asymmetries, congenital anomalies of the root sleeves (e.g., conjoined root sleeves or root cysts), arachnoiditis, obstruction to CSF flow, and cord compression. In patients with sciatica, myelography should only be done when diagnosis is still in doubt after performing CT scan and MRI or if confirmation and localization of intraspinal and extradural pathology is likely to lead to surgical intervention. In this case, postmyelography CT scan should always be done. The combination of myelography and postmyelography CT is superior to MRI alone in the diagnosis of nerve root compromise by bony or soft tissue structures, facet joint disease, neural foramina and central spinal canal stenosis, extent of cauda equina compression, communication of the thecal sac with adjacent cystic structures, and the presence and extent of certain types of spinal vascular malformations. Although relatively safe, postmyelographic side effects such as headache, nausea, vomiting, vasovagal episodes, and leg pain may occur. Other complications of myelography include seizures, hypersensitivity reaction, bleeding, aseptic meningitis, infection, and cardiovascular complications.

D. Discography involves direct injection of contrast material into the intervertebral disk through a needle placed in the disk. Leakage of contrast material out of the nucleus pulposus has been claimed to indicate disk pathology, however, this is vigorously disputed by others. Disk abnormalities, however, may be also found in asymptomatic patients. Provocation testing may be done during the injection to determine if the pain is similar to the patient's usual pain syndrome. Discography is currently not recommended for the diagnosis of disorders of the intervertebral disks. It is neither sensitive nor reliable; false positives are frequent; and findings do not necessarily correlate with other, more reliable, techniques. Moreover, it has the inherent risks of invasive procedures (e.g., disk space infection).

E. Arthrography involves the intraarticular injection of water-soluble contrast media, with or without air, to evaluate articular structures such as cartilage, synovium, and ligaments. Injection of air alone may be used to detect loose bodies. Rare complications include infection and anaphylactic reaction to contrast material. Vasovagal reaction, which may occur during arthrography, should not be mistaken for an allergic reaction. Arthrography has been largely replaced by MRI scanning but may still be used if MRI is contraindicated or if the patient is unable to tolerate MRI due to claustrophobia.

1. **Shoulder arthrography** can be used to diagnose rotator cuff tears, adhesive capsulitis, labral and capsular deformity that may occur after shoulder dislocation, bicipital tendon abnormalities, articular and synovial pathologies, infection, and impingement syndrome.

2. **Elbow arthrography** can be helpful in detecting loose bodies in the joint and in the diagnosis of articular cartilage defects and osteochondral fractures.

3. **Wrist arthrography** is most useful in demonstrating ligamentous disruption in the posttraumatic wrist. It can also be used to detect tears of the triangular fibrocartilage and abnormal synovial communications within the wrist joint.

4. **Hip arthrography** is used in adults to evaluate painful hip prostheses (for loosening of hardware or for infection), synovial proliferative disease (cartilage destruction and loose bodies), osteochondral fractures, and communicating bursae and abscess cavities. In infants and children, it may be used to assess the septic hip (by obtaining aspirate and assessing joint damage) and to evaluate the position of the cartilaginous femoral head with respect to the acetabulum in Legg-Calve-Perthes disease, congenital dislocation of the hip, and coxa vara deformities.

5. **Knee arthrography** is used mainly to diagnose meniscal injuries, but it may also be used to outline collateral and cruciate ligament tears, articular cartilage alterations, synovial processes, masses, and periarticular synovial cysts (popliteal cysts). Postarthrogram CT scans of the knee are helpful in evaluating the mediopatellar plicae and the patellar cartilage.

6. **Ankle arthrography** is useful in the evaluation of acute ligamentous injuries and in assessing chronic osseous and osteocartilaginous abnormalities (e.g., osteochondritis dissecans).

BIBLIOGRAPHY

Firooznia HF, Golimbu C, Rafii M, et al.: *MRI and CT of the musculoskeletal system,* St. Louis, 1992, Mosby.

Merritt JL, Anderson JM, Fisher SV, et al.: Rehabilitation of musculoskeletal and soft tissue disorders. Part 6: Diagnostic tests and examination. *Arch Phys Med Rehabil* Suppl 69:S-146-S-149, 1988.

Nordin BEC, Chatterton BE, Need AG, et al.: The definition, diagnosis, and classification of osteoporosis. *Phys Med Rehabil Clin North Am* 6 (3):395-414, 1995.

Paget S, Pellicci P, and Beary JF, III, editors: *Manual of rheumatology and outpatient orthopedic disorders,* ed 3, Boston, 1993, Little, Brown.

Stein J, editor: *Internal medicine,* ed 4, St. Louis, 1994, Mosby.

CHAPTER 2.4

ELECTRODIAGNOSTIC TESTS

Electrodiagnostic (EDX) studies involve the recording and analysis of responses of nerves and muscles to electrical stimulation. It is most useful in distinguishing between neuropathic versus myopathic origin of peripheral neuromuscular pathology. It can help assess peripheral radiculopathy and determine which root level is involved. This chapter gives a brief overview of EDX. For specific EDX procedures and interpretation, refer to the textbooks listed in the bibliography.

 I. **Nerve conduction studies (NCS) or electroneurography** are recording and analysis of nerve impulses (action potentials) generated in the peripheral nervous system elicited in response to electrical stimulation. Under standardized conditions, normal ranges of latencies (interval [ms] between the onset of the stimulus and the onset of a response), amplitude (the maximum voltage difference [mV or μV] between two points, usually baseline to peak or peak to peak), total duration [ms] of individual potential waveforms (the interval from the beginning of the first deflection from the baseline to its final return to the baseline), the duration of a recurring action potential (the interval from the beginning to the end of the series), and the *maximum conduction velocity* (loosely referred to as *nerve conduction velocity*) can be determined. For reference values of motor and sensory nerve conduction studies, refer to Appendices A-4 and A-5, respectively.

 A. **Maximum conduction velocity (CV) or nerve conduction velocity (NCV)** is the speed of propagation of an action potential along a nerve (motor, sensory, autonomic, or mixed) or muscle fiber. It is calculated from the latency of the evoked potential at maximal or supramaximal stimulation at two different points. The distance between the two points (conduction distance) is divided by the difference between the corresponding latencies (conduction time). The calculated velocity represents the conduction velocity of the fastest fibers and is expressed as meters per second (m/sec).

 B. **Compound sensory nerve action potential (compound SNAP or sensory potential or sensory response)** is evoked from afferent fibers by recording electric activity only from a sensory nerve or from a sensory branch of a mixed nerve, from electrical stimulus applied only to a sensory nerve or a dorsal nerve root, or from an adequate stimulus applied synchronously to sensory receptors. The *sensory amplitude* is measured from the most positive peak to the most negative peak (maximum peak-to-peak voltage). The *sensory latency* (i.e., *onset latency*) is the interval from onset of stimulus to initial deflection. The *peak sensory latency* is measured from the onset of stimulus to the negative peak. The *total sensory duration* is the interval from the first deflection of the waveform from the baseline to its final return to the baseline.

 C. **Compound motor nerve action potential or compound muscle action potential (CMAP)** is evoked from efferent fibers by recording electric activity only from a motor nerve or a motor branch of a mixed nerve or from electrical stimulus applied only to a motor nerve or a ventral nerve root.

   1. **M-wave** is a compound muscle action potential evoked from a muscle by a single supramaximal electrical stimulus to its motor nerve. The recording

electrodes should be placed so that the initial deflection of the evoked potential is negative. Normally, the configuration of the M-wave (usually biphasic) is quite stable with repeated stimuli at slow rates (1-5 Hz). The *motor latency* is the interval from the onset of stimulus to the onset of the first phase (positive or negative) of the M-wave. The *amplitude* of the M-wave is measured from the baseline to the peak of the first negative phase. The *duration* of the M-wave is the interval from the deflection of the first negative phase from the baseline to its return to the baseline.

2. **Late responses** are evoked potential with longer latency than the M-wave. Late responses (F- and H-waves) can be used to evaluate proximal lesions (as impulse travels to spinal cord and returns to distal recording electrode).

   a. **F-wave** is a compound muscle action potential evoked intermittently from a muscle by a supramaximal electrical stimulus to the nerve. Compared with the maximal amplitude M-wave of the same muscle, the F-wave has a smaller amplitude (1-5% of the M-wave), variable configuration, and a longer, more variable latency. The F-wave can be found in many muscles of the upper and lower extremities, and the latency is longer with more distal sites of stimulation. The F-wave is caused by antidromic activation of motor neurons. Abnormal F-wave studies are seen in patients with hereditary motor sensory neuropathy, acute or chronic demyelinating neuropathy, diabetic neuropathy, uremic neuropathy, alcoholic neuropathy, as well as in entrapment neuropathies, amyotrophic lateral sclerosis, and radiculopathies. Reference values for F-wave studies are shown in Appendix A-6. In general, the minimum F-latency is less than 35 ms for the upper limb and less than 60 ms for the lower limb. The side-to-side differences in the minimum F-latency should be less than 2 ms in the upper limb and 4 ms in the lower limb.

   b. **H-wave** is a compound muscle action potential having a consistent latency evoked regularly, when present, from a muscle by an electrical stimulus to the nerve. It is regularly found only in a limited group of muscles, particularly the soleus muscle (through stimulation of the tibial nerve). It is also recordable over the flexor carpi radialis (FCR) muscle (through stimulation of the median nerve), although its onset latency is often obscured by the preceding M-wave. The H-wave is most easily obtained with the cathode positioned proximal to the anode. Compared with the maximum amplitude M-wave of the same muscle, the H-wave has a smaller amplitude, a longer latency, and a lower optimal stimulus intensity. The latency is longer with more distal sites of stimulation. A stimulus intensity sufficient to elicit a maximal amplitude M-wave reduces or abolishes the H-wave, hence a submaximal electrical stimulation must be used. The H-wave is believed to be caused by the H or Hoffman reflex. In the H-reflex, the motor neuron to the muscle is activated through a monosynaptic reflex connection in the spinal cord elicited by the electrical stimulation of the afferent fibers in the mixed nerve supplying the muscle. The H-reflex is similar to the stretch reflex but unlike the stretch reflex which is stimulated via activation of muscle spindles, the H reflex bypasses the muscle spindle by using electrical stimulation.

   The normal latency of H-wave in adults is 28-35 ms when measured from the soleus muscle. The measured H-latency should be within 5.5

ms of the predicted value which can be computed by the Braddom-Johnson formula:

Predicted H-latency (ms) = 9.14 + 0.46 × leg length (cm)
                                      + 0.1 × age (yrs)

If the H-latency is prolonged or if there is clinical suspicion of S1 radiculopathy (e.g., absent ankle jerk), then contralateral H-latency should be measured. Assuming equal leg lengths, a difference of >1.0 ms between the two legs may indicate S1 radiculopathy. If H wave is recorded from the FCR muscle, a difference of >0.8 ms between the two arms may indicate C6 or C7 radiculopathy. Prolonged H-latency has also been reported in patients with early Guillain-Barre Syndrome.

c. **A-wave** is a compound muscle action potential evoked consistently from a muscle by submaximal electrical stimuli to the nerve and is frequently abolished by supramaximal stimuli. The amplitude of the A-wave is similar to that of the F-wave, but the latency is more constant. The A-wave usually occurs before the F-wave, but may occur afterwards. The A-wave is caused by normal or pathologic axonal branching and may be elicited in pressure injuries of the peripheral nerve, peripheral neuropathies, amyotrophic lateral sclerosis, and root injuries. A-waves have limited clinical significance as they may also be elicited in normal subjects.

d. **T-wave** is a compound muscle action potential evoked from a muscle by rapid stretch of its tendon, as part of the muscle stretch reflex.

II. **Electromyography (EMG)** is the use of intramuscular (IM) needle electrodes to evaluate motor units (i.e., the anatomic unit of anterior horn cell, its axon, the neuromuscular junctions, and all of the muscle fibers innervated by the axon). The electrical potential reflecting the electrical activity of a single anatomic motor unit is called the motor unit action potential (MUAP). The following MUAP configuration should be described: peak-to-peak amplitude; total duration (probably the most reliable routine EMG feature to use in distinguishing "neuropathic" versus "myopathic" conditions); number of phases (monophasic, biphasic, triphasic, tetraphasic, or polyphasic [i.e., more than 5 phases]); sign of each phase (negative, positive); number of turns; variation of shape, if any, with consecutive discharges; presence of satellite (linked) potentials, if any. The recruitment characteristics in relationship to the voluntary muscle exertion should also be described. Limb muscles commonly tested in a routine needle EMG session are shown in Table 2.4-1. Motor innervations of upper and lower limb muscles are shown in Appendices B-3 and B-4, respectively.

Most EMG studies are done to evaluate denervation, which demonstrates fibrillation potentials (biphasic waves with initial positive deflection, duration of less than 5 ms, and high-pitched "ticks" that sound like "rain on a tin roof") and positive sharp waves (biphasic waves with primarily sharp positive deflection followed by a small prolonged negative potential, duration of 10-100 ms, and a dull thud sound recurring in a uniform regular pattern usually in response to needle movement). Fibrillation potentials and PSWs represent abnormal spontaneous single muscle fiber discharge caused by increased muscle membrane irritability. They may also be seen in inflammatory myopathies (e.g., polymyositis) and almost any other myopathies (except for, possibly, chronic steroid myopathy or thyroid myopathy), neuromuscular junction disorders (e.g., myastenia gravis), upper motor neuron lesions (e.g., stroke

Table 2.4-1. Limb muscles commonly tested in a routine needle electromyographic procedure (listed in sequential order of testing)

MUSCLE	SPINAL ROOTS*	PERIPHERAL NERVE	TEST MANEUVER
UPPER LIMB:			
Lateral deltoid	**C5**, C6	Axillary	Abduct shoulder
Biceps brachii	C5, **C6**	Musculocutaneous	Flex elbow (with forearm supinated)
Triceps brachii	C6, **C7**	Radial	Extend elbow
Flexor carpi radialis	C6, C7	Median	Flex and radially deviate wrist
Abductor pollicis brevis	C8, **T1**	Median	Abduct thumb (perpendicular to palmar plane)
First dorsal interossei	C8, **T1**	Ulnar	Abduct (or radially deviate) index finger
Extensor indicis propius†	C7, C8	Radial	Extend index finger (with other fingers flexed)
LOWER LIMB:			
Tibialis anterior	**L4,** L5	Deep peroneal	Dorsiflex foot
Peroneus longus	L5, S1	Superficial peroneal	Evert plantarflexed foot
Gastrocnemius	**S1,** S2	Tibial	Plantar flex foot (with knee extended)
Vastus medialis	L2, **L3, L4**	Femoral	Extend knee
Tensor fascia lata	**L4, L5,** S1	Superior gluteal	Abduct thigh (with hip flexed)
Gluteus maximus	**L5, S1,** S2	Inferior gluteal	Extend hip (with knee flexed)
Hamstrings† (e.g., short head of biceps femoris)	L5, **S1,** S2	Sciatic	Flex knee

* A **bold** designation indicates the predominant root supply.
† Optional.

and spinal cord injury), direct muscle trauma, or intramuscular injection or bleeding.

A summary of typical EMG findings in neuropathic and myopathic conditions is shown in Appendix A-7. In general, the MUAPs in neuropathy conditions (in which partial denervation and reinnervation have occurred) have increased polyphasicity, amplitude, and duration; while in myopathic conditions (in which there is loss or impairment of individual muscle fibers), the MUAPs have increased polyphasicity but decreased amplitude and duration. Neuromuscular junction diseases tend to mimic MUAP changes seen in myopathy.

A. Insertional activities are electric activities caused by the insertion or movement of the needle electrode. Their amount may be described as normal, reduced, or increased (prolonged) with a description of the waveform and repetitive rate.

B. Spontaneous activities (e.g., fibrillation potentials and positive sharp waves) are recorded from muscle at rest after insertional activities have subsided in the absence of any voluntary contraction or external stimulus.

C. Involuntary activities are MUAPs that are not under voluntary control. The condition under which they occur should be described (e.g., spontaneous or reflex potentials; or, if elicited by a stimulus, the nature of the stimulus must be described).

D. Recruitment (or interference) patterns are qualitative or quantitative descriptions of the electrical activities recorded from a muscle with needle electrode during maximal voluntary effort. The recruitment pattern may be described as *full* (no individual motor unit action can be clearly identified), *reduced or intermediate* (some of the individual MUAPs may be identified while other individual MUAPs cannot be identified because of overlap), *discrete* (each of several different MUAPs can be identified), or *single* (a single MUAP is identified, firing at a rapid rate during maximal voluntary effort). The force of contraction associated with the recruitment pattern should be specified.

III. Evoked potential studies refer to recording and analysis of electrical waveforms generated in both peripheral and central nervous system in response to electric or physiologic stimuli. There are two systems for naming complex evoked potential waveforms. In the first system, the different components are labeled PI for the initial positive potential and NI for the initial negative potential. The subsequent positive and negative potentials are named PII, NII, PIII, NIII, etc. In the second system, the components are specified by polarity and average peak latency in normal subjects to the nearest millisecond. The first nomenclature principle has been used in an abbreviated form to identify the seven positive components (I–VII) of the normal brainstem auditory evoked potential (BAEP). The second nomenclature principle has been used to identify the positive and negative components of visual evoked potentials (N75, P100) and somatosensory evoked potentials (P9, P11, P13, P14, N20, P23). The problem of the second system is that the latencies of components of evoked potentials depend upon the length of the pathways in the neural tissues. Thus, the components of a somatosensory evoked potential (SEP) recorded in a child have different average latencies from the same components of an SEP recorded in an adult.

A. Somatosensory evoked potentials (SEPs) are elicited by electrical stimulation of peripheral sensory fibers (commonly used nerves are median nerve, common peroneal nerve, and posterior tibial nerve). The normal SEP is a complex waveform with several components that are specified by polarity and average leak latency. The polarity and latency of the individual component depend on subject variables (e.g., age and sex), stimulus characteristics (intensity and rate of stimulation), and recording parameters (e.g., placement and combination of recording electrodes and amplifier time constants). **Short-latency somatosensory evoked potentials (SSEPs)** are portion of a wave form of a SEP normally occurring within 25 ms after stimulation of the median nerve at the wrist, 40 ms after stimulation of the common peroneal nerve at the knee, and 50 ms after stimulation of the posterior tibial nerve at the ankle. The SEPs are used to study brachial plexus injuries and to monitor spinal cord function during spine surgery.

B. Visual evoked potentials (VEPs) or visual evoked responses (VERs) are recorded over the cerebrum and elicited by light stimuli. The VEPs are classified by stimulus rate as transient or steady state VEPs. The normal transient VEP to checkerboard pattern reversal or shift has a major positive occipital peak at about 100 ms (P100), often preceded by a negative peak (N75). The precise range of normal values for the latency and amplitude of P100 depends on subject variables (e.g., age, sex, and visual acuity), stimulus characteristics (type of stimulator, full- or half-field stimulator, check size, contrast, and lumines-cence), and recording parameters (e.g., placement and combination of record-ing electrodes). Abnormal VEPs are seen in optic neuritis (due to multiple sclerosis or other demyelinating disease) with latency prolongation up to 250 ms.

C. Brainstem auditory evoked potentials (BAEPs) or brainstem auditory evoked re-sponses (BAERs, BERs) measure auditory evoked potentials originating between the eighth cranial nerve and the inferior colliculus in response to sound stim-uli. The normal BAEP consists of a sequence of up to seven waves, named I to VII, which occur during the first 10 ms after the onset of the stimulus and have positive polarity at the vertex of the head. It is the most accurate noninvasive procedure in the diagnosis of acoustic neuromas and has the lowest false positive rate.

IV. Special EDX studies

A. Neuromuscular junction (NMJ) studies are used to confirm the diagnoses of myas-thenia gravis (MG), which is caused by antibody destruction or blocking of the postsynaptic acetylcholine (Ach) receptors, and Lambert-Eaton myasthenic syndrome (LEMS), which is caused by autoimmune attack against calcium channels in the presynaptic nerve terminal, resulting in impaired release of Ach quanta.

1. Repetitive nerve stimulation (RNS; formerly known as the **Jolly test)** uses a series of supramaximal stimuli given to a specific nerve in rapid succession to fatigue the NMJ. RNS causes depletion of Ach, thus allowing inspection of the resultant compound muscle action potentials (CMAPs) for consis-tency of amplitude and duration. Although distal nerves (e.g., ulnar or peroneal nerves) can be tested, the proximal nerves tend to have higher diagnostic yields (i.e., spinal accessory, axillary, musculocutaneous, or facial nerves).

In MG, the single-stimulation CMAP amplitudes are usually normal. Using 2-5 Hz stimulation, there is a decrease of more than 10% in the amplitude of the fourth or fifth CMAP as compared with that of the first. A maximum isometric contraction for 10 to 15 seconds or a stimulation of 20 Hz for 10 seconds will usually result in a short-lived (15-30 seconds) increase in the CMAP amplitude (i.e., postactivation facilitation), but no greater than 50% above baseline. The intravenous injection of edrophonium hydrochloride (Tensilon), a short-acting acetylcholinesterase inhibitor, usually reverses the decrement in CMAP amplitude in patients with MG (this may, however, also be seen in some patients with LEMS).

In LEMS, the single-stimulation CMAP amplitudes are usually low. Using 2-5 Hz stimulation, the first response may be increased or there may be a decremental response. With a maximum isometric contraction for 10 to 15 seconds or a stimulation of 20 Hz for 10 seconds, there is an increase in the CMAP amplitude that is usually greater than 50%, often 200-400% above the single-stimulation CMAP.

2. Single-fiber EMG (SF-EMG) examines the relationship of two single-muscle fibers within one motor unit by using a specialized needle electrode. Nor-mally, during depolarization of a motor axon, the action potential travels distally and excites all the muscle fibers within that motor unit at more or less the same time. The variation in the time interval between the excitation of the two fibers is known as the jitter (reported as mean value of the difference between consecutive interpotential intervals). Muscles commonly studied are the extensor digitorum communis and the orbicularis oculi. In patients with NMJ disorders, the jitter is usually prolonged even without overt clinical weakness. SF-EMG is the most sensitive test to demonstrate impaired NMJ transmission (abnormal in 95 to 99 percent of patients with generalized MG). However, SF-EMG, although quite sensitive, is not specific and is typically abnormal in neuropathic and myopathic disease. Hence, SF-EMG should only be reserved for patients with high suspicion of MG whose RNS is negative or equivocal.

B. Blink reflex or blink response is used to evaluate trigeminal and facial nerve function, such as in Bell's palsy, trigeminal neuropathy, and multiple sclerosis. It is obtained by stimulation over the supraorbital branch of the trigeminal nerve (afferent arc), with surface recording over both ipsilateral and contralateral orbicularis oculi (which are supplied by the efferent arc of the facial nerve. Normally, there is an early compound muscle action potential (R1 wave) ipsilateral to the stimulation site with a latency of about 10 ms and a bilateral late compound muscle action potential (R2 wave) with a latency of about 30 ms. In general only the R2 wave is associated with a visible twitch of the orbicularis oculi.

BIBLIOGRAPHY

Braddom RL, Johnson EW: Standardization of H-Reflex and diagnostic use in S1 Radiculopathy. *Arch Phys Med Rehabil* 55:161-166, 1974.

Dumitru D: *Electrodiagnostic medicine*, Philadelphia, 1995, Hanley & Belfus.

Johnson EW, Pease WS, editors: *Practical electromyography*, ed 3, Baltimore, 1997, Williams & Wilkins.

Kimura J: *Electrodiagnosis in diseases of nerve and muscle: Principles and practice*, ed 2, Philadelphia, 1989, FA Davis.

Liveson JA, Ma D: *Laboratory reference for clinical neurophysiology*. Philadelphia, 1992, FA Davis.

Nomenclature Committee of American Association of Electromyography and Electrodiagnosis: AAEE glossary of terms in clinical electromyography, *Muscle and Nerve* Suppl 10 (8S):G1-G60, 1987.

CHAPTER 2.5

MUSCULOSKELETAL AND WORK-RELATED TESTS

Most of the musculoskeletal and work-related tests are affected by psychosocial factors (e.g., motivation, pain, fear avoidance, anxiety related to test situation, conscious symptom magnification or malingering, unconscious symptom magnification or illness behavior, psychological stress, depression, cognitive changes, and active legal cases); physical condition of the subject (e.g., fatigue, cardiovascular capability, general fitness, and training effect); environmental conditions (e.g., nature of the external load, metabolic conditions, pH level, temperature, noise, and number of people present in testing room); biophysical state of the muscles (e.g., fiber composition, physiological cross-sectional area of the muscle, muscle length, rate of change of muscle length, and joint ROM); testing protocol used (e.g., axis placement, posture, feedback, instruction, and test design and sequence); and type of device used (e.g., its attachment and calibration). This chapter gives an overview of the common musculoskeletal and work-related tests used in PM&R. Manufacturers and suppliers of musculoskeletal and work-related testing devices can be found in Appendix G-7.

I. **Range of motion (ROM) and flexibility measurements** in the clinical setting use simple, uniplanar, noninvasive techniques. In general, intratester reliability for ROM testing is higher than intertester reliability, hence the same examiner must be used for successive ROM measurements. Examiners should also use consistent, well-defined testing positions and anatomical landmarks to align the arms of the goniometer.

A. **Visual estimation** can be used to quickly gauge the ROM but is unreliable and, therefore, not acceptable.

B. **Goniometric techniques**

1. **Universal goniometer** consists of a protractor (180- or 360-degree scale) with a stationary arm (aligned parallel to the proximal limb segment), a mobile arm (aligned parallel to the distal limb segment), and an axis (placed as close to the joint axis as possible). The angle between the stationary and mobile arms is the ROM measurement. The universal goniometer can measure any joint ROM (a small version called *finger goniometer* may be used for measuring metacarpophalangeal [MCP] and interphalangeal [IP] joints). It is inexpensive and easy to obtain, transport, and use. Its reliability is generally good to excellent for measuring limb joint ROM, with the upper limb ROM measurement being more reliable than for the lower limb. However, for the measurement of spinal ROM, the use of the universal goniometer has lower reliability than that for the measurement of limb joint. The reliability of the universal goniometer for ROM measurements of the cervical spine is better than that for lumbar spine. In measuring cervical spine ROM, the universal goniometer has good intertester reliability for cervical extension and lateral bending but is difficult to align for neck flexion and extension.

2. **Gravity-dependent goniometers** use gravity's effect on pointers and fluid lev-

els to measure joint position and motion. The device is strapped on the distal limb segment with the proximal limb segment positioned vertically or horizontally. At the end of ROM, the position of the pointer or bubble on the scale is read as the ROM measurement. The advantage the gravity–dependent goniometers have over universal goniometers for limb joint ROM measurement is they do not have to be aligned with bony landmarks (i.e., it is not necessary to align the goniometer with the joint axis), and passive ROM is easily assessed because the examiner does not have to hold the goniometer. For trunk ROM, gravity-dependent goniometers are easier to use and more accurate than universal goniometers. Their disadvantages (compared to universal goniometer, tape measure, and flexible ruler) are they are bulkier, more expensive, not as readily available, and require additional instruction and practice to use properly. Also, they are difficult to use on small joints and in the presence of soft tissue deformity or edema. Moreover, they are difficult to use in measuring transverse plane motion (i.e., rotation) because of their gravity dependence.

a. **Inclinometer** is a pendulum-based goniometer consisting of a 360-degree scale protractor with a counter-weighted pointer maintained in a constantly vertical position. Electronic versions are also available (Cybex electronic digital inclinometer, Orthoranger). The *AMA: Guides to the Evaluation of Permanent Impairment* recommends the inclinometer (in particular the use of double inclinometer technique) for measurement of spinal ROM to determine "true" spinal ROM. In the double inclinometer technique for lumbar ROM measurement, one inclinometer is positioned at T12 and the other one at midsacrum area. The degree of inclination on the sacral inclinometer represents flexion of the hip while the reading on the T12 inclinometer represents total trunk flexion. Their difference is the "true" lumbar flexion. For the thoracic spine, T1 and T12 landmarks are used. The disadvantages of the double inclinometer technique are it is relatively expensive and difficult to manipulate, and it needs a considerable amount of practice time to locate landmarks for instrument placements. Intratester reliability for the double inclinometer technique is only moderate, while intertester reliability ranges from poor to high. The double inclinometer technique does not appear to be superior to the tape measure (e.g., modified Schober's technique) in measuring lumbar flexion and extension.

b. **Fluid goniometer (bubble goniometer or hydrogoniometer)** uses a 360-degree scale in a flat, fluid-filled circular tube, which contains a small air bubble.

3. **Combined compass and gravity-dependent goniometers** have the same advantage and disadvantage listed for gravity-dependent goniometers, except that the addition of the compass makes it easier to measure rotational movements. The OB Myrin goniometer cannot measure the small joints of the hand and foot whereas the Cervical ROM Device is designed specifically for the neck ROM. They have acceptable intratester and intertester reliability. As with gravity-based goniometers, their intertester reliability is higher than that for universal goniometer, tape measure, and flexible ruler.

a. **OB-Myrin goniometer** consist of a fluid-filled ratable container (with ROM scaled in tenths of degrees) mounted on a plate. The container has a compass needle that reacts to the earth's magnetic field (this is used to rotational measure movements in the transverse plane) and an inclination needle that is influenced by gravity (this is used to measure movements in the frontal and sagittal planes).

 b. **Cervical ROM Device** is an instrument consisting of two gravity-dependent goniometers and a compass attached to a frame mounted over the bridge of a subject's nose and ears. The two gravity-based goniometers measure flexion, extension, and lateral bending of the neck. Neck rotation is measured by the compass in conjunction with a shoulder-mounted yoke containing magnetic poles pointing north.

 4. **Electrogoniometer** uses a potentiometer attached to two arms, which are strapped to the proximal and distal limb segments. Movement of the arms causes the resistance in the potentiometer to vary. Variations in voltage can then be calibrated to represent joint ROM. They are expensive and are used mainly in research and occasionally for gait analysis (see section VI.C.1.b).

C. **Tape measures** are used to determine spinal ROM through observation of a change in distance from one segment to another. For ROM measurement of the thoracolumbar spine, the tape measure technique is the least expensive and easiest to obtain, transport, and use.

 1. **Cervical ROM measurements using tape measure** include neck flexion and extension (the distance between chin and suprasternal notch is measured) and side bending (the distance between mastoid process and acromion process is measured).

 2. **Thoracolumbar ROM measurements using tape measure**

 a. **Finger-to-floor (FTF) technique** measures the distance from tip of the middle finger to the floor in either trunk flexion or side bending. This method is inaccurate for spinal motion because it does not differentiate hip from thoracolumbar motion. Also, it is affected by the flexibility of the fingers, wrist, elbow, and shoulder. Despite these, the FTF method is still being used because of its simplicity.

 b. **Skin distraction technique** is used for the thoracic and lumbar spine ROM measurement. The most commonly used method is the **modified Schober's technique.** The tape is aligned at two points in the spine (from a point 10 cm above lumbosacral junction and 5 cm below the lumbosacral junction, a total of 15 cm distance). The subject bends forward or backward and the distance is remeasured and then subtracted from the original 15 cm. Although it conforms to the spinal curvature, the modified Schober's technique does not take into account hip motion, which is the largest component of trunk forward flexion beyond 30 degrees of motion. The modified Schober's technique has good reliability and validity and is easier to use than the double inclinometer method. It is slightly more difficult to use than the FTF because the lumbosacral junction needs to be located.

D. **Flexible ruler (Flexirule or flexicurve)** is a pliable metal band encased in a supple nonelastic plastic covering, which is used for measuring lumbar ROM. It can be contoured onto the lumbar spine to accommodate lordosis in measuring spinal ROM. Flexible rulers demonstrate repeatable measurements but are inaccurate in obese patients because of skinfolds. Their validity is questionable, and they are not generally recommended for clinical use.

E. **Photometric (or video-based) motion analysis systems** use infrared light sources, light-emitting diodes (or reflectors), or laser light attached to the body part to measure relative motions of the segments between each light source. They can either use two-dimensional or three-dimensional optical systems to measure dynamic ROM of the spine and limbs during different tasks (including gait; see also section VI.C.1.a). With the recent advancement of computer and optoelectric technologies, video-based motion analysis (e.g., Computerized Motion Diagnostic Imaging, Motion Analysis Spinetrak, Oxford Metrics VICON System, and Peak Performance Systems) can now be automatically digitized with increasing accuracy to quantify range of motion. Although they have good validity and reliability (i.e., when properly calibrated), they are relatively expensive.

II. **Strength assessment** can be measured either manually (e.g., manual muscle test [MMT]) or using a dynamometer (i.e., an external apparatus onto which the body exerts force or torque). In PM&R, strength measurement can "potentially" be used for prescribing treatment, monitoring treatment progress, and evaluating physical impairment. In the medical-legal field, it can "potentially" be used to test effort consistency, identify maximal exertion, and assess disability. In industry, its "potential" uses are in providing ergonomic and rehabilitation guidelines, and in screening for job preplacement and return-to-work. However most of the above mentioned "potential" benefits (in particular for trunk strength assessment) remain unproved by randomized controlled studies.

   In using dynamometers for strength measurement, the following guidelines are suggested: subject must be educated and informed of the purpose of the machine; maximum voluntary effort must be exerted by the subject; axis of joint motion must be aligned with the axis of rotation of the shaft of the machine; joint must be properly positioned and stabilized to ensure muscle isolation and reproducibility; the uninvolved limb must be tested first; warm-ups must be done before testing; verbal commands should be standardized to ensure test reproducibility; visual feedback, if used at all, must be consistent; angular velocity used for testing should be the same as for rehabilitation; the instrument must be calibrated every 2 weeks to ensure validity; and data generated from one system should not be used on another system.

   In general the upper-body strength of women is 40 to 50% less than that of men, and the lower-body strength is 20 to 30% less than that of men. This holds true for upper-body strength in women even in relation to lean body mass, but the lower-body strength appears equal to that of men in relation to lean body mass. However, there appear to be no differences between the sexes when strength is measured for cross-sectional area of muscle.

A. **Manual muscle testing (MMT)** is traditionally used for determining patterns of muscle weakness in neuromuscular diseases. However, it is inaccurate for testing strength greater than fair or 3/5 (see MMT grading in Chapter 1.1, section II.O.2.c). MMT has also been shown to be insensitive to 20% to 25% changes in strength and to overestimate normalcy of muscle strength. Hence, MMT is inadequate for determination of functional capacity, especially in patients with strength greater than fair or 3/5.

B. **Nondynamometric isotonic strength testing** uses the 10 RM (repetition maximum) value (see Chapter 4.2, section II.B.2.a.1).

C. **Hand strength measurements**

   1. **Grip strength** is measured using a standard Jamar dynamometer, which is recommended because it has extensive normative data (from 6-75 + years), and it is superior to other grip dynamometers (e.g., Digital Jamar Dynamometer, Martin Vigorimeter, and My-Gripper). Its absolute accuracy is within 5%. For pre- and posttesting, the same dynamometer must be used because different versions may vary. Normally grip is strongest in the

dominant upper extremity by about 5 to 10 lb and is greater in the midposition of grip, being weaker with either a narrow or wide grip.

2. **Pinch strength** is measured using a B & L Engineering pinch gauge (0-60 lb), which is recommended because it has an accuracy of $\pm$ 1 percent, and it has extensive normative data (from 6-75 + years) for tip, key, and palmar pinch. It is superior to the Preston pinch gauge.

D. Dynamometry for limb muscle groups

1. **Hand-held dynamometry** provides objective measurement of limb muscle group strength by having the patient exert maximal effort against a portable force-measuring device held by the examiner. Nonelectrical units that use either spring or hydraulic system, display the force exerted on a dial gauge, and electrical units that uses load cells, or strain gauges display the exerted force digitally. The "make test" (wherein the hand-held dynamometer is held stationary by the tester while patient exerts maximum effort against it) is preferred over the "break test" (wherein the tester exerts a force against the subject's limb segment until it gives way) because the break test may require higher force beyond the capability of the dynamometer or the strength of the tester. Subjects are measured either seated or supine, preferably in a gravity-reduced position with proper stabilization. The muscle groups to be tested are placed in the middle of their length ranges and the dynamometer is positioned perpendicular to the limb. If the test is done properly by an experienced tester on a sincere subject, only one trial is needed. Duration of exertion is usually 4 to 5 seconds. Obviously, the hand-held dynamometer can only be used if the tester is stronger than the subject. Commercially available hand-held dynamometers include Nicholas Manual Muscle Tester, Newman Myometer, Penny and Giles Transducer Myometer, Hammersmith Dynamometer, Force Evaluation and Testing System, and Spark Hand-held Dynamometer.

2. **Isometric (static) dynamometry for limb muscle groups** measures static muscle strength without limb joint movement. The muscle length is kept constant by either soft constraints (verbal instruction) or hard constraints (stabilization straps). Isometric dynamometers measure peak and average force, reaction time, rate of motor recruitment of motor units, maximal voluntary exertion, and fatigue. The advantages of isometric testing are its relative safety, its low cost, its simplicity and ease of interpretation. Effective stabilization is easier to attain than in dynamic testing. It also produces less systemic fatigue than dynamic testing devices, hence more muscles can be tested in a given session. It is preferred in conditions in which joint motion causes pain (e.g., contractures).

Its main disadvantage is that it does not correlate with real-life dynamic activities such as lifting and manual materials handling. However, isometric testing can be done at multiple points in the arc of joint range of motion to create a strength curve. Isometric testing should be used with precaution in the presence of acute, active musculoskeletal problems, osteoporosis, significant cardiovascular or respiratory pathology, or structural weakness of the abdominal or thoracic wall (immediate postsurgery; hernia). It is contraindicated in the presence of unsplinted fractures, unhealed torn or sutured tendons, and in uncontrolled hypertension.

Strain-gauge (fixed-load cell) dynamometers are commonly used for testing isometric strength of limb muscle-groups. They use electroconductive materials that are sensitive to loads, i.e., tension, compression, or shear. When the subject pushes or pulls against the dynamometer, the gauge is deformed leading to a change in its electrical resistance and alteration of the current passing through the gauge. The change in voltage can then be calibrated and converted into torque. Most dynamometers used primarily for dynamic testing of muscle performances contain a strain-gauge, which can be used for isometric testing by locking the machine either mechanically or through computer control or both.

3. Dynamic dynamometry for limb muscle groups

a. Isotonic dynamometry for limb muscle groups use constant weights or resistance to measure strength at variable speed. Although ''isotonic'' implies constant tension, this is not true because muscle tension changes as the leverage changes. Commercially available ''isotonic devices'' are not purely isotonic. They can be isokinetic-like, i.e., allowing contraction at an accommodating speed and an accommodating resistance (e.g., Ariel Computerized Exercise System [CES], Physio-Tek, and Tru-Kinetics) or they can have variable speed with accommodating resistance (e.g., Hydra-Fitness Gym).

b. Isokinetic limb muscle group dynamometer measures strength as the joint moves at a constant preselected speed (0-500 degrees/sec). Isokinetic machines provide resistance that accommodates the muscle as its length-tension ratio changes and as the muscle leverage changes throughout the range of motion; therefore, the muscle contracts at its maximal capability at all points throughout the ROM. The joint velocity or rate of shortening or lengthening of the muscle is kept constant, i.e., acceleration and jerk are zero. A more accurate term is probably *isovelocity* or maybe *isokinematics* because it is usually the change in angle at a joint that is set constant.

In isokinetic testing, the reported torque is that produced by the machine to keep the limb from accelerating beyond the preset speed of the machine. If the muscle force is less than the preset speed, then the machine does not register any force and the isokinetic torque is reported as zero. This should not be interpreted as absence of muscle tension. Because zero does not mean absence of torque, isokinetic torque measures are considered as interval-scale, not true ratio-scale. Hence, torque ratios (flexion/extension) should not be computed from isokinetic measures, because they are not ratio-scaled.

The advantages of isokinetic mode are that it can test at different speeds and it is safe (i.e., the resistance provided by the machine is equal to the force exerted, and the subject never meets more resistance than he or she can handle). Its disadvantages are its cost, constraints in motion pattern, and patient's unfamiliarity with the task of moving at a preselected speed. Isokinetic testing cannot accurately measure the full arc of muscle performance because of acceleration artifact at the beginning ROM arc and deceleration artifact at the end ROM arc. Also, it does not simulate real life because human beings don't move at constant velocity.

1) Passive isokinetic systems allow isokinetic concentric exertions only, e.g., Cybex and Universal Merac.

2) Active isokinetic systems allow both isokinetic eccentric and concentric exertions as well as passive ROM testing, e.g., Biodex and Kin-Com.

E. Trunk dynamometry

1. Isometric trunk dynamometers have similar principle, advantages, disadvantages, precautions, and contraindications as limb muscle isometric dynamometers (see II.D.2). Unlike the limb, the trunk has more than one axis of motion, making it more difficult to standardize. For accuracy, the chosen axis of motion (e.g., L3) must be used consistently for within subject and between subject testing. Proper stabilization, especially around the pelvis, is also important for accurate testing.

    a. Cable tensiometers consist of a harness connected to a cable that is attached to a fixed object, e.g., a wall or floor. When the harness (strapped around the individual's chest) is pulled, the cable is stretched. The tension in the cable is then measured in calibrated units on a tension-sensitive gauge. Cable tensiometers are best used to determine peak isometric torques rather than the average torque.

    b. Strain-gauge (fixed-load cell) trunk dynamometers use electroconductive materials that are sensitive to loads (see II.D.2). The MedX Lumbar Extension Machine and MedX Rotary-Torso Machine use a computer-monitored strain-gauge dynamometer designed for testing trunk isometric strength in sitting position. In contrast to the other isometric devices, the MedX machines have better stabilization and are able to test isometric strength at multiple points throughout the full trunk ROM. This allows multipositional isometric training, which has been shown to be effective in increasing lumbar extensor strength. Other dynamometers used primarily for testing dynamic trunk strength usually contain a strain gauge, which can be used for isometric testing by locking the machine either mechanically or through computer control or both.

  2. Dynamic trunk dynamometers

    a. Isokinetic trunk dynamometers have similar principles, advantages, and disadvantages as limb-muscle isokinetic dynamometers (see II.D.3.b). Commercial isokinetic trunk devices include Cybex Flexion/Extension Rehabilitation Unit, Cybex Torso Rotation Rehabilitation Unit, Kin-Com Back Testing Device, and Biodex Back System.

    b. Isoinertial trunk dynamometers measure the torque and velocity of trunk motion as the trunk exerts against a constant inertia or load (isoinertial exertion). The only commercially available isoinertial trunk dynamometer is the Isostation B-200 Triaxial Dynamometer, but this device is no longer manufactured.

 F. Cervical dynamometry usually uses the isometric mode of strength measurement at different points in the cervical ROM arc (e.g., MedX Cervical Extension Machine and MedX Cervical Rotation Machine).

 G. Whole-body dynamometry usually includes isometric and dynamic testing of upper and lower limb strengths as well as trunk strength and lifting strength. They include the ARCON, the Baltimore Therapeutic Equipment (BTE), the ERGASYS, and the ERGOS (from Work Recovery Systems).

III. Lifting capacity tests include measurements of the strength and endurance of muscles of the trunk as well as the upper and lower limbs. Manual lifting analysis, as proposed by the National Institute for Occupational Safety and Health (NIOSH) guide for manual lifting (revised, 1991), should include the weight of the object lifted, the position of load with respect to the body (measured at both the starting and ending points of a lift in terms of horizontal coordinates, i.e., distance of the object from the body, and the vertical coordinates, i.e., the vertical distance over which the object is lifted), frequency of lift (i.e., average lifts/min), and total duration (or period) of lifting. Measured data on weight of object and position of loads are used for comparison with established biomechanical and psychophysical strength limits, and data on lifting frequency and duration are used to predict the metabolic energy requirements of a job and for comparison with established work-capacity norms. Risk of injury increases with heavy or bulky objects, lifting from the floor, or frequent lifting.

The NIOSH isometric lifting guidelines identify two parameters for evaluating potentially hazardous lifting activities. The first parameter is the Action Limit (AL) which sets a maximum lifting load of 39 kg or approximately 39 Newtons (N) if isometric lifting is accomplished in an optimal manner (i.e., the object is held so that its center is 15 cm from the body, the vertical distance lifted is no greater than 25 cm, the maximum height of the lifted object is 75 cm, and the frequency of lifting is no greater than one lift every 5 min). Lifting a load of 39 kg has an equivalent compressive force of 3.4 kN (approximately 760 lb) at the L5-S1 disc. If the AL is exceeded, there is a risk of back injury of 1% for men and 25% for women. The second parameter is the Maximal Permissible Limit (MPL), which is three times the AL, or the equivalent of a compressive load of 6.9 kN (or approximately 1,550 lb) at the L5-S1 disc. If the MPL is exceeded, the relative risk of back injury is 75% for men and 99% for women. For fatigue-producing tasks, the equivalent metabolic costs of the AL and MPL is 3.5 kcal/min and 5.0 kcal/min, respectively. Both AL and MPL may vary up or down with corresponding changes in the "optimal" lifting parameters previously described. Computerized programs based on the NIOSH guidelines for evaluating lifting tasks and for prediction of AL and MPL have been developed by the University of Michigan (i.e., Two-Dimensional or Three-Dimensional Static Strength Prediction Program).

The above NIOSH guidelines do not account for asymmetric lifting (e.g., one-handed lifting, lifting at the side, or any lifting that deviates from two-handed lifting in the midsagittal plane), which results in shear force across the annulus fibrosis or increased compressive force at a particular spinal segment as a result of an increase in asymmetric contraction of trunk muscles. They also do not reflect the dynamic factors (e.g., the speed or rhythmicity) of lifting, i.e., they do not account for the proportionate increase in the load across the L5-S1 motion segment (which is independent of object weight) when the speed of lifting is increased or when the lifting pattern is dysrhythmic or "jerky."

A. **Static or isometric lifting test (tray-lifting strength)** uses a hand dynamometer attached by a cable and pulley system to the bottom of a metal tray. The subject grasps the tray handholds and pulls directly upward. A potentiometer output is displayed on a digital readout after averaging the force sustained from the beginning of the second second to the end of the fourth second of the pull. Isometric lifting tests are easier to standardize than dynamic tests. However, they do not simulate dynamic lifting, and their ability to predict subsequent development of industrial back injuries remains controversial. Variations in isometric lifting tests include whole-body isometric testing in various positions (e.g., leg lift–squat, torso lift–bent back, arm lift–upright) to simulate dynamic activity.

B. **Dynamic lifting capacity tests** are more valid from the industrial perspective but are difficult to standardize. The primary problems are load acceleration and muscle length changes. Commercial devices and protocols for evaluating dynamic lifting capacity are available from Blankenship, EPIC Functional Capacity Evaluation System, Isernhagen Work Systems, Key Functional Assessment, and Work Evaluation Systems Technology (WEST).

   1. **Psychophysical lifting tests** are safe and are essentially patient-controlled submaximal strength tests. They are based on psychophysics, which is a field in psychology that deals with the relationship between sensations and physical stimuli. In psychophysical lifting tests, the person increases the load (mass)

in small increments until reaching subjective maximum exertion (i.e., the dependent variable measured is the person's subjective feelings of fatigue or perception of what load can be sustained for several hours—all of which could be affected by the environmental temperature, noise, or light). As the characteristics of the lift or work environment are varied, the acceptable weight may change. These tests permit a person to evaluate acceptable workload in dynamic tasks, but the results cannot be extrapolated too far beyond the conditions of the test. What is an acceptable load to lift in a well-designed tray with handholds is not necessarily acceptable if the load is unstable or in a container with rough edges. Studies have shown that although psychophysical lifting are not predictive of new cases of low back pain, there is a close association between the perception of work load and the prevalence of low back pain. An example of psychophysical lifting test is the progressive isoinertial lifting evaluation (PILE) test described below.

2. **Progressive isoinertial lifting evaluation (PILE)** is a standardized lifting test protocol that uses both psychophysical and isoinertial lifting characteristics. The lumbar PILE consists of free style lifting from floor to waist height (0 to 30 in), and the cervical PILE is from waist to shoulder height (30 to 54 in). The lifting load for men starts at 13 lb and is increased by 10 lb every 20 seconds, while for women it starts at 8 lb and is increased by 5 lb every 20 seconds. For every 20 seconds, the subject should lift at a rate of four lifting cycles (i.e., one lifting cycle for lumbar test is from floor to waist then back to the floor; for cervical test, one lifting cycle is from waist to shoulder and back to waist). The test is ended when subject reaches any of the following: (1) psychological end-point, e.g., complaints of pain, discomfort, or fatigue, or inability to complete four lifting cycles in 20 seconds; (2) aerobic end-point, i.e., when target heart rate range (THRR) is reached (usually 85% of maximum heart rate or lower for cardiac patients; see Chapter 4.2, section III.A.1 for calculating THRR); or (3) safety end-point, i.e., a predetermined ''safe limit'' of 55 to 60% of body weight is lifted.

After completion of lifting, the parameters computed include the maximum weight lifted, the endurance time to discontinuation of test, the final and target heart rates, total work (TW), and total power (TP) consumption. The TW is computed by adding all the weights lifted and multiplying the total by a total distance of 20 feet for lumbar test or 16 feet for cervical test. The 20-foot distance for lumbar PILE is computed by multiplying the distance from the floor-to-waist-to-floor (i.e., 30 in $\times$ 2 = 60 in or 5 ft) by four, which is the number of lifting cycles in a 20-second interval. The 16-foot distance for cervical PILE is computed in similar fashion by using the waist to shoulder distance of 24 inches or 2 feet multiplied by two (i.e., 4 ft) then multiplied by four lifting cycles. A sample calculation for a woman who reached an end-point after completing 100 seconds of lumbar lifting at 5-lb increments every 20 seconds is TW = [8 + 13 + 18 + 23 + 28] $\times$ 20 = 1800 lb-ft. The TP is computed by dividing TW with the total time (i.e., 1800 lb-ft/100 sec = 18 lb-ft/sec).

3. **Isotonic lifting tests** are easy and relatively inexpensive. Weighted objects such as trays, boxes, push-pull carts, or other objects can be used as test loads. The subjects attempt to move the test objects the desired direction and distance on a trial and error basis. Weight can be added or removed from the containers so that an estimate of the maximum load or effort can be established. The 10-repetition maximum (10 RM value) system may be used. While easy to conduct, isotonic lifting tests are not easy to standardize

because they are easily confounded by the techniques used and the velocity and acceleration of the dynamic movement, which are influenced by the subject's efforts. Useful databases on dynamic efforts have rarely been established due to the high degree of specificity associated with these types of tests.

4. **Isokinetic lifting tests** use an isokinetic device attached to a tray or other object to simulate a lifting task. The force and velocity signals are recorded. During data analysis, the velocity data are integrated to give the displacement data. Thus, during the simulated lifts, a record of instantaneous force at incremental vertical heights can be obtained. Because the isokinetic device eliminates most acceleration, the force generated at a vertical location depends on the force-generating capacity of the body at that position. In these lifts, very large forces are generated at low heights where the lifting capacity is high and the lifter relies on momentum to assist the lift at higher positions. Because the resistance that must be overcome during lifting is frictional as opposed to gravitational, the isokinetic strength testing system is not restricted to vertical force measurements. The system can also be used to profile pushing, pulling, and oblique lifting capacities. The use of an isokinetic testing approach does not eliminate the need for standardization of testing procedures. Of particular importance is the velocity of testing because the force that can be developed by a group of muscles decreases with increasing velocity. Therefore, simulated isokinetic lifting at high velocities results in maximal strength values that are less than those found in tests performed at slower speeds. Although isokinetic testings appear to be more functional, the use of constant speed is not truly physiologic. Few prospective studies have used these parameters as predictors of low back pain.

IV. **Aerobic-work capacity tests** measure the maximum amount of work that can be done when there is enough oxygen to supply the muscles.
   A. **Whole body aerobic capacity tests** use cardiac and cardiopulmonary graded exercise tolerance testing described in Chapter 2.7, sections I.A. and II.A.
   B. **Upper body aerobic capacity tests**
      1. **Arm ergometry** uses a modified bicycle ergometer or an arm ergometer to measure upper body work by arm cranking (see Chapter 2.7, sections I.A.2.b).
      2. **Upper body lifting test.** The weight of the tray is increased in four stages while it is lifted at 2 times per minute around a series of shelves. This test appears to be limited by the discomfort felt at the wrists when the tray is lifted.

V. **Work assessment** consists of **functional capacity evaluation (FCE),** which is a broad term that includes tests of manual material handling capabilities, aerobic capacity, posture and mobility tolerance, anthropometric measurements, activities of daily living (ADLs), energy conservation techniques, and need for adaptive methods or technology. The information obtained from FCE can be used to establish maximal permissible limits for nonrepetitive activities and to delineate safe parameters for repetitive activities in a normal population. However, objective data (including validity) for the injured or disabled population are not yet available. In return-to-work programs, FCE usually refers to physical capacity evaluation and work capacity evaluation, both of which are described in Chapter 5.11, section V.D.

VI. **Gait assessment techniques** can be done qualitatively by informal visual analysis (see Chapter I, section II.P.7) or quantitatively using the techniques described

Table 2.5-1.   Definition of gait variables and determinants

GAIT PARAMETERS	DEFINITION
1. Gait cycle	Period between ipsilateral foot contacts (i.e., two steps or one stride); the functional unit of gait.
2. Spatial variables	
a. Step length	Distance (cm) between foot strikes of contralateral feet; normal range is 37.5 to 50 cm.
b. Stride length	Distance (cm) between foot strikes of ipsilateral feet; normal range is 75 to 160 cm; 1 stride = 2 successive steps = 1 gait cycle.
c. Stride width or base of support	Distance (cm) between the midline of contralateral foot strikes; normal range is 7.5 to 15 cm.
d. Toe out	Angulation of the long axis of the foot (in degrees) to the line of walking progression; the normal range is up to 15°.
3. Temporal variables	
a. Cycle time	Time (sec) of one complete gait cycle.
b. Stance time	Time (sec) that one foot is in contact with the support surface.
c. Single-support time	Time (sec) that one foot is the sole contact with the support surface during one gait cycle.
d. Double-support time	Total time (sec) that both feet have contact with the support surface; double support is absent in running.
e. Step duration	Time (sec) between contralateral foot contacts.
f. Stride duration	Time (sec) between ipsilateral foot contacts.
g. Cadence	Number of steps per unit time; normal cadence ranges from 70 to 130 steps per minute with an energy cost of 100 cal/miles.
4. Gait velocity	Rate (meters/sec) of forward body motion; i.e., (stride length × cadence)/2; comfortable walking speed is 80 m/min or 3 mph.
5. Center of gravity (COG)	Located 5 cm anterior to 2nd sacral vertebra; COG is displaced 5 cm vertically and 5 cm horizontally during an average adult male step.
6. Gait determinants	Mechanisms used by the body to reduce and smooth out the path of the center of gravity for a smooth and efficient gait.
a. Pelvic rotation	Right and left pelvic rotation around a vertical axis about 4° in each direction.
b. Pelvic tilt	Slight (4°) downward drop of pelvis on the side of the swing limb.
c. Knee flexion in stance	Knee flexion at foot strike and at heel-off (or terminal stance).
d. Ankle dorsiflexion in stance	Movement of the tibia over the foot during the foot-flat (loading response) to midstance, and midstance to heel-off phases.
e. Coordinated knee, ankle, and foot motion	The knee flexes, the ankle plantar flexes, and the foot pronates from foot strike to midstance; the knee extends, the ankle plantar flexes, and the foot supinates from midstance to heel-off.
f. Pelvic lateral displacement	The base of support and the tibiofemoral angle (with slight genu valgum) allows the tibia to remain vertical and the feet relatively close together.

Table 2.5-2. Normal gait

	STANCE (60%)						SWING (40%)	
	FIRST DOUBLE SUPPORT (DS) (10%)	SINGLE LIMB STANCE (40%)			SECOND DS (10%)	LIMB ADVANCEMENT		
RLA terms	Initial contact	Loading response	Midstance	Terminal stance	Presswing	Initial swing	Midswing	Terminal swing
Traditional terms	Heel (foot) strike	Foot flat	Midstance	Heel-off	Toe-off	Acceleration	Midswing	Deceleration
Stage of gait cycle	0-2%	0-10%	10-30%	30-50%	50-60%	60-70%	70-90%	90-100%
KINEMATICS								
Pelvis/femur	Internal rotation		External rotation			Internal rotation		
Hip	30° Flexion	20° Flexion	Extending to 0°	10° hyperextension	Neutral	20° Flexion	20-30° Flexion	30° Flexion
Knee	0-5° Flexion	15° Flexion	Extending to 5° Flexion	0-5° Flexion	35-40° Flexion	60° Flexion	30° flexion	0-5° Flexion
Ankle	0-3-5° PF	7-15° PF	From PF to 5° DF	10° DF	20° PF	10° PF	0-2° DF	0 to 3-5° PF

KINETICS

Subtalar	Eversion	Eversion	Maximum eversion	Inversion	Maximum inversion	Neutral	Neutral	Neutral
Iliopsoas	Inactive				Concentric action			
Gluteus maximus	Eccentric action							
Gluteus medius	Eccentric action					Inactive		
Hip adductors	Inactive			Concentric action		Inactive		
Hamstrings	Eccentric action			Inactive		Eccentric action		
Quadriceps	Eccentric action			Inactive		Eccentric action	Inactive	
Pretibial	Eccentric action			Inactive		Concentric action		
Calf muscles	Inactive		Eccentric action	Concentric action		Inactive		

Abbreviations: RLA = Rancho Los Amigos; DF = dorsiflexion; PF = plantarflexion.
Data adapted from: Perry J: *Gait analysis: Normal and pathological function*, Thorofare, NJ, 1992, Slack; Pathokinesiology Service and Physical Therapy Department: *Normal and pathological gait syllabus*, Downey, CA, 1989, Professional Staff Association of Rancho Los Amigos Medical Center, p. 11.; and Mann RA: Biomechanics of the foot. In Bunch, WH, Keagy RD, Kritter, AE, et al, eds: *American Academy of Orthopedic Surgeons (AAOS) Atlas of Orthotics: Biomechanical principles and application*, ed 2, St. Louis, 1985, CV Mosby, p. 112-125.

below. Table 2.5-1 shows the variables and determinants of gait, Table 2.5-2 shows the kinematic and kinetic events in normal gait, and Table 2.5-3 shows abnormal gaits and their probable causes. When analyzing gait, the clinician must be aware of the effect of gait speed on the gait cycle and gait patterns (e.g., slow walking can increase the period of double-limb stance, shorten the swing phase, and increase muscular cocontraction to provide greater stability on the lower limbs). Multiple observations may also be needed (in a natural setting if possible) as the patient's self-consciousness of being observed may also alter the gait pattern.

A. Observational gait analyses are done visually, with and/or without videotaping. The patient is asked to walk, with and/or without shoes (with and/or without orthotic/prosthetic devices or other gait aids, if applicable), on level ground (or on a treadmill) and/or on different surfaces as well as stairs. The gait parameters (see Table 1.1-10 in Chapter 1.1) are then observed from the front, side, and rear. The overall pattern of walking as well as kinematic gait parameters are described and analyzed from the foot and up to the trunk and upper limbs. If a videotape is used, certain aspects of the gait cycle can be viewed repeatedly (in slow motion if needed) for closer analyses.

B. Functional community analyses determine the distances required for independent community ambulation (e.g., going to the post office, bank, doctor's office, supermarket, department store, drug store, as well as in crossing intersections). Typical curb heights and crosswalk times in the patient's neighborhood can also be analyzed. The patient's gait ability as well as endurance are then evaluated (ideally by bringing the patient out on a field trip) to determine the feasibility of community ambulation (with or without gait aids or assistance from another person). If needed, the patient may be recommended a manual or powered mobility system (see Chapter 4.7) for community use.

C. Dynamic gait-analysis systems

1. Motion analysis system

a. Video-based (photometric) motion analysis systems (see section I.E) use high-speed infrared cameras to record relative motion of reflective markers attached to different body parts during ambulation. The information gathered is then digitized by the computer to generate two- or three-dimensional gait kinematic parameters. The system can generate raw data on segment positions that can easily be coordinated with ground reaction forces to compute joint kinetic information. Video-based systems are commonly used in most gait-analysis laboratories but are relatively expensive.

b. Electrogoniometers (described in section I.B.4) may be used to collect single-axial or multiaxial ROM data during ambulation. They are less expensive than video-based motion analysis systems and are useful for remote data-collection protocols (in which the use of a video-based system is impractical). However, they are not commonly used because they are cumbersome to the patient (because of the need for attaching the goniometric arms to the proximal and distal segments of the patient's limbs). Moreover, their data cannot be easily used to compute joint kinetic information (due to difficulty in coordinating goniometric data with ground reaction forces).

2. Foot pressure measurements can be used as aids in gait analyses and also in helping fabricate foot orthoses (e.g., wedges needed to reduce foot pressure in patients with diminished foot sensation).

a. Force-platform systems measure direct pressures at the plantar surface of

Table 2.5-3.   Abnormal gaits and their probable causes

GAIT PATHOLOGY	PROBABLE CAUSES
1. Foot strike to foot flat	
a. Foot slap	Moderately weak dorsiflexors
2. Foot strike through midstance	
a. Genu recurvatum	Weak, short, or spastic quadriceps; compensated hamstring weakness; Achilles tendon contracture; plantarflexor spasticity
b. Excessive foot supination	Compensated forefoot valgus deformity; pes cavus; short limb; uncompensated external rotation of tibia or femur
c. Excessive trunk extension	Weak hip extensor or flexor; hip pain; decreased knee ROM
d. Excessive trunk flexion	Weak gluteus maximus and quadriceps
3. Foot strike through toe-off	
a. Excessive knee flexion	Hamstring contracture; decreased ankle dorsiflexion; weak plantarflexor; long limb; hip flexion contracture
b. Excessive medial femur rotation	Tight medial hamstrings; anteverted femoral shaft; weakness of opposite muscle group
c. Excessive lateral femur rotation	Tight lateral hamstrings; retroverted femoral shaft; weakness of opposite muscle group
d. Increased base of support	Abductor muscle contracture; instability; genu valgum; leg length discrepancy
e. Decreased base of support	Adductor muscle contracture; genu varum
4. Footflat through heel-off	
a. Excessive trunk lateral flexion (Trendelenberg gait)	Ipsilateral gluteus medius weakness; hip pain
b. Pelvic drop	Contralateral gluteus medius weakness
c. "Waddling" gait	Bilateral gluteus medius weakness
5. Midstance through toe-off	
a. Excessive foot pronation	Compensated forefoot or rearfoot varus deformity; uncompensated forefoot valgus deformity; pes planus; decreased ankle dorsiflexion; increased tibial varum; long limb; uncompensated internal rotation of tibia or femur; weak tibialis posterior
b. Bouncing or exaggerated plantar flexion	Achilles tendon contracture; gastrocsoleus spasticity
c. Insufficient push off	Gastrocsoleus weakness; Achilles tendon rupture; metatarsalgia; hallux rigidus
d. Inadequate hip extension	Hip flexor contracture; weak hip extensor
6. Swing phase	
a. Steppage gait	Severely weak dorsiflexors; equinus deformity; plantarflexor spasticity
b. Circumduction	Long limb; abductor muscle shortening or overuse
c. Hip hiking	Long limb; weak hamstring; quadratus lumborum shortening

the foot (under barefoot conditions) as well as forces at the foot-ground interface. They use force plates (either strain gauges or piezoelectric sensors) on a walkway to measure foot pressures and to determine the ground reaction forces (i.e., the vertical, horizontal, and rotatory forces that are transmitted through the lower limb during each step), the ground reaction moments about the platforms' vertical and horizontal axes, as well as the center of pressure and shear forces.

b. **Foot-based pressure measurement devices** determine the pressure at the foot-shoe interface. They can consist of either shoe insoles with embedded load sensor arrays, or individual load sensors, which are applied to the specific areas of the foot that need to be studied.

3. **Dynamic electromyography (EMG)** uses surface or fine-wire electrodes to quantify the muscle recruitment patterns (i.e., timing and intensity of muscle activities in relation to different muscle of the same limb as well as the opposite limb) during ambulation. The EMG data from the electrodes can be transmitted through a telemetry system or through a cable (i.e., hard-wired) system. The EMG data can then be used to determine which muscles need attention during rehabilitation.

4. **Stride analyses** involve the determination of stride and step width, length, and duration as well as cadence and velocity. Toe-drag and symmetry of foot pressure can also be assessed. A simple method is to use footprint analysis (e.g., ink and paper method) and use a stopwatch to time the steps. A more expensive method is to use foot switches or a sensored walkway (similar to the foot-pressure measurement devices described earlier).

5. **Gait energy-expenditure determinations** are used to evaluate the function of the cardiopulmonary system during walking and running activities, with or without orthoses or prostheses. Parameters measured (e.g., oxygen cost, heart and respiratory rate, and blood pressure) are similar to those used for a cardiopulmonary graded exercise tolerance testing (see Chapter 2.7, section II.A.1). The energy expenditure of ambulation using prostheses is shown in Table 4.4-1 in Chapter 4.4, and the energy expenditure of ambulation using gait aids is discussed in Chapter 4.6, section I.

BIBLIOGRAPHY

Amundsen LR, editor: *Muscle strength testing: Instrumented and non-instrumented systems,* New York, 1990, Churchill Livingstone.

Chaffin DB, Andersson GBJ: *Occupational biomechanics,* ed 2, New York, 1991, John Wiley.

Doege TC, editor: *American Medical Association: Guides to the evaluation of permanent impairment,* ed 4, Chicago, 1993, American Medical Association.

Esquenazi A, Keenan MA: Gait analysis. In DeLisa JA, Gans BM, editors: *Rehabilitation medicine: Principles and practice,* ed 2, Philadelphia, 1993, JB Lippincott, pp. 122-130.

Eastman Kodak Company: *Ergonomic design for people at work,* vol. 2, New York, 1986, Van Nostrand Reinhold.

Giallonardo LM: Gait. In Myers RS, editor: *Saunders manual of physical therapy practice,* Philadelphia, 1995, WB Saunders, pp. 1105-1119.

Inman VT, Ralston HJ, Todd F: *Human walking,* Baltimore, 1981, Williams and Wilkins.

Jacobs K: Preparing for return to work. In Trombly CA, editor: *Occupational therapy for physical dysfunction,* ed 4, Baltimore, 1995, Williams & Wilkins, pp. 329-349.

Mayer TG, Barnes D, Kishino ND, et al: Progressive isoinertial lifting evaluation: Part I. A standardized protocol and normative database. *Spine* 13 (9):993-997, 1988.

Mayer TG, Gatchel R, Barnes D, et al: Progressive isoinertial lifting evaluation: Erratum notice. *Spine* 16 (5):5, 1991.

National Institute for Occupational Safety and Health (NIOSH): *Application manual for the revised NIOSH lifting equations* (NTIS Publication No. PB 94-176930 OSM). Springfield, VA, 1991, U.S. Department of Commerce.

Norkin CC, White DJ: *Measurement of joint motion: A guide to goniometry,* ed 2, Philadelphia, 1995, FA Davis.

Pease WA, Quesada PM: Kinematics and kinetics of gait. In Braddom RL, editor: *Physical medicine and rehabilitation,* Philadelphia, 1996, WB Saunders, pp. 83-103.

Perry J: *Gait analysis: Normal and pathological function,* Thorofare, NJ, 1992, Slack.

Saunders JBCM, Inman VT, Eberhardt HD: The major determinants in normal and pathological gait. *J Bone Joint Surg* 35A:543-548, 1953.

United States Department of Labor. *Dictionary of Occupational Titles: The classification of jobs according to worker trait factors,* ed 4, Washington, DC, 1991, U.S. Government Printing Press.

CHAPTER 2.6

PULMONARY FUNCTION TESTS

Pulmonary function testing (PFT) is used to determine the cause of respiratory symptoms (e.g., dyspnea) when it is not clinically apparent, to determine the presence of a suspected pulmonary disease (in patients with high risk factors for respiratory disease), to determine the pattern of pulmonary disease (i.e., obstructive vs. restrictive or combined obstructive and restrictive pattern), to assess severity of respiratory impairment in patients with known disease (e.g., exercise tolerance in asthmatics), to follow the progression or regression of respiratory disease (e.g., neuromuscular diseases that tend to get progressively worse), to assess response to treatment (e.g., bronchodilators), to do preoperative evaluation in patients with pulmonary disease or risk factors, and to assess impairment and disability due to pulmonary problems.

In the PM&R setting, the PFT is usually done with the patient at rest to differentiate between obstructive and restrictive pulmonary disorders and to estimate severity and progression of disease. The patient is usually seated; however, in patients with chronic alveolar hypoventilation (see Chapter 5.12), supine PFT should also be done. The PFT measures lung volume and capacity (see Fig. 2.6-1 and Table 2.6-1), flow rates (forced vital capacity [FVC], forced expiratory volume in 1 sec [FEV_1], FEV_1/FVC ratio, peak expiratory flow rate [PEFR], peak inspiratory flow rate [PIFR], forced expiratory flow rate [FEFR], and maximum voluntary ventilation [MVV]); lung diffusion capacity (lung diffusion capacity using carbon monoxide [D_{LCO}]); and blood gases. Chest wall compliance, maximal inspiratory pressure (MIP), and maximal expiratory pressure (MEP) may be measured in patients with chronic restrictive pulmonary disease (e.g., neuromuscular disorders). Pulmonary function tests can also be done as part of integrated cardiopulmonary exercise tolerance testing (see Chapter 2.7, section II.A). Other special PFTs such as sleep studies and bronchoprovocation inhalation tests are beyond the scope of this book.

After PFT, the measured values are compared to the predicted normal values based on age, sex, height, and weight. Normally, the measured PFT values should be at least 80% of the predicted values. A guide to the interpretation of PFTs is given at the end of this chapter in section V.

I. Tests of ventilation (lung volume and flow rate)

    A. Direct spirometry measures lung capacity, volume, and flow rates using a spirometer (a bell suspended in a container of water). The bell rises and falls in response to the breathing of the patient who inhales and exhales into a tube connected to the spirometer. The proportional movements of the bell are recorded on an electrical potentiometer or a kymograph. The values are then compared with predicted values for a particular age, sex, height, and weight.

        1. Static lung volume and capacity are measured using a bell or electronic spirometer. The subject is told to take regular breaths (tidal volume [TV]), then breath in maximally (inspiratory capacity [IC]) followed by a maximum exhalation (vital capacity [VC]). The parameters of the measured lung volume and capacity are shown in Fig. 2.6-1 and defined in Table 2.6-1.

            a. *Slow vital capacity (SVC)* is a subtype of vital capacity (VC = IC +

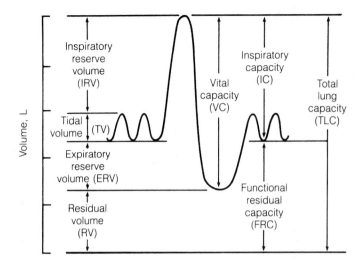

Figure 2.6-1
Spirogram of lung volumes and capacities. *Capacity* refers to two or more volumes.
(From Grippi MA, Metzger LF, Krupinski AV, et al: In Pulmonary function testing.
Fishman AP, editor: *Pulmonary diseases and disorders*, vol. 3, ed 2, New York,
1988, McGraw-Hill, reproduced with permission of the McGraw-Hill Companies).

expiratory reserve volume [ERV]). SVC is the maximum volume of
air that can be expired (or inspired) slowly and completely after a full
inspiratory (or expiratory) effort. It is decreased as restrictive disease
increases in severity.

b. *Inspiratory capacity (IC)* is the maximal amount of inspired air from end-
expiratory tidal volume in normal breathing or from functional residual
capacity (FRC). Changes in IC usually parallel changes in SVC and can
be used to identify lung or chest wall restriction. Most lung diseases do
not affect the IC per se, hence in most PFT interpretation the SVC is
used instead.

c. *Expiratory reserve volume (ERV)* is the maximal amount of air that can
be exhaled from end-expiratory tidal volume in normal breathing. It is
used to identify lung or chest wall restriction. Decreased ERV indicates
a chest wall restriction caused by weak inspiratory muscles or because
of nonpulmonary causes such as elevated diaphragm (seen in pregnancy,
ascites, or obesity), pleural effusion, kyphoscoliosis, thoracoplasty, and
massive cardiomegaly.

2. Dynamic lung volume and flow rate measurements are used to distinguish between chronic obstructive and restrictive pulmonary diseases. However, a
specific diagnosis cannot be made by using these tests exclusively. The
obstructive pulmonary pattern (see Table 2.6-2) generally shows normal
lung volumes but reduced FEV_1/FVC ratio due to reduced flow rate on
inspiration and expiration; whereas the restrictive pulmonary pattern (see
Table 2.6-2) generally shows reduced total lung capacity (TLC) but relatively normal and expiratory flow rate.

Table 2.6-1. Definition of static lung volumes and capacity

STATIC LUNG VOLUME/CAPACITY	SYMBOL	DEFINITION
Tidal volume	TV*	Amount of air normally inspired or expired with each breath during quiet breathing
Inspiratory reserve volume	IRV	Maximum amount of air inspired from the end-inspiratory level of the TV
Expiratory reserve volume	ERV	Maximum amount of air expired from the end-expiratory level of the TV
Residual volume	RV	RV = FRC − ERV; amount of air remaining in the lungs at the end of a maximal expiration
Vital capacity	VC	VC = VT + IRV + ERV = IC + ERV; maximum amount of air that can be inspired from the point of maximum expiration; or the maximum amount of air that can be expired from the point of maximum inspiration; or the maximum amount of air that can be breathed from RV to TLC
Slow vital capacity	SVC	Same as VC but using long, slow breath
Forced vital capacity	FVC	Same as VC but using quick, forceful breath
Inspiratory capacity	IC	IC = TV + IRV; maximum amount of air inspired from the end-expiratory level of the TV or from FRC
Functional residual capacity	FRC	FRC = RV + ERV; amount of air remaining in the lungs at the end of a normal exhalation (i.e., at the end-expiratory level of the TV)
Total lung capacity	TLC	TLC = IC + FRC = RV + VC = IRV + TV + ERV + RV; the sum of all air volumes in the entire lungs after maximum inspiration

* The symbol TV is traditionally used for tidal volume to indicate a subdivision of static lung volume, while the symbol V_T is used in gas-exchange formulas.

a. **Forced expirogram (forced vital capacity or time-volume curve)** is determined by having the subject maximally exhale into a water-sealed spirometer in which volume is measured against time. It records a maximum rapid exhalation after a maximum inhalation against time (Fig. 2.6-2 demonstrates a normal forced expirogram using a bellow or electronic spirometer).

Figure 2.6-2
A normal forced expirogram (forced vital capacity [FVC] or time-volume) curve using a bellow or electronic spirometer. In the top figure, the subject exhales as forcefully and rapidly as possible to indicate the forced expiratory volume (FEV) at intervals of 0.5, 1.0, 2.0, and 3.0 seconds. The bottom figure shows the forced expiratory flow rate from 25% to 75% of FVC ($FEF_{25-75\%}$) which reflects the average airway flow through large airways ($FEF_{25\%}$) and small airways ($FEF_{75\%}$). $FEF_{25\%}$ and $FEF_{75\%}$ may be determined by multiplying the FVC by 0.25 and 0.75, respectively. (From Ruppel GE: *Manual of pulmonary function test*, ed 6, St. Louis, 1994, Mosby-Year Book, pp. 47, 52; with permission)

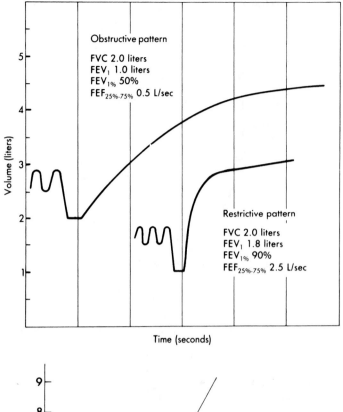

Obstructive pattern

FVC 2.0 liters
FEV_1 1.0 liters
$FEV_{1\%}$ 50%
$FEF_{25\%-75\%}$ 0.5 L/sec

Restrictive pattern

FVC 2.0 liters
FEV_1 1.8 liters
$FEV_{1\%}$ 90%
$FEF_{25\%-75\%}$ 2.5 L/sec

Volume (liters)

Time (seconds)

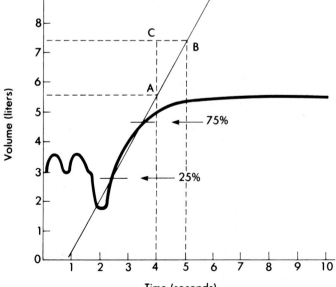

Volume (liters)

Time (seconds)

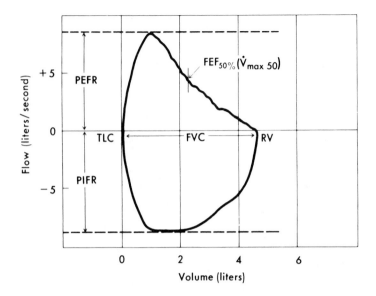

Figure 2.6-3
A normal flow-volume loop generated by successive recording of a forced vital capacity (i.e., expiratory) and a forced inspiratory vital capacity (FIVC) maneuver. In the flow-volume loop, the flow (L/sec) is plotted in the vertical axis; whereas the volume (L) is plotted in the horizontal axis. Abbreviations: PEFR, peak expiratory flow rate; PIFR, peak inspiratory flow rate; TLC, total lung capacity; FVC, forced vital capacity; RV, residual volume; $FEF_{50\%}$, forced expiratory flow rate at 50% of FVC. (From Ruppel GE: *Manual of pulmonary function test*, ed 6, St. Louis, 1994, Mosby-Year Book, pp. 55; with permission)

1) *Forced vital capacity (FVC)* is similar to SVC except that it uses a maximal quick, forceful expiration. Because forceful expiration prematurely closes the terminal airways (in subjects with airway obstruction), the FVC tends to be lower than the SVC. FVC (in conjunction with FEV_1) can be used to differentiate obstructive from restrictive pulmonary diseases.

2) *Forced expiratory volumes in one second (FEV_1)* is the volume of air forcefully expired during the first second after a full breath during the FVC maneuver (see Fig. 2.6-2). It normally comprises over 75% of the VC. In obstructive pulmonary disease, the ratio of FEV_1/FVC is decreased, but in restrictive pulmonary disease, this ratio stays normal (i.e., over 80%) or may be elevated.

b. **Flow-volume curve (flow volume loop; see Fig. 2.6-3)** can be generated from successive recording of a forced vital capacity (i.e., expiratory) maneuver and a forced inspiratory vital capacity (FIVC) maneuver using a pneumotachograph, or by calculating it from a forced expirogram.

1) *Peak expiratory flow rate (PEFR);* see Fig. 2.6-3) is the highest flow rate achieved at the beginning of the FVC and is reported in L/sec. The first one-third phase of the expiratory airflow is through the large

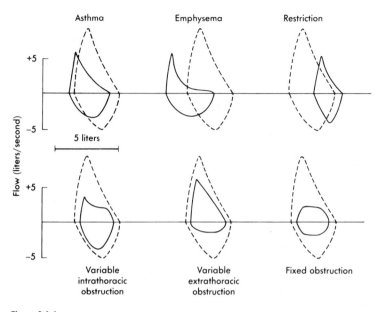

Figure 2.6-4

Flow volume curve patterns of various chronic obstructive and restrictive pulmonary abnormalities plotted in liters per second against the forced vital capacity. The dotted curve represents normal flow-volume loop. (From Ruppel GE: *Manual of pulmonary function test*, ed 6, St. Louis, 1994, Mosby, p. 56; with permission)

airways and is dependent on the subject's expiratory effort. But the last two-thirds phase of the expiratory airflow (i.e., downslope of the expiratory phase of the flow volume loop) is dependent on the intrinsic properties of the small airways. The absence of cartilage and decreased elasticity of the small airways predisposes them to collapse (at the same rate) during forced expiration regardless of the patient's effort. Reduced PEFR with normal inspiratory airflow is seen in weakness of the expiratory muscles, in poor expiratory effort, and in variable intrathoracic airway obstruction (e.g., chronic obstructive pulmonary disease [COPD], intrathoracic malignancy, and tracheomalacia). In *variable intrathoracic airway obstruction* (see Fig. 2.6-4), the trachea widens during inspiration because of the negative pressure created during a maximal forced inspiration (thus, the inspiratory phase remains relatively unaffected); however, during maximal expiration, the abnormal airways are compressed by the markedly positive pleural pressure thus reducing PEFR. The more abnormal and weaker the airways (e.g., terminal bronchioles), the faster is the rate of their collapse during expiration, leading to increased ''scooping'' of the downslope of the expiratory phase of the flow volume loop.

2) *Peak inspiratory flow rate (PIFR)*; see Fig. 2.6-3) is the highest flow rate achieved at the beginning of the forced inspiratory vital capacity (FIVC) and is reported in L/sec. It is dependent on the subject's inspi-

ratory effort. Reduced PIFR with normal expiratory airflow is seen in weakness of inspiratory muscles (e.g., neuromuscular disease), poor inspiratory effort, and variable extrathoracic airway obstruction (e.g., laryngeal dysfunction). In *variable extrathoracic airway obstruction* (see Fig. 2.6-4), the trachea narrows during inspiration (thus reducing PIFR) because the pressure in the extrathoracic area is less than atmospheric pressure; however, during maximal expiration, the expiratory flow rates remain relatively unaffected because the trachea widens as a consequence of the intratracheal pressure being greater than atmospheric pressure (and thus greater than extrathoracic pressure).

If both inspiratory and expiratory airflows are greatly reduced and have no peaks, the flow volume loop has a "boxed" appearance. This is indicative of a *fixed upper airway obstruction* (see Fig. 2.6-4), which can be extrathoracic (e.g., substernal thyroid, tracheal stenosis, tracheal tumor, plugged tracheostomy tube, and foreign body) or intrathoracic (e.g., tumor, rib cage deformity, and sarcoidosis). Although the smaller airways are normal and do not collapse easily, the amount of air getting in and out of the lungs is greatly reduced due to the fixed obstruction.

3) *Forced expiratory flow rate (FEFR)* is the rate of flow at different airway sizes and is thus independent of the subject's effort. It is determined at different percentages of FVC which correspond to different airway sizes. It is decreased in obstructive disease and is usually normal in restrictive disease except in severe cases when it can be reduced. By calculating FEFR at 25%, 50%, or 75% of FVC, the airway obstruction can be localized. Averaging *forced expiratory flow rate* from 25 to 75% of FVC ($FEF_{25-75\%}$) reflects average airway flow through small, medium and large airways (see Fig. 2.6-2).

a) *Forced expiratory flow rate at 25% of FVC ($FEF_{25\%}$)* is decreased in large airway obstruction.

b) *Forced expiratory flow rate at 50% of FVC ($FEF_{50\%}$)* is decreased in medium airway obstruction.

c) *Forced expiratory flow rate at 75% of FVC ($FEF_{75\%}$)* is decreased in small airway obstruction.

3. Maximum voluntary ventilation (MVV) is the maximum amount of air a subject can breathe in 12 seconds (expressed in L/min). It is done for less than 12 seconds to prevent hyperventilation and fainting. It reflects thoracic cage compliance, lung compliance, airway resistance, and the available muscle force. It is reduced in obstructive pulmonary disease, poor neuromuscular control, and poor respiratory effort. In emphysema, it is not only reduced but the baseline is also noted to be gradually rising as the ventilation progresses (this is attributed to air trapping). The MVV can be also be estimated by multiplying the $FEV_1 \times 40$.

B. Indirect spirometric techniques for determining FRC and derivatives

1. Helium dilution or equilibration technique is a closed-circuit method of measuring RV and FRC. The patient is connected to the spirometer containing a known concentration of helium, which is virtually insoluble in blood. After some breaths, the helium concentrations in the spirometer and lung equilibrate (i.e., the amount of helium dilution is proportional to the thoracic gas volume). This is measured as the FRC, which is then used to calculate RV (see Table 2.6-1 and Fig. 2.6-1)

a. *Residual volume (RV)* is the amount of air that remains in the lungs after maximal expiration (RV = FRC − ERV). An increase in RV is seen in obstructive respiratory diseases with air trapping, e.g., emphysema.

  b. *Functional residual capacity (FRC)* is the amount of air left in the lungs after tidal or normal respiration. (FRC = ERV + RV). Changes in the elastic properties of the lungs are reflected in the FRC. A value below 75% indicates restrictive disease, but a value above 125% suggests air trapping consistent with obstructive airway disease.

  c. *Total lung capacity (TLC)* is the total amount of air that is the lungs after maximal inspiration (TLC = VC + RV). A decreased TLC is the hallmark of restrictive pulmonary disease.

 2. Nitrogen washout is an open circuit method in which the patient exhales into the room. It is assumed that room air as well as the lungs have the same concentration of nitrogen (i.e., 80%). If the patient breathes 100% oxygen, nitrogen is washed out or removed from the lungs. The test begins at FRC and continues until the nitrogen concentration of the exhaled gas is below 1.0%. The volume and the nitrogen concentration of the exhaled gases are measured and a proportion is made to calculate the FRC, which is then used to compute RV and TLC.

 C. Body plethysmograph can be used to determine FRC. It is a large airtight box like a telephone booth in which the subject sits. At the end of a normal expiration, the patient (wearing a nose clip) is asked to make inspiratory efforts against a closed shutter over the mouthpiece (the shutter is closed so that the measured mouth pressure equals alveolar pressure). With each inspiratory effort, mouth pressure falls and lung volume increases. Because the plethysmograph is a closed box, the increase in lung volume produces a corresponding increase in box pressure because its gas volume decreases. The pressure and volume changes within the box as well as the intrathoracic lung volume are recorded. Then Boyle's Law is applied to compute the FRC.

II. Tests of pulmonary mechanics

 A. Body plethysmograph (see description in section I.C) can also be used to test for airway resistance and static lung compliance.

  1. *Airway resistance (R_{AW})* is the pressure required to produce a given flow. It can be measured with a body plethysmograph or more commonly by inferring it from dynamic lung volumes and expiratory flow rates.

  2. *Static lung compliance* is defined as the volume change/unit pressure change and reflects lung elasticity or stiffness.

 B. Manometric techniques measure the *maximal inspiratory pressure (MIP)* and *maximal expiratory pressure (MEP)* by having the subject forcibly inhale and exhale through a closed mouthpiece attached to a pressure gauge. Both MIP and MEP reflect the strength of the respiratory muscles. They are reduced in patients pulmonary diseases caused by neuromuscular disorders (see neuromuscular etiologies in Chapter 5.12, section III.B).

III. Measurement of lung diffusion capacity using carbon monoxide (D_{LCO}) is determined as the subject inspires maximally (from RV) a gas containing a small concentration of carbon monoxide, holds his breath for 10 seconds, then slowly exhales back to RV **(single breath D_{LCO} technique).** An aliquot of alveolar gas is analyzed for carbon monoxide and the amount absorbed during that breath is then calculated and expressed in milliliters of carbon monoxide absorbed/min/mm Hg. It assesses the lung for gas-exchange abnormalities arising from alveolar-capillary pathology (i.e., transfer of gas into the blood). The amount of gas transferred across a tissue is in part directly proportional to the tissue area and inversely proportional to the tissue thickness.

The D_{LCO} is reduced in loss of functioning alveolar-capillary bed with decreased lung volume (e.g., lung resection, diffuse interstitial fibrosis, asbestosis, scleroderma, histiocytosis-X, sarcoidosis, and pneumonia), loss of pulmonary capillary bed with relatively normal lung volume (e.g., emphysematous lungs, multiple pulmonary emboli, sarcoidosis, and collagen vascular disease), failure of air to reach alveoli because of poor distribution of ventilation (e.g., severe bronchospasm, pneumonia, foreign body, blocked bronchus, hilar tumor, and pulmonary embolism), and in reduced oxygen binding site due to low RBC (anemia).

Elevated D_{LCO} may be seen in increased pulmonary blood volume (e.g., left-to-right cardiac shunt, left heart failure, alveolar hemorrhage, during exercise, high altitude, and in the supine position) and in increased RBC production (polycythemia).

The D_{LCO} can be used to differentiate different COPD subtypes, e.g., emphysema usually has reduced D_{LCO}, and asthma and chronic bronchitis usually have normal D_{LCO}. Pure restrictive pulmonary diseases with normal pulmonary blood flow and capillary bed (e.g., those caused by neuromuscular disease or chest wall disease) have normal D_{LCO}.

IV. **Measurement of blood gases** are used to determine the adequacy and the efficiency of gas exchange.

  A. **Arterial blood gases (ABG) analysis** at room air is used to measure arterial oxygen tension (PaO_2), hemoglobin saturation (SaO_2), arterial carbon dioxide tension ($PaCO_2$), and alveolar-arterial oxygen tension difference or $P_{(A-a)}O_2$. The PaO_2 is the most sensitive indicator of pulmonary gas-exchange abnormalities of any etiology. A hemoglobin saturation (SaO_2) of less than 90%, which usually corresponds to PaO_2 of less than 60 mm Hg, indicates seriously compromised tissue oxygenation. The $PaCO_2$, which is normally kept within the narrow range of 35 to 45 mm Hg, determines the subject's ventilatory status. Hence hypocapnia ($PaCO_2$ <35) indicates hyperventilation, while hypercapnia ($PaCO_2$ >45) indicates hypoventilation. If hypercapnia is persistent, especially when the patient is asleep, positive-pressure airway mechanical ventilators (see Chapter 5.12, section IV.A.4.a) should be considered during sleep. The $P_{(A-a)}O_2$, i.e., A-a gradient, is another way of measuring pulmonary gas-exchange. $P_{(A-a)}O_2$ is the difference between calculated alveolar oxygen tension (P_AO_2) and measured PaO_2. Normally the $P_{(A-a)}O_2$ is less than 10 to 15 mm Hg. It remains normal when the decreased PaO_2 is solely due to alveolar hypoventilation, a low inspired oxygen tension, or a decrease in respiration. If $P_{(A-a)}O_2$ is increased, it is indicative of impaired diffusion, ventilation-perfusion mismatching, or intrapulmonary shunting.

  B. **Transcutaneous oximetry (pulse oximetry)** can be used to monitor arterial oxygen saturation at rest, during exercise, during activities of daily living, and during sleep. It closely correlates with oxygen saturation obtained by ABGs except during severe peripheral hypoperfusion, during carbon monoxide poisoning, when skin pigmentation is extremely dark, or when saturation is below 70%. As with ABGs, a pulse oximeter reading of oxygen saturation of less than 90%, which usually corresponds to PaO_2 below 60 mm Hg, indicates seriously compromised tissue oxygenation. This is explained by the oxygen-hemoglobin dissociation curve, which shows a steep decline in SaO_2 if PaO_2 is below 60 mm Hg or if the measured oxygen saturation (e.g., by pulse oximeter) is below 90%.

V. **Interpretation of PFTs** is contingent upon the quality of the testing session. The subject should be able to follow instructions for the test and should have given

Table 2.6-2. Patterns of pulmonary function abnormalities in various pulmonary diseases

PATTERNS OF ABNORMALITIES	VC	RV	TLC	FEV₁/FVC	D_LCO
A. Obstructive					
1. Asthma	N or ↓	N or ↑	N or ↑	↓	N or ↑
2. Chronic bronchitis	N or ↓	N or ↑	N	↓	N
3. Emphysema	N or ↓	↑	↑	↓	↓
B. Restrictive					
1. Pulmonary parenchyma	↓	↓	↓	N or ↑	↓
2. Extrapulmonary	↓	↓	↓	N	N
C. Obstructive and restrictive	↓	N or ↓	↓	↓	N or ↓

From Loke JSO: Pulmonary function testing. In Stein J, editor: *Internal medicine*, ed 4, St. Louis, 1994, Mosby, p. 1595, with permission.
VC = vital capacity; RV = residual volume; TLC = total lung capacity; FEV_1 = forced expiratory volume in 1 second; FVC = forced vital capacity; D_{LCO}, = diffusing capacity of carbon monoxide; N = normal; ↓ = decreased; ↑ = increased.

his or her best effort. Although PFT cannot diagnose a specific disease, it can differentiate between obstructive and restrictive patterns of pulmonary disease. Patterns of pulmonary abnormalities in various pulmonary disease states are shown in Table 2.6-2 and Fig. 2.6-4. The degree of severity of the pulmonary disease is determined by the percentage of measured value compared to predicted value (i.e., normal if ≥80%, mild if 65-79%, moderate if 50-64%, and severe if <50% of predicted values). The PFTs for the very young (<20 years old) or very old (>75 years old) subjects should be interpreted with caution due to lack of normative data in these age groups. All PFTs should be correlated with clinical findings.

A. **Obstructive pulmonary disease** (see Table 2.6-2) features reduced inspiratory and expiratory flows but generally normal lung volumes. Because it is an airflow disease, the hallmark is reduced FEV_1/FVC ratio (i.e., <80%). Also, there is scooping of the downslope of the expiratory phase of the flow-volume loop due to increased airway resistance. The TLC, FRC, and RV may be increased. The major cause of reversible obstructive pulmonary disease is asthma. For COPD, the major risk factor is tobacco. A normal FEV_1/FVC ratio excludes obstructive pulmonary disease. A low FEV_1/FVC ratio in the setting of increased FEV_1 and FVC, however, can be a variant of normal (seen in athletes). If the FEV_1/FVC ratio is low with elevated FRC (>125%) or elevated RV, it is indicative of emphysema due to air trapping and lung hyperinflation. If the FEV_1/FVC ratio and the $FEF_{75\%}$ are both low, it is indicative of small airway obstructive disease (e.g., due to bronchospasm in asthma). All patients with obstructive patterns should be tested for reversibility with bronchodilators, i.e., improvement in FVC or FEV_1 of more than 12% or more than 200 ml within 15 minutes of bronchodilator treatment. Lack of PFT improvement after a single bronchodilator treatment should be interpreted with caution because it reflects one particular bronchodilator agent given at that particular time of testing. The agent may not have been administered properly or the patient may have responded only to long-term therapy. In determining bronchodilator responsiveness, the FEV_1/FVC ratio should not be used.

B. **Restrictive pulmonary disease** (see Table 2.6-2) features reduced lung volumes but normal flow rates on inspiration and expiration. Because it is a lung-volume disease, its hallmark is reduced TLC (<80% of predicted TLC) with normal or elevated FEV_1/FVC ratio. Restrictive pulmonary diseases caused by abnormalities of the pulmonary interstitium (e.g., interstitial pulmonary fibrosis, lobectomy, and massive pneumonia) have abnormal D_{LCO}, but those caused by chest wall restriction (e.g., kyphoscoliosis; elevated diaphragm because of obesity, ascites, or pregnancy; massive cardiomegaly; pleural effusion; and neuromuscular disease) have normal D_{LCO}. In general, a normal TLC precludes restrictive pulmonary diseases.

   C. Combined obstructive and restrictive pulmonary disease (see Table 2.6-2) has features of both obstructive and restrictive pulmonary diseases, e.g., low FEV_1/FVC ratio with low TLC.

BIBLIOGRAPHY

Grippi MA, Metzger LF, Krupinski AV, et al.: Pulmonary function testing. In Fishman AP, editor: *Pulmonary diseases and disorders,* vol 3, ed 2, New York, 1988, McGraw-Hill, pp. 2469-2521.

Irvin CG, Corbridge T: Physiologic evaluation of patients for pulmonary rehabilitation. *Seminars in respiratory medicine,* 14(6):417-429, 1993.

Kiss GT: Use and interpretation of pulmonary function tests. In Ferri FF, editor: Practical guide to the care of the medical patient, ed 3, St. Louis, 1995, Mosby, pp. 576-583.

Loke JSO: Pulmonary function testing. In Stein J, editor: *Internal medicine,* ed 4, St. Louis, 1994, Mosby, p. 1590-1596.

Ruppel GL: *Manual of pulmonary function testing,* ed 6, St. Louis, 1994, Mosby.

West JB: *Pulmonary pathophysiology: The essentials,* ed 4, Baltimore, 1992, Williams & Wilkins.

CHAPTER 2.7

EXERCISE TOLERANCE TESTING

Exercise tolerance testing or ETT (also called exercise stress testing) can be used for diagnostic, prognostic, and functional purposes. In the PM&R setting, ETT is mainly used to determine the functional work capacity, which in turn can be used to determine disability as well as guide the cardiac and/or pulmonary rehabilitation (e.g., to determine the intensity of the prescribed exercise or activity). In patients with predominantly cardiovascular diseases (e.g., coronary artery disease or after uncomplicated myocardial infarcts), ETT is primarily used to measure cardiac parameters (e.g., electrocardiogram [ECG], blood pressure [BP], heart rate [HR]). In patients with predominantly pulmonary diseases (e.g., chronic obstructive pulmonary diseases), ETT measures pulmonary parameters (e.g., breathed gas concentrations of O_2 and CO_2; blood gases) in addition to cardiac parameters. This chapter gives an overview of ETT as used in the PM&R setting for determining functional work capacity. Exercise tolerance testing for diagnostic purposes is beyond the scope of this book.

I. **Cardiovascular (CV) ETTs (i.e., ECG exercise test),** for determining functional work capacity as well as for determining prognosis (i.e., risk stratification), are justified only in patients with coronary heart disease and with uncomplicated myocardial infarcts (according to the general consensus of the American College of Cardiology/American Heart Association). Their usefulness for determining functional work capacity in the following conditions remains controversial: (a) apparently healthy men over age 40 who are sedentary and plan to enter a vigorous exercise program, (b) patients with valvular heart disease, and (c) patients with hypertension or cardiac pacemakers who wish to engage in static or dynamic exercise training. The absolute and relative contraindications to ETT in general are listed in Table 2.7-1, and the endpoints for exercise termination are listed in Table 2.7-2.

Prior to ETT, the patient is advised not to drink caffeinated beverages for at least 24 hours and not to eat for at least 3 hours. Patients are also told to wear comfortable, loose-fitting clothes and comfortable walking shoes for the ETT session. Most of the CV-ETT protocols use continuous incremental workloads (i.e., the exercise is uninterrupted and the work load is increased in stages) and are referred to as graded ETT or GXTT. Although some CV-ETT protocols make no allowance for warm-up or cool-down because of the extra time required, it is always prudent to include a warm-up and cool-down period, especially in the PM&R setting in which the CV-ETT is primarily used for determining functional work capacity. The benefits of proper (low-load) warm-up include gradual adjustment of the heart to the increased work demand, reduced incidence of ST-T segment depression during exercise, and reduced incidence of muscular injuries and patient anxiety. The cool-down or recovery period, which should be at least 3 minutes, can help prevent pooling of the peripheral circulation and possible fainting.

A. **CV graded-ETTs (CV-GXTTs)** use continuous incremental workloads, which begin at a low workload and progress to higher workloads until either subjective or objective "maximal" endpoints (see Table 2.7-2) preclude further exercise

Table 2.7-1. Absolute and relative contraindications to exercise tolerance testing

ABSOLUTE CONTRAINDICATIONS	RELATIVE CONTRAINDICATIONS
A. Unstable or severe CV disorders 1. Acute (e.g., <5 days) myocardial infarction (MI) or recent complicated MI 2. Unstable angina 3. ECG parameters: recent (within 4 weeks) changes in resting ECG suggesting MI or acute cardiac events; serious cardiac dysrhythmias (e.g., rapid ventricular or atrial arrhythmias), second- or third-degree atrioventricular block 4. Severe (>70%) left main coronary obstruction 5. Severe valvular (e.g., aortic) stenosis 6. Severe symptomatic left ventricular dysfunctions or obstructions (e.g., severe hypertrophic obstructive cardiomyopathy) 7. Dissecting aortic aneurysm 8. Acute congestive heart failure 9. Resting blood pressure ≥200/≥120 mm Hg 10. Acute myo-, endo-, or pericarditis 11. Acute deep venous thrombosis, thrombophlebitis, or cardiac thrombi B. Pulmonary conditions 1. Blood gas shows: PaO$_2$ <40 mm Hg in room air; PaCO$_2$ >70 mm Hg 2. FEV$_1$ <30% of predicted value 3. Asthma attack 4. Acute pulmonary emboli or infarct C. Noncardiopulmonary conditions 1. Any acute or serious systemic disorders (e.g., fever, infections, severe anemia) 2. Acute psychosis 3. Neurologic or musculoskeletal conditions precluding adequate exercise 4. Drug or alcohol intoxication 5. Inability to cooperate; lack of motivation; patient refusal 6. Inappropriate pretesting documentation or medical indication	A. Stable or less serious CV disorders 1. ECG parameters: severe ST segment depression at rest; frequent or complex ventricular ectopy; tachy- or bradydysrhythmias 2. Suspected or <70% left main coronary obstruction or its equivalent 3. Moderate valvular heart disease 4. Less severe hypertrophic cardiomyopathy (e.g., asymmetric septal hypertrophy) 5. Ventricular aneurysm 6. Chronic congestive heart failure 7. Significant arterial hypertension 8. Significant pulmonary hypertension 9. Fixed-rate pacemaker (rarely used) B. Noncardiopulmonary conditions 1. Uncontrolled metabolic disorders (diabetes mellitus, thyrotoxicosis, or myxedema) 2. Chronic systemic diseases (e.g., hepatitis, AIDS, mononucleosis, malnutrition) 3. Known electrolyte abnormalities (e.g., hypokalemia, hypomagnesemia) 4. Drug effect 5. Neurologic or musculoskeletal conditions that can be exacerbated by exercise 6. Advanced or complicated pregnancy 7. Nonpsychotic psychiatric illnesses

Table 2.7-2.   Endpoints for exercise tolerance testing

DETERMINANT	SPECIFIC ENDPOINTS
Subjective	1. Subject wants to stop 2. Significant and progressive angina 3. Marked fatigue 4. Severe dyspnea 5. Other limiting symptoms (e.g., lightheadedness, headache, blurred vision, confusion, ataxia, pallor, cyanosis, nausea, vomiting, leg claudication, cramps, severe joint pains)

Objective	A. ECG changes
	    1. **Ischemic changes:** >2-mm horizontal or downsloping ST depression or elevation; T-wave inversion; or Q wave
	    2. **Accelerated rhythms:** supraventricular tachyarrhythmias; ventricular tachycardia or fibrillation; premature ventricular complexes or PVCs (increasing frequency; multifocal; in couplets; runs of ≥ 4; R-on-T); atrial tachycardia, fibrillation, or flutter
	    3. **Bradycardias:** unexplained inappropriate bradycardia (i.e., pulse rise slower than 2 SD below age-adjusted normal values); onset of second- or third-degree atrioventricular block
	    4. **Intraventricular conduction abnormalities:** onset of bundle branch block
	B. Blood pressure (BP) and heart rate (HR) parameters:
	    1. **Systolic BP (SBP):** >250 mm Hg, drops > 10-20 mm Hg, or falls below standing SBP
	    2. **Diastolic BP (DBP):** >120 mm Hg or increase >20 mm Hg
	    3. **HR or SBP** drops progressively or fail to rise despite an increase in exercise load after the initial adjustment period
	C. Blood gas parameters:
	    1. **PaO$_2$:** <55 mm Hg or fall of >20 mm Hg
	    2. **PaCO$_2$:** >65 mm Hg or rise of >10 mm Hg

Others	1. Attainment of predicted (i.e., maximal) or targeted (i.e., submaximal) values (e.g., HR or METS [see specific parameters in Chapter 5.13, section IV.A.2.b] or ventilation). 2. Equipment failure (e.g., dislodged ECG leads)

or a predetermined "submaximal" endpoint is reached (e.g., target heart rate [see Chapter 4.2 section III.A.1 for formula] or target workload as specified by the test protocol). The incremental work should last for a reasonable period of time, i.e., a minimum of 8 minutes and a maximum of 18 minutes. During CV-GXTT, there is no rest period at all, thus the patient's peak capacity or endpoint is reached earlier. The graded-exercise protocol is practical and is most commonly used in CV-ETT protocols.

Measured parameters

• **Blood pressure (BP)** of the brachial artery can be determined by using a sphygmomanometer. The predicted rise in BP for sedentary middle-aged men is $\geq 205/\geq 95$. In general, the systolic BP should increase in proportion with the workload, but should not be greater than 250 mm Hg. Likewise, the diastolic BP should not exceed 120 mm Hg or increase by more than 20 mm Hg.

- **Electrocardiogram (ECG) pattern and heart rate (HR)** can be determined by using a 12-lead ECG telemetric monitor. The ECG is taken before the start of the test (in supine and erect positions to ensure that there are no changes in the ECG based solely on position changes), at each stage of the test, and during the recovery period. During GXTT, the following are suggestive but not diagnostic of myocardial ischemia: development of downsloping ST segment depression, development or increase in the number of premature ventricular contractions, and a significant atrial arrhythmia.
- **Workload** can be determined by using a treadmill or a cycle ergometer in accordance with a CV-GXTT protocol (see below). There is a linear relationship between workload and HR up to an age-determined maximum, i.e., the nominal age-adjusted maximum HR of 220 − age in years.
  Calculated parameters
- **Rate-pressure product or RPP (or double product)** is calculated by multiplying HR × systolic BP. The RPP, which is usually a five digit number, is then converted into a three-digit number by dropping the last two digits. The RPP (see Chapter 4.2, section III.A) has a good correlation with myocardial oxygen consumption and is an excellent indicator of aerobic conditioning (i.e., a high RPP indicates poor physical conditioning and vice versa).
- **Metabolic (MET) equivalent** is an estimation of the metabolic or energy demands of a given activity (i.e., the volume of O_2 consumed [VO_2], see description in section II.A). One MET is the amount of oxygen consumed by a seated individual at rest (VO_2 rest) and is equal to approximately 3.5 ml of oxygen per kg/min. Actual measurement of VO_2 (which is impractical

Table 2.7-3. Conversion of treadmill workload at different speed (miles per hour [mph]) and percent grade incline into approximate metabolic equivalents (METs)

% GRADE	MET* LEVEL FOR TREADMILL SPEED (mph) AT DIFFERENT % GRADE INCLINATION					
	1.7 mph	2.0 mph	2.5 mph	3.0 mph	3.4 mph	3.75 mph
0	2.3	2.5	2.9	3.3	3.6	3.9
2.5	2.9	3.2	3.8	4.3	4.8	5.2
5.0	3.5	3.9	4.6	5.4	5.9	6.5
7.5	4.1	4.6	5.5	6.4	7.1	7.8
10.0	4.6	5.3	6.3	7.4	8.3	9.1
12.5	5.2	6.0	7.2	8.5	9.5	10.4
15.0	5.8	6.6	8.1	9.5	10.6	11.7
17.5	6.4	7.3	8.9	10.5	11.8	12.9
20.0	7.0	8.0	9.8	11.6	13.0	14.2
22.5	7.6	8.7	10.6	12.6	14.2	15.5
25.0	8.2	9.4	11.5	13.6	15.3	16.8

Adapted from American College of Sports Medicine: *Guidelines for exercise testing and prescription,* ed 4, Philadelphia, 1991, Lea & Febiger, p. 298, with permission from copyright © holder, Williams & Wilkins.
* 1 MET = 3.5 ml of O_2 consumption/kg/min during rest.

Table 2.7-4. **Conversion of bicycle ergometry workload (in watts) into approximate metabolic equivalents (METs) for different body weights**

	MET* LEVEL FOR WORKLOADS IN WATTS‡ (W) FOR DIFFERENT BODY WEIGHT								
WEIGHT	25 W‡	50 W	75 W	100 W	125 W	150 W	175 W	200 W	250 W‡
50 Kg	3.6	5.1	6.9	8.6	10.3	12.0	13.7	15.4	16.3
60 Kg	3.3	4.3	5.7	7.1	8.6	10.0	11.4	12.9	14.0
70 Kg	3.1	3.7	4.9	6.1	7.3	8.6	9.8	11.0	13.5
80 Kg	3.0	3.2	4.3	5.4	6.4	7.5	8.6	9.6	11.0
90 Kg	2.9	2.9	3.8	4.8	5.7	6.7	7.6	8.6	10.0
100 Kg	2.8	2.6	3.4	4.3	5.1	6.0	6.9	7.7	9.2

Adapted from American College of Sports Medicine: *Guidelines for exercise testing and prescription.* ed 4, Philadelphia, 1991, Lea & Febiger, p. 299, with permission from copyright © holder, Williams & Wilkins.
* One MET = 3.5 ml of O_2 consumption/kg/min during rest.
† One watt = 6 kg-meter/min; thus 50 watts = 300 kg-meter/min = 1.0 Kp-meter/min (kilopond-meter/min)
‡ The MET or VO_2 consumption cannot be estimated with reasonable accuracy for workloads below 50 W and above 200 W.

in most clinical situations) is described in section II.A. To estimate the "maximal" metabolic demand (i.e., "maximal" MET level) from CV-GXTT, the workload must be known. By using Tables 2.7-3 and 2.7-4, the respective "maximal" workloads attained from treadmill and bicycle-ergometer protocols (see below) can be converted into "maximal" MET levels. For example, if the Bruce protocol (discussed in section I.A.2) is used, and the "maximal" exercise level is reached at the treadmill setting of 2.5 mph and 12% grade incline, then the estimated "maximum" MET level is 7 (see Table 2.7-3) i.e., the person is consuming 24.5 ml of oxygen per kg/min or seven times the resting rate of 3.5 ml oxygen per kg/min.

The drawbacks in using the relative MET equivalent from the table of activities include (a) the MET level tables tend to overestimate the MET level for patients with cardiopulmonary problems because most of the data used in constructing the table were derived from normal healthy subjects (b) the maximal MET level obtained during GXTT using lower-limb protocols (e.g., treadmill) may not correlate well the MET level of predominantly upper-limb activities (e.g., carpentry), (c) the MET level tables do not take into account the concomitant emotional or physiological stresses that may add to metabolic demands during performance of an activity in real-life settings. Hence, MET tables should be used with great caution and an awareness of their physiologic limitations.

Interpretation guidelines. The CV-GXTT performed in the PM&R setting is usually used to determine the "maximal" functional work capability of the patient (e.g. for exercise prescription). A CV-GXTT is considered "maximal" only if the limiting signs or symptoms are reflective of the person's functional capacity, e.g., if the test were stopped because of the onset of angina or significant changes in ECG, BP, or HR parameters; however, if the patient requests the test to be stopped (e.g., due to some localized muscle fatigue), the test is considered "maximal-volitional." The HR achieved at the end point of a "maximal" or "maximal-volitional" CV-GXTT test is considered the "maximal heart rate" (MHR), or more accurately the "peak HR," for the purpose of exercise prescription (see Chapter 4.2, section III.A.1 on how to use MHR to compute the target heart rate range used for guiding aerobic exercise intensity). The "maximal" workload attained during the CV-GXTT can also be converted into its "maximum" MET level to estimate the workload's metabolic demand or the VO_2max. The use of MET levels in prescribing aerobic exercise intensity is described in Chapter 4.2, section III.A.2. If a "submaximal" protocol is used, the "MHR" may need to be adjusted because estimates of VO_2max derived from submaximal performance on a GXTT may vary by about 10 to 15% from the actual or measured VO_2max. Another use of the CV-GXTT is to help classify a patient according to functional capacity (see Table 2.7-5) and to use this functional classification in the determination of maintenance levels for cardiac exercise therapy, in advising patients about recreational and occupational activities (see Chapter 4.2, section III.A.2), and in predicting subsequent cardiac events and prognosis for survival.

1. **Treadmill (TM) CV-GXTTs,** which use a motor-driven TM, are the most commonly used protocols for CV-GXTT in the United States.

   Advantage. The advantages of using a TM over a bicycle ergometer include (a) TM permits higher peak cardiopulmonary workload and is a more accurate predictor of VO_2max, (b) walking is familiar to most people, thus less skill is needed, and there is less local fatigue of the leg muscles, (c) TM protocols are quite flexible because the speed and grade of TM walking can be varied independently to change the workload, and (d) TM workloads can be better administered because the patient is forced to keep up with the preset TM speed.

   Disadvantage. TMs are more expensive, occupy more space, are relatively noisier, and not as convenient for recording the patient's BP, HR, and ECG than bicycle ergometry.

   Test Protocols. TM protocols for CV-GXTT vary in terms of percent grade (i.e., TM incline), speed, duration of stages, and size of increments between stages. Although there are variations in the rate of workload increment, most protocols accomplish about the same effect. In general, smaller and more gradual uniform workload increments are preferred for cardiac patients because large, rapid, unequal workload increments tend to result in an overestimation of exercise capacity.

   Among the many validated TM protocols available (see description of common TM protocols in Table 2.7-6), the most widely used is the Bruce protocol because of its ease of administration and economy of time (i.e., it takes a relatively short duration for most subjects to reach maximal effort). However, for most cardiac or cardiopulmonary patients, the standard Bruce protocol is too strenuous. Hence, a less strenuous protocol using 2 to 3 min stages with low speed and one MET increments (e.g., modified Naughton, modified Balke, and modified Bruce protocols; see Table 2.7-6) should be used. The modified Naughton has also been used to extensively classify cardiac patients into high-risk and low-risk categories (i.e., risk stratification; see Table 5.13-3 in Chapter 5.13). The major disadvantage of using a less strenuous protocol is the longer duration of exercise required to achieve maximal effort (hence they are not practical for healthy subjects). The clinician should carefully evaluate the patient's cardiopulmonary status and decide which particular protocol to use (ideally, one that brings the patient to "maximal" effort in 8-12 min) rather than use one protocol for all pa-

Table 2.7-5. Correlation of metabolic equivalent (MET) levels to the functional and therapeutic classification of cardiac or cardiopulmonary impairment/disability and to the U.S. Department of labor classification of work

MET* LEVEL	<2	2	3	4	5	6	7	8	9	10	11	12	13	14	15	16
Clinical status		←Symptomatic→														
Clinical status			Diseased, recovered													
Clinical status						←Sedentary healthy→										
Clinical status									←Physically active→		←I and normal→					
Functional class†‡	IV		III			II				I and normal						
Work classification (see Table 5.11-1 in Chapter 5.11 for details).	Sed§		Light			Medium			Heavy to very heavy							

* One MET (metabolic equivalent) = 3.5 ml of O_2 consumption per kg/min at rest.

† **New York Heart Association (NYHA) classification:**
• **Class I** patients have no limitations as they can perform ordinary physical activity without undue fatigue or symptoms.
• **Class II and III** patients may experience fatigue or symptoms (e.g., dyspnea, anginal pain) with ordinary or lighter than ordinary activity.
• **Class IV** patients have symptoms at rest and cannot perform any physical activity without discomfort.

‡ **Canadian Cardiovascular Society classification:**
• **Class I** (ordinary physical activity such as walking and climbing stairs, does not cause angina. Angina with strenuous or rapid or prolonged exertion at work or recreation);
• **Class II** (Slight limitation of ordinary activity; Walking or climbing stairs rapidly, walking uphill, walking or stair climbing after meals, in cold, in wind, or when under emotional stress, or only during the few hours after awakening; Walking >2 blocks on the level and climbing >1 flight of ordinary stairs at a normal pace and in normal conditions);
• **Class III** (Marked limitation of ordinary physical activity; Walking 1-2 blocks on the level and climbing 1 flight in normal conditions);
• **Class IV** (Inability to carry on any physical activity without discomfort; anginal syndrome may be present at rest).

§ Sed, sedentary

Adapted from Criteria Committee of the New York Heart Association. Diseases of the heart and blood vessels: Nomenclature and criteria for diagnosis, ed 6, Boston, 1953, Little, Brown, and Co, pp. 112-113; Campeau L: Letter to the editor. *Circulation* 54:522, 1976; and U.S. Department of Labor Employment and Training Administration: *Dictionary of Occupational Titles*, vol. II, ed 4, revised, Washington, D.C., 1991, U.S. Government Printing Press, p. 1013.

Table 2.7-6. **Common treadmill protocols for cardiovascular graded-exercise tolerance testing arranged in approximate order of increasing strenuousness**

TREADMILL	PROTOCOL
Modified Naughton	Set speed q 2 min to: 2.0, 2.0, 2.0, 2.0, 2.0, 2.0, 3.0, 3.0 mph* Set % grade q 2 min to: 0, 3.5, 7.0, 10.5, 14.0, 17.5, 12.5, 15 mph Corresponding MET level q 2 min is 2, 3, 4, 5, 6, 7, 8, 9 METs
Cornell	Set speed q 2 min to: 1.7, 1.7, 1.7, 2.1, 2.5, 3.0, 3.4, 3.8, 4.2 mph Set % grade q 2 min to: 0, 5, 10, then increase by 1% Corresponding MET level q 2 min is, 2, 3, 4, 5.5, 7, 8.5, 10, 11.5, 13 METs
Modified Balke	Set speed q 3 min to: 2.0, 2.0, 2.0, 2.0, 2.0, 2.0, then 3.0 mph thereafter Set % grade q 3 min to: 0, 3.5, 7.0, 10.5, 14, 17.5, 12.5, 15, 17.5, 20, 22.5 mph Corresponding MET level q 3 min is 2.5 with 1 MET increase thereafter
Modified Bruce	Set speed q 3 min to: 1.7, 1.7, 1.7, 2.5, 3.4, 4.2, 5.0, 5.5, 6.0 mph Set % grade q 3 min to: 0, 5, 10, 12, 14, 16, 18, 20, 22% Corresponding MET level q 3 min is 2, 3, 5, 7, 10, 13, 16, 19, 22 METs
Naughton-Balke	Set and maintain speed q 2 min to: 3.0 mph Set % grade q 2 min to 2.5, then increase by 2.5% Corresponding MET level q 2 min is 4, 5, 6, 7, 8, 9.5, 10.5, 11.6, 12.6 METs
USAFSAM‡	Set and maintain speed q 3 min to: 3.3 mph Set % grade q 3 min to 0, then increase by 5% Corresponding MET level q 3 min is 4, 6, 8, 10, 13, 15 METs
Standard Bruce	Set speed q 3 min to: 1.7, 2.5, 3.4, 4.2, 5.0, 5.5, 6.0 mph Set % grade q 3 min to 10%, then increase by 2% Corresponding MET† level q 3 min is 5, 7, 10, 13, 17, 20, 24 METs

* mph = miles per hour
† One MET (metabolic equivalent) = 3.5 ml of O_2 consumption/kg/min at rest
‡ USAFSAM = U.S. Air Force School of Aerospace Medicine

tients. The patient's "maximal" workload on the TM can be converted into METs using Table 2.7-3, and the MET level can then be used to determine the patient's functional classification (Table 2.7-5). In general, one MET represents an increment on the treadmill of roughly one mph or 2.5% grade.

2. **Cycle-ergometer CV-GXTTs**

   a. **Upright-bicycle ergometer CV-GXTTs** offer a useful alternative for patients who have difficulty with TM walking because of ambulatory instability or orthopedic limitations. Upright bicycling is preferred because supine bicycling does not significantly change stroke volume and end-diastolic volumes. The peak values for heart rate during upright cycle ergometry have been shown to be similar to TM exercise, although the maximum myocardial VO_2 may be approximately 10% less than for TM exercise. The workload of bicycle ergometers are expressed in units of absolute mechanical power, i.e., watts (W), kg-meter/min (kg-m/min), or kilopond-meter/min (Kp-m/min). These can then be converted into MET levels (by using Table 2.7-4), which in turn can be used to determine the patient's functional classification (see Table 2.7-5). In general, one MET represents an increment on the bicycle ergometer of roughly 20 W (120 kg-m/min) for a 70-kg person.

Advantage. The advantages of upright-bicycle ergometry compared to TM protocols include use of nonweight-bearing exercise and more convenient monitoring of ECG, HR, and BP due to less interference from chest and arm motions. Moreover, bicycle ergometers are cheaper, take up less space, have easy-to-control workload gradations, make less noise than a TM, and allow the patient to voluntarily discontinue the test at any time.

Disadvantage. The disadvantages of bicycle ergometry include myocardial VO_2 is 6 to 25% less than in TM exercise, greater cardiac stress (i.e., BP and RPP tend to be higher), some patients being unfamiliar with bicycling and not learning to use it (e.g., because of incoordination), and a greater tendency of the patient to discontinue the test earlier (i.e., submaximally) due to local fatigue of muscles recruited for the unfamiliar task of bicycling. During bicycle ergometry, the patient should not tightly grip the handlebars as the additional isometric loading of hand gripping can cause exaggerated cardiac response, thus leading to overestimation of the functional capacity by as much as 20%.

Test Protocols. The protocol for upright-bicycle ergometry CV-GXTT, like TM protocols, should bring the patient to "maximal" effort in 8 to 12 minutes (hence it entails careful assessment of the patient's cardiopulmonary status). The seat height of the bicycle ergometer is first adjusted so that there is only minimal (5°) knee flexion when the foot is at its lowest position on the pedal. The patient is then instructed to warm up for 2 to 3 minutes by free-wheeling (i.e., cycling with "no resistance") at a rate of 50 to 60 rpm. This is followed by an initial work load of 10 or 25 watts and subsequent progressive workload increases of 25 to 50 watts (150 to 300 kg-meter/min) every 2 to 3 minutes while the pedaling rate is maintained. Patients with severe deconditioning may use even smaller workload increments of 10 to 25 watts every 1 to 2 minutes. During the test, HR and BP are measured every 1 to 2 min, and an ECG tracing is taken at the end of each 2- or 3-minute stage. Unlike TM protocols, cycle ergometry has no horizontal component because the cycle is stationary. When the endpoint is reached (see Table 2.7-2), the resistance is reduced to zero and the patient cycles at the same rate for at least 3 minutes to cool down.

b. **Arm or upper-limb crank ergometer CV-GXTTs** can be used for patients who are unable to use their lower limbs because of neurological, orthopedic, or vascular impairment of lower limbs or for patients for whom arm excercise is necessary in their occupations or avocations. Peak oxygen uptake (or VO_2max) achieved with upper-limb ergometry is between 60 to 80% of that maximally achieved by the lower-limb exercise, depending on the strength of the arm and the shoulder muscles. Hence, UE-exercise capacity is a poor predictor of lower-limb exercise capacity and vice versa. The maximum cardiac output for upper-limb exercise is lower than for lower-limb exercise, but the attained peak or maximal HR is similar or slightly less in upper than lower-limb exercise. In upper-limb exercise, the RPP is also more elevated due mostly to the greater increase in the systolic BP (SBP) than the HR. The increased SBP has been attributed to increased peripheral vascular tone in the nonexercising vascular beds.

Arm crank ergometry testing can be performed while seated or standing. The standing position generally permits a greater use of trunk and postural muscle groups to achieve higher peak cardiopulmonary workload. After 2 to 3 minutes of ''no-load'' cranking for warm-up, the workload is initially set to 25 to 50 watts and increased in 2- or 3-minute stages by 10 to 25 watts. The typical peak values achieved by men 50 to 65 years old are approximately 100 watts (600 kg-m/min). Blood pressure may periodically be measured in one arm while the other arm cranks at submaximal intensities, or it may be measured immediately after cessation of a 2-minute stage. However, due to the rapid decline of BP immediately after termination of upright arm cranking exercise, the immediate postexercise BP values are most likely lower than the peak-exercise BP. Most patients are unable to tolerate a continuous protocol, hence needing an intermittent testing protocol (see below).

B. CV intermittent-load ETTs include rest periods (which vary from 30 sec to 2 min or longer) between a series of constant workloads, which are repeated at progressively higher intensities. Muscle strength can be restored during rest and greater total stress can be subsequently applied. The ECG and BP can also be recorded with less motion artifact during rest. This approach, however, takes a longer period of time to complete and is not practical for most routine testing in the clinical setting. They are used for arm-crank ergometry ETT (e.g., increments of 25 W for 2 min separated by 1 or 2 min of rest) to improve patient tolerance of the arm-exercise and to permit more frequent measurement of immediate postexercise BP. The intermittent method is also occasionally used for lower–limb exercise testing, in more severely impaired patients who can only perform a constant workload such as unloaded pedaling or walking at a slow pace.

C. CV single-load ETTs

1. Master's test (''2-step test'') is a crude method of determining physical fitness. It has declined in popularity and has been replaced by the CV-GXTT protocols described above in section I.A.

2. Bench-stepping test (or sitting-chair step-test) may be used as a form of CV single-load ETT in patients who are unable to do a formal CV-GXTT (e.g., elderly patients). The following protocol is by Smith and Gilligan (*Phys Sportsmed* 11:91-101, 1983). Patient sits with both feet flat on the floor in a straight-backed chair facing a step (e.g., a bench or a pile of books). The distance of the step to the patient is equal to the length of the patient's extended leg. At the count of one (a metronome set at 120 may be used), the arch of the right foot is brought up to touch the edge of the step; on the count of two, the same foot is returned to the floor. On the next count of three, the arch of the left foot touches the step edge and, on four, returns to the floor. This alternating foot process is continued for a 2- and a

5-minute duration, at a rate of 60 steps/min, using a 6-inch-high step (stage 1; O_2 cost is 2.3 METs), a 12-inch-high step (stage 2; O_2 cost is 2.9 METs), and an 18-inch-high step (stage 3; O_2 cost is 3.5 METs). Stage four (O_2 cost is 3.9 METs) is similar to stage three with the addition of the following arm exercises. The right arm is raised (at the same time the arch of the right foot touches the step) and then extended over the leg; as the right foot returns to the floor, the right arm is lowered so that the hand rests on the knee. This process is alternately repeated on the left and right side for 5 minutes. For each stage, the heart rate is recorded after 2 minutes to determine if the patient should proceed to the 5-minute test. The HR is again recorded after the 5-minute test, and if it is still below 75% of age-adjusted maximum HR (i.e., 220 − age), then the patient proceeds to the next stage.

II. **Pulmonary ETTs** are actually **integrated cardiopulmonary (CP) ETTs** because the pulmonary system is tightly linked to the cardiovascular system. They directly measure cardiac and pulmonary responses while indirectly assessing peripheral gas exchange. In the PM&R setting, they are primarily used to determine functional work capacity in patients with an established pulmonary diagnosis (e.g., for disability evaluation), to evaluate the need for supplemental oxygen during exercise, and to determine the appropriate intensity of prescribed exercise or activity. They may also help provide an objective assessment of complaints of limited exercise capacity and clarify the nature of any limiting factors (e.g., cardiac vs. pulmonary factors in patients in whom history, physical examination, and PFTs are equivocal). In general, CP-ETT are not used for diagnostic purposes because they are time consuming, expensive, and lack specificity (the few conditions in which they have high specificity include psychogenic dyspnea, exercise-induced asthma, deconditioning, myocardial ischemia, and peripheral vascular disease). Their absolute and relative contraindications as well as endpoints for exercise termination are similar to those for CV-ETT (see Tables 2.7-1 and 2.7-2).

A. **Cardiopulmonary graded-ETTs (CP-GXTTs)** use continuous incremental workload for 6 to 14 minutes. They can be done using stationary cycle ergometers or treadmills (see section I.A.1 and I.A.2 for description), allowing the subject to reach the maximal attainable work while measuring the exhaled gas (volume and O_2 and CO_2 concentrations), ventilatory parameters, blood gases, ECG, HR, and BP. Their purpose is to differentiate whether the impairment is due to cardiac disease or due to exercise-induced bronchospasm from pulmonary disease. They can also determine the reasons for exercise-related symptoms and can be used to document the patient's progress during rehabilitation by showing changes in symptom-limited oxygen consumption and other physiologic parameters. Protocols used for CP-GXTT in patients with pulmonary disease are shown in Table 2.7-7.

Measured parameters include the cardiovascular parameters (see section I.A) such as BP, HR, 12-lead telemetric ECG, and the workload provided by the treadmill or cycle ergometer. In addition, they also include the following pulmonary parameters:

• **Breathed gas concentrations of oxygen and carbon dioxide**, i.e., a breath-by-breath determination of the volumes of oxygen uptake (VO_2) and carbon dioxide output (VCO_2), as well as the actual peak oxygen uptake (peak VO_2) or maximum oxygen consumption (VO_2max). The VO_2, VCO_2, and peak VO_2 or VO_2max can be determined by using a headgear with a mouthpiece and a nose clip to collect the necessary gas samples, which are then quantified by a gas analyzer. Although the term *VO₂max* is usually used interchangeably with the term *peak VO₂* (i.e., peak O_2 uptake), they are not

Table 2.7-7. Graded exercise tolerance testing protocols for patients with pulmonary disease

MODE	PROTOCOL
I. Treadmill	
Massachusetts Respiratory Hospital	Set and maintain speed q 2 min to: 1.5 mph
	If FEV_1 is >1 L/s: set % grade q 2 min to 0, then increase by 4%
	If FEV_1 is <1 L/s: set % grade q 2 min to 0, then increase by 2%
Naughton	Set and maintain speed q 3 min to: 2.0 mph
	Set % grade q 3 min to 0, then increase by 3.5%
Balke and Ware	Set and maintain speed q 2 min to: 3.3 mph
	Set % grade q 2 min to 0, then increase by 3.5%
II. Cycle*	
Massachusetts Respiratory Hospital	Begin at 25 W; increase 10 W every 20 sec or 5 W every 20 sec when FEV_1 is <1 L/s
Jones	Begin with 17 W, increase 17 W every min
Berman and Sutton	Begin with 17 W, increase 17 W every min or 8 W every min when FEV_1 is <1 L/s
Jones and Campbell	Begin with 25 W, increase by 15 W every min

Adapted from Brannon FJ, Foley MW, Starr JA, et al: *Cardiopulmonary rehabilitation: Basic theory and application*, ed 2, Philadelphia, 1993, FA Davis, p. 269, with permission.
* Cycle speed is constant at 50 rpm.
mph = miles per hour; FEV_1 = forced expiratory volume at 1.0 second; L/s = liter per second; W = watt; 1 W = 6 kg-meter/min; 25 Watts = 150 kg-meter/min = 0.5 Kp-meter/min (kilopond-meter/min)

exactly the same. Strictly speaking, a true VO_2max can only be established if the patient keeps on exercising at a near maximal exercise level so that there is a VO_2 plateau. Because most PM&R patients are unable to maintain a maximal VO_2 plateau, the *peak VO_2* (which is the point of highest O_2 uptake during the exercise testing) is used instead of *VO_2max*. The VO_2max or peak VO_2, which are expressed in L/min or ml/min/kg, are dependent not only on the circulatory system but also on the number of muscles involved in the task being performed (i.e., the more muscles involved, the higher the possible VO_2max; for example, cross country skiing, which involves the arms and legs, permits the person to reach a higher peak VO_2 or VO_2max than arm cycling).

The predicted VO_2max is highly variable as it depends on several factors such as age, height, genetic body type, physical training, and familiarity with the testing protocol. In general, it is above 2.1 L/min for men and above 1.4 L/min for women. One way of computing for the predicted VO_2max value (ml/min) for sedentary middle-aged men is estimated by **(height in cm − age in yrs) × 21.** It has been reported that a normal person is capable of performing a task for up to 8 hours if the maximal work load of that task needs less than 40% of the worker's peak VO_2 or VO_2max. The actual direct measurement of VO_2max can produce anxiety and is objectionable to most patients (because of the uncomfortable headgear), thus resulting in less than the maximal test with inaccurate VO_2max measurement. Hence, instead of actual VO_2max measurement, the metabolic equivalent (i.e., METs; see description below and also in section I.A above) for the "maximum" workload is usually used to estimate the VO_2max.

- **Tidal volume (TV), ventilatory frequency (f), and maximum exercise ventilation (VE_{max})** can be determined by using a spirometer or pneumotachometer (see Chapter 2.6) before and after the CP-GXTT. Initially, as the exercise begins, there is increasing TV. As the work increases, the f also increases. Ventilation is likely to become a limiting factor in CP-GXTT if (a) the VE_{max} closely approaches within 10 to 15 L/min of the maximal voluntary ventilation (MVV) measured prior to exercise, (b) the exercise TV approaches to within 10% of the resting inspiratory capacity, or (c) the f is more than 50 per minute. If early during recovery there is prompt decrease in HR but no normal prompt decrease in ventilation, it is suggestive of a ventilatory limitation.

- **Blood gases** including arterial oxygen pressure **(PaO_2)**, arterial carbon dioxide pressure **($PaCO_2$)**, and oxygen saturation **(SaO_2)** can be determined by sampling the arterial blood gas (ABG) (see Chapter 2.6 section IV.A). The noninvasive pulse oximetry (see Chapter 2.6 section IV.B) may also be used to measure SaO_2. During heavy exercise, there is a rise in $PaCO_2$, which in turn stimulates ventilation and causes the $PaCO_2$ to decline, thus minimizing the respiratory acidosis. In patients who are limited in ventilatory ability (e.g., because of severe obstructive or, less commonly, restrictive pulmonary disease), a respiratory acidosis is sometimes seen. The PaO_2 should remain at about 90 mm Hg throughout the CP-GXTT.

  Calculated parameters
- **Rate-pressure product or double product,** i.e., RPP = HR × systolic BP (see discussion of RPP in section I.A), which is well-correlated with myocardial oxygen consumption, indicates aerobic conditioning (i.e., the higher the RPP, the poorer the aerobic conditioning).

- **Metabolic (MET) equivalent** is fully described in section I.A. Because one MET is equivalent to the resting VO_2 (i.e., VO_2rest = 3.5 ml of O_2 consumption per kg/min), a given MET value can be determined by dividing the measured peak VO_2 or VO_2max with the 3.5 (i.e., the resting VO_2). However, the actual measurement of VO_2max or peak VO_2 is impractical and can be erroneous due to anxiety and the discomfort caused by the headgear apparatus for VO_2 measurement. Hence, tables of MET equivalents are used instead. These MET equivalent tables (see Tables 4.2-2 and 4.2-3 in Chapter 4.2) were constructed from actual measurements of VO_2max in normal subjects during different activities or exercises. The limitations and disadvantages of using the MET equivalent tables for CP-GXTT interpretation and for exercise prescription are discussed in section I.A and in Chapter 4.2, section III.A.2.

- **Peak O_2 pulse** can be calculated either by dividing peak VO_2 or VO_2max with peak heart rate (i.e., ml O_2 per heart beat) or by multiplying the effective ventricular stroke volume with the difference between the arterial and mixed-venous oxygen contents. In general, the peak O_2 pulse at maximum exercise is greater than 12 ml oxygen per heartbeat in men and greater than 8 ml oxygen per heartbeat in women. During the CP-GXTT, the peak oxygen pulse normally increases in a curvilinear fashion from rest to exhaustion. A smaller than appropriate increase of the peak O_2 pulse indicates dysfunction in oxygen transport and an inefficient cardiopulmonary system. The peak O_2 pulse is reduced if the maximal stroke volume is decreased (e.g., valvular heart disease, coronary artery disease, cardiomyopathy, pulmonary vascular disease, or peripheral vascular disease), the arterial oxygen content is decreased (e.g., anemia, hypoxemia, or carboxyhemoglobinemia), or the mixed-venous oxygen content is increased (e.g., poor peripheral O_2 extraction or inability to increase exercise to higher levels because of the presence of other systemic diseases).

- **Anaerobic threshold (AT) and respiratory quotient (RQ).** During aerobic metabolism, as the workload increases there is a linear increase in ventilation, heart rate, oxygen consumption, and carbon dioxide production. However, during anaerobic metabolism (which is used to supplement energy production when O_2 demand surpasses its supply), this increase becomes nonlinear. The point at which this nonlinear response occurs is called the anaerobic threshold (AT) or lactic acid threshold (LAT). In the average young person, AT occurs at a VO_2 value that is approximately 45 to 60% of the predicted VO_2max. An AT that is less than 40% of the predicted (not the measured) peak VO_2 or VO_2max is abnormal and is indicative of circulatory dysfunction, regardless of age, gender, or body size.

  The AT can be measured directly by determining the lactate level; however, this is invasive and inconvenient. An indirect and convenient method of determining AT is by identifying the point when the RQ is above 1. The RQ is the ratio of the carbon dioxide produced to the oxygen consumed, i.e., VCO_2/VO_2 occurring at the cellular level of metabolism. The equivalent VCO_2/VO_2 at the lung level is called the respiratory exchange ratio or RER. The RQ and RER are usually used interchangeably. In general, carbohydrate produces a RQ of 1.0, protein 0.8, and dietary fat 0.7. During anaerobic metabolism, the excess lactic acid is buffered into carbon dioxide thus raising the RQ to above 1 and causing the blood pH to become acidic. When the breath-by-breath values of measured VCO_2 output versus VO_2 intake values are displayed graphically, the point at which the VCO_2 output surpasses the VO_2 intake can be identified. This intersection point signifies that the RQ is above 1 and the AT has been reached.

  The AT can be used to determine the intensity of an activity or exercise (i.e., activities requiring VO_2 above the AT are considered as heavy or intense, and activities requiring VO_2 below the AT are considered to be less intense). When exercise is done beyond the AT, fatigue (and cramps caused by lactic acid accumulation) usually occurs unless the person is trained to tolerate fatigue and pain. With physical training, both the AT and the peak VO_2 or VO_2max generally increase. Also, the AT/peak VO_2 ratio increases to as high as 0.85 in some highly trained endurance athletes.

- **Ventilatory equivalents (V_E)** denote the efficiency of ventilation related to metabolism. Normally, the resting V_E values for oxygen (i.e., V_EO_2) and for carbon dioxide (i.e., V_ECO_2) are 35 to 60. During exercise near AT level, the V_EO_2 decreases to 23 to 27, while the V_ECO_2 decreases to 28 to 30. If the V_EO_2 and V_ECO_2 do not decline appropriately, it is most likely due to a high dead space volume/tidal volume ratio (VD/TV, see below). When exercising at or above the AT, the resulting metabolic acidosis stimulates further ventilation, thus both V_EO_2 and V_ECO_2 become significantly elevated. Another cause for elevated V_E is unusually low $PaCO_2$ (e.g., in acute hyperventilation, chronic respiratory alkalosis, or chronic metabolic acidosis), thus ABG needs to be checked to rule this out.

- **Dead space volume/tidal volume (VD/TV)** is calculated from the measured mixed expired carbon dioxide, $PaCO_2$, TV, and the dead space of the breathing valve and mouthpiece or face mask. During exercise, as the TV increases and the airspaces are increasingly perfused with high carbon dioxide–laden blood, the VD/TV normally decreases. In normal, sedentary middle-aged men, the VD/TV falls to 0.30 or less at maximal exercise, while in younger men the decrease is even greater. If there is primary or secondary pulmonary vascular disease or severe maldistribution of ventilation to perfusion, the VD/TV does not decline appropriately but may be increased at rest and markedly increased with exercise.

Test interpretation. The use of CP-GXTT for exercise prescription is similar to that for CP-GXTT described above. For specifics on how to use it for prescribing aerobic exercise intensity, see Chapter 4.2, section III.A. The CP-GXTT can also be used to determine the need for supplemental oxygen during exercise (see Chapter 5.12, section IV.A.3 for parameters on the prescription of O_2 supplementation).

1. **Treadmill CP-GXTTs** provide a more accurate functional assessment of the patient with pulmonary disease than does a bicycle ergometer test. For a full discussion on the advantages and disadvantages of TM, refer to section I.A.1. Some of the commonly used TM protocols for CP-GXTT in pulmonary patients are shown in Table 2.7-7. These protocols are extremely low levels (i.e., low speed, low increment, and low MET levels). For less impaired patients in whom these protocols may be too slow, the modified TM protocols for cardiac patients may be used (see Table 2.7-6). In general, the Bruce protocol is rarely indicated in pulmonary patients due to its high workload. To convert the patient's "maximal" workload on the TM into METs, refer to Table 2.7-3.

2. **Bicycle ergometer CP-GXTTs** have the same indications, advantages, and disadvantages as those used for CV-GXTT (see section I.A.2). Some of the low-level bicycle protocols commonly used for CP-GXTT in pulmonary patients are shown in Table 2.7-7. To convert the patient's "maximal" workload on the bicycle ergometer into METs, refer to Table 2.7-4.

B. **Constant workload CP-ETTs** use a series of constant workloads, which can be repeated at progressively higher intensities with rest periods in between. They may take one or more days to complete. Patients using constant workloads can achieve a similar peak VO_2 or VO_2max for a given task as when using the more practical continuous incremental workload. Constant workload CP-ETTs may be used for evaluating the efficacy of oxygen breathing or drug therapy in relieving symptoms or for an accurate measurement of the AT (see AT description in section II.A above).

C. **Timed-walking test** is easy and inexpensive and can be used as an objective way of measuring exercise performance before and after a therapeutic intervention. The patient is asked to walk as far as possible in 12 minutes (may be modified to 6 or even 2 or 3 minutes for some pulmonary patients). The HR, BP, and walking time and distance are then measured. The results of the test, as described by Kenneth Cooper, have been shown to positively correlate with FVC and VO_2max as determined by CP-GXTT (i.e., incremental treadmill or bicycle ergometry test). Additional parameters that may be measured during the timed-walking test are oxygen saturation, ECG, and perceived exertion.

BIBLIOGRAPHY

American College of Sports Medicine: *Guidelines for exercise testing and prescription,* ed 4, Philadelphia, 1991, Lea & Febiger.

Brannon FJ, Foley MW, Starr JA, et al: *Cardiopulmonary rehabilitation: Basic theory and application*, ed 2, Philadelphia, 1993, FA Davis.

Ellestad MH: *Stress testing: Principles and practice*, ed 4, Philadelphia, 1996, FA Davis.

Fardy PS, Yanowitz FG: *Cardiac rehabilitation, adult fitness, and exercise testing*, ed 3, Baltimore, 1995, Williams & Wilkins.

Flores AM, Zohman LR: Rehabilitation of the cardiac patient. In DeLisa JA, Gans BM, editors: *Rehabilitation medicine: Principles and practice*, ed 2, Philadelphia, 1993, JB Lippincott, pp. 934-951.

Hansen JE, Wasserman K: Integrated cardiopulmonary exercise testing. In Demeter SL, Andersson GBJ, Smith GM, editors: *American Medical Association: Disability evaluation*, St. Louis, 1996, Mosby, pp. 318-337.

Myers JN, Froelicher VF: Exercise testing and prescription, *Phys Med Rehabil Clin North Am* 6(1):117-151, 1995.

Salazar-Schicchi J, Haas F, Reggiani JL: Exercise stress testing. In Haas F, Axen K, editors: *Pulmonary Therapy and Rehabilitation. Principles and Practice*, ed 2. Baltimore, 1991, Williams & Wilkins, pp. 121-131.

Stein J, editor: *Internal medicine*, ed 4, St. Louis, 1994, Mosby.

Subcommittee on Exercise Testing: Guidelines for exercise testing: A report of the American College of Cardiology/American Heart Association Task Force on Assessment of Cardiovascular Procedures. *J Am Coll Cardiol* 8:725-738, 1986.

Wasserman K, Hansen JE, Sue DY, et al: *Principles of exercise testing and interpretation*, ed 2, Philadelphia, 1994, Lea & Febiger.

CHAPTER 2.8

FUNCTIONAL ASSESSMENT INSTRUMENTS

Functional assessment instruments are standardized tests used to measure functional performance in self-care such as mobility, feeding, dressing, grooming, bathing, personal hygiene, toileting activities, communication, and social cognition. They can also be used to quantify functional outcome and to indicate the effectiveness of the rehabilitation program. The following are some of the more popular standardized functional assessment instruments.

I. **Functional independence measures (FIM)** (see Fig. 2.8-1) measures 18 items in six categories: self care, sphincter control, mobility, locomotion, communication, and social cognition. Each item is scored on a 7-point ordinal scale (1 = total assistance; 7 = complete independence) with total score ranging from 18 to 126. The score is not a direct observational measure but is based on information provided by the patient and the rehabilitation team. Its interrater reliability is 0.95. The FIM is widely used in the United States and other countries as a measure of disability or for program evaluation of initial rehabilitation programs. Using the Uniform Data System, assessment data from several hundred facilities have been collected. The strength of the FIM is that it measures social cognition and functional communication as well as mobility and activities of daily living (ADL), and it uses a seven-point scale, which is more sensitive compared to other scales. However, it has a "ceiling" and "floor" effect at the upper and lower ends of function.

II. **Barthel Index** measures 10 items: bowel control, bladder control, feeding, personal grooming and hygiene, dressing, bathing, toilet use, transfer, mobility, and stair negotiation. Items are scored according to a weighted numerical system with total scores ranging from 0 (totally dependent) to 20 (totally independent). By multiplying each item score by 5, an equivalent score of 0 to 100 may be obtained. Its interrater reliability is >0.95 and its test-retest reliability is 0.89. It is widely used in the United States to assess disability and rehabilitation outcome in patients with stroke or spinal cord injury (SCI). A maximum Barthel score does not necessary signify independence in all ADL because it does not measure higher level of function (i.e., ADL such as cooking, housekeeping, and socialization are not assessed).

III. **PULSES profile** measures the following: **P**hysical condition or basic health/illness status, **U**pper limb functions, **L**ower limb functions and mobility, **S**ensory components (sight and communication), **E**xcretory function (bowel and bladder control), **S**upport factors (psychosocial, emotional, family, social, financial support). Each section is graded from 1 (no abnormalities) to 4 (severe abnormalities limiting independence) with scores ranging from 0-24. Its scoring system and rating criteria has been modified in 1975. Its interrater reliability is >0.95 and its test-retest reliability is 0.87. It is currently used in detecting functional change before discharge among varying patient populations, especially in patients with stroke or SCI in whom substantial functional improvement is likely to occur. Its limitation is that it lacks subscore detail in discrete ADL variable.

IV. **Klein-Bell ADL scale** consists of 170 tasks in six categories: dressing, elimination,

UDSMR^SM FIM^SM Instrument

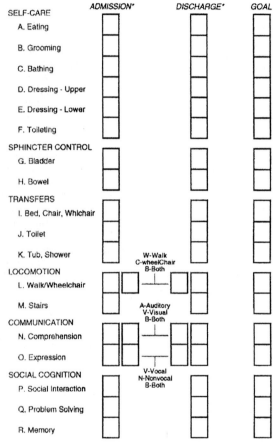

* Leave no blanks. Enter 1 if not testable due to risk.

FIM LEVELS

No Helper

7 Complete Independence (Timely, Safely)
6 Modified Independence (Device)

Helper - Modified Dependence

5 Supervision (Subject = 100%)
4 Minimal Assistance (Subject = 75% or more)
3 Moderate Assistance (Subject = 50% or more)

Helper - Complete Dependence

2 Maximal Assistance (Subject = 25% or more)
1 Total Assistance or not testable (Subject less than 25%)

mobility, bathing/hygiene, eating, and communication. Each task is scored as "achieved" (no physical or verbal assistance) or "failed" (assistance needed). Based on the "achieved" tasks, a percentage score is computed. A 100% level means, the patient is able to perform all self-care skills during the day with no attendant help. The Klein-Bell ADL scale can be used as predictor of independence in self-care, and it has an interrater reliability of 0.92. Although it is one of the most sensitive and carefully designed scales, it has not been extensively validated.

V. Katz index of independence in ADL evaluates the patient's functional independence in bathing, dressing, going to the toilet, transfers, continence, and feeding. Through observation, the rater determines which assistance is needed, that is, active personal assistance, directive assistance, or supervision. Using specific rating criteria, the patient's level of independence is ranked ordinally as A, B, C, D, E, F, G, or other. An A signifies independence in all six functions, while G signifies dependence in all rated functions. Other signifies dependence in at least two functions but not classifiable as C, D, E, or F. Its coefficient of scalability is 0.89. It is used to study results of treatment and prognosis in the elderly and chronically ill (e.g., recovery in stroke, the need for care among rheumatoid arthritis [RA] patients).

VI. Kenny self-care evaluation measures 17 items on the following six categories: bed mobility, transfers, locomotion, dressing, personal hygiene, and feeding. The scoring ranges from 0 (completely dependent) to 4 (independent), the highest score being 24, which indicates maximum independence on the ADL skills assessed. Although it is sensitive to changes in overall function of the patient and can be used to document rehabilitation progress, it is not as widely used as the other scales. No formal reliability coefficients have been reported.

BIBLIOGRAPHY

Christiansen CH, Schwartz RK, Barnes KJ: Self care: Evaluation and management. In DeLisa JA, Gans BM, editors: *Rehabilitation medicine: Principles and practice*, ed 2, Philadelphia, 1993, JB Lippincott, pp. 178-200.

Granger CV, Hamilton BB, Sherwin FS: *Guide for use of the uniform data set for medical rehabilitation*, Buffalo, 1986, Uniform Data System for Medical Rehabilitation.

Guccione AA, Functional assessment. In O'Sullivan SB, Schmitz TJ, editors: *Physical rehabilitation: Assessment and treatment*, Philadelphia, 1994, FA Davis, pp. 193-207.

Katz S, Ford AB, Moskowitz RW: Studies of illness in the aged. The index of ADL: A standardized measure of biological and psychosocial function, *JAMA* 185:914-919, 1963.

◀──

Figure 2.8-1
The adult Functional Independence Measure (FIM) rating form (Reprinted with permission of the Uniform Data System for Medical Rehabilitation, a division of UB Foundation Activities, Inc. (UDS$_{MR}$^{SM}). Copyright 1996. *Guide for the Uniform Data Set for Medical Rehabilitation [including the FIM^{SM} instrument], version 5.0.*, Buffalo, NY 14214: State University of New York at Buffalo; 1996)

Klein RM, Bell B: Self-care skills: Behavioral measurement with Klein-Bell ADL scale, *Arch Phys Med Rehabil* 63:335-338, 1982.

Mahoney FI, Barthel DW: Functional evaluation: The Barthel index, *Maryland State Med J* 14(2):61-65, 1965.

Moskowitz E, McCann CB: Classification of disability in the chronically ill and aging, *J Chronic Dis* 5:342-346, 1957.

Schoening HA, Anderegg L, Bergstrom D, et al: Numerical scoring of self-care status of patients, *Arch Phys Med Rehabil* 46:689-697, 1965.

CHAPTER 2.9

PSYCHOLOGIC TESTS

This chapter gives an overview of the common psychologic tests used in PM&R. They are typically administered by a psychologist or a neuropsychologist. Tests used specifically for determining psychological aspects of pain are discussed in Chapter 5.10, section IV.

I. **Personality tests** provide information about an individual's emotional stability, motivation, interpersonal relations, interests, and attitudes. They usually involve completion of a self-administered questionnaire.

   A. **Minnesota Multiphasic Personality Inventory (MMPI)** is the most widely used and extensively researched objective test of personality. In PM&R it is commonly used to diagnose the presence of conversion disorders in chronic pain patients. Specific scales on the test have been reported to correlate with chronic pain treatment outcome, with particular emphasis on scales 1 (hypochondriasis), 2 (depression), and 3 (hysteria). Chronic pain patients may also have elevated scale 6 (paranoia) and 8 (schizophrenia) because of sensory disturbances, confusion because of medications, or bizarre interpretation of their symptoms. There is also extensive MMPI data on specific disability groups such as spinal cord injury and multiple sclerosis.

   The MMPI contains 556 true-false questions describing one's thoughts, feelings, ideas, attitudes, behaviors, physical and emotional symptoms, and life experiences. Items are grouped into 10 clinical scales on the basis of their ability to distinguish between a criterion group having certain defined characteristics or displaying certain distinctive behaviors and the general population. These clinical scales are interpreted with the help of four validity scales that are effective in identifying malingering attempts and provide a sensitive indicator of unconscious or other subtle distortions of responses. The MMPI provides information on the client's response style, such as literacy, cooperation, tendency toward malingering, comprehension, and use of denial or defensiveness. A score of 70 or greater (98th percentile on general population norms) is traditionally considered suggestive of a pathologic level of the trait in question.

   The MMPI requires a sixth-grade reading level and is appropriate for age 15 and above. It needs 1.5 to 2 hours to complete. A variety of factors such as race, socioeconomic status, unique family circumstances, and ethnic background may distort its profile. New norms include larger samples subdivided by gender and age and exclude individuals with a history of major medical or psychiatric illness. They have been shown to validate the original norms. The new **MMPI-2** provides larger, nationally represented norms and updated item content; however, it requires an eighth-grade reading level (compared to sixth grade for the original MMPI) and is to be used only with adults 18 years of age or older.

   B. **Millon Clinical Multiaxial Inventory II (MCMI-II)** is intended for screening those suspected of significant personality disorders and is inappropriate for the general patient population. It consist of 175 true-false items written at an eighth-grade reading level and is appropriate for persons 17 years old or older.

It requires 30 minutes to complete. The questions are divided into categories that reflect enduring personality characteristics (i.e., Axis II), clinical syndromes (Axis I), and levels of pathologic severity. The MCMI-II is the only clinically oriented personality inventory reflective of Diagnostic and Statistical Manual of Mental Disorders (DSM-III) diagnostic categories.

C. **Strong Interest Inventory (SII)** is the most recent version of the **Strong Vocational Interest Blank (SVIB)**, which is traditionally used to measure vocational interests but can also be used as a valid nonpathology-oriented measure of personality. It asks the respondent to indicate liking, indifference, or dislike for occupations, school subjects, activities, amusements, and types of people. Two subsections ask for preferences between two occupational activities and the self-rated possession of 13 personal characteristics. The test contains 325 items, requires 45 to 50 minutes to complete, and is written at an eighth-grade reading level.

II. **Intellectual ability tests** are used to measure general intellectual ability to help physiatrist set appropriate expectations about the rate and complexity of learning that can be legitimately expected from the patient. They can also be used to determine the presence of organic brain dysfunction and provide guidance for postdischarge vocational and educational planning.

A. **Stanford-Binet Intelligence Test** comprises 142 verbal and nonverbal items assessing language, memory, conceptual thinking, reasoning, numerical reasoning, visual motor, and social reasoning for individuals 2 years old and older. Responses are scored according to established procedures to yield mental age and inteligence quotient (IQ). This is then reported in percentile. The untimed test takes 45 to 90 minutes to complete.

B. **Wechsler Adult Intelligence Scale, revised (WAIS-R)** comprises six subtests for verbal IQ and five subtests for performance IQ for individuals 16 years old and older. Raw scores are converted into scale scores and reported in percentile. The untimed test lasts about 75 minutes. The WAIS-R is commonly used in rehabilitation (e.g., as part of neuropsychological evaluation in patients with traumatic brain injury).

III. **Academic achievement tests** provide insight into the patient's current level of academic achievement and are used to determine patient's educational and vocational needs, especially after discharge from the hospital. Those with low reading and math achievement levels may need special education.

A. **Wide-range Achievement Test, revised (WRAT-R)** provides two levels of difficulty for each of three types of academic achievement: reading, spelling, and arithmetic. Level 2, used with subjects 12 years old and older, is most relevant to adult rehabilitation patients. The test can be completed in 30 minutes, and the results are presented in the form of standard scores, percentiles, and grade equivalents. Although it has adequate reliability and norms, the correct pronunciation of individual words represents a limited index of reading comprehension.

B. **Woodcock-Johnson Psycho-educational Battery-revised (WJ-R)** contains 21 subtests for cognitive ability and 14 subtests for academic achievement. The academic achievement subtests are grouped into reading, arithmetics, written language, knowledge, and skills. Each subtest requires 20 minutes to complete.

IV. **Neuropsychologic battery tests** are standardized scales designed to test relatively pure cognitive skills and, thus, allow assessment of the presence and site of organic neurologic disease. It is commonly requested in the assessment of mental status after brain injury (e.g., traumatic brain injury [TBI], stroke); early diagnosis, assessment of severity, follow-up observation, and counseling in patients with suspected dementia; differentiation of the relative part played by functional and by organic components in disease states; detection and evaluation of cognitive deficits in cases of learning disability, mental retardation, etc.; and counseling of patients and their families about management of acquired cognitive deficits.

    A. Halstead-Reitan Neuropsychological Battery (HRNB) consists of five tests of seven variables selected for their abilities to distinguish frontal lobe dysfunction. The result is presented as the Halstead impairment index, a summary of values computed by dividing the number of test scores in the impaired range by seven. It should be placed in the context of other test data analyzed by inferential methods including level of performance, pattern of performance, and specific behavioral deficits or pathognomonic signs, and by comparison of performance of the right and left sides of the body. Although HRNB can diagnose the presence and type of brain dysfunction, it does not consistently localize lesions and discriminate psychiatric from organically impaired patients.

    B. Luria-Nebraska Neuropsychological Battery (LNNB) has 269 items divided into 14 clinical scales. Performance on each item is scored from 0 (no impairment) to 2 (severe impairment). Total administration time is a maximum of 2.5 hours. The LNNB systematically assesses qualitative aspects of the patient's behavior, especially integrated motor performance. Criticisms involve issues of diagnostic unreliability, confounding of scale content, insufficient scale length, and difficulty in examining gradations of impairment.

V. Aptitude tests, vocational interest tests, and achievement or skill tests measure global skills or interests in an effort to clarify an individual's vocational potential. They are generally used in the rehabilitation of work-related musculoskeletal problems. (Examples are listed in Chapter 5.11, section V.D.2.c.)

VI. Value or attitude tests are used by counselors as a focus for discussion of personal matters and to assist their clients in gaining better self-understanding. Although they enhance communication in counseling and facilitate progress in vocational planning, the information they yield relates more to personality and lifestyle than to vocational choices or to questions of vocational success.

VII. Mood assessment includes tests for depression that assess both psychologic and physical symptoms.

    A. The Beck Depression Inventory (BDI) consists of 21 items with a cumulative scoring system based on questions common in depression, such as sleep disturbance, weight change, fatigue factors, sexual dysfunction, and cognitive components of depressive illness. Patient selects one of four or five statements ranked in order of severity for each item. Scores range from 0 to 63 with high scores indicating greater depression. It requires only 5 minutes to complete. The BDI is commonly used throughout a treatment program for the chronic pain patient as a measure of improvement. It has good validity and reliability.

    B. Zung Self-rating Depression Scale is a 20-item, self-report measure yielding a numerical estimate of depression severity. Patients rank each item on a 4-point scale indicating frequency of occurrence of symptom. The higher the score, the more severe is the depression. It lacks data on retest reliability and on validity with nonpsychiatric patients.

BIBLIOGRAPHY

Aronoff GM, editor: *Evaluation and treatment of chronic pain,* Baltimore, 1992, Williams & Wilkins.

Beck AT: *Beck Depression Inventory: Manual,* San Antonio, 1987, Psychological Corporation.

Butcher JN, Dahlstrom WG, Graham JR, et al: *MMPI-2: Manual for administration and scoring,* Minneapolis, 1989, University of Minnesota Press.

Dahlstrom WG, Welsh GS, Dahlstrom WG, editors.: *An MMPI handbook, vol. I: Clinical interpretation,* revised ed, Minneapolis, 1972, University of Minnesota Press.

Golden CJ, Hammeke TA, Purisch AD: *The Luria-Nebraska Battery manual,* Los Angeles, 1980, Western Psychological Services.

Hansen JC, Campbell DP: *Manual for the Strong Interest Inventory,* ed 4, Palo Alto, CA, 1985, Consulting Psychologists Press.

Jastak S, Wilkinson GS: *Wide-Range Achievement Test diagnostic and technical manual,* Wilmington, DE, 1984, Jastak Associates.

Millon T: *Millon Clinical Multiaxial Inventory II manual.* Minneapolis, 1987, National Computer System.

Reitan RM, Wolfson D: *The Halstead-Reitan Neuropsychological Test Battery: Theory and clinical interpretation.* Tucson, 1985, Neuropsychological Press.

Rohe DE: Psychological aspects of rehabilitation. In DeLisa JA, Gans BM, editors: *Rehabilitation medicine: Principles and practice,* ed 2, Philadelphia, 1993, JB Lippincott, pp. 131-150.

Turner JA, Romano JM: Psychologic and psychosocial evaluation. In Bonica JJ, editor: *The management of pain,* ed 2, Philadelphia, 1990, Lea & Febiger, pp. 595-609.

Wechsler D: *The Wechsler Adult Intelligence Test: Revised manual,* New York, 1983, Psychological Corporation.

Woodcock RW, Mather N: *Woodcock-Johnson Tests of Achievement,* Allen, TX, 1989, DLM Teaching Resources.

Zung WWK: A self-rating depression scale. *Arch Gen Psychiatry* 12:63-77, 1965.

PART THREE

PM&R Differential Diagnoses

CHAPTER 3.1

DIFFERENTIAL DIAGNOSES OF PAIN

As with other fields of medicine, the majority of complaints in PM&R are pain related. This chapter deals with the differential diagnoses of acute and chronic pain problems commonly encountered by the physiatrist in both in- and out-patient settings. These differential diagnoses are to be used as a guide in the diagnostic and therapeutic process of pain problems. Other details on acute and chronic pain (i.e., their neurophysiology, psychosocial factors, assessment, and management) are discussed in Chapter 5.10.

Pain problems may be related to either the neuromusculoskeletal systems or the nonneuromusculoskeletal systems. In making the differential diagnosis of pain, general sources of pain must be determined based on the patient's pain description. *Cutaneous pain* from skin and subcutaneous tissues is usually well localized. *Deep somatic pain* from bone, nerve, muscle, tendon, ligaments, periosteum, arteries, and joints is poorly localized and may be referred to the body surface (as cutaneous pain). *Visceral pain* from body organs in the trunk or abdomen usually corresponds to the dermatomes from which the affected organs receive their innervation. Due to multisegmental innervation, visceral pain is not well localized and is usually referred to the back (generally from organs of the abdomen and pelvis) or shoulder (generally from intrathoracic organs and from the gall bladder). *Referred pain* (either from cutaneous, deep somatic, or visceral structures) is usually well localized but occurs in remote areas supplied by the same (shared) central afferent neurosegment supplying the affected organ. The usual musculoskeletal sites of referred pain are the shoulder, scapula, chest, thoracic spine, lumbar spine, groin, sacroiliac joint, and hip.

I. **Neuromusculoskeletal pain problems.** *Joint pain due to nonsystemic joint dysfunction* is sudden, sharp, occurring after some unguarded joint movement, and is associated with warmth or swelling. It is usually limited to one joint, aggravated by movement, and is reduced by rest. *Joint pain of systemic joint disease* can be deep, aching, throbbing and may be reduced by pressure, or it can be sharp or dull or either constant or occurring in waves. Joint pain of systemic joint disease generally occurs with systemic signs and symptoms (e.g., skin rash, jaundice, fatigue, low-grade fever, and weight loss). *Pain due to musculoskeletal neoplasm* is usually constant, not relieved by changing positions or rest, and awakens the patient at night.

Muscular (or soft tissue) pain is induced by movement of musculoskeletal parts (bones, joints, bursae, tendons) or by mechanical forces (pressure or stretch) and is usually relieved by rest. Muscular pain may occur from accumulation of metabolites (e.g., from anaerobic exercise) or from ischemia (e.g., intermittent claudication). *Fibromyalgia pain*, usually seen in females, is insidious, diffuse, generalized, and occurs symmetrically in muscular and bony areas. *Myofascial pain*, occurs with equal frequency in both sexes, is associated with acute muscle strain or chronic muscle overuse, is limited to muscles, and occurs asymmetrically in isolated or regional muscles. Both fibromyalgia and myofascial pain are associated with stress, poor sleep pattern, fatigue, depression, and negative laboratory and neurologic results.

Radicular pain is felt in a dermatome and myotome and is caused by the direct irritation or involvement of the root of a spinal nerve. If nerve root irritation is caused by compression, the pain may be relieved by decompression, either nonsurgically (e.g., sitting and bending forward may relieve the pain of spinal stenosis) or surgically. If the pain does not occur in a radicular pattern that conforms to a dermatome or myotome, then other diagnoses should be considered, such as diabetic neuropathy, toxic neuropathy, and psychiatric disorders (e.g., hysterical or conversion reactions). Patients with nonanatomic patterns of radicular pain (e.g., glove and stocking pattern or pain in entire leg) in the absence of any objective findings should be considered for further psychological assessment to rule out nonorganic causes especially in the presence of inappropriate or exaggerated illness behaviors.

Nonorganic neuromusculoskeletal pain, which is usually seen in patients with chronic pain includes psychosomatic musculoskeletal pain (e.g., tension syndrome or fibrositis), psychogenic musculoskeletal pain, psychogenic modification of organic musculoskeletal pain, and situational spinal pain (e.g., litigation reaction and exaggeration reaction). The usual symptoms of nonorganic pain are multifocal pain, nonmechanical pain (present at rest), involvement of entire limb, limb "gives way" (i.e., complaints of knee buckling, which patient is able to catch at the last minute), poor response to treatment (e.g., no response to any treatment, "allergic" to treatment, and refusal of treatment), multiple crises, multiple hospital admissions or consultations, and multiple doctors. Signs of nonorganic pain (see Chapter 5.11, section V.B.3.) include superficial tenderness (over skin), nonanatomic pain, positive simulated movement tests, positive distraction tests, weakness or numbness of the entire arm or leg, and an "award-winning" performance.

The following differential diagnoses of neuromusculoskeletal pain problems are classified by syndromes and inferred pathophysiology, by specific body region, and by pattern and distribution of musculoskeletal pain.

A. **Differential diagnosis of pain classified by syndromes and inferred pathophysiology** (based on the classification by Portenoy [see bibliography]; excluding headache and facial pain which are classified under systemic pain problems).

1. **Neuropathic pain** is any acute or chronic pain syndrome in which the sustaining mechanism for the pain is inferred to involve aberrant somatosensory processing in the peripheral or central nervous system (CNS). The following classification is based on inferred predominant pathophysiology rather than on site of the inciting lesion or on the basis of diagnosis. It classifies whether neuropathic pain is primarily sustained by processes in the CNS or by processes in the peripheral nervous system.

a. **Predominating "central" pain generator**

1) **Deafferentation pain (anesthesia dolorosa)** is a descriptive term for pain due to injury of the central or peripheral nervous system. The term does not refer to any specific set of known mechanisms, although the pain is inferred to be due predominantly to a sustaining central mechanism that is independent of activity in the sympathetic nervous system. There is "central sensitization," which is a denervation hypersensitivity of neurons and ectopic foci of spontaneous neuronal activity that develops in the dorsal horn of the spinal cord, thalamus, and perhaps cerebral cortex following an injury to afferent pathways. "Central desensitization" may involve changes in the central neurons that may be structural (e.g., transynaptic and transganglionic degeneration or collateral sprouting) or functional (e.g., lowered threshold

for activation, exaggerated activation, ectopic discharges, enlarging receptive fields, and loss of normal inhibition).

a) Phantom pain. Phantom limb pain, phantom pain following amputations of nonlimb structures (e.g., breast, tooth), and phantom body pain (i.e., pain in regions of the body that are totally denervated but not amputated, such as that which occurs after spinal cord transection or peripheral nerve injury; instead of using the confusing term *phantom body pain,* it is better to call it *central pain* [see below] or nonspecifically as *deafferentation pain*).

b) Avulsion of plexus. Brachial plexus avulsion or lumbosacral plexus avulsion.

c) Postherpetic neuralgia

d) Central pain syndrome includes deafferentation pain syndromes that can occur following injury to the CNS. Some have been named by the location of the lesion (e.g., thalamic pain) or by the inciting injury (e.g., poststroke pain). Most however, do not conform to a named syndrome (e.g., pain associated with syringobulbia), hence it is better to use the term *central pain syndrome.*

   (1) *Spinal cord lesions.* Trauma, focal demyelination, infection, vascular lesions, neoplasms, syringomyelia.

   (2) *Brainstem lesions.* Vascular lesions, trauma, infection, neoplasms, syrinx, focal demyelination.

   (3) *Cerebral lesions.* Vascular lesions, trauma (including surgical), neoplasms, and lesions associated with seizures.

e) Others. Reflex sympathetic dystrophy (RSD)/causalgia (described below) and miscellaneous labels for deafferentation pain (e.g., postsurgical pain syndrome and postthoracotomy pain), which are merely descriptive and do not imply pathophysiology.

2) Sympathetically maintained pain (SMP) (Roberts, 1986; see bibliography) is any pain that is sustained, at least in part, by sympathetic efferent activity. It is usually caused by a partial peripheral nerve lesion (unlike reflex sympathetic dystrophy [RSD] which can be caused by any type of lesion). SMP is hypothesized to be caused by a vicious cycle of nerve injury which results in sensitization (i.e., lowering of pain threshold) of central projection neurons (e.g., wide-dynamic-range neurons in the spinal cord) leading to their enhanced response to low-threshold mechanoreceptors and an increase in adrenergic receptors in the periphery, which may then be activated further by norepinephrine release from sympathetic fibers.

SMP occurs less commonly than RSD. The cardinal symptoms of SMP are spontaneous pain (mostly burning; predominantly superficial; no orthostatic component, i.e., intensity is not dependent on the position of the limb), mechanical allodynia (i.e., pain produced by a normally non-painful stimulus such as light touch, wind, and mild temperature changes), and local hyperalgesia (to cold stimulus). Other symptoms of SMP are autonomic dysregulation (e.g., edema, vasomotor disturbances), involuntary motor response, and trophic changes. The sensory, motor, and autonomic symptoms of SMP are mostly localized to the territory of the affected peripheral or spinal nerve (unlike RSD symptoms which occur independent from the site of the preceding lesion). SMP can usually be alleviated by sympathetic blockade. Unequivocal (and at least temporary) relief of spontaneous and evoked pain after sympathetic blockade confirms the presence of SMP. Examples of neuropathic pain that may have SMP components include RSD/causalgia (see section I.A.1.c), phantom pain, avulsion of nerve plexus, and postherpetic neuralgia.

b. Predominating "peripheral" pain generator include "nerve sheath pain," i.e., activation of "normal" nociceptors (e.g., sensitization of C and A-delta nociceptors following injury, "backfiring" of C-fiber with release of pain mediators, unmodulated pain input because of large-fiber loss, and activation of nociceptive nervi nervorum), and dysesthetic pain, i.e., aberrant activity from injured nerves (e.g., neuroma formation from severed nerve, focal demyelination, or formation of nociceptor ephapses or abnormal connections).

1) Painful polyneuropathies.

a) *Metabolic disorders.* Diabetic neuropathy, neuropathy associated with insulinoma, nutritional deficiency (e.g., alcohol-nutritional neuropathy, thiamine deficiency, niacin deficiency, pyridoxine deficiency, and Strachan's syndrome or Jamaican neuropathy, which may be associated with beriberi or pellagra), hypothyroid neuropathy, uremic neuropathy, amyloid neuropathy, and neuropathy associated with Fabry's disease.

b) *Drugs or toxins.* Isoniazid, hydralazine, nitrofurantoin, metronidazole, phenytoin, disulfiram, gold, vincristine, cisplatin, alcohol, arsenic, cyanide, lead, and thallium.

c) *Neoplasm.* Subacute sensory neuropathy (a subtype of paraneoplastic neuropathy most commonly associated with small cell carcinoma and other carcinomas and lymphomas), nonspecific paraneoplastic sensorimotor neuropathy associated with carcinoma, and sensorimotor neuropathy associated with dysproteinemia (e.g., multiple myeloma, Waldenstrom's macroglobulinemia, cryoglobulinemia, solitary plasmacytoma, and osteosclerotic plasmacytoma).

d) *Connective tissue diseases.* Polyarteritis nodosa, rheumatoid arthritis, systemic lupus erythematosus, and Churg-Strauss disease.

e) *Other causes.* Hereditary neuropathy (e.g., hereditary sensory neuropathy type I), painful polyneuropathy associated with Guillain-Barre syndrome, acute intermittent porphyria, sarcoidosis, AIDS

2) Painful mononeuropathies refer to a diverse group of pain syndromes, all of which are inferred to be associated with a known peripheral nerve injury, and is experienced, at least partly, in the territory of the affected nerve. The pain may follow the injury immediately and then persist, or it may occur days, weeks, months, or rarely, years after nerve injury. The injury may be due to:

a) *Nerve inflammation.* Acute herpetic neuropathy, acute brachial plexus neuropathy (brachial plexitis), lumbosacral plexus neuropathy, and sensory perineuritis.

b) *Nerve trauma* from transection (e.g., surgical), stretch, inflammation, or compression of the nerve. The most common types are those caused by neuroma (e.g., residual limb pain) or compression (e.g., low back pain due to spinal nerve compression by herniated nucleus pulposus and nerve entrapment such as carpal tunnel syndrome).

c) ***Nerve vascular lesion.*** Diabetic mononeuropathy (femoral neuropathy, diabetic amyotrophy, lumbar radiculoplexopathy), cranial neuropathy (e.g., oculomotor neuropathy), thoracoabdominal neuropathies, mononeuritis or mononeuritis multiplex due to vasculitis (e.g., polyarteritis nodosa, rheumatoid arthritis [RA], Sjogren's syndrome, and Churg-Strauss syndrome).

d) ***Nerve neoplasm*** from benign tumors (neurofibroma) or malignant tumors.

e) ***Lancinating neuralgia*** is related to nerve injury and is characterized by brief paroxysmal pain (similar to trigeminal neuralgia).

   (1) ***Cranial neuralgias.*** Trigeminal neuralgia (the most common), glossopharyngeal neuralgia, occipital neuralgia, geniculate (nervus intermedius) neuralgia, supraorbital neuralgia, superior (or vagal) neuralgia. See also headache classification in I.A.4 and I.B.1.

   (2) ***Neuralgia of other sites.*** Intercostal neuralgia, ilioinguinal neuralgia, genitofemoral neuralgia.

c. **Reflex sympathetic dystrophy (RSD)/causalgia** has been ascribed to both central and peripheral processes. Peripheral processes include activity in nociceptive visceral afferents, which travel with sympathetic efferent fibers; processes unrelated to sympathetic nervous system that increase activity in somatic nociceptors (e.g., sensitization following injury, C-fiber "backfiring" with release of pain mediators, and ectopic electrical activity from neuroma or areas of focal demyelination); and processes involving sympathetic-somatic link (e.g., sympathetic hyperactivity that changes peripheral tissues to activate nociceptors in a "vicious cycle;" increased sensitivity of damaged nociceptors to catecholamines released by sympathetic nerves; nociceptor sensitization by prostaglandins released by sympathetic nerve; or formation of sympathetic nociceptor ephapses or abnormal connections). However, recent evidence favors central mechanism as the fundamental process; the most compelling evidence being that the complete isolation of the painful part from the CNS, for example, by neurectomy or rhizotomy, did not reliably eradicate the pain. Other evidence of central mechanism of RSD include the occurrence of classic RSD following damage to the CNS or viscera.

Reflex sympathetic dystrophy/causalgia is known by many other names such as shoulder-hand syndrome, posttraumatic syndrome, symphathalgia, and Sudeck's atrophy. The International Association for the Study of Pain (IASP) proposed the termed *complex regional pain syndrome*. According to the IASP consensus (Janig et al., 1991; see bibliography), RSD is a "complex disorder or group of disorders that may develop as a consequence of trauma affecting the limbs, with or without an obvious nerve lesion. RSD may also develop after visceral diseases, and central nervous system lesions, or, rarely, without an obvious antecedent event. It consists of pain and related sensory abnormalities, abnormal blood flow and sweating, abnormalities in the motor system and changes in structure of both superficial and deep tissues ('trophic' changes). It is not necessary that all components are present. It is agreed that the name 'reflex sympathetic dystrophy' is used in a descriptive sense and does not imply specific underlying mechanisms." Causalgia typically refers to the same syndrome (as RSD) produced by peripheral nerve injury.

The underlying central mechanism of RSD/causalgia can be either sympathetically maintained or caused by deafferentation. Reflex sympathetic dystrophy/causalgia is distinguished from SMP (see section I.A.1.a.2) in that RSD is common, develops in the distal region of the affected limb irrespective of the type and the site of the preceding lesion (e.g., minor trauma, partial nerve lesion, bone fracture, and other lesions such as shoulder trauma, myocardial infarction or even a contralateral cerebrovascular lesion), is usually distally generalized (e.g., glove-like distribution), has common (but not obligatory) spontaneous pain (which has variable character, mostly deep and diffuse, with orthostatic component, i.e., pain is alleviated by elevating the limb and aggravated by lowering it), and has less common incidence of mechanical allodynia than in SMP. The subtype of RSD/causalgia with SMP-features responds favorably to sympathetic blockade.

In general, the symptoms of RSD/causalgia can be classified into: (a) sensory symptoms, that is, deep spontaneous pain, hypo- or hyperalgesia, hypo- or hyperesthesia, movement-related pain, diffuse mechanical allodynia (seen in late cases), and hyperpathia (i.e., pain produced by painful stimuli that appears with a delay, outlasts the stimulus and spreads beyond the site of the stimulus); (b) autonomic symptoms, that is, distally generalized swelling, warm or cold affected limb, marbled, reddish, or cyanotic skin, and hypo- or hyperhydrosis; and (c) motor symptoms, that is, weakness, tremor (postural- or action-related), difficulty in initiating movement, spasm, dystonia, and increased reflexes and tone.

In chronic cases of RSD/causalgia, there is trophic changes (e.g., disturbed nail growth, increased hair growth, palmar or plantar fibrosis, thin glossy skin, and hyperkeratosis) and changes in bone (e.g., diffuse distal osteoporosis). The staging of untreated RSD/causalgia into acute, dystrophic, and atrophic stages do not always conform to the clinical course, and is, thus, not very useful. It is probably more practical to grade the symptoms of RSD/causalgia according to its intensity (i.e., mild, moderate, or severe).

The diagnostic criteria of RSD has been categorized as follows (Kozin et al., 1986; see bibliography): (a) definite RSD, indicated by pain in association with vasomotor instability, edema, and dystrophic skin and nail changes; (b) probable RSD, indicated by pain, vasomotor instability, and edema; (c) possible RSD, indicated by pain, and vasomotor instability or edema; and (d) doubtful RSD, indicated by pain alone. Although this simple diagnostic classification may be helpful in the clinics, empirical evidence is lacking. The treatment of RSD/causalgia is discussed in Chapter 5.10, section VI, and summarized in Table 5.10-2.

2. Musculoskeletal pain

    a. *Inflammatory arthropathies.* Rheumatoid arthritis, seronegative spondyloarthropathies (e.g., ankylosing spondylitis, reactive arthritis, psoriatic arthritis, gut-associated arthritis), infections (e.g., bacterial, postviral).

    b. *Degenerative arthropathies.* Osteoarthritis, aseptic necrosis, neuropathic (''Charcot'') joints.

    c. *Crystal-associated arthropathies.* Gout, calcium pyrophosphate deposition disease (CPDD) or pseudogout.

    d. *Soft tissue rheumatic problems.* Enthesopathies, injury, diffuse (fibromyalgia) and regional (myofascial pain) syndromes (either of which may be superimposed on other pain syndrome).

    e. ***Systemic connective tissue diseases.*** Systemic lupus erythematosus (SLE), vasculitides, systemic sclerosis.

    f. ***Metabolic bone disease.*** Osteoporosis, osteonecrosis, osteomalacia, Paget's disease.

3. Low back pain (based on the classification by Kanner [see bibliography]).

    a. Acute low back pain (see also section I.B.3.b)

        1) ***Acute pain originating in the bony elements.*** Vertebral metastases, osteoporosis, vertebral osteomyelitis, traumatic fractures.

        2) ***Acute pain originating in the muscles, aponeuroses, and nerves.*** Low back strain, locked back syndrome (i.e., slippage of an articular facet with encroachment on the pain-sensitive joint capsule), pain originating in neural structures, radicular pain without spinal pathology, herniated lumbar intervertebral disks.

    b. Chronic low back pain

        1) ***Somatic nociceptive pain.*** Degenerative spine or disk disease, facet disease, spondylolisthesis, fibromyalgia/myofascial pain syndrome.

        2) ***Visceral nociceptive pain.*** Referred from pelvic organ, the retroperitoneal space, the gallbladder, and the pancreas.

        3) ***Neuropathic pain.*** Lateral recess syndrome, spinal stenosis, lumbar arachnoiditis, neoplasm (e.g., neoplasm of the cauda equina, filum terminale, or lumbar dura).

        4) ***Psychogenic pain,*** which may be associated with malingering, "hysterical features," delusional pain, depression, secondary gain (e.g., monetary compensation), and somatization.

    c. Failed low back syndrome is broadly defined as persistent low back pain, despite usually efficacious therapy occurring in a heterogeneous and difficult group of patients. In its most limited meaning, it refers to pain after surgery to correct the presumed cause of the pain. It could be due to incorrect patient selection, incorrect surgery, or complications of surgery.

    d. Noncancer chronic back pain syndrome is pain and disability disproportionate to any recognizable organic cause and is associated with abnormal pain behavior.

4. Headache (HA) and facial pain (see also section I.B.1)

    a. Acute HA

        1) Focal HA

            a) ***Vascular HA.*** Complex migraine HA, cluster HA.

            b) ***HA caused by meningeal inflammation.*** Meningitis, encephalitis.

            c) ***"Traction HA"* associated with** increased ***intracranial pressure (ICP).*** Tumor, subdural hemorrhage (SDH), intracranial bleeding, acute hydrocephalus, cerebral edema, brain abscess, subdural empyema, benign intracranial hypertension (or pseudotumor cerebri).

        2) Nonfocal HA

            a) ***Vascular HA.*** New onset migraine HA, reactive vasodilation HA (e.g., fever, drug-induced, postictal, hypoglycemia, hypoxia, hypercarbia, hyperthyroidism), arterial hypertension (HTN) (diastolic blood pressure above 120), paroxysmal severe HTN (e.g., pheochromocytoma, coital HA), giant cell ("temporal") arteritis.

            b) ***HA caused by meningeal inflammation.*** Subarachnoid hemorrhage, meningitis, encephalitis.

c) *HA and head pain caused by cranial neuralgias.* Trigeminal neuralgia or "tic douloureux," glossopharyngeal neuralgia, occipital neuralgia, supraorbital neuralgia, geniculate (or nervus intermedius) neuralgia, superior (or vagal) neuralgia.

d) *"Traction HA" associated with increased ICP.* Bilateral SDH, dural venous sinus thrombosis.

e) *"Traction HA" association with decreased ICP.* Postlumbar puncture HA.

f) *HA and head pains caused by diseases of eyes, ears, nose, sinuses, teeth, or skull* (e.g., sinusitis, glaucoma, extracranial infections).

g) *HA and facial pain without demonstrable physical findings.* HA of uncertain cause (tension HA, posttraumatic HA).

b. **Chronic/intermittent HA**

1) *HA with demonstrable muscle spasm.* Posturally induced (prolonged computer work, driving), paralesional muscle spasm (cervical spondylosis, cervical disc herniation), psychophysiologic muscular contraction (stress related), "muscle contraction HA," myofascial pain syndrome, temporomandibular (TMJ) syndrome, musculoskeletal HA.

2) *HA and facial pain without demonstrable physical findings.* HA of uncertain cause (tension HA), psychogenic HA (hypochondriacal, conversional, delusional, malingering), facial pain of uncertain cause ("atypical facial pain").

3) *Combined tension-migraine HA.* Episodic migraine superimposed on chronic tension HA, chronic daily HA ("rebound HA" associated with analgesic and/or ergotamine).

4) *Vascular HA.* Arteriovenous malformation.

5) *"Traction HA" associated with increased intracranial pressure (ICP).* Chronic hydrocephalus.

5. **Pain syndromes associated with cancer**

a. **Tumor involvement**

1) *Intracranial tumors* causing headache (see section I.A.4 for headache classification).

2) *Cranial neuralgias.* Painful trigeminal neuropathy, referred facial pain syndrome (e.g., from lung tumor), painful glossopharyngeal neuropathy.

3) *Bony infiltration of the skull.* Orbital syndrome, parasellar syndrome, middle fossa syndrome, jugular foramen syndrome, clivus metastases, sphenoid sinus metastases, odontoid fracture, jaw metastases.

4) *Infiltration of peripheral nerve, nerve root, plexus, meninges, and spinal cord*

5) *Infiltration of hollow viscus,* i.e., intestine, biliary tract, and ureters.

b. **Cancer-therapy related**

1) *Postsurgical.* Pain after radical neck dissection, pain after mastectomy, pain after thoracotomy, phantom pain, residual limb pain, pain after nephrectomy, postsurgical pelvic floor myalgia.

2) *Postchemotherapy.* Painful chemotherapy-related toxicities, painful polyneuropathy, painful plexopathy from intraarterial chemotherapy, corticosteroid-associated pain syndrome (e.g., perineal pain, steroid pseudorheumatism, and aseptic necrosis of the femoral and humeral head), postherpetic neuralgia (e.g., due to immunosuppressive therapies)

3) *Postradiation therapy.* Radiation injury to the brachial plexus (radiation

fibrosis, reversible or transient radiation injury, acute ischemic brachial plexopathy), radiation fibrosis of the lumbosacral plexus, radiation myelopathy, radiation-induced peripheral nerve tumors.

B. Common differential diagnoses of acute pain by specific body region

1. Headache and facial pain (see also section I.A.4) can be associated with cranial
bone; neck (e.g., cervical spine and retropharyngeal tendinitis); eyes (e.g.,
acute glaucoma, refractive errors, and heterotropia); ears; nose and sinuses
(e.g., acute sinus headache); TMJ; mouth; teeth; or other facial or cranial
structures.

2. Neck pain

a. *Acute anterior neck pain.* Trauma (anterior whiplash injury, blunt laryngotracheal trauma), myofascial pain disorder, thyroid or parathyroid disease, esophageal pathology, lymphadenitis, infection, abscess, internal
carotid artery dissection, referred pain (e.g., myocardial infarction [MI]
and coronary insufficiency).

b. *Acute lateral neck pain.* Myofascial syndromes of the trapezius muscles,
sternocleidomastoid muscle trauma or pseudotumor, parotid disorder
(e.g., viral parotitis), salivary duct stone, cervical lymphadenitis, referred
pain (e.g., pleuritis involving the diaphragm), infections, cysts.

c. *Acute posterior neck pain.* Cervical disc degeneration; cervical disc herniation and radiculopathy; disorders mimicking cervical disc herniation
(e.g., cervical osteomyelitis and fracture, transverse myelitis, Lyme disease and radiculitis, myofascial syndrome and referred arm pain, osteoarthritis [OA] of the cervical spine with foraminal narrowing); arthritis-
related cervical subluxation, especially of the atlantoaxial joint (e.g., RA,
ankylosing spondylitis [AS], and juvenile rheumatoid arthritis [JRA]);
trauma (e.g., whiplash injury, cervical spine fracture, or dislocation);
myositis of the posterior neck muscles; occipital migraine/neuralgia; bacterial and viral meningitis; meningismus; coital neck- and head-pain;
acute torticollis; and infection.

3. Back, buttock, and pubic pain

a. *Acute midline thoracolumbar pain.* Pathological vertebral fracture (because
of osteoporosis, metastatic carcinoma, multiple myeloma, and pyogenic
or tuberculous [TB] osteomyelitis), myofascial pain, fractures and soft
tissue injuries, acute transverse myelitis, anterior cord ischemia, epidural
abscess, herpes zoster, referred visceral pain (duodenal ulcer, pancreatitis), pneumothorax.

b. *Acute lumbosacral pain* (see also section I.A.3.a.). Lumbosacral strain and
sprain, disc degeneration (with or without herniation or protrusion), lateral recess stenosis with nerve root compression, spinal stenosis, spondylolysis, spondylolisthesis, facet syndrome (posterior joint syndrome),
locked-back syndrome, trauma (e.g., fractures and subluxations, hyperextension injury), pathologic vertebral fractures (due to osteoporosis, metastatic carcinoma, multiple myeloma, Paget's disease, primary spine
tumor, pyogenic, or TB osteomyelitis), vertebral osteomyelitis, myofascial pain syndrome (gluteus maximus syndrome, quadratus lumborum
syndrome, pyriformis syndrome), referred visceral pain (e.g., diverticuli-
tis of the colon and acute pelvic inflammatory disease [PID]), acute sacroiliitis (due to Reiter's syndrome), anterior cord ischemia, intraspinal
synovial cysts, cauda equina syndrome (due to central disc herniation),
infarction of the conus medullaris, acute epidural abscess, acute nontraumatic epidural hematoma.

c. **Acute buttock pain.** Spondylolisthesis, disc degeneration, myofascial syndrome (gluteus maximus syndrome, quadratus lumborum syndrome), facet syndrome (posterior joint syndrome), hamstring strain or tear, buttock trauma, trochanteric bursitis, nodular fasciitis (episacroiliac lipomas), acute sacroiliitis (e.g., Reiter's syndrome), sacral neuralgia (e.g., genital herpes), furuncle, abscess (injection-related, epidural, anorectal abscess), nontraumatic epidural hematoma, levator ani spasm.

d. **Acute pubic pain.** Pubic fracture, pathologic fracture of the pubic bone (disease-associated), stress fracture of the pubic bone (athletic activity—associated), Paget's disease, osteitis pubis, osteomyelitis of the pubic bone, pyogenic arthritis of the pubic symphysis, pubic osteolysis, postpartum symphyseal pubic pain.

4. **Scapular and upper limb pain**

a. **Acute interscapular and scapular pain.** Myofascial pain, pathological fracture of the spine (due to osteoporosis, metastatic carcinoma, multiple myeloma, and pyogenic or TB osteomyelitis), trauma, cervical radiculopathy (because of disk herniation), transverse myelitis, acute epidural abscess, herpes zoster, viscerogenic (MI, dissecting aortic aneurysm, common bile duct stone, pyelonephritis, pleuritis, pancreatitis).

b. **Acute axillary pain.** Fracture of the proximal humeral, anterior costochondritis with axillary pain radiation, axillary myalgic pain, radicular pain involving T1 root, postaxillary dissection pain, breast disorders in women, axillary abscess, hidradenitis suppurativa, axillary-subclavian venous thrombosis, pleuropulmonary disease, pneumothorax, gaseous gastric distention.

c. **Acute shoulder and upper arm pain.** Calcific tendinitis, subdeltoid bursitis, trauma (proximal humeral fracture, humeral shaft fracture, pathologic fracture of the humerus, anterior or posterior glenohumeral joint dislocation, acromioclavicular separation, clavicular fracture), cervical radiculopathy (C5, C6), neuralgic amyotrophy (brachial neuropathy), acute arthritis (gout or pseudogout of the glenohumeral joint, Reiter's syndrome, Lyme arthritis, septic arthritis, acute rheumatic fever, hepatitis B—associated arthritis), osteonecrosis of the humeral head, bicipital rupture or tendinitis, pectoralis major tendinitis, acute osteomyelitis of the shoulder, acute hemarthrosis of the glenohumeral joint (due to anticoagulant therapy or hemophilia), referred pain.

d. **Acute upper and lower arm pain.** Acute cervical (C6-T1) radiculopathy (due to disc herniation, spondylosis, nerve root avulsion, ligamentous or muscular injuries, fracture or dislocation of the lower cervical spine, osteomyelitis, epidural abscess), brachial plexopathy (acute thoracic outlet syndrome, acute brachial neuropathy or neuralgic amyotrophy, blunt or penetrating trauma), myofascial pain, carpal tunnel syndrome (CTS), acute arthritis (acute RA, acute gout and pseudogout, Reiter's syndrome, Lyme arthritis, septic arthritis, acute rheumatic fever, hepatitis B—associated arthritis), cellulitis, vascular pain, referred pain (e.g., acute MI or acute coronary insufficiency and chest wall pain)

e. **Acute elbow and forearm pain**

1) *Diffuse or generalized elbow and forearm pain.* Simple dislocation of the elbow, forearm muscle strain, fractures (supracondylar fracture of the humerus, transcondylar fracture of the humerus, medial epicondylar fracture of the humerus, intercondylar fracture of the humerus, olecranon fracture, radial head fractures, Monteggia's fracture-dislocation

of proximal third of ulna, radial head fracture with acute distal radioulnar dislocation), acute C8 radiculopathy, impending Volkmann's ischemic contracture (anterior compartment syndrome of the forearm), acute monoarticular arthritis (septic arthritis, disseminated gonococcal infection, gout, pseudogout, hemophilic hemarthrosis), acute polyarthritis with elbow involvement (rubella arthritis, rubella vaccine–induced arthritis, acute rheumatic fever, acute hepatitis-B arthritis, Reiter's syndrome, Lyme disease arthritis), arterial occlusion pain, referred pain (e.g., acute MI or acute coronary insufficiency).

2) *Anterior elbow pain.* Brachialis muscle tear, rupture of the distal biceps muscle tendon, biceps muscle tear, anterior capsular tear, disruption of the annular ligament and anterior radial head dislocation, acute thrombophlebitis.

3) *Posterior elbow pain.* Triceps tendinitis, triceps rupture, valgus extension overload syndrome, stress fracture of the olecranon, olecranon bursitis (septic bursitis, gouty bursitis, traumatic bursitis).

4) *Medial elbow pain.* Medial epicondylitis ("golfer's" elbow), rupture of the flexor forearm, rupture or injury of the medial collateral ligament, medial epicondylar fracture, little leaguer's elbow (partial separation of medial epicondyle apophysis), acute ulnar neuropathy, epitrochlear lymphadenitis.

5) *Lateral elbow pain.* Lateral epicondylitis ("tennis" elbow), rupture of the lateral extensor muscle origin, disruption of the annular ligament and anterior radial head dislocation, entrapment of the musculocutaneous or lateral antebrachial cutaneous nerve, osteochondral fracture of the radial head–capitellum articulation.

f. **Acute wrist pain**

1) *Diffuse or generalized wrist pain.* Neurogenic wrist pain (acute carpal tunnel syndrome, acute ulnar tunnel syndrome), traumatic ulnar translocation of the carpus, acute arthritis of the wrist (septic arthritis, pseudogout, gout, avascular necrosis of lunate, hemophilic arthropathy, idiopathic arthritis), wrist instability radiographic patterns (volar intercalated segment instability, dorsal intercalated segment instability).

2) *Radial wrist pain.* Distal radius fracture (Colles' fracture, Smith's fracture, articular margin fracture of the distal radius and carpal dislocation), scaphoid fracture, trapezium fracture, scapholunate interosseous ligament sprain, radial collateral ligament sprain, noninfectious tenosynovitis (de Quervain's disease, tenosynovitis of the extensor pollicis longus, flexor carpi radialis tendinitis, intersection syndrome, extensor indicis proprius syndrome), infectious tenosynovitis (suppurative flexor pollicis longus tenosynovitis, gonococcal tenosynovitis).

3) *Middorsal wrist pain.* Fractures (capitate fracture, lunate fracture), perilunate sprains and dislocations, volar lunate dislocation.

4) *Ulnar wrist pain.* Distal radioulnar joint disorders (fracture of the distal ulna or radial sigmoid fossa, fracture of the triquetrum or lunate, triquetrum avulsion fracture, dislocation of the distal ulna, dislocation of the lunate or triquetrum, triangular fibrocartilage complex injury, extensor carpi ulnaris subluxation and/or tendinitis, extensor digiti minimi tendinitis), hamate fracture, pisiform fracture, triquetrolunate sprain, tendinitis (flexor carpi ulnaris tendinitis, digital flexor tendinitis), pisotriquetral arthritis, midcarpal instability.

g. Acute hand and finger pain

1) *Diffuse or generalized hand and finger pain.* Entrapment neuropathies (carpal tunnel syndrome, ulnar tunnel syndrome, proximal causes of neuropathic hand and finger pain, double-crush syndrome), RSD, acute polyarthritis with wrist and hand involvement (hepatitis-B arthritis, rubella-associated arthritis, rubella immunization–associated arthritis, acute rheumatoid arthritis, SLE arthritis, acute rheumatic fever, acute traumatic arthritis, arthritis-dermatitis syndrome caused by *Neisseria gonorrhoeae,* acute gout, pseudogout, arthritis associated with inflammatory bowel disease, psoriatic arthritis, septic arthritis), mononeuritis multiplex, vascular hand and finger pain (acute arterial embolism), secondary Raynaud's phenomenon (acute arterial occlusive disease, drug therapy), cutaneous disorders of the hand, infections, bites.

2) *Carpometacarpal and metacarpophalangeal (MP) pain.* Carpometacarpal dislocation, metacarpal shaft fractures, MP joint dislocation and ligament injuries (volar plate disruption, collateral ligament sprain, dorsal capsule injuries, fractures of the metacarpal neck and head).

3) *Proximal phalanx and proximal interphalangeal (PIP) pain.* Fractures of the proximal phalanx, PIP joint area (ligament sprains, volar plate injuries, intraarticular fracture-dislocation, collateral ligament tears, volar dislocations, PIP joint deformities, boutonniere deformity).

4) *Middle phalanx pain.* Fracture, sprain.

5) *Distal interphalangeal (DIP) pain.* Extensor tendon disruption (mallet finger), flexor tendon disruption from distal phalanx, fracture of the distal phalanx, subungual hematoma, dislocation of the DIP joint.

h. Acute thumb pain

1) *Trapeziometacarpal pain.* De Quervain's disease, abductor pollicis longus tendinitis, fractures (Bennett's fracture at the base of first metacarpal, Rolando's fracture at the carpometacarpal joint of the thumb), dislocation.

2) *MP joint pain.* Volar plate injury, ulnar collateral ligament injury, radial collateral ligament injury

3) **Proximal phalanx pain.** Neuropathy of a digital nerve (bowler's thumb), fractures of the proximal phalanx

4) *Interphalangeal joint pain.* Dislocation, fracture of the distal phalanx, extensor tendon disruption (mallet thumb).

5. Lower limb pain

a. Acute thigh and leg pain

1) *Diffuse or generalized thigh and leg pain.* Myalgic pain (e.g., after exercise or associated with fever), iliofemoral thrombophlebitis, iliofemoral arterial embolism or thrombosis, polyarthritis, mononeuritis multiplex, acute spondylolisthesis, sacroiliitis, genital herpes.

2) *Anterior and anteromedial thigh and leg pain.* Radiculopathy of L2, L3, or L4 (from disc herniation, facet joint arthritis, previous L5-S1 fusion operation), lumbar plexopathy (L2-L4), femoral neuropathy (with or without iliacus syndrome).

3) *Posterior and/or posterolateral thigh and leg pain.* Sacral plexopathy (L5-S1), panplexopathy (L2-S1), radicular or "sciatic" pain (acute lateral herniation of L4-L5 or L5-S1 disc, nerve root irritation in a stenotic lateral recess or foramen, or due to osteoarthritis or spondylolisthesis), epidural abscess, cauda equina syndrome, epidural hematoma, midline disc herniation, conus medullaris infarction.

4) *Lateral thigh and leg pain.* Trochanteric bursitis, meralgia paresthetica.

b. Acute thigh pain

1) *Diffuse or generalized thigh pain.* Muscle strain because of overuse, femoral shaft fracture (traumatic or stress), lumbosacral plexus injury, fever-related myalgias, iliofemoral venous thrombosis, idiopathic dermatomyositis or polymyositis, complex anterior and posterior compartment syndromes, pathologic fracture due to bone tumor or cyst, soft tissue sarcoma, infectious polymyositis, rhabdomyolysis and myoglobinuria, thigh infection, sickle cell pain crisis.

2) *Anteromedial thigh and inguinal pain.* Traumatic fractures of the hip and pelvis (femoral neck fracture, intertrochanteric fracture, greater trochanteric fracture, lesser trochanteric fracture, subtrochanteric fracture, central acetabular fracture and fracture-dislocation, fractures at or near the pubic symphysis, impacted fracture of the femoral neck), dislocation and fracture-dislocation of the hip (posterior, anterior), pathologic fracture of the hip (femoral neck, intertrochanteric and femoral shaft), stress fracture of the hip and pelvis, acute arthritis of the hip in adults (septic arthritis, acute gout, acute pseudogout, acute rheumatic fever, acute rheumatoid arthritis of the hips, chronic rheumatoid arthritis with acute noninfectious arthritis of the hip, osteoid osteoma, Reiter's syndrome), acute synovitis of the hip in children and adolescents (transient synovitis of the hip, juvenile rheumatoid arthritis of the hip, Legg-Calve-Perthes disease, slipped capital femoral epiphysis, pubic osteomyelitis), osteonecrosis of the femoral head, iliopsoas muscle disorders (iliopsoas bursitis, iliopsoas tendinitis, iliopsoas abscess), femoral neuropathy, iliofemoral venous thrombosis, inguinal or femoral hernia, inguinal or femoral lymphadenitis, cellulitis, sexually transmitted disease (e.g., syphilis, gonococcal urethritis, genital herpes, chancroid).

3) *Anterior thigh pain.* Femoral shaft fracture (traumatic), quadriceps injury (muscle strain, contusion, or tendon rupture), radicular pain (L2-L4 spinal roots), femoral neuropathy, femoral shaft stress fracture in athletes, sartorius muscle strain of the thigh, anterior compartment syndrome of the thigh, myositis ossificans traumatica, obturator hernia, referred pain, herpes simplex neuritis.

4) *Posterior thigh pain.* Radicular pain (disc protrusion, spinal epidural abscess, spinal epidural or subdural hematoma, conus medullaris infarction), hamstring muscle injury (strain, ischial apophysis avulsion), myofascial pain, pyriformis syndrome, hamstring syndrome (gluteal sciatica), ischial bursitis, lumbar facet joint disease, sacroiliitis (Reiter's syndrome or reactive arthritis, septic arthritis), sacroiliac sprain, posterior femoral cutaneous neuropathy, posterior compartment syndrome of the thigh.

5) *Medial thigh pain.* Adductor muscle strain, iliopsoas muscle strain or avulsion fracture of the lesser trochanter, pubic bone disorders (e.g., osteitis pubis), greater saphenous vein phlebitis.

6) *Lateral thigh and trochanteric pain.* Traumatic fracture of the femoral shaft, trochanteric bursitis, snapping hip syndrome, meralgia paresthetica, acute arthritis of the hip, osteonecrosis of the hip, hip pointer (iliac crest contusion), fracture of the iliac crest apophysis.

c. Knee

1) *Diffuse or generalized knee pain.* Trauma (supracondylar fractures of the femur, patellar fractures, fractures of the proximal tibia, fractures of

the tibial spines or intercondylar eminence), knee dislocation (anterior, posterior, medial, or lateral), patellar dislocation, intraarticular ligament injury (anterior cruciate ligament tear, posterior cruciate ligament tear, multiple ligament and meniscus injuries, "dashboard knee"), reflex sympathetic dystrophy of the knee, mimics of septic monoarthritis (pseudogout, gout, traumatic synovitis, foreign body synovitis, acute leukemic arthritis, acute hemarthrosis due to coagulopathy, juvenile rheumatoid arthritis, acute rheumatic fever, idiopathic monoarthritis, Lyme arthritis, acute rheumatoid arthritis of the knee), acute septic monoarthritis of the knee (gonococcal or nongonococcal), acute polyarthritis involving the knee (gonococcal or nongonococcal septic arthritis involving the knee, reactive arthritis, acute rheumatic fever, crystal-induced polyarthritis, hepatitis B–associated arthritis, acute Lyme arthritis, acute rheumatoid arthritis, rubella arthritis, rubella vaccine arthritis, varicella arthritis, acute juvenile rheumatoid arthritis, referred pain from the hip (e.g., acute synovitis).

2) *Anterior knee pain.* Patellar tendon injury, patellofemoral pain syndrome, patellofemoral tracking disorders, patellar tendinitis ("jumper's knee"), prepatellar bursitis ("housemaid's or miner's knee"), retropatellar bursitis, infratellar bursitis, infrapatellar fat pad injury, Hoffa's disease (hypertrophy and inflammation of the infrapatellar fat pad), osteochondritis dissecans of the patella, osteochondral fracture of the patella, quadriceps tendon rupture, Osgood-Schlatter disease (tibial tubercle avulsion fracture), synovial plica, meniscal disorders.

3) *Posterior knee pain.* Gastrocnemius muscle strain, hamstring muscle strain, hamstring tendinitis, muscle spasms (cramps), posterior cruciate ligament and/or posterior capsule tear, plantaris muscle strain or rupture.

4) *Medial knee pain.* Medial meniscus tear (traumatic or degenerative), pes anserine bursitis, tibial collateral ligament bursitis, tibial collateral ligament injury (sprain, rupture), pes anserine-gastrocnemius-related tendinitis, semimembranosus tendinitis, Hoffa's disease (hypertrophy and inflammation of the infrapatellar fat pad), osteonecrosis of the medial femoral condyle, osteonecrosis of the proximal tibia, extraarticular displacement of the medial meniscus.

5) *Lateral knee pain.* Iliotibial band friction syndrome, lateral meniscus tear, biceps femoris tendinitis, tibiofibular joint disorder, osteochondral fracture of the lateral femoral condyle, lateral (fibular) collateral ligament injury, popliteus tenosynovitis, popliteus tendon rupture.

d. Leg

1) *Diffuse or generalized leg pain.* Fractures of the tibial shaft or fibula (traumatic or pathologic), delayed muscle soreness caused by exercise, acute occlusion of the superficial femoral or popliteal artery, cellulitis, sickle cell crisis pain.

2) *Anteromedial leg pain.* Stress fracture of the tibia, stress microfractures of the tibia, medial tibial stress syndrome (periostalgia), soleus syndrome, distal deep posterior compartment syndrome, greater saphenous vein thrombophlebitis, saphenous neuritis, osteomyelitis of the tibia, shin splints related to systemic disease (e.g., Paget's disease of tibia).

3) *Anterolateral leg pain.* Muscle strain or hematoma in the anterior com-

partment, anterior compartment syndrome, lateral compartment syndrome, compression of the superficial peroneal nerve, fibular fracture, anterior tibial vein thrombosis, pyomyositis.

4) *Posterior leg (calf) pain.* Deep vein thrombosis, mimics of calf vein thrombosis (complications of a baker's cyst, gastrocnemius muscle strain, soleus muscle strain, hematoma of the calf, acute rhabdomyolysis, rupture of the Achilles tendon, acute posterior compartment syndrome, pyomyositis), benign calf muscle cramps (e.g., after exercise, during pregnancy, at night in elderly persons), muscle cramps due to underlying disease (peripheral neuropathy root or plexus lesion, drug-related, metabolic causes).

e. Acute ankle pain

1) *Diffuse or generalized ankle pain.* Acute injuries of the ankle (fracture of the medial or lateral melleolus, disruptions of the medial or lateral ligament of the ankles, fracture of the neck of the talus, fracture of the body of the talus, anterior or posterior ankle dislocation), acute monarthritis of the ankle (septic arthritis, acute gout, acute pseudogout, RA, RSD, hemophilic arthropathy, acute hemarthrosis), ankle arthritis associated with acute polyarthritis (polyarticular septic arthritis, acute rheumatic fever, Lyme arthritis, hepatitis B–associated arthritis, rubella and rubella vaccine–associated arthritis, arthritis associated with inflammatory bowel disease, acute polyarticular gout, pseudogout, Reiter's syndrome, rheumatoid arthritis), osteochondritis dissecans of the talus, acute osteomyelitis, transient migratory osteoporosis.

2) *Anterior ankle pain.* Peritendinitis of the extensor tendons of the foot and toes, cruciate crural ligament (retinaculum) sprain, sprain or rupture of the anterior tibiofibular ligament, fracture of the anterior lip of the distal tibial articular surface.

3) *Posterior ankle pain.* Achilles tendinitis, subcutaneous Achilles bursitis, retrocalcaneal bursitis, partial rupture of the Achilles tendon, complete rupture of the Achilles tendon, fracture of the calcaneal tuberosity.

4) *Medial ankle pain.* Fracture of the medial malleolus, shin splints (stress fracture of tibia, periostitis, and musculotendinous pain), fracture of the sustentaculum tali, deltoid ligament sprain, tibialis posterior tendinitis, tendinitis of the flexor hallucis longus and flexor digitorum communis.

5) *Lateral ankle pain.* Lateral collateral ligament injuries (anterior talofibular, calcaneofibular, and posterior talofibular ligaments), mimics of anterior talofibular ligament sprain (anterior tibiofibular ligament sprain, fracture of the lateral malleolus, fracture of the lateral process of the talus, fracture of the lateral tubercle of the posterior process of the talus, peroneal tendinitis, traumatic dislocation of the peroneal tendons, ganglion cyst, stress fracture of the fibula, calcaneofibular ligament sprain [isolated]).

f. Acute foot pain

1) *Generalized foot pain.* Nerve and root compression syndrome (L5-S1 root compression, superficial or deep peroneal nerve entrapment, sural nerve entrapment, tarsal tunnel syndrome), arthritis (RA, AS, Reiter's syndrome, psoriatic arthritis, gout, pseudogout, acute rheumatic fever, SLE, hepatitis B–associated arthritis, rubella-associated arthritis), sickle cell crisis pain, vascular pain (acute arterial occlusion, nocturnal rest pain, ulcers and gangrene (e.g., due to arterio-sclerosis obliterans, progressive ischemia, vasculitis), RSD, foot cramps, peripheral polyneuropathy (see section I.A.1.b), trauma (crush injury, compartment syndrome, amputation), infection (cellu-litis, necrotizing fasciitis, abscess, osteomyelitis), cold injury (frost-bite, chilblains), bites, cutaneous disorders (e.g., shoe dermatitis, tinea pedis).

2) *Forefoot pain.* Morton's neuroma (plantar interdigital nerve hypertro-phy), inflammatory arthritis of the metatarsophalangeal joint, arterial insufficiency, traumatic metatarsal fractures, forefoot sprain, metatar-salgia due to high-heeled shoes, metatarsalgia due to equinus foot or cavus foot, metatarsalgia due to central-ray overload syndrome, metatarsalgia due to first-ray insufficiency syndrome or Morton's syn-drome (acute march fractures and chronic first-ray insufficiency), Freiberg's disease (osteonecrosis of second and third metatarsal head), second metatarsal space syndrome, idiopathic synovitis of the second MTP joint, bursitis (submetatarsal and interdigital), submetatarsal cysts.

3) *Great toe and medial forefoot pain.* Radicular pain (L5 root), first meta-tarsophalangeal joint injury (sprain, dislocation or sesamoid fracture, "turf" toe), fracture of the great toe, crush injury of the distal toe (soft tissue injury), dislocation of the interphalangeal joint, hallux valgus, bunion of the great toe, hallux limitus or rigidus, first metatar-sophalangeal joint arthritis (septic arthritis and osteomyelitis, podagra due to gout or pseudogout), shoe vamp ulcer and bursitis, gangrene or ulceration of the great toe, subungual hematoma, plantar cutaneous lesions (corns, warts, calluses), nail lesions and infection of the hallux, Joplin's neuroma (of plantar digital nerve of great toe), first-ray over-load syndrome, calcific tendinitis of the flexor hallucis tendons, tu-mors.

4) *Small toe pain.* Dorsal interphalangeal joint area pain and inflammation, trauma (contusions and fractures), arthritis of the small toes, ulcera-tions of the toes (ischemic, neuropathic), hammer toe deformity, mal-let toe deformity, gout tophus, tailor's bunion (bunionette of the fifth toe), Raynaud's disease and phenomenon, plantar cutaneous lesions (corns, warts), tinea pedis, candidiasis, Osler's nodes, subungual tu-mors.

5) *Midfoot pain.* Plantar fascial pain (plantar fasciitis, heel pain syn-drome), longitudinal arch strain, subtalar osteochondral fracture, stress fracture of one or more metatarsal or tarsal bones, osteoarthritis (first metatarsocuneiform joint, cuboideometatarsal joint), tarsometa-tarsal joint trauma (sprain or dislocation or fracture-dislocation), mid-arsal trauma (Chopart's or the transverse tarsal joint), navicular frac-tures (traumatic or stress fractures), fracture of the fifth metatarsal (avulsion fractures, diaphyseal or true Jones fractures), aseptic necro-sis of the navicular bone, tendinitis (flexor hallucis longus tendinitis, peroneal tendinitis), interosseous myositis or strain, osteomyelitis, ac-quired flatfoot (rupture of the tibialis posterior tendon, ligamentous or bone failure), plantar abscess.

6) *Dorsal foot pain.* Acute gout or pseudogout, peripheral polyneuropathy, trauma (metatarsal, tarsal), stress fracture of the metatarsal, OA of the tarsometatarsal joint, tendinitis (extensor hallucis longus muscle,

extensor digitorum longus muscle, tibialis anterior muscle), cruciate crural ligament injury, cellulitis, RSD, peroneal nerve entrapment (superficial or deep), subtalar arthritis or osteochondral fracture, aseptic necrosis of the navicular bone, interosseous muscle strain, acquired pes planus, shoe dermatitis, foot abscess, osteomyelitis, septic arthritis, herpes zoster.

7) *Diffuse or generalized hindfoot pain.* Intraarticular calcaneal fractures, extraarticular calcaneal fractures (fracture of the medial calcaneal process, fracture of the superior portion of the calcaneal tuberosity, fracture of the sustentaculum tali), ischemic necrosis of the heel.

8) *Plantar hindfoot pain.* Heel pain syndrome due to overuse ("plantar fasciitis") or due to systemic disorders (e.g., RA, seronegative arthritis, spondyloarthropathies), fat pad disorders (atrophy, inflammation, fat pad separation from the calcaneus), stress fracture of the calcaneus, rupture of the plantar fascia, entrapment neuropathy of the first branch of the lateral plantar nerve to abductor digiti quinti muscle, flexor tendinitis (flexor hallucis longus tendinitis, flexor digitorum longus tendinitis).

9) *Posterior hindfoot pain.* Achilles tendinitis, retrocalcaneal bursitis, superficial Achilles bursitis ("pump bump"), Achilles tendon rupture, calcaneal periostitis and osteitis, fracture of the posterosuperior calcaneal tuberosity, calcaneal osteomyelitis.

10) *Medial hindfoot pain.* Tarsal tunnel syndrome, tibialis posterior tendinitis, flexor hallucis longus tendinitis, calcaneal fractures (medial calcaneal process or sustentaculum tali), calcaneal branch neurodynia.

11) *Lateral hindfoot pain.* Lateral ankle sprain, peroneal muscle strain, peroneal tendinitis, fracture of the lateral process of the talus, osteochondral fracture of the talar dome, stress fracture of the lateral malleolus, sural nerve entrapment.

C. **Differential diagnosis of musculoskeletal pain by its distribution pattern**

1. **Acute generalized musculoskeletal pain.** Postexertional in normal individuals, fibromyalgia, viral infection (influenza A, Epstein-Barr virus, coxsackievirus, herpes simplex, human immunodeficiency virus [HIV]), therapeutic drugs (lovastatin, clofibrate), postimmunization, electrolyte and mineral deficiencies (hyponatremia, hypokalemia, hypocalcemia, hypomagnesemia, hypophosphatemia), alcohol abuse, drug abuse (amphetamines, cocaine, heroin or its contaminants), endocrine disorders (diabetes mellitus, hypo- or hyperthyroidism, hypoadrenalism, panhypopituitarism, hypoparathyroidism), metabolic muscular disorders, eosinophilia-myalgia syndrome, mimics of the eosinophilia myalgia syndrome (e.g., polymyositis, esosinophilic fasciitis, sarcoidosis, dermatomyositis), polymyalgia rheumatica, seronegative RA.

2. **Acute generalized joint pain.** Reactive arthritis (Reiter's syndrome), rubella-associated arthritis, HIV-associated arthritis, acute seropositive RA, crystal-induced polyarthritis due to gout or pseudogout.

3. **Monoarticular joint pain**

   a. **Acute monoarthritis.** Infectious arthritis (bacterial, Lyme disease), crystal-induced disease such as gout and pseudogout (CPDD), hemarthrosis, which can be due to nontraumatic causes (anticoagulant therapy, dialysis) or trauma, noninfectious inflammatory conditions such as JRA and seronegative spondyloarthropathies (e.g., psoriatic arthritis, Reiter's syndrome), periarticular syndrome (e.g., erythema nodosum, inflammatory bowel disease, acute sarcoidosis), monoarticular presentation of a polyarticular disease (e.g., RA).

   b. Chronic monoarthritis. Infectious arthritis (e.g., pyogenic bacteria, fungal, Lyme, tuberculosis), noninfectious inflammatory conditions such as RA, pauciarticular JRA, sarcoid arthropathy and seronegative spondyloarthropathies (e.g., psoriatic arthritis, Reiter's disease), noninflammatory conditions such as OA, avascular necrosis of bone (osteonecrosis), neoplasia (pigmented villonodular synovitis, synovial chondromatosis), neuropathic ("Charcot") joint.

4. Polyarticular joint pain

   a. Acute migratory polyarthritis. Neisserial infection (e.g., gonorrhea), reactive or postinfectious arthritis (e.g., acute rheumatic fever, Reiter's syndrome, poststreptococcal arthritis), early stage of Lyme disease, viral infection (e.g., rubella, mumps, Epstein-Barr virus), serum sickness (occasionally), acute leukemia, inflammatory bowel disease, familial hypercholesterolemia.

   b. Acute nonmigratory polyarthritis. RA, serum sickness, SLE, polyarticular JRA, acute phase of seronegative spondyloarthropathies (e.g., psoriatic arthritis, Reiter's syndrome, AS, enteropathic arthritis), crystal-induced disease (acute polyarticular gout and pseudogout), sarcoidosis, vasculitis, hematologic disorders (e.g., leukemia, sickle cell disease, lymphoma), serum sickness, viral arthritis (e.g., HIV, Epstein-Barr).

   c. Chronic polyarthritis. RA, SLE, polyarticular JRA, sarcoid arthritis, connective tissue disease (e.g., scleroderma, polymyositis) and overlap syndromes, chronic phase of seronegative spondyloarthropathies (e.g., psoriatic arthritis, Reiter's syndrome, AS), OA, crystal-induced disease (chronic polyarticular gout and pseudogout).

II. Nonneuromusculoskeletal pain-related problems. *Cardiac pain* develops due to ischemia induced by increase cardiac workload resulting from exertion, cold, or emotion. It may subside with rest and relaxation. *Mediastinal pain* is induced by activities of esophagus (swallowing), musculoskeletal movement, or aorta (increased systolic thrust). *Pleural and tracheal pain* is associated with respiratory movements. *Arterial pain*, usually throbbing is seen in arteritis, migraine, and vascular headaches and is aggravated by increased systolic pressure (e.g., exercise, fever, bending over). *Gastrointestinal tract pain* is increased with peristaltic activity (especially if with obstruction, e.g., impacted stool) and is aggravated by eating and may be relieved with fasting or by vomiting or bowel movement. *Pain induced by gastric juice* is related to food intake and may be relieved by food or antacids. *Visceral pain* from abdominal organs (e.g., kidneys, liver, spleen, and pancreas) is intensified by body positions or movements that increase intraabdominal pressure.

BIBLIOGRAPHY

Asbury AK, Fields HL: Pain due to peripheral nerve damage: An hypothesis. *Neurology* 34:1587-1590, 1984.

Bennett JC, Plum F, editors: *Cecil textbook of medicine.* ed 20, Philadelphia, 1996, WB Saunders.

Goodman CC, Snyder TEK: *Differential diagnosis in physical therapy,* ed 2, Philadelphia, 1995, WB Saunders.

Headache Classification Committee of the International Headache Society: Classification and diagnostic criteria for headache disorders, cranial neuralgias, and facial pain. *Cephalalgia* 8 (suppl. 7):1-96, 1988.

Healey P, Jacobson EJ: *Common medical diagnoses: An algorithmic approach*, ed 2, Philadelphia, 1994, WB Saunders.

Isselbacher KJ, Braunwald E, Wilson JD, et al., editors: *Harrison's principle of internal medicine*, ed 13, New York, 1994, McGraw-Hill.

Janig W, Blumberg H, Boas RA, et al: The reflex sympathetic dystrophy syndrome: Consensus statement and general recommendations for diagnosis and clinical research. In Bond MR, Charlton JE, Woolf CJ, editors: *Pain research and clinical management: Proceedings of the VIth World Congress on Pain*, vol. 3, Amsterdam, 1991, Elsevier, pp. 372-375.

Kanner RM: Low back pain. In Portenoy RK, Kanner RM, editors: *Pain management: Theory and practice*, Philadelphia, 1996, FA Davis, pp. 126-144.

Kozin F: Reflex sympathetic dystrophy syndrome. *Bull Rheum Dis* 36: 1-8, 1986.

Macnab I, McCulloch J: *Neck ache and shoulder pain*, Baltimore, 1994, Williams & Wilkins.

Paget S, Pellicci P, and Beary JF, III, editors: *Manual of rheumatology and outpatient orthopedic disorders*, ed 3, Boston, 1993, Little, Brown.

Portenoy RK: Neuropathic pain. In Portenoy RK, Kanner RM, editors: *Pain management: Theory and practice*, Philadelphia, 1996, FA Davis, pp. 83-125.

Roberts WJ: A hypothesis on the physiological basis for causalgia and related pains. *Pain* 24:297-311, 1986.

Stein J, editor: *Internal medicine*, ed 4, St. Louis, 1994, Mosby.

Wiener SL: *Differential diagnosis of acute pain by body region*, New York, 1993, McGraw-Hill.

Wall PD, Melzack R, editors: *Textbook of pain*, ed 3, Edinburgh, 1994, Churchill Livingstone.

CHAPTER 3.2

DIFFERENTIAL DIAGNOSES OF NONPAIN PROBLEMS

This chapter deals with the differential diagnosis of common PM&R problems that do not have pain as the primary feature although pain may play a secondary role in some of them. They are encountered in either the in- or out-patient setting of a PM&R practice. The diagnosis and treatment of many of these problems may not fall within the realm of physiatric practice per se; however, recognizing the potential diagnosis and knowing when to refer them to another specialist is important for good patient care. As in the previous chapter, these problems are divided into the neuromusculoskeletal system and nonneuromusculoskeletal system.

I. Neuromusculoskeletal nonpain-related problems

A. Muscle weakness

1. **Neurogenic causes**
   a. *Upper motor neuron (UMN) and cortical disorders.* Vascular (e.g., stroke, intracranial hemorrhage, and cerebral palsy), demyelinating (e.g., multiple sclerosis [MS]); infectious (e.g., encephalitis, meningitis, Creutz-feldt-Jakob disease, and AIDS), structural (e.g., neoplasm, Arnold-Chiari malformation, syringomyelia, and syringobulbia), exogenous (e.g., traumatic brain injury [TBI], cervical spinal cord injuries, and drug-induced causes).
   b. *Combined upper and lower motor neuron disorders.* Amyotrophic lateral sclerosis (ALS), progressive muscular atrophy, progressive bulbar palsy, primary lateral sclerosis.
   c. *Lower motor neuron (LMN) disorders*
      1) *Motor neurons.* Spinal muscular atrophy, poliomyelitis, postpolio syndrome.
      2) *Peripheral nervous system.* Guillain-Barre syndrome (GBS), plexopathies, radiculopathies, compressive neuropathies, acute intermittent porphyria.
      3) *Neuromuscular junction.* Myasthenia gravis, Lambert-Eaton myasthemic syndrome, botulism.

2. **Myopathic causes** (usually presents with proximal weakness).
   a. *Muscular dystrophy.* Duchenne muscular dystrophy, fascioscapulohumeral dystrophy, limb-girdle dystrophy, myotonic dystrophy, oculopharyngeal dystrophy, congenital myopathies.
   b. *Rheumatologic disorders.* Primary amyloidosis, sarcoid myopathy, dermatomyositis, polymyositis, rheumatoid arthritis (RA), polyarteritis nodosa, systemic lupus erythematosus (SLE), polymyalgia rheumatica (PMR), stiff-man syndrome, fibromyalgia, cervical and lumbar spondylosis, Paget's disease of bone.
   c. *Toxin- and drug-induced myopathies.* Steroid myopathy, hypokalemic myopathy, alcoholic myopathy, drug-induced myopathy (D-penicillamine, colchicine, chloroquine, clofibrate, cimetidine), drug-induced rhabdomyolysis and myoglobinuria.

Chapter 3.2 Differential Diagnoses of Nonpain Problems **125**

d. **Metabolic myopathies.** Familial periodic paralysis, diabetes mellitus (DM), electrolyte imbalance (hypo- or hyperkalemia, hypercalcemia, hypermagnesemia, hypophosphatemia), vitamin D deficiency, renal tubular acidosis, mitochondrial myopathy, McArdle's syndrome, familial myoglobinuria, acid maltase deficiency, carnitine deficiency, other metabolic storage disease.
e. **Endocrine myopathies.** Hypothyroid myopathy, thyrotoxic myopathy, acromegalic myopathy, hyperparathyroidism, Cushing's syndrome.
f. **Infectious myopathy (with myositis).** Viral (poliomyelitis, rabies, coxsackie, influenza, rubella, human immunodeficiency virus [HIV], Epstein-Barr virus), bacterial (staphylococcal, streptococcal, salmonella, clostridial, *Mycobacterium leprae*, *Mycoplasma pneumoniae*), parasitic (trichinosis, toxoplasmosis, *Trypanosoma cruzi, Echinococcus alveolaris*), fungal (*Candida tropicalis*).
g. **Others.** Endogenous depressive psychosis.

B. **Paraplegia or tetraplegia**
1. **Neurogenic causes**
   a. **Upper motor neuron (UMN) and cortical disorders**
      1) **Brain.** Vascular (e.g., bilateral cerebral infarction, ventral pontine infarction, bilateral medullary pyramid infarction, and cerebral palsy), neoplastic (frontal lobe tumor, brainstem glioma, parasagittal tumor [paraplegia]), demyelinating (e.g., MS), hydrocephalus (e.g., Arnold-Chiari malformation).
      2) **Spinal cord.** Trauma (spinal cord injury [SCI]), vascular (e.g., anterior spinal artery thrombosis, spinal arteriovenous malformation, epidural hematoma, hematomyelia, and arteritis), neoplasm (primary intramedullary [ependymoma, astrocytoma] or extramedullary [neurofibroma, meningioma], secondary extradural metastasis), inflammatory (idiopathic transverse myelitis, MS), degenerative (cervical spondylotic myelopathy, intervertebral disc prolapse, vertebral disease with myelopathy, atlantoaxial subluxation [e.g., in RA]), congenital (spina bifida, syringomyelia), infectious (herpes zoster or simplex myelitis, HIV myelopathy, tuberculosis [TB] [Pott's disease], spinal epidural abscess, syphilitic meningomyelitis), nutritional (subacute combined degeneration due to vitamin B_{12} deficiency), granulomatous (sarcoidosis), others (decompression myelopathy in divers, myelopathy of systemic disease, toxin-induced).
   b. **Combined upper and lower motor neuron disorders,** e.g., ALS and primary lateral sclerosis.
   c. **Lower motor neuron (LMN) disorders**
      1) **Motor neurons.** Spinal muscular atrophy, poliomyelitis.
      2) **Peripheral nervous system.** GBS, acute intermittent porphyria, neoplasm, heavy metal poisoning.
      3) **Neuromuscular junction.** Myasthenia gravis, botulism.
2. **Myopathic causes.** Polymyositis, rhabdomyolysis, familial periodic paralysis, electrolyte imbalance (hypo- or hyperkalemia, hypercalcemia, hypermagnesemia, hypophosphatemia).

C. **Hemiplegia or hemiparesis**
1. **Vascular.** Stroke, transient ischemic attacks (TIA), reversible ischemic neurologic deficit (RIND), cerebral palsy, vasculitis.
2. **Trauma.** Traumatic brain injury (brain contusion, subdural hematoma, epidural hematoma).

3. **Brain tumor.** Primary or metastatic.
4. **Demyelinating disease.** Demyelinating disease (MS, acute necrotizing myelitis).
5. **Infections.** Brain abscess, encephalitis, subdural empyema, meningitis.
6. **Other.** Hypoglycemia, migraine syndrome, Todd's paralysis, nonketotic hyperosmolar coma, leukodystrophies.

D. **Gait disorders**
   1. **Pathologic gait**
      a. **Central nervous system disease.** Hemiparetic gait (cerebral palsy [CP], stroke), Parkinson's disease.
      b. **Peripheral nervous system disease**
         1) **Gluteus medius insufficiency.** Poliomyelitis, myelodysplasia.
         2) **Gluteus maximus or lurch gait.** Muscular dystrophy.
         3) **Complete or partial quadriceps paralysis.** Poliomyelitis.
         4) **Paralysis of the anterior compartment of the leg.** Foot drop with hip hike, ALS, lumbar radiculopathy.
      c. **Musculoskeletal dysfunction.** Antalgic pattern, orthopedic problems.
   2. **Wide-based unsteady gait (ataxia)**
      a. **Cerebellar ataxia.** Wernicke's encephalopathy, alcoholic cerebellar degeneration, multiple sclerosis, vertebrobasilar artery ischemia, neoplasms, hemorrhage, abscess, infarct, following hyperthermia, hypoxic encephalopathy, non-Wilsonian hepatocerebral degeneration (posthepatic coma), hypoparathyroidism, congenital, hereditary (ataxic telangiectasia).
      b. **Sensory ataxia** (loss of postural or proprioceptive sense). Polyneuropathy (diabetic), tabes dorsalis, multiple sclerosis, subacute combined degeneration of the spinal cord, vitamin B_{12} deficiency, spinal cord tumor, hereditary (Friedreich's ataxia).
      c. **Others.** Frontal lobe lesions (tumors, thrombosis of anterior cerebral artery, hydrocephalus), labyrinthine destruction (neoplasm, injury, inflammation, compression), parainfectious (GBS, acute ataxia of childhood and young adults), hydrocephalus (normal pressure), paraneoplastic syndromes, hypothyroidism, myopathy, toxins (phenytoin, alcohol, sedatives, organophosphates), Wilson's disease (hepatolenticular degeneration), meningomyelopathy, Creutzfeldt-Jakob disease, hysteria, AIDS, dysequilibrium (see section II.B.5).

E. **Isolated foot drop**
   1. *With sensory deficit.* L5 radiculopathy, lumbar plexopathy, sciatic nerve palsy, peroneal neuropathy (compression or injury at fibular head, diabetes), early GBS, hereditary motor and sensory neuropathy (e.g., Charcot-Marie-Tooth disease).
   2. *Without sensory deficit.* ALS, scapuloperoneal variety of fascioscapulohumeral muscular dystrophy.

F. **Involuntary movement disorders** include tics (Tourette's syndrome), athetosis (e.g., in CP), and the following:
   1. **Dystonia** (sustained abnormal fixed posture).
      a. **Primary generalized dystonia.** Idiopathic torsion dystonia (hereditary or sporadic).
      b. **Secondary dystonia.** Acquired (e.g., CP, poststroke, head trauma, drug induced [neuroleptic, anti-Parkinson], vascular malformation, multiple sclerosis, brain tumor, encephalitis, peripheral trauma), degenerative disorders (e.g., Parkinson's disease, progressive supranuclear palsy, rigid

Huntington's disease, oliovopontocerebellar degeneration), neurologic disorder with identifiable metabolic defect (e.g., Wilson's disease) or suspected metabolic defect (e.g., ataxia telangiectasia).

c. *Focal dystonia.* Blepharospasm, torticollis, spastic dysphonia, writer's cramp.

d. *Stiff-man syndrome.* Associated with diabetes, vitiligo and thyroiditis.

2. **Tremor** (oscillating involuntary movement of the joint).

a. *Tremor at rest (pill-rolling).* Parkinsonian tremor.

b. *Action tremor*

1) *Postural tremor.* Essential tremor, enhanced physiologic tremor, neuropathic tremor.

2) *Intention tremor.* Cerebellar intention tremor.

3) *Task specific tremor.* Primary writing tremor.

c. *Medication-induced tremor.* Thyroid extract (synthroid), epinephrine, amphetamine, phenylephrine, and other sympathomimetics, caffeine, theophylline and other xanthines; nicotine; lithium; phenothiazines; methyl bromide; monosodium glutamate; corticosteroids (in high doses); insulin and oral hypoglycemic agents; alcohol withdrawal; metal intoxication (lead, arsenic, bismuth, mercury, manganese); tricyclic antidepressants.

3. **Chorea** (irregular, brief movements of the limbs and trunk accompanied by facial grimacing, head movements, and a peculiar dancing gait).

a. *Huntington's disease*

b. *Non-Huntington disease.* Acute rheumatic chorea (Sydenham's disease), chorea gravidarum, SLE, chorea acanthocytosis, glutaric acidemia, methylmalonic aciduria, familial calcification of the basal ganglia, acute vascular hemichorea, senile chorea.

4. **Dyskinesia (drug-induced)**

a. *Acute.* Levodopa, bromocriptine, anticholinergics, dopaminergic agonists, antihistamines, oral contraceptives.

b. *Chronic tardive dyskinesia.* Neuroleptic drugs.

5. **Myoclonus** (brief muscle jerk, which can be spontaneous, or evoked by voluntary movement or sensory stimuli).

a. *Physiologic.* Sleep jerks, hiccups.

b. *Essential.* Familial essential myoclonus, sporadic essential myoclonus, startle syndrome.

c. *Epileptic myoclonus*

d. *Symptomatic myoclonus.* Toxic or metabolic encephalopathy, viral encephalitis, spinocerebellar degeneration, basal ganglia degeneration, Alzheimer's disease, Creutzfeldt-Jakob disease, storage disease with progressive myoclonus epilepsy, posthypoxic, focal central nervous system (CNS) damage.

G. **Paresthesia**

1. *Peripheral neuropathy*

2. *Peripheral nerve entrapment, compression, or trauma.* Intervertebral disk herniation, thoracic outlet syndrome, carpal tunnel syndrome.

3. *Arteriosclerotic peripheral vascular disease*

4. *Spinal cord disease.* Spinal cord or nerve root compression, tabes dorsalis, subacute combined degeneration of the spinal cord.

5. *Metabolic imbalance.* Hyperkalemia, hypophosphatemia, hypocalcemia, respiratory alkalosis, hypothyroidism.

H. **Neurogenic dysphagia** (see Chapter 5.6, section IV.A).

II. **Systemic (nonneuromusculoskeletal) nonpain-related problems:** The following are differential diagnoses of common PM&R problems that do not have pain as a primary feature although pain may play a secondary role in some of them:

A. **General problems**

1. **Chronic fatigue**

   a. *Psychogenic origin* (80% of cases). Anxiety states, depression, "chronic fatigue syndrome."

   b. *Fatigue of physical origin* (20% of cases). Infectious disease (febrile states, TB), metabolic disorders (DM, hypothyroidism, hyperparathyroidism, hypopituitarism, Addison's disease), blood dyscrasias (anemia, lymphoma, leukemia), renal disease (acute renal failure, chronic renal failure), liver disease (acute hepatitis, chronic hepatitis and cirrhosis), chronic pulmonary disease, chronic cardiovascular disease, neoplastic disease, neuromuscular disease with weakness.

2. **Fever acquired in the hospital (nosocomial)**

   a. *Infectious.* Sepsis associated with intravascular therapy, urinary catheter–associated bacteriuria, lower respiratory infection (pneumonia), surgical wound infection (deep wound abscess), cardiac bypass (postperfusion syndrome caused by cytomegalovirus or Epstein-Barr virus), upper respiratory infection (sinusitis, pharyngitis, colds), pacemaker and prosthesis infections, skin and soft tissue infections, infections incubating at the time of hospital admission, bacteremia without an apparent source (may be due to endocarditis).

   b. *Noninfectious.* Reactions to therapeutic agents (medications, contrast dyes), surgical procedures, intravascular catheter–induced inflammation without concurrent infection, transfusion of blood products, thrombophlebitis, pulmonary embolism, instrumentation (e.g., angiography, colonoscopy, bronchoscopy, and cystoscopy), therapeutic devices (e.g., nasotracheal intubation), noninfectious illnesses (e.g., arthritis, gout, malignancy, hepatitis, appendicitis, and intracerebral bleeding, etc.), factitious (self-induced) fever.

3. **Anxiety**

   a. *Psychiatric disorder.* Anxiety disorders, depressive illness, schizophrenia.

   b. *Disease of the CNS.* Postconcussion syndrome, vascular disease, degenerative disorders, seizures.

   c. *Endocrine and metabolic disorders.* Hyperthyroidism and hypothyroidism, hyperparathyroidism, hyperadrenocorticism, hypoglycemia, pheochromocytoma.

   d. *Drug effects.* Sympathomimetic agents, corticosteroids, alcohol.

   e. *Drug withdrawal syndromes.* Alcohol, barbiturates.

   f. *Miscellaneous.* Menopause, mitral valve prolapse, porphyria.

B. **Neurologic problems**

1. **Acute confusional states**

   a. *Metabolic dysfunction.* Electrolyte imbalance (hyper/hypoglycemia, hyper/hyponatremia, hyper/hypomagnesemia, hyper/hypocalcemia), hyper/hypothermia, hepatic failure, renal failure, hypoxia, hyper/hypocarbia, endocrinopathies (thyroid storm, myxedema, adrenal dysfunctions), acidosis, alkalosis, porphyria, vitamin deficiencies.

   b. *Drugs and toxins.* Psychoactive medications, alcohol, toxic ingestions, drug and alcohol withdrawal, carbon monoxide poisoning.

   c. *Infections.* Systemic infections, CNS infections (meningitis, encephalitis).

d. *Seizures.* Complex partial seizures, psychomotor and absence seizures, status epilepticus, postictal states.

e. *Brain disease.* Focal brain lesions (right parietal lobe, medial occipital lobes, right frontal lobe), generalized brain lesions (head trauma, concussion, skull fractures, hypertensive encephalopathy, subdural hematoma [SDH], intracranial bleed, space occupying masses, herniation, vasculitis, petechial hemorrhages, brainstem lesions).

f. *Others.* Psychiatric illness, arrhythmia.

2. Dementia

a. *Focal neurologic.* Trauma (cerebral contusion), tumor, chronic SDH, MS, vascular dementia (multiple cerebral infarcts, single cerebral infarcts, lacunar infarcts), Huntington's chorea, Pick's disease, normal-pressure hydrocephalus, Parkinson's disease, progressive supranuclear palsy, olivopontocerebellar degeneration.

b. *Nonfocal neurologic.* Lupus cerebritis, brain abscess, progressive multifocal leukoencephalopathy, acute and chronic meningitis, limbic encephalitis, carcinomatosis, Creutzfeldt-Jakob disease, Whipple's disease, postconcussion syndrome, Alzheimer's disease, senile dementia, Wernicke's encephalopathy, paraneoplastic syndromes.

c. *Metabolic and endocrine abnormalities.* Pernicious anemia (vitamin B_{12} or cyanocobalamin deficiency), pellagra (niacin deficiency), Wernicke-Korsakoff syndrome (thiamine deficiency), hyper/hypocalcemia, hyper/hypomagnesemia, hyper/hypothyroidism, hypoparathyroidism, chronic hypoglycemia, chronic hypoxemia, hepatic encephalopathy, Cushing's disease, Addison's disease, chronic renal disease (uremia), chronic dehydration.

d. *Others.* Depression (pseudodementia), schizophrenia (dementia praecox), syphilis, AIDS encephalopathy, heavy metal intoxication (mercury, lead, aluminum), drug induced (chronic drug toxicity).

3. Seizure must be differentiated from syncope, TIA, migraine, hypoglycemia, paroxysmal vertigo, narcolepsy, and psychogenic spells. The usual causes of seizure includes:

a. *Metabolic.* Hyper/hypoglycemia, hyper/hypomagnesemia, hyper/hyponatremia, hypocalcemia, hypoxia, acid-base disturbance, organ failure (renal, hepatic), drug withdrawal (alcohol, sedatives), drug intoxication (aminophylline, lidocaine, cocaine, amphetamine).

b. *Focal cortex lesion.* Infarction, contusion, concussion, tumor, abscess, meningitis, encephalitis, cerebritis, subdural hematoma, intracranial bleed, postoperative scar.

c. *Cardiovascular.* Hypertension, heart block, MI, brady/tachyarrhythmia.

d. *Congenital (hereditary or acquired).* Idiopathic, perinatal injury, maldevelopment, degenerations.

4. Ill-defined dizziness other than vertigo (see section II.B.6), syncope, or disequilibrium (see section II.B.5). Consider psychiatric disorders such as hyperventilation syndrome, anxiety neurosis, hysterical neurosis, and affective disorders (depression).

5. Disequilibrium (feeling of unsteadiness without rotation).

a. *Multiple sensory deficits* (diminished proprioception with concomitant visual loss, extrapyramidal dysfunction, orthostatic hypotension, or vestibular disturbances).

b. *Cerebellar dysfunction.* Alcoholic cerebellar dysfunction, tumors, infarcts.

c. **Extrapyramidal diseases.** Parkinson's disease, progressive supranuclear palsy.

d. **Schwannomas and other cerebellopontine angle tumors.** Schwannoma, meningioma, epidermoid tumors, other posterior fossa tumors.

e. **Nonfunctioning labyrinths**

f. **Drug-induced disequilibrium.** Anticonvulsants (e.g., barbiturates, phenytoin, ethosuximide, carbamazepine), alcohol (ethanol, methanol) intoxication, salicylates, cinchona alkaloids (e.g., quinine, and quinidine), tranquilizers (e.g., diazepam, lorazepam, and flurazepam), aminoglycoside antibiotics (e.g., tobramycin, amikacin, and gentamicin).

6. **Vertigo and nystagmus** (vertigo is the illusion of motion usually accompanied by nausea, vomiting, nystagmus, and disequilibrium).

a. **Peripheral or labyrinthine.** Otitis media, acute labyrinthitis (bacterial, viral, syphilis), vestibular neuronitis, benign positional vertigo, barotrauma, posttraumatic vertigo (labyrinthine concussion, perilymph fistula), Meniere's disease, cerebellopontine angle tumor (acoustic schwannoma), lesions of the eighth nerve (acoustic neuroma, meningioma, mononeuropathy, metastatic carcinoma), mastoiditis, Cogan's syndrome, ototoxic drugs (alcohol, quinine, salicylates, aminoglycoside antibiotics, such as streptomycin and gentamycin), "physiologic" (motion sickness, vision-induced vertigo, vertigo at heights), temporomandibular joint (TMJ) syndrome.

b. **CNS or central.** Vertebrobasilar artery insufficiency, posterior fossa tumor or other brain tumors (meningioma, hemangioma), infarction/hemorrhage (cerebral cortex, cerebellum, or brainstem), cerebral vasculitis, arteriovenous (AV) malformation, intracranial aneurysm, basilar migraine, multiple sclerosis, CNS infections (viral, bacterial), granulomatous meningitis, herpes zoster oticus (Ramsay-Hunt syndrome), temporal lobe epilepsy (vestibular epilepsy, seizure aura), Arnold-Chiari malformation, syringobulbia, migraine headache (HA), persistent vestibular dysfunction, diplopia.

c. **Others.** Drugs (tranquilizer, antihypertensives, antidepressants), metabolic (hypoxia, anemia, fever), hypotension, severe hypertension, cardiac arrhythmia, functional disorder, psychogenic (hyperventilation, hysteria).

BIBLIOGRAPHY

Bradley WG, Daroff RB, Fenichel GM, et al, editors: *Neurology in clinical practice: Principles of diagnosis and management*, vol 1, Boston, 1991, Butterworth-Heinemann.

Healey P, Jacobson EJ: *Common medical diagnoses: An algorithmic approach*, ed 2, Philadelphia, 1994, WB Saunders.

Isselbacher KJ, Braunwald E, Wilson JD, et al, editors: *Harrison's principle of internal medicine*, ed 13, New York, 1994, McGraw-Hill.

Paget S, Pellicci P, Beary JF, III, editors: *Manual of rheumatology and outpatient orthopedic disorders*, ed 3, Boston, 1993, Little, Brown.

Samuels M, editor: *Manual of neurologic therapeutics*, ed 5, Boston, 1995, Little, Brown.

Samuels MA, Feske S, editors: *Office practice of neurology*, New York, 1996, Churchill Livingstone.

Stein J, editor: *Internal medicine*, ed 4, St. Louis, 1994, CV Mosby.

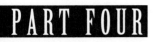

PART FOUR

PM&R Management Tools

CHAPTER 4.1

PHYSICAL MODALITIES

Modalities that use physical energy for their therapeutic effect (called physical modalities) are commonly prescribed in PM&R. They include thermotherapy (heat and cold), hydrotherapy, electrotherapy (including biofeedback), light therapy (ultraviolet radiation, laser), manipulation and mobilization, traction, massage, and acupuncture. Because of the passive nature of most of these modalities, they should not be prescribed indiscriminately. They should only be given for a short period as an adjunct, not as a substitute, to active modalities such as exercise and education.

I. **Therapeutic heat.** Physiologic response of tissue to heat depends on intensity of heat applied (therapeutic range is 40 to 45.5°C or 104 to 113.9°F), time of heat exposure (therapeutic range is 3-30 min), size/volume of area to be heated, and rate of temperature rise in the tissues (i.e., if heat rise is faster than heat dissipation, overheating may occur). Therapeutic heat causes vasodilation, which can either be local or consensual (i.e., distal vasodilation via reflex mechanism). In the subacute and chronic stage, vasodilation can help in resolving inflammatory infiltrates and exudates, and in promoting tissue healing (by increasing nutrient supply to the heated area). Other therapeutic effects of heat include increase in nerve pain threshold, increase in metabolic rate, decrease in firing rate of muscle spindles, and increase in plastic elongation of collagen fibers in connective tissues (i.e., when heat is combined with stretching).

General applications of heat include relief of pain and muscle spasm, reduction of joint stiffness, and increase in joint range of motion. General contraindications and precautions include acute inflammation, trauma, or hemorrhage; bleeding disorders (e.g., hemophilia); insensate skin (e.g., complete spinal cord injury [SCI]); inability to communicate or respond to pain (e.g., coma or dementia); poor thermal regulation (e.g., from neuroleptics); sites of malignancy; areas of ischemia (e.g., arterial insufficiency); atrophic skin (e.g., patients on prolonged steroid regimens); immature scar tissue; edema; and open wounds and infected skin lesions. Use of any form of heat must be supervised, especially in the elderly and the very young, because excessive heat may cause skin burn.

Methods of heat transfer include conduction (via physical contact between two surfaces), convection (through current movements in liquid or gases), and conversion (through absorption of electromagnetic energy, e.g., radiant heat, ultrasound, microwave, and short waves). Therapeutic heating agents can either be superficial or deep.

A. **Superficial heating agents** are used to heat joints with relatively little soft tissue covering (e.g., hand and foot) or to cause a deeper effect (e.g., relief of muscular spasm) through reflex mechanisms. They achieve maximum tissue temperatures in skin and subcutaneous fat.

1. **Conductive heat agents**

a. **Hot moist packs (hydrocollator packs)** are canvas bags filled with hydrophilic silicate and stored on racks in 70 to 80°C (158-176°F) water. The pack is wrapped in six to eight layers of towels and can be applied for 20 to 30 minutes. For home treatment, patients may use electrically controlled, moist heating pack (e.g., Thermophore) or a microwavable gel pack.

  b. **Paraffin** is a mixture of one part mineral oil to seven parts paraffin wax heated to 52 to 54°C (125.6-129.2°F). The mineral oil lowers the melting point of paraffin and the combination has low specific heat, which allows paraffin to be tolerable even at 47 to 54.4°C (118-130°F). Paraffin is most commonly used on irregular surfaces such as distal extremities of patients with rheumatoid arthritis, hand contractures, and scleroderma. It may be applied by dipping the extremity 8 to 10 times followed by wrapping in wax paper or a plastic bag then a covering with a towel to retain heat or by continuous immersion of the extremity in the paraffin bath. Application time is 20 to 30 minutes.

2. Convective heating agents

  a. **Fluidotherapy** uses a device that blows hot air through a container holding fine cellulose particles (made of beads or corn husks) to produce a dry, warm, air-fluid mixture with properties similar to those of a liquid. Temperature ranges from 38.8 to 47.8°C (102-118°F). The limb may be immersed for 20 to 30 minutes.

  b. **Hydrotherapy** (see section III below for details)

3. Radiant heating agent (infrared lamp). Infrared radiant energy is absorbed by the skin and converted to dry, superficial heat. Unlike hot packs, there is no discomfort from the weight of an object; however, only one body surface at a time can be heated. Distance from lamp to skin is usually 45 to 60 cm (18-24 in). Application time is 20 to 30 minutes.

B. Deep heating agents can increase tissue temperature to a depth of 3 to 5 cm or more without overheating skin and subcutaneous tissue. They are used to heat deeper structures such as the hip joint or the belly of the trapezius muscle. Deep heat is produced from the conversion of energy into heat as it penetrates the skin into the ligaments, muscles, bones, and joint capsules. The forms of energy used are high-frequency sound waves (ultrasound), high-frequency currents (shortwave diathermy), and electromagnetic radiation (microwave diathermy). Ultrasound is convenient and is commonly used, but both shortwave and microwave diathermies are cumbersome and are seldom used.

1. Ultrasound (US). Ceramic and quartz piezoelectric crystals are used to convert electric signals to ultrasonic soundwaves (with high frequency of 0.8 to 1.0 MHz), which are propagated through and are absorbed by the tissues and converted to heat. Ultrasound is absorbed and attenuated most in bone followed by, in decreasing order, tendon, skin, muscle, and fat. It is markedly attenuated by air and is totally reflected at the air-tissue interface. At the interface of bone and soft tissue, there is further increase in temperature because of the change in level of absorption and attenuation. Ultrasound, as a thermal agent, is used as an adjunct in the management of soft tissue dysfunctions including joint contracture, scar tissue (keloids), tendinitis, bursitis (calcific bursitis), myositis ossificans, skeletal muscle spasm, musculoskeletal pain, and postherpetic neuralgic pain. It produces temperatures of up to 46°C (114.8°F) in deep tissue (e.g., bone and muscle interface).

   The nonthermal effects of US include cavitation (gas bubble production in a sound field due to turbulence), acoustic streaming (unidirectional movement of compressible material or medium due to pressure asymmetries caused by the traveling ultrasonic waves) and standing waves (superposition of high and low pressure waves at half wavelength interval). Acoustic streaming and stable cavitation are believed to cause wound contraction and protein synthesis. Both thermal and nonthermal effects of US may facilitate tissue healing in dermal ulcers, incision wounds, tendon surgery, bone fractures, and nerve compression injury.

Ultrasound waves can be delivered continuously or in pulses. Usual dosage range from 0.5 to 2.0 watts/cm^2 for 5 to 10 minutes applied daily or every other day for 6 to 12 sessions. It may be applied directly to regular surface skin by stroking in linear or circular sweeps using a coupling medium (e.g., a water soluble gel), or rarely, by a stationary method. In areas with irregular surface (e.g., hand and ankle), both the US transducer and the area to be treated are placed under water at a distance of 1 cm between skin and transducer. The US transducer must be moved constantly to avoid hot spots, unstable cavitation (gas bubbles that continue to grow in size and then collapse), blood cell stasis, or blood vessel (endothelial cell) damage.

In addition to the general contraindications of heat, US should not be applied over fluid-filled cavities (e.g., eyes, testes, and pregnant uterus), the heart, cardiac pacemakers, brain, cervical and stellate ganglia, laminectomized spine, thrombophlebitic sites, growing epiphyses, infected bone, and malignant tumor. Its use in metal implants is controversial. Although studies have shown that metal implants do not concentrate heat energy, US must be used with caution in the presence of metal implants (e.g., screws, plates, or uncemented prostheses). When methylmethacrylate cement is used in joint replacements, however, US should not be used due to the possibility of loosening via unstable cavitation in the cement.

A form of ultrasound in which topical medications (mixed with the US coupling medium) are driven through the skin is called **phonophoresis (sonophoresis)**. Phonophoresis probably induces transdermal migration by increasing cell permeability through the thermal effects of ultrasound. Commonly used topical medications include corticosteroids (e.g., 1% or 10% hydrocortisone and dexamethasone) or local anesthetics (e.g., 1% lidocaine [Xylocaine]). Its main indications include tendinitis (e.g., Achilles, patellar, or bicipital), tenosynovitis, epicondylitis (e.g., tennis elbow), chronic suprahumeral impingement of shoulder, osteoarthritis, bursitis, capsulitis, strains, fasciitis, contracture, scar tissues, neuromas, and adhesions. Common US parameters include 1 or 2 MHz of continuous (or pulsed) ultrasound with an intensity of 1 to 3 W/cm^2 for 5 to 7 minutes per site. It may be given once per day for 3 or 4 consecutive days for a total of 10 days. Prolonged use should be avoided as it may cause tissue (e.g., tendon) weakening. Phonophoresis should not be confused with iontophoresis, which uses direct current to drive medications through the skin (see section V.A.1.a).

2. **Short wave diathermy (SWD)** uses radio waves (usually 27.12 MHz in the United States; other frequencies are 13.56 and 40.68 MHz) to heat the tissue by conversion. These radio waves, delivered either continuously or in pulses by a SWD machine, are transmitted through the area to be treated via a circuit element (i.e., a capacitor or inductor) and tuned as if the patient and the machine were components of a radio transmitter. It raises the temperature up to 15°C in the subcutaneous fat and 4 to 6°C in the muscle. It is applied for 15 to 30 minutes. Clinical indications include

muscle spasm, muscle and joint contractures, and tendinitis or bursitis. In addition to the aforementioned contraindications of general heating, it should not be used in the presence of jewelry, pacemakers, transcutaneous nerve or muscle stimulators, electrophrenic pacers, cerebellar stimulator, urinary bladder stimulator, surgical implants, contact lenses, metallic intra-uterine devices (IUDs), and the menstruating or pregnant uterus. Moist wound dressings, moist clothing, and perspiration can focus the heat and lead to overheating.

3. **Microwave diathermy (MWD)** uses electromagnetic radiation, at frequencies of 915 and 2450 MHz to heat the tissue by conversion. Like SWD, it raises the temperature in the subcutaneous fat (up to 10-12°C) more than muscle (3-4°C). It is applied for 15 to 30 minutes and is used to heat relatively superficial muscles and joints. It is also used to help resolve hematoma and to produce local hyperthermia in cancer treatment. It has the same contraindications as SWD.

II. **Therapeutic cold.** Physiologic effects of cold include local vasoconstriction, distal vasoconstriction (via reflex mechanism), decrease in metabolic rate and in the release of vasoactive agents (e.g., histamine), increase in nerve pain threshold, decrease in motor and sensory nerve conduction, decrease in sensitivity of muscle spindle to stretch (controversial), increase in tissue viscosity with de-creased tissue elasticity (this may increase joint stiffness), and transient increase in systolic and diastolic blood pressure. Methods of cold transfer include con-duction (e.g., using ice pack) and evaporation (i.e., use of volatile liquids, such as fluorimethane, which evaporates upon contact with skin producing a cool steam, which extracts heat from the skin surface). Although therapeutic cold is restricted to superficial application, the physiologic effect lasts longer than that of heat.

General applications of cold include relief of pain and muscle spasm, reduc-tion of spasticity and clonus, and control of inflammation and edema in the acute (within 24-48 hrs) posttraumatic stage. General contraindications and precautions include coldsensitivity symptoms (e.g., Raynaud's phenomenon, cold urticaria, cryoglobinemia, paroxysmal cold hemoglobinurias, and cold in-tolerance), circulatory-compromised areas (e.g., ischemic areas in patients with peripheral vascular disease affecting arterial system), the initial 2 to 3 weeks of wound healing stage, insensate skin (if cold is used, skin must be closely monitored for burns), severe hypertension (if cold is used, blood pressure must be monitored closely), and patients who are unable to communicate or respond to pain (e.g., comatose or demented patients). Use of cold must be closely supervised, especially in the elderly and the very young, because excessive cold may cause skin burn.

Depending on the size of the area to be cooled as well as its accessibility to cold application, one of the following methods of cold application can be used:

A. **Cold packs** are vinyl bags filled with silica gel or a sand slurry mixture stored in a refrigeration unit at −5°C (23°F). The pack is wrapped in moist towels and can be applied for 20 to 30 minutes. For home treatment, patients may use commercial gel packs (stored in a household freezer) or cold packs chemically activated by squeezing or hitting them against a hard surface.

B. **Ice massage** consists of rubbing a piece of ice onto the skin in overlapping strokes. The ice may be frozen in paper cups or onto a tongue depressors, i.e., ice ''lollipops.'' Ice massage is indicated for cooling a small area (e.g., muscle belly, tendon, or trigger point) before deep-pressure massage. Analgesia can be attained in 7 to 10 minutes.

C. Ice towels are terrycloth towels soaked in a bucket of crushed ice or in ice slush mixture, wrung out, and wrapped around a joint. The towel must be changed after 4 to 5 minutes to retain its coldness. This method is impractical.

D. Cold baths are water-filled containers (e.g., iced whirlpool) with temperatures of 13 to 18°C (55.4-64.4°F) into which the distal limb is immersed for cooling. Treatment time is from 20 to 30 minutes.

E. Vapocoolant sprays use volatile liquids such as ethyl chloride or fluorimethane for inhibiting spasms (in combination with "spray and stretch" exercise [see Chapter 4.11, section II.A.1.b], "spray and limber" exercise [see Chapter 4.11, section II.A.1.a]) and for local skin anesthesia. Fluorimethane is less volatile and less flammable than ethyl chloride.

F. Controlled cold compression units use sleeves containing circulating cold water (with adjustable temperature) into which the edematous limb is placed. This sleeve is then attached to an intermittent pump unit.

III. Hydrotherapy is the external use of water for treating physical dysfunctions. This effect is achieved through the physical properties of water (i.e., buoyancy, pressure, relative density, and viscosity), temperature, and agitation. Buoyancy provides assistive exercise (when motion occurs toward the water surface) and resistive exercise (when motion occurs away from the water surface). Hydrostatic pressure helps in circulation and decreases the tendency of blood pooling in the lower part of the body. Relative density (measured in specific gravity) provides support for the body or limb, thus reducing stress on the weight-bearing joint. The viscosity of water is low thus providing little friction with low-speed movements. As speed increases, there is also increase in turbulence (positive pressure) and drag (negative pressure), hence there is greater friction, making movements more difficult. The thermal effects of hydrotherapy are the same as in local heat or cold application except that there is more systemic effect because of immersion of the larger body surface. Cold can decrease heart rate and increase blood pressure by peripheral vasoconstriction. Heat increases heart rate and causes an initial increase in blood pressure, followed by a drop in blood pressure due to vasodilation. Respiratory rate increases in both heat and cold hydrotherapy but less markedly with heat. The methods of heat or cold transfer are by conduction and convection.

The nonthermal (mechanical) effect of hydrotherapy is achieved through water pumps or turbines, which agitate the water and provide massage and debridement. The physiologic effects of water agitation include relief of pain and muscle spasm (through mechanical stimulation of skin receptors, which may act as a counterirritant or as a stimulation to large sensory afferents, thus blocking pain input), mechanical debridement, and facilitation of exercise. If only mechanical effect is desired, water at neutral temperature (33-36°C or 91.4-96.8°F) is well tolerated.

Indications for hydrotherapy include wound and burn treatment, joint mobilization after cast removal, rheumatoid arthritis, and muscle spasm. General contraindications and precautions are the same as in therapeutic heat and cold except that hydrotherapy may be applied on open and infected wounds as long as the tanks are sterilized. For wound treatment, whirlpool disinfecting additives commonly used are povidone-iodine solution, sodium hypochlorite, household bleach, and chloramine-T.

A. Whirlpools are tanks used for partial body immersion. The "limb" tank is used for immersion of one or both upper limbs or the distal lower limb. The "lowboy" and "highboy" tanks are used for lower limb immersion or immersion of the trunk up to the midthoracic level. In the lowboy tank the patient is in the long sitting position and can perform full range-of-motion (ROM) exercises of both knees. In the highboy tank, the patient is seated in chest high water with flexed hips and knees. Usual temperature is 37.8 to 38.9°C (100-102°F) for the lower limbs and 37.8 to 40.6°C (100-105°F) for the upper limbs. Temperatures of 43°C (109.4°F) to as high as 45 or 46°C (113 or 114.8°F) may be applied for 5 to 20 minutes.

B. **Hubbard tanks** are used for whole body immersion. The shape and design of the tank allow for motion of all four limbs and accessibility of the patient to the therapist. Temperatures should be less than 39°C (102.2°F) to avoid systemic problems. For mild heating, 36.7 to 37.2°C (98-98.9°F) may be used, while for more vigorous heating, 37.8 to 38.3°C (100-100.9°F) may be used. Duration of treatment is 10 to 20 minutes depending on cardiopulmonary tolerance. In addition to the general contraindications of hydrotherapy, it should not be used in patients who are incontinent of bowel or bladder, have skin infections, unstable blood pressure, uncontrolled epilepsy, severe mental disorders, acute febrile episodes, upper respiratory infections, and tuberculosis. Caution should be used in pulmonary patients with vital capacities of less than one liter.

C. **Pool therapy** is used to promote patient relaxation, improve circulation, restore mobility, strengthen muscles, provide gait training with reduced stress on weight-bearing joints, and improve psychological and emotional outlook (because patients are usually able to ambulate better in water by using water's buoyancy). Specific clinical indications include rheumatoid arthritis, orthopedic patients with musculoskeletal disorders or joint replacements, patients with neurologic disorders (e.g., multiple sclerosis in nonheated pools and incomplete paraplegia) or those with partial peripheral lesions (e.g., poliomyelitis, polyneuritis), and in mild cases of spastic cerebral palsy (e.g., postrhizotomy). Unlike whirlpool therapy, pool patients must not have open or discharging wounds. General contraindications are the same as for Hubbard tanks. Patients with incontinent bladders may use the pool as long as they are catheterized. For patients with spasticity or for those requiring immersion up to 20 to 45 minutes, lower temperatures of 30 to 34.5°C (86-94°F) are used. Patients with multiple sclerosis require temperatures of 29°C (84°F) or less. Arthritic patients may be immersed for 10 to 20 minutes at higher temperatures of 36 to 37°C (96.8-98.6°F).

D. **Contrast bath** is a special technique of treating the distal limb using the whirlpool tank. It alternates exposure of the limb to heat (38-44°C or 100.4-111°F) and cold (10-18°C or 50-64.4°F) to produce reflex hyperemia. Typical treatment begins with an initial soaking of the limb in the warm whirlpool for 10 minutes and then followed by four cycles of alternate 1- to 4-minute cold soaks (in a basin of water) and 4- to 6-minute warm soaks (in the whirlpool tank). It is used for rheumatoid arthritis, reflex sympathetic dystrophy, joint sprains, muscular strains, mild peripheral vascular diseases, and to toughen amputation stumps. Aside from the general contraindication to heat and cold, it should not be used when patients have small vessel disease caused by diabetes, arteriosclerotic endarteritis, or Burger's disease.

IV. **Light therapy**

A. **Ultraviolet radiation (UVR)** has a wavelength of 2000 to 4000 angstroms (bactericidal wavelength is 2537 A) and can be produced by a small, handheld, low-pressure mercury or "cold quartz" lamp. Ultraviolet radiation interacts with tissue and bacteria, causing nonthermal photochemical reactions and alterations in DNA and cell proteins. Its physiologic effects include bactericidal effect on motile bacteria, increase vascularization at wound margins, hyperplasia and exfoliation (peeling), tanning, increased vitamin D production, and excitation of calcium metabolism. The major clinical indication of UVR today is treatment of wounds (aseptic or septic) and dermatologic conditions such as psoriasis (using Goeckerman technique, i.e., application of coal tar ointment to skin prior to UVR), acne, and folliculitis.

Dosages are determined by exposure time required to produce erythema on the volar aspect of the forearm. Minimal erythemal dose (MED), also called the first-degree erythema, is the exposure time necessary to produce a faint erythema within a few hours in average Caucasian skin. The MED subsides within 24 hours. A 2.5 MED exposure produces second-degree erythema in 4 to 6 hours with pain and subsides in 2 to 4 days, followed by desquamation. A 5 MED exposure produces third-degree erythema in 2 to 4 hours with pain and local edema followed by marked desquamation. A 10 MED exposure produces fourth-degree erythema with superficial blister. Usual UVR prescription doses begin with 1 or 2 MED and are kept to less than 5 MED. It is given 2 to 3 times per week.

Ultraviolet radiation must be used with caution in persons using photosensitizing drugs or cosmetics; in persons with fair complexion, scars, or atrophic skin; or in the presence of acute renal and hepatic failures, severe diabetes, hyperthyroidism, generalized dermatitis, advanced arteriosclerosis, and active, progressive pulmonary tuberculosis (TB). To prevent conjunctivitis and photokeratosis, the eyes of both patient and therapist must be shielded (using UV goggles or cotton pledgets). Contraindications include porphyrias, pellagra, sarcoidosis, and the acute onset of psoriasis, lupus erythematosus, eczema, herpes simplex, and xeroderma pigmentosum.

B. **Low-power cold laser.** LASER is the acronym for Light Amplification by Stimulated Emission of Radiation. Lasers emit photons (energy particles of light) that can interact with biological molecules to produce light-induced thermal or chemical reactions in the body. Laser devices can either be thermal (hot) or nonthermal (i.e., cold, lowpower, or soft). In PM&R, low-power cold laser produced by helium-neon gas (He-Ne lasers) or by gallium-arsenide semiconductors (Ga-As lasers) are commonly used. **He-Ne lasers** deliver a red beam with wavelength of 632.8 nanometer (nm) in a continuous wave and have direct effects in the first 2 to 5 mm of soft tissue and indirect effects up to 10 to 15 mm deep. **Ga-As lasers** are invisible with a wavelength of 904 nm delivered in pulse mode and have direct penetration of 1 to 2 cm and indirect penetration of up to 5 cm.

Physiologic effects of cold lasers include facilitation of wound and ulcer healing by stimulating fibroblasts; increasing tensile strength of laser-treated wound; increasing phagocytosis by leukocytes with bactericidal effects; increasing T and B lymphocyte activities; reduction of edema by decreasing prostaglandin E_2 (PGE_2); reducing scar tissue formation by promoting epithelization with less exudative material and with more regular alignment of collagen; pain reduction by reducing action potential amplitude and decreasing sensory conduction velocity; and promotion of bone healing by bone and articular cartilage remodeling.

Clinical uses include wound and ulcer healing, burns, sprain, strain, contusions, pain (e.g., back and neck pain, osteoarthritis, headache, and neuropathy), and fracture nonunion. For pain treatment, the laser may be applied over acupuncture points or at painful nerve sites or by combining with electrical stimulation.

Contraindications include cancerous tissue, direct stimulation into the eyes (may cause retinal burns), and the first trimester of pregnancy. A temporary increase in pain or syncopal feeling may be experienced during treatment, but these are generally are self-limited.

The usual dose is 0.05 to 0.5 joules per cm^2 for acute conditions and 0.5 to 3.0 joules per cm^2 for more chronic conditions for 3 to 6 treatments. Treatment time is in seconds/cm^2 and varies with the prescribed J/cm^2.

V. Electrotherapy is the therapeutic use of electricity to transcutaneously stimulate the nerve or the muscle or both using surface electrodes. Its physiologic effects include muscle group contraction, which can increase joint ROM, reeducate muscles, retard muscle atrophy, and increase muscle strength; increase circulation with relief of pain and muscle spasm via muscle pumping effect, and release of polypeptides and neurotransmitters (e.g., β-endorphins, dopamine, enkephalins, vasoactive intestinal polypeptides, and serotonin); inhibition of pain fibers via stimulation of large peripheral type A nerve fibers (e.g., gate-control theory and central-biasing theory); wound healing and osteogenesis (via tissue regeneration and remodeling); and for driving medicated ions through the skin (iontophoresis).

Clinical indications include pain management (acute and chronic musculoskeletal pain, chronic neurogenic pain, general systemic pain), joint effusion or interstitial edema (acute and chronic); protective muscle spasm; muscle disuse atrophy; dermal ulcers and wounds; and circulatory disorders (venous insufficiency, neurovascular disorder).

General contraindications include circulatory impairment (e.g., arterial or venous thrombosis and thrombophlebitis), stimulation over the carotid sinus, stimulation across the heart (especially in patients with demand pacemakers), pregnancy, seizure disorders, fresh fractures, active hemorrhage, and malignancy. Direct current and can cause electrochemical burns and should not be used in skin with decreased sensation.

Treatment time per session is variable. It can be 1 to 5 minutes per trigger point in the monopolar treatment of chronic musculoskeletal pain; 10 to 30 minutes for acute pain and circulatory disorders; 30 to 60 minutes for skin ulcers and wounds; 2 to 4 hrs for edema control; and a few to many repetitions for muscle strengthening. It can be once or twice daily or three times per week for a few weeks. For treatment time using transcutaneous electrical nerve stimulators (TENS), see section IV.E.

In PM&R, transcutaneous electrical stimulators (TES) can be classified by the type of current as direct current (DC), alternating current (AC), or pulsed current. It can also be classified by its stimulation effect as subliminal (nonperceived) current, TENS, and neuromuscular electrical stimulator (NMES). Technically speaking, all pulsed and most AC currents (except when used for subliminal or subthreshold stimulation) are *TENS* because they work transcutaneously and excite the peripheral nerve. However, in common usage, *TENS* refers to the small, portable, battery-operated TES unit used for pain relief. The TES used for neuromuscular stimulation of innervated muscles are called NMES.

A. TES classification by type of therapeutic current

    1. Direct current (DC) is an electrical current that flows in one direction for at least 1 sec.

        a. Continuous or uninterrupted low-voltage DC (galvanic current) is used to promote healing of superficial skin ulcers (mainly by changing skin pH and causing reflex vasodilation) and to facilitate union of fracture. It is the current used to drive ions through the skin in **iontophoresis**. Indications for iontophoresis include administration of local anesthetics (e.g., 1% lidocaine) in neuritis or bursitis; reduction of edema in acute and chronic musculoskeletal inflammatory conditions (e.g., bursitis, tendinitis, and ligamentous sprain) using topical corticosteroids (e.g., 1% or 10% hydrocortisone and dexamethasone), sodium salicylate, or hyaluronidase (Wydase); promoting muscle relaxation and vasodilation using magnesium sulfate (Epsom salts); softening scars and adhesions using sodium chloride; and reducing calcium deposits in calcific tendinitis using acetic acid. Iontophoresis can also be used for the treatment of skin conditions like idiopathic hyperhydrosis using tap water, small (<1 cm) open ischemic ulcers using zinc oxide, and fungus infections (*Tinea pedis*) using copper sulfate.

It is contraindicated in persons with previous allergic reaction to the iontophoresis agent and in insensate skin. The intensity of iontophoresis current range from microamperes (more comfortable but takes longer to apply) to 5 mA (or even up to 30 mA). Although transdermal penetration of drugs via iontophoresis or phonoresis has been reported in animal studies, this has not been clearly substantiated in humans. Except for occasional superficial skin blisters caused by iontophoresis, both iontophoresis and phonophoresis are safe, noninvasive, and generally not associated with the systemic side-effects of the medication.

  b. **Modulated DC** can either be reversed, interrupted, or surged (ramped). It is not commonly used because it is uncomfortable and can potentially cause skin burns. It has been used to directly stimulate denervated muscle fibers and to retard atrophy. However, recent studies have shown that electrical stimulation of denervated muscles may be deleterious possibly due to muscle fiber degeneration (with or without associated fibrosis) and retardation of reinnervation.

2. **Alternating current (AC)** is an electrical current that changes the direction of flow (i.e., with reference to the zero baseline) at least once every second.

  a. **Continuous or uninterrupted AC** is a bidirectional current, with no interval between pulses and no modulation. This current is often referred to simply as AC and is the household electrical current used in North America (i.e., 60 Hz AC).

  b. **Modulated AC**

  1) **Time-modulated AC** in burst mode is referred to as **"Russian" current**. It has been used for muscle reeducation. However, it has a fixed-phase duration, uses unnecessarily high total current, is not indicated for strong contraction of small muscles, and is less versatile and less comfortable than symmetric biphasic pulsed current. Studies have shown that pulsed current (i.e., pulsed high-volt monophasic or biphasic currents) are just as effective as ''Russian'' current for muscle reeducation during motor stimulation.

  2) **Amplitude-modulated AC** can be produced by mixing two AC sources with different frequency to generate **interferential current (IFC)**. The IFC has been used for relief of acute superficial pain or chronic deep aching pain from various tissue origins, for vascular conditions (e.g., Raynaud's disease, venous insufficiency, and orthostatic hypotension), and for urogenital dysfunction (e.g., urinary stress inconti-

nence). However, their effectiveness over other forms of current (e.g., pulsed current) remain controversial. Like the "Russian" current, IFC has a fixed-phase duration, uses unnecessarily high total current, and is less versatile and less comfortable than symmetric biphasic pulsed current during motor stimulation.

3. **Pulsed current** is an electrical current conducted as a signal of short duration with each pulse lasting only a few milliseconds or microseconds followed by an interpulse interval. Pulsed current is classified by its waveform as either monophasic (one phase to each pulse) or biphasic (two opposing phases in each pulse).

   a. **Monophasic pulsed current**

      1) **Low-voltage monophasic pulsed current (diadynamic current)** usually has sinusoidal wave and provides direct excitatory responses. It is very uncomfortable and is obsolete.

      2) **High-voltage monophasic pulsed current (HVPC)** is used for wound healing (e.g., decubitus ulcer and postsurgical wounds), pain modulation (e.g., before debriding burns and in hand injuries), edema and muscle spasm reduction (e.g., sprains and strains), muscle reeducation and maintenance of muscle integrity (e.g., disuse atrophy), and prevention of postoperative deep vein thrombosis. Like the modulated AC, HVPC has a fixed-phase duration, uses unnecessarily high total current, is not indicated for strong contraction of large muscles, and is less versatile and less comfortable than symmetric biphasic pulsed current during motor stimulation.

   b. **Biphasic pulsed current**

      1) **Asymmetric biphasic pulsed current (Faradic current)** used to be mistaken as a form of AC. This low-voltage current is not very comfortable and has limited clinical use due to limited current modulation.

      2) **Symmetric biphasic pulsed current** with interphase (also termed *intrapulse*) interval is an optimally designed current, which is comfortable and can be used for stimulating peripheral nerves and for connective tissue regeneration and osteogenesis.

B. **TES classification by stimulation effect**

1. **Subliminal or nonperceived current (microcurrent electrical neuromuscular stimulation [MENS])** is a low-frequency, low-intensity current given below threshold of nerve stimulation ("subliminal"). It has been used in alcohol and drug addiction, acute and chronic pain, protective muscle spasm, inflammation, and in promoting tissue regeneration (connective tissues, bones, nerves). Its efficacy, however, remains controversial.

2. **Transcutaneous electrical nerve stimulation (TENS)** is the transmission of electrical current to stimulate nerve fibers for the symptomatic relief of pain. Its proposed mechanism of pain control is based on the gate-control theory of Melzack and Wall (i.e., stimulation of large A fibers modulates pain-input transmission of small-diameter A-delta and C fibers at the dorsal horn), the "central biasing" or "central control trigger" theory (a modification of the gate control theory wherein large fiber activates central inhibitory mechanisms that descend to modulate pain transmission neurons within the dorsal horns), and the endogenous opiate pain-control theory (e.g., β-endorphin).

   The TENS unit is a portable, battery-powered device the size of a cigarette pack. It transmits current impulses through lead wires and electrodes attached to the patient's skin. Some units offer monophasic pulses,

Table 4.1-1. **Types of TENS stimulation. The frequency and duration are usually preset. The amplitude or intensity is adjusted until the desired level of paresthesia (P) or contraction (C) is reached**

STIMULATION MODES*	FREQUENCY (pps or Hz)	DURATION (μs)	AMPLITUDE (mA)
1. Conventional†	High 50-100 Hz	Narrow 30-75 μs	P = mild C = none 10-30 mA
2. Strong Low Rate‡ (acupuncture-like)	Low 1-4 Hz	Wide 150-200 μs	P = highest tolerable C = rhythmic 30-80 mA
3. Pulse burst a. Low-Intensity	2 bursts/sec 70-100 Hz/burst	Narrow 40-75 μs	P = mild C = none 30-60 mA
b. High-Intensity	2 bursts/sec 70-100 Hz/burst	Wide 150-200 μs	P = mild C = rhythmic 30-60 mA
4. Brief Intense§	High 100-150 Hz	Wide 150-200 μs	P = highest tolerable C = nonrhythmic or tetanic 30-80 mA

Adapted from Mannheimer JS, Lampe GN: Electrode placement sites and their relationships. In JS Mannheimer, GN Lampe, editors: *Clinical transcutaneous electrical nerve stimulation.* Philadelphia; 1984, FA Davis, p. 338, with permission.
* Usual patient preference: conventional > modulated > pulse-burst > strong low-rate > brief intense.
† Conventional mode: onset of relief is within 1-20 minutes with post-TENS analgesia equal to that of stimulation duration or even lasting 1-3 hours or longer; used for all types of pain (especially musculoskeletal pain).
‡ Strong low rate mode, the onset of relief is within 20-30 minutes with post-TENS analgesia lasting 2-6 hours; used in chronic neuropathic pain (e.g., reflex sympathetic dystrophy), deep structural pain, fibrositis/myofascial pain syndrome.
§ Brief intense mode is seldom used except as an adjunct to joint mobilization.

while others offer symmetrical or asymmetrical biphasic pulses; few offer burst or amplitude modulated AC pulses. Some bigger, nonportable TES units, for example IFC units and HVPC units can also be used as a TENS. Short-wave diathermy can be pulsed at a high-frequency (27 MHz) electromagnetic radiation and can be used as a TENS alternative instead of a deep heating device.

Most TENS units have three stimulation parameters: pulse rate, pulse duration, and amplitude (or intensity). The pulse rate and duration are usually preset, but the intensity is adjustable. The four modes of TENS stimulation as described by Mannheimer are listed in Table 4.1-1. In the conventional mode, the onset of relief is within 1 to 20 minutes with post-TENS analgesia equal to that of stimulation duration or even lasting 1 to 3 hours or longer; however, in the strong low-rate mode, the onset of relief is within 20 to 30 minutes with post-TENS analgesia lasting 2 to 6 hours. The prolonged effects could probably be due to the release of endorphins.

In the newer TENS units, the current may be modulated, i.e., one or more parameters (rate, duration, or intensity) can be set automatically to fluctuate according to a preset level, usually within a range of 40 to 100% from the starting level, once or twice each second. The aim of TENS modulation is to improve patient tolerance and prevent nerve accommodation. Among the TENS stimulation modes, patient preference is usually conventional > modulated > pulse-burst > strong low-rate > brief intense. The brief intense mode is seldom used except as an adjunct to joint mobilization.

Treatment duration of TENS is usually 30 minutes to 1 hour per session, with a maximum of 2 hours per session, for a total of 8 hours per day. This is continued for 3 weeks and then gradually reduced in the next 8 to 12 weeks.

3. **Neuromuscular electrical stimulators (NMES)** are TES units used for the stimulation of muscles with intact peripheral nervous system or muscles that are decentralized (i.e., following central nervous system or spinal cord injury). Their use in denervated muscles is controversial due to reports of deleterious effects such as retardation of reinnervation and degeneration of muscle fibers. The NMES is more powerful than the TENS unit and is usually modulated to provide interrupted current for stronger motor excitation.

The NMES is used to strengthen or maintain muscle mass (i.e., retard atrophy) or both during or following periods of immobilization. (The NMES has been shown to increase muscle strength even without voluntary effort by the subject. It can also convert type II fast muscles fibers into type I slow fibers, although this change is reversible after cessation of NMES.) It can maintain or gain joint ROM (in soft tissue joint contractures), enhance voluntary motor control (through facilitation technique or muscle reeducation program), temporarily reduce the effects of spasticity, and act as semipermanent replacement of conventional bracing (e.g., to gain normal shoulder alignment of subluxed shoulders in hemiparetic patients and to assist dorsiflexion in stroke patients with foot drop or in spinal cord injury patients).

In patients with paralysis due to decentralization, NMES can be used for conditioning and strengthening exercises (e.g., computerized NMES to induce coordinated knee flexion and extension so the patient can pedal a bicycle ergometer or exercise using an isokinetic knee dynamometer). When NMES is used to activate multiple muscles in a coordinated sequential manner to attain specific functional goals (e.g., functional ambulation in paraplegics and hand grasp and standing transfers in tetraplegics), it is called **functional electrical stimulation (FES) or functional neuromuscular stimulation (FNS)**.

VI. **Biofeedback (BF)** is the process of monitoring internal physiological events using equipment (usually electronics) that can display these otherwise involuntary or unfelt events in the form of visual and auditory signals. These signals are then fed back to the patients so they learn how to manipulate them and thus regulate their own internal physiological events. It is used in psychotherapy, for relaxation in patients with chronic pain (e.g., tension headache, vascular headache, and chronic neck and back pain), Raynaud's disease, urinary and fecal incontinence, sports medicine, and psychoimmunology. Specific PM&R conditions that might benefit from biofeedback include stroke, SCI, cerebral palsy (CP), traumatic brain injury (TBI), multiple sclerosis (MS), dystonias and dyskinesias, peripheral nerve denervation, and orthopedic disorders. Biofeedback has no specific medical contraindication; however, it should only be prescribed if patients have potential for voluntary control, are well-motivated and cooperative, and are able to follow commands (e.g., no receptive aphasia). In general, biofeedback training is given two to three times per week with each session lasting about 30 to 45 minutes. Between training sessions the patient is given detailed instructions to carry out a program of repetitive, daily, self-administered exercises at home. The length of biofeedback training varies from 3 months up to 2 years. Biofeedback treatment programs must be regularly monitored by the physiatrist to ensure that the patient is benefiting from it.

A. Myoelectric or electromyographic biofeedback (EMG-BF) is the most widely used form of biofeedback in PM&R. It transduces muscle potentials into auditory or visual cues to help patient learn how to increase or decrease voluntary muscular activities. It is used for muscle recruitment in patients with peripheral nerve injury, muscle weakness due to immobilization, joint surgery, deconditioning, pain, antagonists to spastic muscles, muscle-tendon transfers, reeducation of weak or flaccid muscle, and recovery of shoulder control poststroke. It can also be used to help relax patients with stress-related hyperarousal, pain, spasticity, rigidity, and torticollis.

B. Position biofeedback is used to help patients regulate position and movement so they can develop appropriate timing and coordination. It can be used to train for head position control; coordination and control of hand movements in ataxia and following hand surgery; and knee joint position in children with cerebral palsy, adults with hemiplegia, and prosthesis wearers. It can also be used to train muscles that are difficult to isolate (e.g., pronation and supination of forearm) in stroke patients.

C. Pressure or force biofeedback is used to determine the amount of force being transmitted through a body segment or assistive device, for example, training of symmetrical standing gait in hemiplegics, use of a feedback cane to determine amount of force borne by the cane, and gait analysis.

D. Blood pressure biofeedback uses regular plethysmography to train patients how to relax. This is usually used in conjunction with EMG-BF and BF for temperature control of limbs.

E. Sphincteral control training uses perineal EMG-BF with pressure transducers in the anal canal or vagina, for sphincteral training in patients with incontinence.

F. Respiratory biofeedback is used for training breathing functions in patients with respiratory problems, for example, asthma and high level SCI.

G. Temperature and peripheral blood flow biofeedback is used by clinical psychologists usually for relaxation. It is also used for Raynaud's disease.

H. Electroencephalographic (EEG) biofeedback is used mainly for relaxation training.

VII. Spinal traction is a pulling force applied to the cervical or lumbar spine for the following physiological effects: vertebral joint distraction; prevention and loosening of adhesions within the dural sleeves, nerve roots and adjacent capsular structures; reduction of compression and irritation of the nerve root and disc; improvement of the circulation within the epidural spaces of nerve root canals; and reduction of pain, inflammation, and muscle spasm.

The most common clinical indication of spinal traction is to relieve pain from disc herniation, with or without concomitant nerve root compression. In acute lumbar disc herniation, lumbar mechanical traction has been used to keep the patient immobile in bed.

The main reason for spinal traction failure is inadequate pull because of insufficient weight and improper neck or body positioning or both. Hence spinal traction must never be used by anyone with inadequate training. Cervical and lumbar traction are contraindicated in spondylotic myelopathy, malignancy (e.g., lytic lesions), osteopenia, spinal infection (e.g., disciitis and TB), acute soft tissue injury, congenital spinal deformity, hypertension or cardiovascular disease, and in anxious patients who are unable to relax. Additional contraindications for cervical traction are cervical ligamentous instability (e.g., in rheumatoid arthritis, Down's syndrome, or patients with hypermobile joints), atlantoaxial subluxation with spinal cord compromise, vertebrobasilar arterial insufficiency, atherosclerosis of the carotid or vertebral arteries, and acute whiplash injury. Most of these conditions are commonly seen during old age, thus spinal traction must be used with caution in the elderly. In lumbar traction, additional contraindications (due to the use of chest and abdominal harness) include pregnancy, cauda equina compression, aortic aneurysm, active peptic ulcers, hiatal or other hernia, and restrictive lung disease or other breathing disorder.

Prescription of spinal traction depends more on the practitioner's empirical observation than on objective data. The parameters to be considered are positioning, weight to be used, duration, and sustained (static) versus intermittent application. Most importantly, the patient must be comfortable and the traction must not cause nor aggravate pain.

Spinal traction is usually used in conjunction with other modalities for relaxation, such as heat and massage. Patients receiving traction must be given exercises and postural reeducation to maintain the effect of traction. Ideally, mechanical spinal traction should only be started if active modalities or if manual traction has not achieved the desired goal. If the symptoms have worsened or if there is no improvement after six to eight sessions, traction should be discontinued.

A. Cervical traction

  1. Manual cervical traction is a type of spinal manipulation used as a trial before application of mechanical (motorized or home) traction. Patient is positioned in supine with the head supported on the therapist's hand so that the patient's neck is flexed to about 20 to 25 degrees. A tractive force is then applied by the therapist to the patient's occiput (not to the mandible).

  2. Mechanical cervical traction uses free weights and pulley systems to pull the cervical spine. Depending on the patient's size, neurologic symptoms, specific lesions, and comfort, the weight used ranges from 10 to 35 lb applied for 15 to 20 minutes (a 10-lb minimum is necessary to counterbalance the weight of the head) with the patient's neck flexed 20 to 30 degrees in either a seated or supine position. The greater the traction force, the shorter the traction time needed. Treatment is provided three to four times per week for 10 to 15 sessions (or 3-4 weeks).

    a. Intermittent mechanical cervical traction is a motorized traction with adjustable rest periods (in seconds) in between traction pulls. Compared to sustained (static) traction, it is more comfortable and patients can tolerate greater amount of weight. It must be monitored by a physical therapist during treatment, which is both an advantage (because the amount of weight and neck positioned is monitored) and a disadvantage (because patient must come to the physical therapy office for treatment).

    b. Sustained (static) mechanical cervical traction

      1) Motorized static mechanical cervical traction applies a constant level of traction to induce fatigue in the paraspinal muscles so that more pull can theoretically be transmitted to the cervical spine. Compared to intermittent traction, it is less comfortable and most patients can only tolerate a small amount of weight.

2) **Nonmotorized static mechanical cervical traction** is a home-unit traction consisting of a head harness, rope and pulley system, and a counter weight (usually a bag filled with 20 or more pounds of water or sand). They can be applied in a seated position (by attaching the pulley system over the door or onto the wall) or in supine position (by attaching the pulley system to the bed). Home cervical tractions are usually ineffective, probably because of incorrect use (inadequate amount of weight, improper head and neck position) and poor compliance. Hence, a physical therapist must regularly monitor the patient's technique of application by having the patient demonstrate it.

B. **Lumbar traction** needs a great amount of force to attain lumbar distraction (usually between 65 and 200 lb or half the patient's body weight) and is not as effective as cervical traction. There are several home lumbar traction units currently available, but none are shown to be effective.

1. **Manual lumbar traction** is a type of spinal manipulation used as a trial before application of mechanical lumbar traction. Because of the tremendous amount of force needed to separate the lumbar vertebrae, a split table (with a fixed and a mobile segment) is usually needed to decrease frictional forces between the body and the table surface. The patient is either positioned sidelying to provide manual traction to a specific vertebral level or supine for a unilateral leg-pull manual traction.

2. **Mechanical lumbar traction** uses a split table, a nonslip traction harness and a pulley system. The patient is attached to the truncal traction harness and positioned in a neutral spinal position either supine with hips flexed to about 90 degrees or prone. The harness is then connected to the pulley system, which provides traction by weights or by a motorized device.

a. **Intermittent mechanical lumbar traction:**

1) **Traditional intermittent mechanical lumbar traction** uses a motorized pulley system, which provides rest periods (e.g., 5 to 15 seconds) between each traction pull (progressive force of up to 50 lb applied for 7 to 60 seconds). The treatment protocol can either be pre-programmed or patient-controlled. Treatment duration is usually between 20 to 30 minutes. It is better tolerated than sustained mechanical lumbar traction.

2) **Vertebral Axial Decompression (VAX-D) Therapeutic Table** is a recently-developed split-design table that uses a fully automated system to provide gradual intermittent mechanical lumbar traction. The patient lies prone on the table and fixes the upper body by grasping adjustable hangrips, designed to eliminate the use of a chest harness. A pelvic harness applies distraction forces (ranging from 20-100 lb) primarily to the lateral pelvic crests along the natural anatomical lines of the spinal column with minimal anterior-posterior pressures. Treatment consists of a series of 10 to 20 decompression-relaxation cycles administered once or twice daily over a period of 2 to 3 weeks, each session lasting 30 to 45 minutes. The procedure is generally safe as the patient can release the handgrip at any time to end the session.

Intradiscal-pressure studies of five cases showed that the VAX-D effectively decompresses the nucleus pulposus to pressures below minus 100 mm Hg. Uncontrolled clinical trials showed it to be effective in relieving low back pain in selected patients with herniated disks, degenerative disk disease, posterior facet syndrome, and radicular pain. However, further clinical trials (ideally, controlled and randomized) are needed to determine its long-term effectiveness in reducing back pain and disability.

   b. Sustained (static) mechanical lumbar traction uses a steady amount of weight (less than that of intermittent lumbar traction but greater than that of continuous lumbar traction) for 10-30 minutes (or up to 1 hour). It is not as well tolerated as intermittent traction.

   c. Continuous mechanical lumbar traction uses light weights for several hours (up to 20 to 40 hours). It is not effective in distracting the lumbar vertebrae, and its sole use is to enforce bedrest during acute disc herniation.

   3. Autotraction uses a specially designed table on which the patient administers sliding tractive force by pulling with the hands on the grasp bar at the head of the table while a traction belt restrains the pelvis to the table. This active form of traction seems to provide more symptomatic relief than the passive forms of lumbar tractions and has the advantage of having the patient regulate the traction force. Treatment is usually applied every 2 to 3 days for 6 to 10 treatments.

   4. Gravity or inversion traction is a positional traction that uses the weight of the body hanging upside down from a bar to distract the lumbar vertebrae. This is often accompanied by numerous musculoskeletal and other complaints and is contraindicated in patients with hypertension, bleeding disorders, and glaucoma. It should be prescribed with caution, or not at all.

VIII. Manipulation as done in PM&R by either a physiatrist or physical therapist is a skilled passive, mechanical movement applied to a specific joint or to a joint segment to restore its motion or extensibility and to reduce pain. It must be differentiated from massage (applied to soft tissue), mechanical traction (nonspecific), and active exercise. While manipulation may be used alone, it is usually helpful to add short-term nonsteroidal antiinflammatory drugs (see Chapter 4.8, section I.A.3) or other analgesics and to diminish the postmanipulation tissue inflammatory reaction. In acute cases, a brace might be necessary to immobilize the spine. Active modalities, such as exercise and education, must be provided to maintain the effects of manipulation and prevent recurrence.

   Various hypotheses for pain relief achieved with manipulation include mechanical or reflex relaxation of soft tissues due to restoration of vertebral range of motion, normalization of bulging disc by the suction forces created or by stretching the posterior longitudinal ligament, which pushes the disc material anteriorly, away from pain-sensitive structures, and alteration of proprioceptive input to the spinal cord causing the "gate" to close.

   A. Spinal manipulation is the application of passive maneuvers (anterior-posterior glide, lateral flexion tilt, forward flexion tilt, extension tilt, rotation, and distraction) to the spine to restore its normal motion and to reduce pain caused by altered biomechanics. It is indicated in mechanical musculoskeletal pain problems of the back, pelvis, and neck in which loss of vertebral function or localized tenderness on induced motion may be a contributing factor.

   Spinal manipulation should only be done by a skilled practitioner. Depending on its velocity, manipulation can be classified as thrust (using high velocity and low amplitude) or nonthrust (usually using low velocity and high amplitude). In general, the higher the velocity used in manipulation, the more contraindications arise. In nonthrust technique, contraindications include vertebral malignancy, infection or inflammation, cauda equina syndrome, myelopathy, spondylosis, multiple adjacent radiculopathies, vertebral bone disease, vertebral bony joint instability (e.g., fracture or dislocation), and rheumatic disease in the cervical region.

Aside from the above, additional contraindications for thrust manipulation include fixed spinal deformities and anomalies, systemic anticoagulation (disease-related or pharmacologic), severe diabetes, atherosclerosis, severe degenerative joint disease, vertigo or signs and symptoms of vertebrobasilar arterial disease or insufficiency, spondyloarthropathies, inactive rheumatologic disease, ligamentous joint instability or congenital joint laxity and syndromes (e.g., Marfan and Ehlers-Danlos), aseptic necrosis, local aneurysm, osteomalacia, osteoporosis, osteopenia, objective radicular signs, hypermobility, obsessional fixation on pain, absence of any pain-free direction of vertebral motion. In clearly defined root pain without objective signs of radiculopathy, use of manipulation remains controversial.

In many of the aforementioned conditions and even in pregnancy, gentle nonthrust techniques can be used. In muscle energy, some of the absolute contraindications are only relative contraindications (e.g., osteoporosis, diabetes, noncervical rheumatoid disease, degenerative joint disease, joint laxity). One specific contraindication for muscle energy is concurrent myositis (due to patient's active contraction).

Manipulation must only be used on a short-term basis in conjunction with other active modalities such as exercises and patient education. Its treatment duration is determined on an individual basis. Thrusting usually has an immediate effect with improvement within 1 week postmanipulation. Muscle energy effect may take longer. Lack of improvement in objective findings after 2 to 4 weeks suggests the need for reevaluation.

1. **Thrust spinal manipulation (chiropractic "adjustment")** uses high-velocity and low-amplitude maneuvers, delivered at the end of the pathologic spinal ROM ("barrier") either directly (in the direction of the barrier) or indirectly (in the opposite direction of the barrier) with the purpose of increasing passive ROM. The facets of the involved vertebral segments are first "locked" by positioning the patient. The involved vertebral segment is then passively moved to its barrier so that all slack motion is removed. A brief (10 to 100 msec), controlled thrust is applied by the manipulator to increase the passive ROM. This may be associated with an audible "pop" or "click." If the thrust is applied over a spinous or transverse process, it is called short-lever technique. If applied distant from the vertebra through the locked vertebral column, it is called long-lever technique. Although extremely rare, accidents and even death have been reported with the use of thrust manipulation in the neck.

2. **Nonthrust spinal manipulation** consists of gentle, persuasive pressure performed at the end of the pathologic spinal ROM or within its available ROM. Unlike thrust manipulation, it uses relatively slow and controlled movements, hence, there is immediate sensory feedback to the therapist by the patient during the time of application.

   a. **Articulatory technique ("spinal mobilization")** uses maneuvers with high amplitude but low velocity.

      1) **Graded oscillation** technique uses alternate (on and off) oscillatory pressure at different parts of the available ROM. The oscillation amplitude is graded on a scale of 1 to 4. Its vibratory nature activates

the sensory mechanoreceptors to reduce pain and improve proprioception.

    2) Progressive stretch mobilization uses a successive series of short-amplitude, spring-type pressures or a series of short-amplitude stretch movements to overcome mechanical or soft tissue restrictions. It is given at progressive increments and is also graded on a 1 to 4 scale.

    3) Continuous stretch is the application of a sustained, gradually increasing stretch or a pressure without interruption for immediate tissue feedback used to improve mobility in soft tissue contractures.

  b. Muscle energy ("isometrics") is the most common nonthrust form of spinal manipulation. It requires muscle contraction on the part of the patient from a precisely determined position in a specific direction against a distinct counterforce. Its force direction can be direct (in the direction of the barrier) or indirect (in the opposite direction of the barrier). It has 3 phases (contraction, relaxation, and stretch) that are comparable to the contract-relax form of active inhibition exercise (see Chapter 4.2, section I.C.1). As in thrust manipulation, slack motion is first removed. Then the patient exerts moderate forces against the operator (force direction can be direct or indirect) for 5 to 10 seconds, followed by relaxation. The original barrier to movement is then reassessed (there should be less barrier and greater ROM) and the procedure is repeated two to three times. To maintain the gains in ROM, active flexibility exercise must be prescribed.

  c. Functional technique uses active-assistive positioning of a joint away from the motion barrier of restriction (i.e., indirect technique) and into a position of ease to inhibit reflex muscle guarding. The patient is asked to relax by breathing in and out. When muscle relaxation is sensed by the practitioner during expiratory phase, the patient's joint is repositioned into a new position of ease.

  d. Counterstrain (Jones technique) involves application of pressure into the sensitive myofascial trigger point while the muscle and related joint are maintained in the position of maximal relaxation to inhibit reflex muscle guarding and spasm. This pressure is applied for at least 90 seconds and is followed by a slow passive return to neutral so that muscle guarding and spasm does not recur.

  e. Craniosacral therapy assumes that an innate cranial rhythmic impulse (CRI) can be palpated on the body by an experienced practitioner. Part of the CRI causes an ebb and flow of the cerebrospinal fluid (CSF), which can presumably be palpated and manipulated by the practitioner using various techniques (e.g., compression of the fourth ventricle by laying of hands on the occipital condyle). Because the parasympathetic nervous system is situated in the cranial and sacral portions of the nervous system, the therapeutic effects are often attributed to the effects on the autonomous nervous system. Craniosacral therapy is highly controversial.

B. Peripheral joint manipulation and mobilization is the application of passive maneuvers (anterior-posterior glide, lateral glide, distraction, flexion tilt, extension tilt, and rotation) to a limb joint to increase its passive ROM. Clinical indications include painful limb joints with reflex muscle guarding and muscle spasm, reversible joint hypomobility, and joints with progressive limitation and functional immobility. They are contraindicated in joints with hypermobility, effusion, or acute inflammation. Extra caution must be observed in the presence of malignancy (e.g., lytic lesions), osteoporosis, unhealed fracture, excessive pain, or total joint replacement. In patients with inadequate knee flexion after total knee arthroplasty, joint manipulation under anesthesia may be done (usually by an orthopedic surgeon).

1. **Thrust manipulation of peripheral joint** uses high velocity, short amplitude maneuvers at the end of the pathologic limit of the limb joint to alter its positional relationships, to break adhesions, or to stimulate joint receptors. It is indicated in peripheral limb joint with loss of ROM due to immobilization resulting from trauma or adhesive capsulitis. Its capability to realign intrasynovial structures, such as a displaced meniscus, is highly controversial.

2. **Nonthrust manipulation of peripheral joint**
   a. **Peripheral joint mobilization** uses slow and controlled movements which are applied at a speed slow enough that the patient can stop the movement. Depending on the patient's response, a rhythmic oscillation (graded oscillation technique) or a sustained distraction (sustained translatory joint-play technique) may be used. In general, oscillation techniques are used for pain management and sustained techniques are used for loss of joint play with decreased functional range.
   b. **Muscle energy ("isometrics")** can also be done in the peripheral joint (see section VIII.A.2.b).
   c. **Functional technique** can also be done in the peripheral joint (see section VIII.A.2.c).
   d. **Counterstrain** can also be done in the peripheral joint (see section VIII.A.2.d).

IX. **Massage** is the systematic, mechanical stimulation of the soft tissues of the body by means of rhythmically applied pressure and stretching for therapeutic purposes. Physiological effects of massage can either be mechanical (i.e., increase in venous return and lymphatic drainage, breaking of adhesion and softening of scars, loosening of secretions) or reflexive (i.e., increase in circulation via reflex vasodilation, general relaxation and sedative effects, increased perspiration and secretion of sebaceous glands, and decreased pain probably caused by gate control or release of endogenous opiates or neurotransmitters). The ''laying of hands'' also has psychological effects and can promote a sense of general well-being.

Massage is used to reduce excessive fluids in interstitial spaces or joints (e.g., lymphedema), increase circulation to paralyzed muscles, restore tight muscles to normal length, mobilize tissues that are abnormally adhered to surrounding structures, increase tolerance of tissues to pressure, relieve pain and muscle spasm, loosen secretions (e.g., in chronic obstructive pulmonary disease [COPD]), promote specific and general relaxation, and enhance psychological well-being. Massage does not alter the general metabolism and has no effect on obesity, muscle mass, muscle strength, muscle recovery rate, or the rate of atrophy of denervated muscle.

Contraindications include any acute inflammatory conditions of the skin, soft tissues, or joints due to bacterial action (phlebitis, cellulitis, synovitis, abscesses, septic arthritis), open wounds, burns, nerve entrapments (e.g., carpal tunnel syndrome), bursitis, rheumatoid and gouty arthritis, rheumatic fibrositis, panniculitis (subcutaneous fat inflammation), arteriosclerosis, venous thrombosis or embolism, severe varicose veins, clotting disorders (or during anticoagulation), fractures, and malignancies.

Treatment time depends on the size of the area to be treated. It usually takes

15 to 30 minutes for trunk massage (abdomen, back, or neck) and 5 to 15 minutes for the limb massage. Generally, limb massage is done from distal to proximal (centripetally). But if there is swelling (e.g., lymphedema), the proximal part must be massaged before the distal part (''uncorking effect''). Massage should always be used in conjunction with other forms of treatment, preferably active modalities such as exercises. If possible, the patient should be taught self-massage.

A. **Massage using the hands** is more effective than massage using mechanical devices because the hand can assess (through palpation) as well as treat.

   1. **Western massage**

      a. **Classical massage** is the blending of the following strokes (a popular form is the **Swedish massage,** which involves percussion, petrissage, and deep tissue massage):

         1) **Effleurage:** Light gliding strokes over skin without moving deep muscle masses used for muscle relaxation.

         2) **Petrissage:** Kneading manipulations that intermittently lift, press, and roll the muscles under the fingers or hands used for increasing circulation and reducing edema.

         3) **Percussion (tapotement):** Series of brisk alternating blows (e.g., hacking, slapping, beating, pinchment, tapping with finger tips, cupping, or clapping) used to stimulate circulation, desensitize operated sites (e.g., amputee stump), and dislodge secretions (in chest physical therapy).

         4) **Vibration:** Fine tremulous movement made by hand or finger to cause the part to vibrate. It can be soothing when applied gently or stimulating when done more vigorously. It can be used in conjunction with percussion to loosen secretions.

         5) **Friction:** Circular motions of the fingertips with pressure applied so that the therapist's fingers and the patient's skin move as one. It is used to loosen or break up underlying adhesions of healed scar tissue.

      b. **Cross-fiber friction massage** is a deep friction massage applied parallel or perpendicular to the muscle, tendon, or ligament fibers to loosen any adherent fibrous tissue. It can also aid in absorption of local edema or effusions and in reducing local muscle spasm. When done over trigger points, it can have reflex effects.

      c. **Connective tissue massage (CTM) or Bindegewebsmassage** is a series of pulling strokes carried out in the layers of the connective tissue on the body surface to stimulate cutaneovisceral reflex (via autonomic nervous system) and affect visceral organs whose innervation corresponds to cutaneous dermatomes. This claim, however, remains controversial. A variation of CTM, called **Rolfing**, involves vigorous, pounding massage of the deep connective tissue.

      d. **Soft tissue mobilization (STM)** is a forceful form of passive stretching of the muscular and fascial system element through its restrictive direction in a manner and at a speed that are within the ability of the patient to control the movement. It incorporates movement and joint position with the basic application of CTM techniques. It places the fascia and muscle in an elongated rather than a shortened or relaxed position thus exposing the tissue to be treated, stretching the connective tissue, and changing the resting length of the muscle.

      e. **Myofascial release (MFR)** is the application of prolonged light pressure in specific directions into the fascia system to release soft tissues from the abnormal grip of tight fascia. It is a gentle form of passive stretching.

2. **Eastern massage** closely resembles CTM in its claim to affect visceral organs via peripheral manipulation of the nervous system (cutaneovisceral reflex). Like CTM, it remains controversial.

   a. **Acupressure** is a Chinese form of massage that uses finger pressure over acupuncture points or over trigger points to decrease pain. It can supposedly increase endogenous opiates after 1 to 5 minutes of pressure at a single point. Other specific forms of acupressure are **reflexology/zone therapy** (which uses the sole of the foot) and **auriculotherapy** (which uses the ear).

   b. **Shiatsu** is the Japanese form of acupressure.

B. **Massage using mechanical devices** loses the ''laying of hands'' effect and is often not as effective as manual massage.

   1. **Hand-held or hand-strapped devices** usually provide percussion (percussor), vibration (vibrator), and suction (e.g., massage suction-roller). Vibrators with frequency of 100 to 200 Hz and amplitude of 1.5 mm are commonly used for muscle facilitation and muscle reeducation in patients with upper motor neuron lesions and for temporary relief of musculoskeletal pain.

   2. **Stationary massage devices** are not moved during their use. The body part to be massaged is placed upon the stationary device that vibrates (e.g., vibrating pads, vibrating belts or strap, message roller pad).

   3. **Alternating pressure mattresses and pads** (see Chapter 5.2, section VI.B.3.b) uses massage-like actions for the treatment and prevention of pressure sores (by emptying and refilling superficial blood vessels).

   4. **Intermittent compression devices** uses a hollow cuff, sleeve, or boot that is worn around a limb or part of it and then intermittently filled with air or water to provide centripetal rhythmic compression for the relief of lymphedema. The best known is Jobst pneumatic intermittent compression unit, which is mostly used for postmastectomy lymphedema of the upper limb.

   5. **Devices for hydromassage** provide massage by pressure and movement of water, e.g., shower massage, underwater jet massage, whirlpool baths, and Jacuzzi.

X. **Acupuncture** is a neurostimulatory technique that induces analgesia and other neurophysiologic effects by the insertion of small 28 to 36 gauge, 1.25 to 5.0 cm long, solid needles into acupuncture points found on the skin at varying depths, typically penetrating the underlying musculature. Many of the acupuncture points that are distributed along meridians (hypothetical lines through which the life force, i.e., *Chi* or *Qi,* flows) on the surface of the body were found to correspond to motor points. The enhanced sensitivity and reactivity of the acupuncture points may be due to their greater concentration of pain fibers and vascular structures. On the trunk, the points are found at segmental innervation levels where nerves and blood and lymphatic vessels penetrate muscle fascia. On the face and head, they are found near the cranial nerves and blood and lymphatic vessels. On the ear, there appears to be a relationship between the acupuncture points and the cranial nerves and blood vessels, although the traditional postulate is that the body is represented in the ear in the shape of an inverted homunculus. Recent studies show that acupuncture stimulation need not be applied at the points indicated by the traditional acupuncture charts, and it is believed that intense stimulation rather than inserting the needle at the precise site is more crucial to its effectiveness.

Acupuncture has been used as an adjunctive treatment in the management of mild-to-moderate acute and chronic pain syndromes including musculoskeletal pain (e.g., epicondylitis, back and neck pain, fractured ribs, temporomandibular pain, foot pain, osteoarthritis, and headache), neuropathic pain (e.g., post-herpetic neuralgia, trigeminal neuralgia, and phantom limb pain), cancer pain, and other pain syndromes; asthma; gastrointestinal disorders; menstrual problems; chronic stress; obesity; depression; insomnia; withdrawal for addictive substances; and immune dysfunctions.

The mechanism of action of acupuncture remains controversial. Popular Western theories include neuropharmacological theory (e.g., involving opioid system such as the release of endorphins and enkephalins or nonopioid system such as the serotonergic system), neurophysiologic theory (as shown by its effectiveness in increasing heart rate and blood pressure as well as altering gastrointestinal function, blood chemistry, and immunologic reactions), hyperstimulation theory (i.e., central nervous system hyperstimulation "drowns out" pain messages), gate control theory (i.e., stimulation of large- or medium-sized afferent nerve fibers in muscles blocks out the small-fiber input), autonomic nervous system theory, and distraction and counterirritation theory. The placebo effect theory has been proposed but is weakened by studies showing partial analgesia in animals such as monkeys, rats, and mice.

Acupuncture is an invasive therapy and is contraindicated in patients who are anticoagulated, have infection at the site of needle insertion, or have active, blood-borne infection. Potential complications include needle-related complications (e.g., breaking a needle; causing bleeding; creating local infection; transmitting disease, such as hepatitis B, AIDS, or cytomegalovirus; and invading nontargeted tissues causing pneumothorax, paresthesias, or nerve damage) and technique-related problems (e.g., vasovagal reactions and fainting, lack of therapeutic effect, and delay in providing more conventional therapy).

The number of acupuncture points used and the number of treatments provided depend on the practitioner's preference, type of pain, and chronicity and seriousness of the problem. Because acupuncture tends to be cumulative, an average course of treatment before significant results occur may be 2 to 3 times per week for 3 to 6 weeks. The average length of each treatment varies from 20 to 30 minutes. After acupuncture needle insertion, the patient should feel a sensation of warmth, heaviness, soreness, or local fullness. The needle can be left untouched, twirled, or connected to a low-volt current. Studies show that 50 to 80% of patients may exhibit a short-term benefit from acupuncture especially when it is used as a component of a comprehensive treatment program. To date, there are few controlled studies on the clinical efficacy of acupuncture. One of the problems in doing a controlled study on acupuncture is the difficulty in doing an adequate controlled double-blind study (e.g., in the use of sham acupuncture, inserting the needle at an incorrect point may have some pain reduction effect; also, because the acupuncturist is aware of the difference, he or she might transmit his or her expectations to the patient). Recent metaanalyses produced mixed and inconclusive results and do not specify which types of pain problems acupuncture can or cannot alleviate.

BIBLIOGRAPHY

Alon G: Evaluation of clinical electrical stimulators, *Physical Therapy Practice* 1(2):7-19, 1992.

Basford JR: Electrical therapy. In Kottke FJ Lehmann JF, editors: *Krusen's handbook of physical medicine and rehabilitation*, ed 4, Philadelphia, 1990, WB Saunders, pp. 375-401.

Basford JR: Physical agents. In DeLisa JA, Gans BM, editors: *Rehabilitation medicine: Principles and practice,* ed 2, Philadelphia, 1993, JB Lippincott, pp. 404-424.

Basmajian JV: Biofeedback in rehabilitation medicine. In DeLisa JA, Gans BM, editors: *Rehabilitation medicine: Principles and practice,* ed 2, Philadelphia, 1993, JB Lippincott, pp. 425-439.

Basmajian JV, editor: *Manipulation, traction and massage,* ed 3, Baltimore, 1985, Williams & Wilkins.

Geiringer SR, Kincaid CB, Rechtien JR: Traction, manipulation, and massage. In DeLisa JA, Gans BM, editors: *Rehabilitation medicine: Principles and practice,* ed 2, Philadelphia, 1993, JB Lippincott, pp. 440-462.

Han JS, Terenius L: Neurochemical basis of acupuncture analgesia, *Ann Rev Pharmacol Toxicol* 22:193-220, 1982.

Lee MHM, Liao SJ: Acupuncture for pain management. In Lennard TA, editor: *Physiatric procedures in clinical practice,* Philadelphia, 1995, Hanley & Belfus, pp. 49-56.

Lehmann JF de Lateur BJ: Diathermy and superficial heat, laser, and cold therapy. In Kottke FJ, Lehmann JF, editors: *Krusen's handbook of physical medicine and rehabilitation,* ed 4, Philadelphia, 1990, WB Saunders, pp. 283-367.

Mannheimer JS, Lampe GN: Electrode placement sites and their relationships. In JS Mannheimer, GN Lampe, editors: *Clinical transcutaneous electrical nerve stimulation,* Philadelphia, 1984, FA Davis, pp 249-329.

McLean B, Fives HE: Stimulation-induced analgesia. In Warfield CA, editor: *Principles and practice of pain management.* New York, 1993, McGraw-Hill, pp. 413-425.

Melzack R: Folk medicine and the sensory modulation of pain. In Wall PD, Melzack R, editors: *Textbook of pain,* ed 3, Edinburgh, 1994, Churchill Livingstone, pp. 1209-1217.

Michlovitz SL, editor: *Thermal agents in rehabilitation,* ed 3, Philadelphia, 1996, FA Davis.

Nelson RM, Currier DP: *Clinical electrotherapy,* ed 2, Norwalk, CT, 1991, Appleton and Lange.

Prentice W, editor: *Therapeutic modalities in sports medicine,* ed 2, St. Louis, 1990, Times Mirror/Mosby College Publishing.

Ramos G, Martin W: Effects of vertebral axial decompression on intradiscal pressure. *J Neurosurg* 81:350-353, 1994.

Rowlingson, JC, Kessler RS, Dane JR, et al: Adjunctive therapy for pain. In Hamill RJ, Rowlingson JC, editors: *Handbook of critical care pain management,* New York, 1994, McGraw-Hill, pp. 229-249.

Sverdlik SS: Principles of physical medicine. In Goodgold J, editor: *Rehabilitation medicine,* St. Louis, 1988, CV Mosby, pp. 773-786.

Weber DC, Brown AW: Physical agent modalities. In Braddom RL, editor: *Physical Medicine and Rehabilitation,* Philadelphia, 1996; WB Saunders, pp 449-463.

CHAPTER 4.2

THERAPEUTIC EXERCISES

Therapeutic exercise is the prescription of muscular contraction and bodily movement ultimately to improve the overall function of the individual and to help meet the demands of daily living. It involves the positive and progressive application and adjustment of stress and forces of the appropriate type and amount to the body system to correct an impairment, improve musculoskeletal function, maintain a state of well being, or prevent dysfunction without causing injury. Depending on the patient's needs, specific exercises can be employed to achieve different beneficial goals such as to increase or maintain range of motion (ROM), strength, endurance and cardiovascular fitness, coordination and control, and speed, and to promote relaxation.

In general the immediate systemic effects of active rhythmic exercise (i.e., excluding relaxation exercise) include increased blood flow to muscle due to increased demands for oxygen, increased heart rate (HR) (probably through neural influence), increased arterial pressure with heavy exercise (due to increased stroke volume, increased cardiac output, increased HR, and increased peripheral resistance to blood flow), increased oxygen demand and consumption, increased rate and depth of respiration, decreased insulin secretion with increased glucagon secretion to maintain blood glucose level, and increased secretion of catecholamines and other hormones when the exercise is sustained (see Fig. 4.2-1).

As active rhythmic exercise continues at a constant rate, the heart rate, blood pressure, and cardiac output reach a steady state. When this exercise is terminated, there is an initial rapid decrease in heart rate and then a slower return to normal. Abrupt cessation of active rhythmic exercise may cause a sudden drop in blood pressure, hence, a cool-down period is recommended. Likewise, sudden vigorous exercise may cause electrocardiogram (ECG) abnormalities with syncopal episodes, hence, a warm-up period is recommended. If active rhythmic exercise continues beyond the body's ability to maintain it, fatigue and muscle soreness ensue. Muscle soreness usually peaks 48 hours after active rhythmic exercise and lasts 5 to 7 days (up to 2 weeks) probably because of tissue damage as well as subsequent structural changes in the muscle fibers to improve their metabolic capacity. This muscle soreness is greater in eccentric (lengthening) exercises than in concentric (shortening) exercises. The long-term (adaptive) cardiovascular changes that occur in the rhythmic endurance and strengthening exercises are discussed in their respective sections below.

In prescribing therapeutic exercises, the factors to be considered are type of exercise, objectives of exercise (e.g., to increase ROM, strength, endurance, or coordination and to promote relaxation); details of exercise instructions (e.g., frequency, duration, repetitions, types and amount of resistance, sequence of progression, exercise equipment, preferred time of day for exercise, environment, and warm-up and cool-down periods), and other general problems (e.g., time or schedule, pain, medical problems, general contraindication, cost, and motivation). To increase patient compliance, exercises should be simple and enjoyable. They should not be burdensome, and they should not drastically change one's lifestyle. The therapist should explain to the patient what to expect during and after the exercise program. Muscle soreness that is labeled "good pain" should be distinguished

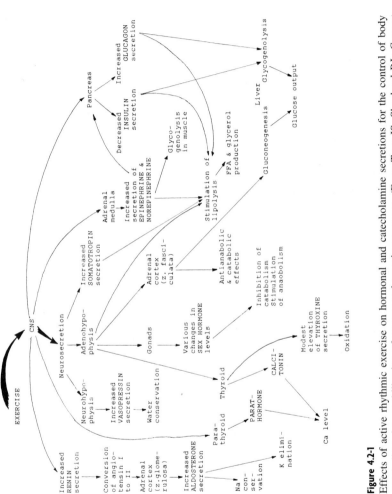

Figure 4.2-1

Effects of active rhythmic exercise on hormonal and catecholamine secretions for the control of body metabolism, i.e., mobilization of energy and protein resources. (From Torg JS, Shephard RJ: *Current therapy in sports medicine*, ed 3, St. Louis, 1995, Mosby–Year Book, p. 504.)

from "bad pain" such as radiating pain. Patients must be supervised closely to make sure the exercise goals are achieved. This should be reinforced with a home program by using either an exercise booklet or customized written or computer-generated instructions and drawings, with an explanation of the purpose of each exercise. Training by using a quota system and by providing positive reinforcement are effective, especially in patients with chronic problems.

This chapter gives an overview of therapeutic exercises. For details on how to design specific exercise programs for different disease process (rheumatic disease, scoliosis, stroke, multiple sclerosis [MS], spinal cord injury [SCI], chronic obstructive pulmonary disease [COPD], peripheral vascular disease, amputation, cancer, total joint replacement, coronary artery disease, etc.), refer to Kisner and Colby's *Therapeutic Exercise: Foundations and Techniques* and Basmajian and Wolf's *Therapeutic Exercise* (see bibliography).

I. **Mobility exercises** are used to maintain or restore the mobility of soft tissues (e.g., muscle, connective tissue, and skin) and joints so the patient can perform normal functional movements. They can be active (performed by the patient without assistance), active-assisted (performed by the patient with assistance by another person or a mechanical device), or passive (performed for the patient by another person or by a mechanical device). Mobility exercises can be performed actively with absent or minimal active muscle contraction such as in Codman's pendular exercise (prescribed for adhesive capsulitis or frozen shoulder) in which the pendular shoulder movement is mainly propelled by gravity rather than muscle contraction. Both active and active-assistive exercises will neither maintain nor increase strength (if muscles are very strong to begin with), and they will not develop skill or coordination (except in the movement patterns used). Both active and active-assistive exercises are contraindicated (or used with precaution) when motion is disruptive to healing (e.g., acute fracture) and when the patient's cardiovascular condition is unstable (e.g., immediately after myocardial infarction). Passive exercises will *not* prevent muscle atrophy, increase strength or endurance, and assist circulation to the extent that active muscle contraction will. In general, passive exercises are contraindicated when motion is disruptive to healing (e.g., acute fracture). Additional contraindications and precautions of passive stretching are discussed below.

A. **Range of motion (ROM) or flexibility exercises** are not synonymous with stretching exercises (see below). Range of motion or flexibility exercises maintain mobility within the available range while stretching exercises increase ROM by lengthening the shortened structures (e.g., muscles and tendon) beyond the available range. Such exercises should be performed slowly with gradual progression to greater ranges of motion to avoid excessive pain and injury. Each ROM or flexibility exercise (done actively if possible) should be repeated 3 to 5 times and performed 1 to 2 times daily for at least three times per week. Patterns in ROM exercises can be done through the anatomic planes of motion, combined patterns of motion (diagonal patterns similar to proprioceptive neuromuscular facilitation [PNF] patterns), or functional patterns (e.g., patterns used in teaching activities of daily living and in instructing the blind in functional activities). Flexibility exercises performed slowly within full ROM with minimal effort are also called limbering exercises. In limbering exercises, elimination of gravity by positioning helps (e.g., performing hip flexion and extension in sidelying position). The ROM or flexibility exercises may be combined with stretching by following the slow dynamic movement with a static stretch held for 10 to 30 seconds, and they can be performed using manual assistance, mechanical assistance, or self-assistance from the patient. The following are commonly used equipment in ROM exercises:

1. **A wand, cane, or wooden stick** may be used in hemiparetic patients with some voluntary muscle control in the involved upper limb but requires guidance or assistance to complete the ROM at the shoulder or elbow. The normal limb is used to move the involved extremity through the ROM.

2. **Finger ladder (wall climbing) device** can motivate the patient to do shoulder ROM by providing objective reinforcement. Patients should not be allowed to substitute shoulder ROM with trunk side bending, toe raising, or scapular elevation.

3. **Shoulder wheel,** which is permanently attached to a wall, can be adjusted to various heights and arm length to motivate the patient to do active shoulder ROM. Resistance can be added to the wheel for strengthening exercises.

4. **Overhead pulleys** are used to assist an involved limb in performing ROM. Two pulleys are attached to an overhead bar or to the ceiling about shoulder-width apart. A rope is passed over both pulleys, and a handle is attached to each end of the rope.

5. **Suspension** is used to free a body part from the resistance of friction while it is moving. The involved part is suspended in a sling attached to a rope that is fixed to an appropriate point above the body segment. In a vertical fixation, the point of attachment of the rope is over the center of gravity of the moving segment. The part can then move like a pendulum, describing an arc. Because of its small ROM, this type of suspension is primarily used for support. In an axial fixation, the point of attachment of all ropes supporting the part is above the axis of the point to be moved. The part moves on a flat plane, parallel to the floor. This allows for maximum movement of a joint (vertical and axial fixation).

6. **Skate or powder board** is a device placed under the involved upper or lower limb to help increase ROM by reducing the effect of friction and gravity on the moving limb.

7. **Reciprocal exercise unit ("restorator")** is used to provide some hip and knee flexion/extension to an involved lower limb by using the strength of the normal lower limb. The device is mobile in that it can be attached to a patient's bed, wheelchair (WC), or standard chair. It can be used for reciprocal patterning, endurance training, and initiating a strengthening program.

8. **Continuous passive movement (CPM) machine** is a mechanical device that passively moves a desired joint continuously through a controlled ROM without patient effort for as long as 24 hours a day. It is effective in lessening the negative effects of joint immobilization following limb surgery. It can prevent development of adhesions, decrease contracture formation, decrease postoperative pain, increase synovial fluid lubrication of the joint, decrease joint effusion and wound edema thus improving wound healing, increase the rate of intraarticular cartilage healing and regeneration, and provide a quicker return of ROM. Its effectiveness in increasing lower limb circulation and preventing DVT remains controversial. It should be used only as an adjunct to other exercise programs because it serves only to maintain ROM without the strengthening component.

B. **Passive stretching** is a therapeutic maneuver to lengthen pathologically shortened structures thereby increasing ROM along the anatomic planes of motion. **Self-stretching** (which may be combined with active inhibition techniques) can be carried out by the patient using body weight as the stretch force. Prior to stretching, the following may be used to elongate both contractile and noncontractile tissues: general relaxation (e.g., Jacobson's progressive relaxation described in section VI.A.2), heat (Chapter 4.1, section I), cold (e.g., ethyl chloride spray; see Chapter 4.1, section II.E), massage (Chapter 4.1, section IX), biofeedback (Chapter 4.1, section VI), warm-up exercise, and joint traction or oscillation. Passive stretching must be used with extreme caution in patients with known or suspected osteoporosis, prolonged immobilization, bone malignancy, excessive pain, hypermobility of associated joints, and total joint replacements. They are contraindicated in presence of the following conditions in the joint to be stretched: hypermobility, effusion, inflammation, hematoma or other trauma, recent fractures, or when contractures or shortened soft tissues are needed to provide joint stability or increased functional abilities (particularly in patients with paralysis or severe muscle weakness).

1. **Manual passive stretching** is the manual application of external force beyond the free ROM so the tissues are elongated beyond their resting length. This is in contrast to passive ROM, which is applied within the unrestricted available range. The stretch force is applied very slowly and gently (to inhibit the stretch reflex and to encourage connective tissue creep, i.e., increase in strain with time under constant load) for at least 15 to 30 seconds and repeated several times within the exercise session. Ballistic stretching (high intensity with very short duration) must be avoided because it facilitates the stretch reflex (increasing the tension in the muscle being lengthened), and it also can cause microtrauma in the muscle. The intensity and duration of the stretch, which are controlled by the therapist, are dependent on the patient's tolerance and the therapist's strength and endurance.

2. **Prolonged mechanical (or positional passive) stretching** is the application of a low-intensity external force (5-15 lb) using a mechanical device for 20 to 30 minutes or longer. A weighted traction and pulley system, a dynamic splint or brace, or serial casts may be used. In noncontractile tissues, plastic deformation occurs; however, in muscles, sarcomeres are added in series.

3. **Cyclic mechanical stretching** is similar in intensity and duration to manual passive stretching. Instead of using an external manual force, however, it uses mechanical equipment in a cyclic mode. The intensity of the stretch, the length of each stretch cycle, and the number of stretches per minute are adjustable.

C. **Active inhibition** is a technique in which the patient reflexively relaxes the muscle to be elongated prior to the stretching. The muscles to be inhibited should be innervated and under the patient's control.

   1. **Contract-relax (or hold-relax)** is also called **"muscle energy"** (see Chapter 4.1, section VIII.A.2.b) by manual therapists. The patient performs an isometric contraction of the tight muscle for 5 to 10 seconds against resistance (the contraction may be maximal or submaximal). The patient then relaxes the muscle and the therapist passively lengthens the tight muscle through the gained range. The prestretch contraction of the tight muscle causes that same muscle to relax as a result of autogenic inhibition.

   2. **Contract-relax-contract (hold-relax-contract)** combines the autogenic inhibition and reciprocal inhibition techniques. The patient performs a contraction and relaxation on the tight muscle (as in contract-relax technique) followed by a concentric contraction of the muscle opposite the tight mus-

cle. Then the patient actively moves his or her own limb through the gained range.

3. **Agonist contraction** technique involves the patient's active contraction of the "agonist" (muscle opposite the tight muscle) against resistance to cause a reciprocal inhibition of the tight muscle (called the antagonist) so that the tight muscle can lengthen more readily as it is stretched. This is effective in tight muscles that are painful (due to muscle spasm) or in the early stages of healing. It is least effective when the ROM is close to normal.

D. Joint mobilization and manipulation (see Chapter 4.1 section VIII).

II. **Strengthening exercises** are primarily used to increase muscle strength (i.e., the capacity to produce motor output such as torque or work by voluntary activation of the muscles), although they may also increase local muscle endurance. In the normal muscle, strength is influenced by the cross-sectional size of the muscle, length-tension relationship, recruitment of motor units, type of muscle contraction, speed of contraction, and motivation of the patient. Strengthening exercises are based on the Hellebrandt's "overload" principle, i.e., increase in strength occurs only if the load that is greater than what the tissue is accustomed is applied to the point of fatigue.

For the first two weeks of training, increase in strength (i.e., peak muscle force) is almost totally due to neural factors (i.e., increased neuromuscular efficiency as shown by the decreased electromyographic [EMG] activities needed for maintaining the same muscle force). Subsequently, there is hypertrophy of the muscle and tendon, and possibly muscle hyperplasia. Strengthening exercises (unlike endurance exercises in section III) have little long-term cardiovascular effects. There is little or no change in resting heart rate (HR), resting blood pressure (BP), resting stroke volume, resting myocardial oxygen consumption, and arteriovenous oxygen difference. Likewise, there is little change in left ventricular wall thickness and mass because the increments of BP are maintained for only a few seconds at a time. However, there is decreased exercise HR, better-sustained exercise stroke volume, slower rate of rise of exercise BP, and reduced myocardial oxygen consumption during exercise. Hemoglobin level may sometimes be increased in hypertrophied muscles.

Among the modes of strengthening exercises, isometric (i.e., static increase in muscle tension without joint movement; see section II.B.1) and isokinetic (i.e., dynamic strengthening exercise with constant velocity; see section II.B.3), strengthening exercises produce the greatest rise in exercise BP. Moreover, isometric strengthening exercises can decrease local blood flow to the contracting muscle leading to complete blood vessel occlusion when performing 70% of maximum voluntary exertion capability. To effectively increase muscle strength, active muscle activation is recommended, although recent studies seem to suggest that neuromuscular electrical stimulation (NMES), a passive modality, can also increase muscle strength as long as the muscle is not denervated (e.g., normally innervated muscles or decentralized muscles; see Chapter 4.1, section V.B.3).

In the presence of muscle or joint inflammation and pain, dynamic strengthening exercises are contraindicated, but static (isometric) exercises may be done gently. Strengthening exercises must be used with caution in patients with cardiovascular problems (e.g., recent myocardial infarction, uncontrolled hypertension, and recent stroke), abdominal surgery or abdominal wall hernia, easy fatigability (e.g., multiple sclerosis, peripheral vascular disease, cardiac disease, and pulmonary disease), osteoporosis, and acute inflammatory conditions (e.g., acute rheumatoid arthritis and polymyositis). Valsalva maneuver must be avoided during strengthening exercises especially in cardiac patients because it causes a temporary fall in stroke volume.

General guidelines in prescribing strengthening exercise include starting at submaximal resistance (e.g., 50% of maximum voluntary exertion capability) with gradual increment towards maximal voluntary exertion capability; using low repetitions, which can be increased up to 12 to 15 times per set for 1 to 3 sets; training 2 to 3 times per week; exercising large muscle groups before smaller groups; exercising in an even manner; and avoiding overfatigue and substitution of motion. When high-intensity exercises for specific muscles are done in high repetitions, the strengthening exercise is called **resistance training**. In resistance training, there is increase in *local* muscle endurance (i.e., local ability of the specific muscle to maintain a predetermined level of motor output over a period of time in contrast to generalized cardiopulmonary endurance produced by total body endurance exercises described in section III) and power (i.e., ability of the specific muscle to do work per unit time) in addition to strength.

A. **Manual strengthening exercise** uses resistance force applied by the therapist to either a static (isometric) or dynamic (isotonic) muscular contraction (see description of isometric and isotonic exercises below). It is carried out in the anatomic places of motion or in diagonal patterns known as proprioceptive neuromuscular facilitation (PNF) patterns. A specific muscle may also be strengthened by resisting the action of that muscle as described in manual muscle testing (MMT) procedures. The direction of resistance is directly opposite to the desired motion. Resistance is usually applied to the distal end of the segment where the muscle to be strengthened is attached to generate the greatest amount of external torque with the least amount of effort from the therapist. In older patients prone to osteoporotic fractures, however, a more proximal lever arm (i.e., resistance applied closer to the joint) must be used. Proper stabilization must be provided to avoid substitution of motion. The resistance is appropriate if maximum pain free effort is done smoothly. Usually 8 to 10 repetitions per set of a specific motion is adequate (as they induce fatigue). The exercise set may be repeated 2 to 3 times per session after an adequate period of rest.

B. **Mechanical strengthening exercise** is any form of strengthening exercise in which resistance is applied by mechanical equipment.

   1. **Isometric (static) strengthening exercise** occurs when tension is generated in the muscle without visible joint movement nor appreciable change in total muscle length. It is most efficient when the exertion occurs at the resting length of the muscle. Its main advantage is that it is easy to perform and requires little time and setup. It is useful when joint motion is contraindicated due to pain, inflammation, or other reasons. Its disadvantage it that isometric strength does not necessarily transfer to dynamic activities (e.g., the increase in strength is joint-angle specific; it has no effect on coordination training) nor does isometric exercise cause hypertrophy. In patients with cardiovascular problems, it must be used with caution because it can cause ventricular arrhythmias and significantly increase blood pressure during exercise.

      a. **Isometric strengthening exercise regimens**

         1) **Brief maximal isometric exercise regimen** (Hettinger and Muller) uses single isometric contraction against fixed resistance, held for 5 to 6

seconds, once per day, 5 to 6 times per week. This protocol has been shown to be ineffective for increasing muscle strength.

2) **Brief repetitive isometric exercise (BRIME) regimen** (Liberson and Asa) uses 5 to 10 brief but maximum isometric contractions (each bout held for 6-15 seconds) performed against resistance 5 days per week. It is more effective than the single brief maximal isometric exercise.

3) **Multiple angle isometric exercise regimen** uses resistance at least every 20 degrees through the ROM. The **"rule of tens"** by Davies uses 10 sets of 10 repetitions of 10 second contractions every 10 degrees in the range of motion.

b. **Equipment used for isometric strengthening exercise** is usually the same as those used for dynamic exercises or testing. The joint is kept from moving by either the use of soft constraints (verbal instructions) or hard constraints (use of stabilization straps or mechanically locking the equipment).

2. **Isotonic strengthening exercise** is a dynamic exercise with a constant load but uncontrolled speed of movement. The constant weight or load is moved through the ROM. The term *isotonic* falsely assumes that the muscle exerts the same force throughout the range of motion. As the muscle lengthens and shorten, however, the lever arm changes and consequently the forces in the muscle changes.

a. **Isotonic strengthening exercise regimens**

1) **Progressive resistive exercise (PRE) (DeLorme technique).** The 10 repetition maximum (RM) is first determined. The 10 RM refers to the greatest amount of weight that can be lifted, pulled, or pushed 10 times through full ROM. The patient then performs one set of 10 repetitions at 50% of the 10 RM, a second set of 10 repetitions at 75% of the 10 RM, and a final set of 10 repetitions at the full 10 RM. All three sets are performed at each session with a brief rest period in between sets. Every week, a new 10 RM is determined as strength increases. The above protocol has been modified by DeLateur by adding a few pounds daily to the initial 10 RM in addition to the weekly determination of the new 10 RM. Another modification by McMorris and Elkins uses 10 repetitions at 25%, 50%, 75%, and 100% of the 10 RM.

2) **Regressive resistive exercise (RRE) (Zinovieff's Oxford technique)** is the reverse of the DeLorme technique designed to diminish resistance as muscle fatigue develops. This principle of strengthening exercise was proved wrong by Hellerandt's overload principle (see explanation in section II).

3) **Daily adjustable progressive resistance exercise (DAPRE) (Knight technique)** was developed to objectively determine when and how much resistance to increase in an isotonic strengthening exercise program. First, determine an initial working weight (e.g., 6 RM). The patient then performs 10 repetitions of 50% of working weight (set no. 1), 6 repetitions of 75% of the working weight (set no. 2), as many repetitions as possible of the full working weight (set no. 3), then as many repetitions as possible of the adjusted working weight (set no. 4). The adjusted working weight is based on the number of repetitions of the full working weight performed during set number 3. The number of repetitions done in set number 4 is used to determine the working weight for the next day. Guidelines for the adjustment of the working weight are in Table 4.2-1. The ideal maximum number

Table 4.2-1. Guidelines for the daily adjustable progressive resistance exercise (DAPRE) (Knight technique)

NUMBER OF REPETITIONS PERFORMED DURING SET #3	ADJUSTMENT TO WORKING WEIGHT FOR SET #4	ADJUSTMENT TO WORKING WEIGHT FOR NEXT DAY
0-2	Decrease 5-10 lb and repeat set	Decrease 5-10 lb
3-4	Decrease 0-5 lb	Same weight
5-6	Keep weight the same	Increase 5-10 lb
7-10	Increase 5-10 lb	Increase 5-15 lb
11	Increase 10-15 lb	Increase 10-20 lb

From Knight KL: Knee rehabilitation by the daily adjustable progressive resistive exercise technique, *Am J Sports Med* 7:337, 1979, with permission.

of repetitions when the patient is asked to perform as many repetitions as possible is 5 to 7. The DAPRE system eliminates the arbitrary determination of how much weight should be added in a strengthening exercise program on a day-to-day basis. This system can be used with free weights or with weight machines.

4) **Circuit weight training** (see also Chapter 5.13, section IV.C.2.b) requires the participant to exercise in short bouts, using light to moderate work loads with frequent repetitions, interspersed with short rest periods. They are carried out in a specific sequence using a variety of exercises for total body conditioning and to challenge both the skeletal muscles and the cardiovascular system. Exercises can be done using free weights or weight training units such as the Universal, Nautilus, or Eagle system. Exercises could include 8 to 10 RMs of bench press, leg press, sit-ups, shoulder press, squats, and curls with a 30-second to 1-minute rest period between each bout of exercise.

b. **Isotonic strengthening exercise equipment**

1) **Free weights** are graduated weights that are hand held or applied to the upper or lower limbs. They include barbells, dumbbells, cuff weights with Velcro closures, sandbags, and weighted boots. Improvised weights may be made from household items, such as the plastic one-gallon milk jug whose weight can be readily adjusted by varying the amount of water or sand it contains.

2) **Elastic resistance devices** include TheraBand and Rehabilitation Xercise tubing, which are cut at different lengths and set up on bed rails or walls so that the upper or lower limbs or trunk can be strengthened. The resistance provided can be increased by using thicker elastics.

3) **Pulley systems** use weights or springs for upper or lower limb strengthening. They include the pulley weight systems (free-standing or wall-mounted) and the Elgin exercise unit. The Elgin unit uses a series of interconnected cables and independent weights and pulleys that make it possible for a patient to perform isotonic or isometric exercises.

4) **Isotonic torque arm units,** such as the N-K unit, provide constant resistance through either a hydraulic force plate friction mechanism or an interchangeable weight-resistance system. They are usually designed for the knee but can be adapted for the hip and shoulders.

5) **Variable resistance equipment** or **dynamic variable resistance (DVR) systems,** such as the Nautilus, Eagle, and Universal DVR systems use a cam shaft device in the weight-cable system to provide maximal load at multiple points rather than at just one point in the ROM as the muscle exerts concentrically and eccentrically. Other variable resistance units (e.g., Keiser Cam II system) use pressurized pneumatic resistance. These machines occupy a great amount of space because multiple units are usually needed to strengthen different muscle groups.

6) **Cycle ergometers (stationary bicycles)** use a friction device to increase resistance and are used to increase lower limb strength and endurance.

7) **Resistive reciprocal exercise units** are used for repetitive reciprocal exercises to improve lower limb endurance, strength, or reciprocal coordination as well as cardiovascular fitness. They can be wall-mounted and adapted for upper limb exercise or they can be attached to a sturdy straightback chair or WC as an alternative for patients who cannot use a stationary bicycle.

3. **Isokinetic strengthening exercise** is a dynamic exercise performed with constant angular joint velocity, i.e., the muscle shortens or lengthens at a constant rate. However, the load or force exerted may be variable. Due to the specificity of exercise, the strength gain is greatest at the speed trained. To increase strength, isokinetic training at slow speed is more effective. Isokinetic resistance is controlled through a dynamometer, which can provide either passive (allowing only concentric actions) or active (allowing both concentric and eccentric actions) modes. The isokinetic machine is quite safe and can provide a computerized record of the torque for analysis; however, it is costly, does not accommodate all muscle groups, and can greatly increase blood pressure during exercise. Patients must be advised to move maximally, because if they move at a speed lower than the preset speed, there is no torque generated and strengthening exercise is not attained. Isokinetic exercise is usually done at five to seven repetitions in three sets. Isokinetic exercise equipments include Cybex (most common), Biodex, Kincom, Lido, Merac, Orthotron II, and Upper Body Exerciser.

III. **Cardiopulmonary endurance exercises (**also known as **conditioning** or **total body endurance exercises)** refer to low-intensity, high-repetition exercises of large groups of muscles to enhance the overall cardiopulmonary fitness of an individual (this is in contrast to resistance training referred to in section II, which improves only local muscular endurance). Cardiopulmonary endurance exercises increase one's ability to perform repeated motor tasks in daily living and to carry on a sustained level of functional activity, such as walking or climbing stairs.

Long-term cardiovascular effects of cardiopulmonary endurance training include decreased HR at rest and submaximal effort (thus the heart rate reserve is increased although the peak HR remains unchanged or is slightly decreased); small (5-10 mm Hg) but clinically useful decrease in BP at rest and submaximal effort, but increased peak BP during ''maximal'' exercise (or ''peak'' exercise because it is difficult to determine if the effort is indeed ''maximal'' especially if the patient voluntarily terminates the exercise session); a 20- to 30-ml increase in peak stroke volume (SV) during ''maximal'' exercise (probably due to increased cardiac preloading caused by plasma volume expansion and decreased afterloading caused by increased ventricular contractility and increased muscle strength); little effect on resting cardiac output with a small decrease in cardiac output during submaximal exercise and an equivalent of 10 to 20% increase of peak cardiac output during "maximal" exercise (due to training-induced increment in peak SV despite absent or slightly reduced peak HR [because cardiac output = SV × HR]); and reduced myocardial oxygen consumption at rest and submaximal effort, but a small increase in peak myocardial oxygen consumption during "maximal" exercise (as reflected by the unchanged peak HR and the potential increase of peak systolic BP).

Cardiopulmonary endurance training can also decrease exercise recovery time (i.e., more rapid return of the above changes to resting levels after exertion), increase coronary blood flow (probably due to longer diastolic phase thus allowing longer period of coronary perfusion), increase the wall thickness and muscle mass (up to 30%) of the left ventricle (thus increasing end-diastolic volume and ejection fraction), increase aerobic enzymatic activity; increase arteriovenous oxygen difference; and increase maximum ventilatory ability. The hemoglobin concentration remains unchanged or may be slightly decreased due to expansion of plasma volume. Overall, there is an increase in oxidative (aerobic) capacity of the muscle.

Another systemic effect of cardiopulmonary endurance exercise is an increased blood cortisol level (see Fig. 4.2-1), which in turn promotes protein catabolism (especially in less active muscle) and suppresses protein synthesis. This catabolic effect (occurring during the exercise session) increases the pool of free amino acids, which, after the exercise session, are eventually used as "building materials" for the adaptive synthesis of structural and enzymatic proteins (probably through the mediation of thyroid hormone, growth hormone, insulin, and/or testosterone). There is also improved thermal regulation capability (i.e., increased sweating, begins at lower temperatures with less salt content); increased lipolysis (see Fig. 4.2-1), which leads to increased free fatty acid and glycerol production; and decreased serum triglycerides (TG) and low-density lipoproteins (LDL) with increased high-density lipoproteins (HDL). The alteration in serum lipid (which lasts for 1 to 2 days after the exercise session) helps reduce the risk of coronary artery diseases in trained individuals.

For a given work load, the increase in blood pressure, heart rate, cardiac output, and oxygen uptake during maximal exercise is greater in cardiopulmonary endurance exercises involving the upper limbs than those involving the lower limbs. The increase in cardiac output in upper–limb exercises is caused by the increased heart rate, not stroke volume. As in strengthening exercises, the overload principle applies to cardiopulmonary endurance exercises, i.e., the body must work close to the point of fatigue (or mitochondrial exhaustion) to increase its metabolic or aerobic capacities.

A. Aerobic endurance exercise encompasses strengthening and cardiopulmonary endurance exercise. It uses large groups of muscles to increase the oxygen consumption gradually (a combination of arm and leg aerobic exercise is the most effective way of producing cardiopulmonary fitness). Depending on the patient's preference and physical condition, the following low-impact aerobics may be recommended: stationary bicycling, cycling, race-walking, calisthenics, low-impact aerobic exercises, swimming, aquatic exercises, rowing, hiking, and cross-country skiing. All aerobic endurance exercises should be controlled and progressive. They must be done using correct technique (i.e., knowledge of the basic rules of the sport), proper equipment, and appropriate protective measures (e.g., wearing appropriate shoes; exercising on non-concrete surfaces; stretching, warming-up, and cooling down). Unless the patient is physically well-conditioned and has good musculoskeletal conditions, the following should be avoided: contact sports (e.g., basketball, football, soccer); sports that involve trunk twisting (e.g., tennis, racquetball, squash, golf); and other high-impact activities (e.g., jogging, running, volleyball, hopping, jumping, rope-skipping, high-impact forms of aerobic dancing, downhill skiing).

Each aerobic endurance exercise session should consist of a 5- to 10-minute warm-up period; followed by 20 to 30 minutes of training at 40 to 60% (low-intensity training), or 60 to 70% (moderate-intensity training), or 70 to 85% (heavy-intensity training) of their maximal functional capacity (see below for methods of determining exercise intensity); ending with a 5- to 10-minute cool-down period. In patients whose functional capacities are below 3 metabolic equivalents (MET) (see below) short sessions of about 5 minutes should be performed several times a day. Patients with functional capacities above 5 MET should exercise 3 to 5 times per week.

Depending on such factors as age, functional capacity, health status, and compliance, the rate of exercise progression generally follows three stages: (1) the initial *conditioning stage*, which involves low-intensity exercise for 10 to 15 minutes (this stage lasts for 4-6 weeks); (2) the *improvement stage*, which involves performing the exercise at the appropriate training intensity (discussed below) with gradual increment in duration until the patient can exercise at least 20 to 30 minutes (this stage lasts 4-5 months); and (3) the *maintenance stage*, which involves regular continuation of the routine acquired in the improvement stage (this stage is usually attained after about 6 months of training).

Aerobic exercise can be used for weight control because of its ability to lower TG and LDL, increase HDL, and increase caloric expenditure. These effects are dependent on the intensity and frequency of the exercise. To control excess body fat, the aerobic activity should use about 300 kcal per exercise session and be performed for at least 20 minutes for a minimum of 3 days per week. Aerobic exercise for longer durations and at lower intensities, performed for 4 or 5 days per week may be prescribed to maximize the weight-controlling effect. In addition to aerobic exercises, the overweight or obese patients should lower caloric intake (generally not <1200 kcal/day to allow for a gradual weight loss of about 2 lb/week); gradually reduce fat intake and increase complex carbohydrate and fiber intake; incorporate behavioral techniques to help manage eating and exercise behavior; and participate in peer social support groups. These patients may find regular counseling from therapists (for about 6 months) as well as periodic physician follow-up helpful.

During aerobic exercise, HR must be monitored to ensure that the maximal safe exercise limit will not be exceeded, especially in situations that naturally increase HR (e.g., hot, humid weather). In addition to HR, the rate-pressure product (RPP) (also called double product) should be monitored. The RPP (i.e., $RPP = HR \times systolic\ BP$; see Chapter 2.7, section I.A), decreases for a given work load as the patient becomes more conditioned during training. The following are techniques commonly used to prescribe and monitor aerobic endurance exercise intensity:

1. **Target heart rate range (THRR) methods.** The THRR can be used to guide aerobic exercise intensity as follows: if the pulse or heart rate exceeds the upper limit of THRR, then the exercise intensity should be slowed down, but if the pulse or heart rate is less than the lower limit of the THRR, then

the exercise intensity should be increased. For a training effect to occur, the exercise intensity must be such that the pulse or heart rate is within the THRR for at least 20 to 30 min.

a. **Karvonen formula** uses the heart rate reserve, which is computed by subtracting the resting HR from the maximal HR. The "maximal" heart rate (MHR) is obtained from an exercise tolerance test (e.g., cardiovascular or cardiopulmonary graded exercise tolerance test described in Chapter 2.7, sections I.A and II.A, respectively); while the resting heart rate is obtained with the subject in a seated position. The THRR using the Karvonen formula can then be computed, **(maximal HR − resting HR) (40-85%) + resting HR = THRR.** The low range (40%) and the high range (85%) of the THRR may be lowered for patients with more impaired cardiopulmonary functions or in the initial phase of cardiac rehabilitation (see Chapter 5.13, section IV.A).

b. **Age-adjusted maximal HR (AAMHR) formula,** which is less accurate, can be used to estimate the THRR in healthy subjects who have not undergone formal graded exercise tolerance testing. The AAMHR is estimated by subtracting the patient's age in years from 220. The THRR using the AAMHR can thus be computed, **(220 − age) (65-85%) = THRR.** Although this method is easier to calculate, it is not generally recommended because it yields significantly lower THRR values. If used at all, the THRR should be adjusted by adding 10 to 15%.

2. **Metabolic equivalents (MET) method.** The use of MET (see description in Chapter 2.7, section II.A.2.a) for prescribing aerobic exercise intensity in patients with cardiopulmonary disease is probably the least accurate and must, therefore, be used with great caution and an awareness of the physiologic limitations. This is partly because most of the experiments used in constructing the table showing the MET equivalent for different activities (see Tables 4.2-2 and 4.2-3) derived their data from normal subjects (e.g., healthy, young men), hence their values tend to be overestimated for patients with cardiopulmonary problems. Moreover, MET levels estimated from an exercise tolerance test using the lower limbs (e.g., treadmill or bicycling test) do not determine the exact MET level that might be achieved during upper–limb exercise, nor does it account for the emotional or physiologic stress that may increase the metabolic demand during actual performance of activities.

When the MET equivalent is used for exercise prescription, it is advisable to begin the exercise program with an initial target range of 50 to 60% of the "maximal" MET level, which is estimated from the cardiovascular or cardiopulmonary graded exercise tolerance test (see Chapter 2.7, section I.A and II.A). For some patients (e.g., elderly or those with severe cardiopulmonary disease), the initial training intensity may be as low as 40% of the "maximum" MET level. As training effects are achieved, the target range can be increased up to 70 to 85% of the "maximum" MET level. Using the table of various activities with corresponding MET equivalents (see Tables 4.2-2 and 4.2-3), the individual may select activities for training that are known to require energy expenditures within the target MET range. Likewise, if the MET equivalent table is used for advising patients about recreational and occupational activities, the recommended activity should correspond to a MET level that is 50 to 80% lower than the "maximum" MET level obtained during exercise tolerance testing. For example, if the "maximum" workload corresponds to a "maximum"

Table 4.2-2.   Classification of self-care or home activities and occupational activities by MET* units

(METs)	SELF-CARE OR HOME	OCCUPATIONAL
1.5-3 (very light)	Self-care (washing, shaving, dressing) Light house work (washing dishes, polishing furniture, washing clothes) Writing at desk	Sitting (desk work, clerical, assembly, computer work, driving car/truck, operating crane, radio and television repair, light woodworking, riding lawn mower) Standing (bartending, standing as a store clerk, janitorial work)
3-5 (light)	House work (mopping or scrubbing floors, cleaning windows, slowly waxing floors, vacuuming) Yard work (raking leaves, hoeing, weeding, pushing light-power mower) Carrying objects (15-30 lb)	Auto repair, machine assembly, stocking shelves (light objects), paperhanging, light carpentry, masonry (plastering, brick laying, pushing wheelbarrow with 100-lb or 45-kg load), welding (moderate load), painting, energetic musician, trailer truck in traffic
5-7 (moderate)	Yard work (easy digging in garden, level hand–lawn mowing) Climbing stairs (slowly) Carrying objects (30-60 lb) Shoveling 10 times/min (4.5 kg or 10 lb)	Carpentry (exterior home building), using pneumatic tools, splitting wood
7-9 (heavy)	Stair climbing (moderate speed) Carrying objects (60-90 lb) Shoveling 10 times/min (5.5 kg or 14 lb)	Digging ditches, sawing hardwood, tending furnace, pick and shovel.
>9 (very heavy)	Climbing stairs (quickly), carrying load upstairs, carrying objects (>90 lb) Shoveling 10 times/min (7.5 kg or 16 lb)	Lumber jack, heavy laborer

Adapted from Fox SM, III, Naughton JP, Gorman PA: Physical activity and cardiovascular health: Part III. The exercise prescription: Frequency and type of activity. *Mod Concepts Cardiovasc Dis.* 41(6):27-28, 1972, with permission and Haskell WL: Design and implementation of cardiac conditioning programs. In Wenger NK, Hellerstein HK, editors: *Rehabilitation of the coronary patient*, New York, 1978, John Wiley, pp. 214-215.

* One MET (metabolic equivalent) = 3.5 ml O_2 consumption/kg/min at rest.

MET level of 12 to 13, then an activity corresponding to a level of 8 MET is recommended, i.e., bicycling at 13 mph or walking at 3.4 mph with 10% grade (see Table 4.2-3).

3. **Borg's rate of perceived exertion (RPE) scale method.** The Borg's RPE scale (see Table 4.2-4) is used by the patient to rate the intensity of exercise. It provides a subjective means of monitoring exercise intensity as patients become more familiar with the "feeling" associated with exercising at the appropriate THRR. A rating of 12 to 13 (somewhat hard) on the 20-

Table 4.2-3. Classification of recreational and physical conditioning activities by MET units for a 70-kg person (See also Table 2.7-3 for determining MET units during treadmill exercise.)

MET	RECREATIONAL	PHYSICAL CONDITIONING
1.5-2	Card playing, flying, knitting, motorcycling, sewing	Standing, walking (1 mph), bed exercise (arm movement, supine or sitting)
2-3	Billiards, bowling, canoeing, golfing with power cart, horseback riding at a walk, powerboat driving, skeet shooting, shuffleboard	Walking (2 mph), level bicycling (5 mph), TM (2 mph, 0% grade = 2.5 MET), very light calisthenics
3-4	Archery, badminton (social doubles), dancing (moderate), fly fishing (standing in waders), golf (pulling cart), horseback riding (trotting), pitching horse shoes, sailing (handling) small boat, softball (excluding pitcher), volleyball (6-person, noncompetitive)	Walking (3 mph), bicycling (6 mph), TM (2 mph, 2.5% grade = 3.2 MET; or 3 mph, 0% grade = 3.3 MET), light calisthenics
4-5	Badminton (singles), ballet, dancing (foxtrot, vigorous), golf (carrying clubs), Ping Pong, tennis (doubles), rowing (noncompetitive)	Walking (3.5 mph), bicycling (8 mph), TM (2.5 mph, 5% grade = 4.6; or 3 mph, 2.5% grade = 4.3 MET), many calisthenics (in general)
5-6	Canoeing (4 mph), horseback riding ("posting" to trotting), skating (9 mph, ice or roller), stream fishing (walking in light current in waders)	Walking (4 mph), bicycling (10 mph), TM (2 mph, 10% grade = 5.3 MET; or 3 mph, 5% grade = 5.4 MET)
6-7	Badminton (competitive), dancing (folk, square), skiing (light downhill, touring at 2.5 mph), tennis (singles), water skiing	Walking (5 mph), bicycling (11 mph), TM (3 mph, 7.5% grade = 6.4 MET), swimming (20 yds/min)
7-8	Basketball, canoeing (5 mph), football (touch), hiking (mountain, no backpack), horseback riding (gallop), ice hockey, paddleball, skiing (vigorous, downhill)	Jogging (5 mph), bicycling (12 mph), TM (3 mph, 10% grade = 7.4 MET)
8-9	Basketball (vigorous), fencing, handball (social), rope skipping, ski touring (4 mph), squash (social)	Running (5.5 mph), bicycling (13 mph), TM (3.4 mph, 10% grade = 8.3 MET), swimming (30 yards/min),
10 +	Handball (competitive), rowing (11 mph = 13.5 METs), ski touring (5 mph), squash (competitive)	Running (6 mph = 10 MET); 7 mph = 11.5 MET; 8 mph = 13.5 MET; 9 mph = 15 MET; 10 mph = 17 MET), TM (3.4 mph, 14% grade = 10 MET), TM (3.4 mph, 18% grade = 12 MET), swimming (>40 yds/min)

Adapted from Fox SM, III, Naughton JP, Gorman PA: Physical activity and cardiovascular health: Part III. The exercise prescription: Frequency and type of activity, *Mod Concepts Cardiovasc Dis.* 41:27-28, 1972, with permission of the American Heart Association.

One MET (metabolic equivalent) = 3.5 ml O_2 consumption/kg/min at rest; TM = treadmill; mph = miles per hour.

Table 4.2-4. Borg's Ratings of Perceived Exertion (RPE) and Category-Ratio (CR-10) scales

RPE SCALE[1]	CATEGORY-RATIO (CR-10) SCALE[2]
6 No exertion at all	0 Nothing at all
7 Extremely light	0.5 Extremely weak (just noticeable)
8	1 Very weak
9 Very light	2 Weak (light)
10	3 Moderate
11 Light	4 Somewhat strong
12	5 Strong (heavy)
13 Somewhat hard	6
14	7 Very strong
15 Hard (heavy)	8
16	9
17 Very hard	10 Extremely strong (almost max)
18	● Maximal*
19 Extremely hard	
20 Maximal exertion	

Note: The RPE scale is commonly used for rating perceived exercise intensity in exercise tolerance testing and in exercise prescription. The scale values of 6 to 20 was chosen to approximate the linear increase in heart rate from 60 to 200 beats per minute as exercise intensity increases. The CR-10 is commonly used for intensity evaluation and has been used to rate angina, aches in the working muscles, and pain from loaded passive joint structures.

* If the intensity rating is greater than 10, the person can choose any large number in proportion to 10 that describes the proportionate increase in intensity, i.e., if it feels 30% more than at the rating of 10, the RPE would be 13.

[1] From: Borg G: Perceived exertion as an indicator of somatic stress. *Scand J Rehabil Med*, 2 (2-3), 92-98, 1970, and Borg G: *An introduction to Borg's RPE scale*, Ithaca, NY, 1985, Movement Publications. Copyright © Gunnar Borg, 1970, 1985, used with permission.

[2] From: Borg G, Holmgren A, Lindblad I: Quantitative evaluation of chest pain. *Acta Medica Scand*, Suppl. 644: 43-45, 1981, and Borg G: A category scale with ratio properties for intermodal and interindividual comparisons. In Geissler HG, Petzold P, editors: *Psychophysical judgment and the process of perception*. Berlin, 1982, VEB Deutscher Verlag der Wissenschaften, pp. 25-34. Copyright © Gunnar Borg, 1981, 1982, used with permission.

point scale corresponds to about 60% of maximum HR, but a rating of 15 (hard) corresponds to about 85%. If the category-ratio (CR–10) scale is used (see Table 4.2-4), these ratings would be between 4 and 5. Denial of perceived exertion (in competitive individuals) limits the practical application of the Borg's RPE scale. The Borg's RPE scale is probably more psychological than physiological. Its use allows an individual to concentrate more on how a particular intensity of exercise feels and still have some assurance that he or she is within the THRR. This ability to use the RPE makes it easier for patients to be independent in their own activities and to wean patients off external monitoring devices. In patients with cardiac transplant (see chapter 5.13, section IV.A.2.a), the RPE is recommended because of denervation of the heart (which decreases the reliability of other parameters such as heart rate).

B. Anaerobic endurance exercises are performed to deplete the glycolytic system, which functions in the first 1 to 2 minutes of exercise. High-resistance, short duration exercises at 80% of maximum exertion capacity are needed. Interval training with intense short duration activity of 1 or 2 minutes has been recommended (e.g., for sprinters).

IV. Motor coordination and skill exercises increase one's ability to regulate muscles simultaneously or in sequence to perform apparently simple or complex activities. It is controlled by the conscious activation of an individual muscle or the conscious initiation of a preprogrammed engram. General principles of coordination exercises include constant repetition of a few motor activities, use of sensory cues (tactile, visual, proprioceptive) to enhance motor performance, and increase in the speed of the activity over time.

A. Frenkel exercises are a series of exercises of increasing difficulty to improve proprioceptive control in the lower limbs. They begin with simple movements with gravity eliminated, then gradually progress to more complicated movement patterns using simultaneous hip and knee motions carried against gravity. They are useful for coordination retraining for proprioceptive or cerebellar dysfunction.

B. Traditional approaches for improving motor control and coordination emphasize the need for repetition of specific movement for learning, the importance of sensation to the control of movement, and the need to develop basic movements and postures, with the assumption that when movement is ''normalized'' then skilled movement would occur automatically (based on the hierarchical theory of motor control wherein development progresses sequentially from lower to higher levels of control). These approach are aimed at permanently reorganizing the central nervous system (CNS). The four traditional systems presented below differ in whether abnormal spinal and brainstem reflexes should (Brunnstrom) or should not (Bobath) be used to elicit movement when the patient cannot otherwise move, whether redevelopment of motor control should be sought in an ontogenetic sequence (PNF and Rood) or in a proximodistal sequence (Bobath and Brunnstrom), and whether conscious attention should be directed toward the movement itself (Brunnstrom and PNF) or only toward the goal of the movement (Rood and Bobath). None of the traditional systems addresses methods of developing skilled movement. They are used in a variety of neuromotor impairments (e.g., spasticity in spinal cord injury [SCI], cerebrovascular accident [CVA], traumatic brain injury [TBI], and cerebral palsy [CP] patients and multiple sclerosis [MS] patients with ataxia). Their clinical effectiveness, however, remains to be proved in randomized controlled studies.

1. Peripheral neuromuscular facilitation (PNF) (Kabat and Voss approach) uses spiral and diagonal components of movement rather than the traditional movements in cardinal planes of motion with the goal of facilitating movement patterns that will have more functional relevance than the traditional techniques of strengthening individual muscle groups. The movement patterns are developmentally sequenced but do not emphasize inhibition of abnormal reflex activities. It uses resistance during the spiral and diagonal movement patterns with the goal of facilitating ''irradiation'' of impulses to other parts of the body associated with the primary movement.

2. **Movement therapy (Brunnstrom approach)** is based on the theoretical concept that damaged CNS has undergone an evolution in reverse and has regressed to phylogenetically older patterns of movement (e.g., limb synergies and primitive reflexes). Thus, synergies, reflexes, and other abnormal movement patterns are seen as normal part of the recovery process before normal movement is attained. Patients are taught to voluntarily control the motor patterns available to them at that point in their recovery process (e.g., limb synergies). These are subsequently modified into simple to complex movement combination patterns. (For details, refer to Brunnstrom S: *Movement therapy in hemiplegia*, New York, 1970, Harper & Row.)

3. **Neurodevelopmental technique (NDT) (Bobath approach)** is based on the theoretical concept that pathologic movement patterns (e.g., limb synergies and primitive reflexes) must not be used for training because repeated use of the pathologic efferent pathways may make it too readily available for use at the expense of normal pathways. This approach is opposite to the Brunnstrom and PNF approaches, in which abnormal reflex activity is reinforced rather than inhibited. The goal of NDT is to normalize tone, to inhibit primitive or "abnormal" reflex patterns, and to facilitate automatic reactions and subsequent normal movement patterns. Patients are taught to use patterns of movement, which are opposite to abnormal patterns (so called "reflex inhibiting patterns") and are guided by the therapist from "key points of control" to inhibit abnormal motor activity and facilitate more normal motor activity. "Key points of control" refer to points on the body, usually proximal such as shoulder and pelvic girdles, which, when handled by the therapist in a specific manner, can be used to influence or reduce abnormal/spastic movements. (For details, refer to Bobath B: *Adult hemiplegia: evaluation and treatment,* London, 1978, W. Heinemann.)

4. **Sensorimotor approach (Rood approach)** uses sensorimotor stimuli to normalize tone and activate purposeful movement and postural responses starting at the patient's current level of development and progressing sequentially to higher levels of control. These sensorimotor stimuli include quick stretch, icing, fast brushing, slow stroking, tendon tapping, vibration, and joint compression to promote cocontraction of proximal muscles.

C. **Contemporary approaches for improving motor control and coordination** are influenced by contemporary skill acquisition and motor development theories. They emphasize motor performance using functional tasks and consider factors other than CNS damage that may affect performance, include remediation of performance components and modification of the environment to improve task performance, stress practice that fits the nature of the task, and reject the assumption of the hierarchical model of motor control and the traditional developmental theories. These approaches are new and need further research.

1. **Motor relearning program (MRP) for stroke patients (Carr and Shepherd approach)** draws heavily from cognitive motor learning theory and is influenced by Bobath's NDT. The patient is considered an active participant whose major goal is to relearn how to move functionally and how to problem solve during attempts at novel tasks. The MRP provides guidelines for evaluating and improving motor control in seven categories of functional daily activities: upper limb function, orofacial function, sitting up over the side of the bed, balanced sitting, standing up and sitting down, balanced standing, and walking. Instead of providing a specific sequence for intervention, MRP recommends an analysis of the task, practice of the missing compo-

nent, practice of the task, and transference of training. The five strategies used are: verbal instruction; visual demonstration; manual guidance; accurate, timely feedback about the quality of performance; and consistency of practice.

Unlike traditional approaches that emphasize repetitive performance of a specific movement for improving skill, MRP teaches general strategies for solving motor problems. In MRP, activities like rolling are not given emphasis as in the traditional approach because MRP does not believe in the hierarchical theory of motor control. Instead of the proximodistal sequence, MRP therapists encourage any active movement in wrist and finger muscles. If possible, hand function is practiced simultaneously with shoulder girdle control and postural adjustments within the context of functional reaching tasks. The therapist's role is to guide the individual in this process and to prevent or remove obstacles that may lead to the use of inefficient compensatory strategies. When the patient can perform activities effectively and automatically in a variety of environmental contexts, then task learning is considered successful.

2. **Contemporary task-oriented approach** uses purposeful activity as the primary treatment modality with the assumption that functional tasks help organize motor behavior. It assumes that after CNS damage or other changes in personal or environmental systems, the patient's behavioral changes reflect attempts to compensate to achieve functional goals, and that occupational performance emerges from the interaction of multiple systems that represent the unique characteristics of the person and the performance context. Another assumption is that personal and environmental systems are heterarchically organized (i.e., no automatic or inherent ordering of the system in terms of their importance or influence on the motor behavior), and that a person needs to practice and experiment with varied strategies to find the optimal solution for a motor problems and develop skill in performance. Treatment goals are to help the patient develop the optimal movement patterns for performing a task, achieve flexibility in task performance by providing practice opportunities in varying contexts, maximize use of personal characteristics and environmental factors that make efficient and effective task performance possible, and facilitate problem solving by the patient so he can identify his own solutions at motor problems in the home and community environments.

V. **Speed training** is of importance in athletes and is believed to be influenced by nervous system control mechanisms. Although increase in strength can cause an increase in velocity, it does not increase absolute speed. Speed training includes rapid load movement or the use of sudden loading with muscle stretch before contraction (i.e., plyometric loading). Isotonic training can also be used to increase the speed of movement against light loads. A high-resistance, high-speed isokinetic protocol has been used by some athletes as it is believed to cause selective hypertrophy of type II fibers without hypertrophy of type I fibers, thus helping the athlete become both faster and stronger.

VI. **Relaxation exercises** are done consciously (with active mental and physical participation from the patient) to induce a ''relaxation response,'' which is a psychophysiologic state of low arousal characterized by generalized decrease in sympathetic nervous system activity and concomitant decreases in respiratory rate, oxygen consumption, heart rate, blood pressure, arterial blood lactate levels, and muscle tension, as well as increases in skin resistance, skeletal muscle blood flow, and electroencephalographic (EEG) α–activity. This ''relaxation response'' has been demonstrated using biofeedback tools (see Chapter 4.1, section VI) in conjunction with relaxation techniques. They are beneficial to most PM&R patients, for example, to help reduce pain perception in patients with acute or chronic pain (see Chapter 5.10, section VI.F.3.b) and to reduce cardiopulmonary stress in patients with cardiac and/or pulmonary problems (see Chapters 5.12 and 5.13). For the relaxation technique to be effective, it must be congenial to the patient, help restore the patient's sense of control, be easy to apply in different settings (i.e., portable), offer relatively immediate reduction of pain, promote other pain-related benefits (e.g., reduced intake of pain medication and increased activity), and be cost-effective.

Relaxation exercises can be performed singly or incorporated into the other exercise sessions (e.g., as part of the warm-up or, more commonly, the cool-down session of aerobic exercise and before or after limbering or stretching exercises). At the beginning of training, relaxation exercises should be done in a quiet semidarkened room with the patient in a comfortable supine or semireclining position. Constricting garments should be loosened, and small pillows may be used (e.g., under the head or under the knees) to promote muscle relaxation. Biofeedback machines (see Chapter 4.1, section VI) may be used during the training period. Eventually, the patient must learn how to apply relaxation techniques in more upright postures such as sitting or standing and during other activities. Patients are encouraged to schedule relaxation sessions at home and at work, and to perform them during stressful periods. The following relaxation exercise techniques can be used singly or in combination (e.g., controlled-breathing exercises, followed by progressive muscle relaxation, and then dissociative visualization while breathing is maintained in a rhythmic relaxing pattern throughout the session):

A. Physiologic relaxation strategies

1. **Controlled-breathing relaxation exercise** involves slow breathing patterns to promote parasympathetic activity and counteract sympathetic activity. Usually, the pattern of breathing used is a **diaphragmatic breathing** (see also Chapter 5.12, section IV.B.2.a.1) in which the abdomen swells out during inspiration so that the lower part of the chest and, finally, the upper chest expands and slightly lifts; then the breath is held momentarily and released slowly as the abdomen is drawn in, the diaphragm is lifted, and the chest relaxes.

   a. **"One" breathing technique,** which is a form of meditation, involves the passive focusing of awareness on the diaphragmatic breathing cycle while silently repeating the word ''one'' with each exhalation. The patient is instructed to maintain a passive attitude and permit (rather than force) relaxation to occur at its own pace. It can be performed for 10 to 20 minutes, one to two times daily.

   b. **Eye-movement breathing technique** involves looking up to the eyebrows (without head movement) during the inspiratory phase of diaphragmatic breathing, then holding the breath for 2 seconds followed by looking down to the chin (without head movement) while breathing out very slowly and completely (as a ''sissing'' sound is produced between the teeth and as the abdomen is drawn in as in diaphragmatic breathing). To promote relaxation, the expiratory phase can be prolonged. The cycle is repeated at least four to five times and is usually used before or after other exercises (e.g., limbering or stretching exercises; see Chapter 4.11, section I.B.3.a) or in synchrony with muscle stretching (e.g., of the trunk, neck, or shoulder).

2. **Progressive muscle relaxation exercise (Jacobson)** consists of systematically learning to tense muscle groups (for about 10 sec) followed by active relaxation (i.e., releasing of tension for 10-15 sec). Usually, about 14 to 16 major muscle groups are sequentially tensed and relaxed. During the tensing and relaxation of each muscle group, the patient is asked to be consciously aware of different feelings associated with tension and with relaxation. To be effective, the patient must be able to recognize or discriminate relaxation from tension, and to voluntarily induce the state of relaxation.

B. **Cognitive relaxation strategies** involve the use of "mental" strategies to induce the "relaxation response." They can be done singly or usually in conjunction with physiologic relaxation strategies such as controlled breathing.

1. **Dissociative visualization** involves passive focusing on some personally meaningful, pleasing, relaxing, and absorbing memory or image. The technique of focusing may be attending to sensory information such as the colors and sounds of the imagery. Practice sessions usually last 15 to 20 minutes.

2. **Autogenic relaxation training,** which is a form of self-hypnosis, relies on a series of self-directed formulas to induce the relaxation response through alterations of proprioception and sensation. The patient is instructed to assume a relaxed position, to close the eyes, and to passively concentrate on a series of six standard autogenic formulas (e.g., my left arm is heavy). Standard formula one focuses on promoting the feeling of heaviness in the limbs, and formula two focuses on promoting the sensation of warmth in the limbs. Formula three and four focus on cardiac and respiratory regulation, respectively. Formula five focuses on promoting the sensation of warmth in the abdomen, and formula six focuses on the feeling of coolness in the forehead. The patient is instructed to practice these formulas daily until such time as a voluntary shift to a state of wakeful low arousal is readily attained. In addition to the six standard formulas that focus on the psychophysiologic aspects of the relaxation response, there are a series of organ-specific formulas, intentional formulas, and meditative formulas.

3. **Other cognitive techniques** include (a) the use of audiotapes or videotapes with instructions or music for relaxation, (b) guided imagery, (c) hypnosis (see Chapter 5.10, section IV.F.3.e.), (d) self-hypnosis (e.g., autogenic relaxation technique described above), and (d) meditation, i.e., focusing on one's experience (e.g., "one" breathing technique; Transcendental Meditation).

C. **Nontraditional (alternative) "psychophysical" techniques** incorporate physiologic and cognitive relaxation strategies as well as postural reeducation techniques. They include the Feldenkrais Method, Alexander Technique, Trager Psychophysical Integration, Tai Chi Chuan, and Hatha Yoga. Although most of the nontraditional techniques are able to induce a "relaxation response," their effectiveness over the more traditional and more cost-effective techniques (e.g., controlled breathing, progressive muscle relaxation, and dissociative visualization) remain controversial and are at best anecdotal.

BIBLIOGRAPHY

Basmajian JV, Wolf SL, editors: *Therapeutic exercise*, ed 5, Baltimore, 1990, Williams & Wilkins.

Brannon FJ, Foley MW, Starr JA, et al: *Cardiopulmonary rehabilitation: Basic theory and application*, ed 2, Philadelphia, 1993, FA Davis.

Ciccone CD, Alexander J: Physiology and therapeutics of exercise. In Goodgold J, editor: *Rehabilitation medicine*, St. Louis, 1988, Mosby–Year Book, pp. 759-772.

DeLateur B: Therapeutic exercise to develop strength and endurance. In Kottke FJ, Lehmann JF, editors: *Krusen's handbook of physical medicine and rehabilitation*, ed 4, Philadelphia, 1990, WB Saunders, pp. 427-464.

Gaupp LA, Flinn DE, Weddige RL: Adjunctive treatment techniques. In Tollison CD, Satterthwaite JR, Tollison JW, editors: *Handbook of pain management*, ed 2, Baltimore, 1994, Williams & Wilkins, pp. 108-135.

Hamill RJ, Rowlingson JC: *Handbook of critical care pain management*, New York, 1994, McGraw-Hill.

Joynt RL, Findley TW, Boda W, et al: Therapeutic exercise. In DeLisa JA, Gans BM, editors: *Rehabilitation medicine: Principles and practice*, ed 2, Philadelphia, 1993, JB Lippincott, pp. 526-554.

Kisner C, Colby LA: *Therapeutic exercise: Foundations and techniques*, ed 3, Philadelphia, 1996, FA Davis.

Pollock ML, Wilmore JH: *Exercise in health and disease*, ed 2, Philadelphia, 1990, WB Saunders.

Torg JS, Shephard RJ. *Current therapy in sports medicine*, ed 3, St. Louis, 1995, Mosby–Year Book.

Trombly CA, editor: *Occupational therapy for physical dysfunction* ed 4, Baltimore, 1995, Williams & Wilkins.

CHAPTER 4.3

ORTHOSES

An orthosis (or brace) is an external device applied to body parts to provide support or stabilization, improve function by restricting or assisting motion, correct flexible deformities, prevent progression of fixed deformities, or reduce pressure and pain by transferring load from one area to another. A temporary orthosis is referred to as a splint. In general, orthoses should be lightweight with reasonable durability, acceptable cosmetically, easy to maintain and clean, easy to don/doff correctly and rapidly, and adjustable to accommodate progression or resolution of disorders. Most importantly, patients should be motivated to wear it. In patients with fluctuating edema, orthoses are generally not recommended. In the presence of fluctuating muscle tones, different sets of splints or orthoses may be prescribed to meet different demands (e.g., a resting splint at night and a wrist cock-up orthosis during the day while undergoing rehabilitation activities that may increase muscle tone). If feasible, active exercises and functional activities should be prescribed together with the orthoses.

Orthoses can be constructed from metal, plastic, leather, synthetic fabrics, or any combination of these basic materials. Metal orthoses are adjustable but are heavy and are not cosmetically pleasing. Commonly used metals include stainless steel and aluminum alloys. Steel is widely used in prefabricated joints, metal uprights, metal bands and cuffs, springs, and bearings. It is relatively inexpensive, easy to work with, and fatigue-resistant (i.e., high strength with high rigidity or ductility); however, it is heavy and needs expensive alloys to prevent corrosion. Aluminum alloys are corrosion-resistant and have high strength-to-weight ratio. It is commonly used in upper limb orthoses because of its lightweight nature. Unfortunately, although its static loading strength is good, aluminum has a lower endurance limit (i.e., unable to withstand repetitive stress without failure) compared to steel. Thus, if loading conditions are known to be great and highly repetitive (e.g., adult lower limb orthoses), steel is superior to aluminum.

The type of leather most commonly used in orthotics are cattle hides, which are vegetable-tanned for texture and to prevent skin irritation. Cattle hides are recommended for shoe construction because they conduct heat well, absorb water from the moist air surrounding the foot, draw perspiration away from points of heavy sweating and redistribute it, stretch as the shoe becomes moist thus preventing constriction of hot or sweaty feet.

Plastic orthoses are used because they tend to be lighter and can provide a closer fit (i.e., it can be molded, extruded, laminated, or hardened into any desired form). Moreover, they are unaffected by fluids (e.g., water, urine, and oils) and are radiolucent. However, they are not adjustable in length and are not as durable as metal (hence not commonly used as joints). Plastics used for orthoses can be classified into thermosetting and thermoplastic materials.

Thermosetting materials develop a permanent shape when heat and pressure are applied; therefore, they cannot be softened when reheated and then be reshaped. Thermosetting plastics are somewhat more difficult to use than thermoplastics and generally cause more body irritation or allergic reaction. Polyester resins are especially useful for laminating purposes in orthotics. Epoxy resins formulated for laminating are noted for their high tensile, compressive, and flexural strength; high-impact resistance; and superior bonding strength. They have good chemical resistance and excellent resistance to weathering. Polyurethane foam is used primarily for cosmetic covers and pads for orthoses or other devices. It can be bonded not only to other plastics but also to metal or plywood.

Thermoplastics soften (and become moldable) when heated and harden when cooled. They can be divided into low-temperature and high-temperature thermoplastics. Low-temperature thermoplastics (Orthoplast, Aquaplast, Bioplastics, Glassona, Hexcelite, Kay-splint, Lightcast, Polysar, Warm-N-Form) can be molded at temperatures just above body temperature (<80°C or <180°F), hence they may be shaped directly to the body without the need for a cast. Closed-cell foam polyethylene materials, such as Plastazote, require higher temperature (110-140°C) for molding, but air convection cools their surface so rapidly that they can be formed safely on the skin, hence they are also considered low-temperature plastics. Low-temperature thermoplastics can be fabricated easily and rapidly (requiring only a supply of hot water, scissors, and a source of hot air, such as a heat gun or an oven) and are mainly used in upper limb orthotics in which low stress activity is anticipated.

High-temperature thermoplastics (acrylic, polyethylene, polypropylene, polycarbonate, acrylonitrile-butadiene-styrene [ABS] and the group of vinyl polymers and copolymers that includes polyvinyl chloride [PVC], polyvinyl alcohol [PVA], and polyvinyl acetate) require up to 150-160°C (300-350°F) to become moldable, hence they must be shaped over a plaster replica (or cast) of the body part. They are creep-resistant (i.e., it does not easily change in shape with continued stress and heat) and are ideal for long-term or permanent use especially when high stress is anticipated (e.g., in lower limb orthoses and in spastic limbs).

In general, orthotic prescription should include medical diagnosis (e.g., compressive peroneal nerve palsy), current impairment and any resulting disability (e.g., flaccid foot drop), type of orthosis (e.g., plastic ankle-foot orthosis [AFO] with flexible ankle held in neutral position), and orthotic goals (e.g., toe clearance during swing-through and prevention of foot slap during early stance). This chapter covers only orthoses primarily used for adults.

I. **Shoes and lower–limb orthoses** are generally used to safely assist gait, reduce pain, decrease weightbearing, control movement, and minimize worsening of a deformity. The prescribed lower–limb orthosis should be properly fitted so the patient can easily don and doff it and either rest the desired segment or stand, sit, and perform the prescribed movement comfortably (throughout all phases of gait) when wearing the orthosis. Any discomfort should be addressed because it could lead to decreased use of orthosis and subsequent loss of function. In patients with decreased sensation or impaired circulation, the skin must be checked regularly for redness, trophic changes, abrasions, and dermatitis. Skin redness should disappear 10 minutes after orthosis removal. The orthosis also must be functionally as well as cosmetically acceptable to the patient.

A. **Shoes** are integral part of the lower limb orthoses. They are worn to protect the feet from the external environment, keep the feet warm, and help transfer body weight to the ground while walking. In persons with orthopedic problems, shoes can be modified to reduce pressure on sensitive deformed structures by redistributing weight toward pain-free areas. Shoes can also serve as the foundation of lower limb orthoses. Parts of three basic shoe types are shown in Fig 4.3-1. Different types and styles of shoes used in PM&R are shown in Fig. 4.3-2. A properly fitted shoe should have adequate room for the foot to expand upon bearing weight. The shoe should be at least 1 cm

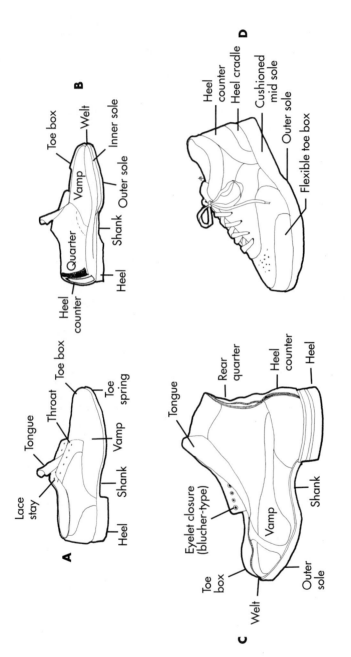

Figure 4.3-1
Parts of 3 basic shoe types. **A,** Low-quarter shoe (external view). **B,** Low-quarter shoe (cut view). **C,** High quarter shoe. **D,** athletic shoe.

Table 4.3-1.   Suggested shoe modifications for common foot problems

FOOT PROBLEMS (GOALS)	SUGGESTED SHOE MODIFICATIONS
Limb shortening (to equalize leg length, improve posture and gait)	Heel elevation (if <1/2 in = internal; if >½ in = external); heel and sole elevation (if >1 in); rocker bar; high quarter shoe
Arthritis, fusion, or instability of ankle and subtalar joints (to support and limit ankle joint motion, improve gait, accommodate deformities)	High quarter shoe; reinforced counters; long steel shank; rocker bar; SACH heel
Pes plano-valgo (to reduce eversion, support longitudinal arch)	Thomas heel with medial high wedge; medial longitudinal arch support with cookie or scaphoid pad
Fixed pes equinus (to provide heel strike, contain foot in shoe, reduce MT head pressure, improve ease of putting on shoe, equalize leg length)	High quarter shoe; heel elevation; heel and sole elevation on other shoe; modified lace-stay for wide opening; medial longitudinal arch support; rocker bar, occasionally
Pes varus (to realign flexible deformity, accommodate a fixed deformity, increase medial and posterior weight bearing on foot)	High quarter shoe; long lateral counter; reverse Thomas heel; lateral shoe and heel wedges for flexible deformity; medial wedges for fixed deformity; lateral sole and heel flanges; medial longitudinal arch support
Pes cavus (to distribute weight over entire foot, restore AP foot balance, and reduce pressure on MT heads)	High quarter shoe; high toe box; lateral heel and sole wedges; metatarsal pads or bars; molded inner sole; medial and lateral longitudinal arch support
Calcaneal spurs (to decrease pain)	Heel cushion; inner relief in heel and fill with soft sponge
Metatarsalgia (to reduce pressure on MT heads, support transverse arch)	Metatarsal or sesamoid pad; metatarsal or rocker bar; inner sole relief
Hallux valgus (to reduce pressure on 1st MTP and big toe, prevent forward foot slide, immobilize 1st MTP, shift weight laterally)	Soft vamp with broad ball and toe; relief in vamp with cut-out or balloon patch; low heel; metatarsal or sesamoid pad; medial longitudinal arch support
Hallux rigidus (to reduce pressure and motion on 1st MTP, improve push-off)	Soft vamp; long steel spring in sole; sesamoid pad; metatarsal or rocker bar; medial longitudinal arch support
Hammer toes (to relieve pressure on painful areas, support transverse arch, improve push-off)	Soft vamp; extra depth shoe with high toe box or balloon patch; metatarsal pad
Unilateral Foot shortening (to fit shoe to foot)	Extra inner sole and padded tongue for difference of <1 size; shoes of split sizes or custom-made
Foot fractures (to immobilize fractured part)	Long steel shank; longitudinal arch support; metatarsal pad; metatarsal or rocker bar

From Ragnarsson, KT: Lower extremity orthotics, shoes, and gait aids. In DeLisa, JA, editor: *Rehabilitation Medicine: Principles and Practice,* 2nd ed, Philadelphia, JB Lippincott, 1993, pp. 499-500, with permission.
Abbreviations: MT = metatarsal; MTP = metatarsophalangeal joint; SACH = solid ankle cushion heel; AP = anteroposterior.

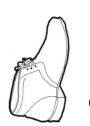

E

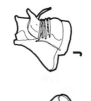

J

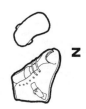

N

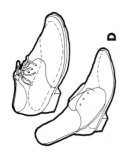

D

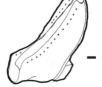

I

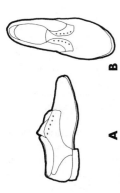

C

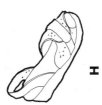

H

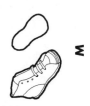

M

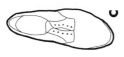

B

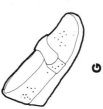

G

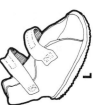

L

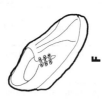

A

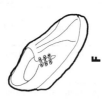

F

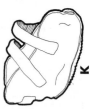

K

longer than the longest toe and the widest part should correspond to the foot's widest part. It should be snug from the heel to the ball of the foot and should fit closely around the anatomic heel. For adults with foot disorders, the most versatile shoe has an extra-depth, Blucher-type upper with a laced or Velcro closure and a low heel (see Fig. 4.3-2.D). Accommodative shoe with spacious toe box is prescribed for patients with hammer toe, claw toe or mallet toe, or bunion. Suggested shoe modification for common foot problems are shown in Table 4.3-1. Most of the current lower-limb orthoses (e.g., plastic leaf spring-type of ankle foot orthoses) use various thermoplastics that can fit inside the shoe. The orthosis is used to position and support the affected lower limb, while the shoe serves only to hold the plastic orthosis in place. For this purpose, individuals may use commercially available shoes with sturdy counters rather than leather oxford or custom-fitted "orthopedic" shoes.

1. **External shoe modifications** (see Fig. 4.3-3), unlike internal shoe modification, do not reduce shoe volume. However, they may erode as the patient walks and can be conspicuous and uncosmetic. The patient is also limited to wearing the same shoe that has been modified.

    a. **Heel modifications**

        1) **Cushioned heel** (see Fig. 4.3-3.A) is a wedge of compressible material inserted into the heel to absorb shock at heel (or foot) strike. It reduces the knee flexion moment by allowing for more rapid ankle plantarflexion and is indicated when the patient wears an orthosis with a rigid ankle.

        2) **External heel flare** (see Fig. 4.3-3.B) can be applied either medially (to resist hindfoot eversion) or laterally (to resist hindfoot inversion). Both medial and lateral heel flares may be used together to provide greater heel stability.

        3) **External heel wedge** (see Fig. 4.3-3.C, H) can be applied either medially (to rotate hindfoot into inversion) or laterally (to rotate hindfoot into eversion). The shoe must have opposite heel counter strong enough to resist the hindfoot from sliding on the wedge incline.

        4) **Extended heel** can project anteriorly either on the medial side (Thomas, orthopedic, S-shaped, or keystone heel; see Fig. 4.3-3.F) or on the

◄───

Figure 4.3-2
Different types and styles of shoes used in PM&R. **A,** Low quarter oxford-type shoe with lacing. **B,** Low quarter oxford-type shoe with Blucher-type lacing (i.e., the lace stays are not stitched to the vamp and remain loose and fully open, thus leaving more room for the entering foot). **C,** Low quarter oxford-type shoe with Bal- or Balmoral-type lacing (i.e., the lace stays meet in front and are stitched to the vamp). **D,** Extra-depth shoe (accomodates severe foot deformities such as hammer-toe deformities and allows for shoe insert). **E,** High-quarter (chukka) shoe with lacing. **F,** Custom-molded shoe (for gross deformities of feet such as diabetic neuropathy). **G,** Plastazote shoe. **H,** Plastazote sandal. **I,** Convalescent shoe with anterior lacing. **J,** Convalescent shoe with posterior lacing. **K,** Orthopedic cast boot (closed toes). **L,** Orthopedic cast boot (open toes). **M,** Pediatric prewalker (for mild residual metatarsus varus or for holding the foot in the desired position after casting). **N,** Pediatric clubfoot shoe (for residual of mild to moderate metatarsus varus or when it is necessary to hold a postsurgically corrected clubfoot).

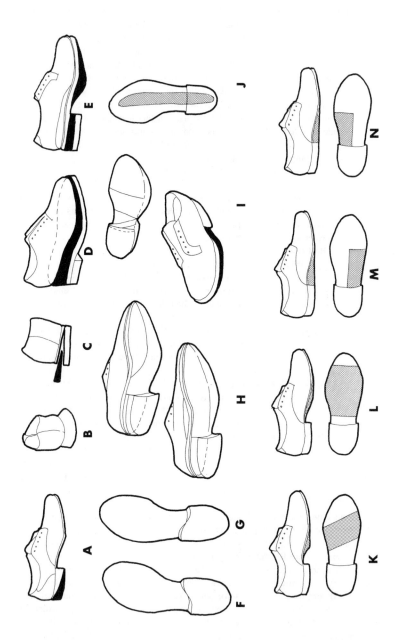

lateral side (reverse Thomas or reverse orthopedic or reverse extended heel; see Fig. 4.3-3.G). The Thomas heel provides additional support and stability to the medial longitudinal arch, while the reverse Thomas heel provides support for the lateral longitudinal arch.

5) External heel elevation (shoe lift; see Fig. 4.3-3.E) is used to compensate for fixed pes equinus deformity or a leg length discrepancy of more than 1 cm or more than 1/4 inch. A leg length discrepancy of less than 1 cm is left uncorrected to aid in swing phase transition. It can be used with a scaphoid pad to reduce tension and pain in plantar fasciitis. It also helps reduce traction force and promote healing of Achilles tendinitis.

b. External sole modifications

1) Rocker bar (see Fig. 4.3-3.E, L) is a convex strip placed across the sole just posterior to the metatarsal heads. It assists rollover by shifting the rollover point posterior to the metatarsal heads, and relieves pressure from the metatarsal heads by transferring load to the metatarsal shafts, e.g., to manage ulcers over the metatarsal head in diabetic patients with peripheral vascular disease. It can also be used in patients with multiple sclerosis to facilitate rollover and decrease demand on the plantar flexors.

2) Metatarsal bar (see Fig. 4.3-3.K) is a simple bar (e.g., a flat strip of leather) placed across the sole just posterior to the metatarsal heads. Because of its flat surface, it does not assist with rollover. Rather, it relieves pressure from the metatarsal heads by transferring load to the metatarsal shaft during late stance, for example, in metatarsalgia.

3) Sole wedge (see Fig. 4.3-3.H) alters mediolateral metatarsal alignment. A lateral wedge tends to pronate the forefoot, while a medial wedge promotes forefoot supination.

4) Sole flare (see Fig. 4.3-3.I) provides greater stability. A medial flare resists eversion, while a lateral flare resists inversion of the foot.

5) Steel bar (see Fig. 4.3-3.J) is inserted between inner and outer soles to prevent motion of the anterior sole and thus reduce stress at phalanges and metatarsals. It is commonly used with the rocker bar to assist rollover.

6) Shank filler can be applied medially (see Fig. 4.3-3.M) for additional support of the medial longitudinal arch or laterally (see Fig. 4.3-3.N) for additional support of the lateral longitudinal arch.

c. Combination external heel and sole modifications (see Fig. 4.3-3.D, E, H) are used to avoid equinus posture when heel elevation is higher than sole elevation.

Figure 4.3-3
Types of external shoe modifications (see text for description). **A,** Cushioned heel. **B,** External heel flare. **C,** External heel wedge. **D,** Combination external sandwich-elevation of the heel and sole. **E,** External heel sandwich-elevation (shoe lift), with rocker bar at the sole. **F,** Thomas heel (with medial heel extension). **G,** Reverse Thomas heel (with lateral heel extension). **H,** Combination medial sole and heel wedging (top shows sandwiching in two sections; bottom shows an overlay unit extending the full length of the sole and feet). **I,** Lateral sole flare. **J,** Steel bar. **K,** Metatarsal bar. **L,** Rocker bar sole. **M,** Medial shank filler. **N,** Lateral shank filler.

2. **Internal shoe modifications** (see Fig. 4.3-4) are inconspicuous, more cosmetically acceptable, and can fit in different shoes; however, they reduce shoe volume, requiring adequate shoe space for comfortable fit.
   a. **Internal heel modifications**
      1) **Heel excavation or heel cushion-relief** (see Fig. 4.3-4.A) is a soft pad with excavation under painful part of the heel (e.g., a calcaneal spur). The excavation is usually filled with a compressible material (e.g., soft Plastazote).
      2) **Internal heel wedge** can be applied medially (see Fig. 4.3-4.B) to rotate the hindfoot into inversion (e.g., in flexible pes valgus) or laterally (see Fig. 4.3-4.C) to evert the hindfoot and relieve pressure on the cuboid (e.g., in flexible pes varus). It also increases plantar-bearing area and can be used in fixed pes varus.
   b. **Internal sole modifications**
      1) **Inner sole excavation** (see Fig. 4.3-4.D) is a soft pad with excavation under one or more painful metatarsal heads. The excavation is usually filled with compressible material.
      2) **Metatarsal pad** (see Fig. 4.3-4.E) is a domed pad glued to the inner sole with its apex under the metatarsal shafts. It reduces stress on the metatarsal heads by transferring load to the metatarsal shafts, for example in metatarsalgia.
      3) **Scaphoid pad (*navicular pad; cookie insole*)** (see Fig. 4.3-4.F) is a rubber, cork, or plastic foam wedge used to provide medial longitudinal arch support to prevent depression of the subtalar joint. It extends from a point 1/2 inch posterior to the first metatarsal head to the anterior tubercle of the calcaneus. Its apex is between the talonavicular joint and the navicular (scaphoid) tuberosity. A semirigid scaphoid pad can be used to realign flexible pes valgus. With heel elevation, it can be used in plantar fasciitis to reduce tension on plantar fascia. It can also be used for foot length discrepancy to support the compromised medial longitudinal arch.
      4) **Toe crest** (see Fig. 4.3-4.G) is a crescent shaped pad placed behind the second through fourth phalanges. It reduces the stress from the toes by filling the void under each proximal phalanx.
B. **Foot orthoses (inserts or inlays;** see Fig. 4.3-5) are internal shoe appliances that usually extend from posterior border of foot to a point just posterior to metatarsal heads. Foot orthoses are generally custom-molded and can be transferred from shoe to shoe. Like shoe modifications, foot orthoses in most instances do not correct foot abnormalities. Instead, they accommodate the abnormal foot to help restore lower-limb biomechanics to as normal as possible.
   1. **University of California Biomechanics Laboratory (UCBL) insert** (see Fig. 4.3-5.A) is used to realign flexible flat foot (pes valgus), especially in runners. It is made of rigid plastic, fabricated over a plaster mold of the foot held in maximum manual correction. It encompasses the heel and midfoot and has rigid medial, lateral, and posterior walls. It provides a very effective longitudinal arch support.
   2. **Heel cup** (see Fig. 4.3-5.B) is a rigid plastic insert that covers the plantar surface of the heel and extends posteriorly, medially, and laterally up the sides of the heel. It is prefabricated and is shorter in length than the UCBL. It is designed to prevent lateral calcaneal shift (calcaneal valgus) in the flexible flat foot.

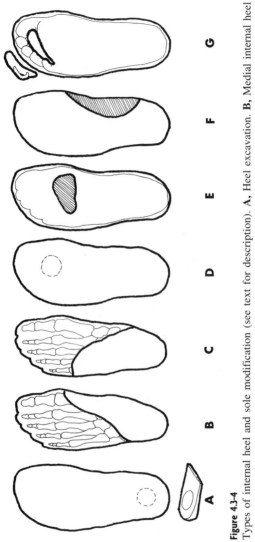

Figure 4.3-4
Types of internal heel and sole modification (see text for description). **A**, Heel excavation. **B**, Medial internal heel wedge. **C**, Lateral internal heel-wedge (extended to fifth metatarsal head). **D**, Inner sole excavation. **E**, Metatarsal pad. **F**, Scaphoid pad (navicular pad, cookie insole). **G**, Toe crest.

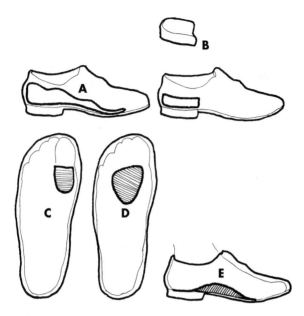

Figure 4.3-5
Types of foot orthoses or inserts (see text for description). **A,** UCBL (University of California Biomechanics Laboratory) insert. **B,** Heel cup. **C,** Sesamoid insert. **D,** Metatarsal insert. **E,** Medial longitudinal arch insert.

    3. Sesamoid insert (see Fig. 4.3-5.C) is a three-quarter length insert with an extension under the hallux to transfer pressure off the first metatarsal head and onto its shaft.

    4. Metatarsal insert (see Fig. 4.3-5.D) has similar function as the metatarsal pad described in section I.A.2.b.2.

    5. Longitudinal arch insert can be applied medially (see Fig. 4.3-5.E) for additional support of the medial longitudinal arch or laterally for additional support of the lateral longitudinal arch.

  C. Ankle-foot orthoses (AFOs) (formerly called **short leg brace** or **below knee orthoses**) encompass the shoe and terminate at some point below the knee. They consist of a foundation (i.e., a shoe and an insert foot plate or a steel stirrup, which is riveted to the shoe), an ankle control component (with the joint usually centered over the tip of the medial malleolus) to limit or assist in dorsiflexion (DF) and plantarflexion (PF), a foot control component to restrict mediolateral motion, and superstructures including the plastic shell or metal uprights and the proximal band. They are usually prescribed to improve gait patterns and ensure safe ambulation in patients with weak or paralyzed ankle dorsiflexors, plantarflexors, invertors, and/or evertors. They can also be used to prevent or correct deformities, reduce hypertonicity, as well as to stabilize and reduce weight bearing in the foot and ankle. Positioning of the ankle indirectly affects the stability of the knee. When the ankle component is positioned in plantarflexion, an extension moment is created in the knee, but positioning the ankle in dorsiflexion provides a knee flexion force, which

Table 4.3-2. Guidelines for prescription of ankle-foot orthoses (AFOs).

PATIENT GROUP	SUGGESTED AFOs
GROUP I • Weakness/absence of dorsiflexors without severe plantarflexor weakness • Good mediolateral stability during stance • Passive ankle dorsiflexion to 90 degrees • Absent to moderate spasticity • Adequate knee stability and strength • Adequate hip strength • Reduced position sense at the ankle	1. Posterior leaf spring AFO 2. Double metal upright AFO with dorsiflexion assist (and plantarflexion assist if needed) 3. Shoe clasp (VAPC) or wire spring AFO
GROUP II • Weakness/absence of dorsiflexors and plantarflexors • Tendency to varus/valgus in stance or mediolateral instability in swing • Absent to moderate spasticity • Adequate knee and hip strength (but may be less than in Group I) • Reduced position sense at ankle	1. Double metal upright AFO with dorsiflexion stop at 90 degrees (in the absence of plantarflexors the ankle tends to hyperdorsiflex, creating a knee flexion moment; dorsiflexion must be stopped at 90 degrees to prevent knee buckling). For increased mediolateral stability, the uprights can be attached to an insert molded to realign the foot, or a T-strap can be used. 2. Spiral AFO prevents footdrop, resists dorsiflexion during stance (thus assisting push-off) to provide a knee extension moment. It also counteracts a valgus tendency because the spiral starts on the medial side of the foot. 3. Hemispiral AFO will counteract a varus tendency as the spiral starts on the lateral side.
GROUP III • Weak/absent dorsiflexors and plantarflexors • Severe spasticity with equinovarus in swing and stance; knee and hip strength adequate for weight bearing • Severe position sensory loss associated with spasticity (may be adequate criteria even without weakness) • Pain on ankle movement (may be single criterion)	1. Solid AFO 2. Double upright metal AFO with no ankle movement and correction strap or shoe insert

Tabulated from Sarno JE: Below knee orthoses: A system for prescription. *Arch Phys Med Rehabil* 54:548-552, 1973, with permission of WB Saunders.

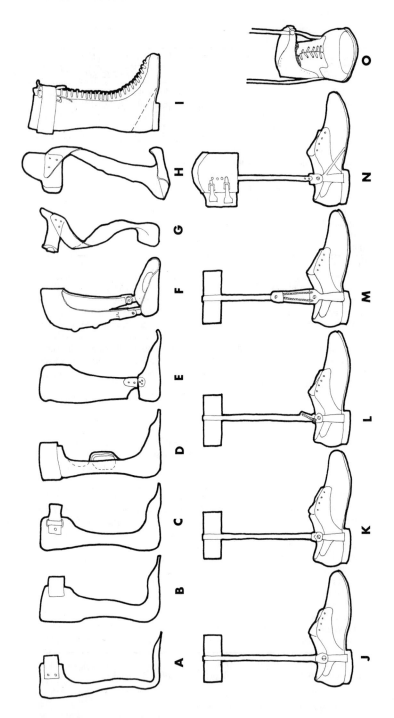

can help control genu recurvatum. Excessive ankle dorsiflexion position of the orthosis should be avoided as it may cause knee buckling.

The AFOs have been shown to reduce the energy cost of ambulation in patients with spastic diplegia (in cerebral palsy), lower motor neuron weakness (in poliomyelitis), and spastic hemiplegia (in stroke). In hemiplegics, AFOs reduced energy expenditure and increased speed of ambulation. Whether wearing AFOs improve the ability of hemiplegics to ascend and descend stairs remains controversial. On the use of metal or plastic AFO, some studies show that they have similar efficiency, but other studies show that spiral and hemispiral AFOs are slightly more efficient than metal AFO (e.g., for foot drop due to lower motor neuron lesion). Other conditions in which AFO may be recommended are peripheral neuropathy (especially peroneal neuropathies), lumbar radiculopathies, multiple sclerosis (MS), and traumatic brain injury (TBI). Guidelines for AFO prescription are shown in Table 4.3-2.

1. **Thermoplastic AFOs** (see Fig. 4.3-6.A to H) consist of three sections: a shoe insert, a calf shell, and a calf strap attached proximally. They are available off-the-shelf or can be custom fitted. Their rigidity depends on the thickness and composition of the plastic and also on the trim lines and shape. They can be worn inside the shoe. They are contraindicated in fluctuating edema (especially the spiral, hemispiral, and solid AFO) and in inadequate hip and knee strength.

   a. **Posterior leaf spring (PLS) or modified AFO** (see Fig. 4.3-6.A) is the most common type of AFO. It has a narrow calf shell and a narrow ankle with trim line below and behind the malleoli. During early stance, the narrow junction between the calf shell and shoe insert is bent backward slightly. As the patient goes into swing phase, the plastic recoils to lift the foot into dorsiflexion. The PLS also resists plantarflexion at heel (or foot) strike and during swing phase (thus preventing foot slapping and toe dragging respectively). Because of its low ankle trimline, it has minimal mediolateral control with the use of shoes. It is indicated in weakness of ankle dorsiflexors, moderate to severe spasticity, mediolateral ankle instability with marked varus/valgus deformity, and fixed ankle deformity with dorsiflexion limited to less than 90 degrees. It may be inappropriate for weak or absent plantarflexors.

   b. **Solid AFO (SAFO)** (see Fig. 4.3-6.C) has similar design as PLS but with wider calf shelf and with trim lines in the ankle area extending anterior to the malleoli. It holds the foot in a predetermined position, prevents dorsiflexion and plantarflexion, and resist any varus/valgus deviation

Figure 4.3-6
Types of plastic (**A** to **H**) ankle-foot orthoses (AFOs) and metal (**J** to **O**) AFOs (see text for description). **A,** Posterior leaf spring. **B,** Semisolid ankle foot orthoses. **C,** Solid AFO. **D,** Solid AFO with flange. **E,** Solid AFO with adjustable hinge. **F,** AFO with adjustable hinge and anterior band. **G,** Spiral AFO. **H,** Hemispiral AFO. **I,** Vannini-Rizzoli stabilizing boot. **J,** AFO with free-motion ankle joint. **K,** AFO with limited motion ankle-joint stop. **L,** AFO with dorsiflexion-assist ankle joint (Klenzak joint). **M,** AFO with dorsiflexion and plantar flexion assists (commonly used as a double-adjustable ankle joint with rigid stops). **N,** AFO with weight relieving brim. **O,** Varus-correction T-strap.

of the hind foot and ankle. It is indicated in structural collapse of foot-ankle, pain because of ankle movement, severe spasticity with sustained clonus, and severe sensory deficit. It should not be used if there is significant functional movement of ankle during gait. Modifications are the **semisolid AFO** (see Fig. 4.3-6.B), which covers part of the malleoli and provides less mediolateral support than solid AFO, and the hinged *SAFO* (see Fig. 4.3-6.E; described below). The semisolid AFO can be trimmed into a PLS.

c. **AFO with flange** (see Fig. 4.3-6.D) has an extension (flange) that projects from the calf shell medially for maximum valgus control and laterally for maximum varus control of the foot and ankle.

d. **Hinged AFOs** (see Fig. 4.3-6.E,F) have adjustable ankle hinges, which can be set to the desired range of ankle dorsi- or plantarflexion. A SAFO (see Fig. 4.3-6.E) is used to provide greater mediolateral stability. The anterior band (see Fig. 4.3-6.F) is used to prevent knee buckling during early stance phase.

e. **Spiral AFO** (see Fig. 4.3-6.G) is a design in which the single upright spirals from the medial aspect of the shoe insert passes around the leg posteriorly, then passes anteriorly to terminate at the medial tibial flare where a calf band is attached. This design allows rotation in the transverse plane while controlling dorsiflexion/plantarflexion and eversion/inversion without eliminating motion. Spiral AFOs are indicated in weakness of ankle dorsiflexors and/or plantarflexors with moderate mediolateral instability and mild motor weakness of knee extensors. They are contraindicated in pronounced imbalance of forces acting on ankle-foot complex, moderate to severe spasticity, severe mediolateral ankle instability, and fixed ankle deformity with dorsiflexion limited to much less than 90 degrees.

f. **Hemispiral AFO** (see Fig. 4.3-6.H) is a design in which the upright starts on the lateral side of the shoe insert and passes up the posterior leg, terminating at the medial tibial flare where the calf band is attached. It makes only half a turn around the leg (whereas the spiral AFO makes a full turn) and provides better control of equinovarus than does the spiral design. It is indicated in motor weakness of ankle dorsiflexors and evertors with moderate to severe lateral instability and/or strong tendency toward equinovarus, internal rotation of foot, and moderate spasticity. It is contraindicated in severe spasticity with sustained clonus, valgus, and fixed ankle deformity with dorsiflexion limited to less than 90 degrees.

g. **Tone-reducing AFO (TRAFO)** is a custom-made plastic orthosis made of a broad foot plate to provide support around most of the foot, extending distally under the toes and up over the foot medially and laterally to maintain the subtalar joint in normal alignment. It is designed to inhibit spasticity by maintaining a neutral foot position or by hyperextending the toes and having pads that apply constant pressure to the plantar flexors and invertors. They are indicated for patients with moderate spasticity (e.g., spastic hemiplegia) with varus instability but whose deformity is not fixed.

2. **Metal and metal-plastic or metal-leather AFOs** (see Fig 4.3-6.J to O) usually consist of two metal uprights (medial and lateral) connected proximally to a calf band (made of leather covered metal or plastic) and distally to the ankle joint mechanism, which is anchored to the shoe or foot attach-

ment. The calf band, which provides reaction point for force application, must be sufficient to distribute forces evenly without exceeding tissue tolerance. A posterior calf band and a plantarflexion stop ankle joint can be used to control knee hyperextension in genu recurvatum. The posterior calf band provides anteriorly directed force on the knee during early stance, while the plantarflexion stop promotes knee flexion during stance phase. Although most AFOs have two uprights, some have only a posterior upright (e.g., Veterans Administration Prosthetics Center [VAPC] design) or a single medial or lateral upright depending on the support needed (e.g., in mild dorsiflexor weakness, single uprights may be adequate). The metal uprights are attached to a sturdy shoe by means of a stirrup (usually steel) or a caliper (a round tube placed in the heel of the shoe, which allows easy interchangeability of shoes). An alternative is to attach the stirrup to a molded shoe insert, which is fitted into the shoe. The mechanical ankle joints prevent mediolateral instability and either control or assist dorsiflexion and plantarflexion by means of stops or assists (springs) or straps. The following are variations in the ankle joint, strap, and weight-bearing brim of metal and metal-plastic or metal-leather AFOs:

a. **Free-motion ankle joint** (see Fig. 4.3-6.J) is a stirrup with a completely circular top that allows free ankle motion and provides only mediolateral control.

b. **Ankle joint stops** are used to limit a predetermined ankle range of motion (ROM). They can be used in Achilles tendinitis to limit mediolateral foot motion and prevent instability caused by painful tendinitis and the plantarflexed posture of the foot. They are prescribed with a shoe with rocker-bar sole in patients with plantarflexor paralysis.

   1) **Plantarflexion (posterior) ankle-joint stop** has a posterior angulation at the top of the stirrup that restricts plantarflexion but allows unlimited dorsiflexion and affects the knee by promoting knee flexion during early stance. It is used in patients with weakness of dorsiflexors (foot drop) and with flexible pes equinus.

   2) **Dorsiflexion (anterior) ankle-joint stop** has an anterior angulation at the top of the stirrup that restricts dorsiflexion but allows full plantarflexion and affects the knee by promoting knee extension during early stance. It is used in patients with weak plantarflexors to achieve late stance.

   3) **Limited-motion ankle-joint stop** (see Fig. 4.3-6.K) has anterior and posterior angulations at the top of the stirrup that limit dorsiflexion and plantarflexion, respectively. The angulation of the cut determines the amount of restricted motion. It is recommended in ankle weakness affecting all muscle groups.

c. **Ankle joint assists** use springs or spring wire or resilient uprights, to assist ankle motion. During stance phase, dorsiflexion assists promote knee flexion. Dorsiflexion assists are used by patients with flexible pes equinus and with weak/paralyzed dorsiflexors (foot drop). They are contraindicated in patients with severe spasticity, paralysis, or joint instability.

   1) **Dorsiflexion-assist spring joint** (Klenzak joint; see Fig. 4.3-6.L) uses coil springs located posteriorly that are compressed following heel (or foot) strike (in stance phase). At heel (or foot) strike, the springs also yield slightly into plantar flexion and help prevent inadvertent knee flexion. During swing phase, the spring rebounds to aid dorsiflexion.

    2) Dorsiflexion/plantarflexion-assist spring joint (see Fig. 4.3-6.M) has an anterior spring that is compressed at midstance and as it recoils, it helps to plantarflex the ankle into push off. It is used in flail ankle.

    3) Spring-wire dorsiflexion assist joint uses light, flexible, easily adjustable spring-wire uprights attached to the shoe. Because of its flexibility, it does not provide any mediolateral stability.

    4) Veterans Administration Prosthetics Center (VAPC) clasp orthosis provides dorsiflexion assist by means of a single, resilient, posterior metal upright that clamps onto the shoe counter.

    5) Bichannel adjustable ankle lock (BICAAL) joint has posterior and anterior receptacles with springs that can be compressed to assist motion. The springs can be replaced by pins to alter the alignment of the joint and thus convert it into adjustable stops.

  d. Weight-relieving brim (see Fig. 4.3-6.N) is used to reduce load on the leg and foot for patients requiring limited weight bearing.

  e. Varus- or valgus-correction straps (T-straps) are leather straps that provide additional stabilization and prevent the foot from deviating in the frontal plane within the shoe. If greater forces are required to correct the varus/valgus, a molded plastic insert with a rigid medial or lateral extension to which a strap is attached can be used.

    1) T-strap for varus correction (see Fig. 4.3-6.O) attaches to the shoe laterally, encircles the ankle, and buckles on the outside of the medial upright to realign flexible pes varus.

    2) T-strap for valgus correction attaches to the shoe medially, encircles the ankle, and buckles on the outside of the lateral upright to realign flexible pes valgus.

3. Vannini-Rizzoli stabilizing boot (see Fig. 4.3-6.I) is a specialized boot with an inner rigid, posterior calf shell continuous with a footplate angled at about 15 degrees of plantarflexion, thus shifting the center of gravity anterior to the ankles and knees. It immobilizes the leg, ankle, and foot and stabilizes the knee in extension. It is used in paraplegic patients with spinal cord injury to achieve standing balance and ambulation by learning how to shift the center of gravity of the trunk and hips while using parallel bars, a walker, or crutches.

D. Knee-ankle-foot orthoses (KAFO) (formerly called **long leg brace** or **above knee orthosis)** consist of an AFO with proximal extension up to the thigh to control knee motion and alignment and to maintain knee stability for weight bearing in patients with paralysis or instability occurring at both the knee and the ankle. If weight bearing needs to be relieved at the knee or ankle, forces can be redistributed to as high as the ischial tuberosity and soft tissues of the proximal thigh. The KAFO can be used to stabilize or support the knee in quadriceps paralysis or weakness (e.g., KAFO with knee lock and anterior leg band); control flexible genu valgum or varum (e.g., KAFO with plastic calf shell extended proximally on the medial side for genu valgum control or on the lateral side for genu varum control); and limit weight bearing of thigh, leg, and foot (e.g., KAFO with quadrilateral or ischial containment brim on which patient can sit on, with a locked knee, limited motion ankle joints, a patten-bottom [see Fig. 4-3-10.D], and a contralateral shoe lift to equalize leg length). In hemiplegic or head trauma patients (with marked quadriceps weakness or hamstring spasticity), AFO is preferred over KAFO because KAFOs are difficulty to don and doff and do not provide functional ambulation. To control genu recurvatum, an AFO (with ankle positioned in dorsiflexion) or a knee orthosis (e.g., Swedish knee cage) is preferred over a KAFO. The orthotic knee joint of a KAFO is usually centered over the medial femoral condyle.

1. Metal-leather and metal-plastic KAFO

a. Double–upright metal KAFO (see Fig. 4.3-7.A) has similar components as the AFO with the addition of two metal uprights connected to a mechanical knee joint. The uprights extend up the thigh and are encompassed by two thigh bands. Knee caps (corrective or anterior pads and straps; see Fig. 4.3-7.N) may be placed in front of the knee to prevent knee flexion within the KAFO. For genu varum or valgum, the knee cap may include a lateral or medial strap, respectively (these buckle around the upright in the same way as ankle straps).

The mechanical knee joint may either be polycentric or single-axis. Polycentric knee joints follow the natural motion of the knee joint more accurately and are indicated if significant knee motion is required during walking. Because most patients needing KAFOs require knee stabilization (rather than increased knee mobility), a fixed or single-axis knee joint is used more commonly. The following are common types of **single-axis knee joints:**

1) Free motion knee joint (see Fig. 4.3-7.G) has unlimited flexion and extension but usually has a stop to prevent hyperextension. It is indicated for patients with a tendency toward genu recurvatum and mediolateral instability but with enough strength to control the knee during weight bearing and ambulation.

2) Offset knee joint (see Fig. 4.3-7.H) is a hinge placed posterior to the knee joint so that the patient's weight line falls anterior to the offset joint, thus stabilizing the knee during early stance phase of gait on level surfaces. It allows the knee to flex freely during swing phase and also allows sitting without the need to manipulate the lock. It should not be used in patients with knee or hip flexion contracture, or with a plantarflexion stop at the ankle. The patient must be careful when walking on a ramp as the knee may flex inadvertently.

3) Locked knee joints are used to prevent knee buckling. To be able to lock the knee joint, the patient must be able to fully extend the knee, either passively or actively. Hence, they are contraindicated in patients with knee contracture (use an adjustable knee lock instead). Although locked knee joints provide maximal knee stability, the gait is awkward and stiff because of lack of knee flexion.

a) Drop-ring locks (see Fig. 4.3-7.I) consist of a ring that can be dropped over the knee joints (by gravity or with manual assistance) while the uprights are fully extended, thus preventing the uprights from bending. For KAFO with bilateral uprights, both medial and lateral joints must be locked for greater stability. A spring-loaded retention button allows the patient or therapist to unlock one upright, then attend to the other one without having the first lock drop. The retention button also prevents inadvertent locking of knee joint in patients who can walk with the knee free but wish to lock the knee joint occassionally. As the patient sits, the retention button can be used to unlock one knee so the patient can grasp the chair with one hand for stability, and use the other free hand to unlock the other upright. For KAFO with unilateral uprights, a spring-loaded pull rod (see Fig. 4.3-7.J) extending to midthigh

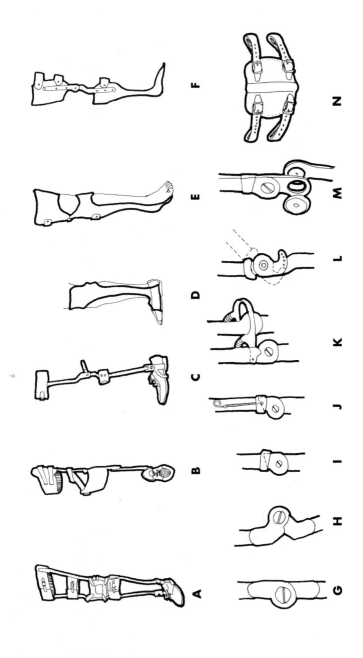

may be added to the drop ring so the patient need not bend to unlock or lock the joint. The spring is used to drive the ring lock down and assist gravity in locking the knee. Drop rings are the most commonly used knee locks to control knee flexion.

 b) **Pawl lock with bail release** (see Fig. 4.3-7.K) consists of a spring-loaded projection (pawl) that fits into a matching recess when the knee is fully extended thus providing simultaneous locking of both uprights. It also has a semicircular lever (bail) attached posteriorly, which easily unlocks both joints with an upward pull on the bail (either manually or by backing up to sit down in a chair). The bail is bulky and can be accidentally released if it hits a rigid object. A variation of the spring-loaded pawl lock is the Swiss or French lock, which uses elastic webbing from the bail to the calf band instead of a spring.

 4) **Adjustable knee joint** has a proximal component consisting of a drop-ring lock and a distal component consisting of an adjustable knee lock, which can either be a fan lock (see Fig. 4.3-7.L), a serrated disk (see Fig. 4.3-7.M), a dial lock, or a ratchet (step-up) lock. The drop ring, which maintains the desired knee position in standing and walking, can be unlocked to permit full knee flexion when sitting. The adjustable knee joint permits locking in different degrees of flexion as the patient's knee is stretched and becomes more extended. Hence, adjustable knee joints are used to provide stability in patients with knee flexion contractures in whom improvement is anticipated with gradual stretching.

 b. **Single lateral-upright metal KAFO** (see Fig. 4.3-7.B) has a lateral upright only, with thigh and pretibial cuffs made of molded plastic. All the other components are the same as in the double upright metal KAFO.

 c. **Scott-Craig metal KAFO** (see Fig. 4.3-7.C) is custom-made for standing and ambulation in adults with paraplegia. It consists of double uprights, a pawl lock with bail release, a posterior thigh band, a hinged pretibial band, a bichannel adjustable ankle lock (BiCAAL) joint (with anterior and posterior adjustable pin stops), and a shoe with cushion heel and embedded with a longitudinal and transverse (T-shaped) foot plate. The longitudinal plate extends from the heel to the metatarsal heads to pro-

◄───

Figure 4.3-7
Types of knee-ankle-foot orthoses (KAFOs) (**A** to **F**) and KAFO locks (**G** to **M**) (see text for description). **A,** Metal KAFO with two uprights and two thigh bands (the distal components are similar to those of AFOs). **B,** Single lateral upright metal orthosis. **C,** Scott-Craig orthosis (double uprights, knee joint with pawl locks and bail control, one posterior thigh band, a hinged pretibial band, an ankle joint with anterior and posterior adjustable pin stops, a cushion heel, and a T-shaped foot plate). **D,** Supracondylar plastic KAFO. **E,** Supracondylar KAFO with conventional metal knee joints and uprights. **F,** KAFO with plastic thigh shell and metal upright. **G,** Free motion knee joint. **H,** Offset knee joint. **I,** Drop-ring lock. **J,** Spring-loaded pull rod. **K,** Pawl lock. **L,** Adjustable fan lock. **M,** Serrated adjustable knee joint. **N,** Knee cap. (Adapted from New York University Prosthetics and Orthotics Staff: *Lower limb orthotics*, New York, 1993, Prosthetic-Orthotic Publications, pp. 140-144, with permission.)

vide a rigid platform, while the transverse plate located at the metatarsal head region provides mediolateral stability. The BiCAAL joint is set in about 10 degrees dorsiflexion so the orthosis and patient's limb lean forward slightly. To attain balance, the patient compensates by hyperextending the hips to bring the center of gravity behind the hip joints and in front of the locked knee and ankle joints thus preventing untoward hip or trunk flexion. With the aid of crutches or a walker, the patient is able to ambulate with a swing-to or swing-through gait. Some patients may be able to use two- or four-point gait by shifting the trunk enough to allow the leg to swing forward in a pendular manner. The Scott-Craig KAFO provides orthotic stabilization of the knee, ankle and foot, and passive or ligamentous stabilization of the hip without recourse to orthotic components at or above the hip. An alternate version substitutes a plastic solid ankle section for the reinforced shoe and metal ankle joints.

2. **Plastic and plastic-metal KAFOs** use thermoplastic materials because they are lighter, more cosmetically acceptable, and can be heated for better contour. Unlike leather, plastic does not absorb perspiration. Plastic and plastic-metal KAFOs are indicated for closer fit and more precise control of pressure and for maximum control of the foot.

   a. **Supracondylar plastic KAFO** (see Fig. 4.3-7.D) is a custom-made plastic orthosis extending from the ankle and foot up to the knee and lower thigh to resist recurvatum forces of the knee without hindering flexion and to provide mediolateral stability. In patients with knee extensor weakness, the ankle and foot component are used to hold the ankle in slight plantarflexion, enough to produce a knee extension moment and eliminate the need for a mechanical knee lock in stance (which could also hinder knee flexion in swing). Its disadvantage is that when the patient sits, the suprapatellar portion protrudes. Also it cannot be used bilaterally because positioning the ankles in plantarflexion interferes with the patient's anteroposterior stability.

   b. **Supracondylar plastic-metal KAFO** (see Fig. 4.3-7.E) has the same function and design as the supracondylar plastic KAFO except that it has conventional metal knee joints and uprights to allow the orthosis to flex while the patient is seated and thus decreasing protrusion above the knee during sitting.

   c. **Plastic shells and metal uprights KAFO** (see Fig. 4.3-7.F) are essentially a posterior leaf spring AFO with double metal uprights extending up to a plastic thigh shell with an intervening knee joint (see section I.D.1.a for different types of knee joints). The proximal contour of the thigh shells are usually quadrilateral in shape to help control rotation and may incorporate an ischial seat for weight bearing.

E. **Knee orthoses (KO)** provide support or control of the knee but not the foot and ankle. Their designs are determined by their function. As with KAFOs, their orthotic knee joint is usually centered over the medial femoral condyle.

   1. **Knee orthoses for patellofemoral disorders** control tracking of the patella as the knee flexes and extends.

      a. **Infrapatellar (Cho-Pat) strap KO** (see Fig. 4.3-8.A) is a foam-padded strap that encircles the knee immediately below the patella. They are worn during periods of activity.

      b. **Palumbo KO** (see Fig. 4.3-8.B) uses an elastic sleeve with patellar cutout, two circumferentially wrapped rubber straps that apply tension to a crescent-shaped patellar pad (placed laterally), and an elastic counter-force strap, which maintains position of the pad and prevents axial rotation of the orthosis. It applies an active medially-displacing force to the lateral border of the patella and maintains constant pressure during flexion, extension, and rotation of the knee.

2. **Knee orthoses for knee control in the sagittal plane** controls genu recurvatum with minimal mediolateral stabilization. They allow almost complete knee flexion.

   a. **Swedish knee cage** (see Fig. 4.3-8.C) is a prefabricated brace, which restricts hyperextension with two anterior straps and one posterior strap held in position by the metal frame medially and laterally. It tends to protrude when the patient sits.

   b. **Three-way knee stabilizer** (see Fig. 4.3-8.D) is similar to the Swedish knee cage, but it has pivotable attachments of the straps, which do not protrude as much in sitting. It has lateral and medial uprights, which provide limited mediolateral stability.

3. **Knee orthoses for knee control in the frontal plane** consist of thigh and calf cuffs joined by side bars with mechanical knee joint. In addition to protecting the knee against mediolateral forces (using the three-point force system), they also provide flexion-extension control by including a hyperextension stop in the mechanical knee joint or by adding a drop lock. The knee joint is usually polycentric to closely approximate anatomic knee motion and contribute better stabilization of the orthosis on the patient's limb.

   a. **Traditional metal-leather KO** (see Fig. 4.3-8.E) has leather thigh and calf cuffs and metal side bars. A pressure pad may be used to apply medial or lateral forces to the knee.

   b. **Miami KO** has side bars and polycentric joints incorporated into the polypropylene calf and thigh shells, which cover the anterior limb surfaces. A suspension wedge is positioned over the medial femoral condyle to prevent downward slippage.

   c. **Canadian Arthritis and Rheumatism Society—University of British Columbia (CARS-UBC) KO** (see Fig. 4.3-8.F) consists of two plastic cuffs (calf and thigh) connected by a telescoping rod, which permits knee flexion. For genu varum, the rod is placed on the medial knee with a pad on the lateral knee while for genu valgum, the rod is placed on the lateral knee with a pad on the medial knee. This three-point pressure system resists varus/valgus forces when the knee is fully extended and is weight bearing. It is difficult to don, interferes with clothing, and does not control axial rotation.

   d. **Supracondylar KO** (see Fig. 4.3-8.G) is similar to supracondylar KAFO (see section I.D.2.a.) except that it does have an ankle or foot extension (hence it cannot hold the ankle in plantarflexion position to produce knee extension moment during stance in patients with knee extensor weakness). It controls genu recurvatum and provides mediolateral knee stabilization. The suprapatellar portion protrudes off the thigh when the patient is seated.

4. **KO for axial rotation control** also provides angular control in the sagittal (flexion-extension) and frontal (mediolateral) planes, in addition to controlling axial rotation. They are used in the prevention and management of sports injuries of the knee (e.g., in patients with anterior cruciate ligament [ACL] injury).

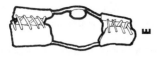

E

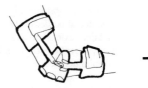

I

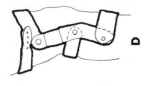

D

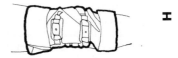

H

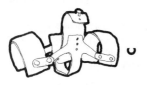

C

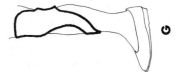

G

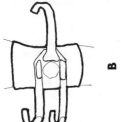

B

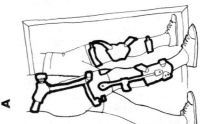

F

A

      a. Lenox-Hill derotation orthosis (see Fig. 4.3-8.H) uses close-fitting cuffs or elastic straps that encircle the thigh and leg.

      b. Lerman multiligamentous knee control orthosis (see Fig. 4.3-8.I) is similar to Lenox-Hill derotation orthosis with the addition of supracondylar pads for additional control of patellar tracking.

F. Hip-knee-ankle-foot orthoses (HKAFO) consist of a KAFO with the addition of a pelvic band and hip joints. They are used to reduce gait deviation caused by faulty control of hip abduction, adduction, and rotation (e.g., in paraplegia caused by spina bifida or SCI). They are more difficult to don than KAFOs, and if the hip joints are locked, they restrict gait to the swing-to or swing-through pattern. Their orthotic knee joint is usually centered over the medial femoral condyle, while their orthotic hip joint is positioned so that the patient can sit upright at 90 degrees.

  1. Pelvic band surrounds the lower trunk and attaches to the upper part of the hip joint. They are likely to be uncomfortable when the patient sits.

      a. Bilateral pelvic band is more commonly used than unilateral pelvic band because most conditions requiring a HKAFO have bilateral involvement. It is made of upholstered metal, which curves posteriorly and downward to contact the most prominent portion of each buttock and continues slightly upward to overlie the sacrum. Its ends are located just anterior to the lateral midlines of the pelvis and are interconnected by a flexible belt.

      b. Pelvic girdle made of molded thermoplastic materials provides maximum degree of control in patients with bilateral involvement. It is similar to the pelvic part of molded plastic thoracolumbosacral orthosis (TLSO) used for scoliosis.

      c. Silesian belt or band attaches to the proximal end of the lateral upright and encircles the pelvis. It has no metal joint or rigid band and cannot control motion in the sagittal plane. It offers mild resistance to abduction and rotational forces at the hip.

      d. Dacron webbing hip rotation strap may be used if the patient requires only control of hip rotation (e.g., toe-in gait). To reduce internal rotation, a strap resembling a prosthetic silesian bandage is used. To reduce external rotation, a strap that passes anteriorly at the groin and connects the lateral uprights of the KAFOs is used.

  2. Hip joints and locks consist of metal hinges that connect the lateral uprights of the KAFO to a pelvic band. By nature of its design, the hip joint also prevents abduction and adduction, as well as hip rotation.

      a. Single-axis hip joint with lock is the most commonly used hip joint. It permits flexion and extension and may include an adjustable stop to

Figure 4.3-8

Types of knee orthoses (KO) (see text for description): **A,** Infrapatellar strap KO. **B,** Palumbo KO. **C,** Swedish knee cage. **D,** Three-way knee stabilizer. **E,** Traditional metal-leather KO with leather thigh and calf cuffs and metal side bars. **F,** Canadian Arthritis and Rheumatism Society—University of British Columbia (CARS-UBC) KO with knee stabilization against genu valgum. **G,** Supracondylar KO. **H.** Lenox Hill derotation orthosis. **I,** Lerman multiligamentous knee control orthosis. (Adapted from New York University Prosthetics and Orthotics Staff: Lower limb orthotics, New York, 1993, Prosthetic-Orthotic Publications, pp. 150-154, with permission.)

limit hyperextension. The flexion-extension capacity can be restricted by a pawl or drop-ring lock similar to those used at the knee joint. The drop-ring lock is useful if hip flexion control is needed, especially in patients with a crouched gait.

    b. **Two-position lock hip joint** can be locked at full hip extension (for standing and walking) and at 90 degrees of flexion (for sitting). It is indicated in patients whose hip spasticity causes difficulty in maintaining a seated position.

    c. **Double axis (flexion-abduction) hip joint** has a flexion-extension axis, which may be free or locked, and an abduction-adduction axis, which includes adjustable stops to place limits on these motions as needed.

G. Trunk-hip-knee-ankle-foot orthoses (THKAFO) incorporates a spinal orthosis attached to the HKAFO to control trunk motion, maintain, or modify spinal alignment, and reduce loads on the spine by elevating intraabdominal pressure. The pelvic band of the spinal orthosis serves as the pelvic band used on THKAFOs. It is indicated in paraplegic patients (e.g., because of SCI, poliomyelitis, spina bifida, and muscular dystrophy) but is seldom worn by patients after discharge from the rehabilitation program because it is heavy, cumbersome, and is very difficult to don. As with HKAFO, their orthotic knee joint is usually centered over the medial femoral condyle; however, their orthotic hip joint is positioned so that the patient can sit upright at 90 degrees. Alternative designs of THKAFO available for paraplegic patients are as follows:

    1. Reciprocating gait orthosis (RGO) (see Fig. 4.3-9) is a THKAFO consisting of a custom-molded pelvic girdle with a thoracic extension and bilateral hip joints, which are connected by one or two metal cables to prevent simultaneous bilateral hip flexion. Both knees are stabilized with knee locks, posteriorly offset knee joints, or pretibial bands and the feet are encased in solid ankle-foot orthoses. For walking, the hip joint can be locked at 180 degrees or set to flex about 25 degrees. As the patient extends one hip, the cable coupling induces hip flexion on the opposite supporting leg or vice versa (i.e., hip extension on one side causes opposite hip flexion). This produces a reciprocal walking pattern not otherwise possible with standard KAFOs or HKAFOs. Using two crutches, paraplegics can slowly ambulate with a stable four- or two-point gait because one foot is always on the floor. When standing, the cable coupling prevents simultaneous hip flexion. For sitting, the cable can be released to enable the hips to flex. An RGO in combination with functional electrical stimulation, can be used for greater aerobic training in paraplegic and possibly tetraplegic (C8) patients.

    2. Hip-guidance orthosis or HGO (Para Walker) is a THKAFO consisting of ball-bearing hip joints, a body brace, and shoes that fit into loops on flat foot plates. The sturdy hip joints guide hip motion in the sagittal plane by using stops that limit hip flexion. Hip extension may be free or may also be limited by a stop. Ambulation is through trunk motion transmitted to the lower limbs through the brace. As the patient shifts weight from side to side during ambulation, the hip joints resist hip abduction and adduction. The gait maneuver is the similar to that used with the RGO.

    3. Pneumatic THKAFO consists of a prefabricated long garment with inflatable tubes both anteriorly and posteriorly. These tubes can be inflated to provide rigidity and deflated to allow flexion of the hips and knees. It is obsolete.

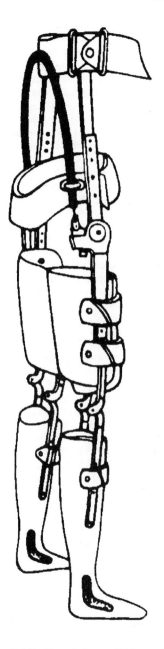

Figure 4.3-9
Reciprocal gait orthosis (RGO). (From Lehmann JF: Lower limb orthotics. In Redford JB, editor: *Orthotics etcetera*, ed 3, Baltimore, 1986, Williams & Wilkins, p. 320, copyright© 1986, Williams & Wilkins, with permission.)

4. Prefabricated pediatric THKAFOs, which include standing frame, swivel chair, and parapodium, are beyond the scope of this book.

H. Hip orthoses consist of hip joints and pelvic bands (described in I.F as part of HKAFOs) with the lower bar of the hip joint terminating on a thigh cuff. The thigh cuff may be extended to the medial femoral condyle to provide additional resistance to adduction as well as internal rotation. It is most commonly used to resist spastic hip adductors in patients with cerebral palsy. It may also be used after total hip arthroplasty to prevent hip dislocation following total hip replacement by limiting adduction and flexion of the hip joint (e.g., a **Postoperative hip-abduction orthosis**). Their orthotic hip joint is positioned so that the patient can sit upright at 90 degrees.

I. Special-purpose lower-limb orthoses

1. Weight-bearing orthoses reduce or eliminate weight bearing through the lower limb. The skin and peripheral circulation on the weight-bearing area should be able to tolerate pressure.

a. Patellar-tendon-bearing (PTB) orthosis (see Fig. 4.3-10.A) has proximal designs similar to the PTB socket used in below knee prostheses (see Chapter 4.4, section I.C.3.a). It supports weight on the patellar tendon and tibial flares with the load being transmitted to the shoe via the metal uprights. It is indicated for unloading the mid or distal tibia, ankle, or foot (e.g., healing os calcis fracture, postoperative ankle fusion, heel with refractory pain, delayed unions or nonunions of fractures or fusion, avascular necrosis of the talar body, degenerative arthritis of the subtalar or ankle joint, osteomyelitis of os calcis, and diabetic ulceration). Because little or no ankle motion is allowed, a cushion heel and a rocker bottom are added to provide smoother gait pattern. A patten-bottom shoe (see Fig. 4.3-10.D) may also be used.

b. Ischial weight-bearing orthosis (see Fig. 4.3-10.B) uses a quadrilateral brim (similar to the quadrilateral socket used in above-knee prosthesis; see Chapter 4.4, section I.D.2.a) or an ischial (Thomas) ring (see Fig. 4.3-10.C) to relieve weight from the femur or knee. The ischial ring is simpler to fabricate but is uncomfortable and less effective in relieving weight because forces are distributed over a smaller area. A patten-bottom shoe (see Fig. 4.3-10.D) may be used.

c. Patten-bottom orthosis (see Fig. 4.3-10.D) uses uprights (with no ankle joint) that terminate in a floor pad distal to the shoe so the foot is freely suspended in midair. It is used in conjunction with a PTB or an ischial weight bearing orthoses so the weight is transmitted directly to the floor pad. A shoe lift on the opposite side is needed to equalize leg length.

2. Fracture orthoses stabilize the fracture site and help promote callus formation by allowing weight bearing and joint movement after an initial rest period to allow pain and edema to subside. They also minimize joint stiffness and reduce complications such as nonunions. Circumferential compression of the soft tissue can be used to prevent undue bony motion at the fracture site.

a. Tibial fracture orthosis (see Fig. 4.3-10.F) consists of anterior and posterior thermoplastic plastic shells fitted over the leg with Velcro straps to ensure compression. Ankle motion is controlled by the distal trimlines, or an ankle joint may be included and may have a stop in either plantarflexion or dorsiflexion. It is used after the tibial and tibial-fibular fractures have been immobilized for about 4 weeks (2 weeks in a long leg cast followed by an additional 2 weeks in a below-knee cast). A

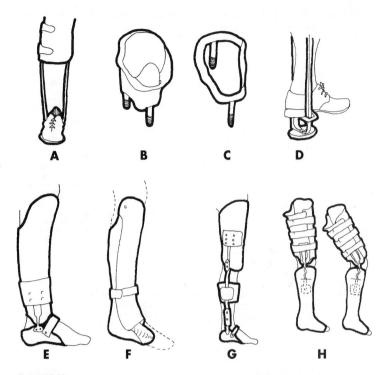

Figure 4.3-10
Types of weight-bearing and fracture lower-limb orthoses (see text for description).
A, Patellar-tendon-bearing (PTB) orthosis. **B,** Ischial weight-bearing orthosis. **C,**
Ischial (Thomas) ring. **D,** Patten-bottom orthosis. **E.** Tibial fracture orthosis with
plastic cable ankle joint. **F,** Tibial fracture orthosis with Velcro straps. **G,** Femoral
fracture orthosis with polycentric metal knee joint. **H,** Femoral fracture orthosis
with flexible plastic knee joint. (Adapted from New York University Prosthetics
and Orthotics Staff: *Lower limb orthotics,* New York, 1993, Prosthetic-Orthotic
Publications pp. 155-158, with permission.)

design variation uses plastic cable ankle joints (see Fig. 4.3-10.E) connected to a plastic heel insert to permit ankle and foot motion while
preventing downward displacement of the orthosis. In a tibial plateau
fracture, stability may be increased by using a plastic thigh section
connected via polycentric knee joints to the distal segment.

b. **Femoral fracture orthosis** consists of a thermoplastic thigh and calf component connected via freely moving metal (see Fig. 4.3-10.G) or plastic
(see Fig. 4.3-10.H) knee joints. The thigh component is quadrilateral
(for rotational stability) with an ischial seat proximally and is similar
to the quadrilateral prosthetic socket. The calf component is attached
to the footplate by ankle joints. It is used in fractures of the middle or
distal third of the femur when there is callus formation and relatively
limited pain, usually after immobilization for more than 4 to 6 weeks.

Table 4.3-3. **Suggested upper-limb orthoses for common hand deformities caused by upper-limb neuropathy**

NERVE INJURY	HAND DEFORMITY	SUGGESTED ORTHOSES
Radial	Wristdrop and drop finger	• Volar wrist-flexion control orthosis (cock-up splint) • MCP extension mobilization orthosis • Wrist mobilization orthosis
Median (distal)	Ape hand*	• Opponens orthosis (C-bar) • Thumb post static orthosis • Dynamic thumb orthosis
Median (proximal)	Active papal sign†	• Prehension orthosis • Buddy splint (taping the index and middle fingers together) may be helpful if middle finger can flex
Median and ulnar	Clawhand (also called Intrinsic minus hand‡)	• Opponens orthoses with MCP block (lumbrical bar) • MCP flexion mobilization orthosis
Ulnar	Ulnar clawing of the 4th and 5th digits (also called benediction hand or static papal sign)	• Opponens orthoses with MCP block (lumbrical bar) to 4th and 5th digits • MCP flexion mobilization orthosis

DIP = distal interphalangeal joint; MCP = metacarpal phalangeal.
* Wasting of the thenar eminence and loss of palmar abduction and opposition of the thumb.
† Loss of DIP flexion of the index and middle fingers due to proximal median nerve lesion, thus the index and middle fingers remain extended when the patient makes a fist.
‡ Unopposed hyperextension at the MCP joints with secondary flexion at the IP joints due to loss of hand intrinsic muscles.

   It is contraindicated in proximal femoral fracture due to difficulty in controlling varus angulation.

   3. Pediatric orthoses include those used for angular and rotational deformities of the leg or foot (e.g., Denis Browne splint, A-frame orthosis, torsion-shaft orthosis, and hip rotation control straps), those that hold the hips in flexion and abduction in congenital hip dislocations (e.g., Pavlik harness, Ilfeld splint, and Von Rosen splint), and those for maintaining the hip in abduction in Legg-Calve-Perthes disease (e.g., Scottish Rite orthosis, trilateral socket hip abduction orthosis [Tachdjian], Toronto hip abduction orthosis or its variation, and the Newington ambulatory abduction orthosis). They are, however, beyond the scope of this book.

II. Upper-limb orthoses are generally used to restore upper limb function by assisting or supporting weak muscles, substituting for paralyzed muscle, protecting painful or deformed parts, correcting (or minimizing) existing deformities or malalignment, permitting controlled directional movement, and allowing attachment of assistive devices (e.g., utensil holders; see section II.A.1.c below). The prescribed upper-limb orthosis should be properly fitted so the patient can easily don and doff it and either rest the desired segment or perform the prescribed movement comfortably when wearing the orthosis. Also, the orthosis must be functionally as well as cosmetically acceptable to the patient. When removed, the skin should be unblemished 10 minutes afterwards. Suggested upper-limb orthoses for common hand deformity because of upper-limb neuropathy are shown in Table 4.3-3. Most wrist and hand orthoses can adequately be held in place using a strap, while other upper-limb orthoses need to be suspended from the torso for ambulatory patients (e.g., shoulder or arm slings described in section

II.C.1.d) or suspended from the wheelchair for wheelchair-bound patients (e.g., balanced forearm orthosis described in section II.C.3.b). Suspension systems commonly used include hoops, shoulder caps, and harnesses.

Traditionally, upper-limb orthoses are classified into *static* (i.e., rigid; gives support without allowing movement) and *dynamic* (also called *functional*; i.e., allows certain degree of movement). Dynamic upper-limb orthoses improve upper limb functions through the use of joints, levers, pulleys, and external power sources (including rubber bands, springs, batteries, and cartridges of compressed gas). The above traditional classification, however, can be confusing because static orthoses are often used to create movement; however, dynamic splints usually have components that restrict motion to create movement at another joint. Another way of classifying upper-limb orthoses is by the anatomical joint covered by the orthosis, for example, FO (finger orthosis), TO (thumb orthosis), WHFO (wrist-hand-finger orthosis), WO (wrist orthosis), WHO (wrist-hand orthosis), EWHO (elbow-wrist-hand orthosis), EO (elbow orthosis), SEWHO (shoulder-elbow-wrist-hand orthosis), SEO (shoulder-elbow orthosis), and SO (shoulder orthosis). This anatomical classification, however, does not indicate function. The following classification, therefore, is used to combine both function and anatomy (based on the classification of upper-limb orthoses of the New York University Prosthetic and Orthotics Faculty published in the *American Academy of Orthopedic Surgeons' Atlas of Orthotics: Biomechanical Principles and Application*).

A. Wrist, hand, and finger orthoses

1. **Assistive and substitutive orthoses** are primarily used to enhance hand function in patients with residual strength (i.e., using assistive orthoses) or absent strength (i.e., using substitutive orthoses). They are usually worn throughout the day.

   a. **Positional orthoses**

      1) **Opponens orthoses and their variations.** Opponens orthoses are primarily used to position the weak thumb in opposition to other fingers to improve hand function by facilitating three-jaw chuck pinch (e.g., in patients with median/ulnar neuropathy, Guillain-Barre syndrome [GBS]; upper motor neuron lesions such as in spinal cord injury [SCI], stroke, traumatic brain injury [TBI], cerebral palsy [CP]. They can also be used to immobilize the thumb to promote tissue healing (e.g., carpometacarpal [CMC] or metacarpophalangeal [MCP] arthritis/synovitis; late-phase of fracture [e.g., scaphoid/thumb]; dislocation, subluxation, or collateral ligament injury of the thumb [e.g., CMC/MCP collateral ligament injury or gamekeeper's thumb]; cumulative trauma disorders [CTD] [e.g., deQuervain's tenosynovitis and thenar tendinitis]; postsurgical thumb [e.g., open reduction internal fixation [ORIF], CMC/MCP fusion, arthroplasty, reconstruction, tendon transfer, tendon/ligament repair, nerve repair, and trapeziumectomy]); to restrict thumb motion and protect it from harmful internal or external stresses during activities (e.g., arthritis, CTD, and in athletes and performing artists).

      a) **Basic opponens orthoses** (see Fig. 4.3-11.A; short opponens splints, C-bar splints, Engen opponens splints, Rancho opponen splints, cone splints, hand-based opponens splints, and static thumb splints) are TOs that consist of a dorsal and a palmar bar that encircles the midpalm, with a thumb abduction bar projecting from the palmar bar.

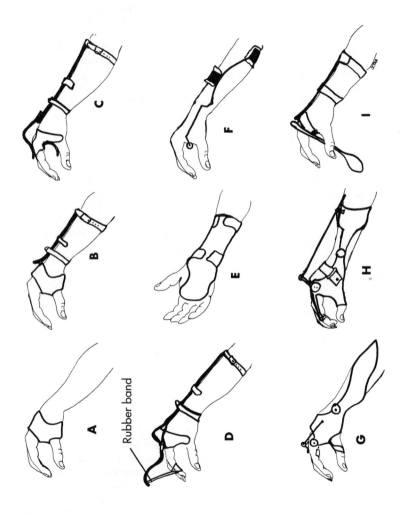

Rubber band

Figure 4.3-11

Assistive and substitutive wrist, hand, and finger orthoses (**A** to **F,** Positional orthoses; **G** to **I,** prehension orthoses). **A,** Basic or C-bar or short opponens orthoses. **B,** Opponens orthoses with wrist control attachments (long opponens orthoses). **C,** Opponens orthoses with lumbrical bar. **D,** Opponens orthoses with finger extension assist assembly (using rubber bands). **E,** Volar wrist-flexion control orthoses (cockup splint). **F,** Wire wrist-extension assist orthoses (Oppenheimer splint). **G,** Finger driven hand prehension orthoses. **H,** Wrist-driven prehension orthoses (tenodesis orthoses). **I,** Utensil holders (universal splints, activities of daily living [ADL] splint).

    b) Opponens orthoses with wrist control attachments (see Fig. 4.3-11.B; long opponens splints and thumb spica splints) are WHFOs that have a forearm bar as well as proximal and distal crossbars for wrist control. In addition to the benefits provided by the opponens orthoses (listed above), they provide the following: (a) the forearm bar maintains the wrist in extension (usually 20°), and prevents wrist dorsi- and volar-flexion contractures and (b) the cross bar helps prevent ulnar or radial deviation deformities (e.g., in rheumatoid arthritic [RA] and systemic lupus erythematosus [SLE]).

    c) Opponens orthoses with lumbrical bar (see Fig. 4.3-11.C; Opponens splints with MCP extension stop assembly, anticlaw splints, hand-based intrinsic-plus splints, clam diggers, and ulnar palsy splints) are FOs that prevent MCP hyperextension but allow full MCP flexion. In addition to the benefits provided by the opponens orthoses (listed above), they (a) prevent clawhand deformity (by preventing MCP hyperextension thus preventing PIP flexion, which could lead to clawhand deformity) in patients with ulnar or combined median and ulnar neuropathy or in patients with upper motor neuron lesions (e.g., stroke and TBI), (b) allow active extension of the proximal interphalangeal (PIP) and distal interphalangeal (DIP) joints in patients with absent or weak intrinsic hand functions (e.g., brachial plexus lesion and GBS), and (c) immobilize the MCP to promote tissue healing and to reduce inflammation (e.g., in trigger finger [i.e., digital stenosing tenosynovitis of the flexor tendon]).

    d) Opponens orthoses with finger extension assist assembly (see Fig. 4.3-11.D) are FOs that assist PIP and DIP extension (e.g., in patients with interphalangeal [IP] flexion contracture, boutonniere deformity, or postsurgical release of Dupuytren's contracture). In addition, they also provide the previously listed benefits of the basic opponens orthoses (see above).

    e) Opponens orthoses with thumb abduction-extension assist assembly are TOs that assist thumb extension and/or abduction, in addition to providing the benefits of the basic opponens orthoses (listed above).

  2) Wrist control orthoses are used to promote slight extension of the wrist or to prevent wrist flexion, thus assisting weak grasp (i.e., via tenodesis effect).

    a) Volar wrist-flexion control orthoses (cock-up splints; see Fig. 4.3-11.E) are WHOs in which the palmar section is extended (usually

20°). They are used to tighten finger flexors (via tenodesis effect) and prevent wrist flexion contracture in patients with radial neuropathy.

    b) Wire wrist-extension assist orthoses (Oppenheimer splints; see Fig. 4.3-11.F) are WHOs prefabricated from spring steel wire and padded steel bands to assist wrist extension by tensing the steel wire, thus aiding finger flexion through tenodesis effect.

b. Prehension orthoses are used to stabilize the thumb while substituting muscle strength from other parts of the body or from an external power source to provide hand grasping, holding, and releasing functions. They are used in patients with severe paralysis of the upper limb (e.g., SCI and polio). The prehension pattern may be a three-jaw chuck or a lateral grasp.

    1) Hand prehension orthoses, such as finger driven hand prehension orthoses (see Fig. 4.3-11.G) are FOs that provide prehension for the index and middle fingers through transmission of active flexion of one or more fingers. Active MCP or IP flexion must be present in at least one finger of the hand.

    2) Wrist-hand prehension orthoses can be anatomically classified as WHFOs.

      a) Finger-driven wrist-hand prehension orthoses (see Fig. 4.3-11.6)substitute for the weakened wrist extensors by means of forearm assembly, thus preventing the fingers from dragging on the table when the patient writes or performs similar tasks.

      b) Wrist-driven prehension orthoses (see Fig. 4.3-11.H; tenodesis orthoses; flexor hinge splints) are used in patients with C6 complete tetraplegia to provide prehension through tenodesis action and maintain flexibility of the hand, wrist, and elbow. They may interfere with manual wheelchair (WC) propulsion. They are rarely accepted by C7 and C8 tetraplegics who prefer to use their residual motor power or utensil holders.

      c) Passive prehension orthoses have the same design as the finger-driven wrist orthoses with the addition of a ratchet assembly (consisting of a notched ratchet bar, spring-operated lever, and push lever), thus converting it into a passively operated orthosis to provide grasp. The term *passive* is used here to describe a mechanism that moves the stabilized fingers by gross motion of the opposite hand or by pushing a lever against a table or similar surface.

      d) Electrically driven prehension orthoses, using a cable, switch, motor, and battery, can be controlled by slight bodily movement (light pressure). They are indicated for high tetraplegics (e.g., C5 lesion).

c. Utensil holders (see Fig. 4.3-11.I; universal splints; activities of daily living [ADL] splints), consist of a handcuff with palmar pocket onto which the utensil can be inserted (see Chapter 4.5, section II.A.3.a.6). Most tetraplegics prefer them over the other complex orthoses.

2. Protective orthoses are used to protect the wrist, hand, and fingers from potential deformity or damage by restricting active function (e.g., to promote tissue healing) while maintaining a desired functional position. Most of them may be worn throughout the day and night to rest the joint.

a. Digital stabilizers

    1) Finger stabilizers

      a) Distal interphalangeal stabilizers (static DIP splints, stax or stack

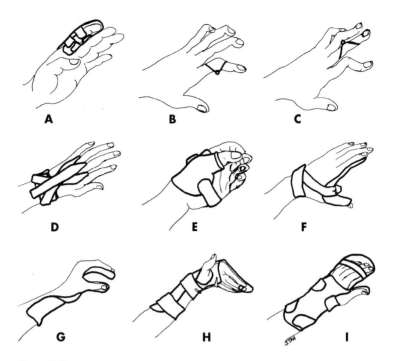

Figure 4.3-12
Protective wrist, hand, and finger orthoses. **A,** IP stabilizer (static finger splints, finger gutter splint). **B,** Swan neck ring (PIP or DIP extension-stop digital stabilizer). **C,** Boutonniere ring (PIP flexion-stop digital stabilizer). **D,** Finger web-space stabilizers (finger web spacers). **E,** Thumb carpometacarpal stabilizers (thumb posts). **F,** Thumb web-space stabilizer (thenar web spacers). **G,** Volar wrist-hand-finger stabilizers (resting hand splint). **H,** Dorsal blocking splint. **I,** Tone-reduction orthosis (Snook splint).

splints, and DIP gutter splints) are FOs covering the tip of the finger to just distal to the PIP volar crease to immobilize the DIP and allow unrestricted PIP movement, e.g., in patients with DIP fracture. When used in patients with distal extensor tendon repair, the DIP should be positioned in slight DIP hyperextension to take tension off repair.

b) **Interphalangeal (IP) (PIP/DIP) stabilizers** (see Fig. 4.3-12.A; static finger splints, eggshell finger casts, and finger gutter splints) are FOs usually used to restrict motions at the PIP and DIP. In general, the IPs are maintained in full extension to keep the collateral ligaments stretched and to prevent IP flexion contractures (unless condition dictates otherwise). They are used to immobilize and promote healing (e.g., phalanx fracture, PIP/DIP dislocation, PIP/DIP collateral ligament injury, and PIP volar plate injury) and to provide prolonged finger stretch (e.g., burns and contractures).

c) Ring stabilizers

(1) Swan neck ring (PIP extension-stop digital stabilizers; see Fig. 4.3-12.B) are FOs that prevent hyperextension of the PIP joint (via a three-point pressure system) while they permit flexion of all joints. They are used in arthritic patients with swan neck deformity or in PIP/DIP volar plate injury.

(2) Boutonniere ring (PIP flexion-stop digital stabilizers; see Fig. 4.3-12.C) are FOs that immobilize the PIP in extension through a three-point pressure system. They should be removed several times a day for ROM exercise. They are used in arthritic patients with boutonniere deformity.

d) Proximal interphalangeal hinged or articulated splints are FOs used to provide mediolateral stability in patients with PIP strains/sprains, PIP volar plate injury (using PIP hinged joint with extension block), or post-PIP surgery.

e) Metacarpophalangeal ulnar-deviation restriction orthoses are FOs used to limit ulnar deviation of the MCP with unrestricted (if possible) MCP flexion/extension in arthritic patients with ulnar deviation of the MCPs. Most patients find these orthoses too cumbersome and, in severe cases, may choose to have MCP arthroplasty instead.

f) Finger web–space stabilizers (finger web spacers; see Fig. 4.3-12.D) are FOs held firmly in the finger web spaces to increase or maintain the space between digits and prevent finger web–space contractures (e.g., burns, postreconstruction of syndactyly, and postrevision of scar).

2) Thumb stabilizers

a) Thumb carpometacarpal stabilizers (thumb posts; see Fig. 4.3-12.E) are TOs that stabilize the first CMC and MCP joints in neutral position to protect the thumb against inadvertent motion. In patients with ''duck-bill'' deformity (the thumb MCP is hyperflexed and the thumb IP extended), thumb posts maintain the thumb in an opposed, abducted position. Thumb posts may be extended distally to the thumb tip for use as an opposition post (e.g., in paralyzed thumb) or proximally over the midforearm to immobilize the wrist.

b) Thumb web–space stabilizers (thenar web spacers; see Fig. 4.3-12.F) are FOs that consist of a rigid C-shaped splint held firmly in the thumb and first finger web space to increase or maintain the thenar space and prevent contractures (e.g., burns and postrevision of scar).

b. Wrist-hand-finger stabilizers (resting hand splints, resting pan splints; static hand splints; functional resting splints) are WHFOs that extend from two-thirds of the distal forearm to the tips of the fingers and/or thumb (sometimes the thumb is left free). They can be volar-based (see Fig. 4.3-12.G), dorsal-based, or circumferential. The wrist is usually positioned in neutral or slightly extended with the digits in an intrinsic-plus position (i.e., the MCPs are flexed at 70-90°, the IPs in full extension, the thumb CMC in palmar abduction, and the thumb MCP/IP in full extension). Intrinsic-plus position is preferred because MCP and IP collateral ligaments are kept stretched, thus minimizing future joint capsule contractures. Also, the thumb position facilitates opposition and three-jaw chuck pinch. Intrinsic-plus position is contraindicated in certain conditions, e.g., after an extensor tendon repair that requires that MCPs be positioned in full extension to minimize tension on the suture site during healing.

Wrist-hand-finger stabilizers are used to immobilize and promote tissue healing (e.g., open wounds, cellulitis, arthritis, cumulative trauma disorders [CTD], flexor/extensor tendinitis, postsurgical conditions of the forearm-wrist-hand such as open–reduction internal fixation [ORIF], tendon/nerve/artery repair, skin graft, Dupuytren's release), to passively maintain ROM of the wrist and hand (often used at night) in patients with upper motor neuron [UMN] lesions (e.g., stroke, TBI, and MS), and to maintain stretch on MCP/IP collateral ligaments (e.g., in amyotrophic lateral sclerosis [ALS], SCI, polio, burns, brachial plexus lesion, and GBS). A variation of the wrist-hand-finger stabilizer is the flexor tendon repair orthoses (e.g., Kleinert splints, Strickland splints, early-controlled motion splints; dorsal blocking splints [see Fig. 4.3-12.H]) which are WHFOs placed on the dorsal forearm, wrist, and hand so that the wrist is in 20 to 45 degrees flexion, the MCPs in 40 to 70 degrees flexion, and the IPs in full extension to protect and promote healing of flexor tendon reconstructions (e.g., in postsurgical flexor tendon repair between DIP and distal volar forearm).

c. Wrist-hand stabilizers

1) Volar wrist-hand stabilizers (resting wrist splints and static wrist splints) are WHOs that extend from two-thirds of the distal forearm to about 1/4 inch proximal to the distal palmar crease to allow unrestricted MCP flexion and maintain the functional position of the wrist and hand. Resting splints are used to rest the wrist and hand (e.g., acutely inflamed RA joints, wrist sprain or contusion, forearm/wrist fractures, flexor/extensor tendinitis, carpal tunnel syndrome [CTS], and postsurgical wrist extensor tendon repair, wrist fusion, or skin grafting), prevent flexion contractures of the wrist and IP joint, prevent extension contracture of the MCP, prevent radial and ulnar deviation of the wrist (e.g., in RA), reduce spasticity and prevent thumb adduction and wrist flexion contractures, and reduce pain from repetitive stress (e.g., CTDs) or from arthritis. For optimal hand function, the wrist is positioned about 15 to 30 degrees of extension (usually 20°). In patients with CTS, there is controversy on whether to maintain the wrist in neutral or up to 20 degree extension (although both positions seem to be beneficial, the neutral position is generally preferred as it can theoretically maximize the carpal tunnel lumen and minimize median nerve compression pressure).

2) Dorsal wrist-hand stabilizers are WHOs that are used to provide the same functions as volar wrist-hand stabilizers as well as greater stabilization (due to the rigid dorsal hand section). However, they are more difficult to fabricate and fit. They are used in patients with severe spasticity but are not suitable for edematous hands because they cover the hand circumferentially.

d. Tone-reduction orthoses are used to reduce spastic flexor tone (e.g., UMN lesions such as stroke, SCI, TBI, MS, and CP). They are typically worn 2 hours on and 2 hours off throughout the day. They can either be hand-based WHOs (e.g., hand-cone splints) or forearm-based WHFOs (e.g., Rolyan preformed antispasticity ''ball'' splints and Snook splints [see Fig. 4.3-12.1]). Forearm based splints are generally more effective because of the extension positioning of the extrinsic finger flexors. An inflatable pressure splint (inflated to a maximum pressure of 40 mm Hg) may be worn for 30 minutes several times a day to reduce spasticity.

e. **Gloves** are worn circumferentially on the hand and wrist. If needed, the tips or whole fingers of the gloves may be cut off.

   1) **Shock absorbing gloves** are used to absorb shock/vibration entering the palm or hand (e.g., CTD and CTS) and to prevent CTDs (e.g., flexor tendinitis, manual WC users, and hypersensitive palmar skin/scars). The palmar aspect of the glove and the volar wrist can be padded with soft materials (e.g., silicone gel).

   2) **Compression gloves** (Isotoner, Tubigrip, and Jobst) are used to reduce edema (e.g., traumatic hand injuries with edema, burns, reflex sympathetic dystrophy, CTD, SCI, and UMN lesions such as stroke and TBI) and to reduce hypertrophic scarring (e.g., maturation phase of burns and scars). For edema reduction, a pressure garment with low to moderate compression of 10 to 15 mm Hg capillary pressure is used; however, for scar reduction, high compression of 15 to 25 mm Hg capillary pressure is used. They may be worn throughout the day (e.g., in scar reduction).

3. **Mobilization (corrective) orthoses** are used to increase passive ROM and alter joint alignment by stretching articular or musculotendinous contractures or adhesions (e.g., burns). In general, a submaximal load is applied for long periods either dynamically using traction (i.e., elastics, coils, or springs) or statically by holding the joint on low tension circumferentially (e.g., eggshell finger casts; serial static splints; buddy splints [i.e., taping or strapping the involved finger to the adjacent relatively normal finger to support and increase IP ROM in the involved finger]). The most commonly used stretching method is dynamic elastic load, specifically rubber bands whose amount of force can be regulated by the rubber tension. Mobilization orthoses are worn for only a specific time during the day.

   a. **Finger mobilization orthoses**

      1) **Interphalangeal mobilization orthoses**

         a) **Interphalangeal extension mobilization orthoses** (see Fig. 4.3-13.A; dynamic IP extension splints, reverse finger knuckle benders, Capener splints, safety pin splints, spring coil assists, eggshell finger extension casts, serial static finger extension splints, and buddy splints) are FOs used to passively extend the PIP joints, for example, in finger IP flexion contracture, boutonniere deformity, and postsurgical release of Dupuytren's contracture.

         b) **Interphalangeal flexion mobilization orthoses** (see Fig. 4.3-13.B; dynamic IP flexion splints, finger knuckle benders, fingernail hook orthoses, eggshell finger flexion casts, IP flexion straps, serial static finger flexion splints, and buddy splints) are FOs used to passively flex the PIP joints, for example, in finger IP extension contractures.

      2) **Metacarpophalangeal mobilization orthoses**

         a) **Metacarpophalangeal-extension mobilization orthoses** (reverse MCP knuckle benders [see Fig. 4.3-13.C]; dynamic MCP extension splints with dorsal outrigger [see Fig. 4.3-13.E]; MCP extension assists; radial nerve splints) are WHFOs or FOs used to extend the MCP joints, for example, in MCP flexion contractures, burns, and post-ORIF of metacarpal fracture. In patients with weak finger extension (e.g., in radial nerve lesion and brachial plexus lesion),

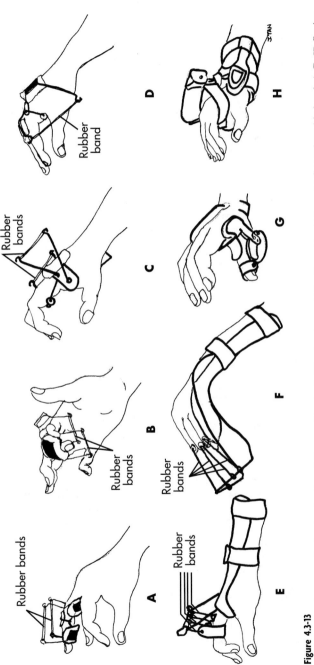

Figure 4.3-13

Mobilization (or corrective) wrist, hand, and finger orthoses. **A,** IP extension mobilization orthosis (reverse finger knuckle bender). **B,** IP flexion mobilization orthosis (finger knuckle bender). **C,** Reverse MCP knuckle bender. **D,** MCP knuckle bender. **E,** Dynamic MCP extension splint with dorsal outrigger. **F,** Dynamic MCP flexion splint with volar outrigger and fingernail hooks. **G,** Dynamic thumb IP extension splints. **H,** Wrist mobilization orthoses.

they may be used to improve hand functions by substituting for lost or weak finger extension.

    b) Metacarpophalangeal-flexion mobilization orthoses (MCP knuckle benders [see Fig. 4.3-13.D]; dynamic MCP flexion splints with volar outrigger and fingernail hooks [see Fig. 4.3-13.F]; MCP flexion assists) are WHFOs or FOs used to flex the MCP joints, for example, in MCP collateral ligament contractures, extensor tendon shortening, median/ulnar lesion, claw hand, postcapsulotomy, or postORIF of metacarpal fracture.

  3) Adjustable wrist hand orthoses (Swanson postarthroplasty orthoses) are used to facilitate controlled MCP as well as PIP and DIP motions as needed after arthroplasty and to selectively stabilize joints so there is undue stretching of unhealed reconstructed tendons and collateral ligaments.

 b. Thumb mobilization orthoses

  1) Thumb extension-mobilization orthoses (see Fig. 4.3-13.G; dynamic thumb IP extension splints and serial static thumb extension splints) are TOs used to passively extend the thumb IP joint, for example, in thumb IP flexion contracture.

  2) Thumb flexion-mobilization orthoses (dynamic thumb IP flexion splints and serial static thumb flexion splints) are TOs used to passively flex the thumb IP joint, for example, in thumb IP extension contracture.

  3) Thumb abduction-mobilization orthoses (dynamic thumb abduction splints and serial static thumb abduction splints) are TOs used to passively abduct the thumb, for example, in thumb adduction contracture.

 c. Wrist mobilization orthoses (see Fig. 4.3-13.H; Ultraflex wrist flexion/extension splints, Dynasplint wrist flexion/extension splints, Phoenix wrist hinge splints, static progressive wrist splints, and turnbuckle wrist splints) are WOs used to passively increase ROM (e.g., in contractures, burns, late-phase of fracture, and postrelease of scar). They can also be used to replace or assist weak wrist extensors to enhance ADLs (e.g., in patients with radial nerve lesions, SCI, brachial plexus lesion, or polio). However, they should not be used on spastic muscles as they may further increase tone.

B. Elbow, forearm, and wrist orthoses

 1. Forearm mobilization (corrective) orthoses (dynamic supination/pronation splints) are elbow-wrist-hand orthoses (EWHOs) consisting of a posterior elbow orthosis and a forearm-wrist or forearm-wrist-hand orthoses. They are used to increase supination or pronation (e.g., in forearm rotational contracture) or increase passive or active-assisted ROM (e.g., upper trunk brachial plexus lesion, or Erb's palsy, and spinal cord injury).

 2. Protective elbow, forearm, and wrist orthoses (sugar-tong splints; see Fig. 4.3-14.A) are EWHOs used to immobilize the elbow, forearm, and wrist to promote tissue healing (e.g., CTDs, forearm fractures, postsurgical elbow arthroplasty, or posttransposition of ulnar nerve).

C. Elbow and shoulder orthoses

 1. Protective elbow and shoulder orthoses are used to hold the joint in the position opposite the anticipated deformity, limit active motion to reduce pain, guard weak ligaments and muscles from untoward stress, and provide optimum environment for newly formed skin (which tend to contract as it heals).

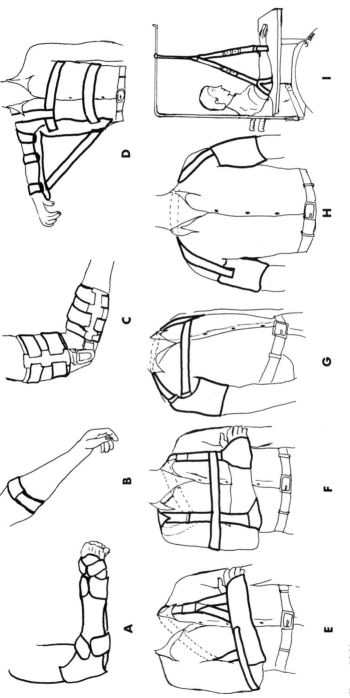

Figure 4.3-14
Protective elbow and shoulder orthoses. **A,** Sugar-tong splint. **B,** Epicondylar strap. **C,** Elbow mobilization orthosis. **D,** Shoulder abduction stabilizer (airplane splint). **E,** Single-strap sling. **F,** Multistrap sling. **G,** Vertical arm sling. **H,** Arm abduction sling. **I,** Arm suspension sling.

a. **Elbow control orthoses** (posterior elbow splints, elbow casts, and elbow air-splint), provide mediolateral elbow and forearm rotational stability, limit range of elbow flexion or extension, or both. They are used to promote tissue healing in medial or lateral epicondylitis, cubital tunnel syndrome, olecranon fracture, burns, and postsurgical repair of the elbow.

b. **Epicondylar straps** (see Fig. 4.3-14.B; tennis/golfer's elbow straps, proximal forearm orthoses, counterforce braces, and forearm bands) are applied circumferentially to the forearm distal to the epicondyles without hindering elbow motion. They are used to reduce pain during activity (e.g., medial or lateral epicondylitis) and to theoretically reduce inflammation and promote tissue healing at the tendinous origin.

c. **Shoulder abduction stabilizers** (airplane splints; see Fig. 4.3-14.D) are SEWHOs that support the upper arm and shoulder, protect the shoulder from adduction contracture, and relieve tension on the superior aspect of the shoulder. It can be used to stretch the internal rotators and relieve tension on the deltoid and rotator cuff. The shoulder can be maintained in abduction for several weeks after a rotator cuff repair to protect the healing tissues. It is used in patients with axillary burns, contractures, shoulder dislocation, and postsurgery (e.g., shoulder fusion, rotator cuff repair, and axillary scar release).

d. **Shoulder or arm slings** are used for patients with shoulder pain or subluxation to protect the shoulder from painful motion (e.g., after injury to shoulder capsule or its supporting muscles). They can be used to promote tissue healing by immobilization (e.g., scapular or humeral fractures, acromioclavicular joint injury, rotator cuff injury, bicipital tendinitis, postsurgical repair of shoulder), prevent overstretching of shoulder muscles or ligaments (e.g., brachial plexus injury), decrease shoulder pain related to arm distraction and shoulder-hand syndrome (e.g., UMN lesions and hemiparesis with subluxation), and keep distal extremity (i.e., hand and forearm) elevated or supported (e.g., edema and cast). They can also be used to protect the flail arm from inadvertent flinging and to place the hand within the patient's immediate visual field. Most arm slings support the forearm with the elbow flexed, arm abducted, and shoulder internally rotated. The use of arm slings in patients with flexion synergy (e.g., hemiplegics) is controversial. They are discouraged by practitioners of neurodevelopmental techniques (see Chapter 4.2, section IV.B.3) as they are believed to encourage flexion synergy, increase flexor tone, and promote contractures.

   1) **Single-strap slings** (see Fig. 4.3-14.E) are used to support the weight of the arm or a forearm cast, elevate and reduce upper-limb edema, protect the upper limb from inadvertent motion, place the hand in the wearer's visual field, and provide minimal glenohumeral support.

   2) **Multistrap slings** (see Fig. 4.3-14.F) have the same functions as single-strap slings but also apply vertical forces (e.g., via figure-of-eight suspension) for additional support of the ipsilateral shoulder.

   3) **Vertical arm slings** (Rolyan hemi-arm slings; see Fig. 4.3-14.G) use a humeral cuff with figure-of-eight suspension to provide vertical upward force to support the humerus and allow the elbow and forearm to be free to extend or flex.

   4) **Arm abduction slings** (hook hemiharness slings; see Fig. 4.3-14.H) consist of bilateral humeral cuffs connected by a posterior yoke. The

yoke provides a diagonal force to support the shoulders in a slightly abducted position while allowing the elbows and forearms to be free.

5) **Arm suspension slings** (see Fig. 4.3-14.I; overhead slings, counterbalance arm slings, deltoid aids, and Swedish slings) are SEWHOs that provide all the functions of the single-strap sling in addition to positioning the arm to allow hand use when shoulder and arm muscles have strength of less than fair (e.g., UMN lesions, proximal myopathy, and GBS); and allowing the arm muscles to be exercised in a gravity-reduced position (e.g., in SCI, muscular dystrophy, and arthrogryposis).

2. **Elbow mobilization (or corrective) orthoses** (see Fig. 4.3-14.C; dynamic elbow splints, Dynasplint elbow splints, Ultraflex elbow splints, static progressive elbow splints, and turnbuckle elbow splints) gently elongate the soft tissues over a long period to attempt to reverse joint malalignment (e.g., contractures, burns, and late phase of fracture). Force are provided by rubber bands, springs, or adjustable mechanisms (e.g., turnbuckles) or by altering the contour of the orthotic frame periodically. They are not used on spastic muscles as they may further increase tone.

a. **Dorsal elbow-extension mobilization orthoses** are used to extend the elbow as well as provide mediolateral elbow stability and rotational forearm stability.

b. **Dorsal elbow-flexion mobilization orthoses** are used to flex the elbow as well as provide mediolateral elbow stability and rotational forearm stability.

3. **Assistive and substitutive elbow and shoulder orthoses** assist in upper arm motion thus making wrist-hand functions more useful. They also protect the upper limb from contracture and from secondary trauma due to inadvertent motion.

a. **Elbow and shoulder articulated orthoses** are used to prevent unwanted motion and to ''lock'' the upper arm in a position necessary for its function. The most commonly used locks are friction locks, ratchet locks (e.g., step-locks), and alternator locks.

b. **Balanced forearm orthoses or BFOs** (see Fig. 4.3-15; mobile arm supports; ball bearing feeders; linkage or friction feeders; or ''gun-slingers'') are SEWHOs that consist of a forearm trough (attached by a hinge joint to a ball-bearing swivel mechanism) and a mount (which can be mounted on the WC, on a table or working surface, or onto the body jacket). The BFOs are used to support the forearm and arm against gravity and allow patients with weak shoulder and elbow muscles (i.e., manual muscle testing of at least trace plus [Tr +] to poor minus [P −]) to move the arm horizontally and flex the elbow to bring the hand to the mouth (e.g., patients with SCI, GBS, polio, muscular dystrophy, and brachial plexus injury). They also allow spastic patients to self-feed by dampening muscle tone through a friction device.

III. **Spinal orthoses and corsets** use external forces to generally stabilize, support, and realign the trunk, as well as to immobilize and protect the spine after acute trauma or spinal procedure. The prescribed spinal orthoses and corsets should be properly fitted so the patient can easily don and doff it; rest the desired segment, as well as sit, stand, and perform the prescribed movement comfortably when wearing the orthosis. Also, the orthosis must be functionally as well as cosmetically acceptable to the patient. When removed, the skin should be unblemished 10 minutes afterwards.

A. **Rigid spinal orthosis** exerts its force via three-point pressure system through

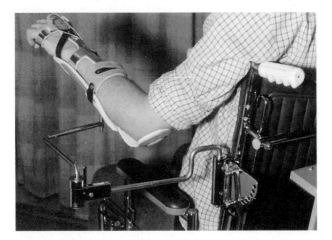

Figure 4.3-15
Balanced forearm orthoses (From Adler C, Pedretti, LW: The balanced forearm orthosis and suspension sling. In Pedretti LW, editor: *Occupational therapy practice skills for physical dysfunction,* ed 4, St. Louis, 1996, Mosby–Year Book, p. 345 with permission.)

the skin, soft tissue, and ribs to restrict motion, stabilize, and realign the spine. Rigid spinal orthoses can also increase intraabdominal pressure (IAP), thereby reducing contraction of the erector spinae and consequently reducing the compression of the intervertebral discs. In addition to the general principles applicable to nearly all orthoses (see the beginning of this chapter), rigid spinal orthoses should allow the patient to sit comfortably while wearing the orthosis, and they must not restrict breathing, digestion, or chewing. Indications include musculoskeletal pain, instability (trauma, degenerative disease, metastasis), osteoporotic compression fracture of the vertebrae, and postoperative spinal support (e.g., after spinal fusion). Although short-term use of rigid spinal orthoses promote reduction of muscle spasm, prolonged use should be avoided because they may promote atrophy, weakness, decreased flexibility, and psychological dependence. The following classification of rigid spinal orthoses are based on the primary function or control provided by the orthoses.

1. **Cervical and cervicothoracic orthoses** are used to reduce pain because of sprain, strain, or arthritis of neck; support the head to allow the patient to see, speak, and eat more easily; and to foster healing of vertebral fracture or surgical arthrodesis. The amount of cervical motion restricted by seven commonly used cervical and cervicothoracic orthoses are shown in Table 4.3-4.
   a. **Cervical flexion-extension (F-E) control orthoses**
      1) **Soft cervical collar** (e.g., Zimmer collar; see Fig. 4.3-16.A) made of polyethylene foam or sponge rubber, limits the least amount of cervical motion. It is fitted high in the back to increase resistance to extension or hyperextension. Through sensory feedback, it reminds the wearer to limit head and neck motions. It also retains body heat,

Table 4.3-4.   Percentage of cervical motion restricted by commonly used cervical and cervicothoracic orthoses

MOTION RESTRICTION (%)	SOFT	THOMAS	PHILADELPHIA	SOMI	YALE	4-POSTER	HALO
Flexion/ extension	26	75*	71	72 NS	87	79	96
Rotation	17	50*	56	66	82	73	99
Side bending	8 NS	75*	34	34 NS	50 NS	54	96

Data adapted from Johnson RM, Hart DL, Simmons EF: Cervical orthoses: A study comparing their effectiveness in restricting cervical motion in normal subjects, *J Bone Joint Surg [Am]* 59:332-339, 1977.
* Data adapted from Hartman JT, Palumbo F, Hill BJ: Cineradiography of the braced normal cervical spine, *Clinical Orthopedics* 109:97-102, 1975.
SOMI = sternooccipital mandibular immobilizer; NS = not significant statistically.

which may help reduce muscle spasm and aid in healing of soft tissue injuries.

2) **Hard cervical collars** provide more restriction to cervical flexion, extension, rotation, and lateral bending than the soft collars. It has similar function as the soft collar. Prolonged use may cause occipital pressure sore.

   a) **Thomas collar** (see Fig. 4.3-16.B) is made of firm plastic with superior and inferior paddings that wrap around the neck and is secured by Velcro.

   b) **Philadelphia collar** (see Fig. 4.3-16.C) is made of two pieces of polyethylene foam (Plastazote) secured by Velcro and is reinforced by rigid anterior and posterior plastic struts. It encompasses the lower jaw and occiput and terminates inferiorly at the proximal thorax. It can be loosened when patient is eating.

b. **Cervical flexion-extension-rotary (F-E-R) control orthoses (sternooccipital mandibular immobilizer [SOMI]**; see Fig. 4.3-16.D) is a poster-type cervicothoracic orthosis in which the uprights supporting the occiput arise anteriorly from a sternal plate. Therefore, it can easily be applied to the supine patient. The mandibular support can be removed so the patient can eat, wash, or shave while supine.

c. **Cervical flexion-extension-lateral-rotary (F-E-L-R) control orthoses**

   1) **Poster-type cervicothoracic orthoses** (see Fig. 4.3-16.E) have mandibular and occipital plates connected to sternal and thoracic plates by two-, three-, or four-posters. They provide greater motion limitations and can hold the head in extension or flexion by adjusting the length of anterior and posterior posters. They are cooler than cervical collars but are bulkier.

   2) **Custom-molded cervicothoracic orthoses** are designed to markedly restrict all neck as well as thoracic motions. They are not frequently used. Instead, a halo-vest orthosis is used for maximum neck motion control.

      a) **Minerva cervicothoracic orthosis** (see Fig. 4.3-16.F) encloses the entire posterior skull, includes a band around the forehead, and extends downward to the inferior costal margin.

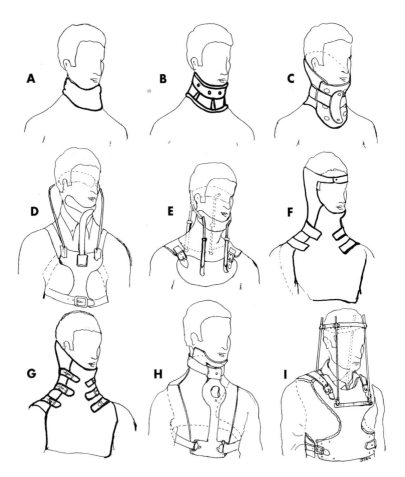

Figure 4.3-16
Cervical orthoses. **A,** Soft cervical collar. **B,** Hard (Thomas) collar. **C,** Hard (Philadelphia) collar. **D,** Sternooccipital mandibular immobilizer (SOMI). **E,** Poster-type cervicothoracic orthoses. **F,** Minerva cervicothoracic orthosis. **G,** Cuirass-type cervicothoracic orthosis. **H,** Yale cervicothoracic orthosis. **I,** Halo-vest cervicothoracic orthosis.

      b) Cuirass-type cervicothoracic orthosis (see Fig. 4.3-16.G) extends superiorly over the chin, mandible, and occiput.

   3) Yale cervicothoracic orthosis (see Fig. 4.3-16.H) is similar to an extended Philadelphia collar with rigid plastic struts extending down the anterior and posterior thorax with Velcro strapping beneath the axillae.

   4) Halo-vest cervicothoracic orthosis (see Fig. 4.3-16.I) consists of a rigid halo secured to the skull with four external fixation pins. The halo supports four-posters that terminate in hardware attached to the front and back of the vest. It provides the greatest control of all cervical motion and is used in patients with high cervical fractures. Its most common complications are pin loosening, pin-site infection, and pressure ulcers. Less common complications are reduced vital capacity, neck pain, brain abscess, and psychological trauma. It is cooler and lighter than the Minerva orthosis. A wrench for quick dismantling of the halo-vest must be taped to the front of the vest in case the patient needs cardiopulmonary resuscitation.

2. **Thoracolumbosacral orthoses (TLSO)** extends from the sacrum to above the inferior angle of the scapulae and are used to support and stabilize trunk (e.g., truncal paralysis, postspinal fusion, and post-scoliotic surgery) and to prevent progression of moderate scoliosis (20-45°) until patient reaches skeletal maturity. Except for the TLS flexion-control orthoses, TLSOs can increase IAP and consequently reduce compression of the intervertebral discs, thus decreasing low back pain (e.g., in spondylolisthesis, and in intervertebral disc disease). TLSOs are usually worn for 3 months after scoliosis surgery.

   a. **The TLS flexion-extension (F-E) control orthosis** (Taylor brace; see Fig. 4.3-17.A) consists of two TLS posterior uprights attached inferiorly to a pelvic band. An interscapular band stabilizes the uprights and serves as an attachment for axillary straps. Anteriorly, there is a full-front abdominal support. It decreases trunk flexion and extension and increases IAP. The control of extension is at a higher level (at thoracolumbar junction) and not at the lumbosacral junction, thus there is less decrease in lordosis.

   b. **The TLS flexion-extension-lateral (F-E-L) control** (Knight Taylor brace; see Fig. 4.3-17.B) is similar to the Taylor brace except for the addition of lateral uprights and a thoracic band to restrict lateral bending.

   c. **The TLS flexion-lateral-rotary (F-L-R) control orthosis** (Cowhorn brace; see Fig. 4.3-17.C) consists of pelvic and thoracic bands connected by a pair of LS posterior uprights and a pair of lateral uprights with abdominal support. The thoracic band extends and curves anteriorly to two subclavian pads to restrict rotation and flexion. It restricts extension at the lumbar area but not thoracic area.

   d. **The TLS flexion (F) control orthosis** has anterior metal plates that restrict trunk flexion. It does not increase IAP nor decrease lordosis. It encourages an hyperextension posture, increases lumbar lordosis, and tends to stabilize the spine to resist lateral and rotary movements.

      1) **Jewett or Becker TLSO** (see Fig. 4.3-17.D) has a sternal plate, a dorsolumbar plate, lateral uprights, and a suprapubic plate. The suprapubic plate is unacceptable in women because it presses on the bladder. A boomerang band, which applies force on iliac crest, is used for women instead.

      2) **Cruciform anterior spinal hyperextension (CASH) TLSO** (see Fig. 4.3-18.A) has a cross-shape anterior vertical and horizontal metal uprights. The vertical upright joins the sternal and suprapubic plates, while the horizontal uprights connects the dorsolumbar plates.

   e. **The TLS flexion-extension-lateral-rotary (F-E-L-R) control (TLS jacket;** see Fig. 4.3-18.B) is made of relatively thick rigid or semirigid polyethylene plastics. It is used for maximum orthotic immobilization, for example, in unstable fracture involving the posterior vertebral elements.

   f. **Boston TLSO** is a symmetrical rigid plastic jacket fitted with interior pads used in moderate scoliosis.

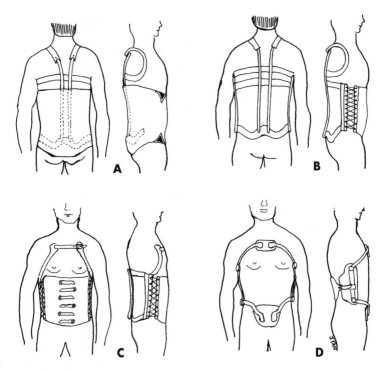

Figure 4.3-17
Thoracolumbosacral (TLS) orthoses. **A,** TLS flexion-extension (F-E) control orthosis (Taylor brace). **B,** TLS flexion-extension-lateral (F-E-L) control orthosis (Knight Taylor brace). **C,** TLS flexion-lateral-rotary (F-L-R) control orthosis (Cowhorn brace). **D,** TLS flexion (F) control orthosis (Jewett or Becker orthoses).

3. **Cervico-thoraco-lumbosacral orthoses (CTLSO)** are plastic TLS jacket that extend upward to the mandible and mastoid. The Milwaukee brace, which is a type of CTLSO used for scoliosis, has a rigid plastic pelvic girdle connected to a neck ring over the upper thorax by one anterior and two posterior uprights. Pads strapped to the uprights apply forces to correct the scoliotic curve.
4. **Lumbosacral orthoses (LSO)** extend from the sacrum to the inferior scapular angle

Figure 4.3-18
Thoracolumbosacral orthoses (TLSO). **A,** CASH or cruciform anterior spinal hyperextension TLSO (TLS flexion [F] control orthosis). **B,** TLS flexion-extension-lateral-rotary (F-E-L-R) control orthosis (TLS jacket). (From Bunch, WH, Keagy RD, Kritter, AE, et al: *American Academy of Orthopedic Surgeons (AAOS) atlas of Orthotics:Biomechanical principles and application*, ed 2, St. Louis, 1985, Mosby–Year Book, p. 245, 249 with permission.)

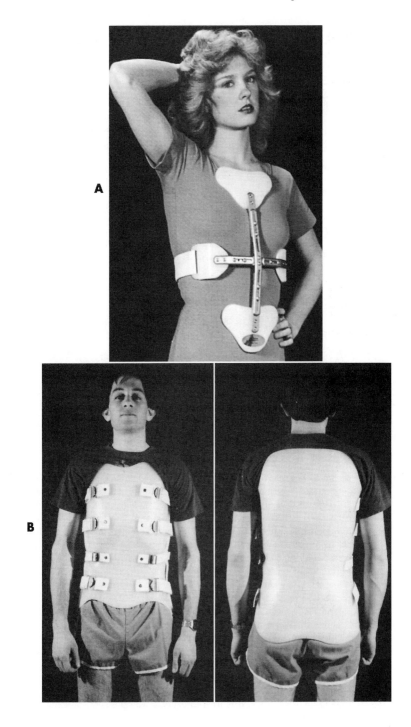

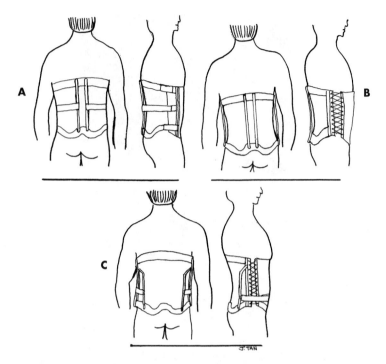

Figure 4.3-19
Lumbosacral (LS) orthoses. **A,** LS flexion-extension (F-E) control orthosis (Chairback orthosis). **B,** LS flexion-extension-lateral (F-E-L) control orthosis (Knight spinal orthosis). **C,** LS extension-lateral (E-L) control orthosis (William's brace).

a. **The LS Flexion-extension (F-E) control orthosis** (Chairback orthosis; see Fig. 4.3-19.A) consists of two LS posterior uprights attached inferiorly to a pelvic band and superiorly to a thoracic band. A full-front abdominal support is fastened to the posterior uprights by means of straps. It increases IAP, restricts flexion-extension, and flattens lumbar lordosis.

b. **The LS flexion-extension-lateral (F-E-L) control orthosis** (Knight spinal orthosis; see Fig. 4.3-19.B) is similar to the LS F-E control orthosis with the additional restriction of lateral motion by lateral uprights. It has a nonelastic abdominal support.

c. **The LS extension-lateral (E-L) control orthosis** (William's brace; see Fig. 4.3-19.C) consists of pelvic and thoracic bands joined by a pair of lateral uprights, which are pivotally attached to the thoracic bands but not attached to the pelvic band. It has elastic abdominal support. It increases IAP, decreases lordosis, and decreases extension and lateral bending but does not restrict flexion.

d. **The LSO with hip spica or thigh cuff** may be used to limit hip motion on one side. It locks the hip joint in extension making it difficult to walk and to climb stairs. It is used in patients with postsurgical screws or fusion of L4 to S1 fractures.

e. **The LS jacket** (Boston overlap brace) is made of semirigid plastic with Velcro straps. It encases the lower trunk and controls all lumbosacral motion.

B. **Corsets (flexible spinal orthoses)** are made of fabric with pouches for vertical stays. The vertical staves can be made of rigid (steel) or flexible materials. Corsets are considered flexible (nonrigid) spinal orthoses because the vertical stays are not connected by horizontal bars (i.e., there are no pelvic nor thoracic bands). Hence, although corsets create similar forces as in rigid spinal orthoses, they do not restrict motion nor realign the spine as much as rigid spinal orthoses do. Corsets increase IAP more than rigid spinal orthoses because the body part is covered snugly without space between corset and skin. Two commonly used corsets are thoracolumbosacral and lumbosacral corsets for patients with low back pain due to minor spondylolisthesis (grade I without neuropathy). In patients with skin irritations, corsets are contraindicated. As with any spinal orthoses, prolonged used of corsets should be discouraged. The efficacy of corsets remains controversial.

1. **The TLS corset** extends anteriorly below the xiphoid process to above the symphysis pubis and posteriorly from the midscapular level to just below the apex of the gluteal bulge for men and lower down to the gluteal fold for women. It can restrict spinal motion at the thoracic and the lumbar spine and can increase IAP, which consequently reduces intradiscal pressure during lifting. Mainly, it is used to remind the wearer to avoid abrupt trunk motion and to lift properly.

2. **The LS corset** (Richard's corset) is the most commonly used corset. It has the same design as TLS corset except that posteriorly it extends to below the inferior angles of the scapulae instead of the midscapular level. It has the same function as the TLS corset but does not restrict thoracic spinal motion.

3. **Sacroiliac (SI) corsets**

   a. **Sacroiliac corset** extends superiorly from the iliac crest level to the symphysis pubis anteriorly and to the apex of the gluteal bulge posteriorly. It is not effective in restricting motion, but it assists in elevating IAP and may be useful for postpartum and posttraumatic stabilization of sacroiliac and symphysis pubic joints. It is also occassionally used temporarily in low back pain patients with sacroiliac pain.

   b. **Sacroiliac belt** encircles the pelvis between the iliac crests and the trochanters with perineal straps to prevent upward displacement. The belt passes below the anterior superior iliac spine but should not encroach on the rectus femoris during hip flexion. It is used for patients with postpartum or traumatic separation of the SI or symphysis pubis or following resection of the symphysis.

   c. **Elastic sacroiliac corset (binder) with plastic insert** is similar to SI corset but has thermoplastic insert contoured to the patient's body and fitted into a posterior pocket with Velcro closure. It is mainly used to remind the patient to correct back posture. It can also increase IAP.

BIBLIOGRAPHY

Bunch, WH, Keagy RD, Kritter, AE, et al: *American Academy of Orthopedic Surgeons (AAOS) atlas of orthotics: Biomechanical principles and application,* ed 2, St. Louis, 1985, Mosby–Year Book.

Edelstein JE: Orthotic assessment and management. In O'Sullivan, SB, Schmitz, TJ, editors: *Physical rehabilitation: Assessment and treatment,* Philadelphia, 1994, FA Davis, pp. 655-684.

Edelstein JE: Orthoses. In Myers RS, editor: *Saunders manual of physical therapy practice,* Philadelphia, 1995, WB Saunders, pp. 1183-1227.

Hennessey WJ, Johnson EW: Lower limb orthoses. In Braddom RL, editor, *Physical medicine and rehabilitation,* Philadelphia, 1996, WB Saunders, pp. 353-358.

Irani KD: Upper limb orthoses. In Braddom RL, editor: *Physical medicine and rehabilitation,* Philadelphia, 1996, WB Saunders, pp. 321-332.

Lehmann JF, editor: Orthotics; *Phys Med Rehabil Clin North Am* 3(1):1-247, 1992.

Faculty of Prosthetics and Orthotics, New York University School of Medicine and Post-Graduate Medical School: *Lower-limb orthotics,* New York, 1986, Prosthetic-Orthotic Publications.

Ragnarsson, KT. Lower extremity orthotics, shoes, and gait aids. In DeLisa JA, Gans BM, editors: *Rehabilitation medicine: Principles and practice,* ed 2, Philadelphia, 1992, JB Lippincott, pp. 492-506.

Redford JB, editor: *Orthotics etcetera,* ed 3, Baltimore, 1986, Williams & Wilkins.

Redford JB, Basmajian JV, Trautman P, editors: *Orthotics: Clinical practice and rehabilitation technology,* New York, 1995, Churchill Livingstone

Sarno JE. Below-knee orthoses: A system for prescription. *Arch Phys Med Rehabil* 54:548-552, 1973.

Sipski ML, Sipski ML, Tolchin RB: Spinal and upper extremity orthoses. In DeLisa JA, Gans BM, editors: *Rehabilitation medicine: Principles and practice,* ed 2, Philadelphia, 1992, JB Lippincott, pp. 477-491.

Chapter 4.4

PROSTHESES

A prosthesis is an artificial substitute for a missing body part. This chapter deals only with prostheses for missing upper and lower limbs. Lower-limb amputations are 10 times more common than upper-limb amputations. The most common causes of lower-limb amputations in persons older than 50 years are ischemia (e.g., foot gangrene) caused by peripheral vascular diseases (which may result from diabetes mellitus, arteriosclerotic disease, thromboangiitis, venous dysfunction, or a combination of these as well as other vascular problems). Infection (e.g., chronic osteomyelitis) and severe burns may occassionally cause amputations. In younger adults and adolescents, the most common cause is trauma due to motor vehicle accidents, work-related injuries, or high-risk recreational activities. Other major causes of lower-limb amputation are malignancy, such as osteosarcoma and chondrosarcoma (peaking in adolescence), and congenital limb (skeletal) deficiency.

Like orthoses, prostheses should be lightweight with reasonable durability, acceptable cosmetically, easy to maintain and clean, easy to don and doff correctly and rapidly, and adjustable to accommodate progression or resolution of concomitant disorders. Most importantly, patient should be motivated to wear it. Patients perceive their prosthesis as "light" if it fits snugly and allows them to sit, stand, and move comfortably. In patients with decreased sensation or impaired circulation, the *residual limb* (formerly called stump) must be checked regularly for redness, trophic changes, abrasions, and dermatitis. Skin redness should disappear 10 minutes after prosthesis removal. Areas that are sensitive to high pressure (e.g., bony prominences) should be accommodated with a concavity within the socket, called a *relief.* In contrast, pressure-tolerant tissues (e.g., patellar tendon) can accept greater loading and should be provided with convexities, called *build-ups* (or *bulges*), within the socket. Selection of the optimal prosthetic component should consider the patient's level of amputation (see Fig. 4.4-1), cardiopulmonary condition, cognitive status, motivation, anticipated vocational and avocational activities, as well as the financial and technical resources available. The energy cost and loss of speed during ambulation using prostheses are shown in Table 4.4-1.

I. **Lower-limb prostheses** substitute for the missing lower limb segment to restore the amputee's appearance of bodily symmetry and usually perform a major role in ambulation. Except for partial-foot prostheses, all lower-limb prostheses include a foot-ankle assembly. For amputations below the knee (transtibial), the prostheses also include shank, socket, and suspension systems. For amputations above the knee (transfemoral), a knee unit is added. Although gait may be asymmetrical, especially in unilateral amputees, it should not deviate significantly from normal gait. Basic prosthetic training includes caring for the residual limb and the prosthesis, instruction in donning the prosthesis correctly, transferring from various chairs, walking, and climbing stairs, ramps, and curbs. An interim (temporary) prosthesis is usually made prior to a definitive (permanent) prostheses, which is cosmetically finished. The interim prosthesis consists of a socket designed to accept full weight bearing, attached to a pylon and foot. It allows early prosthetic fitting before the residual limb volume is stabilized. It helps in shrinking and shaping the residual limb, allow early gait and functional

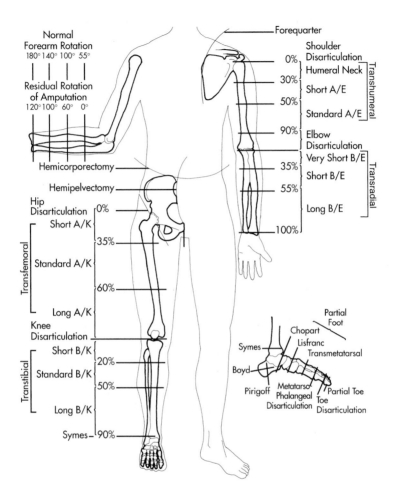

Figure 4.4-1.
Levels of upper and lower-limb amputations. The right upper limb shows the comparison of residual rotation in different levels of amputated forearm vs. normal forearm.

training with the prosthesis, and allow fine tuning of the prosthetic alignment as the amputee's gait progresses.

A. **Partial-foot prosthesis** is used to restore foot function (particularly walking) and forefoot contour. Small toes amputation does not significantly affect gait and requires only toe fillers made of cork or plastic foam. Loss of the great toe reduces push-off force during the late stance phase, thus requiring a resilient toe filler and also a molded insole with an arch support to maintain the alignment of the amputated foot. In transmetatarsal amputation (TMA) (see Fig. 4.4-1), the hindfoot tends to assume equinus position, thus requiring a molded socket connected to a rigid sole plate, which extends to a point just

Table 4.4-1. **Energy cost and speed of ambulation among lower-limb amputees compared to normal subjects walking at a comfortable speed of 80 m/min or 3 mph**

WALKING PARAMETERS	BK	BK + BK	AK + CRUTCH	AK	BK + AK	AK + AK
% increase in Ee/unit distance	23	41	92	99	118	186
% decrease in CWS	20	20	51	51	56	60

Data from multiple sources recalculted and summarized in Gonzales EG, Corcoran PJ: Energy expenditure during ambulation. In Downey JA, Myers SJ, Gonzalez EG, et al: *The physiological basis of rehabilitation medicine,* ed 2, New York, 1994, Butterworth-Heinemann, p. 431, with permission.
BK = below-knee or transtibial amputation; AK = above-knee or transfemoral amputation; Ee/unit distance = energy expenditure per unit distance; CWS = comfortable walking speed = 80 m/min or 3 mph

posterior to the normal toe break, with a distal padding, a toe break, and a toe filler. If the calcaneus is in varus or valgus position, the molded socket with rigid plate could be extended posteriorly and proximally to encompass and stabilize the heel. For Lisfranc amputation (see Fig. 4.4-1) at the tarso-metatarsal junction, the prosthesis used is similar to that for TMA. In midtarsal amputation (Chopart's amputation; see Fig. 4.4-1), only the calcaneus and talus remains, thus the prosthesis should extend to the calf in the form of a plastic calf shell strapped around the leg. An alternative is to strap the residual foot to a posterior leaf spring ankle-foot orthosis (AFO) and add a toe filler. Sensitivity of the distal end is common in partial foot amputation, thus shoes should have low heels to prevent the stump from sliding forward. Also, a rocker bottom sole may be used to promote rollover and protect distal residual limb from pressure.

B. **Syme prosthesis** is used for Syme ankle disarticulation (see Fig. 4.4-1), which is a supraarticular or transmalleolar amputation in which all foot bones are removed and the calcaneal fat (heel pad) is attached to the anterior skin flap to cushion the distal end of the lower limb. It consists of a socket strapped onto the calf usually terminating just below the tibial tuberosity or can be higher (e.g., patellar tendon-bearing [PTB] socket) if more proximal weight-bearing is needed. If the residual limb is bulbous, the socket needs a removable medial or posterior section to facilitate donning. Otherwise, a nonfenestrated socket may be worn.

1. **Original Syme prosthesis** consist of a leather socket, steel sidebars, and a single-axis prosthetic foot. It is rarely used nowadays.

2. **Canadian Syme prosthesis** (see Fig. 4.4-2.A) consists of a plastic laminated socket attached to a modified solid-ankle cushioned-heel (SACH) foot (see section I.C.1.a.1.a) with a removable posterior wall (retained by a strap) to allow donning of the bulbous residual limb.

3. **Removable-window design** or **Veterans Administration Prosthetics Center (VAPC) Syme prosthesis** (see Fig. 4.4-2.B) is made of a plastic laminated socket with a window cut on the medial aspect to increase prosthetic strength. The window allows donning of the bulbous distal end and can be closed by two straps, thus retaining the residual limb without any additional suspension.

4. **Flexible posterior build-up Syme prosthesis** (see Fig. 4.4-2.C), designed for less bulbous residual limb, consists of a nonfenestrated plastic laminated socket

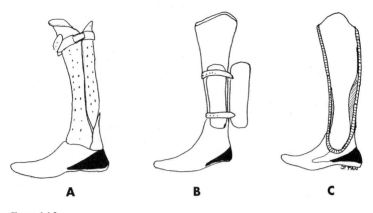

Figure 4.4-2.
Types of Symes prostheses. **A,** Canadian Syme prosthesis. **B,** Removable-window design (Veterans Administration Prosthetics Center [VAPC]) Syme prosthesis. **C,** Flexible posterior build-up Syme prosthesis.

in which all circumferences are equal to that of the distal residual limb. The void between the socket and the residual limb is filled with relatively soft, flexible build-ups that are either located in the socket or provided in the form of an insert that the amputee dons before slipping into the prosthesis. This design is stronger, but not heavier, than the Canadian or VAPC design because it uses one-piece lamination with unbroken exterior.

C. **Transtibial (below-knee) prostheses** are used for amputations above the Syme's site with 5 cm (2 inches) or more of residual tibia. It has four parts: foot-ankle assembly, shank, socket, and suspension.

1. **Foot-ankle assembly** should resemble the shape of the anatomic foot and provide the basic functions required in walking, i.e., shock absorption during heel strike, ankle plantarflexion in early stance, a stable base of support during midstance, and metatarsophalangeal hyperextension (toe-break action) in late stance to propel the body up and forward. The prosthetic foot yields passively in response to the direction of load applied by the amputee. Some models, however, also move in the transverse and frontal planes. Components called **rotators** (or **shank torque-absorber rotator units**) can be placed above the prosthetic foot to absorb shock in the transverse plane and protect the residual limb from chafing, which would occur if the socket is allowed to rotate against the skin. Rotators are not indicated for most transtibial amputees but may be used in those using thigh corsets or who are active athletes encountering discomfort.

   a. **Nonarticulated prosthetic feet** are the most popular types of prosthetic feet. They have streamlined appearance, are relatively lightweight, and have no moving parts that could loosen or become noisy.

      1) **Nonenergy storing prosthetic feet**

         a) **Solid ankle cushion heel (SACH) foot** (see Fig. 4.4-3.A) has a rigid longitudinal keel posterosuperior part of which is attached to the shank, has no definite ankle joint, and has a posteroinferior compressible rubber heel wedge, which simulates plantarflexion during

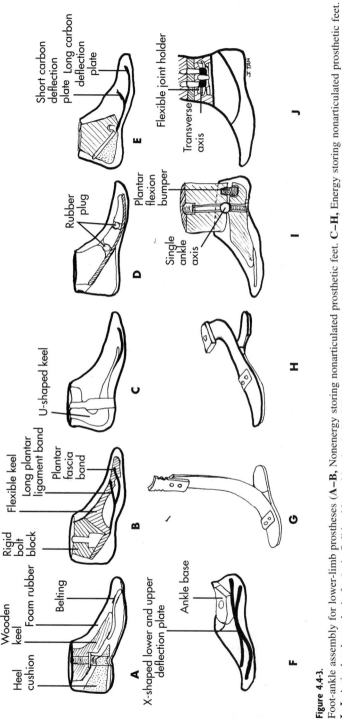

Figure 4.4-3.
Foot-ankle assembly for lower-limb prostheses (**A-B**, Nonenergy storing nonarticulated prosthetic feet. **C-H**, Energy storing nonarticulated prosthetic feet. **I-J**, Articulated prosthetic feet). **A**, Solid ankle cushion heel (SACH) foot. **B**, Stationary attachment flexible endoskeleton (SAFE) foot. **C**, Seattle foot. **D**, STEN (STored ENergy) foot. **E**, Carbon copy II foot. **F**, Quantum modular foot. **G**, Flex-foot. **H**, Flex-walk. **I**, Single-axis prosthetic foot. **J**, Multiple-axis prosthetic foot.

early stance. The distal end of the keel permits hyperextension of the foot during late stance. The keel terminates at the site of the metatarsophalangeal joints. It is covered with rubber, which continues distally to form the toe section. During heel strike, the heel wedge compresses up to 3/4 to 1 inch, plantar flexing the foot, thereby absorbing shock and stabilizing the patient's knee. The heel also compresses on application of medial or lateral loading, such as experienced when walking on uneven terrain. Unlike the normal foot, the SACH version does not dorsiflex at midstance. In late stance, weight advancement causes the foot to hyperextend at the junction between the keel and the toe. The lack of an articulated ankle provides the lever arm to propel the body forward at the end of stance phase.

b) **Stationary attachment flexible endoskeleton (SAFE) foot** (see Fig. 4.4-3.B) has a rigid ankle block attached to the shank, without a definite ankle joint; the anterior part of the block terminates at a 45-degree angle, abutting a more flexible keel, to permit inversion and eversion and accommodate more readily to irregular surfaces. The distal end of the keel permits hyperextension of the foot during late stance. The heel is cushioned (like a SACH foot) to absorb shock and permit plantarflexion during early stance. It is heavier than a SACH foot.

2) **Dynamic response (or energy-storing) prosthetic feet** have keels that deform slightly during midstance, thus storing potential energy. The stored energy is then released during pushoff as the keel recoils to its original shape. Their mechanical efficiency provide significant improvement in the level of function, gait pattern, and overall quality of life of the active amputee. Vigorous amputees are able to run and jump using dynamic response feet (e.g., Flex foot). However, dynamic response feet have not been shown to reduce metabolic energy consumption when compared to other feet (e.g., SACH) especially during normal walking speed.

a) **Seattle foot** (see Fig. 4.4-3.C) has a cantilevered plastic spring keel and Kevlar reinforced toe pad encased in a human-looking polyurethane mold. Body weight after midstance compresses on a U-shaped keel, which acts as a compressed spring. The stored energy is released at push-off. The Seattle foot is wide and heavy and has a relatively high arch, which may interfere with medial-lateral stability. It is useful for the young and middle-aged transtibial and transfemoral amputee.

b) **Seattle light foot** provides a dynamic response similar to the Seattle foot at half the weight. The foot has a less pronounced medial arch and a slim profile. This combination provides the patient with some degree of plantar- and dorsiflexion and the option of a lightweight endoskeletal system. This foot-ankle system is indicated in the geriatric population.

c) **The STEN (STored Energy) foot** (see Fig. 4.4-3.D) uses a modified SACH mold with a dual, articulated wooden keel and a double-reinforced belting system that permits a smoother transition from midstance to push-off. It weighs and costs more than the SACH foot. The STEN foot is not recommended by the manufacturer for transfemoral amputees because of the soft forefoot, which may cause knee instability.

d) Carbon Copy II foot (see Fig. 4.4-3.E) consists of a solid-ankle rigid posterior bolt block made of reinforced nylon/Kevlar and combined with two flexible anterior deflection plates, which permit energy storage in accordance with activity level. It is encased in a realistic-looking Elastomer shell. The foot is as light as a geriatric SACH foot. Because the sole of this foot is flat, it improves mediolateral stability. The cost is higher than that of the Seattle foot. It is an excellent foot to be used by active unilateral transtibial and trans-femoral amputees. It is 50% lighter than Seattle foot.

e) Quantum modular foot (see Fig. 4.4-3.F) consists of a long sole spring, a secondary spring, and an ankle base that are inserted in a hollow cosmetic foot module. It has anterior and posterior deflector plates shaped like an X, a multiple-axis ankle system, and a mecha-nism inside the cosmetically designed foot. The foot is assembled from stock components, which are chosen according to the patient's foot size, weight, and level of activity. Because it is modular, the foot and knee units are easy to interchange. The system is in the same price and weight range as the Carbon Copy II. At this time it is only available for endoskeletal systems.

f) Flex-foot (see Fig. 4.4-3.G) is made from graphite composite to store energy during stance and to release it at toe-off. The Flex-foot keel extends to bottom of the transtibial socket. Shank is also compressi-ble thus more energy storing. The foot is custom designed and fabricated for each amputee taking into consideration body weight and level of activity. This foot is light and is indicated for very active unilateral or bilateral transtibial amputees. It is best for run-ners. Its alignment can be cumbersome and the cost is high.

g) Flex-walk (see Fig. 4.4-3.H) is a shorter version of the Flex-foot. It is lighter, less expensive, and ideal for less active individuals.

b. Articulated prosthetic feet

1) Single-axis prosthetic feet (see Fig. 4.4-3.I) consists of separate foot and distal shank sections joined by a fixed metal axle around which the foot rotates into plantar- and dorsiflexion. Ankle excursion is limited by a resilient plantarflexion bumper posteriorly and a moderately firm dorsiflexion stop anteriorly. Toe hyperextension occurs in a manner similar to the SACH foot. It is indicated for transtibial amputees who go up and down stairs and ramps and for transfemoral amputees.

2) Multiple-axis prosthetic feet (see Fig. 4.4-3.J) provides slight mediolat-eral (inversion/eversion) and transverse (rotation) motion in addition to sagittal movement. It is used by active individuals who run and have to ambulate in uneven terrain. Amputee may feel unstable with it because the foot is controlled by the rubber in the prosthesis and not by the patient. It is more complex, heavier, and costlier than the single-axis foot. It needs to be maintained at least every 6 months. Examples are Greisinger Ankle-foot System, D.A.S. Multiaxial Rota-tion System, McKendrick Ankle-foot System, Multiflex Ankle-foot (Endolite) System, Graph-Lite, and College Park Ankle-foot System.

2. Shank is the rigid portion of the prosthesis that connects the socket to the prosthetic foot. It restores leg length and shape, and transmits the amputee's body weight from the socket to the foot.

a. Endoskeletal shank (see Fig. 4.4-4.A) is a rigid metal or plastic pylon usually fitted with an adjustment mechanism to enable making slight changes in prosthetic alignment. The pylon can be covered with foam

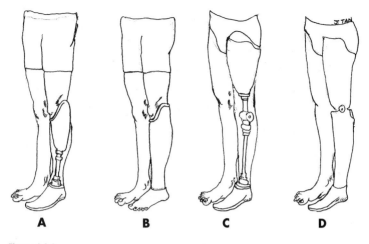

Figure 4.4-4.
Endo- vs. exoskeletal lower-limb prostheses. **A,** Endoskeletal transtibial prosthesis (covered with soft rubber foam). **B,** Exoskeletal transtibial prosthesis. **C,** Endoskeletal transfemoral prosthesis (covered with soft rubber foam). **D,** Exoskeletal transfemoral prosthesis.

   rubber shaped to resemble the contralateral limb. It is more attractive and lighter but less durable than an exoskeletal shank.

 ✓ **b. Exoskeletal (crustacean) shank** (see Fig. 4.4-4.B) is made of rigid material (either plastic foam or hollowed wood) carved to the shape of the contra-lateral leg and covered with a thin layer of waterproof (polyethylene) plastic laminate finish.

 3. Transtibial socket is a receptacle that receives the transtibial residual limb. It can be molded entirely of rigid plastic with or without a resilient liner. Sockets lined with polyethylene foam liners (Pelite inserts) are used in elderly amputees with poor tissue covering of the residual limb or in amputees with continuing vascular problems, sensitive tissue, or fluctuating residual limb volume. The socket may be unlined (hard socket) for amputees who sweat profusely or whose residual limb is matured and has good tissue covering. An alternative socket design is to mold it from a thin, flexible plastic and nest it in a rigid padded frame (Icelandic-Swedish–New York University [ISNY] design, see Fig. 4.4-5.B). The ISNY socket conforms more closely to the amputated limb but is not as durable.

 a. Total contact (patellar tendon bearing [PTB]) socket (see Fig. 4.4-5.A) is the most commonly used socket for transtibial amputation. It is a custom-molded plastic socket, which distributes weight through convex build-ups (bulges) on pressure-tolerant areas (see Fig. 4.4-6.A to C) of the transtibial residual limb (i.e., patellar ligament or tendon, belly of the gastrocnemius, popliteal fossa, area of the pes anserinus, proximomedial tibia, pretibial muscle mass between the tibial crest and the fibula, lateral surface of the fibular shaft, and inferior surface of the medial tibial condyle). Although called PTB socket, the patellar tendon only bears moderate load. The socket also provides concavities or reliefs over pres-

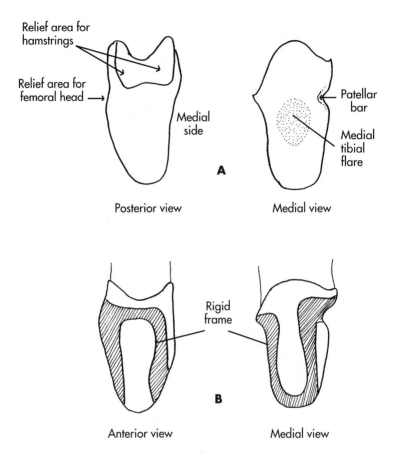

Figure 4.4-5.
Transtibial sockets. **A,** Patellar tendon-bearing (PTB) socket. **B,** Icelandic-Swedish-New York University or ISNY socket (molded from a thin, flexible plastic and nested in a rigid padded frame). (From Kapp S, Cummings D: Prosthetic management. In Bowker JH, Michael JW, editors: *American Academy of Orthopedic Surgeons (AAOS) atlas of limb prosthetics: surgical, prosthetic, and rehabilitation principle,* ed 2, St Louis, 1992, Mosby–Year Book, pp. 454, 456 with permission.)

sure-sensitive areas (see Fig. 4.4-6.D to F; i.e., patella, tibial crest, anterior tibial tubercle, distal end of tibia, anterodistal tibia, fibular head, lateral distal end of the fibula, common peroneal nerve, and hamstring tendons). The socket is aligned on the shank in slight flexion (about 5°) to enhance loading on the patellar ligament, prevent genu recurvatum, resist the tendency of the residual limb to slide down the socket, and facilitate contraction of the quadriceps muscles. The socket is also aligned with a slight lateral tilt to reduce pressure on the fibular head. The intimate total-contact fit helps prevent edema, provides some additional support, and probably provides greater sensory feedback.

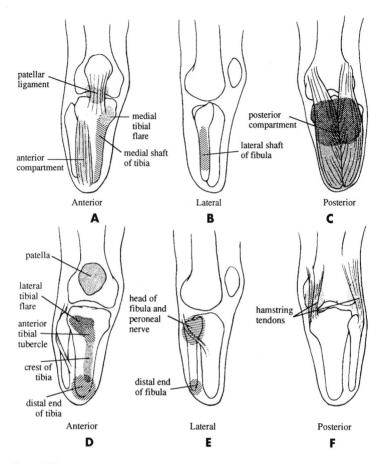

Figure 4.4-6.
Pressure-tolerant (**A–C**) and pressure-relief (**D–F**) areas in a patellar tendon-bearing (PTB) socket. (From Kapp S, Cummings D: Prosthetic management. In Bowker JH, Michael JW, editors: *American Academy of Orthopedic Surgeons (AAOS) atlas of limb prosthetics: Surgical, prosthetic, and rehabilitation principle,* ed 2, St Louis, 1992, Mosby–Year Book, p. 468 with permission.)

b. **Total surface-bearing socket** is less frequently used. It customizes pressure distribution within the socket through careful and extensive checking and adjustment of socket fit using a transparent socket (also called **check socket**). Although theoretically better than the PTB socket, its goals are difficult to attain because the skin-socket interface pressure is constantly changing during active use of the prosthesis. Also, the residual limb can change in size and shape due to weight gain or loss, edema, and muscle function.

4. **Transtibial suspensions** are used to retain the prosthesis on the residual limb during swing phase.

a. **Supracondylar cuff suspensions**
   1) **Supracondylar cuff suspension (without fork strap or waist belt)** (see Fig. 4.4-7.A) is made of adjustable leather or fabric strap that grips over the proximal patella anteriorly and wraps circumferentially around the thigh immediately above the femoral epicondyles. It is indicated in early prosthetic fittings when effective suspension is essential to protect the skin from shear forces during gait; in new amputees that need adjustable suspension or in whom residual limb shrinkage is anticipated; and in limited ambulators who spend majority of time sitting (because the supracondylar cuff is comfortable during sitting). It is contraindicated in patients with severely arthritic hands or limited vision who have difficulty engaging the buckle closure or pressure loop (Velcro) closure of the cuff; in patients who find straps cosmetically unacceptable; in patients with mediolateral knee instability or short residual limbs where problems with mediolateral knee control are anticipated; and in fleshy residual limbs with poor bony definition, hence making it difficult to attain suspension over the patella or femoral condyles.
   2) **Supracondylar cuff with fork strap and waist belt suspension** (see Fig. 4.4-7.B) is essentially a supracondylar cuff with a fork strap attached to the prosthesis distally and to the waist belt proximally. A part of the fork strap is always elastic to allow for the knee to flex during ambulation while maintaining tension for suspension at all times. It is indicated for active amputees with vigorous activities needing additional suspension during athletic activities and for amputees who climb ladders or participate in activities during which the prosthesis is unsupported by the ground for long periods.
b. **Brim suspension** retains the prosthesis by rigid extension of the socket brim proximally to cover the femoral epicondyles. It is easy to don and looks good when the wearer sits but is more difficult to fabricate, more expensive, and is not adjustable. It is difficult to suspend if the femoral condyles are not well-defined.
   1) **Supracondylar (SC) brim suspension** (see Fig. 4.4-7.C) has medial and lateral walls that extend above the femoral epicondyles to increase mediolateral knee stability of the prosthesis. The anterior area is cut out to accommodate the patella. The medial wall can either have a removable brim (see Fig. 4.4-7.D) or it can have a removable plastic wedge (see Fig. 4.4-7.E), which is inserted between the medial epicondyle and proximomedial socket wall to retain the prosthesis snugly on the residual limb. Instead of a removable medial brim or wedge, a compressible foam wedge build-up may be incorporated into the soft liner.
   2) **Supracondylar/suprapatellar (SC/SP) brim suspension** (see Fig. 4.4-7.F,G) is similar to the SC brim suspension with the addition of a high anterior socket margin ("quadriceps bar") that ends above the patella. It is used in transtibial amputation with short residual limb, which has short lever arm and poor resistance of knee forces. It has more effective suspension and mediolateral knee control than SC socket and also helps control genu recurvatum. However, the anterior socket bulk interferes with kneeling and looks conspicuous when sitting.
c. **Sleeve suspension** (see Fig. 4.4-7.H) uses sleeves of neoprene, latex, or other elastic material either as the primary suspension system or in con-

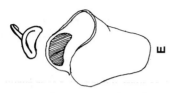

E

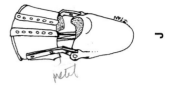

J

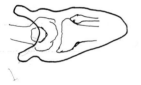

D

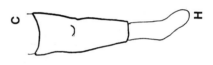

I

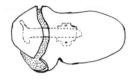

C

H

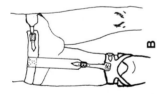

B

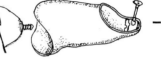

G

Quadriceps
bar

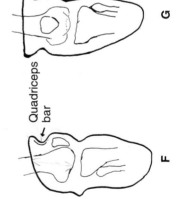

A

F

junction with another suspension (e.g., SC suspension). The distal sleeve is rolled over the prosthetic socket, whereas the proximal end of the sleeve is rolled up over the thigh (extending a few inches above the prosthetic sock). This creates a smooth silhouette when the patient stands and sits. Sleeve suspension is accomplished through a combination of longitudinal tension in the sleeve and negative pressure during swing phase, which results in suction type effect. It is indicated as an auxilliary suspension when added security is desired, control of positioning is essential, or high activity levels create higher suspension demands. It may be used as a primary suspension with standard PTB trim lines for the same population that benefits from a supracondylar cuff. It is contraindicated as a primary suspension with standard PTB trim when mediolateral knee stability is questionable, hyperextension control is required, and when residual limb is short. It should not be used if the patient has a fleshy thigh, perspires excessively (may cause skin irritation), and lacks bimanual dexterity or strength to manipulate the sleeve.

d. **Suction suspension** (see Fig. 4.4-7.I) uses a flexible, molded silicone liner rolled directly onto the residual limb and secured to the outer rigid socket by a distal transverse rod or pin. It provides snug suspension without any prosthetic component contacting the thigh skin. Suspension is accomplished through longitudinal tension in the sleeve, tension between the sleeve and the residual limb, and negative pressure during swing phase, which results in suction type effect between the limb and the liner. The liner may be incorporated into a socket with a soft interface material or a hard socket. Prosthetic socks are worn over the liner to accommodate changes in socket fit. Standard PTB trim lines are commonly used, which allow for the combination of a secure suspension with relative freedom of knee movements. It is indicated in amputees with greater suspension demands because of high activity levels, with short residual limbs for which suspension may be difficult, with residual limbs whose skin integrity is susceptible to shear forces and would thus benefit from a secure inherent suspension, and for whom standard PTB trim lines are adequate for knee stability. It is contraindicated in amputees with stability problems who would benefit from an alternative socket design with higher proximal socket walls and who lack the hand dexterity or strength to manipulate the silicone liner and the distal pin.

e. **Joint and thigh corset suspension** (see Fig. 4.4-7.J) uses a leather thigh

Figure 4.4-7.
Knee suspension for transtibial prostheses. **A,** Supracondylar cuff suspension (without fork stap or waist belt). **B,** Supracondylar cuff with fork strap and waist belt suspension. **C,** Supracondylar (SC) brim suspension. **D,** Removable brim. **E,** Removable plastic wedge. **F,G,** Supracondylar/suprapatellar (SC/SP) brim suspension. **H,** Sleeve suspension. **I,** Silicone suction suspension (3 S; Residual limb with silicone liner is attached to the socket by a shuttle lock system). **J,** Joint and thigh corset suspension. (From Kapp S, Cummings D: Prosthetic management. In Bowker JH, Michael JW, editors: *American Academy of Orthopedic Surgeons (AAOS) atlas of limb prosthetics: surgical, prosthetic, and rehabilitation principle,* ed 2, St Louis, 1992, Mosby–Year Book, p. 457, 459-462, with permission; Figure I, silicone suction socket, reproduced with courtesy of Fillauer, Inc.)

corset connected to the prosthesis through metal joints and side bars. Suspension is achieved through the corset by its grip over the proximal patellar area or with the use of auxiliary suspensions (e.g., fork straps and waist belts). The metal uprights provide maximum mediolateral stability while the leather corset increases weight-bearing area. It can shunt 40 to 60% of the body weight from the residual limb to the thigh situations via the thigh corset and is used when the patellar tendon cannot tolerate weight bearing or when the knee joint is painful or unstable. It is also used to control moderate to severe mediolateral knee instability and to control moderate to severe genu recurvatum by limiting knee extension. However, lacing or strapping the corset complicates donning and continued use can cause atrophy of the thigh muscles.

D. Transfemoral (above-knee) prosthesis uses the same types of prosthetic feet and shank described under transtibial prosthesis. Prosthetic feet that are stable (e.g., single-axis or SACH-type feet) and shanks that are light (endoskeleton; see Fig. 4.4-3.C) are commonly prescribed for the transfemoral amputee. The socket and suspension components for transfemoral amputees differ from those used in transtibial amputees. In addition, prosthesis for transfemoral amputees also requires a knee unit. A **rotator** (or **shank torque-absorber rotator unit**) may be placed between the knee unit and the socket to absorb shock in the transverse plane and protect the residual limb from chafing in active transfemoral amputees.

1. Knee units provide stability during walking (particularly during early stance) and allow the knee to bend when the patient sits and, in most cases, during swing phase.

    a. Knee-unit axes

        1) Single-axis knee unit for transfemoral prosthesis is in the form of a transverse bolt that allows knee flexion and extension. It is simple to maintain, less costly, and has minimal noise.

        2) Polycentric axes knee unit has multiple (usually four-bar) linkage, which constantly shifts the knee axis so that the instantaneous center of rotation remains behind the weight line. Compared to single-axis knee, it is more stable but is heavier, more costly, and needs more maintenance. It is indicated in amputees with short transfemoral residual limb, knee disarticulation, or weak hip extensors.

    b. Friction mechanisms are devices used in **swing-control knee** to dampen the pendular action of the prosthetic knee during swing phase to reduce the incidence of high heel rise in early swing and decrease terminal impact in late swing.

        1) Constant friction knee unit applies uniform resistance throughout swing phase by using a sleeve or split bushing and clamp that slide around the knee bolt. The friction can be adjusted by tightening or loosening the sleeve or bushing. It is the most commonly used friction mechanism because it is simple, low in cost, lightweight, quiet, and easy to adjust and maintain. However, it only allows one cadence and if the amputee walks faster or slower than the preset cadence, the swing becomes asymmetrical.

        2) Variable friction knee unit applies greater friction at the beginning and at the end of swing phase and less friction during midswing. It tends to be noisier, more costly, and to require more maintenance.

            a) Sliding friction is applied by contact of two solid structures that resist motion by moving against each other, such as a clamp on the knee bolt. It is rarely used.

  b) Fluid friction consists of an oil-filled hydraulic friction or air-filled pneumatic friction cylinder in which a piston connected to the knee hinge moves up and down. Fluid friction knee units automatically compensate for changes in walking speed, increasing friction when the wearer walks faster.

 c. Mechanical stabilizers increase the stability of the prosthetic knee unit by using a manual lock or a friction brake.

  1) Manual lock is a spring-loaded pin that automatically locks when the amputee stands and extends the knee. The knee is kept extended throughout the gait cycle to increase stability. Because of lack of knee flexion, the prosthesis usually needs to be shortened by 1 cm to allow gait clearance. It is indicated for amputees who need utmost stability because of muscular weakness or poor coordination, for active amputees whose job requires prolonged standing, and for new unstable amputees temporarily. To sit, the amputee raises the pin manually so that the knee can flex.

  2) Weight-activated friction brake (stance-stabilized knee, safety knee) commonly uses a spring-loaded wedge that is forced into a groove upon transfer of body weight to the prosthesis thus resisting knee flexion during early stance when the knee is flexed less than 25 degrees. It is indicated in amputees with poor control of their residual limb. It can also be used by amputees in training but who are young and capable of ambulating. Several fluid friction units incorporate stance phase controls (e.g., Mauch Hydraulic Swing and Stance [SNS] unit) and are equipped with locking or braking action. The brake does not interfere with swing phase nor sitting, but the unit is relatively heavy. Although durable, it must be maintained every 3 to 6 months.

 d. Extension aids are additional mechanical assistance that stretch during early swing as the knee flexes and recoil in late swing to aid knee extension and make heel contact more secure. It also helps restrain heel rise.

  1) Internal extension aid uses an elastic webbing or an extension lever with compression spring or tension spring attached inconspicuously within the knee unit. It does not protrude when the amputee is seated but can be noisy and difficult to adjust in some knee models.

  2) External extension aid (fork strap, kick strap) consists of an elastic strap (can be fork-shaped) placed externally in front of the knee and connected to a waist belt. It is simple, easy to adjust, and low in cost and maintenance.

2. Transfemoral socket can be molded in rigid plastic or, in the ISNY design (i.e., molded in flexible plastic worn in a rigid frame). The flexible ISNY transfemoral socket is more comfortable, has adaptable shape, provides greater sensory input, and is cooler because body heat dissipates through the thin plastic walls. However, they are more expensive and are not as durable as the rigid socket. Virtually all sockets have a total contact configuration with two basic socket shapes: quadrilateral and narrow mediolateral shape.

 a. Quadrilateral (ischial-gluteal bearing) socket (see Fig. 4.4-8) has four distinct sides and corners. It is narrow from anterior to posterior and relatively wide mediolaterally. The posterior socket wall has a proximal brim lying directly under the ischial tuberosity and buttock and is intended for the majority of the weight bearing thus relieving weight-bearing tasks from the distal pressure-sensitive areas of the residual limb. The anterior wall is higher than the posterior to apply posteriorly directed forces to maintain the position of the ischial tuberosity on the posterior brim. There is a prominent bulge over Scarpa's femoral triangle for wide-pressure distribution. Reliefs are located over the sensitive adductor longus and hamstring tendons and greater trochanter. Extra room is provided for expansion of the gluteus maximus when the muscle becomes tense. Although the design is based on sound anatomical and biomechanical principles, it has several problems including skin irritation at ischium and pubis from proximal brim, tenderness on anterior distal femur, discomfort while sitting from either the anterior proximal brim or the rigid posterior socket wall, poor cosmesis with gapping of lateral socket wall during stance, and frequent lateral lurch when walking.

b. Narrow mediolateral (narrow ML) or ischial containment (IC) socket (see Fig. 4.4-8) has a mediolateral dimension that is narrower than the anteroposterior measurement. The ischial tuberosity (which lies outside the socket in the quadrilateral design) is contained within the narrow ML (or IC) socket. Weight bearing, therefore, is focused primarily through the medial aspect of the ischium and the ischial ramus instead of the ischial tuberosity. The ischial tuberosity is locked in the socket and the resulting "bony lock" between ischium, trochanter, and lateral distal aspect of the femur gives more stable mechanism for acceptance of perineal biomechanical forces, thus providing increased comfort in the groin and better control of pelvis and trunk. The narrow ML design is intended to maintain the femur in adduction although this may not always be feasible if the amputee has uncorrectable deformity because of poor surgical technique. By keeping the femur in relative adduction during the stance phase, the hip abductors are kept in more stretched and efficient position. The narrow ML socket can decrease neurovascular bundle compression and can be fitted to short residual limb. It is more expensive and more difficult to fabricate than the quadrilateral socket. First-time prosthetic wearers may accommodate to the narrow ML design more readily than a longtime quadrilateral socket wearer. The narrow ML socket design developed by Ivan Long is called the Normal Shape-Normal Alignment (NSNA) socket while the narrow ML socket design developed by John Sabolich is called the Contoured Adducted Trochanteric-Controlled Alignment Method (CAT-CAM) socket.

3. Transfemoral suspension mechanism

a. Suction suspension (see Fig. 4.4-9.A):

1) Total suction suspension is equipped with a one-way valve at the distal end of the socket that permits air to escape in stance phase. Thus, pressure within the socket is less than atmospheric pressure so the socket remains on the thigh during swing phase. It requires a snugly fitted socket worn without any sock because socks interfere with the airtight seal. A donning sock (open-ended stockinette) may be used to help in the donning process by applying it around the residual limb, putting the end of the stockinette through the valve hole. As the residual limb is inserted into the socket, the stockinette is removed by pulling it through the valve hole. An alternative way of donning is to lubricate the thigh and socket with hand creams or lotion. In most

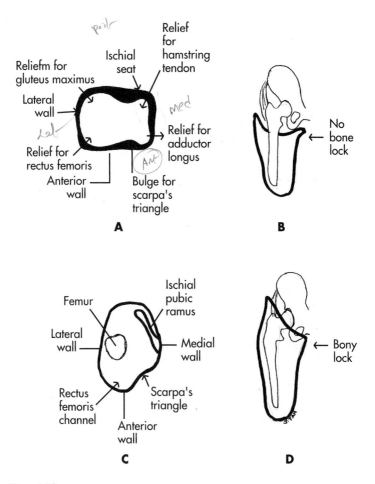

Figure 4.4-8.
Transfemoral sockets. **A, B.** Quadrilateral transfemoral socket, top and anterior view; **C, D.** Ischial containment (or narrow ML [mediolateral]) transfemoral socket, top and anterior view. The ischial containment socket has bony lock. (Adapted from: New York University Prosthetics and Orthotics Staff: *Lower limb prosthetics.* New York, 1993, Prosthetic-Orthotic Publications, p. 140; Sabolich J: Contoured adducted trochanter-controlled alignment method. *Clin Prosthet Orthot* 9:13, 17, 1985; Pritham CH: Biomechanics and shape of the above-knee socket considered in light of the ischial containment concept. *Prosthet Orthot Int* 14:14-15, 1990.)

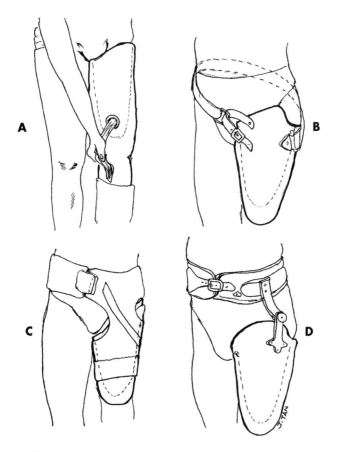

Figure 4.4-9.
Transfemoral suspension. **A,** Suction suspension. **B,** Silesian belt. **C,** Total elastic suspension (TES) belt. **D,** Pelvic band and belt suspension with metal hip joint.

cases, the total suction suspension eliminates the need for wearing any belt around the torso (a silesian belt may be used in a very active individual), thus providing greater control of the prosthesis (particularly in rotation and abduction); increased use of the remaining musculatures; and better cosmesis. It also decreases piston action between limb and socket and is more comfortable. It is indicated in young, active amputees with well-shaped, fairly strong residual limb. It is unsuitable for the elderly amputee due to the relative difficulty of donning, and it is unsuitable if the residual limb fluctuates in volume.

2) **Partial suction suspension** refers to a socket with a suction valve, but one that is worn with socks, which can be added or removed to accommodate limb volume fluctuations. The use of socks reduces the intimate airtight fit, hence an auxiliary suspension (usually a silesian belt or occasionally a rigid plastic or metal and leather pelvic band) is

necessary to prevent the prosthesis from dropping off the limb during swing phase. It is used by amputees who cannot tolerate total suction suspension because of difficulty in donning the prosthesis, are unable to tolerate the prosthesis without a sock, or have residual limbs that fluctuate in volume.

b. **Nonsuction or belt suspension** is provided by a socket that has no suction valve, (it may have a distal hole that is plugged in case it needs to be converted to suction type), hence one of the following pelvic belts is needed.

1) Soft belts

a) Silesian belt or bandage (see Fig. 4.4-9.B) are made of leather, cotton webbing, or Dacron materials. It is attached to the socket in the area of the greater trochanter and passes as a belt around the back and opposite iliac crest, where it achieves most of its suspension. It then attaches anteriorly to the socket at either one or two points. It is simple to use, comfortable, and washable.

b) Total elastic suspension (TES) belt (see Fig. 4.4-9.C) are made of elastic neoprene materials and fits around the proximal 8 inches of the prosthesis and then around the waist and fastens anteriorly with Velcro. It enhances rotational control of the prosthesis and is quite comfortable; however, it retains body heat and has limited durability.

2) Pelvic band and belt suspension (see Fig. 4.4-9.D) made of rigid metal or semirigid plastic with leather or fabric strap is connected to a metal hip joint at the lateral superior aspect of the socket. It is indicated for amputees who need rotational and mediolateral pelvic stability; obese amputees or those with significant redundant tissue that is difficult to stabilize; amputees with weak abductors or with short, weak, or poorly shaped amputation limbs. It is heavy and bulky, and tends to interfere with sitting comfort. The hip joint can be noisy, tear clothing, have maintenance problems, and contribute to excessive piston action of the thigh in the socket. The leather belt may absorb perspiration and cause skin problems.

E. Disarticulation prostheses

1. **Knee disarticulation prosthesis** is not commonly used in the United States because knee disarticulation accounts for only 1 to 2% of all lower-limb amputations. Prosthetic feet are similar to those described for transtibial prosthesis. The socket design is traditionally leather with a laced or buckled anterior opening to facilitate donning if the limb is bulbous. More modern sockets are made of molded polyester laminates with a window to accommodate donning of bulbous residual limb. If the limb is not bulbous, it can fit readily into a nonfenestrated socket with plastic liner or compressible build-ups, or a removable insert may be used. The shape of the socket is usually quadrilateral to minimize rotation. Ordinarily, the knee disarticulation prosthesis requires no special provision for suspension other than snug fitting of the socket around the bulbous, irregular contour of the distal residual limb. If the residual limb can tolerate full end bearing through the femoral shaft, the socket does not have to extend to the ischium. To control shank motion during swing phase, older style prostheses use either sidebars with single-axis knee joints and an extension aid or a conventional knee unit distal to the socket. New designs use compact fluid friction (hydraulic or pneumatic) units housed in the hollow shank so it doesn't protrude when the patient sits. A polycentric four-bar linkage axis may be used to provide knee stability. The polycentric hinges enable the shank to move behind the thigh section slightly to improve sitting appearance.

2. **Hip disarticulation and hemipelvectomy prostheses** use the "Canadian" design to achieve stance phase stability while allowing flexion at the hip and knee during swing phase. It is made of a molded plastic socket, which encloses the ischial tuberosity for weight bearing, extends over the iliac crest to provide suspension during swing phase, and encases the contralateral pelvis to provide mediolateral trunk stability. The socket is attached to a mechanical hip joint, which is a hinge placed on the anterodistal aspect of the socket so that simple downward weight bearing stabilizes the joints against buckling. A posterior hip bumper is used to resist hyperextension. Any type of knee, shank, and foot may be used. The hip joint and the knee unit may each have an extension aid. An endoskeletal shank and thigh are customarily used to save weight.

II. **Upper-limb prostheses** are used either as cosmetic replacement (if it includes a prosthetic hand), or as a functional assistive device, or both depending ultimately on the realistic goals of the amputee. For cosmetic purposes, the prosthetic hand should ideally imitate the color, size, and contour of the anatomic hand during activities and at rest. For functional purposes, a hook may be used instead of a hand. For both cosmetic and functional purposes, a mechanized hand with acceptable grasp force may be used. Because prostheses do not provide sensory feedback, many unilateral upper-limb amputees learn to do all their activities of daily living (ADLs) with their good hand and choose to function without any prostheses at all. As with lower-limb prostheses, the upper-limb prostheses should be lightweight, durable, easy to don and doff, comfortable when worn, capable of performing the prescribed function, and capable of providing total contact socket. Upper-limb prostheses should only be prescribed for patients who are motivated and have realistic expectations as to what the devices can do. The skin should be unblemished 10 minutes after prosthesis removal.

Functional upper-limb prostheses may be body-controlled with body power (using cables and harness), myoelectrically controlled with electric power, or a combination of the two (hybrid, e.g., body control with electric power). Body-powered devices use proximal muscles to move the prosthesis through cables and harnesses. Myoelectric-operated devices are controlled by electromyographic signals from intact proximal muscles. Because the majority of acquired upper-limb amputations are caused by traumatic work injuries, most of these active amputees are initially fitted with a body-powered prosthesis to accomplish manual work and outdoor activities. After their residual limb has matured, a myoelectric-controlled elbow or hand may be considered for unilateral, proximal arm amputees with white collar jobs. For the bilateral upper-limb amputee, a myoelectric-controlled elbow with hooks are usually used. However, a body-powered prosthesis should also be available for backup in case of electrical component malfunction in bilateral upper-limb amputees.

Components for above-elbow (see Fig. 4.4-10) and shoulder disarticulation prostheses include a terminal device (hand or hook), a wrist unit, mechanical elbow unit, socket, suspension, upper arm cuff or pad, and harness and control elements. A below-elbow prosthesis has basically the same components as an above-elbow prosthesis, except that instead of a mechanical elbow unit, it may have an elbow hinge. A wrist disarticulation prosthesis does not have any elbow components at all.

A. **Partial hand prosthesis** is prescribed to restore a more normal appearance, protect

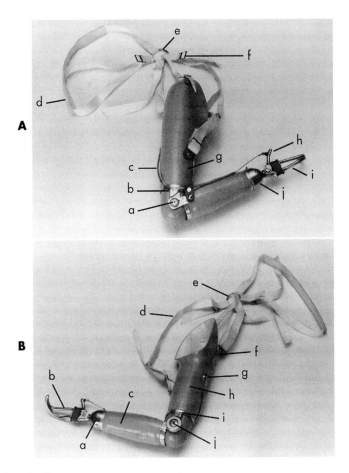

Figure 4.4-10.
Transhumeral (above-elbow) prostheses. **A,** Lateral side of transhumeral prosthesis:
a, Elbow unit; b, Turntable; c, Control cable; d, Adjustable axilla loop; e, Harness
ring; f, Figure-of-eight harness; g, Elbow lock cable; h, Terminal device (TD)
thumb; i, Hook TD; j, Wrist flexion unit. **B,** Medial side of transhumeral prosthesis:
a, Wrist unit; b, Hook TD; c, Forearm; d, Harness; e, Harness ring; f, Control cable;
g, Baseplate and retainer; h, Socket; i, Turntable; j, Spring-loading device. (From
Rock LM, Atkins DJ: Upper extremity amputations and prosthetics. In Pedretti
LW, editor: *Occupational therapy practice skills for physical dysfunction,* ed 4,
St. Louis, 1996, Mosby–Year Book, p. 573, with permission.)

hypersensitive or fragile areas (e.g., neuroma and grafted skin), and to improve grasp (prehension). A cosmetic hand or finger also serves an important functional role by providing opposition to a remaining mobile finger or by lengthening a residual finger that is too short. Partial prostheses used to restore grasp can have static or dynamic configurations. Static devices are nonarticulated and are constructed to perform specific task under rugged conditions of factory work or manual labor (e.g., handling shovels or rakes). Dynamic devices are articulated and powered by residual motions at the wrist or palm to enhance grasp.

B. **Transradial (below-elbow) prosthesis and wrist disarticulation prosthesis**
  1. **Terminal devices (TDs) or hand substitutes** are used in all upper-limb prostheses for amputation at the wrist level and above (see levels of upper-limb amputation in Fig. 4.4-1).
     a. **Passive TDs** have no functional mechanism and do not provide grasps. Whether prefabricated or custom-made, they should be relatively lightweight.
        1) **Passive hand** is intended for cosmetic effect only. It can be covered by a cosmetic glove, which can be custom made or, more often, selected from models manufactured in a wide range of skin tones.
        2) **Flexible passive TDs** are mitt-shaped TDs used to absorb shock and store and release energy during ball sports and other activities. It is manufactured by Therapeutic Recreations Systems (Super Sport series).
     b. **Active TDs** are used to replace the grasp (prehension) function of the hand. The active TD, however, is unable to manipulate objects because of the absence of sensory feedback and absence of individual control of individual fingers of the prosthetic hand. In a unilateral amputee, the active TD is used as a helper and is not usually required for intricate movements, which can be done with the good hand. The TDs that voluntarily open are more commonly used than the voluntary closing TDs.
        1) **Hooks** consist of two fingers made of aluminum lined with synthetic rubber (e.g., neoprene) or of steel, in split-hook design that is either canted or lyre-shaped. It provides lateral prehension and is slender enough to be used in restricted areas. It is superior for grasping small objects because it does not obstruct the amputee's visual feedback as much as do the bulkier insensate fingers of the prosthetic hand. It is lighter in weight, more durable, has lower cost, and is easier to maintain than a hand TD. Manufacturers of hooks include Dorrance, Army Prosthetic Research Laboratory (APRL), and Sierra. Newer, more functional designs include the Grip TD and the Adept TD (both by Therapeutic Recreation Systems), the Utah TD (by University of Utah, and the CAPP (Child Amputee Prosthetics Program) TD.
           a) **Voluntary-opening (VO) hook** is a curved and split hook in which sturdy rubber bands maintain the closed position. The pinch force is determined by the number and type of rubber bands (each rubber band provides about one pound of pinch force). The amputee uses cable-control powered by proximal muscles to open the hook fingers against the force of the rubber band. The rubber band then acts as a spring to close the hook. In myoelectrically controlled hook, the electric motor turns in opposite direction to close the hook.
           b) **Voluntary-closing (VC) hook** is maintained in an open position and

has to be closed voluntarily by cable-control or myoelectric control. It is seldom used because it is heavier and less durable than the VO hooks. Most models have a lock to keep it closed (for cosmetic reasons) when not in use. Some models (e.g., Sierra VC hook) has a self-locking feature that automatically locks the hook in the grasp position as soon as the amputee relaxes, enabling the patient to hold on to an object without exerting continued force. This makes it suitable for fine work. However, it has durability and maintenance problems.

2) **Hands** provide palmar prehension by allowing the amputee to move the thumb, index, and middle finger through body power (using cable) or myoelectric control with electric power. The ring and little fingers remain passive. Compared to hooks, hands are more cosmetic and can be used for grasping a large or round object or just the handle of a tool. However, they are bulkier and heavier than the hooks. The myoelectrically controlled hand initiates palmar tip grasp by contraction of residual forearm flexor musculatures and releases the hand by contraction of residual forearm extensor musculatures. Hence, it is preferred by many patients because it does not require any external harness as in cable-controlled hands. Manufacturers of VO hands are Dorrance, Sierra, Otto Bock, and Becker and Robins Aid.

   a) **Voluntary-opening hand** operates on the same principle as the VO hooks, i.e., springs in the hand close the fingers and produce modest grasp force.

   b) **Voluntary-closing hand** provides control of prehension with automatic locking in various grasp positions.

3) **Nonhand, nonhook (Stanford) design** that can either be voluntarily opened or voluntarily closed and with improved aesthetics are being developed.

2. **Wrist units** are metal devices used for attaching TDs (hooks or hands) to anatomic wrist area at the distal end of the socket. They position the TD into the best position for accomplishing a desired activity and also permit interchange of TD from hook to a hand and vice versa. Wrist units can be positioned passively (by using the sound hand or by pushing the TD against any part of the body or any surface) or by electric-power (e.g., Otto Bock Electric Wrist Rotator, Sierra Wrist Flexion Unit, Hosmer Flexion-Friction Wrist, and United States Manufacturing Company [USMC] E-Z Flex Wrist).

   a. **Wrist friction (rotation) units** hold the TD in the desired pronation or supination position by means of friction resistance provided by a rubber washer or a bushing.

   b. **Quick disconnect/locking wrist units** allow the amputee to quickly interchange TDs. They are useful in amputees who use more than one TD or are routinely performing activities that require the elimination of any unwanted wrist rotation during functional performance. Some models have a locking feature that prevents inadvertent rotation of the TD in the wrist unit when a heavy object is grasped. The lock, however, complicates prosthetic use, because the amputee must lock and unlock whenever repositioning the TD.

   c. **Wrist flexion units** allow the TD to flex and are used on the dominant side (i.e., the side of the longer residual limb regardless of previous dominance) of the bilateral upper-limb amputees for activities close to the midline of the body (e.g., for buttoning and shaving). The hook on the nondominant side is used to position the unit in 0, 25, or 50 degrees of wrist flexion. Wrist flexion units are not useful for unilateral amputees because they generally prefer to use their good hand.

3. **Socket designs** for transradial amputation and wrist disarticulation are determined by the type of suspension desired and the length of the residual limb. All transradial and wrist disarticulation socket designs have "double wall" construction with the inner wall (the socket per se) providing a snug, total-contact fit, including the distal end of the residual limb. The outer wall is shaped and sized to match the contours and length of the contralateral forearm. The socket extends proximoposteriorly to the olecranon and proximoanteriorly to the elbow crease. The shorter the residual limb is, the closer is the trimline to the crease. For wrist disarticulation or for long transradial residual limb (see Fig. 4.4-1 for levels of upper-limb amputation), the volar and dorsal walls of the inner socket are compressed distally so as to capture and transmit as much pronation and supination as possible (see Fig. 4.4-1 comparing residual rotation of amputated forearm vs. normal forearm). An alternative socket design is the ISNY flexible socket, which is made of thin translucent polyethylene with a rigid frame consisting of slender medial and lateral laminates. The thin flexible ISNY socket provides increased function, comfort, and sensory feedback.

   a. **Harness-suspended socket design** uses a harnessing system to suspend the socket from the involved and uninvolved shoulders. The harness is connected to an upper arm half-cuff or a triceps pad, which is then connected to the elbow hinge and socket. The arm half-cuff or triceps pad help provide socket suspension and stability in addition to serving as an anchor for the control cable reaction point. The **arm half-cuff** is used in short transradial fittings, while the **triceps pad** is used with long transradial, wrist disarticulation, and transmetacarpal prosthesis.

   b. **Self-suspended socket design** is less cumbersome and more popular than the harness-suspended socket design. Although harness (usually figure-of-nine harness) is seldom used for suspension, it may still be used for control of TD.

      1) **Suprastyloid suspension** uses silicone bladder, or window/door suspension with elasticized closure, or soft removable inserts that grip the styloids. It is indicated for wrist disarticulation amputations with prominent styloids.

      2) **Sleeve suspension** either uses latex rubber to provide atmospheric pressure suspension, elastic sleeves to provide a skin traction suspension, or neoprene to provides a combination of atmospheric pressure and skin traction suspension.

      3) **Supracondylar brim suspension** retains the prosthesis by enclosing and capturing the humeral epicondyles and the posterior olecranon. It does not allow forearm rotation and sacrifices range of motion for power and stability (i.e., the lesser the ROM allowed, the greater power it has).

         a) **Munster supracondylar socket** is used for short transradial amputation.

         b) **Northwestern University socket** is used for midlength transradial amputation.

         c) **Modified supracondylar brim with olecranon cutout** is used for long transradial amputations.

Table 4.4-2. **Recommended elbow hinges for wrist disarticulation and transradial amputations**

UPPER LIMB AMPUTATIONS	RECOMMENDED ELBOW HINGES
Wrist disarticulation	Flexible elbow hinge
Long transradial (55-90%)	Flexible elbow hinge
Short transradial (35-55%)	Single-axis rigid elbow hinge May use flexible elbow hinge for longer residual limb
Very short transradial (<35%); or if elbow range-of-motion is limited	Polycentric rigid-elbow hinge; or split socket with step-up and locking rigid-elbow hinge

      d) Floating brim suspension is used for long transradial and wrist disarticulation amputations.

    c. Split socket is a special design that consists of a total-contact segment encasing the residual limb and connected by hinges to a separate forearm shell to which the wrist unit and TD are attached. Split socket is used for very short residual limbs so that special elbow hinges (e.g., step up elbow hinge and locking elbow hinge) can be used.

4. Elbow hinges connect the socket to a cuff or a pad on the upper arm and are important for suspension and stability. Their selection depends primarily on the site of amputation and the residual function (see Table 4.4-2).

  a. Flexible elbow hinge (see Fig. 4.4-11.A) can be made out of triple-thickness Dacron webbing or flexible metal cable and is used primarily to suspend the forearm socket. It is used where sufficient voluntary pronation and supination (as well as elbow flexion and extension) are available, i.e., in wrist disarticulation and long transradial amputation.

  b. Rigid elbow hinge is used for short transradial amputation where normal elbow flexion is present but little or no voluntary pronation-supination is available and additional stability about the elbow is needed.

    1) Single-axis rigid elbow hinge (see Fig. 4.4-11.B) is used to provide stability when socket rotation around the very short transradial residual limb becomes a problem.

    2) Polycentric rigid elbow hinge (see Fig. 4.4-11.C) uses a gear that has mating teeth to impart a displacing action to the socket during elbow flexion and provide clearance for bunching of flesh in the crook of the elbow of amputees with fleshy arms.

    3) Step-up elbow hinge (see Fig. 4.4-11.D) uses a gear or double-pivot arrangement that permits the residual limb to drive the prosthetic forearm through an increased ROM. It is connected to a socket with split-socket design and is indicated in amputees with very short transradial residual limb.

      a) Gear-type step-up elbow hinge has step-up ratio of 2 : 1, i.e., the forearm shell of the split socket flexes 2 degrees for every 1 degree of residual limb flexion. Although the ROM is doubled, the energy cost is also doubled also, hence cutting the strength in half.

      b) Double-pivot type step-up elbow hinge has an averages of 3 : 2 step-up ratio.

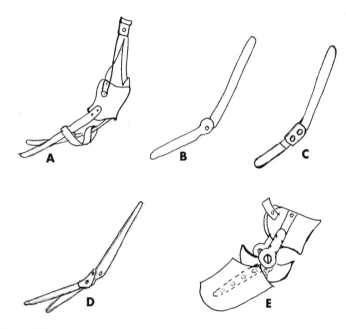

Figure 4.4-11.
Elbow hinges for transradial prostheses. **A.** Flexible elbow hinge; **B.** Rigid elbow hinge, single axis; **C.** Rigid elbow hinge; polycentric; **D.** Step–up elbow hinge; **E.** Residual–limb activated locking elbow hinge.

    c. Residual limb-activated locking elbow hinge (see Fig. 4.4-11.E), together with a split socket (see II.B.3.c) prosthesis and a dual control system, is used for amputees with very short transradial residual limbs and very limited ROM or lifting force. The cable that operates the TD is used to lift the forearm to the desired position whereupon the elbow is locked by a small amount of residual limb motion. Once the elbow is locked, the cable can then be used to operate the TD.

5. Harness suspension and control systems for transradial and wrist disarticulation prostheses are used to suspend the prosthesis from the shoulders so the socket is held firmly onto the residual limb and transmit force from shoulder and scapular motion via a cable system to operate the TD. The harness is usually unnecessary with passive and myoelectrically controlled prostheses with self-suspended socket.

    a. Figure-of-eight harness (see Fig. 4.4-10.A) is the most commonly used harness in prosthesis with harness-suspended socket. It has an axilla loop worn on the sound side, which acts as a reaction point for the transmission of the body force to the TD. The upper strap of the axillary loop runs diagonally across and down the back towards the posterior part of the prosthesis; while the lower strap runs diagonally across and up the back and over to the anterior shoulder of the amputated limb where it connects to the prosthesis via an inverted Y-suspensor strap. This front support strap carries most of the axial loads. The crossing point of the two diagonal straps on the back (which can be connected by an O-shaped metal ring) should be below C7 and slightly to the sound side.

b. Cross chest-strap harness with shoulder saddle consists of a shoulder saddle on the side of the amputated limb, which is connected to a chest strap looped around the opposite axilla. The shoulder saddle is connected to a loop suspensor, which is then connected to the socket through an arm half-cuff or triceps pad. It is used in amputees who cannot tolerate axillary pressure from an axilla loop or in amputees who do a great deal of heavy lifting. This hardness tends to rotate upon the chest when excessive forces are applied to the control cable.

c. Figure-of-nine harness consists of an axillary loop on the sound side with a diagonal strap that runs across and down the back and attaches to a control strap on the prosthetic limb. It is lighter and provides greater freedom and comfort by the elimination of usual front support strap, triceps pad or cuff, etc. It is used in self-suspended transradial socket that requires a harness only for controlling the TD.

6. TD control system for transradial prostheses can either be body-powered or electric-powered. Body-powered units have moderate costs, are moderately lightweight, are most durable, and provide the highest sensory feedback. However, they require the most body movement and the most harnessing to operate, and they are the least cosmetically pleasing. On the other hand, electric-powered units require the least body movement with moderate or no harnessing to operate and provide more function at proximal levels and moderate cosmesis. However, they are heavy, expensive, delicate, hard to maintain, and have limited sensory feedback.

a. Body-powered (cable-activated) TDs uses forces from the shoulder and scapula transmitted via harnesses and cables to operate the TD. The cable system used is the **single-control (Bowden control) cable system,** which consists of a single continuous flexible stranded stainless steel cable, which can slide inside a flexible tube or housing. This housing has terminal fittings that connect one end of the cable to a harnessed body-control point and the other end to a point of operation of the TD. When the amputee flexes the ipsilateral shoulder (or abducts the scapulae for functions close to the body midline), the motion tenses the cable attached proximally to the harness and distally to the TD. The length of the control cable is maintained constant by the cable housing, thus the same amount of body motion is required to operate a TD regardless of elbow joint angle.

b. Electric-powered TDs are controlled by switches or myoelectric signals and are powered with energy supplied from external batteries (e.g., rechargeable nickel cadmium batteries, which can be mounted on or within the prosthesis). The electric-powered TD can be handlike (Otto Bock System Electric Hands and Steeper Electric Hand) or nonhandlike in appearance (Otto Bock System Electric Greifer, Hosmer NU-VA Synergistic Prehensor, and Steeper Powered Gripper).

1) Myoelectric-controlled TD uses surface electrodes placed on the muscles of the residual limb. Myoelectric signals from the muscles are picked up by the surface electrodes, amplified into volts to activate an electric switch (myoswitch), and cause electricity to flow from a battery to an electric motor, thus activating the TD. The TD function (i.e., speed and force) can be controlled either in a constant manner or in proportion to the amplitude of the myoelectric signals (i.e., strength of muscle contraction).

    a) Two-site, two-function myoelectric controller uses two sites for attachment of the electrodes (e.g., the wrist extensors and wrist flexors of the residual limb) to open and close the TD. It is used in Otto Bock Myoelectric Hand, Steeper Electric Hand, Otto Bock System Electric Greifer, Hosmer NU-VA Synergistic Prehensor, and Steeper Powered Gripper.

    b) One-site, two-function myoelectric controller ("double channel") uses myoelectric signal from one muscle to control both opening and closing of the TD, depending on the amplitude with respect to one of two thresholds (e.g., weak contraction closes the TD and strong contraction opens the TD). It is used in Otto Bock Myoelectric Hand, Steeper Electric Hand, Otto Bock System Electric Greifer, Steeper Powered Gripper, and University of New Brunswick controller.

    c) One-site, one-function myoelectric controller are used if the amputee does not have two good myoelectric sites or in very young limb-deficient children. It is used in Cookie Crusher Hand and Steeper Powered Gripper. The NYU-Hosmer Prehension Actuator uses a single-site, single-function myoswitch to open a cable-actuated VO split hook.

  2) Microswitch controlled TD uses either a push-button electromechanical switch, which can be activated by a bony prominence, or a pull-switch, which is incorporated in a harness or cable. It is used in the Otto Bock System Electric Hands and Otto Bock System Electric Greifer.

C. Transhumeral (above-elbow) prosthesis and elbow disarticulation prosthesis (see Fig. 4.4-10) uses the same TD and wrist units described under transradial (or below-elbow) prostheses. However, the socket, harness, and control systems differ from those used in transradial prostheses. In addition, transhumeral prostheses require an elbow unit. Most upper-limb prostheses are exoskeleton. When active function is not a significant goal, however, an endoskeletal prostheses may be used to improve cosmesis and conserve weight. The endoskeletal prosthesis consists of a TD, a wrist module, and a lightweight forearm and humeral pylon covered with a cosmetic foam interconnected by a manually controlled, ratchet locking elbow unit. The following components are for active and functional transhumeral and elbow disarticulation prostheses.

  1. Sockets for transhumeral and wrist disarticulation prostheses have similar double construction as the transradial sockets. The lateral socket wall extends up to the acromion (or higher in case of unusually short transhumeral residual limbs), while the medial socket wall is flattened below the axilla to help prevent inadvertent socket rotation. Elbow disarticulation prostheses have sockets that are flat and broad distally to conform to the anatomic configuration of the epicondyles of the distal humerus and provide the amputee with active control of humeral rotation. An alternative socket design is the ISNY flexible socket (see section I.C.3).

  2. Elbow units consist of hinge and cable systems, which can be locked to position and maintain the prosthesis in various elbow-flexion angles. Most have an alternator lock, in which one pull of the cable locks the hinge and the next pull unlocks it. The pulling movement used to lock or unlock the unit is usually a combination of shoulder depression, extension, and abduction. The amputee unlocks the elbow unit and selects the desired angle of flexion by exerting tension on the elbow flexion cable. The elbow unit is then locked so that the same cable can be used to activate the TD. Most elbow units also provide passive humeral rotation to enable the TD to be positioned for a desired function. This is accomplished by means of a turntable between the elbow unit and the upper arm shell or socket. As with wrist units, friction between the elbow unit and the turntable allows control of the rotation to maintain the desired plane of elbow operation.

a. Elbow flexion-locking system

1) External flexion-locking elbow is used with the elbow-disarticulation prosthesis because there is not enough space for the internal locking mechanism.

2) Internal flexion-locking elbow is used for transhumeral and shoulder prostheses. An internal spring-assist for elbow flexion may be used by amputees who have difficulty flexing their prosthetic forearms.

b. Elbow and TD control system (see section II.B.6 for the advantages and disadvantages of body-powered vs. electric-powered control systems)

1) Body-powered (cable-activated) elbow units transmit forces from the shoulder and scapula via harnesses and cables to lock and unlock the elbow, flex the elbow, and operate the TD. The cable control used consists of two separate cable systems. The first cable system (single-control cable) is used to lock and unlock the elbow, while the second cable system uses a **dual-control** (or **fair-lead control) cable,** which consists of one cable with two functions (i.e., to flex the elbow unit when the elbow is unlocked and to operate the TD when the elbow is locked). The usual sequence of cable-control is as follows: the unlocked elbow is flexed to the desired position using the dual-control (fair-lead) cable; then the first single-control cable system is used to lock the elbow (by any two combinations of the following shoulder motions: extension, abduction, and depression; usually shoulder extension and abduction are used). When the elbow is locked, the TD can be activated via the dual-control cable system by either shoulder flexion or scapular abduction or chest expansion. When the desired TD function is accomplished, the elbow can be extended by unlocking it using the single-control cable (the same shoulder movement combination for locking the elbow unit is used to unlock the elbow).

2) Electric powered elbow units are powered from a battery and controlled by myoelectric signals or microswitches.

a) Myoelectric-controlled elbow units uses amplified myoelectric signals picked up from surface electrodes placed on the residual arm. Example are the Utah Elbow and the Utah Arm, which use the biceps and the triceps for two-site, two-function, proportional control of the elbow.

b) Microswitch controlled elbow units uses push buttons for activation by a bony prominence or a pull switch, which is incorporated in a harness. It is used in Boston (Liberty Mutual) Elbow and NY-Hosmer Electric Elbow.

3) Hybrid control system combines electric- and body- (cable-) control system. The hybrid control/power approach has reasonable proprioceptive qualities and allows simultaneous coordinated control of elbow and prehensor function.

a) Hybrid cable-controlled elbow with myoelectric TD is used for long transhumeral or elbow disarticulation prostheses. Although it has increased TD pinch, the electric TD adds weight to the forearm making it harder to lift.

b) Hybrid electric elbow with cable-controlled TD uses the Boston (or Liberty Mutual) Elbow in conjunction with a cable-control (body-actuated) TD. The cable-controlled TD requires less maintenance but has lower pinch and is uncosmetic.

c) Hybrid cable-controlled elbow with motorized locks is used in the Steeper Electric Elbow Lock, but myoelectric or microswitches are used to lock the cable-actuated elbow.

3. **Transhumeral harness and control** suspends the prosthesis from the shoulders and transmit power from the shoulder to flex the prosthetic elbow, to lock and unlock the elbow unit and to operate the TD. It uses modifications of the basic figure-of-eight harness or a shoulder saddle with chest strap patterns similar to the ones used for the transradial prostheses.

D. **Shoulder disarticulation prostheses and forequarter prostheses** have similar prosthetic TD and elbow units as the transhumeral prostheses. However, their socket and harness/control systems differ from the transhumeral prostheses. In addition, they have a shoulder unit. Although functional shoulder disarticulation and forequarter prostheses are available, most amputees prefer a cosmetic shoulder cap or an endoskeletal prostheses, which can be passively positioned by the opposite hand. This is due to the lack of proximal muscles for cable operation on the involved side and the complexity of actions required for the shoulder prostheses to be functional.

1. **Sockets** for shoulder disarticulation and forequarter prostheses extend onto the thorax to suspend and stabilize the prosthesis. They are also suspended by chest straps attached anteriorly and posteriorly to the socket.

a. **Enclosed socket** are made of plastic laminate to encircle the shoulder and are formed to its contours.

b. **Frame socket** uses padded metal strips (or stiff, carbon-reinforced laminates) to form a frame that encompasses the shoulder and the trunk, extending down to the fifth rib. It provides structural mounting points for the prostheses and location and reference points for a variety of controls.

2. **Shoulder unit**

a. **Motionless shoulder unit** consists of a monolithic construction in which the humeral section and shoulder socket are laminated together, and no motion between these components is possible.

b. **Friction-controlled passive-motion shoulder unit** allows passive positioning of the shoulder joint in flexion-extension and abduction-adduction. Passive abduction of the humeral section is convenient for dressing and for sitting in a chair with arms. Abduction-flexion joint allows abduction and flexion, while the universal shoulder joint can be used to permit motion in all the planes.

3. **Harness suspension and control system** for shoulder prosthesis has a chest strap that is attached to the anterior and posterior aspects of the laminated shoulder section. An elastic suspensor strap helps to stabilize the shoulder section and permits movement of the shoulder girdle. The harness and control assembly usually includes a waist band with a strap connected to the elbow lock control cable. The waist band stabilizes the distal end of the elbow lock control strap so that shoulder elevation can work the elbow lock.

4. **Control system** for shoulder prostheses commonly uses shoulder girdle flex-

ion (i.e., biscapular abduction) for elbow flexion and TD operation and shoulder elevation for elbow locking and unlocking. Other control mechanism for operation of elbow lock includes pulling with the good hand or by using a ''chin-nudge'' button.

a. Cable-control (body-powered) system

1) Dual-control (or fair-lead control) cable system similar to the one used in transhumeral prosthesis is traditionally used for body-powered control of the elbow unit and TD in shoulder prostheses.

2) Triple-cable system is a newer alternative in cable control for shoulder prostheses. It uses three cables, each providing a distinct function. One cable, attached to the forearm shell and an axilla loop, provides active elbow flexion when the contralateral shoulder is flexed. A second cable, attached to the chest strap and the TD, provides TD opening with chest expansion. The third cable, attached to the elbow lock and a nudge control, locks and unlocks the elbow when the nudge control is depressed by the chin or contralateral hand.

b. Electric powered control systems are usually used because it is difficult to provide body-powered control motion of sufficient strength.

BIBLIOGRAPHY

Bowker JH, Michael JW, editors: *Atlas of limb prosthetics: surgical, prosthetic, and rehabilitation principles—American Academy of Orthopedic Surgeons,* ed 2, St Louis, 1992, Mosby–Year Book.

Faculty of Prosthetics and Orthotics, New York University School of Medicine and Post-Graduate Medical School. *Upper–limb prosthetics*, New York, 1986, Prosthetic-Orthotic Publications.

Leonard Jr., JA, Meier III, RH: Upper and lower extremity prosthetics. In DeLisa JA, Gans, BM, editors: *Rehabilitation medicine: principles and practice*, ed 2, Philadelphia, 1993, JB Lippincott, pp. 507-525.

Wilson, Jr., AB: *Limb prosthetics*, ed 6, New York, 1989, Demos.

Chapter 4.5

ADAPTATIONS FOR ACTIVITIES OF DAILY LIVING

Functional independence in the performance of activities of daily living (ADL) can enhance the positive self-image and quality of life of the disabled person. Its attainment can be limited by various conditions that cause limitations in range of motion (ROM), strength, endurance, coordination, dexterity, balance, sensation, vision, cognition, and perception. The detailed evaluation of these functional limitations (see Chapter 2.8 for functional scales) as well as their specific ADL adaptations are typically done by an occupational therapist (except in certain aspects of ADL, e.g., transfers and functional ambulation, in which the physical therapists are primarily involved) with input from other members of the interdisciplinary rehabilitation team.

The goals for ADL adaptation are generally to improve living space, minimize costs of self-care independence, and decrease the time and energy required to safely perform ADLs. Any ADL adaptation must maximize the patient's function within the constraints of limited time, money, and the patient's potential for improvement. Factors to consider in the long-term selection of adaptive or assistive devices include effectiveness in improving ADL and in attaining functional independence, affordability (aside from the purchase cost, also consider the costs of maintenance or repair), operability (i.e., is it easy to use or don and doff? does it respond adequately to demands?), dependability (i.e., does it operate with predictable levels of accuracy under conditions of reasonable use?), and, ultimately, the patient's motivation or desire to use it.

This chapter includes the general and specific principles for ADL adaptation as well as specific adaptations for basic ADLs (i.e., self-care tasks) and the more advanced instrumental ADLs (i.e., tasks beyond caring for oneself that involve complex interaction with the physical and social environment, including occupational adaptations). Activities of daily living adaptations include disposable medical products, for example, medical, nursing, and urinary supplies, prosthetic devices (see Chapter 4.4), orthotic devices (see Chapter 4.3), durable medical products, such as wheelchairs (WC) (see Chapter 4.7), gait aids (see Chapter 4.6), bathing equipment, accessibility products (e.g., lifts, ramps, and hand controls), and self-care adaptive or assistive devices described in this chapter. For details on ADL adaptations, the reader is referred to any major textbook in occupational therapy (see bibliography). Selected resources for disabled persons (including major catalogs listing adaptive devices, electronic resources/bulletin boards, and organizations for the disabled) are provided in the Appendices G-3, G-4, and G-5. For a more comprehensive listing of addresses of vendors of adaptive devices, associations, and other resources for disabled persons, refer to *The complete directory for people with disabilities,* Greyhouse Publishing, Pocket Knife Square, Lakeville, CT 06039, tel. (800) 562-2139 or (860) 435-0868.

I. Principles for ADL adaptation

A. General principles for ADL adaptation

1. Modification of the task, the method of accomplishing the task, and the environment.

   2. Instruction and training on joint and energy conservation.
   3. Safe use of assistive devices (i.e., devices that gives support or aid) or adaptive devices (i.e., devices that are made fit or suitable, often by modification).
B. Specific principles for ADL adaptation
   1. Adaptations for limited ROM include using adaptations to increase reach, eliminate the need to bend over, and compensate for limited grasp; storing frequently used items within reach; and using joint protection techniques (e.g., in patients with rheumatoid arthritis). From an upright wheelchair sitting position, the vertical range of reach is from 20 to 48 inches (50.8-121.9 cm) and the maximum functional horizontal reach is considered 18 inches (45.7 cm) from the edge of a desk or work surface. In general, patients with good trunk control have greater reaching capacity.
   2. Adaptations for weakness include using lightweight objects, utensils, and tools; allowing gravity to assist; using adaptive equipment or methods to replace lost functions such as grasp; using powered tools and utensils; using biomechanical principle (e.g., improving leverage in body mechanics and increasing friction to decrease the power needed for pinch or grasp); and using of two hands. For hemiplegics, specific principles for ADL adaptations include providing substitution for the stabilizing or holding function of the involved upper limb and adapting bilateral activities so they can be done unilaterally.
   3. Adaptations for low endurance include using energy conservation methods, pacing work to prevent fatigue, using principles listed for weakness that reduce workload (e.g., lightweight utensils and powered equipment), matching activity demands to ability, avoiding stressful positions (e.g., bending over, reaching overhead, isometric contractions such as pushing, pulling, and maintained grasp), and environmental stressors (e.g., hot humid environment and overexertion). Energy conservation techniques (see also Chapter 5.12, section IV.B.7) include planning ahead and organizing work; combining tasks to eliminate extra work and eliminating unnecessary tasks; preparing and obtaining all the required equipment before starting a task; using electrical appliances to conserve personal energy; using lightweight utensils and tools; working with gravity assisting, rather than resisting; sitting down when working; and resting before fatigue sets in.
   4. Adaptations for incoordination or poor dexterity include stabilizing the object being worked on; stabilizing proximal limb segments so that control can be concentrated on the distal limb segments; adding weight to the distal segments; using heavy utensils, cooking equipment, tools, etc.; using adaptive equipment that reduces slipperiness and provide stability; and using adaptations that substitute for lack of fine motor skills.
   5. Adaptations for limited vision include organizing so everything is kept in its proper place; using Braille labels to distinguish canned goods, clothing colors, etc.; using techniques and devices that magnify words or images or provide high contrast; and using adaptive equipment that provides auditory, tactile, or kinesthetic feedback to compensate for low vision or blindness.
   6. Adaptations for decreased sensation include protecting the anesthetic part from abrasions, bruises, cuts, burns, and decubiti; substituting vision for poor awareness of limbs and limb movement or to detect texture change; and directing attention to the affected part on a regular basis (e.g., using a long-handled mirror for skin inspection or using a specialized timer that beeps every 15 minutes to remind a person to perform a pressure relief).

7. Adaptations for cognitive and perceptual deficits are discussed in Chapter 5.5, sections I.B and II.

II. Classification of ADLs and their specific adaptations

A. **Basic ADL (B-ADL)** includes mobility, self-maintenance activities (i.e., feeding, grooming, dressing, bathing, personal hygiene, toileting, menstrual care, and skin management), communication, and sexual expression. Driving, which can be considered a component of mobility, is not described here as it involves more advanced skills (see community living skills under instrumental-ADL in section II.B.2.f.2).

  1. **Positioning** in bed (e.g., when resting or sleeping) or chair (e.g., WC) is important in preventing pressure ulcers, contractures, dislocations, and other deformities. Positioning is also important as preparation for other ADLs (e.g., transfers, dressing, sexual acts, sports, work, etc.), exercises, and other interventions. Specifics on different positioning orthotics are discussed in Chapter 5.2, section VI.B.1.

    a. **Bed positioning adaptations** include hour-glass shaped foam leg spacers (e.g., for maintenance of the lower limb and spine alignment in sidelying positions), supporting wedges for the back or limbs, triangular-shaped hip abduction wedge cushions (with straps), modified pillows (e.g., pillows with recessed center or head cradles and neck rolls), blanket cradles to protect sensitive skin (e.g., healing skin grafts) from weight of the blanket, and modified mattresses and other limb positioner or supporters for the prevention of pressure ulcers (discussed in Chapter 5.2, section VI.B).

    b. **Seating positioning adaptations** include abductor wedge cushions (with or without straps), padded knee or leg spreaders (made of metal or flexible plastic), and WC seating adaptations (discussed in Chapter 4.7, section I.A.3.b).

  2. **Mobility** is the ability to move from one position in space (whether sitting, lying down, standing, etc.) to another position in space regardless of the distance between the two positions. For independent bed mobility and transfers, patients may use webbing loops (applied around legs or thighs so they can be lifted by the upper limbs).

    a. **Bed mobility** is the ability to turn over in bed (i.e., rolling side to side), to scoot up, down, or toward either edge of the bed, or to come to a sitting position at the edge of the bed. In addition to motor planning skills, the patient should have adequate head control as well as upper limb strength and endurance.

      1) **Overhead trapeze bars** can be used to assist in scooting up or down in bed and in helping the patient come to a sitting position at the edge of the bed. Trapeze bars can be attached onto the bed through an orthopedic frame or can be mounted on the wall for home use.

      2) **Loops** can be attached along the edge of the bed or bed railings to help the patient with inadequate trunk strength to use the upper limbs to pull himself or herself to either side when rolling. Ladderlike loops have rungs spaced for progressive hand or arm placement when the patient is pulling himself or herself up from supine.

      3) **Electric beds** can be used to raise or lower the head of the bed and assist the patient in coming to a sitting position.

    b. **Transfers** refer to short-distance movements from one surface to another (e.g., to and from bed and WC or commode and to and from WC and tub or car seat). If another person is needed to assist transfers, a transfer or ambulation belt (with or without handles) may be looped around the patient's waist for easy grasping by the assisting person.

1) **Stand-pivot transfer (SPT)** is indicated if weight bearing on the lower limbs is possible or permitted in patients with adequate hip and knee extension and good sitting balance. The patient rises from a seated to a standing position and pivots to the adjacent surface to sit down. This can be done independently or with the supervision or assistance of another person. Prior to SPT, a step stool may be used as an intermediate step between the bed and the floor. If the patient is unable to stand up fully, a variation called **bent-pivot transfer** may be used in which the patient is kept in a bent-knee position to maintain equal weight bearing as the assisting person provides optimal trunk and lower limb support during the pivot transfer. Adaptations to assist in **sit-to-stand transfers** include: cushions to raise up seat height, air or spring cushions that expand posteriorly as the patient leans forward thus assisting patient rise, side rails (home models are also available), and bilateral push-up frames.

2) **Sit-pivot transfer (depression transfer)** is indicated in patients who are unable to bear weight on their lower limbs but have strong upper limbs enabling them to depress their scapulae (and extend elbows) to lift their buttocks off one surface onto another surface without coming to a standing position. The patient should have good sitting balance.

3) **Swivel-trapeze transfer** is indicated in patients who are unable to bear weight on their lower limbs but whose upper limbs are strong enough to lift half of their body weight. The patient holds onto the swivel trapeze bar (attached onto the bed via an orthopedic frame or wall-mounted for home use), pulls himself or herself off the bed, then swings his body onto another surface. This may be done independently or with the assistance of another person (to swing the lower part of the body).

4) **Sliding board transfer (SBT)** is indicated in patients who are unable to bear weight on their lower limbs but whose upper limbs are not strong enough to lift their buttocks off the sitting surface. It uses a sliding board to bridge the gap between transfer site. The basic sliding board is usually made of a flat, sturdy, smooth wood or rigid plastic, which can either be short (if used for toilet transfers) or long (if used for WC to car transfers). Some modifications of the basic sliding board include slots for easy gripping; notches on one end, which can be secured to WC armrest for stability; the addition of rolling balls or sliding or rotating discs for ease of transfer; or offset designs that are shaped to fit around the wheel on the WC when the armrest is removed. Once the sliding board is positioned securely between the surfaces, the patient positions his or her buttocks on one end of the board, and, with the aid of the upper limbs (or another person), scoots across the board to the new surface. If strong enough, the patient may do a series of small shoulder depressions instead of "sliding." The patient should have good sitting balance.

5) **Lift transfer** is indicated if the patient is unable to move at all. It may be done with the assistance of one person (e.g., logroll transfer or one-person carry transfer), or more than one person (e.g., two- or

three-person carry transfer). It may also be done by using a sling-style lift with a mechanical jack (e.g., Hoyer lift or Trans-Aid lift) or hydraulic lift.

6) **Floor transfer (e.g., WC-to-floor or floor-to-WC)** is indicated for WC users with sufficient upper limb strength for transferring to and from the WC and the floor (e.g., for floor mat exercises or in case of a fall). This may be accomplished independently or with the assistance of another person. If necessary, a small bench may be used as an intermediate step between the wheelchair seat and the floor.

c. **Wheelchair mobility** is used for attaining functional independence in the community for patients who can not ambulate or can ambulate only for short distances. Proper positioning in the WC, good sitting tolerance, strength, endurance, and cognitive skills are necessary for efficient and safe WC mobility. Wheelchair and seating prescriptions are described in Chapter 4.7.

d. **Functional ambulation** refers to walking with an aid (e.g., walker) to accomplish a task (e.g., putting clothes into the closet). It is described in Chapter 4.6.

3. **Self-maintenance tasks** include feeding, dressing, grooming and personal hygiene, bathing, and toileting. The following sections list the adaptations commonly prescribed for patients with limited ROM, weakness, incoordination, poor dexterity, and/or low endurance. Most patients need lightweight utensils or devices, except patients with incoordination who need weighted or heavy equipment to maintain steadiness. Plastic or unbreakable materials are preferred. Specifications for environmental adaptations related to self-maintenance tasks (i.e., barrier-free architectural designs of bathroom, toilet, sinks, countertops, closets, etc.) are described in section II.B.1.

a. **Feeding** requires adequate upper limb ROM, coordination, and strength to scoop and bring the hand to the mouth from a surface while grasping a utensil or cup. It also requires the ability to manipulate utensils and to cut food, as well as the ability to suck, to close the lips around the utensil, to manipulate the bolus with the tongue, and to chew and swallow the food (for dysphagia care, see Chapter 5.6)

1) **Spoon and fork adaptations** include modified handles to improve grip (e.g., built-up handles with foam; plastic-molded, nylon-coated, or polypropylene handles; flexible or adjustable handles; swivel handles; curved handles; long extension handles; handles with palmar cuffs; handles that fit easily onto utensil holders), spoon-fork combinations or sporks (e.g., regular, offset, or swivel type) for patients with limited wrist supination and radial deviation, weighted utensils for patients with incoordination, spatula spoons with flat shallow bowls for soft foods, and holders that grip sandwiches (which can be inserted onto a utensil holder).

2) **Knife adaptations** include modified knives (e.g., rocker knife, which cuts food by rocking down on food, rather than the traditional sliding method, which requires stabilization of the food with a fork in the opposite hand, or roller knife or pizza-cutter knife for one-handed use); knife and fork combinations (e.g., rocker knife with fork edges or fork with cutting edge on the side prong); modified knife handles to improve grip (e.g., nonslip handles, wooden handles, or cuff-handle); and serrated knife to facilitate cutting.

3) **Dish adaptations** include scoop dishes, which are deep bowl-like dishes

that prevent food slippage (e.g., round or oval scoop dish, high-sided scoop dish, scooper bowl, scoop plate, plate with inside edge, divided or partitioned scoop dish or scoop plate, scoop dish with lid and bowl, and scoop dish with suction cups or nonskid mat) and food guards, which are C-shaped plastic or stainless steel attachments that can be clipped onto a shallow plate to prevent food slippage.

4) Drinking utensil adaptations include lid adaptations for oral weakness (e.g., lids with snorkel or spout or nipple-shaped lids); drinking utensils with a cutout for the nose so a person can drink without neck extension; drinking utensils adapted to assist grasp (e.g., T-shaped handles, bilateral handles, or foam insulation); weighted drinking utensils (for uncoordinated patients); drinking utensil holders, which can be clipped onto the WC; base extensions to prevent tipping of drinking utensils (e.g., when drinking with straws); straws (one-way straws, long straws, reusable straws, or disposable straws); and straw holders.

5) Self-feeders include electric self-feeders with elevated setups for plate and spoon (which can be activated by slight head movement) for bilateral upper limb weakness, balanced forearm orthoses (also called mobile arm supports, ball bearing feeder or linkage feeder; see Chapter 4.3, section II.C.3.b), and suspension arm slings (see Chapter 4.3, section II.C.1.d.5), which support the forearm and arm to assist horizontal arm movement and elbow flexion in patients with weak (at least Tr+ to poor P−) shoulder and elbow muscles.

6) General feeding adaptations include utensil holders, that is, splints that can be attached to various utensils, for example, universal cuffs with straps, webbings with straps, splints (e.g., long opponens splints or externally powered splints for C5 tetraplegics) with utensil slots, palmar clips or palmar cuffs with utensil pockets, and wrist supports with palmar clips and utensil pockets. General feeding adaptations also include feeding accessories such as plate stabilizers (e.g., nonskid mats, suction bases, or damp dishtowels) and food or crumb catchers (e.g., terry cloth, vinyl, or disposable materials).

b. Dressing involves putting on and taking off clothing, along with managing fasteners (i.e., buttons, zippers, and snaps) and handling accessories such as belts and shoes. It is contraindicated in patients with unstable spines; pressure ulcers or a tendency for skin breakdown during rolling, scooting, and transferring; uncontrollable muscle spasms in legs; and 50% or less vital capacity (especially for lower-limb dressing).

The minimum criteria for upper-limb dressing include: (1) fair to good muscle strength in the deltoids, upper and middle trapezii, shoulder rotators, rhomboids, biceps, supinators, and radial wrist extensors; (2) ROM of 0 to 90 degrees in shoulder flexion and abduction, 0 to 80 degrees in shoulder internal rotation, 0 to 30 degrees in shoulder external rotation, and 15 to 140 degrees in elbow flexion; (3) adequate sitting balance in bed or WC, which may be achieved with the assistance of bedrails, an electric hospital bed, or WC safety belts; and (4) adequate finger prehension, which may be achieved by using tenodesis grasp or wrist-driven flexor-hinge orthosis.

For dressing of the lower limbs, the following are needed in addition to the minimum criteria for upper-limb dressing: (1) adequate balance and strength to pull up underwear, pants, or skirt (i.e., fair to good muscle strength in pectoralis major and minor, serratus anterior, and rhomboid major and minor muscles); (2) adequate ROM to reach the feet to don shoes and socks (i.e., ROM of 0-120° in knee flexion, 0-110° in hip flexion, and 0-80° in hip external rotation); (3) adequate body control for transfer from bed to WC with minimal assistance; (4) ability to roll from side to side, balance in sidelying, or turning from supine to prone position and back; and the ability to lift the buttocks to allow items to be pulled to the waist; and (5) vital capacity of 50% or more. For tips and techniques to make dressing easier in people with disabilities, refer to: *Dressing tips and clothing resources for making life easier,* 933 Chapel Hill Road, Madison, WI 53711, (608) 274-4380.

1) **Dressing material adaptations** include touch fasteners (e.g., Velcro), button hooks (i.e., wire loops, which hook around the button and are then pulled through the button holes; and various handles available including built-up foam handles), large buttons, zipper pulls (hook that attaches to zipper tab, zippers with loops or rings on the tab), combination buttoner-zipper pulls (loops attached to bendable metal cuffs that can be contoured to fit the palm), cuff and collar button extenders, and modified shoelaces (e.g., elastic shoelaces, which are similar to the regular cloth laces except the laces do not need to be untied or retied each time because they stretch as a person places the foot in the shoe; clipped-on shoe fastener unit, which tighten or loosen laces by pinching the unit; shoe buttons on which lace can be wrapped to maintain tightness; and lace locks through which laces can be threaded and tightness can be adjusted by sliding a plastic knob to lock the shoelace in position).

2) **Dressing style adaptations** include front-fastening garments (e.g., bra with front closure), cardigan or pull-over garments instead of slip-on garments in patients with adequate over-head shoulder movement, buttoned items in patients with inadequate over-head shoulder ROM but with fine motor skills to manipulate buttons, large or loose-fitting clothes to facilitate donning and doffing, pants and shorts with elastic waistbands and cuffs, garments with Velcro closures (e.g., bra or trousers), clip-on ties, and slip-on or loafer shoes.

3) **General dressing adaptations** include reachers or grabbers (which are extended sticks, usually made of lightweight aluminum, with a grasping unit at the end, which is operated by squeezing the handle activating the gripper position to open and close; they may be adapted for tetraplegics by using a special orthosis that can activate the reacher through wrist tenodesis), dressing sticks or wands (i.e., long sticks with a hook at the end), trouser pulls (webbing loops that can be hooked onto trouser belts), modified shoehorns (e.g., long-handled or spring-action), and stocking or pantyhose or sock aids (i.e., flexible plastic cores or fabric frames that can hold stockings or pantyhose or socks open, so they can be pulled up the legs via cords attached to the plastic core or fabric frame).

c. **Grooming and personal hygiene** consist of grooming (e.g., shaving; hair combing or brushing; caring for nails; application of facial makeup such as face powder, lipstick, and mascara; and application of antiperspirant, cologne, or perfume) and oral hygiene (e.g., brushing of teeth or dentures and flossing) activities. To perform grooming and hygiene skills, a person must have adequate upper-limb ROM and strength, adequate coordination and hand function, and adequate trunk control and sitting balance.

1) **Grooming adaptations** include shaving aids (e.g., electric shavers, universal electric-shaver holders, razor holders with cuffs that can be contoured to the palm, and clamp-on shaving cream dispenser handle), hair grooming aids (e.g., extension comb and hairbrush, hairbrush with Velcro handles, and straps with Velcro fasteners, which can be attached to hairbrushes), nail grooming aids (e.g., nail clippers, files, or brushes which can be stabilized, attached to a board with suction cups; and long-reach angled toenail scissors), facial makeup aids (e.g., spray powder, long handled powder puffs, and weighted wrist-cuffs for steadiness in makeup application), and modified mirrors (e.g., portable mirrors with suction cups, magnification mirrors, and adjustable mirrors with gooseneck).

2) **Oral hygiene adaptations** include toothbrush aids (e.g., electric toothbrush, self-rotating toothbrush with horizontal palm handle, and toothbrush attached to a base with suction cups), toothpaste dispenser aids (e.g., toothpaste pumps with large handles, which dispense a fixed amount of toothpaste; and tube squeezers), floss aids (e.g., large handle base that holds the floss upright), disposable foam tips for oral hygiene, and WaterPiks.

3) **General grooming/personal hygiene adaptations** include universal cuffs or custom-made palmar cuffs, splints with slots for hygiene care devices, adjustable grooming extenders (e.g., long handles attached to washcloths, combs, or hairbrushes), a cord attached to grooming or hygiene care products (e.g., razor, lipstick, soap, and toothbrush) for easy pickup when dropped, use of spray mechanism (e.g., spray deodorant, spray cologne, hair spray, spray powder, or spray perfume), adapters with large handles for aerosol cans, use of large roll-on deodorants (instead of sprays or creams), short reachers, and balanced forearm orthosis (see Chapter 4.3, section II.C.3.b) or suspension arm slings (see Chapter 4.3, section II.C.1.d.5) for patients with weak (at least Tr+ to poor P−) shoulder and elbow muscles.

d. **Bathing** includes body cleaning or washing (e.g., using showers, bathtubs, sponge baths, or body cleaning by the sink), hairwashing or shampooing, and drying after washing. To use the shower or bathtub, the patient needs to perform gross motor mobility skills (i.e., patient needs adequate upper-limb ROM/strength, fine motor coordination, and transfer/sitting balance to get in and out of the bathtub or shower safely, to sit or stand for the activity, and to do the cleansing activity itself) in a slippery environment. Environmental adaptations (see section II.B.1.b.3) that assist with bathing and safety include placement of grab bars outside and inside the bathing area, placement of nonskid strips inside the tub, extended handles on faucets, and automatic water temperature controls. For patients with a roll-in shower, a WC commode or shower chair is recommended.

1) **Bathing mobility adaptations** include tub transfer bench, which has two legs in the tub and two legs outside the tub for safe means of transfer to and from WC; a cushion inflated with water, which can form a rigid support for transfer; a bath chair, stool, or seat with suction feet; a wheeled shower chair; a bath board, which can be fitted onto the tub for seating; safety rails; wall grab bars; tub grab bars; and nonskid mats.

2) **Body washing and shampooing adaptations** include long-handled bath sponge or bath brush (the handle may be flexible, straight, or curved); soap aids (e.g., soap-on-a-rope for easy pickup of dropped soap; bath

mitt with soap pocket; soap grippers, i.e., finger cuffs with suction cups attached to the soap; pump dispensers); bath mitts (e.g., sponge, mesh, or terrycloth mitts); hair shampoo aids (e.g., pump dispensers, sink trays for shampooing while seated in WC, and shampoo basin for bedside hair washing); finger ring brushes for scrubbing the scalp or hair; a hand-held shower head, which may have a flexible hose or a built-up handle, which may be placed on the side of the tub for easy access; lever-type faucet handles or tap-turning devices; bath supports to hold the person steady in the tub; and inflatable bed baths.

    3) Drying adaptations include towel with loops, terry cloth robes, adjustable hair dryers (e.g., with gooseneck), and hands-free hair-dryer holders.

  e. Toileting include skills necessary to perform bowel and bladder care, that is, mobility and transfer skills (e.g., transferring on and off the toilet), sitting balance, upper-limb ROM and strength, hand function (e.g., pinch and grasp), coordination, and lowering or raising of clothing (see dressing skills in section II.A.3.b). It also includes menstrual care. For specific environmental adaptations (e.g., grab bars, toilet seat height), see section II.B.1.b.3.

    1) Toileting adaptations include raised toilet seats (with or without armrests) for patients unable to sit and arise from a low commode; toilet safety frame with arm rests to assist in transfers; high-back toilet supports; commode chairs and potty chairs, which can be used if the patient has difficulty with standard toilets; chair or bed male urinals; female urinals with collector bags; and snap-on toilet paper holders.

    2) Bowel-care adaptations include toilet paper holders (e.g. wiping tongs, spring clip holders, and extended holders), bidet, digital bowel stimulators, and suppository inserters.

    3) Bladder-care adaptations include positioning aids for catheterization (e.g., labia spreaders and knee spreaders with mirrors), dynamic splints or catheter inserters, modified catheter clamps, pneumatic or electric leg bag clamps, modified leg bag emptiers, modified condom catheter holders (to secure condom catheters), and modified strapping for urinary drainage bags.

    4) Incontinence adaptations include disposable underpads or diapers, reusable incontinent garments with easy access (e.g., Velcro), brief or panty liners, waterproof mattress protectors, and absorbent pads or draw sheets.

    5) Menstrual-care adaptations include the use of sanitary pads that stick to the undergarments instead of tampons.

4. Communication is a process by which information is exchanged among individuals. It is discussed in detail in Chapter 5.5. For electronic assistive technologies, the alternative output strategies may include speech synthesis, tactile output, enlarged character display, or telecommunications. Its input strategies may be done via switches (see classification in section II.A.5.a) or via standard or alternate keyboards or a computer mouse.

  a. Writing adaptations include modified pens or pencils (e.g., with built-up foam handles, weighted, enlarged, or special grips; triangular- or round-shaped grips; or with permanent attachment to a base for stabilization), pen or pencil holders (e.g., slip-on palmar cuffs; wrist supports or stabilizing bar; and figure-of-eight writing splints), and paper stabilizers (e.g., stabilized clipboard, paperweights, and the use of tape to hold the paper to the writing surface).

b. Typing adaptations include electric typewriters (may have self-correcting ribbons), word processors or computers, typewriter holders, modified typing sticks (e.g., mouthsticks, long handle sticks, head-pointer sticks, and splints with a slot or vertical holder for a typing stick), alternative keyboards (e.g., expanded keyboard or a small keyboard), keyguards and a key latch (to facilitate accuracy), and modified switches (see section II.A.5.a).

c. Book-handling and reading adaptations include modified sticks with suction cup ends which stick onto the book page (e.g., mouthstick or head wand or stick), book holders, electric page turners, magnifying readers, prism glasses that allow reading while lying flat, and nonslip plastic or rubber stabilizing sheets (e.g., Dycem).

d. Telephone-use adaptations include speaker phones (may have a quick dial feature), portable cordless phones, headsets, phone holders (e.g., gooseneck holders and clip holders), push-button phones (e.g., use of large button for uncoordinated patients), and mouth sticks for dialing.

e. General communication adaptations include modified mail handlers (e.g., electric letter openers or letter openers with modified handles), armrests, balanced forearm orthosis (see Chapter 4.3, section II.C.3.b) or suspension arm slings (see Chapter 4.3, section II.C.1.d.5) for patients with weak (at least $Tr+$ to poor $P-$) shoulder and elbow muscles, and environmental control units (see section II.A.5.a.3).

5. **Environmental hardware** include switches, faucets, and door hardware (e.g., doorknobs and keys). Environmental modifications for attaining barrier-free architectural designs for the physically handicapped are discussed in section II.B.1.b.

   a. Switch adaptations for household appliances

   1) **Physical-contact switches** include pneumatic switches (e.g., Sip-and-Puff and air cushion); switches requiring contact, no pressure, or slight movement (e.g., P-switch or sensor, mercury or tilt switches, electromyography, or electrooculography switches); and pressure switches (e.g., joystick, light touch, tongue, pillow, lead, wobble, plate, tread, rocker, grasp, or mat switches).

   2) **Nonphysical-contact switches** include eye movement or gaze switches (e.g., infrared sensors), light-sensitive switches (e.g., light-activated, photoelectric, infrared reflex, and blink switches), voice- or sound-activated switches, electromagnetic switches (e.g., remote radio transmitters), magnetic-finger switches, and switches activated by proximity (e.g., heat-sensitive) or a capacitive sensor.

   3) **Environmental control units (ECUs)** refer to a centralized panel that allows easy operation of multiple devices such as televisions, radios, lights, telephones, intercoms, and hospital beds.

   b. Faucet adaptations include extended or built-up handles on faucets, and faucets controlled by infrared sensors.

   c. Door hardware adaptations include door knob adaptations (e.g., lever-type, extended, or covered with rubber or friction tape), vehicle door openers (lever type), automatic door openers, lock system adaptations (e.g., push button and voice- or card-activated locks), and key aids (key holders that are rigid and offer more leverage for turning the key; key lever).

6. **Sexual expression** (e.g., masturbation) is an often neglected part of B-ADL (it may also be considered a more advanced ADL as it may involve tasks beyond caring for oneself with complex interaction with the social environment). Issues related to human sexuality are discussed in Chapter 5.9.

B. **Instrumental activities of daily living (I-ADL)** refer to more advanced problem-solving skills, and more complex environmental interactions including home management, community living skills, health management, safety preparedness, leisure, and work. It also includes environmental adaptations for home and community access (i.e., barrier-free architectural design for the physically handicapped) as well as transportation adaptation and driving.

1. **Home management** requires gross motor mobility skills as well as fine and gross motor coordination, strength, and endurance of the upper limb for the performance of household activities (i.e., meal planning, preparation, service, and clean-up; household maintenance including cleaning and bed-making; clothing care including laundry and sewing; and childcare). When limitations exist, assistive devices can be used in conjunction with work simplification and energy conservation techniques. Environmental adaptations to improve home accessibility can also be made.

a. **Household activities adaptations**

1) **Meal preparation, service, and cleanup adaptations** include cooking appliances, storage, dishwashing, and kitchen utensils. See section II.B.1.b for barrier-free designs of kitchen, for example, floor, countertop, and sink.

a) **Cooking-appliance adaptations** include electric appliances (i.e., stoves, ovens, and blenders); countertop appliances (e.g., broilers and microwave ovens); push button controls at the front of appliances; appliances with side doors (rather than top doors), pull-out shelves, burn-proof counters, and insulation of areas that can potentially cause burns; oven-cleaning adaptations (e.g., self-cleaning ovens; covering the oven with aluminum foil, which can easily be peeled and replaced; and using a hand-held cordless vacuum cleaner); push-pull sticks for oven racks; and mirrors angled above the stove to see into the contents of the pots if patient is WC-bound.

b) **Dishwashing adaptations** include electric dishwashers (i.e., front-loading, front-panel controls with pullout shelves), rubber mats at sink base, air drying, bottle brushes or scrub brushes with suction bases attached to the sink, soap dispensers, and terry cloth or sponge mitts.

c) **Storage adaptations** include two-door, side-by-side model refrigerator and freezer with self-defrosting and automatic ice dispenser features, pull-out shelves or drawers, turntables (e.g., Lazy Susans), storing items vertically (to avoid the need to lift off top items to retrieve bottom items), and easy-to-open plastic containers for food storage.

d) **Kitchen-utensil adaptations** include electric appliances (e.g., choppers, blenders, food processors, mixers, and can openers), one-handed appliances (e.g., can or jar openers, rolling pins, egg-beaters, grapefruit sectioners, and garlic presses), modified openers (e.g., jar lid openers, can openers, soda tab-grabbers, bottle openers, nonslip stabilizing plastic sheets such as Dycem, plastic bag openers, box top opener, and carton openers), modified scissors for opening packages (e.g., electric scissors, quick-clip scissors, and loop-scissors), modified knives (e.g., rocker knives, roller knives or pizza-cutting wheels, right angle knives, and serrated knives), modified paring or cutting board (e.g., with spikes or corner guards to keep food from sliding away or with suction bases for anchoring), peelers, bagel slicers, graters, adjustable strainers, pan holders or stabilizers, tongs (instead of fork, spatula, or serving spoon), jugs with plastic lids (rather than cartons for milk or juice), carton holders, box toppers, clear beakers with clear markings for measuring liquids, and kitchen timers.

e) **General adaptations for meal preparation and service** include modified transporting of items (e.g., wheeled carts, lap apron, basket or apron with large pockets, and wheeled tabletop disks with handles for moving hot pans or dishes), reachers, using convenience and prepared foods, lightweight utensils (except in uncoordinated patients who need heavy utensils for stability), unbreakable utensils, modified handles (e.g., bilateral, built-up, loop, extended, and rubber or plastic covered handles), stability adaptations (e.g., utensils with suction base, and plastic or rubber stabilizing mats or sheets), protective rubber mats or mesh mattings, and well-lit counters that are open underneath.

2) **Household maintenance adaptations** include general housecleaning (see section II.B.1.a.1.a for oven-cleaning) and bedmaking. See also section II.B.1.b for barrier-free designs of living rooms, bedrooms, etc.

a) **Cleaning adaptations** include vacuum cleaners (e.g., upright vacuum, self-propelled vacuum, cordless vacuum cleaner, and central vacuum cleaning system); carpet sweeper; modified handles (e.g., extended, flexible, built-up, and cuff for easy grasping) for dustpans, feather duster, mops, and brooms; dust cloth with rubber band over a top broom; duster mitten; self-wring mops or sponge mops with squeeze lever on the handle; use of furniture with casters for easy moving; wheeled utility carts for transporting several items at once; lightweight utensils (except for patients with incoordination, who need heavy utensils for stability); nonslip mats; and reachers.

b) **Bedmaking adaptations** include modified fitted sheets with touch fasteners or Velcro; lightweight blankets and spreads, satin pillow cases, and quilt covers.

3) **Clothing care adaptations** include laundry (collecting and transportation of clothes; washing, drying, and folding of clothes) and sewing.

a) **Laundry adaptations** include automatic washer and raised dryer (top loading for ambulatory patients, or front-loading for WC-bound patients); a mirror to see into the tub and a reacher to pull out clothes for front-loader for patients in WCs; push-button controls or large knobs; turning handles for adaptation; premeasured detergents, bleaches, and fabric softeners; heat-resistant pads (so iron does not need to be stored vertically); cord holders; adjustable tables for sorting and folding; WC lapboards; hampers lined with plastic bags with handles; utility carts for transporting several items at once; reachers; and the use of no-iron or permanent-press fabrics.

b) **Sewing adaptations** include electric sewing machines (with foot or knee controls), embroidery hoops, and pin cushions or bar of soap to hold needle for threading.

4) **Child-care adaptations** include feeding, diapering/dressing, bathing, lifting and carrying, and child-safety measures.

a) **Feeding adaptations** include breastfeeding (medically preferred and is generally easier than bottle-feeding); modified feeding bottles (e.g., lightweight plastic bottles with screw-on lids, disposable bottle-liners, and premeasured formulas); pillows for supporting the arms and the baby; sturdy highchairs with swing-away trays, one-hand release mechanisms, and safety straps; electric dish warmers; plastic aprons; bibs with pockets and Velcro closures; and rubber-coated spoons to protect the baby's gums and teeth.

b) **Diapering/dressing adaptations** include touch fasteners (e.g., Velcro), disposable diapers, loose clothing with full-length openings, changing tables with straps to secure infant, and padded dressing tables.

c) **Bathing adaptations** include foam-rubber bath aids, infant bath seats, child's bath support, terry cloth apron, and use of the kitchen sink or portable plastic tubs.

d) **Lifting and carrying adaptations** for ambulatory parents include bassinet on wheels or reclining strollers, carriage carts, or cloth infant-carriers; and for WC-bound parents, the child may be placed on the parent's lap supported by soft pillows or strapped to the armrest by touch fasteners to prevent slippage. The side of the crib may be adapted so the child can easily be lifted in and out of the crib.

e) **Safety adaptations** include harnesses to keep the child from wandering away, safety devices to protect the child from accidents, reachers (to pick up clothing and toys), nonslip mats, and the use of a playpen to confine the child to a safe environment.

b. **Home accessibility adaptations** can range from simple modifications (e.g., rearranging the furniture and placing commonly used items within reach) to complex modifications, that is, adaptation of a barrier-free architectural design for the physically handicapped. As with any adaptive equipment, factors to be considered for home or building modifications include support system (are there neighbors or family members who can help or does patient live alone?); financial and physical resources available to implement the modifications (whether the patient owns or rents the home may also dictate the level of modification possible); condition of the patient (is it static or progressive? any aging changes?); type of adaptation (e.g., does the patient need furniture rearrangement, structural modification, or relocation?); and patient's preference, desire, and ability to be independent. If possible, any suggested modification should be tried (e.g., in a simulated setup) before actual implementation at home. The following recommendations are based on the American standards for buildings and facilities (i.e., *American National Standard for Building and Facilities—providing accessibility and usability for physically handicapped people,* published by American National Standards Institute, 1430 Broadway, New York, NY 10018, tel. [212] 642-4900) and on the publications of the United States Architectural and Transportation Barriers Compliance Board ["Access Board"], 1331 F Street, NW Suite 1000, Washington, DC 20004-1111 (800) USA-ABLE). For other resources on accessibility for the disabled, see Appendix G-1.

1) **Access routes** must consist of at least two accessible routes for entrances and exits with emergency evacuation plans.

a) **Stairs** for ambulatory patients must have uniform steps of 4 to 7 inches (10.2-17.8 cm) height with depth of 11 inches (27.9 cm) and nonskid surface; stair nosings or "lips" of 60° from horizontal with a maximal protrusion of 1.5 inches (3.8 cm), or, if possible, it must be removed; and continuous handrails (bilateral if feasible) with height of 34 to 38 inches (86.4-96.5 cm), situated 1.5 inches (3.8 cm) from the wall, with circular cross section of 1.25 to 2 inches (3.2-5.1 cm), and with at least one handrail extending 12 inches (30.5 cm) beyond the top and bottom of the ramp runs.

b) **Ramps** for WC users must have an incline or slope of 12 inches for each inch of vertical rise or the least possible slope; a width of at least 36 to 48 inches (91.4-121.9 cm); continuous bilateral hand rails with measurements as described for stairs; a landing of 5 × 5 feet (60 × 60 inches or 152.4 × 152.4 cm) if the door swings out, or 5 feet wide (60 inches or 152.4 cm) by 3 feet deep (36 inches or 91.4 cm) if the door swings in; and a nonskid surface, which is protected from the elements if possible. In a long or curved ramp, there must be level rest platforms at 10-foot intervals.

c) **Mechanical lifts** for WC users may be installed when space for a ramp is not available. A WC lift must have clear floor space of 30 × 40 inches (76.2-101.6 cm) with a stable, firm, slip resistant surface; a forward approach of 36 inches (91.4 cm) or a parallel approach of 60 inches (152.4 cm); gratings of less than 1.5 inch (less than 3.8 cm) in one direction; operable parts within reach ranges; and enclosing walls and interlocked gates. If a vertical lift is used, an upper landing (dimensions as described for ramps) is often needed. If an inclined platform lift is used, it can be post-mounted on tracks along the stairs or on the wall(s) or stairs themselves. **Chair lifts** with built-in seats may be installed for patients who are not WC users but have difficulty climbing stairs.

d) **Elevators** may be installed in the house if the patient can afford them. They must have call-buttons centered 42 inches (106.7 cm) above the floor (maximum height of 60 inches or 152.4 cm) with minimum button size of $\frac{3}{4}$ inch (1.9 cm); hall signals that are audible and visible (with minimum size of 2.5 inches or 6.35 cm and located 72 inches [182.9 cm] above the floor); automatic doors, which remain open for a sufficient duration (at least 20 sec) and which reopen when a person or object exerts sufficient force at any point on the door edge; emergency communication systems; sufficient space to enter (at least 32 inches or 81.3 cm for WC users); and sufficient space inside the elevator car for WC maneuvers (minimum dimension for 180° WC turn is 60 inches or 152.4 cm diameter).

e) **Doors and doorways** must have clear width of at least 32 inches or 81.3 cm (for WC users) with level threshold (or if threshold is raised, it must be beveled and have maximal height of 0.5 inch or 1.27 cm); hardware situated 3 feet (36 inches or 91.5 cm) high; and if the door is weighted for easy closing, it should be less than 8 lb (<3.6 kg) with opening force of about 5 lb (2.3 kg). Doors can be hinged (regular or fold-back), pocket-sliding, sliding, and folding (accordion type) with automatic or pulley-operated openers and closers. Door knobs must be easy to grasp (e.g., rubber-covered door knobs or door knobs that use lever-operated, push-type or U-shaped mechanisms). For patients unable to use keys, an alternative lock system may be used (e.g., voice or card-activated or push-button system). Kickplates may be positioned 12 inches (30.5 cm) from the bottom of the door or remote controls may be installed. Doors in series should have adequate space between them to permit door swing into space.

f) Hallways for single WC user must have a minimum of 3 feet (36 inches or 91.4 cm) with adequate turning space at the beginning and end of each hallway customized for different WC. For a 180-degree WC turn, the minimum dimension should be a clear space of 60-inch or 152.4-cm diameter or a T-shaped space within a 60-inch or 152.4-cm square with arms 36 inches (91.4 cm) wide and 60 inches (152.4 cm) long and sufficient toe and knee clearance.

2) General living space

a) Ground and floor surfaces should be stable, firm, slope-resistant, and nonskid (options for nonskid surfaces include wood, vinyl, and specifically treated tile). If there is a change in level of a walking surface greater than 0.25 inch (0.64 cm), a slope or edge treatment is needed. If the floor is carpeted, it must have a level loop or textured loop with level-cut pile or pile texture no greater than 0.5 inch (1.3 cm). If possible, avoid thick carpeting and throw rugs. Gratings must have openings no greater than 0.5 inch (1.27 cm) with long openings placed perpendicular to the dominant direction of travel.

b) Windows should be easy to operate and open outward when possible. In general, it is easier to operate double-hung and horizontal-sliding windows than casement or awning windows that have cranks.

c) Controls for lights, drapes, fire alarms, emergency power (fuses and circuit breaker), windows, and heating, ventilating and air conditioning systems should be placed 18 to 48 inches (45.7-121.9 cm) above the floor. Remote control or an alternative control system (e.g., voice-activated, proximity-activated, or pressure-sensitive switches) are available from hardware stores or could be used from an environmental control unit.

3) Bathrooms and toilets

a) Floor space must have clear and unobstructed WC-turning space of at least 60-inch (152.4 cm) diameter and must be nonskid (bathmats may be used).

b) Toilets should have a height of 15 to 19 inches (38.1-48.3 cm) from floor to the top of the toilet seat and should be mounted adjacent to the side wall or partition with at least 18-inch (45.7 cm) clearance to and from centerline of toilet to sink and at least 48-inch (121.9 cm) clear space in front of the bowl and from side wall. Flush controls and toilet paper dispenser should be within reach.

c) Countertops and sinks for WC users must have clear floor space of at least 30 × 48 inches (76.2 × 121.9 cm) in front with maximum of 19 inches (48.3 cm) depth underneath. Countertop should be mounted with a height of 28 to 34 inches (71.1-86.4 cm) from the floor to the countertop and a knee clearance of at least 29 to 30 inches (73.7-76.2 cm) from the floor to bottom of the front edge of the countertop. Sink should have a maximum bowl depth of 6.5 inches (16.5 cm) and same height as for countertops. Built-in sinks should be placed close to the front edge of the countertop. Any exposed pipes and surfaces should be covered to prevent burns.

d) **Cabinets** (e.g., medicine cabinet) should be located 36 to 44 inches (91.4-111.8 cm) from the floor to cabinet bottom.

e) **Water controls** should have a maximum activation force of 5 lb (2.3 kg), valves with single-handle control and a lever blade shape that mixes the water to control temperature and adjust flow, and pressure balance and thermostatic controls.

f) **Shower areas** can be transfer-type showers (with or without a fixed bench of 17-19 inches [43.2 − 48.3 cm] height) with a clear floor space of at least 36 × 48 inches (91.4 × 121.9 cm), or it can be a roll-in shower with a clear floor space of at least 36 × 60 inches (91.4 × 152.4 cm). The maximum threshold height should be 0.5 inch (1.27 cm). For roll in showers, there should be grab bars on the three walls of the shower; whereas for transfer-type showers, there should be grab bars across the control wall and on the back wall to a point 18 inches (45.7 cm) from water-control wall. Water controls should be at 38 to 48 inches (96.5-121.9 cm) above the floor mounted on side wall opposite seat for transfer type showers and on back wall for roll-in showers. The shower spray unit, which can be fixed or hand-held, should have a hose of a least 60 inches (152.4 cm) long and an angle-lever type handle.

g) **Bathtubs** should have clear floor space of at least 30 × 60 inches (76.2 × 152.4 cm) in front for parallel approach or at least 48 × 60 inches (121.9 × 152.4 cm) for forward approach or at least 30 × 93 inches (76.2 × 236.2 cm) when in-tub seat is provided at the head end of the tub and rim height of 17 to 19 inches (43.2 − 48.3 cm) from floor to top of rim. Grab bars should be provided on three walls (back wall, head-end wall, and foot-end wall). Tub benches, bathtub seats, portable seats, built-in seats, and hydraulic seats may be used to facilitate transfer into the bathtub. Water controls should be 33 to 36 inches (83.8 to 91.4 cm) above the floor located between rim of tub and grab bar at foot of tub.

h) **Grab bars** should be 24 to 42 inches (61-106.7 cm) long, 1.5 inches (3.8 cm) in diameter, secured to withstand 250 lb (113.6 kg) of pressure, and mounted at 33 to 36 inches (83.8-91.4 cm) above the floor depending on the patient's transfer style, body mechanics, and equipment used.

i) **Accessories** such as dispensers, hand dryers, towel racks, or other fixtures should be 33 to 48 inches (83.8-121.9 cm) above the floor and should not impede movement. Mirrors should be full length (bottom edge of reflecting surface with maximum of 38 inches or 96.5 cm above the floor) or tilted downwards.

4) **Kitchens**

a) **Floors** should have a clear space of at least 30 × 48 inches (76.2 × 121.9 cm) and should have smooth, nonskid surface. A U- or L-shaped kitchen design is often most efficient for a wheelchair user.

b) **Work surface** should be at least 30 inches (76.2 cm) wide, at least 24 inches (61 cm) deep, and with a height of 28 to 36 inches (71.1-91.4 cm) from the floor.

c) **Countertops, sinks, cabinets, and water controls** have the same specifications as those described for bathrooms. There should be at least

40 inches (101.6 cm) clearance between counters. All storage space should be within the patient's reach. Hardware (e.g., cabinet door handle) and drawers should be easy to operate.

5) Bedrooms should have convenient access to the bathroom.

a) Beds should be stationary and positioned to provide sufficient space for transfers. Bed stability may be improved by placing the bed against a wall or in the corner of the room (except when the patient plans to make the bed). The height of the sleeping surface must facilitate transfer activities (if needed the height can be adjusted by using wooden blocks with routed depressions to hold each leg). The mattress should provide a firm, comfortable surface (to increase firmness, a bed board may be inserted between the mattress and the box spring).

b) Closets should be large, have wide entry, have open or pull-out shelves, and have low hanging rods hung at a maximum of 54 inches (137.2 cm) from the floor for WC users or adjustable clothes rod (42-72 inches or 106.7-182.9 cm) for ambulatory patients. The shelf height should be at waist level (up to 45 inches or 114.3 cm) in ambulatory patients or about 28 to 32 inches (71.1-81.3 cm) for WC users. Wall hooks may be useful addition to the closet area and should be placed 40 to 56 inches (101.6-142.2 cm) from the floor.

2. Community living skills include shopping, handling of money and finance, safety preparedness (i.e., fire safety awareness, ability to call 911, response to smoke detectors, and identification of dangerous situations), and personal health care (i.e., handling medications, self-monitoring, making medical appointments, and management of home attendant). They also include community mobility, that is, barrier-free architectural designs for handicapped accessibility to public buildings, transportation accessibility, and driving. Most of these skills require intact cognition and perception.

a. Shopping adaptations include modified shopping and transport carts (e.g., carts that attach to the WC, motorized carts, and heavy carts, which can be used for support), lightly packed plastic grocery bags with handles, reachers, use of proper body mechanics, use of shopping lists, and shopping at nonpeak hours.

b. Money and finance adaptations include modified writing or typing devices to handle paperwork (see section II.A.4.a).

c. Personal health care adaptations

1) Medication handling adaptations include pillbox with alarm to remind patient of medication schedule, handy compartmentalized storage units containing weekly medications with labels on lids (e.g., Mediplanner and Multi-Med Organizer), pill crusher, pill splitter, push-button pill dispenser, premeasured liquid medicines, premeasured injection shots (e.g., insulin), and one-handed auto-injectors;

2) Self-monitoring adaptations include electronic pulse or blood pressure digital monitors (e.g., self-inflating and deflating cuff and finger monitoring), digital thermometers, modified scales (e.g., large digital display, voice readout, and sitting scale), auto-lancet finger lancing devices, and electronic glucometers (e.g., One-Touch).

d. Safety-preparedness adaptations include prominent display of emergency numbers or emergency exit signs, auto-dial phones, a loud alarm for smoke detectors, Medicalert bracelets, provision of at least two accessible routes for entrance and exit, fire exits, and emergency evacuation plans.

e. Community accessibility adaptations include environmental modifications (i.e., barrier-free architectural designs) of public buildings that provide access for the physically handicapped into social, religious, educational, cultural, entertainment, medical, employment, and shopping facilities. For information resources on accessibility for the disabled, see Appendix G-1.

1) External building accessibility

a) Parking space should be at least 96 inches (243.8 cm) wide, with an access aisle 60 inches wide (152.4 cm) by 20 feet long (240 inches or 609.6 cm) adjacent and parallel to the vehicle pull-up space for loading and unloading. The minimum vertical clearance should be 114 inches (289.6 cm or 9.5 ft). For vans, the parking space should be at least 98 inches (248.9 cm) high and have an access aisle width of 96 inches (243.8 cm). The surface slope should not be steeper than 1 : 48 in all directions (i.e., 1 inch rise for every 48 inches surface length). The location should be reserved and clearly marked as a parking area for the handicapped.

b) Curbs must be beveled with textured cuts, which should meet the street surface with as little lip as possible.

c) Other access routes such as ramps, stairs, doors and doorways, elevators, have similar specifications as for home (see section II.B.1.b.1). Any entrance doors that are not accessible should have appropriate directional signs to the nearest accessible entrance. Automatic revolving doors can be built with sufficiently large space to accommodate a WC. Automatic sliding or swinging doors are also useful.

2) Internal building accessibility (access routes have essentially the same specification as for home described in section II.B.1.b.1.).

a) Corridors should be at least 48 inches wide (121.9 cm) and be free of obstructions such as supporting columns and decorative plants. There should also be adequate WC turning space (see section II.B.1.b.1.f). The floor should have a nonslip hard surface or low pile carpet (see section II.B.1.b.2.a). Path of travel in all areas (e.g., between desks) should be at least 3 feet (36 inches or 91.4 cm).

b) Rest rooms that are WC accessible should be provided at least one each for men and women. There should at least be 48 inches (121.9 cm) between inside wall and partitions enclosing toilet. The entrance to the cubicle should at least be 48 inches (121.9 cm), and there should be adequate turning space in the main area of the rest room (6 × 6 feet or 72 × 72 inches or 183 × 183 cm). Specifications for functional access (e.g., grab bars, toilet flush, sink, etc.) are described in section II.B.1.b.3.

c) Water fountains should not be higher than 36 inches (91.4 cm) from the floor to the level of water flow. They should have buttons or levers for easy activation.

d) Public telephones should have at least one that is WC accessible (mounted not higher than 48 inches or 121.9 cm) with push-button dialing.

e) Identifying signs and labels should be easy to view (i.e., of sufficient size and color contrast). Tactile letters and numbers and Braille letters as well as auditory signals in elevators should be provided to identify floor level. Stairs and corridors should have adequate lighting.

f. Community mobility adaptations refer to commuting (by public transportation or by driving) to visit social, religious, educational, cultural, entertainment, medical, employment, and shopping facilities. Community organizations (e.g., Arthritis Foundation, National Easter Seal Society, Multiple Sclerosis Society, Chamber of Commerce, Veterans Administration, or the school's or campus' disabled student services office) may provide information on transportation services available to the disabled residents.

1) Public transportation adaptations include modified buses (e.g., kneeling buses equipped with a hydraulic unit, which lowers the entrance to curb level for easier boarding or buses equipped with hydraulic lifts to allow direct entry by a wheelchair user), elevator access to subway trains, and door-to-door cab and van service.

2) Driving is a complex task that requires continuous integration of visual, motor, cognitive, and perceptual skills at a high level of functioning. Because driving carries a high potential for harm to the driver and other people, persons with physical handicaps require a predriving clinical screening, a comprehensive driving evaluation (i.e., stationary and behind-the-wheel performance test and vehicular selection and adaptations). Specifics on evaluation programs vary from state to state and must be obtained through the Department of Motor Vehicles and Licensing for each state. A partial listing of adaptive driving resources and association is provided in the Appendix G-2.

a) Predriving screenings are generally done by physicians to medically clear patients and to identify problems related to driving. The patient's desire to drive should be tempered with an acknowledgment of his or her mental, physical, or emotional limitations. Moreover, the patient's family and support system should be supportive and firm. The history and physical examination should include the following (if the physician has any concern, it must be documented in the evaluation form):

(1) *History of physical impairment* including its nature, etiology, and progression. The patient should be under the care of a regular physician and should be stable or improving. Patients with spinal fusion need enough mirrors to provide a 360-degree field of vision.

(2) *Medication history* including drug type, side effects, and reason for use. The patient must show excellent drug compliance and be aware of potential adverse drug effects.

(3) *Social history.* Patients should not be recreational drug or alcohol abusers.

(4) *History of temporary loss of consciousness (LOC)* because of epilepsy, diabetes, etc. Diabetic patients should have good control of blood sugar and should be taught how to prevent, recognize, and treat symptoms of hypoglycemia. Epileptic patients should not have had LOC or seizure episodes (including petit mal) for 6 to 24 months (this prerequisite varies from state to state). Both epileptic and diabetic patients must be under strict medical supervision and must submit proof of medication compliance (e.g., therapeutic range of medication in the blood or normal level of glycosylated hemoglobin for diabetics).

(5) *Functional skill examination,* including musculoskeletal skills (i.e., ROM, strength, endurance, coordination, muscle spasms, deformities, reaction time, upper and lower limb mobility skills, hand grip and dexterity, transfer skills, and sitting tolerance) and the ability to use gait aids, prostheses, orthoses, and WCs. The patient must be able to maximize his or her self-reliance in these functional skills. If available, functional assessment may be done in a simulated environment using a mock-up vehicle.

(6) *Vision examination* including acuity, peripheral fields, scanning, color discrimination, glare recovery, depth perception, visual accommodation, and visuospatial perception (including visual organization, visual search and scanning, spatial relations, directionality, and visual processing speed). Evaluation methods for visual-perceptual skills include observation, functional task performance, pencil and paper tasks, computerized assessment programs and paper tasks. Vision and visual-perception skills must meet safety criteria for safe driving (e.g., visual acuity must have a cutoff point of 20/40 to 20/50, depending on the state law) as determined by the State's Department of Motor Vehicles.

(7) *Communication and hearing examination* including dysarthria, aphasia, and hearing impairment. The patient must meet safety criteria for safe driving as determined by the State's Department of Motor Vehicles.

(8) *Psychologic examination* including problem-solving skills, decision-making skills, selective and divided attention (distractibility), safety judgment (impulsivity), memory, sequencing, ability to plan ahead, recognition of signs and symbols, number recognition, confusion, agitation, hostility, and suicidal ideation. Patient must be rational, have good judgment, have the ability to recognize signs and symbols, and be emotionally stable (i.e., patient's behavior should not be physically or verbally explosive, aggressive, hostile, paranoid, or suicidal).

b) **Vehicular setup** must be done prior to predriving or behind-the-wheel assessment to determine optimal driver positioning and ability to manipulate *primary controls* (i.e., steering wheel, accelerator, and brake) and *secondary controls* (i.e., ignition, turn signals, horn, windshield wiper and washer, headlights, headlight dimmer, heater and air-conditioning, power windows, power door locks, electric mirrors, door and lift controls, electric gear selector, electric parking brake, emergency flashers, and electric WC lockdown). In general, recommendations for adaptive equipment should be made only when a driver can demonstrate the ability to use the same general type of device in a behind-the-wheel assessment.

(1) **Vehicular selections** include a car or a van (full size or minivan). A car is appropriate for patients (e.g., low-level paraplegics) who can enter or exit the vehicle independently and load the mobility equipment. The standard car recommendation is a two-door sedan with power steering, power brakes, automatic transmission, and, if needed, modified car seat or safety harness system. The car should be large enough to allow WC storage behind the front seat or if the patient cannot independently load and unload the WC, it can be modified with a cartop carrier that automatically loads and unloads the WC. The van is appropriate for patients who need to drive from their own WC due to inability to transfer themselves and their WC independently and safely into the vehicle (e.g., tetraplegic or high-level paraplegic patients using motorized WCs or scooters). The width of the van door and roof clearance should accommodate the motorized WC or scooter. Entry into the van can be accomplished by a hydraulic lift (e.g., swing-away style or fold-out platform style), which can be mounted onto the rear or side of the van, or by a portable ramp (for safety reasons, the WC or scooter has to be pushed or driven up the ramp by someone other than the user). WC restraint systems (e.g., manually-operated on electric tie-downs) are also available for vans.

(2) Primary-controls adaptations include modified steering wheels for one-handed use or for weak grip (e.g., use of steering aids such as spinner-knobs, V-shaped grips, tri-pins which use three adjusted pins in a triangular arrangement, universal or palmar cuffs, or amputee rings onto which a prosthetic hook can be inserted); modified gas and brake controls, which include pedal extensions (to increase reach), pedal relocation (e.g. left-sided accelerator pedal for right hemiplegia), hand controls for paraplegics (e.g. rotary, push-pull, push-twist, push-right angle pull, push-pull down, or side-to-side motions for manipulating controls), or high-tech adaptations (e.g., operated by vacuum, pneumatic, or computer). All primary controls may be integrated into a single lever (joystick) system for patients with severe disabilities, such as C5 tetraplegics.

(3) Secondary-controls adaptations include quad key holders, elbow switches, head control switches, and touch pads (instead of toggle) switches which may be built up.

(4) Other modifications include a raised roof, mirrors for rear, side, or 360-degree vision; expanded doorway widths and heights; modified seat belts (and, if needed, chest straps for control of weak trunks); air conditioner (especially for patients with multiple sclerosis); two-way radio; and cellular phones.

c) Stationary (predriving) assessment include the evaluation of the following tasks: moving or transferring to the vehicle, inserting and turning a key (or using "keyless" entry operation or remote control), opening and closing the door, entering and exiting the vehicle, loading and unloading mobility devices (cane, walker, WC), adjusting the driver's seat, adjusting the mirrors, and fastening the seat belt (and chest strap if needed). Adaptive devices include special key holders, vehicle door lever-type openers, loops for lower-limb management, a WC strap to extend reach for WC loading, modifications for independent seat belt retrieval, and use of hydraulic lifts or ramps.

d) Behind-the-wheel assessment can either be simulated or on-the-road. A driving simulator uses a mock-up vehicle to test the patient's defensive driving skills, hazard perception, and emergency procedures as he or she steers and reacts to the simulated driving situation displayed on a movie screen. However, the optimal industry standard of driving competence remains the on-the-road driving test.

3. **Occupational activities** are age-specific, for example, a preschool child's occupation may be play and learning, whereas a school-age child's occupation is school activity and play, and an adult's occupation is work and leisure activity.

   a. **Leisure** refers to unoccupied time (free from work and self-care activities) during which a person may indulge in rest and recreational activities. Benefits of participating in recreational activities include physical, emotional, and social well-being through enjoyment, exercise, competition, and socialization. Leisure activities can be used with therapeutic intent (e.g., using principles of reflex maturation and neurophysiology) to help develop skills needed for the patient's occupation or other ADL tasks. It uses a fun-based setting to encourage patients to use their remaining abilities to compensate for their mental limitations and physical disabilities. Adaptations for leisure activities include the use of high and low technology aids and devices, as well as modification of the physical environment. There are many organizations that provide programs (e.g., camps and WC-adapted basketball, rugby, tennis, or other sports) especially designed for the disabled (see partial listing in Appendix G-6). This information can also be obtained from the local parks and recreation departments, churches, and other disability-related organizations (see partial listing in Appendix G-4). The following are examples of some common adaptations used for indoor and outdoor recreations.

   1) **Indoor recreation adaptations** include bowling (e.g., bowling ball ramp, spring loaded bowling ball, bowling ball holder mounted to WC), knitting (e.g., embroidery hoop, and knitting needle holder), board games (e.g., enlarged game pieces and weighted pieces for uncoordinated patients), card games (e.g., card holders, automatic card shufflers, and magnetic playing cards and boards), toy modifications (e.g., switch-activated, modified handles, and stabilizing surface), spring-loaded cue stick, and indoor photography (e.g., pneumatic-control camera and camera tripod holder, which can be mounted to the WC).

   2) **Outdoor recreation adaptations** include trigger-release archery; raised gardening beds; modified frisbees (e.g., Quad-grip); electric-retrieve fishing reels; upper limb-propelled bicycles (for paraplegics); tricycles with footplates, straps, trunk supports, and extended seats; modified saddles; outrigger skis; modified swings (i.e., swing that can be propelled by pushing and pulling on the handles or using the arms); and outdoor photography (same as for indoor adaptations).

   3) **General recreation adaptations** include universal cuffs, splints with slot or vertical holders, Velcro straps and grips, built-up handles (e.g., for tennis rackets and paint brush), mouthsticks (e.g., for painting), clamp frames, recreation belts, and chest straps or body harnesses.

   b. **Work** refers to activities or tasks done to provide meaning and support to the self, family, and society. It is learned through the process of socialization, is influenced by one's cultural tradition, and is motivated by one's intrinsic urge to be effective in the environment. Work is used by most people to provide their source of livelihood. It is discussed in Chapter 5.11.

BIBLIOGRAPHY

Hopkins HL, Smith HD, editors: *Willard and Spackman's occupational therapy,* ed 8, Philadelphia 1993, JB Lippincott.

Kent H, Redford JB: Adaptive driving modifications. In Redford JB, Basmajian

JV, Trautman P, editors: *Orthotics: clinical practice and rehabilitation technology,* New York, 1995, Churchill Livingstone, pp. 219-234.

Kohlmeyer K: Adaptations in and to the home environment. In Redford JB, Basmajian JV, Trautman P, editors: *Orthotics: clinical practice and rehabilitation technology,* New York, 1995, Churchill Livingstone, pp. 235-255.

Mix CM, Specht DP: Achieving functional independence. In Braddom RL, editor: *Physical medicine and rehabilitation,* Philadelphia, 1996, WB Saunders, pp. 514-530.

Pedretti LW, editor: *Occupational therapy practice skills for physical dysfunction,* ed 4, St. Louis, 1996, Mosby–Year Book.

Trombly CA, editor: *Occupational therapy for physical dysfunction,* ed 4, Baltimore, 1995, Williams & Wilkins.

CHAPTER 4.6

GAIT AIDS AND GAIT PATTERNS

The ability to ambulate (with or without aid) greatly affects a person's level of functional independence. As defined in Chapter 4.5, section II.A.2.d, functional ambulation refers to walking with an aid (e.g., walker) to accomplish some task (e.g., putting clothes into the closet). To become independent in functional ambulation, the patient must have adequate strength, range of motion (ROM), balance, coordination, and cognitive skills (for safety and timing). If the patient has limitation in any of these areas, PM&R intervention is needed. For example, patients may be taught energy- and time-efficient physical compensations (through physical and occupational therapy), and if needed, they may be prescribed orthoses (see Chapter 4.3), wheelchairs (see Chapter 4.7), gait aids, or any combination of these. This chapter deals with gait aids and gait patterns commonly prescribed by physiatrists. Selected resources of adaptive equipment and disability–related products (including gait aids) are provided in Appendix G-3.

I. **Gait aids** (see Fig 4.6-1) are prescribed to improve balance and stability (by redistributing and widening the weightbearing or support area), provide sensory feedback, provide small propulsive forces to assist acceleration during locomotion, and reduce lower limb pain (by decreasing load on musculoskeletal structures). Because they are considered to be an extension of the upper limb, good upper limb strength and coordination are needed. The important muscle groups include shoulder depressors (latissimus dorsi, lower trapezius, pectoralis minor), shoulder flexors, elbow and wrist extensors, and finger flexors. Trunk muscles also are necessary to improve balance and endurance. Strengthening and coordination exercises of these muscle groups should be started while the patient is nonambulatory or preoperatively if surgery is elective.

A gait aid and gait pattern should be prescribed according to the patient's general functional ability, ability to maintain the body erect, and the amount of balance and weightbearing assistance needed. In general, walkers provide the most stability, crutches provide moderate stability, and canes provide the least stability. Walkers are prescribed for patients with more significantly decreased balance, strength, or coordination. The body weight transmitted away from the affected lower limbs are: axillary crutches, up to 80%; nonaxillary crutches, 40 to 50%; and canes, 20 to 25% (i.e., in unilateral canes used opposite the affected side). When compared to normal unassisted gait, the energy expenditure per unit distance is about 18-36% greater for partial weight-bearing gaits using either crutches (axillary or forearm) or a cane and 41-61% greater for non-weight-bearing gaits using either axillary or forearm crutches. All patients should be trained on the proper use of the gait aid. In general, crutch ambulation needs more skill than the other gait aids.

A. **Walkers** (see Fig. 4.6-1M to R) are made of lightweight, durable, tubular aluminum or other tubular metal, with plastic handgrips, and four rubber-tipped legs. They are relatively easy to use, provide greater support and safer gait than canes and crutches, and are often used in the early phase of gait training (e.g., in hemiplegic or ataxic patients) to help patient gain more balance and confidence prior to progressing to crutches or canes. In patients

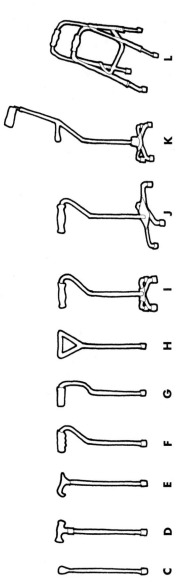

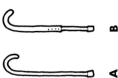

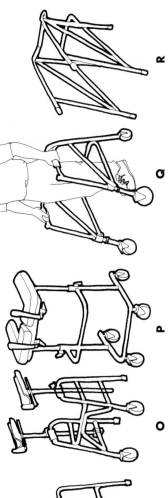

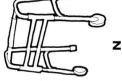

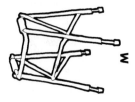

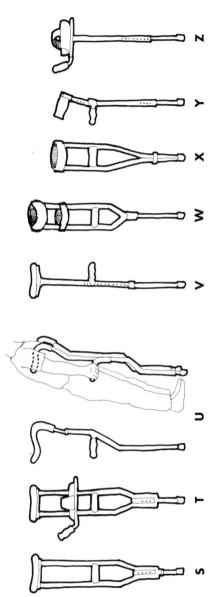

Figure 4.6-1.
Gait aids. **A,** C-handle (J-handle or crook-top) wooden straight cane. **B,** C-handle adjustable aluminum straight cane. **C,** Ball-top straight cane. **D,** Functional grip cane. **E,** Slant-handled straight cane. **F,** Curved-top straight cane. **G,** Adjustable offset cane (e.g., Ortho-cane). **H,** Shovel-handle (stirruplike) straight cane. **I,** Narrow-based quadruped ("quad") cane. **J,** Wide-based quadruped ("quad") cane. **K,** Forearm quad cane. **L,** Walk-cane or Hemi-walker or side-stepper cane. **M,** Non-folding standard walker (folding type not shown). **N,** Rolling or gliding walker. **O,** Bilateral platform walker. **P,** Rolling triceps walker. **Q,** Reverse rollator or posture-control walker. **R,** Stair-climbing walker. **S,** Adjustable axillary crutch (aluminum or wooden). **T,** Axillary crutch with platform. **U,** Ortho-crutch. **V,** Telescoping underarm (axillary) aluminum crutch. **W,** Triceps crutches (e.g., Canadian Elbow Extensor Crutches). **X,** Forearm crutch with closed cuff (e.g., Kenny stick). **Y,** Adjustable forearm crutch (Lofstrand crutch). **Z,** Platform crutch or forearm support crutch.

with lower limb incoordination but good upper limb strength, weights (e.g., sandbags) may be added to the crosspieces of the walker for greater stability. The main disadvantages of walkers are they cause a slow and awkward gait, and, in prolonged use, patients may assume bad posture and walking habits. Also, in most cases, the use of walker is limited to indoor activities. Unless patients are strong enough to use a stair-climbing walker, they are unable to climb stairs using walkers. Walkers are made in several sizes, both for pediatric and adult groups. A walker is fitted by placing it about 10 to 12 inches in front of and partially surrounding the patient. The proper height is set with the patient standing straight, shoulders relaxed, and elbows flexed to between 15 and 20 degrees.

1. **Standard walkers** (see Fig. 4.6-1M) have telescopic or adjustable legs, and the height can be adjusted to most individual patients. Some models fold for easy transportation (e.g., via car trunk). For very tall patients, a tall design may be necessary. The patient needs good standing balance and upper limb strength to lift the walker to advance it forward. The patient should also have sufficient hand strength and range of motion to grip the walker.

2. **Rolling or gliding walkers** (see Fig. 4.6-1N) have wheels on the front legs to help facilitate movement of the walker for patients who lack coordination or strength in the upper limbs and trunk (hence, with difficulty in lifting and advancing crutches or standard walkers). By slightly raising the back legs off the floor, patients may be able to push this walker; however, the wheels may provide some instability, and patients may require supervision.

3. **Platform walkers** have a platform type of forearm support, which can be attached to either a standard walker or a rolling walker (see Fig. 4.6-1O). It is used in patients with flexion contracture of the elbow or pain or deformities of the wrist and hand; however, they are generally quite heavy.

4. **Rolling triceps walker** (see Fig. 4.6-1P) is four-wheeled walker with padded platforms. It is used by persons with limited upper limb strength and range of motion. The patient's forearms, which rest on the pads, accept the patient's weight as the lower limbs take steps. The wheels allow the walker to be pushed forward without lifting.

5. **Reciprocal walker** has swivel joints allowing reciprocal action as each side of the walker moves alternately. It allows a longer stride and a less awkward gait. It is commonly used by patients with bilateral hip replacements.

6. **Reverse walker** (see Fig. 4.6-1Q) is used to facilitate extension posture by a person who tends to maintain a flexed posture while standing. It is commonly used in spastic cerebral palsy children with crouched gait.

7. **Stair-climbing walker** (see Fig. 4.6-1R) has a U-shaped front extension with extra supports to provide stability in stair climbing. It is useful primarily in well-motivated patients with good balance and superior strength in their upper limbs, such as young paraplegics.

B. **Crutches** (see Fig. 4.6-1S to Z) have two points of contact with the body and thus provide better stability than canes. Crutches have rubber tips for absorbing shock and preventing slippage. The clinician must make sure that the crutch tips are not worn out. If needed, special crutch tips (e.g., for rainy and icy conditions) may be prescribed. Padded hand grips are used to reduce pressure on the hands and to help prevent slippage of grip. Crutches should only be prescribed to patients with enough strength to extend the elbows and raise the body 1 to 2 inches off the floor.

1. **Axillary crutches** (see Fig. 4.6-1S to V) provide better trunk support than nonaxillary crutches. They are prescribed for short-term use by patients with good balance and coordination. Patients using axillary crutches can free their hands for opening doors by leaning on the shoulder piece. However, they should be instructed to refrain from leaning their axilla against the axillary pads for prolonged periods as this may cause compressive radial neuropathy leading to "crutch palsy." Other compressive neuropathies (e.g., median and ulnar) may occasionally occur in the upper arm or in the hand and wrist. To measure crutch length (from the top of the axillary pad to the crutch tip) with the patient supine, take the distance from the anterior axillary fold to the heel (without shoes) and add 2 inches. To measure crutch length with the patient standing erect with the shoulders relaxed, take the distance from anterior axillary fold to a point 6 inches anterior and 6 inches lateral to the fifth toe. The hand bars are adjusted in each case to give about 30 degrees of elbow flexion with the wrist in maximal extension, and the fingers forming a fist. This is measured after the total crutch length is determined with the crutch 3 inches lateral to the foot.

   a. **Standard axillary crutches** (see Fig. 4.6-1S) have double uprights with a shoulder piece and handgrip or bar. They can be made of wood or tubular aluminum and their length can be adjusted. They can also be adapted for patients with poor handgrip by attaching a forearm platform (see Fig. 4.6-1T).

   b. **Single-upright crutches** can either be straight (e.g., telescoping underarm [axillary] aluminum crutch; see Fig. 4.6-1V) or have a curved upper half (e.g., Ortho-crutch; see Fig. 4.6-1U). They usually have a contoured underarm piece and an adjustable hand piece. Some patients find the Ortho-crutch to be more comfortable than standard axillary crutches.

2. **Nonaxillary crutches (forearm or arm canes;** see Fig. 4.6-1W–Z) are prescribed for long-term use in patients with good trunk balance and confidence in ambulation (e.g., paraplegics who may require bracing with ambulation).

   a. **Lofstrand crutches** (see Fig. 4.6-1Y) are the most popular nonaxillary type. They are made of tubular aluminum with a padded hand bar and forearm cuff. The forearm cuff (which is open at the front or side) helps to stabilize the forearm and wrist during weight bearing to make ambulation easier and safer. They are most often used bilaterally and provide less support than axillary crutches for ambulation. They are more useful than bilateral canes because they allow the patient to free a hand (without dropping the crutches) to perform certain tasks such as grasping a stair rail, opening a door handle, or adjusting clothes. The Lofstrand handpiece is measured as described above for axillary crutches, with the elbow flexed 20 degrees and the patient standing upright. The proximal portion of the Lofstrand crutches is also angled at 20 degrees for a comfortable, stable fit.

   b. **Platform crutches** (see Fig. 4.6-1Z) have a platform on the top level of the crutch on which to rest the forearm and a vertical handgrip at the distal end of the platform. They are often used by arthritic patients with flexion contracture of the elbow and also by those with weak grip because of pain and deformities of the hand and wrist. Velcro straps around the forearm may assist in holding the crutch in those with poor grip. Their advantage is that the body weight is borne mostly on the forearm instead of the hand. The handgrip can also be contoured to adapt to the deformities. It is measured by having the patient stand upright with the shoulders relaxed and the elbows flexed 90 degrees. The distance from the ground to the forearm rest is the proper length.

    c. Forearm crutches with closed cuff (Kenny Stick; see Fig. 4.6-1X) are similar to the Lofstrand crutches except that instead of an open cuff, they have a closed leather band, which ensures that the patient (more so than with the Lofstrand forearm orthosis) will not drop the crutches. They were designed for polio patients who had satisfactory proximal upper limb musculature but who may have been weak distally and unable to effectively hold and control the crutches. They are prescribed for children who need total contact around their forearm.

    d. Triceps crutches (or **Canadian Elbow Extensor Crutches;** see Fig. 4.6-1W) have a single shaft attached to bilateral uprights, which extend above the elbow. They resembles the style of standard axillary crutches, but they end proximally at the mid-arm level. They have two cuffs, one above and one below the elbow, that support the arm with the elbow extended (thus preventing elbow buckling) during gait. They are useful for patients with triceps weakness (e.g., poliomyelitis patients).

C. Canes (see Fig. 4.6-1) have only a single point of contact with the body and provide less support than other gait aids. Hence, it is not appropriate in patients needing more than partial weight relief or support. The cane is held in the hand on the side of the unaffected lower limb to widen the base of support and reduce the load on the affected hip as well as to simulate a more physiological gait (i.e., in normal walking the opposite leg and arm move together). Without a cane, the load on the hip is increased by four times the body weight during stance phase of the gait because of the gravitational forces and the gluteus medius and minimus force exerted across the weightbearing hip. With the use of a cane, the upper limb exerts force on the cane thus minimizing pelvic drop on the side opposite the weightbearing lower limb and shifting the center of gravity to the unaffected side. This results in decreased work of the gluteus medius-minimus complex and reduced load generated across the affected hip joint. The length of the cane is measured with the patient in an upright position (and the elbow is flexed about 20 to 30°) so that the highest point of the cane is at the level of the greater trochanter. A short cane will tend to hold the elbow in complete extension (hence reducing support during stance phase), and a long cane will force the elbow into too much flexion (hence increasing fatigue by putting excessive demands on the triceps and shoulder muscles).

    1. Regular (straight tip) canes can be made of wood or aluminum. The aluminum canes have adjustable notches (see Fig. 4.6-1B) while the wooden cane needs to be cut to the patient's height. There are several variety of cane handles. The C-handle cane (crook top cane or J-cane; see Fig. 4.6-1A and B) is the most commonly used. A functional grip cane (shaped to fit the approximate contour of a gripping hand; see Fig. 4.6-1D) may offer the patient a more comfortable grip than that of the C-cane for some patients. Other straight cane handles include ball-shaped (see Fig. 4.6-1C), slant-handled (see Fig. 4.6-1E), and shovel-handle (or stirrup-like; see Fig.

4.6-1H). Canes with curved-staff at the top, are claimed to provide better balance for the patient (Fig. 4.6-1F and G). The Ortho-cane (see Fig. 4.6-1G), which has a plastic palm grip and a curved staff at the top, was designed to provide better grip in addition to better balance for the patient.

2. **Quad canes** (Fig. 4.6-1I and J) have four prongs at the base and are prescribed for patients (e.g., hemiplegics) who need more stability than that provided by other canes. The gait of patients using quad cane is relatively slow. However, this slowing is negligible in most patients (e.g., hemiplegics) whose gait is slow to start with. The quad cane's base of support can either be narrow (Fig. 4.6-1I) or wide (Fig. 4.6-1J). In using the quad cane, the lateral two prongs should be directed away from the body. A variation of the quad cane is the forearm quad cane (Fig. 4.6-1K), which is essentially a Lofstrand crutch with four-prong base.

3. **Walk-canes (hemi-walkers** or **side-steppers;** Fig. 4.6-1L) combine the features of a walker and quad cane. They are made of tubular aluminum and are foldable (hence more compact than the quad cane). Their bases of support are wider than that of quad canes and provide significantly better lateral support. They are used by hemiplegics who no longer need parallel bars but are not ready to use the quad cane.

II. Basic gait patterns using gait aids for level ground should emphasize normal heel-to-toe progression of the affected limb. The choice of gait pattern depends on the patient's strength, balance, coordination, and on the walking surface. Each patient should be trained with more than one type of gait pattern.

A. Walker gait patterns are more stable than that of crutch or cane. The patient should pick up and place down the walker on all four legs simultaneously (without tipping the walker on two legs) to achieve maximum stability.

1. **Full-weight-bearing walker gait** sequence is walker is lifted and moved forward, one foot is moved forward, then the other foot is advanced past the first foot.

2. **Partial-weight-bearing walker gait** sequence is walker is lifted and moved forward, the affected lower limb is moved forward, weight is shifted onto the walker (through the upper limbs) and partially onto the affected lower limb, then the unaffected lower limb steps past the affected limb.

3. **Nonweight-bearing walker gait** sequence is walker is lifted and moved forward (the affected lower limb, which does not bear any weight, may be advanced together with the walker or following the walker), weight is shifted through the upper limbs to the walker, and the unaffected lower limb steps forward.

B. Crutch gait patterns

1. **Point gaits**

   a. **Four-point gait** sequence is right crutch, left foot, left crutch, right foot. This is a very stable gait because three points are always in contact with the floor. It is used by patients with ataxia and by those with marked lower limb weakness. However, the gait is relatively slow, and it is more difficult to learn than the other gait patterns.

   b. **Three-point gaits** have only three points of support in contact with the floor and generally require good balance. They are commonly used by patients with lower limb fractures or amputations.

   1) **Nonweight-bearing crutch gait** sequence is both crutches are advanced (the affected lower limb, which does not bear any weight, may be advanced together with the crutches or following the crutches), weight is shifted onto the crutches, and the unaffected lower limb steps forward.

2) Partial weight-bearing crutch gait sequence is both crutches are advanced (the affected lower limb may be advanced together with the crutches or following the crutches), weight is shifted onto the crutches and partially to the affected lower limb, then the unaffected lower limb steps past the crutches.

c. Two-point gait or two-point alternate gait sequence is simultaneous advancement of right crutch and left foot, followed by simultaneously advancement left crutch and right foot. This is faster than the four-point gait and is fairly stable. It is used by ataxic patients and for reduction of weight bearing on the lower limbs.

d. Tripod (drag-to) gaits are initially used by paraplegic patients. When they improve their balance, they progress to a swing gait. Tripod gaits are stable but slow and laborious.

1) Tripod alternate gait sequence is right crutch, left crutch, then both lower limbs are dragged to the crutch level.

2) Tripod simultaneous gait sequence is both crutches are advanced simultaneously, then both lower limbs are dragged to the crutch level.

2. Swing gaits

a. Swing-to gait sequence is both crutches are advanced simultaneously, then the arms push down, and both lower limbs lift and swing *to* the level of the crutches. It is easy to learn and are used by most paraplegic patients.

b. Swing-through gait sequence is both crutches are advanced simultaneously, then the arms push down, and both lower limbs lift and swing *beyond* the level of the crutches. It is the fastest gait (even faster than able-bodied walking) but is very energy-demanding and difficult to do. The patient needs good trunk balance (with functional abdominal muscles) and good strength in the upper limbs.

C. Cane gait patterns uses only point gaits. When only one cane is used, it should be held contralateral to the affected lower limb. The patient should always have the relatively "good" or unaffected lower limb assume the first full weightbearing step.

1. One-cane gait sequence is the cane and affected lower limb are advanced simultaneously, weight is shifted onto the cane (through the upper limb) and partially onto the affected lower limb, then the unaffected lower limb is advanced.

2. Two-cane gaits are similar to the point gaits used in crutch walking (see section II.B.1).

III. Gait patterns using gait aids for elevation activities involve stair climbing with stair-climbing walker, crutches, or cane. Any gait aids may be used for negotiating ramps or curbs, although cane and crutches are more maneuverable than the walker. In general, the sequence for going up stairs or curb is to lead up with the unaffected ("good") lower limb followed by both the gait aid and the affected lower limb. When going down stairs or curb, the sequence is reversed, that is both the affected ("bad") lower limb and gait aid are simultaneously lowered first, followed by the good or unaffected lower limb. The mnemonics is the "good" goes up to heaven and the "bad" goes down to hell.

IV. Gait training program should be individualized based on patient's diagnosis, contraindications, and goals. Some of the following activities may be contraindicated for some patients (e.g., leg-crossing activities that involve hip adduction should not be used by patients with total hip replacements).

A. Preambulation programs are used to improve strength, coordination, and ROM;

facilitate proprioceptive feedback; develop postural stability; develop controlled mobility in movement transitions; and develop dynamic balance control and skills. **Standing aids** may be used for passive standing to control orthostatic hypotension and altered sense of body balance, to facilitate antigravity muscle action, to inhibit spasticity, to improve psychologic state, to decrease lower limb contractures, to prevent or retard osteoporosis, and to provide positioning for functional activities. Several designs of standing aids (stationary or mobile) exist including tilt tables, standing frames, and parapodiums.

1. **Basic mat activities** in different postures use the following progression: sidelying and rolling; prone-on-elbows and prone-on-hands; hooklying and bridging; quadruped; short and long sitting; kneeling and half-kneeling; modified plantigrade (modified standing position with trunk slight flexed so weight is supported on both hands resting on the table or plinth and on both feet standing on floor; the hips are slightly flexed, knees extended, and ankles dorsiflexed); and standing (if patient has postural or orthostatic hypotension, tilt table may be needed [see section IV.A]).

2. **Concurrent activities** include strengthening and coordination exercises, transfer training, and WC management and mobility.

B. **Parallel bars activities progression**

1. **Basic parallel bars activities.** Moving from sitting to standing and reverse, standing balance and weight-shifting activities, hip-hiking, standing pushups, stepping forward and backward, forward progression, use of appropriate gait pattern, and turning.

2. **Intermediate parallel bars activities** (if activities are not feasible within the parallel bars because bar width is not adjustable, these activities may be done outside and next to the parallel bars for added security). Moving from sitting to standing, and reverse, with assistive device; standing balance and weight shifting activities with assistive device; and use of assistive device (with selected gait pattern) for forward progression and turning.

3. **Advanced parallel bars activities** include walking sideward (sidestepping), walking backward, proprioceptive neuromuscular facilitation (PNF) braiding (combination of crossed and sidestep progression), and resisted forward progression (i.e., therapist provides manual resistance on the patient's pelvis or shoulder as patient walks forward) activities.

C. **Indoor progression** includes instruction and training use of assistive device for ambulation on level surfaces; elevation activities, including climbing stairs (if crutches or canes are used for stair climbing, handrails, if present, should be used), and if available indoors, negotiating ramps and curbs; opening doors and passing through doorways (including elevators) and over thresholds; and falling techniques (generally included for active ambulators requiring long-term use of assistive device).

D. **Outdoor progression** includes instruction and training in opening doors and passing through thresholds that lead outdoors; use of assistive device for ambulation on outdoor surfaces and uneven terrain; elevation activities, including climbing stairs, and negotiating ramps and curbs; crossing a street within the time allocated by a traffic light; and getting in and out of private and public transportation.

BIBLIOGRAPHY

Hennessey WJ, Johnson EW: Lower limb orthoses. In Braddom RL, editor: *Physical medicine and rehabilitation*, Philadelphia, 1996, WB Saunders, pp. 353-358.

Nash DL, Thompson JM: Ambulatory aids. In Sinaki M, editor: *Basic clinical rehabilitation medicine*, St. Louis, 1994, Mosby–Year Book, pp. 462-470.

Ragnarsson KT: Lower extremity orthotics, shoes, and gait aids. In DeLisa JA, Gans, BM, editors: *Rehabilitation medicine: principles and practice*, ed 2, Philadelphia, 1993, JB Lippincott, pp. 504-506.

Schmitz TJ: Preambulation and gait training. In O'Sullivan SB, Schmitz TJ, editors: *Physical rehabilitation: assessment and treatment*, Philadelphia, 1994, FA Davis, pp. 251-276.

Varghese G: Crutches, canes, and walkers. In Redford JB, editor: *Orthotics etcetera*, ed 3, Baltimore, 1986, Williams & Wilkins, pp. 453-463.

CHAPTER 4.7

MANUAL- AND POWERED-MOBILITY SYSTEMS

Wheeled mobility systems can be manually propelled (manual wheelchairs [WC] and attendant-propelled WCs) or externally powered (e.g., powered WCs, scooters). From a 1992 survey, there were more than 1 million users of wheeled mobility systems in the United States, 75% of whom used manual WCs. Standards for wheeled mobility systems performance and safety have been established by the Rehabilitation Engineering Society of North America (RESNA), 1700 North Moore Street, Suite 1540, Arlington, VA 22209-1903, Tel. (703) 524-6686, and can be accessed from publications by National Rehabilitation Information Center (NARIC), 8455 Colesville Road, Suite 935, Silver Spring, MD 20910-3319, tel. (800) 346-2742 or (301) 588-9284 or through assistive-technology databases such as ABLE-DATA, tel. (800) 227-0216 or (301) 608-8998. This chapter gives an overview of wheeled mobility systems and seating systems for adults. Information resources on the manufacturers and suppliers of WCs and scooters can be found in Appendices G-8, G-9, and G-10.

I. **Manual WCs** are designed to be manually propelled by a patient with sufficient strength in both upper limbs (e.g., paraplegic or lower-limb amputee patients) or in at least one upper or lower limb (e.g., hemiplegic patients who can be taught to use foot-drive or one-hand-drive WC). They are indicated for patients whose ambulation is either *inadvisable* (e.g., when lower limbs are contraindicated from weight bearing or from assuming dependent positions such as during fracture healing; when prolonged walking is contraindicated because of poor endurance from various cardiopulmonary neuromusculoskeletal conditions; when walking is unsafe because of lower limb or postural instability) or *not functionally possible* (e.g., conditions involving loss of lower limb function such as spinal cord injury [SCI], bilateral amputation, multiple sclerosis [MS], stroke, trauma brain injury [TBI], cerebral palsy [CP], poliomyelitis, muscular dystrophy, arthritis, etc.).

  Absolute contraindications to manual WCs include ischial pressure ulcers, blindness, and poor judgment. Other **relative contraindications** include surgical or postoperative conditions of the pelvis or proximal femur, vertebral fractures, disc and nerve root compression, truncal weakness, and postural defects. If the WC is contraindicated because of ischial pressure ulcers, a gurney (adapted for self-propulsion in prone position) might be considered.

  Complications of manual WCs include back pain and deformities (can be prevented by proper positioning or seating), pressure ulcers (can be prevented by frequent weight shifting or reclining WCs), lower-limb contractures (can be prevented by frequent stretching of tight structures around pelvis, hips, and knees), and dependent lower-limb edema (can be prevented by elevating the legs and using compression garments).

  Wheelchair and seating prescriptions should be done with a team approach that includes the patient, the patient's family or support system, the physician, physical and occupational therapists, orthotist, rehabilitation engineer, rehabilitation technology supplier, social worker, case manager, nurse, and other allied health care professionals. The factors to consider in the prescription of manual WCs and seating systems include:

- The patient's diagnosis and residual abilities (including endurance, vision, cognition, intelligence level, judgment, perception, and motivation), that is, need for attendant-propelled WC, manually propelled WC, or powered mobility systems;
- The patient's expected duration of disability to determine if the WC should be purchased or rented (consider renting if the patient is expected to regain ambulation ability within a short period, e.g., 9 to 12 months, or if the patient only needs the WC periodically such as for prolonged trips);
- The patient's bodily dimension, i.e., need for a standard, heavy, lightweight, or ultralight WC;
- The patient's active or sedentary life-style as well as vocation and avocation;
- Proposed use of the WC, that is, as a primary means of mobility at home, school, work, and community, or as a backup system such as when bilateral leg prostheses are in for repair or when leg prostheses cannot be worn because of residual-limb ulcer, or for use only when showering, toileting, or when the walking terrain is hazardous (e.g., icy sidewalk);
- The need for WC portability, that is, folding versus nonfolding, or lightweight versus standard weight WC;
- Environmental accessibility in home, office, school, and recreational or other community facilities; consider the entrance, door width, turning radius in bathroom and hallways, floor surface, workspace design, etc. (see Chapter 4.5, section II.B.1.b and II.B.2.e for environmental adaptations for WC accessibility);
- Financial resources, that is, bottom of the line versus top of the line WC; and
- Other factors such as availability of WC parts, WC repair, and WC trial opportunity.

If the manual WC is prescribed for temporary use, patients must be encouraged to learn to walk when indicated (with appropriate braces, prostheses, crutches, and hard work) so as not to make them dependent on the WC. Unlike prescription of WCs for children, growth in length is no longer an important factor; however, adult WCs may need adjustability for changes in girth or progression of disease (e.g., amyotrophic lateral sclerosis [ALS], or multiple sclerosis). Two other major considerations in manual WC prescription are proper WC fitting (see Fig. 4.7-1 for critical WC measurements) and proper WC seating and positioning.

Goals of proper WC seating and positioning include prevention of deformities and pressure ulcers, tone normalization, promotion of function (e.g., promote efficient use of upper limbs for propelling a manual WC or for activating switches of a power WC), increasing sitting comfort and tolerance, optimizing respiratory function, and provision of proper body alignment not only for propelling the manual WC or for moving within the WC, but also for keeping the patient alert and comfortable. For details on WC seating and positioning prescription, refer to textbooks by Letts or Mayall and Desharnais (see bibliography).

Manual WC checkout and training. Prior to writing the WC prescription, it is advisable to have the patient try a comparable WC (both indoors and outdoors) to evaluate his or her ability to learn to use the WC and to help the patient decide whether that particular type of WC is appropriate. After the prescribed WC is delivered, the clinician must test drive the WC to check the WC's performance as well as the function and safety of its parts. If everything meets the approval

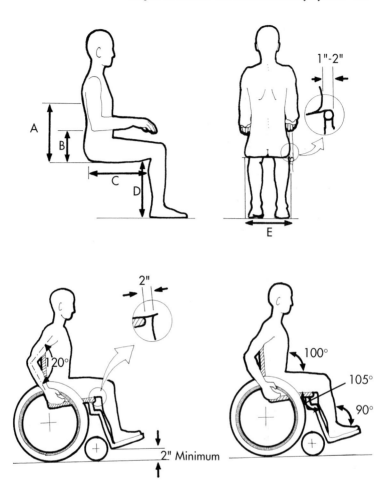

Figure 4.7-1

Critical measurements for wheelchair prescription. **A,** Back height (from seat) = distance from bottom of buttocks to level of scapulae. **B,** Arm height = distance from bottom of buttocks to olecranon with elbow fixed to 90°. **C,** Seat depth = distance between popliteal and back of buttocks (add 1-2 inches so that popliteal fold is clear from anterior edge of seat; alternative method for providing clearance of popliteal fold is to adjust the back cushion or footrest). **D,** Seat height (from floor) = length of leg from bottom of heel to popliteal fold (add 2 inches to provide clearance of footrest when approaching slopes and ramps; alternative method for providing clearance of footrest is to adjust seat cushion or footrest). **E,** Seat width (between uprights) = widest distance across hips (add 1-2 inches to take into account the patient's clothing or braces). The bottom figures show proper elbow, hip, knee, and ankle angles as well as proper footrest and popliteal clearance. (Adapted from Wilson A: *Wheelchairs: a prescription guide,* New York, 1992, Demos, with permission.)

of the prescribing physician, the patient tests the WC and necessary modifications can be made. The patient and caregivers are then trained in the safe use of the newly prescribed WC both indoors and outdoors (including traffic situations if appropriate), transfer techniques, WC transport (e.g., WC assembly and disassembly), WC maintenance (e.g., regular lubrication and cleaning of moving parts, bearing replacements, brake or lock adjustments, caring for batteries of power mobility systems, putting power mobility systems out of gear when not in use), and troubleshooting of common WC problems.

Some important biomechanical and ergonomic principles of WC design and propulsion include:

• *Rolling resistance* refers to the inherent resistance of rolling, which is affected by the weight distribution between the front and the rear wheels (i.e., rolling resistance is reduced by moving the seat [the center of gravity] rearward or by moving the wheel axle forward), type of tire (i.e., solid tires have lower rolling resistance than pneumatic tires; narrower tires have less rolling resistance than wider tires), wheel alignment (i.e., symmetric toeing error with a malalignment of as little as 2 degrees can increase rolling resistance quite dramatically; see section I.A.2.a for description of "toe-in" vs. "toe-out"), and type of floor or ground surface (i.e., a flat, hard surface provides the lowest rolling resistance, while carpeting, rough terrain, and even small inclines or slopes greatly increase rolling resistance and the energy cost of WC propulsion).

• *Propulsion efficiency* is improved by positioning the user more rearward (so the center of gravity is closer to the axle and the elbows are flexed at about 120 degrees during propulsion; see Fig. 4.7-1). This minimizes energy consumption and uses gravity to aid the recovery phase of propulsion, thus making the return to the starting position of the stroke more horizontal and more efficient. In contrast, in WCs in which the user is positioned more anteriorly, the propulsion stroke is predominantly downward, and the user requires excessive internal rotation, extension, and elevation of the shoulders during the recovery phase to grab the rim for the next stroke of the wheel.

• *Downhill-turning tendency (side-slope effect)* refers to the tendency of the WC to turn downhill when the WC moves longitudinally along an inclined surface such as on a slightly tilted sidewalk (this is ever prevalent because most outdoor surfaces have a 1- to 2-degree slope to aid in drainage). A 2-degree slope results in a nearly twofold increase in effort required for forward propulsion. This increased propulsion effort can be reduced by moving the seat and center of gravity rearward relative to the rearwheel axle and also by widening the camber (see description below).

• *Yaw-axis control (maneuverability)* refers to the ease of altering the direction of the WC and involves overcoming the polar moment of inertia of the WC (i.e., the greater the moment of inertia, the more difficult it is to change WC direction). To increase yaw-axis control, the moment of inertia can be reduced by moving the seat rearward, thereby decreasing the distance from the main axis to the center of gravity (i.e., by providing a shorter lever arm).

• *Pitch-axis control (wheelie control or dynamic stability)* refers to rotation at the axle in an anterior and posterior direction, thereby affecting the ease of tipping the WC backward during propulsion or while "popping wheelies." Wheelies, which are performed by the WC user (e.g., when negotiating curbs), refer to the lifting of the front casters off the ground while balancing and/or turning on the rearwheels. During wheelies, the WC user leans the trunk forward to counterbalance the backward tipping force. The ease of performing wheelies can be increased by moving the seat rearward, however, this also increases the backward tipping tendency of the WC, which can be detrimental to users with poor trunk balance and control.

- *Static stability* refers to the tipping angle or stability in the forward-to-rear and side-to-side directions while the chair is stationary (both with and without the wheels locked). The side-to-side static stability can be determined by the camber (see below), while the forward-to-rear static stability can be determined by the relation of the seat or center of gravity to the rearwheel axle. The longer the distance between the rear wheel axle and the center of gravity (i.e., by placing the seat in a relatively forward position), the greater the forward-to-rear static stability. In contrast, placing the seat in a relatively rearward position decreases forward-to-rear static stability. For active users with good trunk balance and control, a rearward seat position is recommended (despite the decrease in static stability, which is easily compensated by leaning forward) because it improves pitch-axis control and decreases angular displacement.

- *Camber* refers to a position in which the bottom parts of the propelling wheels are further apart than the top parts of the wheels (see Fig 4.7-3 H). The camber of a standard WC is 7 degrees (range of 3-9°), but in sports WCs, the camber is usually widened (i.e., tilt angle is increased) by adding different camber washers. A wider camber leads to increased side-to-side as well as the forward stability of the WC, increased ease of WC rolling at higher speeds (camber has little or no effect on rolling resistance at regular speed), decreased WC turning radius (i.e., increased WC maneuverability), reduced downhill-turning tendency, and also increased protection of the user's hands from doorways or other players in sports. The disadvantages of a wide camber include greater wear and tear on the tires and wheel bearings; the need for a wider track, which may cause difficulty in tight spaces; increased tendency of WC to toe-out during a wheelie in proportion to the wheelie angle (even if the wheels are perfectly aligned when all four wheels are on the ground); and decreased rear stability. The decrease in rear stability is associated with a 3.9-fold increased risk of injuries because of instability unless compensatory measures are done (e.g., moving the rear wheel axle rearward, positioning loads closer to the front, or using antitipping devices).

- **Weight/Portability.** The weight of the WC can be heavy (>50 lb or 23 kg), standard (40-50 lb or 18-23 kg), lightweight (20-40 lb or 9-18 kg), and ultralight (15-20 lb or 7-9 kg, e.g., ''sports'' WCs; see section I.B.4). Wheelchair weight is important when considering WC transportability, but it does not have a significant effect on the overall energy cost of wheeling when propelling on a flat surface. When propelling uphill, however, WCs with lighter weight are more energy efficient. Other factors such as weight distribution in the WC and efficiency of propulsion have a greater impact on WC function than simply considering the overall weight of the WC. Although lighter WC models are generally technologically superior and more energy efficient, they tend to be more expensive and are not indicated for every WC user. The standard WC is indicated for temporary use, short-distance dependent mobility, or for some part-time users who have some walking ability. The heavy WCs are indicated for persons over 250 lb (>114 kgs) or needing more than 20 inches (>51 cm) WC width.

A. Parts and subtypes of manual WCs (see Fig. 4.7-2)

1. Frame

a. Folding (X-shaped) frame WCs are the most common frames for manual

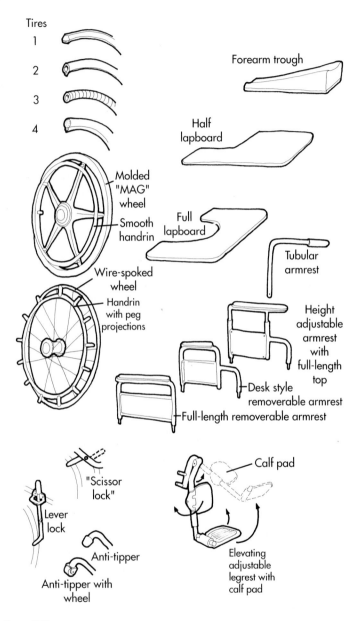

Figure 4.7-2.

Parts of a manual wheelchair. Types of pressure-relief seat cushions: **A,** Contoured foam (Veterans Administration Spinal Injury Orthosis [VASIO]); **B,** Contoured foam base with gel-filled pad (Jay cushion); **C,** Viscoelastic foam with casing; **D,** Polyurethane foam; **E,** Gel enclosed in a nonbreathing plastic casing; **F,** Air-filled villous ROHO cushion; **G,** Water-filled seat cushion. Types of tires: **1,** Solid hard-

CUSHIONS

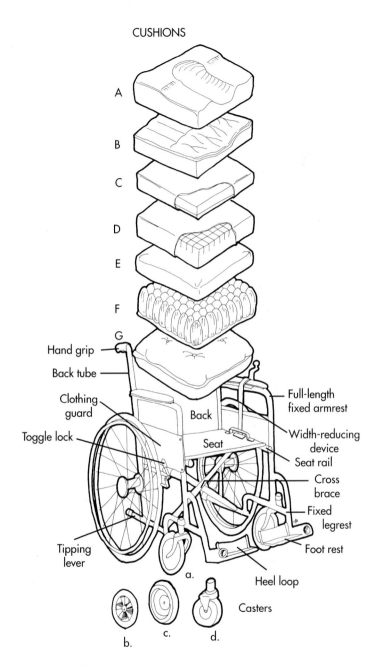

Figure 4.7-2. cont'd
rubber tire; **2,** Pneumatic inner tube; **3,** Semipneumatic tire with coil-reinforced
zero pressure tire (ZPT) inner tube; **4,** Semipneumatic tire with solid foam ZPT
inner tube. Types of casters: **a,** Standard 8-inch diameter with solid rubber tire; **b,**
8-inch diameter with semipneumatic tire; **c,** 8-inch diameter with pneumatic tire;
d, 5-inch diameter with solid rubber tire.

WCs because they are easy to fold and transport. They also provide a smoother ride than rigid-frame WCs because their greater flexibility make it more likely that all four wheels will remain in contact with uneven terrain. However, they have more moving parts and are thus heavier and less energy efficient (because propelling energy is lost or wasted to the torque in the crossframe) than rigid frame WCs. The folding WC can be made narrower temporarily by a few inches by turning the crank of the narrowing (or width-reducing) device (see Fig. 4.7-2) which through a gear mechanism provides the necessary force to slightly fold the WC frame.

b. Rigid-frame WCs are nonfolding and are thus more difficult and cumbersome to transport (despite models with quick-release wheels and a fold-down back). Rigid-frame WCs are commonly used in institutions and are used in "sports" WCs (see section I.B.4) because of their energy efficiency (i.e., compared to X-frame WCs, the wheels of rigid WCs are easier to align precisely thus resulting in less rolling resistance and in greater propelling efficiency). The applied forces (for propulsion and turning) are also not damped because of the WCs rigidity.

2. Propulsion

a. Propelling wheels. The diameter of the propelling wheels of rearwheel-drive WCs is usually 24 inches (61 cm). To decrease the WC height, smaller diameter propelling wheels (e.g., 20- or 22-inch [51- or 56-cm] rear wheels) can be used. The alignment of the propelling wheel also affects the WCs function. The propelling wheel can either be "toed-in" (i.e., the front parts of the wheels are closer to each other than the back parts) or "toe-out" (opposite of "toe-in"). A symmetric toeing error increases rolling resistance, while nonsymmetrical toeing error may cause the WC to deviate persistently to one side. In WCs with axle adjustment plates, the toeing error can be corrected by adding washers under the front or back bolts, but in WCs with axles housed in a tube of fixed alignment, the tube can be rotated.

1) Wheel placement

a) Rearwheel-drive WC (see Fig. 4.7-3), which has propelling wheels placed at the rear (behind the casters) are the most common type of manual WC propelling wheels.

b) Frontwheel-drive WC (unjustifiably known as the "traveler" or "indoor" WC; see Fig. 4.7-3), which is typically used indoors (especially in small rooms, but may also be used outdoors if there are no curbs), has the advantage of being 1 to 3 inches (2.5-7.5 cm) shorter in length (thus requiring less space for turning) and being better balanced posteriorly (thus decreasing the risk of tipping backwards, especially in lower-limb amputees) than the rearwheel-drive WC. The large propelling wheels of the frontwheel-drive WC, which usually have a diameter of 26 inches (66 cm), help overcome the irregularities of streets and roads leading to a smoother WC ride with less vibration; however, when compared to rearwheel-drive WCs, they tend to veer from side to side and, in general, are much more tiring to propel and more difficult to maneuver (for the occupant as well as for the person pushing it) when used over curbs and particularly over stairs.

2) Wheel construction (see Fig. 4.7-2)

a) Molded (plastic-molded) wheels, also called "mag" wheels, because

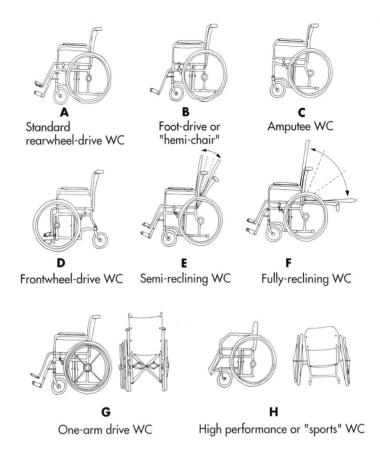

A
Standard
rearwheel-drive WC

B
Foot-drive or
"hemi-chair"

C
Amputee WC

D
Frontwheel-drive WC

E
Semi-reclining WC

F
Fully-reclining WC

G
One-arm drive WC

H
High performance or "sports" WC

Figure 4.7-3

Types of manual wheelchair (WC). Foot-drive or hemi-chair (**B**) has about 2-inch lower seat than standard WC (**A**) and has only one front rigging. Amputee WC (**C**) has rearwheels moved about 1.25 to 2 inches (3-5 cm) toward the rear to compensate for the posterior shift of center of gravity of seated bilateral amputees. The front-wheel drive WC (**D**) is typically used indoors. The semireclining WC (**E**) has back upholstery 5 inch (13 cm) higher than that of a standard WC, and the wheel is set back 1.25 inch (3 cm) toward the rear. Fully reclining wheelchair (**F**) has back upholstery 7 inches (17 cm) higher than that of a standard WC, and the wheel is set back 5 inches (12 cm) toward the rear. The (**G**) one-hand drive WC (WC in illustration is left-hand drive) has driving wheels interconnected so that either or both can be controlled from one side through a dual set of handrims. The high-performance or ''sports'' WC (**H**) is very light and has wider camber (i.e., lower part of wheel is tilted outwards).

they were originally made out of magnesium, are the most commonly used wheels in nonsports WCs. They are heavier but more durable and need less maintenance than spoked wheels.

b) **Wire-spoked wheels** are lighter (preferred in most sports WCs), less durable (because the spokes tend to bend with heavy use), need greater maintenance (e.g., to tighten loosened spokes), and are less safe for elderly patients whose fingers may get caught in the spoked wheels.

b. **Rear-wheel axles.** The rearwheel axles can be fixed or adjustable. In patients who are expected to progress in their rehabilitation, an adjustable rearwheel axle is preferred because the optimal site of axle placement may change as the patient improves. Axle placement can be adjusted either in the vertical direction (i.e., up or down to vary WC height, improve positioning, and allow the user to reach the floor with the "good" foot [e.g., in WCs used by hemiplegics]) or in the horizontal direction (i.e., anterior or posterior placement). The horizontal adjustment of the axle relative to the seat or the center of gravity determines the WC's stability and efficiency. The most important factor to consider in axle placement is safety, in addition to the height, weight, build, and functional abilities of the WC user. An inappropriate axle position relative to the center of gravity can lead to accidental WC tipping and falls; this in fact accounts for the majority of WC accidents (which happen to 3.3% of wheelchair users each year).

1) **Posteriorly placed axle** (i.e., the seat or center of gravity is relatively anterior). This increases WC rear stability (advantageous for the elderly or patients with poor trunk stability, for amputees, and for reclining or posterior tilting WCs). However, there is a tradeoff of increased WC rolling resistance, greater turning radius (i.e., decreased WC maneuverability), increased downhill turning tendency, and decreased ease of doing wheelies (due to difficulty to tilt the WC backwards).

2) **Anteriorly placed axle** (i.e., the seat or center of gravity is relatively posterior). This increases WC anterior stability and leads to decreased rolling resistance, decreased turning radius (i.e., greater maneuverability), and decreased downhill turning tendency; however, it increases the tendency of the WC to tip backwards when accelerating quickly or going up ramps. Anteriorly placed axles are advantageous for active paraplegics with good trunk balance and control who do wheelies to negotiate curbs; however, they are undesirable for patients with bilateral LE amputations, because the lack of forward-placed LE weight puts the sitting center of mass farther backward and makes it even easier for the WC to tip backward.

c. **Handrims** (see Fig. 4.7-2), which are used for selfpropulsion of the WC, are smaller in diameter than the propelling wheel and are attached slightly lateral to the propelling wheel to permit WC control without soiling the hands. Handrims can be modified for patients with poor handgrip by increasing the handrim's thickness (disadvantage of adding weight and width to the WC); adding rubberized coatings to the handrim (disadvantage of the coating wearing off with time, discoloring the hands, or becoming rough, thus causing hand injuries); or attaching knobby projections (pegs or lugs; see Fig 4.7-2) to the handrim with varied spacing and angle (e.g., vertical or oblique) for easy gripping and handrim control by patients with tetraplegia or hand deformities. In most cases, the best way to improve handrim grip is simply by having the patient wear a pair of sports gloves.

1) **Large handrim diameters** make it easier to propel the WC and are used in most WCs because they provide greater power and maneuverability. However, more arm strokes are required to cover a given distance.

2) **Small handrim diameters** are used in sports WCs to maximize the distance covered with each stroke (although more force is required to propel them).

d. **Casters** (see Fig. 4.7-2) are the small steering wheels found on the front of the rearwheel-drive WCs or on the back of frontwheel-drive WCs. Front casters on rearwheel-drive WCs are easily damaged, have downhill-turning tendencies, and tend to flutter (shimmy) at higher speeds. Caster flutter (shimmy) is not only annoying but can also increase rolling resistance and may cause an unintentional change in WC direction. Caster shimmy at normal rolling speeds can be reduced by decreasing the size and weight of the caster, increasing the caster trail (i.e., the distance on the ground between the two casters), or increasing the proportion of the weight on the casters.

1) **Large and wide casters.** For most purposes, 8-inch (20-cm) diameter caster of relatively wide configuration are optimal because these are easier to use on rougher outdoor terrain. Larger diameter casters also make it easier to climb curbs but have more of a tendency to flutter or shimmy. However, large and wide casters provide increased rolling resistance on smooth, level surfaces.

2) **Small and narrow casters.** Casters of 5-inch or 13-cm diameters (often used in sports WCs) and narrow widths are easier to maneuver and are suited for smooth, level surfaces. However they perform poorly on rough outdoor terrain, as they can get stuck on uneven terrain or soft ground, thus causing the chair to tip forward.

e. **Tires** (see Fig 4.7-2) refer to wheel parts fitted onto the rims of the propelling wheels and casters. Narrow tires have less rolling resistance and are suitable for use on hard, flat, indoor surfaces but require much more force to propel through uneven surfaces and are thus not suited for outdoor use. Wide tires are easier to propel on uneven outdoor surfaces but have greater rolling resistance.

1) **Solid (hard rubber) tires** (see Fig. 4.7-2) with smooth treads are very durable and have a low rolling resistance, especially on flat, smooth, and hard indoor surfaces but are relatively heavy and yield a harsh ride when used on uneven, outdoor terrain. They are recommended if the WC is to be used mostly indoors (e.g., in the hospital or nursing home) because the cushioning provided by pneumatic tires is not required for indoor use.

2) **Pneumatic tires** (see Fig. 4.7-2), which use an outer tire casing with an air-filled innertube, are relatively lighter and provide the cushioning needed for outdoor use on uneven terrain not only to give a smooth comfortable ride but also to reduce the wear and tear on the WC when used under normal outside conditions. If treaded pneumatic tires (''clincher'' tires) are used, they also improve traction. The ''all-terrain'' tire has a wider tire with a different tread. The disadvantages of pneumatic tires include high rolling resistance on flat, smooth surfaces and also the tendency to develop a ''flat'' tire. To minimize this ''flat'' tire problem, thorn-resistant innertubes may be used.

3) Semipneumatic tires (see Fig. 4.7-2) uses flat-free inserts (zero-pressure tubes or ZPTs), which eliminate the flat tire problem. The ZPTs can either be a coil type of soft rubber, latex gel, or a solid innertube of foam (see Fig. 4.7-2), which replaces the innertubes. They provide slightly rougher rides than that of pneumatic tires and also add weight to the WC.

3. **Seating systems:** Fig. 4.7-1 shows the critical measurements needed for WC fitting. The usual measurements for a standard adult WC are seat height above the ground (19.5-20.5 inches or 49.5-52.0 cm), seat width (16-18 inches or 41-46 cm), and seat depth (16-18 inches or 41-46 cm). If orthotics are worn, a clearance of 1-2 inches (2.5-5.0 cm) is required on each side. Seat depth is important because if it is too short, the thighs are poorly supported and the area over which forces are distributed is reduced thus causing more pressure; however, if it is too deep, pressure ulcers may develop in the popliteal space, or the patient may tend to slide forward thus increasing sacral pressure and promoting kyphotic postures. The seat-plane angle (i.e., angle of the seat plane relative to the horizontal plane), which is usually 1 to 4 degrees higher in front, may be increased to reduce spasticity, exaggerated lumbar lordosis, and the tendency of the patient to slide forward on the seat. However, it puts more pressure on the ischial tuberosities and makes transfers more difficult.

a. **Seat types**

1) **Sling (hammock) seats** consist of a tautly stretched flexible upholstery suspended between the WC seat rails (see Fig. 4.7-2). They are the most commonly used WC seats and can be considered a ''planar seating'' because they provide a flat seating surface in contact with the body. They are lightweight and easy to fold but provide little support, cannot adequately stabilize the pelvis, and thus can cause an increased incidence of posterior pelvic tilt (because of the tendency of the hips to slide forward), pelvic obliquity, internal rotation, and adduction at the hips (a position generally to be avoided by patients with total hip replacement as it may lead to hip dislocation). The upholstery commonly used is vinyl, which is inexpensive, durable, easy to clean, and comes in a number of colors; however, vinyl tends to cause heat build-up and promote perspiration. Alternatives to vinyl are Dacron and nylon, which are lighter in weight and more breathable, but are less easy to clean.

2) **Solid seats** are usually indicated for posture control. The solid seat design can be planar or linear (i.e., use of flat support surfaces such as flat foam seats), contoured (i.e., use of seats with human contours [e.g., buttocks] shaped by carving or sculpting foams, building with pads and blocks, or using preformed shapes based on research about human contours), modular (i.e., use of prefabricated planar or contoured designs with adjustable and removable components for positioning and stabilization), or custom-molded (i.e., use of seats created from the casted shape or mold taken from the person's body contours; indicated for patients with complex seating and positioning needs; may utilize CAD-CAM, i.e., **C**omputer-**A**ssisted **D**esign and **C**omputer-**A**ssisted **M**anufacturing).

a) **Removable solid seats** can consist of a firm foam insert with a convex lower surface, a flat upper surface, and a cushion on top, or, alternatively, a cushioned plywood base. They are often placed on top of the sling seat to provide better support and decrease sling sagging.

b) Nonremovable solid seats may be used, but they are not easily modified and they also add weight to the WC. They can have a folding design for easy transportability.

c) Drop seat base (drop-hook seats) are used to lower a solid seat surface below the level of the seat rails (usually up to a maximum of 5 cm or 2 inches) so as to provide a level base of support and prevent buildup of the seat height when cushions are added. Suspension hooks may be used to lower the seat base.

b. Pressure-relief seat cushions (see Fig. 4.7-2) are designed to counteract or to minimize stresses that act perpendicular to the skin (i.e., loading pressure) as well as stresses that act parallel to the skin (i.e., shear forces or stresses), both of which may lead to pressure ulcers. The common causes of pressure ulcers in WCs include patient's inability to shift weight; minimal adipose tissue and/or loss of muscle mass over the buttocks; pelvic obliquity (seen in "wind-swept" deformities in which one hip is abducted and one hip adducted causing the legs to appear unequal in length) caused by the "hammock effect" of sling seats, which leads to shearing forces; slumped sitting postures (i.e., sacral sitting) or posterior pelvic tilt, which can cause increased sacral pressure; and poor health or nutritional status. Aside from patient factors (e.g., bowel or bladder continence or presence of spasticity or flaccidity), other important factors to consider in cushion selection include moisture resistance (especially in incontinent patients or in places with hot, humid weather), ease of cushion maintenance and cleaning, weight of the cushion (if it is necessary to transport the cushion), and the cushion's durability and cost.

The design of pressure-relief cushions can either be total contact (to equalize or redistribute weight bearing over a maximal surface area), or specific pressure relief (achieved by carving out the cushion under bony prominences), or a combination of both. Static as well as dynamic pressure-relief cushions are available (see Chapter 5.2, section VI.B.3.a) for descriptions, advantages, and disadvantages). The standard WC cushion is a foam cushion; however, for wheelchair users with high risk of developing pressure ulcers, the two most commonly used static pressure-relief cushions are air- or fluid-filled cushions. At present, studies have shown that no single type of cushion is superior at relieving all types of pressure ulcers for all patients. Each cushion has its own advantages and disadvantages, which should be considered before prescribing any particular type of cushion. The decision about the cushion to be used should be made early because it affects other dimensions of the WC (e.g., backrest, armrest, and seat height). The following are some of the common static pressure-relief WC seat cushions, which can be customized to provide optimal pressure distribution while helping to control posture:

1) Foam seat-cushions (see Fig. 4.7-2) are used in standard WCs because they are lightweight, inexpensive, and have breathable coverings. However, they are not washable, they wear out faster than other types of cushion, and they are not good dissipators of heat (because foams are heat insulators). Foam cushions are usually made of 7.5-cm (3-inch) medium-density polyurethane foams. They can also be made of viscoelastic foams (see Fig. 4.7-2C) which are less resilient than polyurethane foams (see Fig. 4.7-2D). The shape of foam cushions can be modified by placing a ramp on the anterior part of the cushion or by using a wedge-shaped foam cushion anteriorly (to promote hip flexion as well as transfer weight from the sacral, coccygeal, and ischial regions to the thighs for a better pelvic position, control, and stability, which may be beneficial in patients with spasticity); by using a preischial bar (to counteract forward sliding and transfer pressure from the sacral, coccygeal, and ischial regions to the thighs); by using cut-out designs in the areas underlying bony prominences to relieve pressure; or by coating it and contouring it to the shape of the buttocks to decrease skin-to-cushion interface pressures. An example of contoured foam is the Veterans Administration Spinal Injury Orthosis (VASIO) (see Fig. 4.7-2A), in which foams of two different densities are combined and contoured to meet the needs of the paraplegic patient. The use of a foam coating increases the foam cushion's durability and ease of cleaning but also increases heat build-up and are more expensive. Wedge-shaped foam cushions attached to a solid plywood base are also commercially available (e.g., KSS Seat Base).

2) **Gel-filled seat cushions** consist of a firm emulsion (gel) enclosed in a ''nonbreathing'' plastic casing (see Fig. 4.7-2E). They are used to decrease peak pressures over bony prominences, accommodate movement and position shifts of the user, and provide postural stability. The most popular commercial brand is the Jay cushion (see Fig. 4.7-2B), which consists of a contoured foam base (that can incorporate medial and lateral thigh as well as hip support) and a fluid-filled pad (which pockets into the depression created for the ischial tuberosities and is covered with a washable cover). The gel of the newer Jay-2 cushion has a ''memory'' that provides optimal conformation. Jay cushions can also be fitted with modular components. They are durable, easy to maintain and clean, and have high heat capacity (because fluids are moderate conductors of heat) thus helping dissipate skin heat buildup (and decrease the risk of skin breakdown due to overheating). However, they are expensive; tend to be heavy (weight varies from 8-35 lb), which may hinder portability; and some patients may find difficulty with transfer techniques because of the contouring that it provides.

3) **Air-filled villous (ROHO) seat cushions** (see Fig. 4.7-2F), consist of multiple balloonlike air cells, which the patient sits ''in'' to assure maximum skin contact and conformity. The high-profile ROHO cushion (with 10-cm or 4-inch high air cells) is the cushion of choice in preventing and healing pressure ulcers in long-term or high-risk sitting. The low-profile ROHO cushion (with 5-cm or 2-inch high air cells) is used for active patients with less potential for development of pressure ulcers. ROHO cushions can also be custom contoured for asymmetric patients (e.g., unilateral amputees). ROHO cushions are lightweight, easy to clean, and easy to transport. They are expensive, however, and do not provide good seating stability. They are, thusly, not recommended for patients who tend to slide forward in their WC or who have a poor sitting position due to increased extensor tone. The ROHO seating stability can be improved by decreasing air-cell inflation. Patients (especially those with decreased lateral stability due to trunk

weakness) may have difficulty transferring sideways to another surface because of the ROHO's soft and freely moving surface. The ROHO air pressure needs to be maintained regularly for skin protection and seating stability. In terms of their ability to control heat and moisture collection, air cushions are rated between fluid and foam cushions.

4) **Water-filled seat cushions** (see Fig. 4.7-2G) consist of a plastic or rubber membrane filled with chemically treated water or other liquid. The overall effect varies with the amount of water used. They adjust to body movements, are easy to clean, and can decrease temperature on the support surface. They may, however, leak if punctured and are relatively more heavy and difficult to transport.

5) **Combination air- and fluid-filled seat cushions (e.g., Bard Flotation cushion)** consist of a water-filled cushion (to assure even pressure distribution) and an air-filled frame (which prevents sacral sitting and sliding forward in the WC by maintaining the femurs parallel to the seat). They are effective in preventing sacral sliding when 100 degrees of hip flexion cannot be achieved due to mild extension contractures or when patients have increased extensor tone or extensor spasm in the lower limbs or of the whole body. However, they are relatively heavy and difficult to transport.

c. **Seat support and positioning aids** include antithrust designs, pelvic wells, pelvic stabilizers, pelvic bars, pelvic belts, lateral pelvic supports, anterior pelvic supports, medial thigh supports, lateral thigh supports, thigh troughs, abductor wedges, medial knee blocks (abductor pommels), and lateral knee blocks (adductor cushion). A key goal in WC seating is to stabilize the pelvis because, during upright seating, 80% of the trunk weight is borne directly by the pelvis. Patients with pelvic obliquities or other deformities may need special custom-molded seats. Often the seat can be designed to place the patient in a position in which gravity helps stabilize the trunk and the head into the contours of the seat. Although firmer cushions generally provide a better base of support, they may be inappropriate in some patients who are insensate.

4. **Head and neck support and positioning systems** include foam headrests (flat, curved, three-piece, occipital supports, circumferential collars, horseshoe collars, customized), hook-on headrests (i.e., backrest extensions), telescopic headrests, pillow headrests, crown head supports (with headbands), and commercially available head and neck support systems (e.g., QA2 Headrest, KSS Neck Support, and Otto Bock Head and Neck Supports). A reclining WC (see section I.B.5) or tilt-in-space WC (see section I.B.6) may be used to hold the head back.

5. **Trunk support system**

a. **Primary trunk supports (backrests)** can be slings attached to the WC back frame posts (i.e., back tubes; see Fig. 4.7-2). They are made of similar upholsteries as those used in sling seats (described in section I.A.3.a.1). They can also be solid (i.e., removable and placed over sling seats or folding), adjustable (i.e., in height and tension), or customized. The frame posts for the backrests are usually fitted with push handles to allow another person to propel and maneuver the WC. Some WC users, however, prefer not to have push handles because they connote a certain amount of dependence. The backrest height determines the WC user's desired level of control and mobility, that is, higher backrests give more support (to the spine and also to the head) but less freedom of mobility. Lower backrests, however, provide greater freedom of movement to the upper body and trunk but give almost no spinal or head support at all and can lead to a slumped "sacral seating" posture with a tendency toward development of thoracic kyphosis.

An ideal backrest height should provide sufficient support to the user, maintain good posture, and prevent fatigue over an extended time, while affording as much movement as possible without forcing the user into poor posture. In all cases the backrest should provide good support for the lumbosacral spine. In a standard WC, the backrest height is usually 16 to 16.5 inches (41-42 cm) with about 8 degrees of backward tilt from the vertical. This backrest height reaches up to the midback at about 1 to 2 inches (2.5-5 cm) below the inferior angles of the scapulae to minimize scapular irritation from rubbing during propulsion. The backrest width is similar to the seat width. In general, tetraplegic patients require higher backrest heights, but paraplegic patients (with normal trunk control, strong arms, and no spinal deformity) usually do well with a standard or lower backrest height. Wheelchair users with varying needs through-out the day can be given WCs with adjustable backrest heights.

b. Secondary trunk positioning and support aids include foam side cushions, hook-on headrests, padded chest restraints (with or without shoulder straps), chest belts, Posey "Y" WC safety belts, Otto-Bock sternal supports, Otto-Bock spherical side thoracic supports, lateral supports with padded arm rests, padded lateral supports, back cushions, lumbar backrest cushions, soft T-foam back cushions, firm contoured back supports (e.g., Jay Active Back, KSS Back, QA2 Seatback with thoracic support, Jay Back, Jay Care Back, and Avanti Personal Back), modular back supports (e.g., Jay Modular Back), and sacral supports. A reclining WC (see section I.B.5) or tilt-in-space WC (see section I.B.6) may be used to support the back. Wheelchair restraints for maintaining posture and stability should only be used as a last resort as they make it almost impossible to do weight-shifting maneuvers for pressure relief.

6. Upper-limb support and positioning systems
   a. Primary arm support (armrests) are used to provide not only support for the patient's arms in a resting attitude (for maintaining balance and stability) but also to provide lateral support as well as serve as points of pushoff for weight shifting (to assist in transfers or for relief of buttock pressure). The WC armrest height should be such that the WC user does not lean to either side when using the WC armrest, and it should not interfere with arm movement, hand function, manual propulsion of the WC. These conditions are easily met by using adjustable height armrests (although they weigh more than any other armrests). The armrest height of the standard adult WC is 9 inches (23 cm). Prior to specifying the WC's armrest height, the thickness of the seat cushion must be taken into account. Some models of sports WCs have lightweight tubular armrests (see Fig. 4.7-2) or no armrests at all. The following are different types and styles of armrests, which can be combined to produce at least 12 different styles (except, obviously, for the "fixed style with adjustable height" combination).
      1) Fixed versus nonfixed armrests
         a) Fixed armrests (see Fig. 4.7-2) are continuous parts of the WC frame and are not detachable. They are inexpensive and cannot be lost;

however, they make WC fitting more difficult, limit the proximity of the WC to the table or desk surface, and prohibit side transfers (thus they are impractical if the patient is unable to stand for a brief period). They are usually found in WCs used in airports or train stations or for hospital transport and are rarely found in prescription WCs (except in some sports WC models).

b) Nonfixed armrests

(1) Removable armrests (see Fig. 4.7-2) are commonly used because they can be detached to allow for side transfers (in patients who are unable to stand up for transfers) and to increase the proximity of the WC to the table or desk surface. However, they increase the WC weight as well as WC width (the simplest type of removable armrest adds nearly 2 inches or 5 cm to the overall width of the standard WC). Removable armrests (see Fig. 4.7-2) are usually height-adjustable and can have either full-length or desk-style designs. To reduce the WC width, an offset design or a wrap-around design may be used.

(2) Flip-up (or swing-away) armrests have the same features as removable armrests except that instead of detaching the armrest, it is swung away or flipped up when performing side-approach transfers.

(3) Wrap-around (or space-saver) armrests reduce the width of the WC by attaching the armrest behind the backrest frame rather than next to the seat. They can generally be swung away or detached for transfers. They also allow the rear wheels to be placed closer to the WC frame thus narrowing the outside width of the WC without narrowing the seat width. The single functional disadvantage of the wraparound design is that the desk-style armrest cannot be reversed or turned end-for-end.

2) Full-length versus desk-style armrests. Both are available in fixed, nonfixed, or adjustable-height models.

a) Full-length armrests (see Fig. 4.7-2) extend from the backrest to the front of the WC. They are indicated when the patient needs the full height of the front of the armrest to provide the leverage required to stand up from the WC or when lordosis, obesity, or some other physical factors make it necessary to use the front part of the armrest for support while the patient is sitting in the WC. However, they interfere with the ability to maneuver the WC close to table or desk surfaces.

b) Desk-style armrests (see Fig. 4.7-2) extend forward only partially (i.e., it is foreshortened at the forward one-third part) to allow the user to get close enough to a desk or table top for good working conditions. The removable desk-style armrests, which are the most popular, are usually reversible, i.e., they can be used to provide the desk-style feature, or turned end-for-end to the reversed position (i.e., with the foreshortened part at the back) to allow sit-to-stand transfers or provide better access of the arms to the wheels for propulsion. However, when desk-style armrests are used in the reversed position, there is no lateral support of the trunk through the armrests.

3) Fixed-height versus adjustable-height armrests:

a) Fixed-height armrests (see Fig. 4.7-2) are found in WCs with fixed armrests and nonfixed armrests (full-length or desk-style models). Their main disadvantage is their inability to accommodate individuals of different sizes.

   b) Adjustable-height armrests (see Fig. 4.7-2) generally have adjustments ranging 5 to 12 inches above the seat to accommodate arm positioning needs of individuals of different sizes. They are usually found in nonfixed armrests (full-length or desk-style models).

   b. Secondary arm support and positioning aids include arm troughs (see Fig. 4.7-2), which hold the forearms in place (arm troughs can be padded, flat, elevated [to control edema], and molded), swinging armrests (e.g., Otto-Bock Armrests and balanced forearm orthosis), shoulder support (anterior, posterior, superior), and elbow supports (elbow blocks).

   c. Laptrays or lapboards are table-like surfaces (half- or full-size; see Fig. 4.7-2), which are either attached to the armrests or used as a substitute for regular armrests. They are usually detachable or may have swing-away capabilities. They can be used for eating, reading, writing, and other activities as well as for holding objects (e.g., a communication board or a daily schedule) and for supporting the upper limbs and preventing shoulder subluxation (e.g., in hemiplegic patients). When properly adjusted for height, they promote good posture (particularly when the patient would otherwise have to lean forward to reach a working surface). Laptrays can be made of wood (e.g., plywood), opaque plastic, or clear plastic (to allow visualization of the lower limbs, the front rigging of the WC, and the floor, thus helping to reduce the possibility of traumatizing the feet or toes). For certain activities, a laptray with an extra shelf may be useful. Laptray use in frontwheel-drive WCs makes WC propulsion slightly more difficult.

7. Lower-limb support and positioning systems. Optimal lower-limb support and positioning (see Fig. 4.7-1 for proper angulation of the hips, knees, and ankle joints) play important roles in improving the distribution of pressure over the sacrum and ischial tuberosities. In an upright seated position, the forces produced at the weight-bearing surfaces of the buttocks are equal to the body weight minus the supporting forces provided by the footrests or floor. The lower legs (calves) usually do not require direct support if there is proper support of the thighs (seating surface) and feet (foot rest). In most WCs, the knees are positioned at a maximum of 60 to 70 degrees flexion. However, some WC models allow the knees to be hyperflexed (at >90° flexion) to provide tighter turns, get closer access to objects (counter, bathtub, or bed), protect the feet, ease transport of the WC, and inhibit spasticity. Some of the disadvantages of a hyperflexed knee position include difficulty in accommodating users with long legs, a need for smaller caster diameters to avoid the footrests hitting the swiveling casters when changing direction, and decreased effectiveness of the footrests as forward antitipping devices.

   a. Primary lower-limb support (front rigging). *Front rigging* is a collective term for legrest and footrest. Aside from supporting the lower limbs, the front rigging acts as a forward antitipper (i.e., it increases rearward stability). It may consist of fixed bars (nondetachable and nonelevating; see Fig. 4.7-2) that are continuous with the WC frame. Fixed front riggings have no "elevating legrest" but have footrests that may consist of footplates with heel hoops or may simply consist of a single horizontal bar with heel loops (as seen in sports WCs). Although fixed front riggings generally make the WC lighter and allow more freedom of movement of the lower limb for propulsion or other function, they may interfere with transfers and WC portability. Most WCs have nonfixed front riggings, which consist of the following:

1) **Legrests.** Legrests (see Fig. 4.7-2) refer to "elevating legrests" and the calf pads, which support the legs when the legrests are elevated. Legrests usually consist of elevating support brackets with swing-away or detachable mechanisms so they can be moved aside or detached when needed (e.g., for transfers; WC transport; and getting closer to a counter, bathtub, or bed). Some medical or surgical conditions that require leg elevation include dependent lower-limb edema, postsurgery of lower limb (e.g., to allow knee arthrodesis to fuse), knee contracture (i.e., elevating the legrest may help extend the knee), and casted leg. By elevating the legrests, there is decreased forward static stability (because the center of gravity is shifted forward), increased rolling resistance, and more difficulty maneuvering in tight places. The legrests may be elevated up to the level of the seating surface (i.e., a low pivot-point style) or they may project higher than the seat (i.e., goose-neck style). The goose-neck style is less desirable as it can interfere with transfers and provides a point of pressure contact with the leg.

2) **Footrests.** Footrests (see Fig. 4.7-2) consists of foot plates that can be swung up 90 degrees so that they are vertical to the floor to permit easy access to the chair by patients who can stand. They keep the feet off the floor (with the ankle in the neutral position), and they hold the posterior aspect of the distal thighs of paralyzed patients at a height above the front edge of the seat to maintain lower-limb circulation. The lowest point on the footrests (see Fig. 4.7-1) should be at least 2 inches (5 cm) above the floor to avoid being caught on obstacles and on incline transitions. Footrests should not be positioned so high above the floor as to force more weight backward onto the ischial tuberosities and increase the risk of ischial pressure ulcers; nor should they be positioned so low (or removed) as to increase the pressure at the distal thighs, increasing the chance for posterior pelvic tilt, and providing less support for forward leaning. The distance between the footplates and that front edge of the seat can be adjusted to alter the distribution of the loads over the thighs and buttocks.

b. **Secondary lower-limb support and positioning aids** include anterior knee supports, anterior leg supports, knee protectors for elevating legrests, legrest panels, board supports on legrests (legrest board, leg and footrest board), padded wooden legrests, amputee cushions, knee abductors, elevating blocks on foot plates, foot plate extensions, heel straps, foot positioners, wooden foot supports with posterior extensions, foot straps (figure-eight foot straps, ankle straps), ankle positioning aids (ankle positioning blocks, foot plates with adjustable angle sitting), and heel loops (heel loops, instead of calf supports of the legrest units, are often used in sports WCs as they reduce WC weight).

8. **Safety components**

a. **Parking locks (wheel locks)** are devices that put pressure on the propelling wheels or tires (or occasionally including casters for greater stability) to lock them into position (while parked) and prevent unintended rolling of the WC, either on an incline or during transfers. Parking locks should not be used nor be erroneously referred to as "brakes" because they are not intended to slow down a moving WC (this not only subjects the tires to unnecessary wear and tear but may cause sudden stopping and overturning of the WC). If the moving WC needs to be slowed down, the "brake" should be applied by the hand(s) on the handrim(s). Parking locks are usually attached to the sideframe of the WC and are available in either a push-to-lock or a pull-to-lock mechanism. Either mechanism has no distinct advantage as whatever is pushed to lock needs to be pulled to unlock and vice versa. In some WC models, the lock may be placed in the rear of the chair where the it can be activated only by an attendant or caregiver and not by the patient with cognitive deficits. Parking locks can be mounted in a high position with long handles for easy access (e.g. hemiplegic patients), or they can be mounted in a low position with short handles (preferred by active WC users because they do not interfere with their long pushing strokes or get in the way during transfers).

1) Toggle locks (see Fig. 4.7-2), which are used in most WCs, have a preset locking "power," which is turned on or off by moving the activating toggle. The activating toggle can consist of a vertical handle bar, or it can consist of a flat horizontal bar (i.e., a scissors-type lock [see Fig. 4.7-2] used in sports WCs as they present less hazard to the thumbs and hands during vigorous pushing).

2) Lever locks (see Fig. 4.7-2) can be set at different notches to provide varying degrees of holding power. They are advantageous for parking on steep inclines, but their use require greater upper limb control and strength.

b. Grade aids (or "**hill holders**") are spring-loaded devices that are activated only on uphill inclines to prevent the WC from rolling backward but do not interfere with forward motion. They are useful for patients with poor strength or endurance when propelling uphill (because they prevent the WC from rolling backwards between forward thrusts). Grade aids should not be used by active, strong WC users because they can become accidentally activated while the user is performing a wheelie, thus causing a backward tipping fall.

c. Antitip bars (antitippers; see Fig. 4.7-2) are extensions for the lower rail installed in the rear of the WC to prevent at-risk patients (e.g., above-knee amputees with a more posterior center of gravity) from falling backward in the WC. They can be fixed, removable, or can be turned to the "up" position (to help the WC user in negotiating curbs or incline transitions where the device might interfere or "ground" the WC). Antitippers may have wheels at their end, which will come in contact with the floor upon tipping, thus avoiding a sudden deceleration. Antitippers are generally not used by active WC users who practice wheelies to climb up curbs. The front rigging of the WC can be considered an antitipping device (as this increases rear stability). To prevent the WC from tipping forward, antitipping devices may be attached to the front rigging.

d. Seat belts, safety vests, and harnesses are described above under seat support and positioning systems as well as secondary support and positioning systems for the trunk and extremities.

B. Classification by WC user needs

1. The standard (conventional or basic) adult WC (see Fig 4.7-3) is typically made of steel tubings with a sling seat and back; has two large wheels in the rear, each fitted with a concentric handrim, which is turned by the WC user; has two small swiveling wheels (casters) in front; has a front rigging (with legrest and footrest); has a back height of 16 to 16.5 inches (41-42 cm), a seat depth and seat width of 16 to 18 inches (41-46 cm), a seat height of 19.5 to 20.5 inches (49.5-52 cm) from the floor, a weight of about 18 to 23 kgs (40-50 lb.), and usually an X frame that allows for folding of the WC. The standard WC is generally indicated for temporary use, short-distance dependent mobility, or for some part-time users who have some walking ability.

2. **Hemiplegic or one-arm amputee WCs**
   a. **One-arm-drive (or mono-drive) WCs** (see Fig 4.7-3) are designed to be operated with one arm, either right or left. Both handrims are typically mounted on one side. The first handrim is the usual handrim close to the wheel with which it is connected directly. The second handrim is mounted outside the first but is connected by an axle to the wheel on the other side. Turning both handrims moves the WC straight ahead, while turning one or the other handrim steers the WC. An alternative to this design is the use of a single hand-lever propulsion mechanism. The disadvantage of one-arm drive chairs is their increased width and weight. They are rarely used successfully by hemiplegic or one-arm amputee patients, as propelling them requires a fairly high degree of strength and coordination. However, some two-handed patients may find them useful when it is important to have one hand free (e.g., for work) while the other propels the chair.
   b. **Foot-drive (or low-seat) WCs** or **"hemi-chairs"** (see Fig 4.7-3) are practical alternatives to one-arm drive WCs (which are difficult to propel). The hemiplegic patient uses one handrim and one ''good'' foot (both feet may be used if feasible) to help propel and steer the WC. For the foot or feet to reach the ground, the seat is lowered by 2 inches or 5 cm (thus the seat height from the floor is about 17.5-18.5 inches [44.5-47 cm]), and one or both of the front riggings is removed. Lowering of the seat height can be accomplished by using 22-inch (56-cm) diameter wheels (which lower seat height by 1 inch) or by using drop-hook seats (see above section I.A.3.a.2.c).

3. **Lower-limb amputee WCs** (see Fig 4.7-3) are indicated for patients who have lost both lower-limbs (or significant parts of them) or for those whose lower limbs are significantly atrophied. The center of gravity of a bilateral lower-limb amputee in the seated position, even with lower-limb prostheses (which are usually lighter than the amputated extremities), is at least an inch further to the rear than for nonamputees. To maintain stability and compensate for the loss of weight in the absent or atrophied lower limbs, the rear axle and the propelling wheels of the lower-limb amputee WCs should be moved further posteriorly (usually by 1.25 to 2 inches or 3-5 cm). By moving the rearwheel posteriorly, the WC turning radius is increased slightly, but this is compensated when the front rigging is removed for those not wearing lower-limb prostheses. Other alternatives to moving the rearwheel axle posteriorly are to put 10 to 15 pounds (4.5-6.8 kg) of sandbags on the front rigging of a standard WC to reestablish the lost counterweight or to attach two special axles (amputee attachments) behind the original ones.

4. **High-performance WCs** (see Fig 4.7-3) are light-weight (20-40 lb or 9-18 kgs) or ultralightweight WCs (15-20 lb or 7-9 kgs) WCs. The ultralightweight

WCs are generally known as **sports WCs,** and although they are typically used by athletic paraplegics, they can also be used by nonathletic patients. Sports WCs have rigid frames of high strength and durability, fixed front riggings (usually consisting of a horizontal bar with heel loops rather than footplates), lower and firmer backrests (may be detachable), lower armrests (may use detachable tubular armrest or have no arm rest at all), lower and firmer seats positioned more rearward in relation to the rearwheel axle, spoked wheels that are cambered, small-diameter handrims, and small and narrow casters. They are much more energy efficient during propulsion (i.e., they require about 17% less energy to propel than standard WCs) and are not as easy to transport and store as the X-frame WCs. There are different sports WCs for specific sporting events (e.g., racing or basketball).

5. **Reclining WCs** cause an increase in the sagittal angle of the backrest in relation to the seat surface via the use of either manual controls (operated by an attendant caretaker) or motorized controls (may be activated by the patient). As the backrest is lowered during a recline maneuver, the leg rests generally elevate at the same rate as the descent of the backrest. Reclining WCs are used to improve trunk control and spinal alignment, reduce ischial pressure in proportion to the extent of the recline (especially useful for patients who cannot adequately shift their own weight), reduce orthostatic hypotension, increase mobilization of pulmonary secretions, alleviate back pain (because of the decreased effect of gravity on the spine), facilitate catheterizing a patient in the WC, reduce the need for additional transfers during the day for rest periods, and allow some patients with insufficient hip flexion who might not otherwise fit into a WC to "sit" in a WC.

The disadvantages of reclining WCs include increased WC weight, width, and bulk; increased difficulty of WC transportation; reclining may trigger spasticity due to the change in the relative positions of the user's body parts; and reclining may cause increased shear stress over the back and sacrum during position changes (this is particularly true when simple hinge-reclining WCs are used because the mechanical axis of the backrest with variable recline is usually below and behind the anatomic axis of the user's hip joint). If the shear force is not minimized, the process of reclining and resuming the upright posture tends to slide the patient forward onto the seat and into a poor sitting position (especially when there is significant spasticity). To minimize this shear force (particularly for persons at risk for pressure ulcers), any or all of the following measures may be done: slide the seat of the WC anteriorly while reclining; slide the back of the chair downward while reclining; align the axis of movement of the reclining back with the anatomic axis of hip flexion and extension; use a special low-shear or zero-shear reclining WC (which consists of a double-back arrangement that allows the user to adhere to the forward-most back of the chair, while shear-force is concentrated between the "front" and 'rear" backs of the chair); or use a tilt-in-space WC (see below).

a. **Semireclining WC** (see Fig 4.7-3) reclines about 30 degrees from vertical and locks in several positions. It has a back upholstery, which is 13 cm (5 inch.) higher than a standard adult WC; a detachable 25-cm (10-inch) telescopic headrest; and rearwheels set back 3 cm (1.25 inches) to maintain good balance and stability of the WC. Its armrests and legrests must provide support for the limbs in all positions. The semireclining WC relieves part of the pressure from the ischia but not from the sacrum where shearing forces can still lead to sacral pressure ulcers.

    b. Fully reclining WCs (see Fig 4.7-3) may be locked in any position between the vertical and horizontal and, therefore, permit conversion from a wheelchair to a stretcher. These have a back upholstery, which is 17 cm (7 inches) higher than a standard adult WC; detachable 25-cm (10-inch) telescopic headrests; and rearwheels set back 12 cm (5 inches) to maintain WC stability and balance. These provide better relief of pressure from the ischia and sacrum than semireclining WCs.

   6. Tilt-in-space WCs provide alternatives to the reclining WCs. They use a system (usually hydraulic, sometimes manual or motorized) by which the entire seat and back are tilted posteriorly as a single unit in the sagittal plane (thus the angle between seat, backrest, and leg or foot rest remains the same in all positions, and the relative position of the user's body parts remains unchanged). Like reclining WCs, they improve trunk control and spinal alignment, as well as reduce spinal and ischial pressure (in proportion to the extent of the tilt), reduce orthostatic hypotension, and allow for increased mobilization of pulmonary secretions. The advantages of tilt-in-space WCs over reclining WCs include lack of shear stress during tilting movements, less likelihood of triggering spasticity in patients with increased tone or spasticity problems, and better repositioning when the upright position is resumed. However, they tend to be unstable (with large persons), require a higher seating position, do not allow the patient's body to straighten toward the supine position, and are difficult to transport.

   7. Stand-up WCs allow the patient to stand within the frame of the WC. They are used for medical reasons (e.g., to provide weight-bearing benefits on bone or provide pressure relief) as well as other reasons such as improved psychological outlook and increased work access. They are usually available in both motorized and manual versions. Their main disadvantages are increased weight, width, cost, and complexity.

   8. Manual WCs with add-on power-pack units, although technically considered a motorized WC (see section III.A), are classified under manual WCs because they are mainly indicated for manual WC users who are progressively losing strength or who occasionally need power assistance for long distance travel or rough terrain. The add-on power-pack units (which consists of a pair of drive motor and battery, or set of batteries, and a proportional joy stick–type control) are attached to a manual WC (which can either have a folding or a rigid frame) to convert it into a motorized WC. Because the power-pack units can easily be removed, the transportability of the manual WC is retained. Although they are less expensive (especially if the patient already owns a manual WC), they are also less durable, provide less power (due to the smaller batteries), and are less adaptable than other motorized WCs.

II. Attendant-propelled WCs are designed to be pushed by another person because of the patient's short- or long-term inability to propel a manual WC or operate a powered-mobility system in a functional or safe manner. Attendant-propelled WCs may be used on a short-term basis for long-distance transportation in the community or when the patient's power-mobility system is being repaired or cannot be used due to space constraints (e.g., in airline aisles). An example of a long-term indication for attendant-propelled WCs includes demented patients who are unable to walk due to various medical conditions (e.g., lower limb contractures and deformities). The attendant-propelled WCs can be full sized WCs with four small wheels (e.g., posture-care chairs or ''geri-chairs''), or frontwheel-drive manual WCs (used for their maneuverability in limited indoor spaces such as in nursing homes; see above section I.A.2.a.1.b), or they may be smaller and created for use in limited spaces (e.g., folding stroller-type WCs). Many rearwheel-drive manual WCs (see section I.A.2.a.1.a), such as standard-sized manual WCs, can also serve as attendant-propelled WCs. Factors to consider in ordering an attendant-propelled WC include not only the fit and comfort of the patient but also accommodating the person pushing the WC.

III. Powered mobility systems

A. **Manual WCs with add-on power-pack units** are described in section I.B.8 under manual WCs.

B. **Powered or motorized WCs (integral-power mobility systems)** refer to WCs with integrated power-drive systems (direct- vs. belt-drive; see below), battery power sources, and user-operated controls, in addition to other similar features essentially found in manual WCs, such as seating systems, positioning and support systems, and safety components.

Indications. They are indicated for patients with physical limitations not compatible with manual wheelchair propulsion, i.e., those who cannot propel a WC using either the hands or feet because of limb absence, paralysis, deformity, or other neuromusculoskeletal problems and those with poor endurance (because of cardiopulmonary or neuromusculoskeletal conditions) who must conserve their energy for other functions (e.g., vocational work). Some common conditions that might warrant powered WCs include high-level spinal cord injury (e.g., C4 and above); advanced muscle weakness because of amyotrophic lateral sclerosis, multiple sclerosis, or muscular dystrophy; and poor coordination in all limbs (e.g., cerebral palsy). Powered WCs are usually indicated for outdoor use (rarely for indoor use) in patients of all ages who have to travel long distances (usually without help) and who tire easily. Patients with powered WCs generally need standard WCs for indoor use and as backups when their powered WCs are being repaired or cannot be transported. The indoor use of manual WCs also provide beneficial exercise for many patients.

User requirements. To safely use a powered WC, patients must have at least one reproducible movement (using the upper limb or other part of the body) to access the control system; a basic understanding of cause and effect and directionality; sufficient vision, perceptual ability, and judgment to permit movement through the environment; and proper motivation. Even children as young as 2 to 3 years old can be taught to safely operate a powered WC. Potential candidates (even those with severe physical disabilities or cognitive limitations) must be given a trial with a similar powered WC, not necessarily to assess whether the patient can drive the system but to determine the patient's ability to learn to use it.

Potential benefits of powered WCs include an increased independence level at school and work, increased efficiency of mobility, sparing of the upper limb joints (especially shoulder joints) from repetitive stress injury induced by manual WC propulsion or from premature deterioration (e.g., musculoskeletal complications such as arthritis of the upper limb joints), and, possibly, improved self-esteem generated by greater independence.

The *potential disadvantages* of powered WCs include the following: relatively high cost, heavy weight, transportation difficulty, relatively high maintenance, technological dependence, and limited environmental accessibility. Patients also don't get as much needed exercise as manual WC users.

Contraindications to powered mobility systems include inability to securely execute the motions of the control lever or switch, involuntary motions or inattention which might result in activating the controls unintentionally, blindness, lack of judgment, and irresponsibility—all of which count much more than in a manually propelled chair.

Prescription guidelines for a powered WC are based on the same general WC prescription principles described above (see introduction to this chapter) but with greater emphasis on the safety (of the user and of others) and performance of the powered WC. Although it uses the same seating and positioning principles as those described for manual WCs, the positioning of the upper limbs or other body parts is critical for placement of the WC control system. The main factors to consider in powered WC prescription include

- Primary use, i.e., usually for outdoor use; consider the type of terrain and the need for "all-terrain WCs";
- Stability, i.e., lower seat and wider WC base have more stability;
- Overall weight and portability, i.e., ease of assembly and disassembly, if appropriate; the weight, size, and transportability of each disassembled part;
- Availability of adapted vehicles for WC transportation, e.g., vans with ramps or hydraulic lifts;
- Environmental barriers, i.e., need for extensive environmental modifications; dimensions required for turning (in small spaces, short-based WCs are easier to maneuver);
- Battery life, i.e., the range (or distance capability) of the powered WCs based on a single battery charge;
- Power adjustability, e.g., speed, acceleration, and deceleration (high acceleration or deceleration may cause problems in persons with poor trunk control);
- Type and placement of the WC control system, e.g., joystick on the rightside armrest or Sip-and-Puff controls on the leftside mouth angle;
- Safety features, e.g., brakes, parking locks, safety harnesses, and antitippers;
- Availability of other equipment and features, e.g., communication aids, powered recliners, and platforms for respiratory aids;
- Durability, i.e., consider WC maintenance requirements as well as availability of parts and technical support;
- Other factors, e.g., cost (financial resources), noise factors, and ride quality.

The following are essential components of powered WCs that are not found in manual WCs:

1. **Power-drive systems**
   a. **Direct-drive powered WCs (or power-base WCs)** consist of a rigid mainframe (that contains the batteries and drive mechanisms); a seat, which is positioned directly above the power base on a pedestal attached to the rigid mainframe; and four small balloon tires (diameter of 8-10 inches or 20-25 cm and width of 3 inches or 7.6 cm; some newer models have slightly larger wheels in the rear). They are durable and better suited for rough terrain (because of their low center of gravity and wider tires). However, they are less maneuverable indoors or on carpets, and the large caster wheels have a tendency to wrinkle and roll carpeting, especially small rugs.
   b. **Belt-driven powered WCs** have comparable rigid mainframe and seating system as direct-drive WCs but usually have two large rear wheels and two small front casters (the wheels of belt-driven powered WCs look almost like those of manual WCs). They are more versatile (i.e., their frames are better suited to modification and the addition of different

components), more stable, and are generally capable of reaching greater speeds than direct-drive WCs; however, they tend to be less durable.

2. **Control systems** can be activated by any reproducible movement of the body such as those involving the upper extremity (i.e., hand, wrist, arm, fingertip, or upper limb residual limb) or non-upper limb body parts (e.g., head, chin, mouth, lips, tongue, and lower limbs). The activating devices commonly used include joysticks (i.e., a small pressure-sensitive stem attached to a control box; joystick-stem modifications include T-bar handles, knobs, long extension handles, mouthstick, etc.), chin- or head-pressure controls, and pneumatic controls (e.g., Sip-and-Puff, which uses soft or intense inspiration [sip] or expiration [puff]). Other special controls include the leaf switch, touch plate, toggle switch, voice-activated switch, myoelectric control switch, proximity sensing system, and scanning system (i.e., a control option that presents grouped or single choices one at a time until the user selects it by activating a switch). In general, the controls have a high and low range as well as options to increase power (e.g., when negotiating carpeted floor, grassy ground, or rough terrain). If possible, the control system of the powered WC should be compatible with the patient's environmental control unit (see Chapter 4.5, section II.A.5.a.3).

   a. **Primary controls** are used for changing WC direction and speed, as well as for braking.

      1) **Proportional controls** respond to pressure in similar fashion as a car accelerator, i.e., an increase in the amount (or direction) of pressure applied to the control mechanism (most commonly a joystick) proportionately increases such WC parameter as speed, acceleration, or direction change (i.e., forward, reverse, right, left, and all variations in between). They give the greatest degree of WC control and provide the smoothest ride; however, the user must have fair to good motor control.

      2) **Nonproportional (momentary or latching) controls** use microswitch controls, which operate by the all-or-none principle (i.e., the switch is either "on" or "off" like a light switch). The user applies any degree of pressure and as soon as the switch is activated, the system operates at the preset speed and/or direction (i.e., forward, reverse, right, and left). Multiple switch controls (e.g., a series of Sip-and-Puff switches) may be used. They are less responsive than proportional controls and generally require fewer skilled movements to achieve control (although learning to use such controls is not simple).

   b. **Secondary controls** usually consist of nonproportional (on/off) controls (e.g., scanning systems) for operating reclining or tilt-in-space WC functions, call signals, communication aids, environmental control units, or personal computers.

3. **Battery systems** can either be made of gel or lead. The recommended battery is usually a deep-cycle lead acid battery, either wet or sealed cell type. Most batteries are based on a 12- or 24-volt electrical systems (24-volt power is used for outdoor WCs), which need charging on a daily basis. The battery life determines the range (or distance capability) of the wheelchair, which is approximately 20 miles during the course of a day for most batteries. The range in turn depends on the user's driving habits (e.g., fast vs. slow; use of frequent quick starts), type of terrain covered (rough vs. flat), and adequacy of tire inflation. The batteries should be conveniently

placed for easy access (e.g., for removal when transporting WC) and should have indicators showing when the charge is low.

4. **Brake and parking lock systems.** Most powered WCs have an electromechanical brake (which slows down the moving WC; the braking speed may be adjusted for patients with unsteady balance) and a parking lock (which holds the WC still when it comes to a stop). Both must be easily activated (either manually or through an automatic switch).

5. **Special features** include reclining or tilt-in-space mechanism and standing mechanisms for WCs that can negotiate uneven surfaces and stairs.

C. **Electric carts (Scooters)** differ from powered WCs by their use of a front tiller or steering column (which has forward, reverse, turning, and stop controls) and their seat design, which is usually a bracket-type seat (with or without armrests) mounted on a central pedestal, which can be easily adjusted in height or swiveled for easy transfers and for working at a desk. Unlike other types of WCs, they have less "custom fitting" flexibility and generally do not have as good a seating position. Also they have a tendency to be top-heavy and can easily topple, especially when operating at high speed. Compared to powered WCs, they are generally easier to mount and dismount, have better cosmetic appearance, have good suspension and power for travel over rough terrain, and have longer service range. Some units are large, heavy (weighing between 225-250 lb [102-114 kg] or more), and difficult to transport. Others, however, are modular and can be disassembled and loaded in the trunk of a car or back of a station wagon (however certain parts could be as heavy as 50 lb or 23 kg and usually require a hydraulic lift to load and unload). They are indicated for patients who can ambulate, transfer, and perform most activities of daily living but who need the scooter for traveling long distances outside the home (in urban environments) because of lack of endurance or inability to use a manual wheelchair. They are also for patients who must avoid overuse of their limbs.

Scooter users (e.g., patients with rheumatoid arthritis, severe cardiac or degenerative disease, or early stages of multiple sclerosis or motor neuron or neuromuscular junction disease) are generally less disabled than the users of the other power-mobility systems. In general, the user must have good sitting balance, good eye-hand coordination, adequate spatial and figure-ground perception, and good judgment. Although reduced endurance and strength (especially of the LEs) are the main indications, the user must have good control of the upper trunk and at least one upper limb to manually steer the unit. Scooters are usually used in conjunction with walkers, canes, or manual WCs. Like golf carts, they may not be absolutely necessary, but they can help save the user's energy and provide an element of pleasure and fun.

1. **Three-wheeled scooters** have three 6-inch (15-cm) diameter wheels (two wheels in the rear and a third wheel in the front). A rearwheel-drive type (more powerful but bulkier, heavier, and less maneuverable in tight spaces) is generally recommended for outdoor use, while a frontwheel-drive type (lighter, smaller, and more maneuverable in tight spaces but less powerful) is recommended for indoor use. In both types, the controls and steering of the scooters are the same (i.e., the tiller is located above the front wheel). Three-wheeled scooters are generally indicated for users who are less disabled than users of the other types of WCs.

2. **Four-wheeled scooters** are available in both rearwheel- and frontwheel-drive models (with the same tiller mechanism, advantages and disadvantages as

similar three-wheeled models). They are more stable than the three-wheeled models but are less compact and less portable. They are indicated for patients who are more disabled then the users of the three-wheeled models.

D. Adapted vans and cars can be considered sources of powered mobility systems for the disabled patients and their WC or scooter. The driver's seat of the van may be removed so that it can be substituted with the patient's WC or scooter for driving. Selection of vehicles is described in Chapter 4.5 section II.B.2.f.2.b.

BIBLIOGRAPHY

Adler C, Tipton-Burton M: Wheelchair assessment and transfers. In Pedretti LW, editor: *Occupational therapy practice skills for physical dysfunction*, ed 4, St. Louis, 1996, Mosby–Year Books, pp 507-525.

Bergen AF: The prescriptive wheelchair: An orthotic device. In O'Sullivan, SB, Schmitz, TJ, editors: *Physical rehabilitation: assessment and treatment*. Philadelphia, 1994, FA Davis, pp 685-706.

Brittell CW: Wheelchair prescription. In Kottke FJ, Lehmann JF, editors: *Krusen's handbook of physical medicine and rehabilitation*. ed 4, Philadelphia, 1990, WB Saunders, pp 548-563.

Buschbacher R, Adkins J, Lay B, et al.: Prescription of wheelchair and seating system. In Braddom RL, editor: *Physical medicine and rehabilitation*. Philadelphia, 1996, WB Saunders, pp 381-400.

Currie DM, Hardwick K, Marburger, RA, et al.: Wheelchair prescription and adaptive seating. In DeLisa JA, Gans BM, editors: *Rehabilitation medicine: principles and practice*, ed 2, Philadelphia, 1993, JB Lippincott, pp 563-585.

Deitz J, Dudgeon B: Wheelchair selection process. In Trombly CA, editor: *Occupational therapy for physical dysfunction*, ed 4, Baltimore, 1995, Williams & Wilkins, pp 599-609.

Enders A, Hall M, editors: *Assistive technology source book*. Washington, DC, 1990, RESNA.

Gettel AH, Redford JB: Wheelchairs and wheeled mobility. In Redford JB, Basmajian JV, Trautman P, editors: *Orthotics: clinical practice and rehabilitation technology*, New York, 1995, Churchill Livingstone, pp 171-217.

Kirby RL: Manual Wheelchairs. In O'Young B, Young MA, Stiens SA, editors: *PM&R secrets*, Philadelphia, 1997, Hanley & Belfus, pp 117-120.

Letts RM, editor: *Principles of seating the disabled*. Boca Raton, 1991, CRC Press.

Mayall JK, Desharnais G: *Positioning in a wheelchair: a guide for professional caregivers of the disabled adult*, ed 2, Thorofare, NJ, 1995, Slack.

Miller NE: Wheelchair prescriptions and types of wheelchairs. In Sinaki M, editor: *Basic clinical rehabilitation medicine*, St. Louis, 1994, Mosby–Year Book, pp 449-461.

Redford JB: Seating and wheeled mobility in the disabled elderly population, *Arch Phys Med Rehabil* 74:877-885, 1993.

Trudel G, Kirby RL, Ackroyd-Stolarz A, et al.: Effects of rear-wheel camber on wheelchair stability, *Arch Phys Med Rehabil* 78(1):78-81, 1997.

Warren CG: Powered mobility and its implications. In Todd SP, Gianini MJ, editors: Choosing a wheelchair system, *J Rehabil Res Dev* 25 (suppl 2):74-85, 1990.

Wilson A: *Wheelchairs: a prescription guide*, New York, 1992, Demos.

CHAPTER 4.8

PHARMACOLOGIC AGENTS

Drug prescriptions should include the name, age, and address of the patient; date; name of the drug; dosage; route of administration; amount dispensed; dosage schedule instructions; and license (and Drug Enforcement Agency [DEA]) number and signature of the physician. The number of refills should be limited (especially in patients who appear to be self-injurious). For controlled substances, refills should be written in both number and word, for example, disp. #30 (thirty), refills 2 (two). In general, the physician should know the metabolism, route of excretion, and major adverse effects associated with each drug used. Adverse drug reactions (ADRs) may be allergic, idiosyncratic, or dose-related extensions of known effects. The ADRs occur frequently and the rate of occurrence increase in proportion to the number of drugs taken. Drug dosages should be individualized according to the patient's age and weight as well as kidney and liver function.

In the clinical setting, half-life is usually the most relevant pharmacokinetic parameter. It generally takes about 4 to 5 half-lives to reach a steady-state plasma level and about the same time for the drug to be eliminated after drug discontinuation. Hence, a loading dose is usually needed for drugs with long half-life (unless such a dose produces intolerable side effects). Also, if possible, any drug with a long half-life should be avoided in the elderly because it takes longer for the drug to be eliminated in case of toxicity. Drug effects generally continue to increase in intensity until steady-state plasma level is achieved (the relationship between drug effect and plasma level varies in different individuals). In some drugs (e.g., tricyclic antidepressants or nonsteroidal antiinflammatory agents), the drug effect may continue to increase for days to weeks after achieving steady-state plasma levels (thus, clinicians should wait for at least 1 to 2 weeks longer before further drug titration or drug discontinuation). To increase compliance and ensure adequate therapeutic trials, patients must be educated about the titration process, delay in clinical benefit, and anticipated side effects.

I. **Analgesics** are used to temporarily relieve pain and help improve patient's function. Because pain is subjective, analgesic therapy should be individualized. When possible, nonopioid preparations should be used. In patients with chronic pain refractory to analgesics, nonpharmacologic modalities (e.g., nerve blocks, sympathectomy, and relaxation therapy) should be considered (see Chapter 5.10, section VI).

A. **Nonopioid (or nonnarcotic) analgesics** (see Tables 4.8-1 and 4.8-2)

1. **Acetaminophen** (see Table 4.8-1) has antipyretic and analgesic properties similar to aspirin (see section I.A.3.a) but does not inhibit platelet function. Its antiinflammatory effect is probably insignificant. Although its mechanism of action (MOA) is unknown, its primary action appears to be in the central nervous system (CNS). Acetaminophen is approximately equianalgesic with aspirin, but unlike aspirin and other nonsteroidal antiinflammatory drugs (NSAIDs), it does not cause gastric toxicity (although chronic use can cause dyspepsia) or renal toxicity (except in prolonged use). Also, it does not exacerbate encephalopathy or congestive heart failure. In patients with bleeding diathesis or with renal insufficiency who

Table 4.8-1. Recommended dosage of acetaminophen, tramadol, and salicylate NSAIDs

GENERIC	SELECTED BRANDNAMES	AVAILABLE PREPARATIONS (mg)	DOSAGE (mg), ROUTE, FREQUENCY	MDD (mg)
1. Acetaminophen	Tylenol, Tylenol ES, Panadol, Tempra, Anacin-3	*tab* 160, 325, 500, 650; *chew tab* 80; *cap* 325, 500; *supp* 120, 325, 650; *elix* (per 5 ml) 120, 160, 320; *liq* 160/5 ml, 500/15 ml; *drop* 80 mg/0.8 ml	650-1000 po/pr q4-6h	4000
2. Tramadol	Ultram	*tab* 50	50-100 po q4-6h	400
3. Acetylated salicylate				
Aspirin*	ASA; Bayer Ascriptin Ecotrin Empirin	*tab* 81, 325, 500, 600, 650, 800, 975; *cap* 325, 500	325-650 po q4-6h	6000§
4. Nonacetylated salicylate*				
Choline Mg trisalicylate	Trilisate	*tab* 500, 750, 1000; *liq* 500 mg/5ml	750-1500 po bid/tid; 3000 po qd	3000§
Diflunisal	Dolobid	*tab* 250, 500	1000 po initially, then 250-500 po q8-12h	1500
Salsalate‡	Disalcid Salflex	*tab* 500, 750; *cap* 500	500-750 po bid/tid	3000§

MDD = maximum daily dose; ES = extra strength; tab = tablet; chew tab = chew tablet; supp = suppository; elix = elixir; liq = liquid; cap = capsule.
* Plasma half life for ASA is 9-16 hours.
† Plasma half life for choline Mg trisalicylate is 9-17 hour, for diflunisal is 8-12 hrs, and for salsalate is 3-16 hour.
‡ Analgesia indication is not listed by manufacturer.
§ Determined by measurement of serum salicylate level. For optimal antiinflammatory effects, blood levels between 20 and 30 mg/dl and a total daily dose of 3-6 gm are usually required.

need nonopioid analgesics, acetaminophen is safer than other NSAIDs (long-term use of acetaminophen should be avoided by patients with renal pathology). Acetaminophen should be used cautiously by patients with liver pathology (fatal hepatic necrosis has been reported in acute acetaminophen overdosage, i.e., 10-15 g). Acetaminophen is available in oral and suppository forms. When combined with NSAIDs (see section I.A.3) or opioids (see sections I.B), it provides greater pain relief than acetaminophen or the other agents alone. Patients should be advised to refrain from alcohol intake while taking acetaminophen.

2. Tramadol (Ultram) (see Table 4.8-1) is a centrally acting oral synthetic nonopioid analgesic agent. It probably acts by binding weakly to opioid receptors (i.e., μ–receptors) and by inhibiting reuptake of norepinephrine and serotonin. It is one-tenth as potent as morphine and is used in moderate to moderately severe pain. Adverse drug reactions include dizziness, somnolence, nausea, constipation, sweating, pruritus, occassionally orthostatic hypotension, and seizure. Compared to morphine, it causes less respiratory depression, does not cause histamine release, and has milder physical tolerance with less severe withdrawal symptoms. It has no effect on heart rate, left ventricular function, or cardiac index. It can be given without regard to food intake. It is contraindicated in persons with hypersensitivity to tramadol and acute alcohol intoxication. It must be used with caution in patients taking hypnotics, central acting analgesics, opioids, or psychotropic drugs.

3. **Nonsteroidal antiinflammatory drugs,** which are the most widely used drugs in the world, exhibit antiinflammatory, antipyretic, and analgesic activities. They are primarily used for treating inflammatory conditions of the musculoskeletal system (particularly rheumatoid arthritis and other autoimmune arthritides, as well as osteoarthritis, which may be associated with an inflammatory component). Selected drugs have also been formally approved for the treatment of shoulder bursitis/tendinitis (e.g., naprosyn, indomethacin, and sulindac), dysmenorrhea (e.g., ibuprofen, diclofenac, and mefenamic acid), postoperative pain (e.g., intramuscular [IM] ketorolac), and other conditions. A number of NSAIDs have primary indications as analgesics (see Table 4.8-2) and have been used on pain associated with noninflammatory conditions (e.g., neuropathic pain), with chronic or frequently recurrent headache, and with cancer pain (particularly bone pain related to cancer). The NSAIDs are also used to supplement a primary analgesic agent (e.g., morphine) to decrease the required dosage of opioid, and thereby minimize the opioid side effects.

   Mechanism of action. The major MOA of NSAIDs is the inhibition of the synthesis of prostaglandin (PG), specifically PGE_2 via the blocking of cyclooxygenase (COX), which is the enzyme that converts arachidonic acid into PG (see Fig 4.8-1). Prostaglandins do not themselves activate nociceptors, but they lower the threshold to noxious stimulation, i.e., they sensitize the nociceptors to the actions of other noxious endogenous substances (e.g., bradykinin, histamine, substance P, and serotonin). In soft tissues, PGE_2 causes pain and inflammation. In the gastrointestinal (GI) tract, PGE_2 is cytoprotective, that is, it increases secretion of mucus and bicarbonates and decreases secretion of gastric acids and digestive enzymes; whereas in the kidney, PGE_2 enhances renal salt and water excretion by acting as a vasodilator of small arterial blood vessels. Other possible MOAs of NSAIDs are inhibition of lipooxygenase activity and leukotriene production, membrane stabilization, and a supraspinal (central) analgesic effect, which is separate and distinct from the action in the inflamed peripheral tissues. In the arachidonic cascade (see Fig. 4.8-1), the COX enzymes can be subdivided into COX-1, which is responsible for PGE_2 production in the GI tract and the kidney, and COX-2, which is responsible for inflammatory PG synthesis during tissue injury. However, there is controversy in determining COX-1 or COX-2 selectivity due to lack of standardization of the methods for evaluating relative COX-2/COX-1 inhibitory activity. It is generally believed that glucocorticoids selectively block COX-2 and have less ulcerogenic side effects. Acetylsalicylic acid (ASA), however, causes irreversible inhibition of both COX-1 and COX-2 and is ulcerogenic. Most of the other NSAIDs serve as reversible, competitive inhibitors of cyclooxygenase activity, and either nonselectively inhibit the COX-1 and COX-2 enzymes or have selectivity for the COX-1 isoform; hence, they are all ulcerogenic. The possible exceptions are etodolac (Lodine) and nabumetone (Relafen), both of which seem to preferentially inhibit COX-2 and hence have less (but not absent) ulcerogenic side effects.

   Adverse drug reactions. All NSAIDs have similar ADRs. These include gastrointestinal (GI) intolerance in 10% of NSAID users (e.g., nausea or dyspepsia); GI ulceration (i.e., gastric and also duodenal) in 2% of NSAID

Table 4.8-2. Selected nonsalicylate NSAIDs classified by half-life duration

GENERIC	SELECTED BRANDNAMES	AVAILABLE PREPARATIONS (mg)	DOSAGE (mg), ROUTE, FREQUENCY	MDD (mg)
I. Short half-life†				
Diclofenac	Cataflam IR Voltaren DR	*IR tab* 50 *DR tab* 25, 50, 75	*DR/IR*: 50 po bid/tid *DR*: 75 po bid; or *DR*: 25 po qid + hs	150
Fenoprofen*	Nalfon	*cap* 200, 300; *tab* 600	200-600 po tid/qid	2400
Flurbiprofen	Ansaid	*tab* 50, 100	50-100 po tid	300
Ibuprofen*	Motrin, Medipren, Advil, Nuprin, Rufen	*tab* 200, 300, 400, 600, 800; *liq* 100 5ml	200-800 po tid/qid	3200
Indomethacin	a) Indocin, Indocid b) Indocin SR	a) *cap* 25, 50; *supp* 50; *susp* 25 5ml b) *SR cap* 75	a) 25-50 po tid, pc; 50, pr, bid; b) *SR*: 75 po qd/bid	150
Ketoprofen*	a) Orudis b) Oruvail	a) *cap* 25, 50, 75 b) *cap* 100, 150, 200	a) 25-75 po q4-8h; b) 200 po qd	300
Ketorolac*	Toradol	*tab* 10 *inj* 15, 30, 60	10 po q4-6h; 30-60 IM initially, then 15- 30 IM/IV q6h	*tab* 40 *inj* 120
Meclofenamate*	Meclomen	*cap* 50, 100	50 po tid/qid	400
Mefenamic acid*	Ponstel	*cap* 250	500 po initially, then 250 po q6h	1000
Tolmetin	Tolectin	*tab* 200, 600; *cap* 400	200-600 po tid	1800
II. Intermediate half-life‡				
Etodolac*	a) Lodine b) Lodine XL	a) *cap* 200, 300, 400 b) *tab* 400, 600	a) 200-400 po bid/qid b) 400-1000 po qd	1200
Sulindac	Clinoril	*tab* 150, 200	150-200 po bid, pc	400
III. Long half-life§				
Naproxen*	Naprosyn, Aleve; EC-Naprosyn	*tab* 200, 250, 375, 500; *susp* 125 5ml	500 po initially, then 250-500 po bid	1025
Naproxen Na*	a) Anaprox b) Naprelan CR	a) *tab* 275, 550 b) *tab* 375, 500	275-550 po bid; 750- 1000 po qd	a) 1375 b) 1500
Nabumetone	Relafen	*tab* 500, 750	500-750 po bid; 1000 po qd/bid	2000
Oxaprozin	Daypro	*cap* 600	1200 po qd	1200
Piroxicam	Feldene	*cap* 10, 20	20 po qd	20

MDD = maximum daily dose; DR = delayed release; IR = immediate release; SR = sustained release; CR = controlled release; ER or XL = extended release; EC = enteric coated; DS = double strength; tab = tablet; cap = capsule; susp = supension.
† Short half-life = <6 hr; ‡intermediate half-life = 6-10 hr; §long half-life = >10 hr.
* NSAIDs with primary indications as analgesics. Their slow- or extended-release forms (i.e., those with once-a-day dosing) or enteric-coated forms (e.g., EC-Naprosyn) have delayed time-to-peak concentration and are not recommended for primary analgesic use.

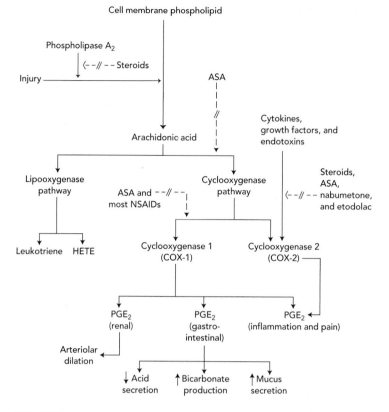

Figure 4.8-1

Effects of steroids and NSAIDs on the arachidonic cascade. There are two major routes of metabolism of arachidonic acid: the lipooxygenase pathway, which leads to the production of leukotrienes and HETE; and the cyclooxygenase pathway, which leads to the production of prostaglandins, specifically PGE_2. The PGE_2 responsible for inflammation as well as for renal and GI protection is activated by the COX-1 pathway, which in turn is blocked by ASA and most NSAIDs. The PGE_2 responsible for inflammation and pain (but not for GI protection nor kidney arteriolar dilation) is activated by the COX-2 pathway. COX-2 is induced by cytokines, growth factors, and endotoxin, and is blocked by glucocorticoids, ASA, and some NSAIDs (nabumetone, etodolac). Therefore, drugs that selectively block the COX-2 receptor cause less GI ulceration. ASA, on the other hand completely blocks the cyclooxygenase pathway and has relatively higher incidence of GI ulceration. Note that aside from acting on the cyclooxygenase pathway, steroids also inhibit arachidonic acid formation by blocking phospholipase A_2. Broken lines (--//--) indicate inhibitory effects.

users; inhibition of PG-mediated renal function, that is, inhibition of anti-diuretic hormone, increased renal reabsorption of chloride, and enhanced reabsorption of K^+ (thus fluid retention in patients with congestive heart failure [CHF], hepatic cirrhosis with ascites, chronic renal disease [analgesic toxic nephropathy with medullary ischemia], hypertension [HTN] or hypovolemia, and hyperkalemia); renal injury (interstitial nephritis, papillary necrosis, or, rarely, acute renal failure); bleeding (due to inhibition of platelet aggregation or gastric erosion and ulceration); inhibition of uterine smooth muscle motility (prolongation of gestation); hypersensitivity reaction; and a vague sense of dizziness and confusion especially in elderly patients. Although not contraindicated, NSAIDs must be used with caution in the elderly and in patients with impaired renal or hepatic function.

Hepatic toxicity. The risk factors for hepatic toxicity include advanced age, decreased renal function, multiple drug use, higher drug dosages, and increased duration of therapy. Agents with high hepatotoxic risk include diclofenac, sulindac and phenylbutazone; while those with lower risk include ibuprofen and ketoprofen. Hence, with institution of a new agent, it is advisable to monitor liver function during the first 4 to 6 weeks in patients with increased risk of hepatotoxicity.

Renal toxicity. Risk factors for NSAID nephrotoxicity include age over 60 years with atherosclerotic cardiovascular disease and concurrent diuretic therapy, renal insufficiency (serum creatinine above 2.0 mg/dl), and states of renal hypoperfusion (e.g., sodium depletion, diuretic use, hypotension, nephrotic syndrome, and congestive heart failure). High-risk patients should be hydrated and treated with the lowest effective dose of the least potent renal cyclooxygenase inhibitor (e.g., sulindac or a nonacetylated agent), and the creatinine and electrolyte levels must be monitored at baseline and after 5 to 7 days of treatment.

Gastrointestinal (GI) toxicity. Nonsteroidal antiinflammatory drug therapy is associated with upper GI symptoms in 25% of patients, causes ulcers or erosions in 40% of patients, increases risk of ulcer bleeding or perforation three- to four-fold, and increases rate of hospitalization or death from a GI complication fivefold. It also causes lower GI complications (i.e., 10-15% of NSAID users experience diarrhea). In spite of the high frequency of ulceration, the risk of developing GI complications while taking an NSAID remains relatively low (1-5% per year). Gastrointestinal irritation, erosion, and mucosal ulceration are thought to be due to the NSAID inhibition of PGs (see Fig. 4.8-1). Prostaglandins are known to provide GI cytoprotection by suppressing gastric acid secretion and maintaining the mucosal barrier. An increased risk of developing GI ulcer from NSAIDs has been strongly associated with a history of either ulcer disease or previous GI complications from NSAIDs, elderly patients (over 70 years old), and concomitant administration of corticosteroids or anticoagulants. Other factors include the use of high NSAID doses, history of cardiac disease, and history of rheumatoid arthritis. Smoking and/or alcohol consumption, in the absence of other risk factors, have been suggested as risk factors of NSAID-induced ulceration but these remain controversial.

In patients with high-risk for GI toxicity who needs NSAID therapy, the following are recommended: A) use of the lowest effective dosages of NSAIDs, B) avoidance of NSAIDs with high levels of enterohepatic recirculation (e.g., indomethacin, sulindac, and meclofenamate), C) use of a nonacetylated salicylate when possible, and D) concomitant use of a GI cytoprotectant such as misoprostol (Cytotec), initially at 100 μg, po, qid after meals, then gradually increased to 800 μg/day (gradual titration is used to prevent diarrhea). Misoprostol, a PG analog, is the only drug that is approved by the FDA for use in prevention of both NSAID-induced gastric and duodenal ulcers. It has been shown to reduce the risk of serious NSAID-induced ulcers to less than 1.5% (after 3 months of NSAID therapy) without reversing the desired antiinflammatory and analgesic effects. However, its long-term use can be costly, thus it should only be considered in patients with high risk for GI toxicity (as listed in the previous paragraph) or in patients who are unable to tolerate a GI complication (e.g., presence of severe comorbid conditions). Misoprostol is contraindicated in pregnant women because it may induce spontaneous abortion.

In patients with NSAID-induced ulcers, the treatment of choice is NSAID discontinuation (which in most cases will lead to ulcer healing). During this period, other analgesic (e.g., acetaminophen or opioids) or antiinflammatory (e.g., corticosteroid) agents may be used. Patients are usually given antiulcer therapy, although its effectiveness in speeding ulcer healing has not been proved. In patients requiring continued NSAID therapy, initial ulcer treatment is similar to that for peptic ulcer disease. Short-term therapy (usually 4-8 weeks) using acid-reduction agents, are effective for NSAID-induced duodenal ulcers. Acid-reducing agents include histamine-2 or H_2 blockers (e.g., nizatidine [Axid], 150 mg, po, bid/qd) and proton-pump inhibitors (e.g., omeprazole [Prilosec], 20 mg, po, qd). In patients with gastric ulcer, higher doses and/or prolonged therapy (e.g., up to 8-12 weeks) using acid-reducing agents may be needed. Sucralfate (Carafate, 1 g, po, 1 hour before meals, and qhs), which may be effective for duodenal ulcers when the NSAID is stopped, is, however, not effective for prophylactic therapy (i.e., during continued use of NSAIDs). Antacids, which may help relieve NSAID-induced dyspepsia, have not been shown to be effective in preventing NSAID-induced ulcers. If GI symptoms persist for more than 2 weeks or if patients have evidence of complication (e.g., iron deficiency anemia, GI bleeding, unexplained weight loss, and dysphagia), endoscopic evaluation is indicated.

Nausea and abdominal pain raise concern about the potential for ulceration, but are actually poor predictors. To decrease GI distress, NSAIDs should be taken with food or milk, and, in some cases, antacids may be used. The use of pro-drugs (which need to be metabolized in the liver to become active) and enteric-coated drugs as well as the concomitant use of acid-reducing agents can decrease local GI injury effects of NSAIDs, because the gastric or intestinal mucosa is not exposed to high concentrations of its active metabolite during oral ingestion. However, local injuries such as superficial gastritis and submucosal hemorrhage, are not predictive of symptoms, are rarely clinically significant, and may resolve with continued NSAID use. As the drug is activated and becomes available systemically, it can eventually cause GI ulceration especially in long-term use. Clinical evidence seems to indicate that parenteral or rectal administration of NSAIDs can produce the same GI complications as oral administrations. Patients with NSAID-induced nausea, can be given hydroxycine (Atarax,

Vistaril), 25 to 50 mg, po, q4-6h. Hydroxyzine is an antihistamine agent, which not only acts as an antiemetic but also as a coanalgesic (see section VI.A).

Contraindications and precautions. The NSAIDs are contraindicated in patients with aspirin or NSAID allergies, active bleeding, high coagulation time, peptic ulcers, as well as in women who are pregnant (may cause palate deformities in the fetus). For lactating women, some NSAIDs such as ASA should be used with caution, while others, such as ibuprofen and naproxen, can be safely used because their drug level in the milk is negligible. (For more information about which drugs are safe for pregnant or lactating women, see Briggs G, Freeman R, Yaffe S: *Drugs in pregnancy and lactation,* ed 4, Baltimore, 1994, Williams & Wilkins.) In patients with known ''triad'' symptoms (aspirin hypersensitivity, rhinitis/nasal polyps, asthma), NSAIDs can cause bronchospasm, laryngeal edema, and urticaria. The NSAIDs are protein-bound after absorption and may displace other drugs or be displaced themselves, thereby potentiating the effects of protein-bound drugs such as oral hypoglycemics (sulfonylureas), warfarin, digoxin, anticonvulsants (phenytoin), methotrexate, and sulfonamides. Thus, the combination of most NSAIDs with warfarin and some NSAIDs with oral hypoglycemic agents should be used with extreme caution or avoided if possible. Other drug-drug interactions include increased GI toxicity when NSAIDs are used with ethanol, increased lithium concentration with concomitant NSAID use, and decreased NSAID excretion with the use of probenecid. Moreover, the use of PG-inhibiting NSAIDs can decrease the antihypertensive (anti-HTN) and diuretic effects of diuretic drugs (e.g., thiazides and furosemide). They can also decrease the anti-HTN effects of β-blockers and angiotensin-converting enzyme (ACE) inhibitors.

Drug administration guidelines. Optimal NSAID selection should be based on the therapeutic goals and the actual need for peripheral antiinflammatory effect versus central analgesia. The NSAIDs such as mefenamic acid, ketorolac, and etodolac have insufficient peripheral antiinflammatory activity (hence are not indicated in the treatment of rheumatoid arthritis) but have significant central analgesic properties (hence are useful for pain relief). Generally, NSAIDs with a longer half-life (see classification in Table 4.8-2) allow better patient compliance, but do not afford as quick an analgesic effect after the dose is taken. Although the half-life itself does not increase the inherent toxicity of the NSAIDs, use of NSAIDs with long half-lives is more likely to result in excess accumulation and serious ADRs.

The dose-response relationship for the NSAIDs is characterized by a ceiling dose for analgesia, i.e., doses higher than the ceiling do not provide additional analgesia but presumably increase the risk of dose-related toxicity. The ceiling dose as well as the minimal effective dose and toxic dose of different NSAIDs have large individual variations. This, in combination with the fact that the recommended therapeutic doses of NSAIDs are based on dose-ranging studies in relatively healthy populations, suggests the need for individual titration of NSAIDs in the clinical setting. The same NSAID should be considered if the patient had favorable response to its previous use for similar indications because of interindividual variability in NSAID response. Although the use of NSAIDs can be titrated against symptoms, around-the-clock dosings are usually more effective than "as needed" (prn) dosings.

For patients with mild to moderate pain and for those with a relatively increased risk of NSAID toxicity (e.g., the elderly, or those on multiple drugs or with renal insufficiency), a relatively low starting dose of NSAID should be given (i.e., one-half to one-third of the recommended dose). For patients with acute severe pain, an initial loading dose of 1.5 to 2 times the conventional starting dose may be given (e.g., when giving ketorolac for postoperative pain). In most other patients, conventional starting doses can be used. The NSAID dose is gradually titrated with at least one week (or up to a few weeks) of observation period between dose adjustments. Dose titration should stop when analgesia is adequate, the ceiling dose is reached (i.e., there is no increased analgesia after the dose is titrated), side effects occur, or the dose approaches a conventionally accepted maximum (usually 1.5 to 2 times the average recommended starting dose). To minimize dose-related side effects, the dose may be lowered to the previous level prior to the ceiling dose level. If the patient is unable to achieve balance between analgesia and side effects at a dose below the maximal safe dose, the drug should be discontinued and another NSAID (even from the same chemical class) should be tried because there is a marked variation in the response of individuals to different but closely related NSAIDs.

There is no indication for the use of two NSAIDs simultaneously (e.g., aspirin and another NSAID or two nonaspirin NSAIDs), as there is no additive effect. Moreover, the addition of a second NSAID increases cost and the incidence of side effects. Because most NSAIDs are equipotent, the only justification for choosing a more costly drug is the convenience of dosing, or if the drug is better tolerated and has better efficacy for that given patient. (Note that while all NSAIDs have antiinflammatory effects, not all are effective as primary analgesics; see Table 4.8-2 to determine which NSAIDs have primary analgesic indications.) In long-term NSAID therapy, the following tests should be monitored regularly: occult fecal blood, hemoglobin, hepatic function, and renal function (blood urea nitrogen [BUN]/creatinine). The frequency of monitoring ranges from every few months (e.g., 1-2 months) for most patients, to more frequent monitoring (e.g., monthly or bimonthly) for patients who are predisposed to side effects and who are receiving relatively high doses of NSAIDs.

a. **Salicylate NSAIDs** (see Table 4.8-1) have analgesic, antipyretic, and antiinflammatory effects. In addition to the ADRs common to other NSAIDs, salicylates can also cause tinnitus, hearing loss, vertigo, metabolic acidosis, and hyperglycemia. In patients receiving concomitant corticosteroids, salicylate toxicity may occur during tapering of corticosteroids.

1) **Acetylsalicylic acid (ASA) or aspirin** is the most commonly used salicylate NSAID. Aspirin is indicated as an analgesic and antiinflammatory agent (for rheumatoid arthritis, osteoarthritis, and related rheumatic disorders) as well as an antiplatelet agent (see section VII.B.2). It produces more gastrointestinal toxicity and less antiinflammatory effect than the other NSAIDs (except for a few, e.g., piroxicam, which has relatively more GI toxicity than ASA). Although ASA does not generally cause liver damage in healthy adults, it may exac-

erbate preexisting liver disease. It has been implicated in Reye's syndrome and is, therefore, not recommended in children. It may also exacerbate preexisting kidney disease and cause salicylate toxicity, especially among the elderly. For optimal antiinflammatory effect, a total daily dose of 3 to 6 g of ASA with blood levels between 20 and 30 mg/dl is usually needed. The maximum tolerated dose must be reached slowly, often with 1 week between alteration in dosage. However, for relief of mild to moderate pain in nonarthritic patients, its optimal dose may be less than the 650 mg given every 3 to 4 hours. At dosages above 1 g, the analgesic effect does not increase although toxicity rises dramatically. To avoid toxicity, the interval between doses should be increased as the dose is increased. Aspirin has the additional effect of inhibiting platelet aggregation and in low doses can be used for stroke prophylaxis. Buffered ASA tablets (containing either absorbable bicarbonate or nonabsorbable antacids) are not necessarily associated with reduced GI bleeding. Enteric-coated ASA tablets often cause less dyspepsia and less occult GI blood loss, but their absorption rates are more variable than either buffered or nonbuffered tablets. Time-release ASA tablets have delayed absorption and possibly more sustained plasma levels.

  2) **The nonacetylated salicylates** produce minimal PG inhibition and minimal platelet effects. They also have less potential for GI ulceration than other NSAIDs.

    a) **Salsalate (Disalcid)** is indicated for use in rheumatoid arthritis, osteoarthritis, and related rheumatic disorders. It has been used to relieve mild to moderate pain, although analgesia is not listed by the manufacturer as a primary indication.

    b) **Diflunisal (Dolobid)** is indicated for use in rheumatoid arthritis and osteoarthritis and as an analgesic for mild to moderate pain. It is longer acting and has more auditory side effects than other salicylates.

    c) **Choline magnesium trisalicylate (Trilisate)** is indicated for use in rheumatoid arthritis and osteoarthritis, and as an analgesic for mild to moderate pain (e.g., acute painful shoulder).

b. **Nonsalicylate NSAIDs** can generally be subdivided into six chemical classes. They are available in many oral preparations and are available in injectable and suppository forms (see Table 4.8-2).

  1) **Indole and indene acetic acid NSAIDs**

    a) **Indomethacin (Indocin)** is primarily indicated for acute gout, rheumatoid arthritis, osteoarthritis, ankylosing spondylitis, and acute painful shoulder (bursitis/tendinitis) but is not approved as a primary analgesic. It can be given orally, as a suppository, and intravenously. The oral form is also available as a sustained-release capsule (this form is not recommended for acute gout). The intravenous (IV) form is only indicated for closure of patent ductus arteriosus. Indomethacin has high GI toxicity and has a higher incidence of headache than other NSAIDs.

    b) **Sulindac (Clinoril)** has the same indications as indomethacin. It is also not approved as an analgesic. It has half the potency of indomethacin but is longer acting and may have lesser renal toxicity than indomethacin. It is a pro-drug with less GI toxicity in short-term use; however, in long-term use (more than 5-14 days), it may increase the risk of GI toxicity.

c) **Etodolac (Lodine; Lodine XL)** is indicated for use in rheumatoid arthritis and osteoarthritis. The short-acting form, Lodine, which is also approved for analgesic use, has been shown to produce analgesia approximately 30 minutes after oral administration with relief lasting 4 to 6 hrs (this is comparable to aspirin and acetaminophen with codeine). Etodolac has lower risk of producing GI complications (less than 0.1%) probably due to selective inhibition of COX-2. Etodolac seems to be well-tolerated, especially by the elderly patients.

2) Arylpropionic acid NSAIDs

a) **Fenoprofen (Nalfon)** is used in rheumatoid arthritis and osteoarthritis, as well as an analgesic. It has greater renal toxicity than other NSAIDs and is therefore contraindicated in patients with impaired renal function.

b) **Flurbiprofen (Ansaid)** is used in rheumatoid arthritis and osteoarthritis but is not approved for analgesic use.

c) **Ibuprofen (Motrin, Advil, and others)** has the advantage of causing less epigastric pain, less GI occult blood loss, and less hepatotoxicity. Ibuprofen (and also diclofenac) have the lowest risk for GI ulceration and bleeding. Aside from its indication for rheumatoid arthritis and osteoarthritis, it is also used as an analgesic for mild to moderate pain and is effective in dysmenorrhea.

d) **Ketoprofen (Orudis, Oruvail)** is indicated for use in rheumatoid arthritis and osteoarthritis. The short-acting form, Orudis, is also approved for analgesic use and for dysmenorrhea. The controlled-release preparation, Oruvail, which can be given once a day, is not recommended for acute pain. Oruvail is pH-dependent and is released in the intestine, thus minimizing gastric irritation. Ketoprofen is reported to have less hepatotoxicity.

e) **Naproxen (Naprosyn, Anaprox, Alleve, Naprelan)** has a long half-life and is more potent than the other propionic acid NSAIDs. It is indicated for rheumatoid arthritis, osteoarthritis, ankylosing spondylitis, juvenile arthritis, acute gout, and for mild to moderate pain (e.g., for dysmenorrhea, bursitis, and tendinitis). The controlled-release form, Naprelan can be given once daily. All formulations (including Naprelan) are recommended for analgesic use in acute pain except the enteric-coated form (EC-Naprosyn) because of its delayed absorption.

f) **Oxaprozin (Daypro)** has a 40 to 50 hour half-life and can be given once a day. It is approved for use in rheumatoid arthritis and osteoarthritis but not as an analgesic.

3) Heteroaryl acetic acid NSAIDs

a) **Diclofenac (Voltaren, Cataflam)** is more potent than the indole and proprionic acid NSAIDs. It is available in a delayed-release (enteric-coated) form (Voltaren) and in an immediate-release form (Cataflam). Both are primarily indicated for rheumatoid arthritis, osteoarthritis, and ankylosing spondylitis, whereas only Cataflam has the additional indication as an analgesic and for dysmenorrhea. In addition to the other ADRs of NSAIDs, diclofenac can cause hepatic toxicity, hence liver enzymes should be monitored in the first 8 weeks of treatment. Diclofenac has a relatively low risk for bleeding GI ulcers.

b) Tolmetin (Tolectin), which is primarily indicated for rheumatoid arthritis and osteoarthritis in adults, is also indicated for children (over 2 years old) with juvenile rheumatoid arthritis. It is not approved as an analgesic.

c) Ketorolac (Toradol) is a potent analgesic but is only moderately effective as an antiinflammatory drug. It is available in both oral and intramuscular (IM) forms (in the United States, ketorolac is the only available injectable nonsalicylate NSAID). It is indicated for short-term use in the relief of acute pain (up to 5 days for the IM form; up to a week for ''prn'' use of the oral form). Intramuscular ketorolac is effective in relieving moderate to severe pain. Thirty mg of ketorolac is equipotent to 12 mg of morphine sulfate or 100 mg of meperidine.

4) Fenamate (anthranilic acid) NSAIDs include **meclofenamate (Meclomen)** and **mefenamic acid (Ponstel).** Both are comparable to aspirin and are primarily indicated as analgesics for moderate pain and for dysmenorrhea (mefenamic acid being more effective). They should not be used for more than 1 week because prolonged use may increase GI toxicity.

5) Enolic acid NSAIDs include phenylbutazone and **piroxicam (Feldene).** Phenylbutazone is no longer used because it can cause death because of aplastic anemia and agranulocytosis. Piroxicam has the longest half-life (50 hours) and can be given once a day. It is approved for use in rheumatoid arthritis and osteoarthritis but not as an analgesic. It has high GI toxicity (greater than ASA).

6) Alkanone NSAIDs include **nabumetone (Relafen)** which, like sulindac (see section I.A.3.b.1), is a pro-drug. Nabumetone has a long half-life (24 hours) and can be given once a day. It has lower risk of producing GI complications (less than 0.1%) probably because of selective inhibition of COX-2. It is approved for use in rheumatoid arthritis and osteoarthritis but not as an analgesic.

4. Nonnarcotic analgesic combinations. Caffeine is added to some of the NSAID combinations to increase the analgesic potency and enhance mood.

a. Acetaminophen with caffeine is used for migraine headaches. A common combination is 325 mg acetaminophen, 50 mg butalbital, and 40 mg caffeine (**Fiorecet, Esgic**), 1 to 2 tabs, po, q4h.

b. Acetylsalicylic acid with caffeine can also used for migraine headaches. Examples are Fiorinal (ASA/butalbical/caffeine 325/50/40 mg), 1 to 2 tabs, po, q4h; Norgesic (ASA/orphenadrine/caffeine 385/25/30 mg), 1 to 2 tabs, po, tid/qid; and Norgesic Forte (ASA/orphenadrine/caffeine 770/50/60 mg), 0.5 to 1 tab, po, tid/qid.

c. Acetylsalicylic acid with muscle relaxants are used to relieve pain in patients with muscle spasms. Examples are Robaxisal (ASA/methocarbamol 325/400 mg), 2 tabs, po, qid and Soma Compound (ASA/carisoprodol 325/200 mg), 1 to 2 tabs, po, qid.

B. Opioid (or narcotic) analgesics refer to drugs that are pharmacologically similar to opium or morphine. They provide analgesia without antipyretic or antiinflammatory action. They are indicated for short-term use in patients with acute severe or moderate-to-severe pain (e.g., postsurgical or posttraumatic pain or acute phase of myocardial infarct) and for long-term use in cancer patients with chronic pain. Their use in noncancer chronic pain remains controversial (see Chapter 5.10, section VI.E.1.b). If possible, they are used in combination with a nonopioid analgesics (e.g., NSAIDs) to reduce the need for the opioid and minimize the opioid side effects. For details on guidelines for the use of opioids in pain management, refer to Chapter 5.10, section VI.E.1.b. Aside from their primary use as analgesics, opioids can also be used clinically to provide sedation, suppress coughs (e.g., in intubated patients), and control diarrhea.

Mechanism of action. All opioid drugs bind to opioid receptors and produce analgesia and other effects by mimicking the actions of endogenous opioid compounds at opioid receptors. These opioid receptors are highly concentrated on the second and third layers of the substantia gelatinosa and are in the cerebral cortex, hypothalamus, medial thalamus, amygdala, extrapyramidal regions, and sympathetic preganglionic neurons. In humans, the opioid receptors have been classified according to their pharmacologic effect and their location into 1) μ–*receptors,* primarily distributed in the brain and spinal cord and associated with supraspinal analgesia (they are further subclassified into μ-1 *receptors*, which mediate somatic and visceral analgesia and the μ-2 *receptors*, which are associated with respiratory depression, bradycardia, decreased GI motility, euphoria, and dependence); 2) δ–*receptors,* which modulate mu activity and mediate somatic (but not visceral) analgesia as well as some respiratory depression; 3) κ–*receptors,* which function at the spinal and supraspinal levels, where they have some direct (and primarily visceral) analgesic function in addition to sedation; 4) σ *receptors*, which are associated with dysphoria, psychotomimetic effects, and other excitatory phenomena (e.g., tachycardia, tachypnea, mydriasis, and hypertonia); and 5) ε–*receptors,* which are not well-defined but appear to be stimulated by β-endorphin and are possibly involved in the control of heat-related antinociception.

Opioid classification. Based on their effect on the opioid receptors, exogenous opioids can be classified into pure-agonist opioids, agonist-antagonist opioids, and pure antagonist opioids. Pure agonist opioids bind and activate μ-receptors. Examples are the opium-related alkaloids (i.e., morphine and codeine) and their semisynthetic (e.g., hydrocodone, hydromorphone, oxycodone, oxymorphone, and dihydrocodeine) as well as synthetic derivatives (e.g., methadone, meperidine, lovorphanol, fentanyl, sufentanil, alfentanil, and propoxyphene). The pure-agonist opioids are preferred over the agonist-antagonist opioids in the management of pain, because the pure agonists do not have a ''ceiling'' effect, and their analgesic effect can accrue until side effects limit their dosage. In contrast, the agonist-antagonist opioids have a ''ceiling'' effect for analgesia (i.e., increasing the dose above a certain level will not produce increased analgesia), this then limits efficacy for pain management, especially for severe pain.

The agonist-antagonist opioids can be subclassified into partial agonists (e.g., buprenorphine) and mixed agonist-antagonists (e.g., butorphanol, nalbuphine, pentazocine, and dezocine). The partial-agonist buprenorphine has limited analgesic efficacy because it partially stimulates the μ-receptor to a level below its maximum level. The mixed agonist-antagonist opioids act simultaneously on different subtypes, with the potential for agonist action on one or more subtypes (e.g., agonists at κ–receptors) and antagonist action on one or more subtypes (e.g., antagonists at δ receptors and weak antagonists at μ–receptors). The selective action of agonist-antagonist opioids at the opioid receptors is responsible for producing less respiratory depression and lowering the risk of abuse (because they do not produce euphoria). Their selective actions can also be responsible for their weak-to-moderate analgesic effect and, except possibly for dezocine, for their increased psychotomimetic side effects (e.g., hallucination and dysphoria). Although agonist-antagonist opioids have lower abuse potential in addict populations, they still can produce withdrawal symptoms or pain recurrence in opioid-dependent patients (because of their antagonistic effects). The lower abuse potential of agonist-antagonist opioids is of little clinical significance because most patients who have no prior history of substance abuse have very low risk of this outcome regardless of the opioid chosen. Hence, the only apparent advantage to agonist-antagonist opioids in pain management is their possible use in patients with substantial pulmonary compromise and the availability of unique routes of administration for patients who cannot tolerate oral or other routes (e.g., intranasal butorphanol for acute headache).

The pure-antagonist opioids, which competitively displace the opiate agonists from the μ, κ, δ, and σ–receptors, are not analgesics but are clinically used to reverse the life-threatening adverse effects (e.g., respiratory depression and hypotension) caused by overdosage from other opioid drugs. Opioid antagonists should not be used to reverse non-life-threatening effects such as confusion or sedation because opioid reversal can result in acute withdrawal, which may be complicated by excruciating pain and seizures. It has recently been hypothesized that stress-induced release of endorphins and the resultant decreased sympathetic output are reversed by opioid antagonists (thus suggesting a possible application in the treatment of ischemic or traumatic neurologic injury, Alzheimer's disease, schizophrenia, intractable pruritus, and thalamic pain syndromes). Examples of pure opioid antagonists are naloxone (Narcan), naltrexone (ReVia, Trexan), and nalmefene (Revex). Naloxone is used to reverse life-threatening side effects (e.g., respiratory depression; see below under Adverse Drug Reactions); whereas naltrexone and nalmefene, which can be given orally, are used as an adjunct to the maintenance of the opioid-free state in detoxified formerly opioid-dependent patients.

Adverse drug reactions. Opioids do not produce major organ toxicity from acute or chronic administration (except isolated cases of pulmonary edema in severely ill patients). Adverse drug reactions include CNS effects (e.g., sedation, dysphoria, confusion, sleep disturbances, and seizures), respiratory depression (rarely occurs except in opioid-naive patients and those with significant pulmonary disease), cardiovascular effects (e.g., hypotension, orthostatic hypotension, dysrhythmias, and bradycardia), gastrointestinal effects (e.g., constipation, nausea and vomiting, and toxic megacolon in patients with inflammatory bowel disease), genitourinary effects (e.g., increase in the tone of the bladder, ureter, and sphincter; and urinary retention), and others (e.g., meiosis, dry mouth, pruritius, skeletal muscle rigidity, sexual dysfunction, inappropriate secretion of antidiuretic hormone, and physical dependence). True hypersensitivity reactions to opioids (e.g., urticaria, rash, and anaphylaxis) are rare. If patients experience such reactions, it is often possible to administer an opioid from another subclass safely, i.e., from the phenanthrene derivatives (e.g., morphine, codeine, hydromorphone, and oxycodone) to phenylpiperidine derivatives (e.g., meperidine and fentanyl) or to diphenylheptane derivatives (e.g., methadone). Drugs that potentiate the adverse effects of opioids include phenothiazines, antidepressants, benzodiazepines, alcohol, and other psychotropic drugs.

The opioid side effects can be managed as follows:

- For mild constipation, increase dietary fiber and use a mild osmotic laxative (e.g., milk of magnesia); for severe constipation, use daily oral hyperosmotic agents (e.g., lactulose) or stimulant laxatives plus stool softeners (e.g., senokot plus docusate) or stimulant suppositories (e.g., bisacodyl). See Chapter 5.8, section VI.B.3.a.5.a.2 for details;

- For persistent opioid-induced sedation, try to reduce the opioid in each dose and increase the dosage frequency to decrease the peak concentration in the blood and brain while maintaining the same total dose. In some patients, switching to another opioid may reduce the sedation. If the above strategy is ineffective, add a psychostimulant drug, for example, caffeine; methylphenidate (Ritalin), 5 to 10 mg, po, bid/tid; dextroamphetamine (Dexedrine), 2.5 to 7.5 mg, po, bid; or pemoline (Cylert), 18.5 to 37.5 mg, po, qd;

- For nausea associated with early satiety, give metoclopramide (Reglan), 10 mg, IV/IM, q2-3h or 5 to 20 mg, po, tid/qid; for nausea associated with vertigo or if markedly exacerbated by movement, give antivertiginous drug, e.g., scopolamine (Transderm Scop), one patch (0.5 mg) behind ear, q72h, meclizine (Antivert), 25 mg, po, q6h, or dimenhydrinate (Dramamine), 50 mg po/IM/IV, q4h; in other cases of nausea, try an antihistamine agent, e.g., hydroxycine (Vistaril), 25 to 100 mg, IM, q4-6h or a dopamine antagonist drug, e.g. prochlorperazine (Compazine), 10 mg, po/IM, tid/qid, or 25 mg, PR, q12h, chlorpromazine (Thorazine), 10 mg, po/IM, bid/tid/qid, haloperidol (Haldol), 1 to 2 mg, IM/po, bid/tid. If the patient complains of nausea after opioid administration has begun, it is often helpful to give an antiemetic on a fixed schedule for several days, after which as-needed dosing is usually adequate. Depending on the antiemetic chosen, patients should be monitored for the possibility of increasing sedation.

- For respiratory depression, give naloxone (Narcan), 0.01 mg/kg or 0.4 to 2.0 mg or more, IV/IM/SC or via endotracheal route. Naloxone should be given incrementally in doses that improve the respiratory function but do not reverse analgesia. A dilute solution of naloxone (0.4 mg in 10 ml of saline) may be given as 0.5 ml (0.02 mg) boluses every minute. Alternatively, an infusion of 2 ampules (total of 0.8 mg) in 250 ml of 5% dextrose in water may be continually titrated toward this goal.

- For pruritus, an antihistamine, e.g., diphenhydramine (Benadryl), 25 to 50 mg, IV/IM/po, q6h may be used.

Physical dependence. With chronic opioid use, tolerance and physical dependence may occur even after as little as a few days of therapy. When the drug is abruptly stopped, physically dependent patients can develop withdrawal or abstinence syndromes (e.g., anxiety, nervousness, agitation, narcotic craving, tachycardia, hypertension, GI distress, temperature instability, diffuse musculoskeletal pain, piloerection, pupil dilation, diaphoresis, lacrimation, and rhinorrhea). Likewise, if an opioid antagonist (e.g., naloxone) has been given, the patient may go into withdrawal even after only 3 days of opioid therapy. Withdrawal or abstinence syndromes are rarely life-threatening, and once withdrawal is complete, dependence ceases. To minimize abstinence syndromes, opioids should be tapered slowly over 3 to 5 days, for example, taper by 50%, then decrease further by 25% q2d; once the dose is tapered to equianalgesic oral morphine dose of 0.6 mg/kg/day for patients above 50 kg, or 30 mg/day for patients below 50 kg, then the opioid can be stopped. If a faster dose reduction is required, sympathetic overactivity during withdrawal can be blocked by coadministration of an α_1-adrenergic blocker, e.g., clonidine (Catapres), 0.1 mg, po bid, or 0.1 to 0.2 mg/day transdermally.

Contraindications and precautions. Opioids are contraindicated in patients with known hypersensitivity to the drug or the component of its vehicle. They are generally not used if the pattern and degree of pain are important diagnostic signs in the acute stage of the disease (e.g., in patients with traumatic brain injury [TBI] or abdominal pain). They should be used with caution in the elderly, neonates, and in patients with impaired renal or hepatic function, respiratory disease (e.g., chronic obstructive pulmonary disease [COPD], asthma, kyphoscoliosis, severe obesity, and chronic cor pulmonale), head injury (increased opioid sensitivity due to alterations in blood-brain integrity), hydrocephalus, hypothyroidism, Addison's disease, hypopituitarism, anemia, severe malnutrition, or debilitation. They must also be used with caution (because of the potential for addiction) in patients with a prior history of drug abuse or severe personality disorder.

Drug administration guidelines. The use of opioids or other analgesics should always be done in conjunction with adjunctive pharmacologic and nonpharmacologic therapies (see Chapter 5.10, section VI). The dose, drug, and route of administration of opioids are chosen according to the severity of the pain, location, cause, risk of potential side effects, and the patient's psychophysiologic condition. Oral administration is as effective as parenteral in appropriate dosages and should be used whenever oral medications are tolerated. In patients with dysphagia, emesis, and decreased GI absorption, opioids may be given rectally (used as if dose is equianalgesic to oral dose) or parenterally. Intravenous (IV) or subcutaneous (SQ) administration is the parenteral route of choice for opioids (e.g., after major surgery). This may be accomplished by bolus or by patient-controlled analgesia (PCA) using special infusion pumps (which can deliver opioid intravenously, epidurally, intrathecally, or subcutaneously). Although effective, epidural and intrathecal administration should be monitored as they may result in delayed, significant respiratory depression. Patient-controlled analgesia has been shown to improve pain relief, decrease anxiety, and allow less total drug to be given in postoperative patients and in cancer patients. The old standard, intramuscular (IM) administration, should be avoided as it is painful and drug absorption is unreliable. Opioids for long-term pain management (e.g., in cancer patients) can also be given transdermally (available for fentanyl).

The type of opioid used should preferably be a pure-agonist opioid. The initial dose should be the lowest recommended dose (see Tables 4.8-3 and 4.8-4 for recommended starting dose for treating severe pain in patients who are opioid-naive or with limited prior opioid exposure). The initial dose can be increased gradually until a favorable balance between analgesia and side effects is attained. After 24 hours, if the pain is not 90% controlled, the opioid dose can be increased by 50%. The absolute opioid dose is immaterial and is considered right for the patient if it provides adequate relief for 4 hours without unacceptable adverse effects. Drug treatment for side effects (see above, under Adverse Drug Reactions) such as nausea, sedation, and constipation, may enhance patient comfort and allow opioid dose escalation

Table 4.8-3.   Commonly used pure-agonist opioids for management of pain

PURE AGONIST OPIOIDS	SELECTED BRANDNAMES	AVAILABLE PREPARATIONS (mg)	DOSAGE (mg), ROUTE, FREQUENCY
I. Short half-life*			
Morphine sulfate	a) MSO$_4$ injection b) MS-IR c) Roxanol	a) *inj* 1, 5, 8, 10, 15/ml b) *tab or cap* 15, 30; *sol* 10, 20/5 ml; 10, 20/ml c) *liq* 20, 100/5 ml; 10/2.5 ml; 30/1.5 ml; 20/ml *supp* 5, 10, 20, 30	a) 0.1-0.2/kg up to 15 IV/SQ/IM q3-4h; 10-30 po q3-4h; b) and c) 10-30 po q3-4h
Morphine sulfate (sustained release)	a) MS-Contin, b) Oramorph c) Kadian	a) *tab* 15, 30, 60, 100, 200 b) *tab* 30, 60, 100 c) *cap* 20, 50, 100	1 tab or cap po q8-12h
Hydromorphone	Dilaudid	*inj* 1, 2, 4, 10/ml *tab* 1, 2, 3, 4 *supp* 3	1-1.5 IM/SQ/IV q3-4h; 2-8 po q3-4h; 3 pr q4h
Meperidine†	Demerol	*inj* 25, 50, 100/ml *tab* 50, 100; *liq* 50/5 ml	1-1.8/kg up to 150 or 50-150 SQ/IM/po q3-4h
Codeine‡	Codeine	*inj* 30/ml; 60/ml *tab* 15, 30, 60	0.5-1/kg up to 60 po/IM q3-4h
Oxycodone	a) Roxicodone b) Oxycontin	a) *tab* 5; *liq* 5/5 ml b) *tab* 10,20,40	a) 0.2/kg up to 20 po q3-4h b) 10-40 po q12h
Oxymorphone	Numorphan	*inj* 1, 1.5/ml *supp* 5	0.02/kg or 1-1.5 IM/SQ/IV q3-4h 5 pr q4h
Propoxyphene	Darvon	*tab* 65	65 po q4h
Fentanyl§	Duragesic TD patch	25, 50, 75, 100µg/hr	1 patch q72h (maximum of 300 µg/hr/day)
II. Long half-life			
Levorphanol	Levo-dromoran	*inj* 2/ml *tab* 2	0.02-0.04/kg up to 2-4 po/SQ q6-8h
Methadone	Dolophine	*inj* 5, 10/5 ml *tab* 5, 10	0.1-0.2/kg IM/SQ q6-8; 10-20 po q6-8h

* Hydrocodone and dihydrocodeine, both of which have short half-lives, are available only in combination with NSAIDs (ASA or acetaminophen). See section I.B.2.a and I.B.2.b for recommended dosage.

† Meperidine may be useful for brief courses (e.g., few days) to treat acute pain and to manage rigors (shivering) induced by medication but should be avoided for pain management due to necessary repeated dosings, which can lead to CNS toxicity (tremor, confusion, dysphoria, or seizure).

‡ Codeine doses above 65 mg are often not appropriate due to diminishing incremental analgesia with increasing doses and continually increasing nausea, constipation and other side effects; IV codeine can cause hypotension.

§ Transdermal fentanyl (Duragesic TD Patch) is used in more chronic (not acute) pain. Doses above 25 µg/hr should not be used in opioid-naive patients.

IR = immediate release; liq = liquid; supp = suppository; MS = morphine sulfate; TD = transdermal; inj = injection; sol = solution.

Table 4.8-4. **Recommended starting dose (oral and parenteral) of opioids in (A) adults over 50 kg body weight and (C) children (excluding babies under 6 months old) or adults under 50 kg body weight**

OPIOID AGONISTS	EQUIANALGESIC ORAL DOSE	EQUIANALGESIC PARENTERAL DOSE	STARTING DOSE§ (ORAL)	STARTING DOSE§ (PARENTERAL)
I. "Strong"*				
Morphine	30 mg q3-4h (ATC); 60 mg q3-4h (single dosing)	10 mg q3-4h	A: 30 mg q3-4h C: 0.3 mg/kg q3-4h	A: 10 mg q3-4h C: 0.1 mg/kg q3-4h
Hydromorphone	7.5 mg q3-4h	1.5 mg q3-4h	A: 6 mg q3-4h C: 0.06 mg/kg q3-4h	A: 1.5 mg q3-4h C: 0.015 mg/kg q3-4h
Levorphanol	4 mg q6-8h	2 mg q6-8h	A: 4 mg q6-8h C: 0.04 mg/kg q6-8h	A: 2 mg q6-8h C: 0.02 mg/kg q6-8h
Methadone	20 mg q6-8h	10 mg q6-8h	A: 20 mg q6-8h C: 0.2 mg/kg q6-8h	A: 10 mg q6-8 h C: 0.1 mg/kg q6-8h
Fentanyl†	N/A	100 μg q30 min–1h	N/A	A: 25-75 μg q30min C: 0.5-1.5 μg/kg q30min
II. "Weak"*				
Codeine‡	130-200 mg q3-4h	75-130 mg q3-4h	A: 60 mg q3-4h C: 1 mg/kg q3-4h	A: 60 mg q2h (IM/SQ) C: NR
Hydrocodone	30 mg q3-4h	N/A	A: 10 mg q3-4h C: 0.2 mg/kg q3-4h	N/A
Oxycodone	30 mg q3-4h	N/A	A: 10 mg q3-4h C: 0.2 mg/kg q3-4h	N/A
Oxymorphone	N/A	1 mg q3-4h	N/A	A: 1 mg q3-4h C: NR
Meperidine	300 mg q2-3h	100 mg q3h	NR	A: 100 mg q3h C: 0.75 mg/kg q2-3h

Adapted from Acute Pain Management Guideline Panel: *Acute pain management in infants, children, and adolescents: operative and medical procedures. Quick reference guide for clinician.* AHCPR Pub. No. 92-0020, Rockville, MD, 1992, Agency for Health Care Policy and Research, US Department of Health and Human Services, with permission.

ATC = around the clock; N/A = not available; NR = not recommended

* Classification of opioids into "weak" opioids (for use in mild to moderate pain) and "strong" opioids (for use in moderate to severe pain) is made principally on the grounds of common patterns of use and not on any pharmacological differences (i.e., there is no pharmacological differences between a high dose of codeine and an equianalgesic low dose of morphine).

† Available as transdermal patches (Duragesic) in four sizes (25, 50, 75, or 100 μg/hr) given q72h for chronic pain use.

‡ Codeine doses above 65 mg is often not appropriate due to diminishing incremental analgesia with increasing doses and continually increasing nausea, constipation, and other side effects; published equianalgesic doses varies.

§ Recommended starting doses do not apply to patients with renal or hepatic insufficiency or other conditions affecting drug metabolism or kinetics.

into an effective range. If possible, opioids should be supplemented with a coanalgesic to help decrease the need for opioids and minimize the opioid side effects (especially in patients with a significant risk of hypoxia and who are at increased risk of respiratory depression or sedation, e.g., patients with morbid obesity, sleep apnea, intrapulmonary shunts, or who are ventilator-dependent). The coanalgesic can either be a nonopioid analgesic (e.g., NSAIDs) or an antihistamine agent (e.g. hydroxycine, which also has anti-emetic properties; see section I.B). It has been reported that regularly scheduled NSAIDs for only 72 hours can significantly reduce opioid requirement in the acute postoperative or postraumatic phase.

In patients with constant pain, continuous (around-the-clock) analgesia is indicated with a supplementary or "prn" dose (also called the "rescue" dose) for breakthrough pain (i.e., pain that occurs in between regularly scheduled analgesic regimen, which may be associated with activity or treatments). The rescue opioid could be another weak or strong opioid, usually one with rapid onset and short half-life (e.g., parenteral hydromorphone; or if using slow-release oral morphine, an immediate-release oral morphine or injectable morphine sulfate could be used as the rescue opioid). The rescue dose is given q2h or more frequently at a dose equal to 5 to 15% of the total daily opioid requirement. If the patient requires frequent "rescue" doses, then the regular dosage should be increased or the interval between doses should be decreased. In patients receiving continuous opioid infusions, the rescue dose is usually 50 to 200% of the continuous hourly rate. If there is inadequate relief and no significant toxicity noted, then the rescue dose may be increased by 50% increment. If 6 or more rescue doses are needed in 24 hours, then the infusion rate should be increased by using the rescue doses taken in the previous 24 hours, i.e., 10×5 mg rescues $\times$ 24 hrs divided by 24 = rate of increase in infusion by mg/hr, or the infusion may be increased by 50%.

If the maximum recommended dose of one narcotic is attained without adequate analgesia, or if the side effects are intolerable, then another opioid preparation should be used. It is inadvisable to prescribe simultaneously two weak opioids or two strong opioids. If changing from a short half-life opioid to another short half-life opioid, start at 50% of the equianalgesic dose and titrate to the desired response (except in circumstances such as severe pain and absence of CNS side effects, which may necessitate starting at 100% of the equianalgesic dose). If changing from a short half-life to a long half-life opioid, start at only 25% of the equianalgesic dose and titrate to the desired response. The equianalgesic dose, which is shown in Table 8.4-4, does not indicate the efficacy of the drug, but is useful to know when one is switching opioid drugs or routes of administration. Published tables vary in the suggested doses that are equianalgesic to morphine. The criterion that must be applied for each patient is the clinical response, which needs to be titrated for each patient. If the patient feels that he or she does not need the prescribed amount of medication, the dose should be reduced. Also, if the cause of the pain is eliminated or lessened (e.g., after cordotomy), the opioid dose should be lowered because patients who previously appeared to be tolerant to adverse opioid effects can suddenly develop adverse drug reactions.

The following is a classification of clinically useful opioid analgesics, i.e., pure-agonist opioids and combination opioid-NSAID drugs. Heroin (Di-amorphine), which is also a pure-agonist opioid, is illegal in the United States and is not discussed. As mentioned before (under opioid classification), the agonist-antagonist opioids are of little benefit in pain management in the PM&R setting and are therefore not discussed below (except for pentazocine, which is available orally in combination with NSAIDs).

1. **Pure-agonist opioids**
   a. **Opium alkaloids (phenanthrene derivatives)**
   1) **Morphine** is the standard against which all other opioids are often compared. It is classified as a ''strong'' opioid analgesic (see Table 4.8-4) and is indicated for use in patients with moderate to severe pain. Its potency is the basis for the construction of the equianalgesic table (see Table 4.8-4), which helps facilitate appropriate dose adjustment when another opioid of different potency is used. Morphine is available in oral (MS-IR, Roxanol), suppository (Roxanol), and injectable (Morphine Sulfate) forms. When given parenterally, the subcutaneous or intravenous route of morphine is preferred because the rate of absorption from the intramuscular route is variable and unreliable. The oral form is also available in slow-release form (MS-Contin, Oramorph SR). Although the slow-release preparations do not increase the bioavailability of the morphine, they play a significant role in the relief of chronic and malignancy-related pain. Because of the advent of the slow-release morphine, there is now less reason for choosing an opioid other than morphine on the grounds of longer duration of effect.

   2) **Codeine or methylmorphine** is usually administered in combination forms with NSAIDs, e.g., Tylenol with codeine, Fiorecet with codeine, Empirin with codeine, and Soma compound with codeine (see section I.B.2.b.1.c). Codeine is classified as a ''weak'' opioid and is indicated for use in mild to moderate pain (Table 4.8-4). Codeine doses above 65 mg are often not appropriate because of diminishing incremental analgesia, continually increasing nausea, constipation, and other side effects with increasing doses.

   b. **Semisynthetic pure-agonist opioids** include hydromorphone (Dilaudid), oxymorphone (Numorphan), oxycodone (Roxicodone, Oxycontin), hydrocodone, and dihydrocodeine. Both hydrocodone (Vicodin, Lortab, Anexsia, Zydone) and dihydrocodeine (Synalgos-DC) are available only in oral forms in combination with NSAIDs (see section I.A.3). Oxycodone is also available as controlled-release single-formulation (Oxycontin) and in combination with NSAIDs (e.g., Percocet, Percodan, Tylox). All semisynthetic pure-agonist opioids are classified as ''weak'' opioids and are indicated for use in mild to moderate pain except hydromorphone, which is a ''strong'' opioid indicated for use in moderate to severe pain (Table 4.8-4). Hydromorphone has a shorter duration and more sedation but produces less euphoria than morphine. It is available in oral, parenteral, as well as suppository forms. Hydromorphone can be used in cases of morphine toxicity in patients with renal disease. The other semisynthetic pure-agonist opioid available in suppository form is oxymorphone, which is also available in injectable but not in oral forms.

   c. **Synthetic pure-agonist opioids** include levorphanol (Levor-Dromoran), methadone (Dolophine), propoxyphene (Darvon), and the phenylpiperidine opioids, which consist of meperidine (Demerol), fentanyl (Sublimaze, Duragesic), and the two fentanyl derivatives, sufentanil (Sufenta) and alfentanil (Alfenta). Sufentanil and alfentanil, which are both intravenous drugs with rapid onset and short duration, are primarily used in general anesthesia. They play no role in physiatric pain management. Among the synthetic pure-agonist opioids, levorphanol, methadone, and fentanyl are classified as a "strong" opioid analgesic drugs (Table 4.8-4) and are indicated for use in patients with moderate to severe pain; whereas meperidine and propoxyphene are classified as "weak" opioid analgesic (Table 4.8-4) and are used in patients with mild to moderate pain.

Levorphanol and methadone are two of the pure-agonist opioids with the longest half-life (12-16 hrs and 15-40 hrs, respectively). Because of their long half-lives, they must be used with caution as they can accumulate and cause delayed respiratory and CNS depression. However, because biologic half-lives do not always correspond to analgesic half-lives, methadone and levorphanol can have much shorter analgesic duration despite the long elimination half-life. They are both available in oral and injectable forms. Oral methadone is the drug of choice for the suppression of narcotic withdrawal symptoms and is a good choice for patients with chronic intractable pain.

Fentanyl is available in an IV form (Sublimaze) and in a transdermal form (Duragesic). The IV form is primarily used in general anesthesia. Transdermal delivery bypasses GI absorption and has been shown to be an effective, noninvasive route, which can reach the same peak concentrations in the blood as with IV administration. Each Duragesic patch contains a 72-hour supply of fentanyl, which is passively absorbed through the skin over this period. Fentanyl, which has high lipid solubility is deposited in the subcutaneous tissue and subsequently absorbed into the systemic circulation. Over a period of 12 to 18 hours after patch placement, the fentanyl levels in plasma rise slowly (this can continue even after patch removal because of subcutaneous deposition). The prolonged time between patch application and the achievement of adequate serum levels producing analgesia makes it inappropriate for use in acute pain. Transdermal (TD) fentanyl should only be considered when patients already on opioid therapy have relatively constant pain and infrequent episodes of breakthrough pain such that rapid increases or decreases in pain intensity are not anticipated. As with other long-acting analgesics, all patients should be provided with oral or parenteral opioids (rapidly acting with short duration) to manage breakthrough pain. The maximum daily dose of TD fentanyl is 300 μg/hr. If patients require larger doses, they should be switched to an equianalgesic dose of an oral or subcutaneously administered opioid. The most commonly reported ADRs of TD fentanyl administration are nausea, mental clouding, and skin irritation. Fentanyl is not available in an oral form because of low oral bioavailability caused by its high hepatic clearance.

Propoxyphene is clinically equivalent to codeine when given regularly but is structurally related to methadone (which is a diphenylheptane derivative). Propoxyphene is available orally as a single formulation or in combination with NSAIDs (Darvocet-N, Wygesic, Darvon compound). Its analgesic efficacy is minimal (with an analgesic potency equivalent to 600 mg of aspirin), and it may be useful as an analgesic for mild pain that is not responsive to aspirin alone. Like meperidine and codeine, it is not indicated in the management of more severe pain because of relatively increased toxicity at higher doses.

Meperidine (Demerol) has a short duration of action and may be useful for brief courses (e.g., a few days) to treat acute pain and to manage rigors (shivering) induced by medication; however, it should not be used if continued opioid use is anticipated. Its active metabolite (normeperidine) can accumulate in patients given repeated dosing for pain control or in patients with renal failure or those taking monoamine oxidase (MAO) inhibitors. This can lead to CNS toxicity, which causes tremor, confusion, dysphoria, or seizure. Moreover, meperidine is difficult to titrate to a steady state because of large fluctuations in plasma concentrations. Meperidine is available in both oral and injectable forms.

2. **Opioid-NSAID combinations** are available in oral preparations and are recommended if optimal analgesia is not attained by NSAID use alone. The combination enhances the analgesic efficacy by combining two analgesics with different MOA and by reducing ADRs (i.e., adequate analgesia can often be achieved while keeping the dose of each constituent below the threshold that causes adverse effects). They should not be given in quantities that exceed the maximal safe amount of the nonopioid coanalgesics (e.g. 4 g of acetaminophen per day). Caffeine is added in some of the opioid-NSAID combinations to increase the drugs's analgesic potency and to enhance mood. All of the following are pure-agonist opioids except pentazocine, which is a mixed agonist-antagonist opioid.

a. **Opioids with acetaminophen combination**
   1) **Codeine**
      a) **Tylenol with codeine** (acetaminophen 300 mg + codeine 15 mg [#2], 30 mg [#3], 60 mg [#4]): 1 to 2 tabs, po, q4h; pediatric elixir (acetaminophen 120 mg and codeine 12 mg per 5 ml): 5 ml/dose if 3 to 6 years old; 10 ml/dose if 7 to 12 years old.
      b) **Fioricet with codeine** (acetaminophen/butalbital/caffeine/codeine 325/50/40/30 mg): 1 to 2 tabs, po, q4h.
   2) **Hydrocodone**
      a) **Anexsia** (hydrocodone/acetaminophen 5/500 mg): 1 to 2 tabs, po, q4-6h; (7.5/650): one tab, po, q4-6h.
      b) **Lortab** (hydrocodone/acetaminophen 2.5/500; 5/500; 7.5/500 mg): 1 to 2 tabs, po, q4-6h; elixir (2.5/167 mg per 5 ml): 15 ml, po, q4-6h.
      c) **Lorcet** (hydrocodone/acetaminophen 5/500; 7.5/650; 10/650 mg): 1 to 2 tabs, po, q4-6h.
      d) **Vicodin** (hydrocodone/acetaminophen 5/500 mg): 1 to 2 tabs, po, q4-6h; **Vicodin ES** (7.5/750 mg): 1 tab, po, q4-6h.
      e) **Zydone** (hydrocodone/acetaminophen 5/500 mg): 1 to 2 caps, po, q4-6h.
   3) **Oxycodone**
      a) **Percocet** (oxycodone/acetaminophen 5/325 mg): 1 tab, po, q6h.
      b) **Tylox** (oxycodone/acetaminophen 5/500 mg): 1 tab, po, q6h.
   4) **Propoxyphene** is available as propoxyphene hydrochloride (Darvon, Wygesic) and propoxyphene napsylate (Darvocet-N). The napsylate form is more stable in liquid and tablet formulations. Because of the difference in molecular weight, however, a dose of 100 mg of propoxyphene napsylate is needed to supply an amount of propoxyphene equivalent to that present in 65 mg of propoxyphene hydrochloride (HCl).

   a) **Darvocet N-50** (propoxyphene napsylate/acetaminophen 50/325 mg), 2 tabs, po, q4h; **Darvocet N-100** (100/650 mg), 1 tab, po, q4h.
   b) **Wygesic** (propoxyphene HCl/acetaminophen 65/650 mg), 1 tab, po, q4h.
   5) **Pentazocine: Talacen** (pentazocine/acetaminophen 25/650 mg): 1 tab, po, q4h.
  b. **Opioid with aspirin (ASA) combination**
   1) **Codeine**
    a) **Empirin with codeine** (ASA 325 mg and codeine 30 mg [**#3**], 60 mg [**#4**]: 1 to 2 tabs, po, q4h.
    b) **Fiorinal with codeine** (ASA/butalbital/caffeine/codeine 325/50/40/30 mg): 1 to 2 tabs, po, q4h.
    c) **Soma compound with codeine** (ASA/carisoprodol/codeine 325/200/16 mg): 1 to 2 tabs, po, q6h.
   2) **Oxycodone: Percodan** (oxycodone/ASA 5/325 mg): 1 tab, po, q6h.
   3) **Propoxyphene: Darvon compound** (propoxyphene HCl/ASA/caffeine 65/389/32.4 mg): 1 tab, po, q4h.
   4) **Dihydrocodeine: Synalgos-DC** (dihydrocodeine/ASA/caffeine 16/356.4/30 mg): 2 caps, po, q4h.
   5) **Pentazocine: Talwin compound** (pentazocine/ASA 12.5/325 mg): 2 tabs, po, q6-8h.
 C. **Adjuvant analgesics** (i.e., drugs primarily approved for the treatment of conditions other than pain but are analgesic in selected circumstances) are described in Chapter 5.10, section VI.E.2.
II. **Skeletal muscle relaxants** refer to "antispasmodic" drugs, which are indicated for short-term relief of acute musculoskeletal pains, some of which are characterized by "muscle spasms," which may result in pain or discomfort or be counterproductive to physical rehabilitation. Their use in the treatment of chronic pain remains controversial (see Chapter 5.10 section VI.E.2.f). The "muscle spasms" that occur in the setting of nerve or muscle (or myofascial) injury represent focal areas of increased muscle activity associated with tenderness and splinting of the painful part. This should be distinguished from the terms *spasticity* and *spasms*.

   Spasticity (see Chapter 5.4) is a component of the upper motor neuron syndrome characterized by a velocity-dependent increase in muscle tone with exaggerated tendon jerks; whereas spasms are spontaneous uncontrolled movements (such as painful flexor or extensor spasms, which in turn may precipitate or aggravate spasticity) or other hyperactive spinal reflexes (e.g., such as cramps, dystonia, and rigidity). The antispasticity drugs (e.g., baclofen, dantrolene, and clonidine), which are discussed in Chapter 5.4, section III.D.1, are not indicated in the "muscle spasms" for which the "skeletal muscle relaxants" are indicated. Likewise, the "skeletal muscle relaxants" are not indicated for the treatment of spasticity. The only drug that qualifies both as "antispasticity" and truly as a "skeletal muscle relaxant" is diazepam. To add to the above confusion, all the drugs commonly referred to as "skeletal muscle relaxants" (except perhaps for diazepam) have not been proved to actually relax the skeletal muscles of human beings in the clinical setting.

   Mechanism of action. The precise MOA of "skeletal muscle relaxants" remains unknown, although it is likely related to a central depressant effect with little or no direct effect on skeletal muscles. In animal models, these drugs have been shown to inhibit polysynaptic spinal myogenic reflexes, but the relationship between these actions and any possible analgesic effect is unknown.

It is unclear if these drugs have analgesic effects that are selective for musculo-skeletal pain problems or if relaxation of the "muscle spasm" is a necessary condition for their analgesic effectiveness.

Adverse drug reactions. At the doses used clinically, the "skeletal muscle relaxants" are generally well tolerated. The most common side effects include drowsiness, dizziness, ataxia, tremor, headache, and changes in temperament. They are usually transient and resolve as the patient develops tolerance to them. Other ADRs include rash, hypotension, dyspnea, chest pain, and syncope. Additional ADRs are discussed under each specific drug.

Contraindications and precautions. They are contraindicated in patients with known hypersensitivity to the drug or the component of its vehicle. Because of the side effect of drowsiness, they should be used with caution by patients for whom mental alertness is required (e.g., machinery operators or drivers). Patients should also refrain from concurrent intake of alcohol or other CNS depressants. Additional precautions and contraindications are discussed under each specific drug.

Drug administration guidelines. "Skeletal muscle relaxants" should be started at a low dose and gradually increased (up to the recommended maximum daily dose) if the response is inadequate and side effects minimal. If treatment is ineffective or if side effects are intolerable with one drug, it is reasonable to switch to another drug. Use should ideally be limited to 10 to 14 days (or up to 3 weeks) because of their potential for abuse (reported in some patients with noncancer chronic pain). Also, long-term effects have not been fully evaluated.

"Skeletal muscle relaxants" are marketed alone and in combination with other compounds (usually with aspirin or codeine).

A. Single formulations

1. **Cyclobenzaprine (Flexeril)** probably exerts its effects centrally, primarily in the brain stem and not in the spinal cord. It is chemically related to the tricyclic antidepressants (see section V.A.1) and possesses many of their adverse effects, including CNS depression, anticholinergic effects, and GI effects (e.g. nausea, vomiting, altered taste, constipation or diarrhea, anorexia, and abdominal pain). It has been reported to be effective in patients with fibromyalgia (see Chapter 4.11; Chapter 5.10, Table 5.10-1). Its use is contraindicated in many forms of heart disease (e.g., acute myocardial infarction) and in patients with hyperthyroidism, symptomatic prostatic hypertrophy, or narrow angle glaucoma. It should not be used concurrently or within 2 weeks of monoamine oxidase inhibitor (MAOI) use. The starting dose is 10 mg, po, tid, which can be increased up to a maximum of 60 mg/day. Flexeril is available only in oral form (10-mg tablets).

2. **Carisoprodol (Soma)** probably acts by blocking interneuronal activity in the descending reticular formation and spinal cord (thus causing CNS depression). It has a rapid onset which lasts for 4 to 6 hours. Idiosyncratic drug reactions include extreme weakness, transient tetraplegia, temporary vision problems, mydriasis, dysarthria, agitation, euphoria, confusion, and disorientation. It must be used with caution in patients with hepatic and renal impairments. It is contraindicated in acute intermittent porphyria. Soma is available only for oral use (350-mg tablets) at a dose of 350 mg, po, tid/qid. It is also available in combination with ASA and/or opioids (see below).

3. **Chlorzoxazone (Parafon Forte)** probably acts at the spinal cord and subcortical levels, by inhibiting multisynaptic reflex arcs that may be associated with

painful muscle spasms. This drug is usually well-tolerated with rare ADRs. The starting dose is 250 to 500 mg, po, tid/qid, which can be increased up to 750 mg, po, tid/qid. Parafon Forte is available only in oral forms (250- and 500-mg caplets).

4. **Methocarbamol (Robaxin)** probably exerts its effects by generalized CNS depression. It is available in both oral (500- and 750-mg tablets) and parenteral forms (100 mg/ml in 10 ml single-dose vial). The initial oral dose is 1500 mg qid, which can be maintained at 1000 mg qid. It is usually given at 6 g/day for the first 48 to 72 hours, then reduced to 4 g/day. Maximum daily oral dose for severe conditions can be as high as 8 g. The oral form is also marketed in combination with opioids and/or ASA (see below). The injectable form contains polyethylene glycol in the vehicle, which is contraindicated in patients with renal pathology (because polyethylene glycol can increase preexisting acidosis and cause urea retention). Intravenous injections have also been reported to cause seizures. The parenteral form can be given 1 g, IM/IV, q6h as needed (maximum rate of IV injection is 3 ml/min; maximum dose is 3 g/day).

5. **Orphenadrine (Norflex)** probably acts in the reticular formation of the brainstem. It is also classified as an antihistaminic agent and has mild anticholinergic effects (dose-related). Its use is contraindicated in patients with glaucoma, pyloric or duodenal obstruction, stenosing peptic ulcers, prostatic hypertrophy or obstruction of the bladder neck, cardiospasm (megaesophagus), and myasthenia gravis. Norflex is available in both oral (100-mg tablet) and parenteral (60 mg/2 ml ampule) forms. The oral dose is 100 mg, po, bid; while the parenteral dose is 60 mg IM/IV, q12h. Oral orphenadrine is also available in combination with ASA and/or opioids (see below).

6. **Metaxalone (Skelaxin)** probably exerts its effects by generalized CNS depression. Additional ADRs include GI upsets (nausea, vomiting), leukopenia, hemolytic anemia, and jaundice. It is contraindicated in patients with significant renal and hepatic impairment, as well as the known tendency to drug-induced hemolytic or other anemia. It is available only for oral use (400-mg tablet) at a dose of 800 mg, po, tid/qid.

7. **Diazepam (Valium)** is discussed in section V.C.1.b.1. It can be used to relieve muscle spasm at a dose of 2 to 10 mg, po, tid/qid.

B. **Combinations with ASA, opioid, or both.** The analgesic effect of ASA and/or opioid can be potentiated by combining them with ''skeletal muscle relaxants.''

   1. **Carisoprodol. Soma Compound** (carisoprodol/ASA 200/325 mg), 1 to 2 tabs, po, qid; **Soma compound with codeine** (carisoprodol/ASA/codeine 200/325/16 mg): 1 to 2 tabs, po, q6h.

   2. **Orphenadrine. Norgesic** (orphenadrine/ASA/caffeine 25/385/30 mg): 1 to 2 tabs, po, tid/qid; **Norgesic Forte** (orphenadrine/ASA/caffeine 50/770/60 mg): 0.5 to 1 tab, po, tid/qid.

   3. **Methocarbamol: Robaxisal** (methocarbamol/ASA 400/325 mg), 2 tabs, po, qid.

III. **Corticosteroids** are one of the two steroids (the other being androgen) synthesized by the adrenal cortex. There are two kinds of corticosteroids: glucocorticoids and mineralocorticoids. In human beings, the main glucocorticoid is hydrocortisone (cortisol), and the main mineralocorticoid is aldosterone. The corticosteroids referred to in this chapter are mainly glucocorticoids. Glucocorticoids have potent antiinflammatory, hormonal, and metabolic effects. They are capable of suppressing many disease manifestations, both articular and systemic. In the PM&R setting, they are primarily used in treating neuromuscular diseases, rheumatic and collagen disorders, and cerebral edema (e.g., after brain surgery, head injury, or stroke). Their possible role as an analgesic is discussed in Chapter 5.10 section VI.E.2.J.

Mechanism of action. Corticosteroids suppress inflammation by blocking phospholipase A_2 thus inhibiting the formation of arachidonic acid, which is the precursor of prostaglandins (see Fig 4.8-1). They also inhibit humoral and cell-mediated immune processes as well as stabilize lysosomal membranes.

Adverse drug reactions. Corticosteroids provide multisystem benefits and likewise cause multisystem ADRs. The ADRs and complications are time- and dose-related, hence long-term or high-dose corticosteroid therapy should be avoided unless it produces a definite advantage. The possible ADRs of corticosteroids include:

- Fluid and electrolyte disturbances, e.g., fluid retention (with weight gain), congestive heart failure, hypertension, and hypokalemic alkalosis;
- Musculoskeletal effects, e.g., muscle weakness and atrophy, tendon rupture, steroid myopathy, osteoporosis, vertebral compression fracture, aseptic necrosis of femoral and humeral heads, and pathologic fracture of long bones;
- Gastrointestinal effects, e.g., peptic or gastric ulcers with possible bleeding (for GI protection, see section I.A.3 under GI toxicity), ulcerative esophagitis, pancreatitis, abdominal distension, and nausea;
- Dermatologic effects, e.g., impaired wound healing, thin fragile skin, petechiae, ecchymoses, acne, hirsutism, striae, purpura, and suppression of reactions to skin tests;
- Endocrine effects, e.g., cushingoid state, manifestations of latent diabetes mellitus, glucose intolerance, increase need for hypoglycemics, growth arrest, secondary amenorrhea, impotence, and suppression of the hypothalamic-pituitary adrenal axis;
- Ophthalmic effects, e.g., cataract, glaucoma, and exopthalmos;
- Neurologic and psychological effects, e.g., convulsions, increased intracranial pressure, vertigo, headache, behavior disturbance, and steroid psychoses;
- Immune system effects, e.g., increased susceptibility to infection, and activation of old infection (e.g., tuberculosis or amebiasis);
- Other effects, e.g., thromboembolism, changes in leukocyte and lymphocyte count, protein catabolism, myocardial rupture following recent myocardial infarction, malaise, and increased appetite.

Contraindications and precautions. Corticosteroids are contraindicated in patients with systemic infection (especially fungal) and patients with known hypersensitivity to the drug or the component of its vehicle. It must be used with caution in patients with diabetes mellitus, hypertension, pregnancy, psychotic tendencies, renal impairments, osteoporosis, active or latent peptic ulcer, ulcerative colitis, and ocular herpes simplex. The steroid effects are enhanced in patients with cirrhosis and in those with hypothyroidism.

Drug administration guidelines. In general, nonsteroidal agents are tried before corticosteroids are begun. When possible, less hazardous agents should be used concurrently to allow the lowest possible dose of corticosteroid. The concurrent use of NSAIDs, however, is not recommended because of the high risk of GI toxicity. In long-term corticosteroid therapy, periodic determinations of blood sugar, electrolytes, complete blood counts, stool guaiacs, blood pressure, and body weight should be obtained. Drug dosage varies widely according to the specific disease, its severity, as well as the corticosteroid preparation and the patient's response. The route of systemic corticosteroid therapy can be oral or parenteral (IM/IV). Dosages of oral and parenteral preparations are generally comparable. High-dose parenteral therapy is often used for severe illnesses. IM administration may provide a sustained or depot action, which can be used to supplement or replace initial oral therapy. Some corticosteroid preparations (e.g., triamcinolone [Aristocort Forte] or dexamethasone [Decadron-LA]) may be effective from 4 to 7 days up to 3 to 4 weeks when given as a single IM dose 4 to 7 times the daily oral dose in selected noncompliant patients. Corticosteroids can also be administered locally by topical applications, by iontophoresis (see Chapter 4.1, section V.A.1.a) or by injecting it into the lesion (e.g., keloids), soft tissues, or joints (see Chapter 4.9). Local corticosteroid administration may be absorbed systemically and cause systemic ADRs. Also, repeated intraarticular or soft tissue injections of corticosteroid may lead to disruption and weakening of cartilage and supporting soft tissue structures as well as possibly causing a crystal-induced transient synovitis.

Daily regimen guidelines. Corticosteroids can be given daily in divided doses or in a single morning dose. In most illnesses, the therapeutic effect of a single morning dose is the same as daily divided doses. For short treatment (<1 month), the dosage schedule does not matter. However, when chronic daily therapy is required, the single morning dose is preferred. This is because of the diurnal rhythm of the hypothalamic-pituitary-adrenal axis (HPAA), i.e., there is maximal activity of the adrenal cortex between 2 AM and 8 AM and minimal activity between 4 PM and midnight. Hence, exogenous corticosteroids suppress the HPAA the least when given at the time of maximal activity (i.e., in the morning). Also, it probably does not increase susceptibility to infection (as does daily divided doses). However, neither single nor divided daily doses have been shown to prevent iatrogenic Cushing's syndrome in long-term therapy. Only short- or intermediate-acting corticosteroids are suitable for single morning-dose therapy because long-acting corticosteroids (i.e., dexamethasone and betamethasone) constantly suppress adrenal activity and do not allow a sufficient period of low steroid level in the blood to prevent side effects.

Alternate-day therapy (ADT) guidelines. In the ADT schedule, corticosteroid is given twice the amount of the daily dose on alternate mornings. This is indicated in patients requiring long-term corticosteroid therapy because it minimizes certain adverse effects such as HPAA suppression, iatrogenic Cushing's syndrome, corticoid withdrawal symptoms, and growth suppression in children. There is also evidence that ADT does not increase the susceptibility to infection. As with single morning-dose therapy, long-acting corticosteroids (i.e., dexamethasone and betamethasone) are not suitable for ADT. If an acute flare-up occurs during ADT, it may be necessary to return to a full suppressive daily divided dose for control. Once control is reestablished, ADT may be reinstituted. To change from a daily single dose to ADT, the dosage can be increased gradually on one day, while the dosage is reduced by the same amount on the alternate day. In the case of divided daily doses, the frequency of the dose is reduced until the whole dose is given in the morning.

Discontinuation guidelines. When chronic corticosteroid therapy is discontinued, the following problems may arise: suppression of the adrenal gland or HPAA yielding corticosteroid withdrawal symptoms and acute exacerbation of the underlying disease. Suppression of HPAA should be considered in any patient who has received more than 10 mg of prednisone or its equivalent for longer than 1 week. With doses closer to the physiologic level, HPAA suppression may not occur for a month. Complete recovery from HPAA suppression may take from months up to a year. These patients usually need no replacement

Table 4.8-5. Selected oral and parenteral (IV/IM) glucocorticoid preparations classified according to half-lives. For intraarticular preparation, see Table 4.9-1

GENERIC	SELECTED BRANDNAMES	AVAILABLE PREPARATIONS (mg)	INITIAL DAILY DOSE (mg) AND ROUTE[d]	EQUIV-DOSE[e]	GLUCO-POTENCY[f]	MINERAL POTENCY[g]
A. short[a]						
Cortisol or Hydrocortisone	a) Hydrocortone b) Solu-cortef	a) *tab* 10, 20 b) *inj* 100, 250/2 ml; 500/4 ml, 1000/8 ml	a) 20-240 po b) 100-500 IV/IM q2-6h prn	20	1	1
Cortisone	Cortone	*tab* 25 *inj* 50/ml	25-300 po/IM	25	0.8	0.8
B. Intermediate[b]						
Prednisone	a) Prednisone b) Liquid Pred	a) *tab* 1,2.5, 5, 10, 20, 50 b) *liq* 5/5 ml	a) and b) 5-60 po	5	4.0	0.8
Prednisolone	a) Pediapred b) Prelone c) Hydeltrasol	a) *liq* 5/5ml b) *liq* 15/5ml c) *inj* 20/5ml	a) and b) 5-60 po c) 4-60 IV/IM	5	4.0	0.8
Methylprednisolone	a) Medrol b) Solumedrol[h] c) Depomedrol	a) *tab* 2, 4, 8, 16, 24, 32 b) *inj* 40/ml, 125/2ml, 500/4ml, 1g, 2g/8ml c) 20, 40, 80/ml	a) 4-48 po b) 10-40 IM/IV[h] c) 4-48 IM/day or 40-120 IM q1-4wk	4	5	0

Triamcinolone	Aristocort	tab 1,2,4,8 inj 40/mo (Forte)	4-48 po/M	4	5	0
C. Long[c]						
Dexamethasone	Decadron; Decadron LA[i]	tab 0.25, 0.5, 0.75, 1.5, 4, 6; liq 0.5/5ml; inj 4/ml, 24/ml (IV only), 8/ml (LA).	0.75-9 po; 0.5-9 IM/IV; LA 8-16 IM q1-3 wks as needed	0.75	20-30	0
Betamethasone	Celestone	inj 6/ml	0.5-9.0 IM	0.6	20-30	0

[a] Short half-life = 8-12 hr.
[b] Intermediate half-life = 12-36 hr.
[c] Long half-life = 36-72 hr.
[d] Dose varies widely according to the specific disease and its severity as well as the patient's response.
[e] Equivalent antiinflammatory dose (in mg).
[f] Relative glucocorticoid potency.
[g] Relative mineralocorticoid potency.
[h] Solumedrol may be given in high-dose therapy at 30 mg/kg, IV over at least 30 min, repeated q4-6 h for 48 h (e.g., within the first 48 hr of spinal cord injury).
[i] LA = long-acting; tab = tablet; inj = injection; liq = liquid

therapy but may require corticosteroid supplementation during periods of stress (e.g., acute infection, other illness, or surgery).

Corticosteroid withdrawal symptoms include anorexia, nausea, vomiting, lethargy, headache, fever, arthralgia, myalgia, and weight loss, which may occur after chronic treatment is discontinued. It is treated symptomatically and/or with small doses (10 mg) of cortisol for several weeks.

Acute exacerbation (flare-ups) of the underlying disease can be prevented by very gradual dose reduction. The rate of corticosteroid taper is determined by the disease activity. Monitoring of the HPAA is usually not necessary. If symptoms consistent with adrenal insufficiency develop, the rate of tapering can be decreased or glucocorticoid replacement can be empirically reinitiated.

Classification. Oral or parenteral corticosteroid preparations can be classified according to their biological half-lives (see Table 4.8-5). Table 4.8-5 also shows the equivalent antiinflammatory dose, as well as the relative glucocorticoid and mineralocorticoid potency of each agent. The short-acting fludrocortisone (Florinef) is not included among the glucocorticoids because it is used only for its mineralocorticoid effects (although it also has glucocorticoid effects). For short-duration oral administration, prednisone is commonly used; however, the inactive prednisone (and also cortisone) needs to be activated in the liver. In patients with liver impairment, therefore, the active parenteral forms (prednisolone or cortisol) should be used instead. Methylprednisolone (Solumedrol) is used for exacerbations of multiple sclerosis and in the first 24 hours after acute spinal cord injury. The long-acting dexamethasone (Decadron), which has slight or absent mineralocorticoid effect (i.e., no sodium retention effect), is used in patients with cerebral edema.

IV. **Anticonvulsants** are used in the PM&R setting for seizure prophylaxis/treatment (e.g., in patients with head trauma, brain tumor, or stroke) and for treatment of chronic neuropathic pain (see Chapter 5.10, section VI.E.2.c).

Mechanism of action. Anticonvulsants control seizures by stabilizing neuronal membranes, i.e., by suppressing spontaneous paroxysmal neuronal discharges and their spread from the site of origin, as well as by reducing neuronal hyperexcitability. Analgesia is probably via the same mechanism because aberrant electrical activity has been recorded from various sites along the neuraxis in humans with neuropathic pain and experimental models of nerve injury.

Adverse drug reactions. Common ADRs (mostly dose-related) include CNS effects (e.g., somnolence, confusion, dizziness, ataxia, slurred speech, tremors, and vision difficulties, such as nystagmus and diplopia) as well as GI effects (e.g., nausea and vomiting). Other rare but serious ADRs include blood dyscrasias, bone marrow depression, and hepatic toxicity. Because anticonvulsants rely on hepatic metabolism for elimination, they may accumulate and lead to toxicity in patients with hepatic impairment. Additional ADRs are listed below under each specific drug.

Contraindications and precautions. As with any drug, anticonvulsants should not be used in patients with known hypersensitivity to the drug or the component of its vehicle. Specific contraindications and precautions are listed below under each drug. They should be used with caution in patients simultaneously taking another anticonvulsant or other drugs (as listed below under the specific drug).

Drug administration guidelines. Phenytoin, phenobarbital, carbamazepine, and primidone are indicated in generalized tonic-clonic seizures and partial seizures. Valproic acid is indicated in absence, photosensitive, atonic, akinetic, myoclonic, and tonic-clonic seizures. Clonazepam is indicated for myoclonic, atonic, absence, and akinetic seizures. Ethosuximide is indicated in absence seizures.

Felbamate is only used as a last resort in severe, refractory seizures because of the increased risk of aplastic anemia. Gabapentin is used as adjunctive therapy in partial seizures with or without secondary generalization. Diazepam, phenytoin, and phenobarbital are used in the treatment of acute seizures. Parenteral diazepam and phenytoin are used in status epilepticus. Diazepam, 1 to 2 mg/min IV, can be given slowly to a total dose of 5 to 10 mg to abort prolonged seizure episodes while other longer-acting anticonvulsants are being administered.

Anticonvulsants should be maintained in their therapeutic range, whether used for prophylaxis or in active treatment. They should not be abruptly withdrawn (especially in patients with a history of seizures) as doing so may precipitate status epilepticus. Patients who are maintained on anticonvulsants should undergo periodic monitoring of blood parameters (complete blood count and differential count) as well as regular medical evaluations. Drug dosage should be raised slowly to build tolerance to side-effects (except anticonvulsants used for acute seizure therapy).

The following discussion concentrates on phenytoin, carbamazepine, valproic acid, and clonazepam—all of which have also been used by physiatrists as adjunctive analgesics in chronic neuropathic pain. Other anticonvulsants used for different types of seizures, e.g., ethosuximide (Zarontin), primidone (Mysoline), felbamate (Felbatol), and gabapentin (Neurontin) are not discussed in this book. Sedatives used as anticonvulsants, e.g., phenobarbital (Luminal) and diazepam (Valium), are discussed under section V.D.1. The possible analgesic roles of the newer anticonvulsants, e.g., felbamate and gabapentin, are discussed in Chapter 5.10, section VI.E.2.c.

A. Phenytoin (Dilantin) is indicated in generalized tonic-clonic seizures, partial seizures, and for seizure prophylaxis as well as in the treatment of acute seizures. Prolonged use can cause gingival hyperplasia, hypertrichosis, maculopapular rash, systemic lupus erythematosus, a Stevens-Johnson syndrome, lymphadenopathy, progressive encephalopathy, osteomalacia and, rarely, permanent cerebellar degeneration. Blood dyscrasias (some fatal) have also been reported, thus warranting periodic blood parameter monitoring.

Some common drugs that affect phenytoin levels are drugs that may *increase* serum phenytoin level (acute alcohol intake, chlordiazepoxide, diazepam, estrogens, fluoxetine, H_2 antagonists, isoniazid, methylphenidate, phenothiazines, salicylates, sulfonamides, tolbutamide, trimethoprim, trazodone), drugs that may *decrease* serum phenytoin level (carbamazepine, chronic ethanol abuse, folic acid, reserpine, rifampin, sucralfate), and drugs that may increase or decrease serum phenytoin level (phenobarbital, valproic acid). Phenytoin may impair the efficacy of the following drugs: corticosteroids, digitoxin, doxycycline, estrogens, furosemide, levodopa, oral contraceptives, quinidine, rifampin, theophylline, thyroid hormones, vitamin D, and warfarin.

The initial dose of phenytoin is 300 mg/day (usually in bid/tid dose; if to be taken once a day, the extended release preparation is preferred; suspension requires more frequent dosing every 6 hours). It is then adjusted to maintain a blood concentration of 10 to 20 μg/ml. When dosage exceeds 300 mg/day, it should be increased at intervals of 2 weeks or more. Phenytoin levels have been reported to rise from subtherapeutic to toxic with as little as a 50-mg/day increment. Dilantin is available in both oral forms (50-mg tablets; 30- and 100-mg extended capsules; 30- and 125-mg per 5 ml suspension) and parenteral forms (50 mg/ml in 2- and 5-ml vials). Intravenous phenytoin is used for controlling status epilepticus and should be given slowly (not to exceed 50 mg/min).

B. **Carbamazepine (Tegretol)** is indicated for generalized tonic-clonic seizures and partial seizures with complex symptomatology (psychomotor or temporal lobe), as well as for trigeminal neuralgia. Serious ADRs include leukopenia and thrombocytopenia (in approximately 2% of patients) and, rarely, aplastic anemia. Other rare adverse effects of carbamazepine include hepatotoxicity, inappropriate secretion of antidiuretic hormone, and cardiovascular effects (e.g., congestive heart failure, arrhythmias, and orthostatic hypotension) and hypersensitivity reactions. Carbamazepine should not be used in patients with previous bone marrow suppression or in patients taking concurrent MAOI drugs. Because carbamazepine is structurally related to the tricyclic antidepressants of the imipramine class, caution similar to the other tricyclics should be exercised (see section V.A.1). Drugs that may increase serum carbamazepine levels include calcium channel blockers, cimetidine, erythromycin, fluoxetine, isoniazid, and propoxyphene.

Baseline complete blood count (CBC), differential count, and liver and renal function tests need to be monitored before drug therapy. Complete blood count and differential counts should be repeated 2 to 3 weeks after initiation of therapy, and monthly for 3 months, followed by biannual counts if there is no evidence of bone marrow suppression. A leukocyte count below 4000 cells/mm^3 is a contraindication to treatment. After therapy is begun, the drug should be discontinued if the white blood cell count falls below 3000 cells/mm^3, the absolute neutrophil count declines below 1500 cells/mm^3, or if there is significant thrombocytopenia or if other blood elements become abnormal. Liver and renal function tests should be monitored periodically.

The initial dose of carbamazepine is 100 to 200 mg, po, bid, which can be titrated up by 100 to 200 mg every 3 to 7 days until the usual dose (given tid or qid) of 400 to 800 mg/day for pain control or 800 to 1200 mg/day for seizure control. The maximum daily dose in most adults is 1200 mg or up to 1600 mg in rare instances. Common ADRs can be obviated by starting at 100 mg bid and slowly titrating up in 100-mg doses. Plasma levels can be used for monitoring compliance and for adjusting dosage (therapeutic range is 4 to 12 μg/ml for antiseizure and analgesic response). Tegretol is available only in oral forms (100- and 200-mg tablets; 100-mg/5 ml suspension)

C. **Valproic acid (Depakene)** is indicated in the treatment of absence seizures as well as generalized tonic-clonic seizures. It may also provide relief for some patients with phantom limb pain syndromes, lancinating neuropathic pain (trigeminal neuralgia), and postherpetic neuralgias. Idiosyncratic reactions include hepatotoxicity (with reports of fatalility), encephalopathy, dermatitis, alopecia, and a rare hyperammonemia syndrome. Liver function tests (LFTs) should be monitored before starting therapy and at frequent intervals thereafter, especially during the first 6 months. In addition, patients should be monitored for serum ammonia, which can be elevated without abnormalities in the LFTs. It is contraindicated in patients with significant liver dysfunction.

The initial dose of valproic acid is 15 mg/kg/day in two or more divided doses, which can be titrated by 5 to 10 mg/kg/day until either seizure control or pain relief is achieved or the patient experiences side effects. Pain relief may be felt at doses lower than those required to achieve the therapeutic anticonvulsant serum concentrations of 50 to 150 μg/ml. Depakene is available only in oral forms (250-mg capsules, 250-mg/5 ml syrup).

D. Clonazepam (Klonopin) is a benzodiazepine (see section V.C.1), which is primarily indicated for absence, myoclonic, and akinetic seizures. It has also been reported to be effective in chronic neuropathic pain (see Chapter 5.10 section VI.E.2.c) and has anxiolytic and sedative effects, which may be beneficial in chronic pain patients with anxiety or insomnia. Rare idiosyncratic reactions include dermatitis, hepatotoxicity, and hematologic effects (blood dyscrasias). Clonazepam should not be used in patients with allergy to benzodiazepines. As with other benzodiazepine drugs, it should not be discontinued abruptly (especially at high doses) as doing so may lead to a withdrawal syndrome. The initial dose is 0.5 mg, po, tid, titrated up by 0.5 to 1 mg every 3 days until seizure or pain is controlled or side effects limit use. Maximum daily dose is 20 mg. As with other anticonvulsants, periodic blood count and LFTs are advisable in long-term use. Klonopin is available only in oral forms (0.5-, 1-, and 2-mg tablets).

V. Psychotropic drugs

A. Antidepressants are used in PM&R primarily as an adjunct to psychotherapy in patients with secondary depression (e.g., associated with stroke, multiple sclerosis, spinal cord injury, head injury, and Parkinson's disease) and as a multipurpose adjuvant analgesic (see Chapter 5.10, section VI.E.2.a) in patients suffering from chronic pain including neuropathic pain (e.g., postherpetic neuralgia, central pain syndromes, phantom pain, reflex sympathetic dystrophy, and painful polyneuropathies or mononeuropathies including diabetic neuropathy), musculoskeletal pain (e.g., fibromyalgia, myofascial pain syndromes, chronic osteoarthritis, chronic low back pain, and mixed arthritic disorders), headaches (e.g., migraine, cluster, or tension headaches), chronic facial pain, cancer pain, postraumatic encephalopathies, and psychogenic pain. The only chronic pain syndrome that possibly does not respond well to antidepressants is pure lancinating neuropathic pain (e.g., trigeminal neuralgia), which has been shown to respond better to anticonvulsant therapy.

Mechanism of action. Antidepressants increase the availability of neurotransmitters (e.g., serotonin and norepinephrine), which are reported to be decreased in patients with depression and chronic pain. Most of them block the reuptake of the neurotransmitters at the neuronal membrane, except probably for monoamine oxidase inhibitors (MAOIs), which enhance neurotransmitters (i.e., dopamine, serotonin, and norepinephrine) through a different pathway involving the inhibition of the monoamine oxidase enzyme. The enhancement of neurotransmitter availability elevates the mood and improves depression. Mood elevation in patients with concomitant pain may also contribute to the analgesia; however, analgesia can occur independent of mood elevation because the primary analgesic dose occurs at a dose lower than that required to treat depression.

Other suggested mechanisms of analgesia include raising the pain threshold, allowing improved sleep, and altering the perception of pain. The sedating effects of some antidepressants (e.g., tricyclic antidepressants) probably help in improving the disturbed sleep cycle of patients with depression and/or chronic pain (e.g., in patients with fibromyalgia). Antidepressants also potentiate the analgesic effectiveness of concomitant opioids and NSAIDs. Other proposed and less commonly accepted mechanisms of analgesic action of antidepressants include an anticonvulsant mechanism, an antiinflammatory mechanism, and an antispasmodic mechanism.

Classification. Antidepressants can be classified according to the pathway in which they increase neurotransmitters (i.e., non-MAOIs vs. MAOIs). The

Table 4.8-6. Relative frequency of adverse drug reactions* (ADRs) of antidepressant drugs commonly used for management of depression and chronic pain

DRUG	ANTI-CHOLINERGIC†	DROWSINESS	INSOMNIA/ AGITATION	SEIZURES	ORTHOSTATIC HYPOTENSION	CARDIAC ARRHYTHMIA	GI DISTRESS‡	WEIGHT GAIN§
A. Tertiary amine TCAs								
Amitriptyline	+ + +	+ + +	+ + +	0/+	+ +	+ + +	+ + +	0/+	+ +
Clomipramine	+ + +	+ + +	+ +	0/+	+ + +	+ +	+ + +	+	+
Doxepin	+ +	+ +	+ + +	0	+ +	+ + +	+ +	0/+	+ +
Imipramine	+ +	+ +	+ +	0/+	+ +	+ +	+ + +	0/+	+ +
Trimipramine	+ + +	+ + +	+ + +	0/+	+ +	+ +	+ + +	0/+	+ +
B. Secondary amine TCAs								
Amoxapine	+	+	+	0/+	+ +	+ +	+ +	+	+
Desipramine	+	+	0/+	0/+	+	+	+ +	0/+	+
Nortriptyline	+	+	+	0/+	+	+	+ +	0/+	+
Protriptyline	+ +	+ +	0/+	0/+	+ +	+	+ + +	0/+	+
C. SSRIs								
Fluoxetine	0/+	0/+	+	+ +	0/+	0/+	0/+	+	0

Paroxetine	0/+	+	++	0	0/+	0	++	0
Sertraline	0/+	+	++	0	0/+	0	++	0
D. Others:								
Bupropion	0/+	0	++	++++	0/+	0/+	0/+	0
Maprotiline	++	++	0/+	+++	++	++	0/+	+
Nefazodone	0/+	+++	+	0	+	0/+	+	0/+
Trazodone	0/+	+++	0	0	++	0/+	0/+	+
Venlafaxine	0/+	++	+	0	0/+	0/+	+	+
E. MAOI‖								
Phenelzine	0/+	+	++	0/+	+++	0	++	+
Tranylcypromine	0/+	+	++	0	++	0	++	+

* 0 = negligible; 0/+ = minimal; + = mild; ++ = moderate; +++ = moderately severe; ++++ = severe. This table should not be used to predict ADR incidence.

TCA = tricyclic antidepressant; SSRI = selective serotonin reuptake inhibitor; MAOI = monoamine oxidase inhibitor.

† Urinary retention, constipation, blurred vision, glaucoma aggravation, dry mouth.
‡ Nausea, diarrhea, vomiting.
§ Weight gain >6 kg.
‖ All MAOIs can have potentially fatal interaction with vasoconstrictors, decongestants, meperidine, methyldopa, levodopa, other antidepressants, other narcotics (possibly), and dietary substances (e.g., tyramine).

non-MAOIs can be subclassified into tricyclic antidepressants (TCAs), selective serotonin reuptake inhibitors (SSRIs), and other antidepressants. The non-MAOI antidepressants (especially the TCAs) interact with other types of receptors (e.g., acetylcholine and histamine receptors). Their inhibition of acetylcholine receptors probably contributes to the analgesic as well as anticholinergic effects of TCAs. Some antidepressants are more selective towards the blockade of serotonin reuptake (e.g., selective serotonin reuptake inhibitors) whereas others are selective toward norepinephrine blockade (e.g., TCAs with secondary amines). Other antidepressants also block dopamine in addition to serotonin and norepinephrine (e.g., amoxapine, buproprion, and the MAOIs). In general, the TCAs with secondary amines and SSRIs are less sedating than the TCAs with tertiary amines. The SSRIs have lesser anticholinergic effects and also less potent analgesic effects (both probably due to their significantly diminished inhibitory effects on acetylcholine receptors) than the TCAs. The ''other'' antidepressants are unrelated and pharmacologically distinct from the remaining classes of antidepressants but also enhance serotonin, norepinephrine, and dopamine availability.

Adverse drug reactions. The side-effect profiles for different antidepressants are summarized in Table 4.8-6. In general, ADRs of antidepressants include anticholinergic effects (e.g., dry mucous membranes is the most common; other more serious but less common anticholinergic effects include urinary retention, precipitation of acute angle-closure glaucoma, obstipation, and delirium), cardiovascular effects (e.g., arrhythmia, hypotension, orthostatic hypotension, and reflex tachycardia), CNS effects (e.g., excessive sedation, insomnia, agitation, anxiety, confusion, tremor, seizure, and occasional development of extrapyramidal symptoms), and other effects (e.g., GI distress, weight gain or loss, respiratory depression, hematologic disturbances, transient elevation in serum transaminase levels, jaundice, hepatitis, endocrine effects, sexual dysfunction, and hypersensitivity reactions). Their orthostatic hypotensive effect probably contributes to the high incidence of hip fractures due to fall in patients taking antidepressants (especially amitriptyline). Many drugs (e.g., norepinephrine, alcohol, and barbiturates) may potentiate toxicity of the antidepressants. The occurrence of serious ADRs during antidepressant therapy is relatively rare, particularly at the low doses typically used to treat pain. Moreover, many patients develop tolerance to the ADRs within several weeks after treatment is initiated.

Contraindications. Concurrent use of any antidepressant with a MAOI antidepressant is contraindicated because their interaction can lead to hyperpyretic crises, severe convulsions, and even death. Patients taking MAOI must discontinue use for at least 2 weeks prior to starting another class of antidepressant. All antidepressants (except possibly SSRIs) should be avoided by patients with recent myocardial infarction, heart failure, left bundle branch block, or other significant cardiac conduction abnormalities. Antidepressants are also contraindicated in patients with symptomatic prostatic hypertrophy, narrow-angle glaucoma, or known hypersensitivity to the drug or the component of its vehicle.

Drug administration guidelines. Start at a low dose and gradually titrate upwards until a therapeutic response is reached with the least amount of side effects. Only one drug should be added or titrated at a time. For use as an analgesic, the dosing guideline of amitriptyline is discussed in Chapter 5.10, section VI.E.2.a. Due to variability in patient response to different antidepressants, sequential trial of different antidepressants (even within the same class) is justified. Because of the arrhythmic effects of tricyclic antidepressants (TCAs), patients who have no known heart disease but are older than 50 years should have a baseline electrocardiogram (ECG) prior to starting TCAs. Older patients should undergo serial ECG if doses are increased to relatively high levels (e.g., at least 150 mg of amitriptyline per day). To further reduce the risk of adverse effects associated with unexpectedly high levels (even with low dose in some elderly patients), the plasma drug concentration and its primary metabolite should be monitored if available (e.g., nortriptyline, desipramine, amitriptyline and its metabolite, and imipramine and its metabolite). Cardiovascular status should also be monitored closely for hypotensive or orthostatic hypotensive effects. Bedside evaluation of the depth of the anterior chamber (to determine narrow angle glaucoma) should be considered before starting TCAs. Prescription of TCAs should be limited to a total of 1 g, without any refills, in the early stages of therapy especially when the patient appears to be suicidal. It is also advisable to check laboratory tests (e.g., complete blood count, differential count, and liver and renal function tests) before starting treatment and periodically thereafter.

1. **Tricyclic antidepressants** (see Table 4.8-7 for dosage), aside from their use in patients with depression, are the most common nonanalgesic medications used in the treatment of chronic pain. The most widely studied TCA in the management of chronic pain is amitriptyline.

   a. **Tricyclic antidepressants with tertiary amines** generally block norepinephrine as well as serotonin reuptake.

      1) **Amitriptyline (Elavil, Endep)** is available in both oral and parenteral (IM) forms. It is indicated for depression and in the treatment of most chronic pain syndromes (e.g., fibromyalgia, chronic low back pain, arthritis, postherpetic neuralgia, central pain, phantom pain, painful diabetic neuropathy, migraine and other types of headache, and psychogenic pain) except lancinating neuropathic pain (where its effectiveness is variable, and where anticonvulsants are more effective). The initial dose for treatment of depression is 75 to 100 mg titrated up to 150 to 200 mg/day or more. For pain management, the dose is lower, that is, starting dose is 10 mg in the elderly or 25 mg in younger patients, then titrated up to 25 to 100 mg/day. It usually takes an average of about 2 to 4 weeks before the analgesic effect is felt (the delay is probably longer for its antidepression effect). Dosing guidelines for amitriptyline in chronic pain management are given in Chapter 5.10, section VI.E.2.a.

      2) **Doxepin (Adapin, Sinequan)** is given orally for either antidepressant or analgesic effects. It is effective in patients with headache, low back pain, and in pain with coexisting depression. It can also be used as an anxiolytic (see section V.A.C.2.e) especially in anxiety accompanied by symptoms of depression.

      3) **Imipramine (Tofranil)** is indicated for depression and nocturnal enuresis. It has also been reported to be beneficial in patients with chronic osteoarthritis, rheumatoid arthritis, low back pain, headache, and painful diabetic neuropathy. It is available in both oral and injectable forms.

      4) **Clomipramine (Anafranil)** has been reported favorably in both neuropathic and nonneuropathic pain syndromes. Aside from its use in patients with depression and pain, it is indicated in patients with obsessive-compulsive disorders. It is available in an oral form.

Table 4.8-7. Selected antidepressants used for treating depression and chronic pain

GENERIC	SELECTED BRANDNAMES	AVAILABLE PREPARATIONS (mg)	INITIAL DOSAGE (mg), ROUTE, FREQUENCY	MDD (mg)
A. Tertiary amine tricyclics*†				
1. Amitriptyline	Elavil, Endep	tab 10,25,50,75,100,150 inj 10/ml	10-75 po qhs or 25 po tid; 20-30 IM qid	300
2. Clomipramine	Anafranil	tab 25,50,75	25 po qd	300
3. Doxepin	Sinequan, Adapin	tab 10,25,50,75,100,150 liq 10/ml	10-25 po tid, or 75 po qhs	300
4. Imipramine	Tofranil	tab 10,25,50	75 po qhs	300
5. Trimipramine	Surmontil	tab 25,50,100	25 po tid	300
B. Secondary amine tricyclics*†				
1. Amoxapine	Asendin	tab 25,50,100,150	25-50 po bid/tid	400
2. Desipramine	Norpramin	tab 10,25,50,75,100,150	10-50 po qhs	300
3. Nortriptiline	Aventyl, Pamelor	cap 10,25,50,75 liq 10/5ml	25 po tid/qid, or 30-50/day (may divide)	150
4. Protriptyline	Vivactil	tab 5,10	5 po tid	60
C. SSRI*				
1. Fluoxetine	Prozac	tab 10,20; liq 20/5 ml	20 po qd	80
3. Paroxetine	Paxil	tab 20,30	20 po qd	50
4. Sertraline	Zoloft	tab 50,100	50 po qd	200
D. Others*				
1. Bupropion	Wellbutrin	tab 75,100	100 po bid	450
2. Maprotiline	Ludiomil	tab 25,50,75	50-75 po qd	225
3. Nefazodone	Serzone	tab 100,150,200,250	100 po bid	600
4. Trazodone	Desyrel	tab 50,100,150,300	50 po tid	600
5. Venlafaxine	Effexor	tab 25,37.5,50,75,100	25 po tid, or 37.5 po bid	375
E. MAOI‡				
1. Phenelzine	Nardil	tab 15	15 po qd	90
2. Tranylcypromine	Parnate	tab 10	10 po qd	60

SSRI = selective serotonin reuptake inhibitors; MAOI = monoamine oxidase inhibitor; MDD = maximum daily dose; tab = tablet; inj = injection; cap = capsule; liq = liquid.
* All non-MAOI antidepressant has potentially fatal drug interaction with MAOI.
† TCAs have potentially fatal drug interaction with antiarrhythmics.
‡ All MAOI have potentially fatal interaction with vasoconstrictors, decongestants, meperidine, methyldopa, levodopa, other antidepressants, other narcotics (possibly), and dietary substances (e.g., tyramine).

    5) Trimipramine (Surmontil), which is available in an oral form, is primarily used for depression.
    b. The TCAs with secondary amines include **desipramine (Norpramine), nortriptyline (Pamelor, Aventyl), protriptyline (Vivactil),** and **amoxapine (Asendin).** They are selective in inhibiting norepinephrine reuptake (except amoxapine, which additionally blocks dopamine receptors) and have relatively fewer anticholinergic effects than TCAs with tertiary amines.

They can be used in patients with significant risk for anticholinergic effects (e.g., symptomatic prostatism and narrow-angle glaucoma) or in patients who are unable to tolerate the side effects of tertiary amines (e.g., drowsiness and orthostatic hypotension). Among the TCAs, desipramine (which has the least sedative effect) and nortriptyline have better side-effect profiles and are commonly used particularly for chronic pain patients with depression. Desipramine has been reported to be effective in postherpetic neuralgia, while nortriptyline, in combination with fluphenazine (Prolixin), has been reported to be effective in treating painful diabetic neuropathy. Nortriptyline is also effective in treating secondary depression (e.g., stroke and parkinsonism). Protriptyline, which is primarily used for depression, also has activating properties that make it particularly suitable for withdrawn patients. Amoxapine is indicated for depression accompanied by anxiety and agitation. All are available in oral forms.

2. **Selective serotonin reuptake inhibitors** include **fluoxetine (Prozac), paroxetine (Paxil),** and **sertraline (Zoloft).** They consist of straight-chain phenylpropylamines, which are unrelated and pharmacologically distinct from other antidepressants. They interact minimally with α-adrenergic, histaminic, and acetylcholinergic receptors and, thus, have relatively fewer anticholinergic and sedative effects. They also have absent or rare cardiac arrhythmic effects and infrequent orthostatic hypotension effects. The following side effects, however, are relatively common: CNS stimulation (e.g., insomnia and agitation), GI distress (e.g., nausea and diarrhea), headache, and weight loss. To avoid insomnia, they should be taken early in the day. The SSRIs are primarily indicated for depression (fluoxetine is also indicated for obsessive compulsive disorders) and are used by patients with significant risk for anticholinergic effects (e.g., symptomatic prostatism). Paroxetine has been reported to have analgesic benefits in patients with painful polyneuropathy, while studies on fluoxetine and sertraline did not show any analgesic effects. However, because of their relatively low incidence of sedative effects, SSRIs may be useful in chronic pain management of depressed patients already taking opioid analgesics. The SSRIs are available in oral forms. See Table 4.8-7 for dosage.

3. **Monoamine oxidase inhibitors,** including **phenelzine (Nardil)** and **tranylcypromine (Parnate),** are mainly used for treatment of atypical depression unresponsive to other antidepressants. They have also been reported to be of some benefit in patients with headache, atypical facial pain, or pain complicated by depression (especially atypical depressions). Although generally not first-line medications for pain or depression, they may be worth trying in treatment-resistant problems or with patients in whom the other antidepressants may be contraindicated. However, because of their potentially fatal interaction with other medications (e.g., other antidepressants) and dietary substances (e.g., tyramine), they generally are not recommended. The MAOIs should not be used in unreliable patients who cannot follow a diet, those who consume alcohol, and those with severe cardiovascular, hepatic or renal disease, or pheochromocytoma. See Table 4.8-7 for dosage.

4. **Other antidepressants** (see Table 4.8-7 for dosage). Most of these drugs are relatively new and still lack clinical studies on their analgesic effects (except perhaps for trazodone and maprotiline). All of the following are available only in oral forms.

a. **Maprotiline (Ludiomil)** is a tetracyclic amine, which mainly enhances the effect of norepinephrine. It is indicated for the treatment of depressive neurosis, and manic-depressive illness and major depression. It can also be used for relieving anxiety associated with depression. The analgesic efficacy of maprotiline was suggested in controlled studies that evaluated patients with idiopathic pain and postherpetic neuralgia. Maprotiline is contraindicated in patients with known or suspected seizure disorder and in the acute phase of myocardial infarction.

b. **Bupropion (Wellbutrin)** is an aminoketone, which enhances the effects of dopamine and possibly norepinephrine. It is indicated for depression. It has been reported to cause a higher incidence of seizures than other antidepressants, especially in patients with bulimia or anorexia nervosa.

c. **Nefazodone (Serzone)** is a phenylpiperazine, which enhances serotonin and is indicated for depression.

d. **Trazodone (Desyrel)** is a triazolopyridine, which enhances serotonin and is indicated for depression with or without anxiety. It can also be used as a sedative (see section V.D.2.d). It has been shown to be effective in patients with poststroke depression, head injury, and cancer pain. However, a well-controlled trial in patients with dysesthetic pains due to traumatic myelopathy failed to demonstrate favorable effects.

e. **Venlafaxine (Effexor)** is a cyclohexanol, which enhances both serotonin and norepinephrine. It is mainly indicated for depression. It has been associated with sustained hypertension.

B. **Neuroleptic drugs** are used in psychiatry to treat psychotic disorders and as tranquilizers. In the PM&R setting, they are used in the management of refractory chronic pain (see Chapter 5.10, section VI.E.2.b); for controlling nausea, vomiting, and intractable hiccups; for sedating or calming patients with organic brain syndrome and in patients with sundown syndrome (i.e., confusion in the evening); and for controlling severe refractory aggression in head injured patients.

Mechanism of action. Their MOA is unknown. They probably act by postsynaptic blockade of dopaminergic receptors, which may lead to the development of extrapyramidal (parkinsonism) reactions. They also act by blocking cholinergic receptors, histamine receptors (producing sedation), and α-adrenergic receptors (producing hypotension). Some neuroleptics (e.g., prochlorperazine and Haldol) provide antiemesis by inhibiting the chemoreceptor trigger zone in the CNS.

Adverse drug reactions. Although addiction does not occur and overdosage rarely results in death, the following ADRs are common: sedation, orthostatic hypotension, dizziness, and anticholinergic effects (e.g., dry mucous membranes and precipitation of acute angle-closure glaucoma, obstipation, and urinary retention). In some cases, they can also cause neuroleptic malignant syndrome (i.e., hyperthermia, rigidity, autonomic instability, and encephalopathy, which is potentially lethal; dantrolene and bromocriptine may be required to treat severe cases) and extrapyramidal reactions including acute dystonic reactions, akathisia, parkinsonism, and possibly irreversible tardive movement disorders (e.g., dyskinesia, dystonia, tics, and myoclonus). Rare idiosyncratic reactions such as blood dyscrasias, dermatoses (e.g., photosensitivity, urticaria, and maculopapular rashes), hepatic damage (e.g., cholestatic jaundice), and galactorrhea have also been reported. Management for the extrapyramidal reactions include benztropine (Cogentin) or diphenhydramine (Benadryl) for acute dystonic reaction, benzodiazepines for akathisia, and antidopaminergic drugs (e.g., bromocriptine [Parlodel]) for tardive dyskinesia. At the first signs of any tardive syndrome (which usually develop after months or years of treatment but can occur at any time during treatment), the drugs should be tapered and discontinued. It is advisable to check laboratory tests (e.g., complete blood count, differential count, and liver and renal function tests) before starting treatment and periodically thereafter.

Contraindications. They should not be used in patients who are comatose, with Parkinson's disease, or who have known hypersensitivity to the drug or the component of its vehicle. They can be used with caution in patients with cardiovascular instability or a history of seizures or abnormal electroencephalogram activity (because of its effect on lowering the seizure threshold). In addition, phenothiazines should be used with caution in patients with impaired hepatic or renal function.

The following are neuroleptics with possible use in the PM&R setting:

1. **Phenothiazines.**

   a. **Chlorpromazine (Thorazine),** is used for the relief of intractable hiccups at a dose of 10 to 25 mg, PO, q4-6h or if symptom persists for 2 to 3 days. Give 25 to 50 mg IM q3-4h or 25 to 100 mg rectal suppository q6-8h. It can also be used for controlling nausea and vomiting at 10 mg, po/IM, bid/tid/qid, prn. There is no evidence that this drug has any analgesic effect.

   b. **Prochlorperazine (Compazine)** is mainly used as an antiemetic. It also has mild analgesic properties. It is rarely used for the treatment of anxiety, agitation, and delirium due to its high incidence of extrapyramidal reactions. For the treatment of nausea and vomiting, the dose is 5 to 10 mg, po/IM, tid/qid, or 25-mg rectal suppository q12h. It is usually given prn.

   c. **Methotrimeprazine (Levoprome)** has been shown to have unequivocal analgesic properties and may be used in patients with refractory chronic pain and cancer pain (see Chapter 5.10, section VI.E.1.b). It also has antiemetic and anxiolytic effects.

   d. **Fluphenazine (Prolixin),** has mild analgesic properties and, when combined with a tricyclic antidepressant (e.g., amitriptyline), has been reported to be beneficial in patients with deafferentation pain (see Chapter 5.10, section VI.E.2.b).

2. **Butyrophenone,** e.g., **haloperidol (Haldol),** is used for managing patients with agitated delirium or with sundown syndrome at a starting dose of 0.25 mg, po/IM, which can be titrated up as needed at 20 to 30 minutes intervals until the desired level of calmness is reached. It also has antiemetic use (1-2 mg, po/IM, bid/tid) and has been suggested to have coanalgesic properties (given at 0.5-1.0 mg, po, bid/tid). At these low doses, it rarely causes excessive sedation, hypotension, or cardiovascular compromise, and it can be given safely to the elderly. Once the condition has stabilized, haloperidol can be tapered over 2 to 5 days before being discontinued. Although low-to-moderate doses of Haldol may be used in acute aggression, its usefulness in the management of chronic aggression in patients with head injury has recently been surpassed by newer, shorter-acting, and more efficacious agents (e.g., buspirone [Buspar] described in section V.C.2.a; see also section V.F for antiaggression drugs).

C. **Anxiolytics** (Table 4.8-8) are primarily indicated for the management of anxiety disorders (which may be part of the symptom complex seen in major depression, panic disorders, metabolic disturbances, and drug toxicity or

Table 4.8-8. Selected anxiolytics used in PM&R and their dosages

GENERIC	SELECTED BRANDNAMES	AVAILABLE PREPARATIONS (mg)	INITIAL DOSAGE (mg), ROUTE, FREQUENCY	MDD$ (mg)
I. Benzodiazepines (short half-life)*				
Alprazolam	Xanax	*tab* 0.25,0.5,1,2	0.25-0.5 po bid/tid	4
Lorazepam	Ativan	a) *tab* 0.5, 1, 2 b) and c) *inj* 0.5/ml; 2/ml; 4/ml	a) 1-3 po bid/tid b) 0.05/kg IM c) 0.044/kg IV	a) 10 b) 4 c) 2
Oxazepam	Serax	*tab* 15 *cap* 10, 15, 30	10-15 po tid/qid	120
II. Benzodiazepines (long half-life)†				
Chlordiazepoxide	Librium, Libritabs	*cap* 5, 10, 25 *inj* 100/5 ml	5-10 po bid/tid/qid 15-100 IM/IV then 25-50 tid/qid prn	300
Clorazepate	Tranxene Tranxene SD	*tab* 3.75, 7.5, 15 *SD-tab*: 11.25, 22.5	*tab* 3.75-15 po tid *SD*: 11.25-22.5 po qd	90
Diazepam	a) Valium b) Valrelease	a) *tab* 2, 5, 10 *inj* 5/ml b) *cap* 15	a) 2-10 po bid/qid 2-10 IM/IV q3-4h prn b) 15-30 po qd	80
III. Nonbenzodiazepines				
Buspirone	BuSpar	*tab* 5,10	5 po tid	60
Chlormezanone	Trancopal	*cap* 100, 200	100-200 po tid/qid	800
Doxepin‡	Adapin Sinequan	*tab* 10,25,50,75,100,150 *liq* 10/ml	10-25 po tid 75 po qhs	300
Hydroxyzine	a) Atarax b) Vistaril	a) *tab* 10, 25, 100; *liq* 10/5 ml b) *cap* 10, 25, 100; *liq* 25/5 ml; *inj* 25, 50/ml; 100/2ml	25-100 po/IM qid	400
Meprobamate	Miltown	*tab* 200, 400, 600	1200-1600/day po in divided doses	2400

* Short half-life <20 hr.
† Long half-life >40 hr.
‡ Dosages given for doxepin are initial dose which may be titrated up or down.
$ MDD = Maximum daily dose for anxiolytic use (may be higher in closely monitored patients or for other uses).
tab = tablet; inj = injection; cap = capsule; SD = single dose

withdrawal) as well as reactionary agitation seen as part of the total "pain" problem in patients suffering from trauma (e.g., head trauma) and acute illness. They can also be used to calm down (and sedate) patients during imaging procedures (e.g., prior to computed tomography or magnetic resonance imaging) as well other diagnostic (e.g., endoscopy) and therapeutic (e.g., cardioversion) procedures. The antegrade amnesia effect of anxiolytics (i.e., benzodiazepines) may be beneficial in patients undergoing procedures because it diminishes the patient's recall of the procedure. Most anxiolytics (especially those belonging to the benzodiazepine class) also have sedative-hypnotic effects (which can be beneficial if patient also has insomnia), as well as the potential for physical dependence and abuse. Whenever possible, nonpharmacologic treatments (e.g., behavioral methods, relaxation training, biofeedback, and cognitive restructuring) should be tried first, adding anxiolytics as an adjunct if these methods are unsuccessful. Anxiolytics generally do not produce sustained improvement in patients with chronic, nonspecific anxiety. It is best to treat the underlying cause of the anxiety.

1. **Benzodiazepines** can be used primarily as anxiolytics or as sedative-hypnotics (discussed in section V.D.1). Their role in pain management (acute musculoskeletal pain and chronic pain) is discussed in Chapter 5.10, section VI.E.2.g.1. In general, they play a very limited role in pain management unless anxiety is the overriding clinical symptom. They are generally not indicated for patients with traumatic brain injury (TBI) except for those whose anxiety is associated with muscle tension and insomnia. The role of some benzodiazepines as anticonvulsants (e.g., diazepam and clonazepam) is discussed in section IV.

   Mechanism of action. Benzodiazepines act as CNS depressants, probably by directly potentiating the inhibitory effects of the gamma-aminobutyric acid (GABA) neurotransmitters throughout the CNS. Studies seem to indicate that they deplete serotonin and can theoretically increase pain perception. They generally do not cause autonomic blockade nor do they produce extrapyramidal side effects (except transient ataxia at high doses).

   Adverse drug reactions. Elderly and critically ill patients are especially at risk for ADRs, because a reduction in renal or hepatic function increases the potential for drug toxicity. Benzodiazepine ADRs include CNS effects (e.g., excessive sedation, morning drowsiness or hangover, incoordination or ataxia, confusion, dizziness, fatigue, anterograde amnesia, and impairment of cognitive and motor behavior), paradoxical excitation (e.g., irritability, agitation, anxiety, auditory and visual hallucinations, delirium, or hostility), respiratory depression (especially in large doses given to elderly patients and those with chronic pulmonary disorders), cardiovascular effects (e.g., hypotension, bradycardia, and even cardiac arrest, especially with IV administration), and other adverse effects (e.g., blurred vision, myalgias, nausea and hiccups, constipation, changes in urination patterns, urticaria, rash, photosensitivity, thrombophlebitis, jaundice, and blood dyscrasias). The effect (and toxicity) of benzodiazepines may be potentiated by concurrent intake of alcohol, other CNS depressants (e.g., opioids, phenothiazines, barbiturates, MAOIs, and other antidepressants), and possibly cimetidine. Although ADRs may occur with initial doses, they diminish as tolerance develops with continued therapy. If ADRs are intolerable, the dose may be decreased or an alternative agent may be used instead. All benzodiazepines have the potential for habituation and may be difficult to withdraw in chronic use.

   Physical dependence. Prolonged use of benzodiazepines (usually at least 4 weeks) can lead to tolerance and physical dependence. When the drug is abruptly stopped in physically dependent patients, withdrawal or abstinence syndromes (see section I.B under Opioid Physical Tolerance) may begin within 1 to 10 days and may last for several weeks. Likewise, patients given benzodiazepine antagonists (e.g., flumazenil [Romazicon]) may also go into withdrawal syndromes. The probability and intensity of the withdrawal effects are greatest with short-acting drugs and least with long-acting preparations. Withdrawal syndromes can be prevented in chronic benzodiazepine users by decreasing the dose by 5 to 10% every

5 days. Those taking long-acting benzodiazepines can be tapered more quickly.

Contraindications and precautions. Benzodiazepines are contraindicated in patients with acute narrow-angle glaucoma (because of possible mydriatic effects) and during the first trimester (because of increased risk of congenital fetal malformations). As with any drugs, they should not be used in patients with known hypersensitivity to the drug or the component of its vehicle (e.g., propylene glycol found in most injectable forms). They are also not recommended in patients with primary depressive disorders, psychosis, or patients in confusional states (as they make the existing delirium worse). Patients whose mental alertness is required for safety (e.g., machinery operators and drivers) should be warned about the possibility of psychomotor impairment even after a single dose of benzodiazepine. Patients should also refrain from concurrently taking alcohol or other CNS depressants.

Drug administration guidelines. Benzodiazepines should only be used for short-term treatment. Aside from greater abuse potential and increased incidence of ADRs, the long-term use of most benzodiazepines (i.e., more than 4 months) has not been assessed by clinical studies. Patients treated with benzodiazepines should be followed regularly to reassess their drug need and to gradually taper off the drug as soon as possible. Dosing must take into account the patient's degree of daytime sedation from the medication or from the insomnia itself. In general, benzodiazepines with long half-lives and/or active metabolites should be avoided by the elderly (or patients with hepatic or renal impairment) because of greater ADR potential because of drug accumulation by repeated dosing (made worse by the fact that drug half-lives may be increased two- to fourfold in these patients). Periodic laboratory tests (e.g., complete blood count and liver function tests) are advisable during prolonged treatment due to occasional reports of blood dyscrasias and jaundice. Serum BUN/creatinine or urinalysis may be done also to determine kidney function (responsible for drug elimination).

a. **Short-acting anxiolytic benzodiazepines** (with half-lives of less than 20 hours) have a delayed onset of action when compared with the long-acting anxiolytic benzodiazepines listed below (hence may not be as useful in acute agitation). However, lorazepam and oxazepam have no active metabolites and are generally safer in patients with liver impairment and in the elderly (i.e., if given at its lowest possible dose; see section V.D.1.a for advantages of short-acting benzodiazepines).

1) **Lorazepam (Ativan)** is also indicated for anxiety associated with depressive symptoms. It has inactive metabolites and is generally well-tolerated by the elderly. The initial dosage in the elderly should not exceed 2 mg to avoid oversedation. It is available in both oral and injectable forms. The injectable form contains propylene glycol and should be administered intravenously at a maximum rate of 2 mg/min.

2) **Oxazepam (Serax)** is also indicated for anxiety associated with depressive symptoms and anxiety associated with alcohol withdrawal. It has inactive metabolites and has been found to be particularly useful in the management of anxiety, tension, agitation, and irritability in elderly patients (at a dosage of 10 mg, po, tid). Hypotension may

occur in rare cases, and Serax must be used with caution by elderly patients prone to it. It is only available in oral form.

3) **Alprazolam (Xanax)** is also indicated for anxiety associated with depression and for panic disorders (with or without agoraphobia). Unlike lorazepam and oxazepam, it produces active metabolites and, in patients with liver disease, its half-life can be prolonged (up to 65 hours). It has possible analgesic effects in cancer patients with neuropathic pain (see Chapter 5.10, section VI.E.2.g) and in patients with fibromyalgia (see Chapter 5.10, Table 5.10-1). It is only available in oral form.

b. **Long-acting anxiolytic benzodiazepines** (with half-lives of 48-96 hours) have rapid onset of action and can be used for the acutely agitated patient. These drugs produce active metabolites and must be used with caution (i.e., lowest dose and longest interval possible) in patients with liver impairment and in the elderly (see section V.D.1.b for disadvantage of long-acting drugs).

1) **Diazepam (Valium)** is also used as an sedative-hypnotic (see section V.D.1), anticonvulsant (i.e., in acute treatment of status epileptics; see section IV), "skeletal muscle relaxant" (see section II.A.7), and antispasticity agent (see Chapter 4, section III.B.2.c), as well as in minimizing the effects of acute alcohol withdrawal. Diazepam has the disadvantage of producing several active metabolites with long elimination half-lives and should be used with caution by the elderly. It is available in oral forms (short-acting and slow-release) and injectable forms. The injectable form contains propylene glycol and should be administered intravenously at a maximum rate of 5 mg/min. Parenteral diazepam is usually used as an adjunct in status epilepticus (see section IV), as a premedication prior to procedures, and in controlling severe anxiety.

2) **Chlordiazepoxide (Librium, Libritabs)** is also useful in managing delirium tremens and early signs of alcohol withdrawal. Unlike other benzodiazepines, it is not listed as being contraindicated in patients with acute, narrow-angle glaucoma. It is available in both oral and injectable forms. The oral form is marketed either as a single agent (Librium, Libritabs) or in combination with amitriptyline (Limbitrol).

3) **Clorazepate (Tranxene)** is also indicated for symptomatic relief of acute alcohol withdrawal and as an adjunct in the management of partial seizures. It is available only in an oral form.

2. **Nonbenzodiazepines anxiolytics**

a. **Buspirone (BuSpar)** is an azapirone, which has high affinity for serotonin receptors and moderate affinity for D_2-dopamine receptors. It has no significant affinity for benzodiazepine receptors and does not affect the GABA neurotransmitter. It is an anxiolytic agent with few side effects (and lesser cognitive effects than benzodiazepines); however, its clinical benefit may not be evident until after weeks of drug administration. Buspirone is less sedating than other anxiolytics and does not produce significant functional impairment. It has limited interaction with ethanol. There is no evidence that it causes either physical or psychological dependence. Although it binds to dopamine receptors, it has not been shown to cause extrapyramidal symptoms. Its ADRs include dizziness, nausea, headache, nervousness, lightheadedness, diarrhea, excitement, paresthesias, and sweating. The only contraindication of buspirone is in patients with hypersensitivity to the drug.

Buspirone is more effective when anxiety is associated with anger and hostility or with depression. In TBI patients, it is preferred over benzodiazepines or haloperidol in managing anxiety disorders (with no accompanying muscle tension or insomnia). It is also effective in managing TBI patients with aggression (see section V.F). Buspirone is not cross tolerant with benzodiazepines, hence it does not prevent benzodiazepine withdrawal. Switching from benzodiazepine to buspirone can be done safely by adding buspirone at 5 mg tid and then gradually tapering the benzodiazepine. Buspirone is only available in oral forms. It is given at 5 mg, po, tid, increasing by 5 mg every 2 days to a maximum of 50 to 60 mg/day.

b. **Hydroxycine (Atarax, Vistaril)** are antihistamines (see section VI), which are also indicated for anxiety associated with psychoneurosis and other organic disease.

c. **Chlormezanone (Trancopal)** is indicated for the treatment of mild anxiety (MOA is unknown). Its common ADRs include drowsiness, drug rash, dizziness, flushing, nausea, depression, edema, inability to void, weakness, excitement, tremor, confusion, and headache. Rare cases of erythema multiforme, Stevens-Johnson syndrome, toxic epidermal necrolysis, and cholestatic jaundice have been reported. It is contraindicated in patients with known hypersensitivity to the drug. It is only available in an oral form.

d. **Meprobamate (Miltown)** is an anxiolytic whose mechanism of action is unknown (it acts at multiple sites in the CNS of animals). The ADRs include CNS depression (e.g., drowsiness, ataxia, dizziness, and slurred speech), GI disorders (e.g., nausea and diarrhea), cardiovascular effects (palpitations and hypotension), and other allergic or idiosyncratic reactions (e.g., Stevens-Johnson syndrome and blood dyscrasias). It can cause physical dependence and can cause potentiation of CNS depression with alcohol or other CNS depressants. It is contraindicated in patients with acute intermittent porphyria or patients with hypersensitivity to the drug or related compound (e.g., carisoprodol). It is only available in an oral form.

e. **Doxepin (Adapin, Sinequan)** is an antidepressant also indicated for anxiety (with or without depression) in patients with organic disease or those with alcoholism. It is discussed in section V.A.1.a.2.

f. **Propranolol (Inderal)** may be used to control somatic symptoms of anxiety (e.g., tachycardia and performance anxiety). It is described under anti-aggression drugs (see section V.F).

g. **Phenothiazines** such as **prochlorperazine (Compazine)** and **trifluoperazine (Stelazine)** have anxiolytic properties but are not recommended because of potentially serious ADRs (e.g., extrapyramidal reactions; see section V.B).

D. **Sedative-hypnotics** (Table 4.8-9) are primarily indicated for the treatment of insomnia characterized by complaints of difficulty in falling asleep, frequent awakenings, and morning awakenings. They are beneficial in hospitalized patients who frequently complain of insomnia because of hospital noise, frequent monitoring and medication administration by the staff, and unfamiliar surroundings. In a rehabilitation ward, sedative-hypnotics given at bed-

Table 4.8-9. Selected sedative-hypnotics used in PM&R and their dosage

GENERIC	SELECTED BRANDNAMES	AVAILABLE PREPARATIONS (mg)	DOSAGE (mg), ROUTE, FREQUENCY	MDD‡ (mg)
I. Benzodiazepines (short half-life)*				
Estazolam	Prosom	*tab* 1,2	0.5-2 po qhs	2
Temazepam	Restoril	*cap* 7.5, 15, 30	7.5-15 po qhs	30
Triazolam	Halcion	*tab* 0.125, 0.25	0.125-0.25 po qhs	0.5
II. Benzodiazepines (long half-life)†				
Fluorazepam	Dalmane	*cap* 15, 30	15-30 po qhs	30
Quazepam	Doral	*tab* 7.5, 15	7.5-15 po qhs	15
III. Nonbenzodiazepines				
Chloral hydrate	Chloral hydrate Noctec Aquachloral supp	*cap* 500, 1000 *liq* 500, 1000/10 ml *supp* 325, 650	500-1000 po qhs	1000
Ethchlorvynol	Placidyl	*cap* 200, 500, 750	200-750 po qhs	1000
Zolpidem	Ambien	*tab* 5, 10	5-10 po qhs	10

* Short half-life <20 hr.
† Long half-life >40 hr.
‡ MDD = maximum daily dose for sedative-hypnotic use (may be higher in closely monitored patients); tab = tablet; cap = capsule; liq = liquid; supp = suppository.

time can be helpful in keeping the insomniac patient from feeling drowsy during daytime rehabilitation sessions. All insomniac patients must be evaluated for a variety of underlying medical or psychiatric disorders (e.g., depression) for which there is a more specific treatment. As with anxiolytics, non-pharmacologic treatments (e.g., behavioral methods, relaxation training, and biofeedback) should be tried, whenever possible, before drug therapy is initiated. If sedative-hypnotics are used, they must be used for a short period (less than 1-2 weeks) and if possible, a nonbenzodiazepine should be used to avoid the potential for abuse common among benzodiazepine users. They must be used with caution in the elderly, or in patients with CNS insults or who are already drowsy or lethargic from surgery. They should not be prescribed in quantities exceeding one month's supply. They should be ingested prior to going to sleep (generally within 30 minutes).

1. **Benzodiazepines** are discussed in section V.C.1. The MOA, ADR, contraindications and precautions of the following sedative-hypnotic benzodiazepines are essentially similar to those of anxiolytic benzodiazepines. They are all available in oral forms.

   a. **Short-acting sedative-hypnotic benzodiazepines** have elimination half-lives of less than 20 hours. They include **temazepam (Restoril), triazolam (Halcion), and Estazolam (Prosom).** They are primarily used for the short-term treatment of insomnia (generally 7-10 days). The advantage of a short half-lives is that drug and metabolites are cleared before the next dose is ingested, hence daytime sedation and performance impairment are minimal or absent (in short-term use). Both temazepam and triazolam have inactive metabolites but estazolam has an active metabolite. In the rehabilitation ward, temazepam (Restoril) is one of the commonly used benzodiazepine sedative-hypnotics. Elderly patients on temazepam should be started at a low dose (7.5 mg) to avoid oversedation.

b. **Long-acting sedative-hypnotic benzodiazepines** have elimination half-lives of more than 40 hours. They include **fluorazepam (Dalmane)** and **quazepam (Doral)**, both of which have active metabolites. They can be used briefly in patients with recurring insomnia or poor sleeping habits, and in acute or chronic medical conditions requiring restful sleep. The disadvantage of long half-lives is that the drug and its metabolites may accumulate during repeated dosage intervals of less than 24 hours and may be associated with impairments of cognitive or motor performance during waking hours. Also the possibility of interaction with other psychoactive drugs or alcohol will be enhanced. In the elderly in whom the half-life may be increased two- to fourfold, benzodiazepines with long half-lives are generally not indicated.

2. **Nonbenzodiazepine sedative-hypnotics**
   a. **Zolpidem (Ambien)** is indicated for the short-term treatment of insomnia (generally 7-10 days). It probably acts by interacting with the inhibitory neurotransmitter GABA. In contrast to the benzodiazepines, which nonselectively bind to and activate all types of GABA receptors, zolpidem is more selective, which probably accounts for its lack of myorelaxant and anticonvulsant effects. It has a short elimination half-life and its metabolite is inactive. The more common ADRs include daytime drowsiness, dizziness, headache, nausea, vomiting, diarrhea, amnesia, confusion, vertigo, incoordination, visual disturbance, palpitations, and dry mouth. As with benzodiazepines, zolpidem can cause physical dependence and should not be withdrawn abruptly after prolonged use. To date, zolpidem has no known contraindication. It has not been shown to accumulate in elderly patients following nightly oral doses of 10 mg for 1 week. This gives an adequate safety margin for the recommended bedtime dose of 5 mg in the elderly. Zolpidem is only available in an oral form. It is one of the most commonly used sedative-hypnotics in the rehabilitation ward (possibly because of its general lack of residual next-day effect during rehabilitation sessions).
   b. **Chloral hydrate (Noctec)** is a rapidly effective hypnotic that may be useful because it has little effect on normal sleep cycles. Its specific mechanism of action remains unknown, although it appears to induce a general depression of CNS functions. In routine doses, it has relatively less adverse respiratory and cardiovascular effects than benzodiazepines. It also seldom produces excitement or hangover. However, in high doses and in long-term administration, it may cause CNS effects (excessive or prolonged sedation, headache, dizziness, ataxia, hallucinations, malaise, and paradoxical excitation), cardiovascular effects (e.g., supraventricular and ventricular arrhythmias following the ingestion of toxic quantities), GI effects, (e.g., nausea, vomiting, hemorrhage, necrosis, and perforation of the stomach), skin reactions (e.g., rash), and other effects (e.g., leukopenia, eosinophilia, ketonuria, apnea, and laryngospasm). Tolerance and physical dependence may also be seen with chronic ingestion. There have been reports of fatal interaction with ethanol and a short-term increase in the effect of warfarin. It is contraindicated in patients with significant hepatic or renal impairments and in those with hypersensitivity to the drug.

c. Ethchlorvynol (Placidyl) is indicated for the short-term treatment of insomnia of up to one week. Its mechanism of action is unknown. The ADRs include hematologic effects (e.g., thrombocytopenia, with one case of fatality), GI effects (e.g., nausea and vomiting), neurologic effects (e.g., dizziness and facial numbness), miscellaneous effects (e.g., blurred vision, hypotension, and mild "hangover"), and other idiosyncratic responses. It can also cause physical dependence and should not be withdrawn abruptly. It is contraindicated in patients with known hypersensitivity to the drug and in patients with porphyria. Ethchlorvynol is only available in an oral form.

d. Trazodone (Desyrel), 50 to 300 mg (up to a maximum of 600 mg/day), po, qhs has been found to be beneficial in TBI patients whose insomnia is attributed to "racing thoughts" as they lie down and try to sleep. Trazodone, which is primarily indicated for the management of depression is discussed in section V.A.4.d. The manufacturer does not include sedative-hypnotic as its major effect, although sedation is listed as one of its major side effects.

e. Diphenhydramine (Benadryl) can be given at 25 to 50 mg, po, qhs for periodic sedation although sedation is only listed as its side effect (not a primary indication). See section VI.B for details about diphenhydramine.

f. Barbiturates have low therapeutic indexes and are not recommended as sedative-hypnotics or anxiolytics. They induce sleep that is deficient in rapid-eye-movement (REM) periods, resulting in inadequate rest. They also have high potential for adverse effects (e.g., respiratory depression, hypersensitivity reactions, cardiovascular depression, paradoxical excitement, and increased sensitivity to pain). Their usefulness as sedative-hypnotics (and also as anxiolytics) have been surpassed by other safer drugs described above (nonbenzodiazepines and benzodiazepines). Barbiturates such as **phenobarbital (Luminal)** or **mephobarbital (Mebaral)** are generally used as anticonvulsants (see section IV), while other barbiturates such as **secobarbital (Seconal), pentobarbital (Nembutal), thiopental (Pentothal),** and **methohexital (Brevital)** are generally used for preoperative or procedural sedation.

E. Psychostimulants are used to improve attention and concentration (which in turn can probably help improve memory and learning) and to counteract the sedatives effects of other drugs (e.g., opioids; see section I.B). They may be beneficial in patients with cognitive communication impairments (e.g., TBI; see Chapter 5.5, section I.B for details on cognitive communication impairment). They should be used only as an adjunct to nonpharmacological measures (i.e., psychological, educational, and social). They should not be given at high doses (may impair performance) and should not be stopped abruptly (may cause withdrawal symptoms).

1. Amphetamines are noncatecholamine, sympathomimetic amines with CNS stimulant activity. Peripheral sympathomimetic effects include hypertension and weak bronchodilator and respiratory stimulant actions.

Mechanism of action. The exact MOA for producing the mental and behavioral effects is unknown. They probably act via direct release of dopamine and norepinephrine, blockade of catecholamine reuptake, and reduction in catecholamine turnover.

Adverse drug reactions include CNS effects (e.g., overstimulation, restlessness, dizziness, insomnia, euphoria, dyskinesia, dysphoria, tremor, headache, psychotic episodes, and exacerbation of tics), GI effects (e.g., dry mouth, diarrhea, constipation, and anorexia), and other effects (e.g., urticaria and impotence). Amphetamines cause tolerance and physical dependence and have been extensively abused.

Contraindications and precautions. Amphetamine use is contraindicated in patients with advanced arteriosclerosis, symptomatic cardiovascular disease, moderate to severe hypertension, hyperthyroidism, glaucoma, agitation, history of drug abuse, concurrent intake of MAOIs, and known hypersensitivity or idiosyncrasy to sympathomimetic amines.

Drug administration guidelines. Patients should initially be monitored for tachycardia, hypertension, anorexia, dysphoria, and insomnia. Prolonged use should be avoided because of abuse potential.

a. **Dextroamphetamine (Dexedrine)** is indicated for narcolepsy and in attention deficit disorder with hyperactivity. There is some evidence of its short-term effects on cognitive and behavior sequelae of patients with TBI. If given in moderate dose, it can probably improve long-term memory, attention, distractibility, disorganization, and impulsivity seen after TBI. Although not listed as an indication by its manufacturer, it has also been used (and abused) as a weight-loss pill in obese patients. It is available in an oral form (5- and 10-mg tablets and 5-mg/5 ml elixir). Its dosage is 2.5 to 5 mg, po, bid (administered morning and at midday) and gradually increased up to 30 to 60 mg/day.

b. **Methamphetamine (Desoxyn)** is indicated for attention deficit disorder with hyperactivity and for short-term use in exogenous obesity. It is available in an oral form (5- and 10-mg tablets) and is given at 5 mg, po, qd/bid (administered morning and at midday) and gradually increased weekly up to 20 to 25 mg/day.

2. **Methylphenidate (Ritalin)** is a mild CNS stimulant whose exact MOA is unknown (probably similar to that of amphetamines except for the increased catecholamine turnover). It is indicated for narcolepsy and in attention deficit disorder with hyperactivity and may be helpful in improving attention and concentration in TBI patients (especially if with hypoarousal). Its ADRs include CNS effects (e.g., nervousness, insomnia, dizziness, headache, drowsiness, dyskinesia, psychotic episodes, and exacerbation of tics), GI effects (e.g., nausea, anorexia, and abdominal pain), cardiovascular effects (e.g., tachycardia, palpitations, increased or decreased blood pressures, and cardiac arrhythmias), hypersensitivity and idiosyncratic reactions (e.g., rash, urticaria, leukopenia, and cerebral arteritis or occlusion). It should not be abruptly stopped as it may cause a severe withdrawal syndrome. It can be potentially abused in emotionally unstable patients. It is contraindicated in patients with marked anxiety, tension, agitation, glaucoma, severe depression, motor tics, Tourette's syndrome, concurrent intake of MAOIs, and known hypersensitivity to the drug. Methylphenidate is available only in an oral form (5-, 10-, or 20-mg tablets and 20-mg sustained-release tablets). It can be given at 5 to 10 mg, po, bid/tid (may be increased up to 40-60 mg/day). Patients should initially be monitored for tachycardia, hypertension, insomnia, and anorexia. Periodic complete blood count and differential count are advisable.

3. **Pemoline (Cylert)** is a CNS stimulant with minimal sympathomimetic effects. It is unrelated to dextroamphetamine and methylphenidate. Its exact MOA is unknown (probably acts on dopaminergic receptors and decreases catecholamine turnover). It is indicated in patients with attention deficit

disorder with hyperactivity. It may be helpful in improving attention and concentration in TBI patients. ADRs include hepatic effects (hepatitis, jaundice, rare cases of hepatic-related fatalities), CNS effects (insomnia, convulsive seizures, exacerbation of tics, hallucinations, dyskinesia, nystagmus, mild depression, dizziness, increased irritability, headache, drowsiness), GI effects (anorexia, nausea, stomach ache), other effects (e.g., aplastic anemia, increased acid phosphatase, and growth suppression in children). It is contraindicated in patients with hepatic impairment and known hypersensitivity to the drug. It has the potential of being misused in emotionally unstable patients. It is available only in an oral form (18.75-, 37.5-, and 75-mg tablets). It can be given at 37.5 mg qd (in the morning), which can be increased by 18.75 mg at 1 week intervals up to a maximum of 112.5 mg/day. Its clinical benefit may not be evident until the third or fourth week of drug administration. Patients should be monitored for liver function tests (LFTs) before starting the drug, and LFTs and CBC should be monitored periodically.

4. **Other drugs** that may possibly improve attention as well as memory and learning include tricyclic antidepressants (e.g., **protriptyline** or **desipramine** may be used for mildly impaired patients with attention difficulties; see under Tricyclic Antidepressants in section V.A.1), **physostigmine** (2 mg, po, tid, increased over 1 week to 3.5-4.0 mg tid; its mechanism of action is probably via decreased destruction of acetylcholine; may improve retrieval of long-term memory), **amantadine** (50 mg, po, bid, increased weekly to a maximum of 400 mg/day; may be helpful in TBI patients with low energy or with depression and may improve cognitive function in selected TBI patients during early recovery stages based on its effects on agitation; however, seizures have been reported in TBI patients taking amantadine), **tacrine (Cognex,** 10 mg, po, qid titrated up to a maximum of 160 mg/day; a reversible cholinesterase inhibitor used in the treatment of mild to moderate dementia of Alzheimer's type; hepatotoxic), **ergoloid mesylate (Hydergine,** 1 mg, po, tid; indicated for patients over 60 years old with symptomatic decline in mental capacity), nootropics or "cognitive activators" (e.g., **pramiracetan,** 400 mg, tid; available only experimentally; probably increases turnover of acetylcholine in the hippocampal cholinergic nerve terminals; may be effective in treating memory and other cognitive problems in patients with long-term stable losses in memory and cognition); **gangliosides** (probably induces neural regeneration; experimental); and **thyrotropin-releasing hormones.**

F. **Antiaggression drugs** may be used as an adjunct to nonpharmacologic measures (e.g., behavioral therapy) in patients with aggression (e.g., TBI patients). A drug commonly used in the PM&R setting for controlling chronic aggression in TBI patients is **buspirone (Buspar)** because of its favorable side-effect profile (see section V.C.2.a); however, it takes weeks of daily administration before its clinical benefits become evident. The most widely studied antiaggression drug is **propranolol (Inderal),** a β-blocker that is used for controlling chronic aggressive behavior. Its dose is 60 mg/day, which can be increased by 60 mg every 3 days to a maximum of 420 mg/day. The clinical benefit of propranolol may not be evident until after 6 to 8 weeks of drug administration. It is contraindicated in patients with asthma, pulse less than 60/min, hypotension, conduction defects, diabetes, and patients on concurrent intake of MAOIs. Another β-blocker used for controlling chronic aggression is **pindolol (Visken),** which can be given at 5 mg, po, bid up to a maximum of

60 mg/day. Pindolol has the same contraindications as propranolol. It causes less hypotension and bradycardia than propranolol but may cause excitement and agitation.

Other drugs used in chronic aggression include: **anticonvulsants** (e.g., **carbamazepine, valproic acid;** or low-dose **clonazepam** combined with clonidine; see section IV for details on anticonvulsants); **antidepressants** (e.g., **trazodone, amitriptyline**; see section V.A); **neuroleptics** (e.g., low-to-moderate doses of **haloperidol [Haldol]** which can be used to calm down acutely aggressive or agitated patients; see section V.B.2); **benzodiazepines** (e.g., **lorazepam**; see section V.C.1.a.1); **psychostimulants** (e.g., **methylphenydate; dextroamphetamine;** see section V.E); **verapamil (Calan; Isoptin;** see section IX.B), a calcium-channel blocker which can be given at 40 mg, po, tid/qid up to 240-320 mg/day; **clonidine (Catapres);** see section IX.A.1); and **amantadine** (see section V.E.4). Toxic drugs such as lithium are best avoided because of the high potential for serious adverse effects.

VI. **Antihistamines** are generally indicated for allergy, pruritus, and for periodic sedation. Some also have antiemetic, antianxiety, and nonspecific analgesic effects. Due to their low potency, they are often used in conjunction with other therapies. Their usefulness is often limited by adverse effects.

Mechanism of action. Antihistamines act by blocking histamine release through competitive inhibition at histamine H_1 receptors. Many antihistamines also possess anticholinergic effects.

Adverse drug reactions. The ADRs include CNS effects (e.g., excessive sedation, dizziness, ataxia, headaches, and muscle weakness), paradoxical excitation (e.g., restlessness, insomnia, tremors, delirium, and possibly seizures), respiratory depression (secondary to generalized CNS depression after administering large drug doses), cardiovascular effects (e.g., hypotension, hypertension, tachycardia, and other arrhythmias; overall incidence is low), and other adverse effects (e.g., nausea, vomiting, changes in bowel habits, hypersensitivity, flushing, dryness of the mouth, dysuria, urinary retention, impotence, vertigo, blurred vision, and tinnitus). Tolerance to these adverse effects frequently occurs after repeated use.

Contraindications and precautions. Antihistamines with pronounced anticholinergic activity, should be used with caution in patients with narrow-angle glaucoma, cardiovascular instability, difficulty with urination (e.g., symptomatic prostatism), or myasthenia gravis. They are contraindicated in patients with hypersensitivity to the drug or the component of its vehicle.

A. **Hydroxyzine (Atarax, Vistaril)** has antihistaminic with anticholinergic, anxiolytic, sedative, antispasmodic, and antiemetic effects. It also has some analgesic effects (see Chapter 5.10, section VI.E.2.g.2) either alone or in combination with morphine. The combination of an NSAID or opioid with hydroxyzine (25-50 mg q4-6h) given orally on a regular basis is useful in controlling moderate pain and the nausea often associated with NSAID (see section I.A) or opioid use (see section I.B). Hydroxycine is available in oral forms (Atarax, Vistaril) and parenteral forms (Vistaril IM solution, 25- and 50-mg/ml vials and 100-mg/2 ml vials). To provide sedation and anxiolytic effects, a dose of 50 to 100 mg, po/IM, qid may be given.

B. **Diphenhydramine (Benadryl)** has antihistaminic with anticholinergic, sedative, antiparkinsonism, and antimotion-sickness effects. Additional ADR include thickening of bronchial secretions with wheezing and nasal stuffiness (thus it should be used with caution in asthmatic patients). Diphenhydramine is available in both oral forms (25 and 50 mg capsules) and injectable forms

(50 mg/ml ampule or syringe). The oral dose is 25 to 50 mg, po, tid/qid, and the parenteral dose is 10 to 50 mg (or up to 100 mg), IM/IV, q4h (up to a maximum of 400 mg/day).

VII. Hematological agents commonly used in PM&R are antithrombotic agents (anti-coagulant and antiplatelet drugs), which interrupt the progression of the thrombotic process. Thrombolytic agents (Streptokinase, Urokinase, and tPA) which actively resolve the thrombus are not discussed in this book because their use is beyond the expertise of most physiatrists. In PM&R, drugs used for treating thromboembolic disease are unfractionated heparin (given IV) and warfarin. For prevention of thromboembolic disease, low molecular weight heparin (LMWH), low doses of unfractionated heparin (given SQ), warfarin, or antiplatelet drugs may be used. Treatment recommendations on anticoagulation and antiplatelet therapy given in this book are derived from the Fourth American College of Chest Physicians (ACCP) Consensus Conference on Antithrombotic Therapy (*Chest* 108:supplement, 1995).

A. Anticoagulant therapy is indicated in patients with atrial fibrillation, deep venous thrombosis (DVT) (see Chapter 5.3, section IV.B.1 and V.A), pulmonary embolism (PE) (see Chapter 5.3, section VI.A.3), vertebral basilar insufficiency, stroke caused by cardiogenic embolus, prosthetic heart valves (especially mechanical valves or complicated bioprosthetic valves; anticoagulant therapy is controversial in uncomplicated bioprosthetic valves), and unstable angina and acute myocardial infarction (especially anterolateral wall). It is also indicated in patients who have cardiac surgery under cardiac bypass; in those who have vascular surgery; during and after coronary angioplasty; in patients with coronary stents; and in selected patients with disseminated intravascular coagulation (DIC).

It is absolutely contraindicated in patients with subarachnoid or cerebral hemorrhage, serious active bleeding (postoperative, spontaneous, or associated with trauma; except selected cases of DIC); severe thrombocytopenia, recent brain, eye or spinal cord surgery; and malignant hypertension. It is relatively contraindicated in other conditions with increased danger of bleeding, that is cardiovascular conditions (severe hypertension, subacute bacterial endocarditis), surgical conditions (during and immediately following spinal tap, spinal anesthesia, or surgery other than those listed under absolute contraindications), hematologic conditions (thrombocytopenia, hemophilia, and some vascular purpuras), gastrointestinal conditions (bleeding due to ulcerative lesions of the stomach or small intestines), and other conditions (menstruation, liver disease with impaired homeostasis, and severe renal failure). It must be used with extreme caution in patients prone to falling (e.g., elderly or debilitated patients) and those with poor compliance. During anticoagulation, the following must be monitored regularly: coagulation time (PT/aPTT), CBC (Hct/Hgb, platelet), urinalysis (hematuria), and stool guaiac. Invasive procedures and intramuscular injections should be minimized and NSAIDs avoided.

1. Warfarin (Coumadin, Panwarfin; see Chapter 5.2, sections IV.B.1.a and V.A.2) is the most widely used oral agent for long-term anticoagulation. It prevents the activation of prothrombin in the coagulation cascade by acting in the liver to deplete and inhibit the production of four vitamin K–dependent clotting factors (II, VII, IX, X) and at least two vitamin K–dependent anticoagulant factors (proteins C and S). Warfarin's anticoagulation effect is not immediate because time is needed to clear the normal coagulation factors already present in the plasma and to replace them

Table 4.8-10. Classes of drugs that can potentially interact with warfarin

EFFECT ON WARFARIN	DRUG CLASS
Potentiation (i.e., causes increased INR)	Adrenergic stimulants (central); alcohol abuse reduction preparations; analgesics; anesthetics (inhalation); anticoagulants; antimalarial agents; antiparasitic drugs; antiplatelets; beta-adrenergic blockers; bromelains; cholelitholytic agents; diabetic agents (oral); gastrointestinal (ulcerative colitis) agents; gout treatment agents; hemorrheologic agents; hepatotoxic drugs; hyperglycemic agents; hypertensive emergency agents; monoamine oxidase inhibitors; narcotics (prolonged use); nonsteroidal antiinflammatory drugs; psychostimulants; pyrazolones; salicylates; steroids (anabolic); thrombolytics; thyroid drugs; uricosuric agents; vaccines
Inhibition (i.e., causes decreased INR)	Adrenal cortical steroid inhibitors; antacids; antianxiety agents; antihistamine; antipsychotic drugs; barbiturates; enteral nutritional supplements; immunosuppressives; oral contraceptives (estrogen-containing)
Potentiation or inhibition	Antiarrhythmics; antibiotics; anticonvulsants; antidepressants; antineoplastics; antithyroid drugs; diuretics; fungal medications (systemic); gastric acidity and peptic ulcer agents; hypnotics; hypolipidemics; steroids (adrenocortical); tuberculosis agents; vitamins

Data adapted from *Physicians' desk reference*, ed 51, Montvale, NJ, 1997, Medical Economics Co, pp. 942-943.

with newly synthesized dysfunctional vitamin K–dependent proteins. Depending on the dose given, the delay in anticoagulation may range from 2 to 7 days.

Warfarin is bound to plasma proteins and can be easily displaced by other medications (see Table 4.8-10 for classes of drugs that can interact with warfarin). Many endogenous conditions can potentiate warfarin including a vitamin K–deficient diet, diarrhea, steatorrhea, hypermetabolic states (fever, hyperthyroidism), liver disease, cancer, collagen disease, and congestive heart failure. Endogenous conditions that can inhibit warfarin are edema, hyperlipidemia, hypothyroidism, and hereditary warfarin resistance. Because patients may be exposed to the above factors, their response to warfarin may be unpredictable. Hence warfarin administration must be monitored regularly using the prothrombin time test, which reflects the warfarin dose given 24 to 48 hours earlier.

The standard reporting of prothrombin time is in international normalized ratio (INR). The recommended INR is 2.0 to 3.0 for all indications except for patients with mechanical prosthetic heart valves in which case an INR of 2.5 to 3.5 is recommended. If the INR is above therapeutic range, refer to the ACCP guidelines described in Table 5.3-3. Duration of warfarin treatment varies from 3 to 6 months (e.g., patients with slow-resolving risk factors, such as prolonged immobilization) to a lifetime (e.g., patients with chronic atrial fibrillation). Warfarin (Coumadin) is available in 1-, 2-, 2.5-, 5-, 7.5-, and 10-mg tablets and is given once a day (usually at bedtime). Adverse drug reactions include bleeding and, rarely, cutaneous microvascular thrombosis (with subsequent skin necrosis). Warfarin crosses the placenta and should not be used during pregnancy, particularly during the first trimester. When anticoagulation is needed in pregnancy, heparin is preferred.

Although commonly practiced, starting warfarin therapy with a loading dose is unnecessary. If a rapid anticoagulant effect is needed, an initial dose of IV heparin (see section VII.A.2) should be used and overlapped with warfarin for at least 4 days (during which time both anticoagulants are given in combination). The heparin can be discontinued when the INR has been in the therapeutic range for 2 consecutive days. If anticoagulation is not urgent (e.g., chronic stable atrial fibrillation), it is safer to start with an estimated maintenance dose of 4 to 5 mg/day of warfarin, which usually results in the patient reaching an INR of 2.0 in about 4 or 5 days and achieving a steady-state anticoagulant effect in about 14 days.

Prothrombin time (INR) is monitored daily until therapeutic range has been achieved and maintained for at least 2 consecutive days, then two to three times weekly for 1 to 2 weeks. Thereafter, if the INR remains stable, the interval of testing can be reduced to weekly or biweekly and eventually to once every 4 to 6 weeks. If dose adjustments are required, then the cycle of more frequent monitoring is repeated until a stable dose response is again achieved. Unexpected fluctuations in dose response could be attributed to changes in diet (e.g., high vitamin K-diet) or undisclosed drug use (see Table 4.8-10 for drug and food interaction), inaccuracy of prothrombin time testing, poor patient compliance, surreptitious self-medication, or intermittent alcohol consumption.

2. **Heparin (unfractionated heparin;** see Chapter 5.2, sections IV.B.1.b and V.A.1) enhances the activity of antithrombin III which in turn inactivates factor IIa (thrombin) and, to a lesser degree, factors Xa and IXa. It also inhibits the activation of factors V and VIII by thrombin. It is prescribed in units (U) and can be given either by IV or SQ routes. Adjusted high-dose heparin (25,000-35,000 U/day) is given IV (or SQ) for treatment of established PE or DVT or to prevent recurrent thrombosis; while fixed, low-dose heparin (10,000-15,000 U/day or 5,000 U q8-12h) is given SQ for the prevention of DVT. The anticoagulation effect of SQ heparin is delayed for about 1 hour and peak levels occur at about 3 hour. If the SQ route is selected, a high initial dose should be used (35,000 U/24 hours in two divided doses) to overcome the poor bioavailability of moderate doses, or if immediate anticoagulation is needed, the SQ injection should be preceded by an IV bolus of 5,000 U. The anticoagulation effect of heparin is monitored q6h after injection using the activated partial thromboplastin time (aPTT) test, which is sensitive to the inhibitory effects of heparin on thrombin, factor Xa, and factor IXa. Fixed, low-dose SQ heparin does not require aPTT monitoring. Routine CBC is needed in all patients receiving heparin to detect bleeding and thrombocytopenia.

Adjusted-dose unfractionated heparin (ADUH) by IV infusion is the drug of choice when a rapid (immediate) anticoagulant effect is needed and for the treatment or prevention of PE and DVT. Adjusted-dose unfractionated heparin is usually indicated for short-term anticoagulation. Long-term ADUH is occasionally used (e.g., when anticoagulant therapy is needed in pregnancy and in the rare patient who develops recurrent venous thromboembolism while being treated with appropriate doses of warfarin). Length of ADUH anticoagulation is 5 to 10 days with warfarin administered jointly with heparin for 4 to 5 days. When the INR is therapeutic, ADUH may be discontinued. Administration of ADUH must be monitored and its dosage adjusted as needed. (See Table 5.3-4 for ADUH dose adjustment using body weight or Table 5.3-5 for ADUH dose adjustment without using body weight.) A commonly used alternative method is to load 5,000 U of IV ADUH then infuse 25,000 U in 250 ml 5% dextrose in water or normal saline (NS) (i.e., 100 U/ml) at 800 to 1000 U/hour (8-10 ml/hour) and adjust at the rate 100 U/hour as needed until the therapeutic dose (aPTT of 1.5 to 2.0 times the normal value) is reached.

Adverse drug reactions of heparin include bleeding, hematoma at subcutaneous injection sites, thrombocytopenia (incidence is 1-5%; usually benign and reversible; more common with bovine than porcine heparin; heparin should be stopped if platelet count is <100,000/ml), paradoxical thrombotic events, skin lesions (urticarial lesions, erythematosus papules and plaques, and skin necrosis), osteoporosis, hypersensitivity reactions, and increases in transaminases (59% incidence). If bleeding occurs (e.g., GI or CNS), protamine sulfate, 10 to 50 mg IV over 10 minutes (0.5-1 mg protamine sulfate neutralizes about 100 U heparin) is used to reverse the anticoagulation.

3. **Enoxaparin (Lovenox;** see Chapter 5.2, sections IV.B.1.c and V.A.3) is a LMWH that weighs about one-third of the unfractionated heparin, i.e. about 4500 to 5000 dalton versus 15,000 for unfractionated heparin. It was developed in an attempt to reduce the risk of major bleeding that accompanies treatment with unfractionated heparins. Because of its low molecular weight, it does not inhibit thrombin (IIa); however, it retains its ability to inhibit factor Xa and is, therefore, factor Xa specific. With more predictable anticoagulant responses, LMWH has a longer plasma half-life (4.6 hours) than standard unfractionated heparin (2.9 hours). Hence LMWH can be given twice daily and without laboratory monitoring (except for routine CBC to check for thrombocytopenia).

Low molecular weight heparin effectively reduces (by 60-90%) the relative risk of venous thrombosis in stroke, SCI, and other high-risk patients. This beneficial effect occurs with lower incidence of bleeding complications than standard unfractionated heparin. Its side effects (bleeding being the major ADR) are similar to unfractionated heparin, but the incidence is generally lower. Like unfractionated heparin, it does not cross the placental barrier and thus can be used in pregnancy. The only LMWH commercially available for DVT prophylaxis (in musculoskeletal or neurologic conditions) is enoxaparin (Lovenox) given at 30 mg, SQ, bid. Use of LMWH for the treatment of acute thromboembolism is still under investigation. Enoxaparin is usually given within 24 hours after surgery or 48 hours poststroke for 7 to 14 days (both the onset and duration of treatment remains controversial).

B. Antiplatelets

1. **Dextran-40 solution** (10%) is a low molecular weight (40,000 dalton) polysaccharide originally used as a plasma volume expander, but it was found to have antithrombotic effects related to its ability to decrease platelet adhesion and fibrin polymerization. It also forms a coating on the endothelial walls, thereby inhibiting nidus formation. It is ineffective in preventing DVTs in stroke patients. In other high-risk patients (e.g., after total hip or knee replacement), its antithrombotic effects are controversial. Adverse

drug reactions include increased risk of congestive heart failure risk, volume overload, anaphylaxis (hence, test dose must be done), renal insufficiency, phlebitis from IV insertion, and about 14% incidence of postoperative bleeding (e.g., GI bleeding and wound hematomas). It is given intravenously at 20 ml/kg up to 500 ml.

2. **Aspirin** (see section I.A.3.a) interferes with platelet activity. Aspirin is indicated in patients with stable angina, unstable angina, acute myocardial infarction, transient cerebral ischemia, thrombotic stroke, and peripheral arterial disease. It is also indicated in patients with atrial fibrillation in whom warfarin is contraindicated. A dose of 75 to 100 mg/day of ASA should be used chronically for all indications, although an initial dose of 160 to 325 mg should be used in acute settings. For patients with cerebrovascular disease, a dose of 75 mg/day is effective. (Whether higher doses are more effective awaits the results of clinical trials.) A dose of 100 mg/day may be combined with warfarin in patients with mechanical prosthetic heart valves who develop systemic embolism while on warfarin. For DVT prophylaxis, ASA is generally not recommended because it is not as effective as other DVT prophylaxis methods.

3. **Dipyridamole (Persantine)** is a platelet inhibitor, which, at 225 mg/day, is indicated as an adjunct (not as sole therapy) to warfarin anticoagulation in the prevention of thromboembolism in patients with prosthetic heart valves who develop systemic embolism while on warfarin and who cannot tolerate aspirin. It has also been used together with ASA for stroke prophylaxis (although there is no convincing evidence that this combination is more effective than ASA alone). Dipyridamole has not been shown to be effective (and is thus not recommended) in DVT prophylaxis. The ADRs include dizziness, abdominal distress, headache, and rash. It is available in oral forms (25-, 50-, and 75-mg tablets) and is given at 75 to 100 mg, po, tid/qid.

4. **Ticlopidine (Ticlid)** inhibits platelet aggregation by inhibiting adenosine diphosphate–induced platelet-fibrinogen binding and subsequent platelet-platelet interaction. This inhibitory effect is delayed for 24 to 48 hours, thus it may not be used when a rapid antiplatelet effect is required. Ticlopidine is indicated instead of aspirin in ischemic stroke patients with aspirin allergy or aspirin intolerance and in patients who develop recurrent thromboembolism despite aspirin. The ADRs include GI complaints, reversible neutropenia, rash, and abnormal LFTs (hence CBC and LFTs must be done regularly). It is available in 250-mg tablets and is given at 250 mg, po, bid with food.

VIII. **Bone-metabolism regulators** are used in conjunction with other nonpharmacologic treatment of osteoporosis, including exercise.

A. **Anti-bone-resorption agents** act by decreasing the rate of bone resorption through inhibition of bone osteoclasts. They are generally useful for the type I (''high-turnover'' or involutional) type of osteoporosis (e.g., postmenopausal osteoporosis).

1. **Estrogen replacement** is the most effective preventive strategy in the management of postmenopausal osteoporosis (PMO) in women, whether the menopause is natural or surgically induced (e.g., oophorectomy before age 50). It has been shown to inhibit bone resorption, slow the loss of bone mass, and partially reduce (i.e., by 50%) the risk of fractures in postmenopausal women. Also, for the most part, bone that has already

been lost after menopause cannot be replaced (despite retardation of bone loss). Estrogen replacement also reduces the risk of myocardial infarction, stroke, cardiovascular death, and death from all causes.

Mechanisms of action. Estrogen decreases bone response to parathyroid hormone (PTH); promotes synthesis of calcitonin; and enhances availability of vitamin D. It probably also acts directly on specific estrogen receptors in osteoblasts.

Adverse drug reactions. The ADRs of estrogen replacement include menstrual bleeding, weight gain, nausea, headache, and breast tenderness—all of which can be alleviated by a reduction in estrogen dose. Estrogen replacement can also increase the risk of endometrial cancer and possibly breast cancer (these risks can be reduced or eliminated by cyclic therapy with added progestin; however, the coronary artery disease risk of adding progesterone is unknown). There is no evidence of hypertension or increased risk of thromboembolism in postmenopausal estrogen replacement.

Contraindications and precautions. Contraindications to estrogen replacement include a history of breast or endometrial cancer, recurrent thromboembolic disease, acute liver or gall bladder disease, and unexplained vaginal bleeding. Relative contraindications include fibrocystic disease of the breast, uterine myomata or fibroids, endometriosis, or a family history of breast cancer.

Drug administration guidelines. Estrogen replacement is indicated for all women with premature menopause and no contraindications. Patients who have had a hysterectomy may take estrogen daily without cycling with progesterone.

In postmenopausal women without hysterectomy, a cyclic regimen including estrogen and a progesterone should be used, giving estrogen on days 1 to 25 of each month with the addition of progesterone (e.g., medroxyprogesterone [Provera], 10 mg, po, qd) started between days 12 and 15 through day 25 of each monthly cycle. Estrogen preparations and their doses include conjugated estrogens (Premarin), 0.625 mg, po, qd; ethinyl estradiol, 20 μg, po, qd; or estradiol, 1 mg, po, qd. In women who have side effects at these doses, conjugated estrogen, 0.3 mg, po, qd, may be tried. Patients on estrogen replacement should be given calcium supplements (1500 mg/day; see section VIII.A.4). An alternative to oral estrogen replacement is transdermal estradiol (0.05-0.10-mg patch twice a week), which bypasses the GI system and circumvents the possible GI ADRs but still adequately delivers to the skeletal system. If noncycled estrogen without progesterone is used in a women with an intact uterus, endometrial biopsy should be done regularly (at least every 2 years).

Estrogen replacement should begin as soon as possible after the menopause to delay the rapid phase of bone loss; however, therapy may be beneficial as late as age 70 (beyond this age, there is little evidence to support its usage). The optimal duration of therapy is not established, but there is consensus that it should continue for at least 10 years (or up to age 70). Women with premature menopause should be treated at least until the time of normal menopause (about age 50). Regular evaluation should include breast examinations, annual mammography, and prompt evaluation of unexpected vaginal bleeding with endometrial biopsy.

2. **Calcitonin (Calcimar, Miacalcin)** can be used in women over 70 years of age (because estrogen is ineffective in women over 70), postmenopausal

women in whom estrogen is contraindicated, women or men with established osteoporosis (especially "high-turnover" osteoporosis), women with medical or chemical oophorectomy, persons with low bone mass, amenorrheic athletes, painful vertebral crush fractures, and lytic disease of weight-bearing bones. Calcitonin also has analgesic properties (e.g., in cancer patients with bone pain or in elderly patients in whom CNS side effects from analgesics are contraindicated; see Chapter 5.10, section VI.E.2.m). The role of calcitonin in osteoporosis prevention is under investigation. Calcitonin has not been shown to reduce the risk of fracture.

Mechanisms of action. Calcitonin is a polypeptide hormone with receptors in osteoclasts that decrease bone resorption, inhibit osteoclasts, and may be helpful in rapid bone losers. Aside from its direct action on bone, it also has direct renal effects and actions on the GI tract.

Adverse drug reactions. Side effects include nausea, flushing, and, rarely, allergic reactions (e.g., urticaria and local reactions at injection sites). These may diminish or disappear after continued administration or may be alleviated by an antiemetic or antihistaminic agent.

Contraindication. It is contraindication in patients with hypersensitivity to the drug or the vehicle of its component.

Drug administration guidelines. There are three forms of injectable calcitonin: salmon calcitonin (Calcimar, Miacalcin), human calcitonin (Cibacalcin), and eel calcitonin. To date, only salmon calcitonin is FDA-approved for postmenopausal osteoporosis. It has high activity, low antigenicity, and costs less than the other preparations. Salmon calcitonin (Calcimar or Miacalcin, 200 IU/ml in 2-ml vials) is given at 50 to 100 IU, IM or SQ, qd or qod for at least 1 to 3 months. Prior to administration, skin testing for allergy should be done. When an adequate response is achieved (usually after several months), the dosage is decreased to 50 IU, SQ, 3 times a week for at least 3 to 6 months (it is not clear if treatment beyond a total of 12-18 months is beneficial). Aside from injectable forms, salmon calcitonin is also available as a nasal spray (i.e., Miacalcin nasal spray, 200 units intranasally daily in alternate nostrils; patient should be monitored for nasal ulcers or rhinitis). If resistance to salmon calcitonin develops, human calcitonin (Cibacalcin), 0.5 mg, SQ or IM, qd or qod, is often effective. Patients on calcitonin needs adequate vitamin D (e.g., 400 IU/day; see section VIII.A.5) and calcium intake (1500 mg/day; see section VIII.A.4) to prevent progressive loss of bone mass in postmenopausal osteoporosis. Periodic urinalysis for sediments or casts is also recommended.

3. **Biphosphonates** can be used instead of calcitonin in women over 70 years of age, postmenopausal women for whom estrogen is contraindicated, and women and men with established osteoporosis. It can also be used in Paget's disease and in heterotopic ossification. Biphosphonates inhibit bone turnover by interfering with the function of osteoclasts and the dissolution of hydroxyapatite. In high doses, however, it can impair bone mineralization as well as promote osteomalacia as prevent the formation of heterotopic ossification (see section VIII.A.3.b).

   a. **Alendronate (Fosamax)** is a new biphosphonate which is 200 times more potent than etidronate. Because of its high potency, it provides effective inhibition of bone resorption at doses that do not impair mineralization. Hence it is indicated for chronic treatment regimens in patients with postmenopausal osteoporosis and Paget's disease of bone. The ADRs include GI upset, musculoskeletal pain, and headache. It is contraindicated in patients with severe renal dysfunction (creatinine clearance of less than 35 ml/min). However, for less severe renal insufficiency, it may be given without dose adjustment. Its recommended dose is 10 mg, po, qd for postmenopausal osteoporosis and 40 mg/day for 6 months for Paget's disease (may repeat treatment after 6 months evaluation if serum alkaline phosphatase is still increased). Patients taking alendronate need adequate intake of vitamin D (e.g., 400 IU/day; see section VIII.A.5) and calcium (e.g., 1500 mg/day; see section VIII.A.4). Alendronate must be taken with plain water on an empty stomach 30 minutes before any other beverage or medication to maximize its absorption. Also, patients should avoid recumbency for 30 minutes after intake. It is available only in oral form (10- and 40-mg tablets).

  b. Etidronate (Didronel) is primarily indicated for the management of heterotopic ossification and Paget's disease. It is given in high doses for prevention of bone mineralization in patients predisposed to heterotopic ossification (see section VIII.C). In Paget's disease, it is given at a dosage of 5-10 mg/kg/day for a period not to exceed 6 months (which may be repeated after 90 days if Paget's disease is still active and symptomatic). Etidronate has also been experimentally shown to be beneficial for PMO, as it increases vertebral bone density and decreases the rate of vertebral fracture. For PMO, it can be given intermittently in a 12-week cycle at 400 mg, po, qd for 2 weeks, followed by 10 weeks of calcium supplementation, and repetition of the cycle. The ADRs, contraindications, precautions, preparations, and administration guidelines for etidronate are given in section VIII.C.

  c. Pamidronate (Aredia) is a biphosphonate mainly used in patients with hypercalcemia due to malignancy. It is also used as an adjuvant analgesic in cancer patients with bone pain (see Chapter 5.10, section VI.E.2.m).

4. **Calcium** is the major inorganic component of bone. It structures the human skeleton along with collagenous fibers, and it regulates many cellular activities. It also decreases the effect of PTH on bone resorption. Foods high in calcium include milk, buttermilk, yogurt, cheese, ice cream, sardines (with bones), shrimp, salmon, broccoli (cooked), tofu (bean curd), and turnip greens (cooked). The intestinal absorption of dietary calcium is reduced as the person ages and in women with estrogen deficiency. The recommended calcium intake for premenopausal women and men is 1000 mg/day and for postmenopausal women, 1500 mg/day. To achieve this level of intake, most women need calcium supplements, 500 to 1000 mg/day. Calcium supplementation can slow loss of bone mass in postmenopausal women with low calcium intake. Side effects of calcium supplementation include dyspepsia, constipation, and hypercalciuria. It can also cause digitalis toxicity. It is contraindicated in patients with kidney stones or those who are prone to form kidney stones. Among calcium preparations, calcium carbonate (e.g., Os-Cal, 250 or 500 mg elemental calcium per tablet, Tums Extra-strength, 400 mg elemental calcium/5 ml, or various generics) is probably the best and least expensive. Calcium citrate (Citracal) may also be used.

5. **Vitamin D** allows increased calcium absorption from the GI tract. While some studies found it useful in maintaining bone mass, others suggest that it can actually accelerate bone loss. Hence it should only be supple-

mented if the patient has vitamin D deficiency (shown by testing serum 25-hydroxy vitamin D). Dietary vitamin D deficiency can initially be treated with vitamin D, 50,000 IU po weekly for several weeks to replete body stores, followed by long-term therapy with 400 to 800 IU/day. If vitamin-D deficiency is caused by malabsorption, the dose ranges from 50,000 IU po weekly to daily. For both dietary deficiency and malabsorption deficiency, the dose should be adjusted to maintain serum 25-hydroxy vitamin D levels within the normal range. Calcium supplements (e.g., 1500 mg/day; see section VIII.A.4) are usually required during vitamin D supplementation. Vitamin D preparations include calcium supplements containing vitamin D (e.g., Os-Cal + D, 125 IU/250- or 500-mg tablet), many multivitamins (400 IU/tablet), and vitamin D drops (200 IU/drop or 8000 IU/ml). The combination calcium/vitamin D tablets (e.g., Os-Cal + D) should be used with caution because the ratio may lead to vitamin D toxicity.

Elderly people may tolerate two to three times the recommended daily allowance of vitamin D if cutaneous generation of vitamin D, mediated through sun exposure, is reduced. Some clinicians advocate that 5 to 10 minutes of sunshine 3 times per week rather than supplementation. If the patient does not respond to high doses of vitamin D, calcifediol (Calderol, 20 or 50 μg/capsule), 20 to 100 μg, po, qd, may be better absorbed (the dose is then reduced depending on serum 5-hydroxy vitamin D levels). Patients on vitamin D supplementation should be monitored every 3 to 6 months for serum 25-hydroxy vitamin D, serum calcium, and 24-hour urine calcium.

B. Bone-formation agents stimulate bone growth and are generally useful in type II (or "low-turnover" or senile) osteoporosis.
  1. **Vitamin D** stimulates bone growth and prevents bone resorption. It is described in section VIII.A.5.
  2. **Fluoride** stimulates osteoblastic cells to form new bone and increases trabecular bone density (but not cortical bone density). Its effect on the incidence of fracture is controversial and might be dose dependent (i.e., larger doses result in bones with impaired mineralization, which are more likely to fracture). Although used in Europe, fluoride use in osteoporosis has not been formally approved in the United States. It may be indicated for the treatment of established vertebral osteoporosis with symptomatic fractures that will not respond to other therapies. The ADRs include GI problems (gastric irritation, nausea, recurrent vomiting, and peptic ulcer); rheumatologic problems (e.g., plantar fasciitis, synovitis, arthralgias, and questionable increased risk of hip fractures), and anemia. It may be given as sodium fluoride (e.g., Luride, 2.2 mg/tablet or 1.1 mg/ml) at 25 mg, po, qd with food, increasing slowly to 25 mg tid as tolerated over a few weeks. It should be given with calcium (1500 mg/day) and vitamin D (400 IU/day).
  3. **Anabolic steroids (androgens)** can increase bone mass perhaps by increasing bone formation; however, their prolonged use in osteoporotic patients is generally not recommended because of their androgenic (virilizing) effects as well as adverse effects on carbohydrate, lipid metabolism, and liver function. Studies have shown that 10 to 20% of men with osteoporosis have partial or complete hypogonadism of various causes. In osteoporotic men with low plasma testosterone, androgen (e.g., testosterone enanthate) may be used under the supervision of an endocrinologist.

C. **Anti bone-mineralization agents** are used in preventing heterotopic ossification (HO). Heterotopic ossification is characterized by metaplastic osteogenesis and can be associated with traumatic conditions (e.g., SCI, TBI, burns, severe thigh bruises, as well as surgical trauma such as total hip replacement [THR]) or nontraumatic conditions (e.g., infection of the CNS and peripheral neuropathy; association with various benign and malignant neoplasms). The biphosphonate etidronate (see section VIII.A.3), when given in high dose, prevents or retards HO by inhibiting bone mineralization through chemical absorption of calcium hydroxyapatite crystals and their amorphous precursors, thus blocking the aggregation, growth, and mineralization of these crystals. Etidronate is indicated in the prevention and treatment of HO (e.g., after THR and SCI). Studies show that in patients with THR, etidronate does not promote loosening of hip prostheses or impede trochanteric reattachment; and in SCI, it does not inhibit fracture healing or stabilization of the spine. The ADRs of etidronate include GI problems (e.g., diarrhea and nausea) and rarely blood dyscrasias. The GI problems can be usually alleviated by dividing the daily total dose. Etidronate is contraindicated in patients with hypersensitivity to the drug and with clinically overt osteomalacia. It should be used with caution in patients with renal impairment.

Etidronate disodium (Didronel) is available orally in 200- and 400-mg tablets. It is given as a single oral dose (may be divided if patient has GI upset) on an empty stomach to maximize absorption. Food should be avoided within 2 hours of dosing (especially high calcium food such as milk; or vitamins with mineral supplement or antacids). Patients also need to have adequate intake of vitamin D (see section VIII.A.5) and calcium (see section VIII.A.4). For the prevention and treatment of HO in THR patients, the dose is 20 mg/kg/day for 1 month before and 3 months after surgery (4 months total). For the prevention and treatment of HO in SCI patients, the dose is 20 mg/kg/day for 2 weeks followed by 10 mg/kg/day for 10 weeks (12 weeks total). Treatment should begin prior to any evidence of HO because etidronate does not affect mature HO. Ideally it should be started in the hypervascular precursor phase (demonstrated when the flow and pool phases of a three-phase bone scan are positive).

IX. **Cardiovascular drugs** prescribed by physiatrists for noncardiac indications include
A. **Adrenergic drugs**
1. **Centrally acting adrenergic agonists,** which include **clonidine (Catapres), methyldopa (Aldomet),** and **guanabenz (Wytensin),** are primarily used as antihypertensive agents. Among these drugs, only clonidine is described as it is a multipurpose drug commonly used in the PM&R setting. Clonidine is an α_2-adrenergic agonist as well as an α_1-adrenergic blocker. It is used in the management of pain (see Chapter 5.10, section VI.E.2.i), spasticity (see Chapter 5.4, section III.D.1.d), aggression (see section V.F), and sympathetic overactivity during opioid withdrawal (see section I.B) or autonomic dysreflexia (see Chapter 5.7, section V.F). Its ADRs include cardiovascular effects (e.g., hypotension, syncope, dizziness, palpitation, bradycardia, and rarely arrhythmias), CNS effects (e.g., sedation, mental depression, agitation, nervousness, vivid dreams, and nightmares), GI effects (dry mouth, constipation, nausea, vomiting, and anorexia), and other effects (e.g., weight gain, malaise, rash, decreased sexual activity, and weakness).

The risk of serious adverse cardiovascular effects appears to be low in younger patients without a significant associated medical disorder. In the elderly, there is higher risk of serious adverse cardiovascular effects especially those predisposed to hypotensive effects, those receiving other drugs with additive effects on blood pressure, and those with concurrent diseases such as renal or cardiac failure. Clonidine is contraindicated in patients with hypersensitivity to it or a component of its vehicle (e.g., contact sensitivity to the transdermal patch). Clonidine is available in oral and transdermal forms at 0.1-, 0.2-, and 0.3-mg strength. The oral form is taken twice daily, and the transdermal patch is changed every week. Currently, no data suggest better efficacy of one versus the other route, and the choice is based on patient preference. The starting dose of 0.1 to 0.2 mg per day is gradually titrated up (every few days for oral route and every 1 to 2 weeks for transdermal route) to a usual dose of 0.2 to 0.6 mg/day and a maximum of 2.4 mg/day depending on patient's response (especially blood pressure). For oral route, the higher dose should be taken at bedtime to minimize transient effects of dry mouth and drowsiness. Prior to discontinuation, tapering is required to prevent rebound hypertension.

2. **Peripherally acting adrenergic blockers,** e.g., **guanethidine (Ismelin)** and **reserpine (Serpasil)** are primarily used as hypertensive agents; however, their parenteral forms (available only for experimental use) can also be used as ganglionic blocking agents for IV regional sympathetic blocks in patients with reflex sympathetic dystrophy (see Chapter 4.10, section IV.B.4).

3. **Selective α_1-adrenergic blockers,** for example **prazosin (Minipress), terazosin (Hytrin),** and **doxazosin (Cardura)** are primarily used as antihypertensive agents but can also be used to improve bladder-emptying function (see Chapter 5.7, section IV.D.4.a). Prazosin has also been used as an adjunct analgesics in patients with neuropathic pain (see Chapter 5.10; section VI.E.2.i).

4. **Nonselective α_1- and α_2-adrenergic blockers,** for example **phenoxybenzamine (Dibenzyline),** are primarily used to control hypertension in patients with pheochromocytoma but have been reported to be effective in selected cases of reflex sympathetic dystrophy (see Chapter 5.10; section VI.E.2.i.3).

5. **Nonselective β_1- and β_2-adrenergic blockers,** which are primarily used as antihypertensive agents, can also used in the management of pain (see Chapter 5.10; section VI.E.2.i), aggression (see section V.F), and anxiety (see section V.C.2.f). They include **propranolol (Inderal)** and **pindolol (Visken),** both of which are described in section V.F.

B. **Calcium-channel blockers,** which are primarily used as antihypertensive, antiischemic (or antianginal), and antiarrhythmic agents include **verapamil (Calan, Isoptin), diltiazem (Cardizem), isradipine (DynaCirc),** and **nicardipine (Cardene). Nifedipine (Procardia, Adalat),** is also a calcium-channel blocker but is primarily used as an antiischemic agent for the emergency management of hypertensive crises (e.g., in autonomic dysreflexia; see Chapter 5.7, section V.F) and for management of reflex sympathetic dystrophy, causalgia, and Raynaud's phenomenon (see Chapter 5.10, section VI.E.2.i.5). Among the other calcium-channel blockers, verapamil is used in the PM&R setting as an antiaggression agent (see section V.F) and as an adjunct analgesic in patients with neuropathic pain (see Chapter 5.10, section VI.E.2.i.5). The ADRs of verapamil include cardiovascular effects (e.g., hypotension, syncope, dizziness, palpitation, bradycardia, atrioventricular block, angina pectoris, myocardial infarct, and congestive heart failure), CNS effects (e.g., headache, sedation, insomnia, paresthesia, confusion, equilibrium disorders, stroke, and psychotic symptoms), GI effects (dry mouth, constipation, diarrhea, nausea, and gingival hyperplasia), and other effects (e.g., rash, impotence, blurred vision, and fatigue). Verapamil is contraindicated in patients with severe left ventricular dysfunction; hypotension (systolic blood pressure below 90 mm Hg) or cardiogenic shock; arrhythmias such as sick sinus syndrome, second- or third-degree atrioventricular block (except in patients with a functioning artificial ventricular pacemaker); atrial flutter or fibrillation; accessory bypass tract (e.g., Wolff-Parkinson-White and Lown-Ganong-Levine syndromes); and known hypersensitivity to verapamil or a component of its vehicle. Verapamil is available in oral (immediate and sustained release) and parenteral forms. It is usually started at 40 mg, po, tid/qid, and titrated up to 240 to 320 mg/day.

C. **Antiarrhythmic drugs** can also be used as local anesthetics in the management of chronic pain (see Chapter 5.10, section VI.E.2.d). They include intravenous local anesthetics (e.g., **lidocaine [Xylocaine], procaine [Procan]**) and oral local anesthetics (e.g., **mexiletene [Mexitil], tocainamide [Tonacard],** and **flecainide [Tumbocor]**). Lidocaine is also used as a topical anesthetic agent (e.g., **EMLA;** see Chapter 5.10, section VI.E.2.e) and an iontophoresis agent (see Chapter 4.1, section V.A.1.a)

X. **Gastrointestinal drugs** for bowel problems (i.e., antidiarrheal and laxative drugs are both described in Chapter 5.8, section VI.A.2 and VI.B.3, respectively).

Other GI medications are discussed in different sections of this chapter, for example, antiemetic drugs used to treat nausea in patients taking opioids (see section I.B. under Adverse Drug Reactions), and antiulcer drugs used for GI protection when taking NSAIDs (see section I.A.3 under GI Toxicity).

XI. **Neurourologic drugs** commonly used in treating voiding dysfunction are described in Chapter 5.7, section IV.D. They include anticholinergic, cholinergic, α-adrenergic agonist, and α-adrenergic blocking agents.

XII. **Pulmonary drugs** are primarily used in patients with COPD (see Chapter 5.12).

BIBLIOGRAPHY

Acute Pain Management Guideline Panel: *Clinical practice guideline: acute pain management,* AHCPR Pub. No. 92-0032, Rockville, MD, Feb, 1992, Agency for Health Care Policy and Research.

Aronoff GM, editor: *Evaluation and treatment of chronic pain,* Baltimore, 1992, Williams & Wilkins.

Bjorkman DJ: Nonsteroidal anti-inflammatory drug-induced gastrointestinal injury, *Am J Med,* 101 (suppl 1A): 25S–32S, 1996.

Brooks PM, Day RO: Nonsteroidal antiinflammatory drugs—differences and similarities, *N Engl J Med,* 324:1716-1725, 1991.

Cardenas DD, McLean A, Jr: Psychopharmacologic management of traumatic brain injury, *Phys Med and Rehab Clin N Amer* 3(2):273-290, 1992.

Consensus Development Conference: Diagnosis, prophylaxis, and treatment of osteoporosis, *Am J Med* 94:646-650, 1993.

Dean BZ, Williams FH, King JC, Goddard MJ: Pain rehabilitation. 4. Therapeutic options in pain management, *Arch Phys Med Rehabil* Suppl 75:21-30, 1994.

Hamill RJ, Rowlingson JC, editors: *Handbook of critical care pain management,* New York, 1994, McGraw-Hill.

Hardman JG, Limbird LE, editors: *Goodman and Gilman's The pharmacological basis of therapeutics,* ed 9, New York, 1996, McGraw-Hill.

Hirsch J, Dalen JE, Deykin D, et al: Oral anticoagulants: mechanism of action, clinical effectiveness, and optimal therapeutic range. *Chest* 108 (4) suppl: 231S–246S, 1995.

Hirsch J, Dalen JE, Fuster V, et al: Aspirin and other antiplatelet drugs: the relationship among dose, effectiveness, and side effects. *Chest* 108 (4) suppl: 247S–254S, 1995.

Mysiw WJ, Jandel, ME: The agitated brain injured patient. Part 2: Pathophysiology and treatment, *Arch Phys Med Rehabil* 78:213-220, 1997.

Physicians' desk reference, ed 51, Montvale, NJ, 1997, Medical Economics.

Portenoy RK, Kanner RM, editors: *Pain management: theory and practice,* Philadelphia, 1996, FA Davis.

Wall PD, Melzack R, editors: *Textbook of pain,* ed 3, Edinburgh, 1994, Churchill Livingstone.

CHAPTER 4.9

JOINT AND SOFT TISSUE INJECTIONS

Joint and soft tissue injections should be considered adjuncts to the overall management of musculoskeletal disorders. They are performed only after other conservative methods (e.g., physical modalities, oral analgesics, or antiinflammatory agents) have failed. They are relatively safe procedures when performed judiciously by a skilled practitioner. This chapter deals with joint and soft tissue injections for diagnostic purposes (e.g., arthrocentesis and joint arthrography) as well as for therapeutic purposes (e.g., injection of corticosteroid or combination of corticosteroid with local anesthetic agents into the joint, bursa, and tendon for the relief of inflammation and pain and for the restoration of joint functions). Most injection therapies do not have well-controlled trials but are based on anecdotal and empirical evidence.

I. Supplies

A. "Intraarticular" corticosteroids are suspensions of insoluble particles whose antiinflammatory effect is profound only where the material is deposited. It can be injected into acutely inflamed joints or soft tissues (e.g., synovitis, bursitis, tenosynovitis, epicondylitis, and adhesive capsulitis) of patients with rheumatoid arthritis, spondyloarthropathies, gout, pseudogout, systemic lupus erythematosus (SLE), and other forms of arthritis. Their usefulness in patients with osteoarthritis (OA) remains controversial. Many clinicians believe that they are beneficial in OA patients in whom an effusion can be identified or from whom synovial fluid can be aspirated.

Mechanism of action (MOA). The exact MOA by which corticosteroids inhibit local joint or soft tissue inflammation is not fully known. Pharmacologically, corticosteroids are known to inhibit the process of chemotaxis, decrease capillary permeability, decrease vasodilation, prevent release of arachidonic acid and its metabolites, decrease fibroblast and collagen deposition, stabilize lysosomal membranes, and inhibit macrophage function. For details about the MOA of corticosteroids, see Chapter 4.8, section III.

Adverse drug reactions (ADRs). The injection of corticosteroid into joints or soft tissues seldom causes permanent deleterious effects when performed using accepted guidelines. The ADRs (and prevalence) include postinjection flare (2-5%; attributed to the microcrystalline structure of the steroids or joint trauma of injection; joint appears inflamed or even infected within 2-4 hours after injection and subsides spontaneously in 24-72 hours; give supportive care, ice, and NSAIDs); steroid arthropathy of weight-bearing joints (0.8% occurring after multiple steroid injections; can lead to aseptic osteonecrosis); tendon rupture (less than 1%); facial flushing (less than 1%); benign but uncosmetic skin changes (less than 1%; e.g., depigmentation, scarring, and skin depression due to atrophy of the underlying subcutaneous tissues; may remit over 5 years); and infection (less than 0.1%; avoided by sterile technique). Rare complications include transient paresis of the injected limb, hypersensitivity, asymptomatic periarticular calcification in finger joints, and sickle cell crisis. If injections are frequently repeated (especially using long-lasting corticosteroids) or if the patient is receiving concomitant oral corticosteroid therapy, there is the possibility of systemic corticosteroid effects and suppression of the pituitary-adrenal axis (see Chapter 4.8, section III for the systemic effects of corticosteroids).

Contraindications and precautions for corticosteroid injections include infection (systemic and local), bleeding diathesis, uncontrolled brittle diabetes, extreme obesity, severe joint destruction (e.g., osteoporosis) or soft tissue destruction, traumatic arthritis secondary to fracture through the joint, unstable joints, joint prosthesis, inaccessible joints, soft tissue or bony tumors at or near the underlying joint, failure to respond to previous injections, and hypersensitivity to the corticosteroid or its vehicle. Patients taking an anticoagulant may be injected carefully after checking the prothrombin time and informing the patient of its risks and benefits.

Drug administration guidelines. The "intraarticular" corticosteroid preparations are shown in Table 4.9-1. They have low hormonal side effects and do not dissipate rapidly from the joint. None of these preparations appear to have any superiority over another; however, triamcinolone hexacetonide (Aristospan) is the least water-soluble preparation with the longest duration of action within the peripheral joint space (it also causes less postinjection flares). The choice of a particular corticosteroid preparation depends on its duration of action, solubility, potency, onset of action, and intended purpose. The more insoluble the preparation, the longer is its duration of action, but the longer is the delay in its onset of action. To overcome the lack of immediate response, some clinicians combine short-acting with delayed-acting steroid preparations, and others suggest the addition of a short-acting anesthestic agent (e.g., lidocaine) to form insoluble materials. The combination of corticosteroid and anesthetic agents, however, has been associated with crystal-like formations in the joint, which can cause postinjection flares. Crystal-like formations are attributed to the preservatives (e.g., methylparaben, propylparaben, and phenol) in the anesthestic agents reacting with the steroid; hence, preservative-free anesthestic agents must be used.

For long-term suppression of an inflammatory process such as rheumatoid arthritis, the low-solubility and intermediate- to long-acting triamcinolone hexacetonide (Aristospan) would be preferable. If the patient's condition requires a long-acting agent with faster relief of symptoms, the betamethasome phosphate and acetate preparation (Celestone Soluspan) would be preferable. The short onset from the phosphate preparation and the long duration from the acetate preparation make this a desirable choice. For more rapid onset of therapy, the shorter acting methylprednisolone acetate (Depo-Medrol) would be the drug of choice. Aristospan and Celestone seem to remain within the joint cavity longer than Depo-Medrol, and their systemic effect is limited because of their low serum levels and release over a prolonged period of time.

The number of injections per joint or soft tissue should be limited so as to avoid joint damage (steroid arthropathy) and soft tissue damage. Large (e.g., weight-bearing) joints should not be injected more than 3 times per joint per year up to a maximum of 10 cumulative injections. Small joints should be injected less often, i.e., not more than 2 times per joint per year up to a maximum of four cumulative injections. Although multiple joint injections interfere with normal cartilage protein synthesis, it has been shown that patients with long-standing rheumatoid arthritis who do not receive intraarticular corticosteroids have joint disuse and decreased function much sooner than those who receive the injections. For pain reduction in osteoarthritis as well as an adjunct in the mobilization of the adhesive capsulitis, injections

Table 4.9-1. Corticosteroid preparations for joint and soft tissue injection and their dosages for different joints

"INTRAARTICULAR" CORTICOSTEROIDS (BRANDNAME)	SOLUBILITY	PREPARATION (mg/ml)	HIP (mg)	KNEE/SHOULDER (mg)	WRIST/ELBOW/ANKLE (mg)	SMALL JOINTS (mg)
I. Short-acting*						
Hydrocortisone acetate (Hydrocortone)	Low	25	30-40	25-40	12.5-37.5	10-25
II. Intermediate-acting†						
Prednisolone sodium phosphate (Hydeltrasol)	Intermediate	20	15-20	10-20	5-10	5
Methylprednisolone acetate (Depo-Medrol)	Intermediate	20, 40, 80	40-100	20-80	10-40	4-10
Triamcinolone diacetate (Aristocort)	Low to intermediate	25, 40	30-40	20-40	10-25	5-15
III. Intermediate to long acting‡						
Triamcinolone hexacetonide (Aristospan)	Low	20	15-20	10-20	5-10	1-5
IV. Long-acting§						
Dexamethasone acetate (Decadron-LA)	Intermediate	8	4-6	2-4	1-2	0.5-1.5
Betamethasone phosphate and acetate (Celestone Soluspan)	High	6	6-12	6-9	3-6	3

* Short-half-life = 8-12 hr
† Intermediate half-life = 12-36 hr
‡ Intermediate to long half-life = 12-72 hr
§ Long half-life = 36-72 hr

at the rate of one every 4 to 6 weeks for a maximum of three injections is the most commonly accepted regimen.

B. Local anesthetics without epinephrine are usually combined with "intraarticular" corticosteroids for injection into the joint and soft tissues. This combination provides a larger volume of injectable material with which to bathe the joint more adequately, in addition to providing immediate (although temporary) pain relief. Some clinicians prefer to use corticosteroids alone without anesthetic agents because the anesthetic effect can obscure the exact site of the needle tip (on which these clinicians rely to determine the point of maximal tenderness for injection of the corticosteroid).

The local anesthetic commonly used in combination with corticosteroids include short-acting agents (e.g., 0.5, 1.0, or 2% lidocaine [Xylocaine] or procaine [Novacain]) and longer-acting agents (e.g., 0.25 or 0.5% bupivacaine [Marcaine, Sensorcaine]). Lidocaine and bupivacaine may be combined to obtain an early onset of action with prolonged anesthesia. The anesthetic dosages vary widely with the size of the joint. Usually, the smaller joints such as the acromioclavicular, sternoclavicular, and elbow joints would take 1 to 2 ml of 1% lidocaine combined with the corticosteroid. The glenohumeral, knee, and hip joints would take 2 to 4 ml of anesthetic agent. Bupivacaine is often preferable for nonweight-bearing joints, such as the shoulder, elbow, acromioclavicular, and sternoclavicular joints, as long as these joints can be somewhat immobilized for several hours. Lidocaine injection is preferred for weight-bearing joints, such as the knee, because its duration is much shorter and thus, the joint is subject to less postinjection trauma by noncompliant patients. Longer-acting anesthetics should not be used on noncompliant patients as they may "feel cured" and proceed to use the anesthetized joint indiscriminately. The ADRs, contraindications, and precautions of local anesthetics are discussed in Chapter 5.10 section VI.E.2.d.

C. Sterile needles range from gauge 16 to 24 (for hip, knee, and shoulder joints), gauge 20 to 22 (for wrist, ankle, elbow, and facet joints), and gauge 25 to 27 (for small and superficial joints). For aspiration of inflamed joint or soft tissues with thick fluids, a large-bore needle may be necessary.

D. Sterile syringes range from 3 to 50 ml. Choice of syringe depends on the joint and amount of effusion to be tapped.

E. Other supplies include aseptic skin preparation materials (sterile gloves, Betadine solution, alcohol solution, sterile gauze pads, and Band-Aids) and tubes for synovial fluid analysis (e.g., chemistry tube for glucose, hematology tube with ethylene-diamine-tetra-acetic acid [EDTA] for cell and differential count, sterile tube for cultures and smears, heparinized tube for crystal analysis, and cytology bottle if neoplasm is suspected). Make sure that the heparinized tubes do not use powdered anticoagulants as they may interfere with crystal identification.

II. General injection techniques

A. Medication preparation. Single-dose vials are preferred as they eliminate the possibility of contamination from previous withdrawal of steroid or anesthetic from the vial. When an anesthetic and steroid are given together, the mixing should be done in the injection syringe. If multiple-dose vials are used, draw the steroid first, followed by the anesthetic so the anesthetic will not be introduced inadvertently into the vial of steroid. The mixture must be used immediately and any unused portion discarded.

B. Skin preparation. Use universal precautions by wearing gloves to prevent contact with bloodborne pathogens. Select the site of injection based on available bony landmarks. Bony landmarks are used because they are more stable than soft tissue landmarks. Using an indelible felt pen, carefully outline the site with a circle (as a target) at least 3 cm in diameter. A less preferable alternative (if a felt pen is unavailable) is to use skin markings made by fingernail pressure. Clean the area with three swipes of povidone-iodine (Betadine) and one swipe of 70% isopropyl alcohol, taking care not to erase the markings. The presence of hair should not alter the method of skin decontamination. Hair shaving should be avoided as it increases wound infection rate (if absolutely necessary, hair may be clipped or depilatory cream may be used). After skin decontamination, the prepared area should not be touched. With this technique, no drapes or sterile room is required.

C. **General injection techniques.** Inject an anesthetic (e.g., 1% lidocaine [Xylocaine]) into the epidermis (creating a small wheal) using a 0.75- to 1.0-inch, 25- to 30-gauge needle with 1 ml syringe. If the patient is particularly apprehensive about the injection procedure, topical anesthetics such as vapocoolant spray (e.g., ethyl chloride or fluorimethane) or EMLA cream (see Chapter 5.10, section VI.E.2.e.2; EMLA cream must be applied at least 1 hour before injection) may be applied on the skin. If the joint is distended with fluid or if the joint is superficial (e.g., acromioclavicular, sternoclavicular, and interphalangeal joints), use a topical anesthetic rather than raising a skin wheal for skin anesthesia. After raising a skin wheal, use another needle (e.g., 1.5-inch, 18-22 gauge) attached to an anesthetic-filled syringe and insert it through the wheal. Stop and aspirate every 0.5 cm and, if no clear or bloody aspirate is drawn up, inject another small bolus of anesthetic.

When the joint capsule is entered (or when the needle is placed at the tender site of soft tissues), the hub of the needle should be clasped securely with a clean (or sterile) hemostat. The anesthetic-filled syringe is then removed, and it is replaced with an aspirating syringe (for arthrocentesis) or a syringe with the injectate (for soft tissue injections). For arthrocentesis, the joint may be "milked" by using steady pressure with the opposite hand on the joint itself and kneading the skin toward the site of aspiration. After all of the available fluid is aspirated, a separate syringe containing the injectate is attached to the needle. The hub of the needle should not be grasped for syringe exchange with the fingers so as to prevent needle shaft contamination.

When depositing the injectable material, use slow, steady pressure on the plunger. If resistance is met during the time of the injection, the needle should be redirected under the skin surface without removing or pulling the needle out of the skin. The syringe is then reaspirated (to make sure that it does not pierce a blood vessel) prior to reinjection. If corticosteroid is injected, a slight amount of lidocaine is used to flush the needle before withdrawal to avoid leaving a needle tract of cortisteroid through the adipose tissue and skin, which may cause depigmentation or subcutaneous necrosis. After the injection, the needle is quickly withdrawn and mild pressure is applied with a sterile gauze pad followed by a Band-Aid to prevent bleeding. Before getting up, the patient is assessed carefully for vasovagal response, and appropriate measures are taken to prevent any secondary harm, e.g., falling as a result of transient hypotension. Patients should also be advised to rest the joint (especially weight-bearing joints) for at least 1 day to prevent joint destruction because of premature resumption of vigorous exercise.

III. **Specific injection techniques**
A. **Joint injection techniques** for arthrocentesis and for therapeutic intraarticular injections are the same. In arthrocentesis the joint is aspirated and the synovial

fluid is sent for analysis as part of the initial evaluation and to rule out superimposed infection versus crystal-induced arthritis in an already diseased joint (especially in patients with monoarthritis). If joint infection is strongly suspected (e.g., purulent synovial fluid), corticosteroid should not be injected until the final culture report is back. However, if the possibility of joint infection is slight, steroid injection may be given after aspirating the joint for culture (injecting an infected joint may delay the diagnosis but not necessarily cause increased joint damage). The aim of therapeutic joint injection is to relieve pain by drainage of an effusion, installation of medication, and drainage of aseptic joints or hemarthroses (after first correcting coagulation disorders).

1. **Upper limb**
   a. **Glenohumeral joint.** The patient is seated with hands in the lap and the shoulder muscles relaxed.
      1) **Anterior approach.** Palpate the glenohumeral joint by placing one's fingers between the coracoid process and the humeral head. Internally rotate the shoulder to feel the inward turning of the humeral head and the joint space, which can be felt as a groove just lateral to the coracoid. Insert a 20- or 22-gauge needle lateral to the coracoid and avoid the thoracoacromial artery (which runs on the medial aspect of the coracoid). Direct the needle dorsally and medially into the joint space, then slightly superiorly to avoid the neurovascular bundle.
      2) **Posterior approach.** Place the patient's ipsilateral hand on the opposite scapula (as if hooking a bra) to maximally internally rotate the shoulder. Place a finger posteriorly along the acromion and insert a 20- or 22-gauge needle about 1 cm inferior to the posterolateral tip of the acromion and direct it anteriorly and medially (aimed toward the coracoid process, which can be anteriorly marked with the index finger). This approach is usually used for adhesive capsulitis and synovitis or chronic osteoarthritis.
   b. **Acromioclavicular (AC) joint.** With the patient sitting or supine and the shoulder propped on a pillow, locate the tip of the distal clavicle and insert a 25-gauge needle either from a superior angle or an anterosuperior angle into the AC joint space (located about 0.5 cm medial to the tip of the acromion). The AC joint may be injected for diagnostic purposes (using local anesthetics) to delineate the source of pain in the shoulder. If the pain is refractory to a trial of local anesthetics (e.g., lidocaine), corticosteroids may be used. A vapocoolant spray or EMLA cream may be used for superficial skin anesthesia.
   c. **Sternoclavicular (SC) joint.** The patient is supine or seated. The SC joint is palpated just lateral to the sternal notch where the clavicle attaches to the sternum. It cannot be readily entered by a needle, hence a 25- or 27-gauge needle is superficially inserted adjacent to it (taking care not to hit the brachiocephalic veins, which are immediately posterior to the SC joint). A vapocoolant spray or EMLA cream may be used for superficial skin anesthesia (the EMLA cream must be applied at least 1 hour before injection).
   d. **Elbow joint.** Do not use the medial approach (because of potential of ulnar nerve injury) or the anterior approach (because of hazard to the biceps tendon, brachioradialis tendon, median nerve, radial nerve, and branches of the radial artery). The position of the elbow is between 50 to 90 degrees of flexion with the palm facing the patient.

1) Posterolateral approach. Palpate the triangular bony landmark consisting of the olecranon process, the head of the radius, and the lateral epicondyle. Insert a 22-gauge needle perpendicular to the elbow joint just anterior to the center of this triangle and posterior to the head of the radius.

2) Posterior approach. Palpate the posterior olecranon and the lateral olecranon groove located just posterior to the lateral epicondyle. Insert a 22-gauge needle above the superior aspect of and lateral to the olecranon.

e. Wrist joint. The hand and wrist are relaxed in a slightly flexed position (e.g., over a rolled towel). The approach used should be based on the area of maximal point tenderness or site of inflammation and specific anatomic structures underlying the region to be infiltrated. After joint injection, medication diffusion can be facilitated by range-of-motion exercises.

1) Radial or dorsal approach. Palpate the joint space at the distal edge of the radius just medial to the extensor pollicis longus tendon and insert a 22-gauge needle perpendicularly into the joint space from the dorsal aspect (midpoint of radius and ulna). The dorsal or radial approach is preferred to avoid any major arteries, veins, and nerves.

2) Dorsal snuffbox approach. Palpate the joint space between the edge of the distal radius and the carpal bones. Then insert a 22-gauge needle into the joint space dorsally and just medial to the anatomic snuffbox.

3) Ulnar approach. Palpate the joint space just distal to the lateral ulnar margin and insert a 22-gauge needle directed in a volar and radial direction.

f. Intercarpal joints. Connect an imaginary line between the ulnar and radial styli to define the proximal row of carpal bones. Insert a 22-gauge needle into the intercarpal joint space at the point of maximal tenderness. Fluoroscopic guidance may be needed for precise location of a specific carpal joint, which has its own synovial cavity.

g. Carpometacarpal (CMC) joint of the thumb. Hold the thumb in slight flexion and insert a 25-gauge needle into the point of maximal tenderness from the dorsal aspect of the radial side of the CMC joint. Avoid the radial artery and the extensor pollicis brevis tendon.

h. Metacarpophalangeal (MCP) joint of the thumb and fingers. Have the patient make a fist so the knuckles protrude. Palpate the MCP joint, which is distal to the apex of the knuckles. Insert a 25-gauge needle into the joint space distally at about a 60-degree angle (not directly laterally or directly superiorly) to avoid the digital nerve, artery, and vein and the extensor tendon apparatus on the superior aspect of each digit.

i. Interphalangeal joints (proximal and distal). Use a vapocoolant spray or EMLA cream for superficial skin anesthesia. Palpate the dorsal borders of the interphalangeal (IP) joint (just distal to the skin crease) and insert a 25- or 27-gauge needle from the dorsal aspect and directed slightly distally into the area just beyond the apex of the IP joint. Inject less than 2 ml of medication into the adjacent subcutaneous tissue where it can eventually be transported into the inflamed capsule and synovium. Postinjection splinting of the affected joint may be needed for resolution of the inflammation.

2. Facet joint injection. The patient is prone (with pillow under the hip). Insert a 22-gauge, 3.5-inch needle into the appropriate facet joint under fluoroscopic or computed tomography (CT) scan guidance. Inject 1 to 2 ml of local anesthetic followed by 20 to 25 mg of triamcinolone diacetate (Aristocort).

3. Lower limb

a. Hip joint. Fluoroscopic guidance is necessary to confirm needle placement because the hip joint is deep and difficult to infiltrate or aspirate. To verify needle placement in the hip joint bursa, a small injection of radiopaque dye may be necessary. A 18 to 20 gauge, 3 to 4 inch long needle is used, and depending on joint integrity, 2 to 4 ml of medication may be injected. A major potential complication of hip injection of corticosteroid is avascular necrosis.

1) **Anterior approach.** The anterior approach is preferred. Position the patient in a supine position with the lower limb externally rotated. Palpate the area 2 cm distal to the anterior superior iliac spine and 3 cm lateral to the palpated femoral artery at a level corresponding to the superior margins of the greater trochanter. Insert the needle at an angle 60 degrees posteromedially through the tough capsular ligaments into the bone, then slightly withdraw it.

2) **Lateral approach.** The patient lies on the uninvolved side with the leg externally rotated. Insert the needle just anterior to the greater trochanter of the femur and walk it medially along the neck of the femur until the joint is reached.

b. Sacroiliac (SI) joint. The SI joint may be injected at the point of maximal tenderness or preferably under fluoroscopic guidance.

c. Knee. The patient is supine with the knee comfortably extended to relax the quadriceps muscle (a small pillow may be used under the knee). Grasp the patella and rock it gently side to side to determine adequate relaxation. A 19-gauge needle (or a larger bore needle if the effusion is thick) is inserted at the point of maximal effusion or through one of the following approaches:

1) **Medial approach.** The medial approach is generally easier for aspiration. Slightly displace the patella laterally to increase the medial gap between the patella and femur. The traditional route of entry is through the medial side of the patella in a direction parallel to the plane of the posterior surface of the patella midway between the superior and inferior margins of the patella. However, this traditional point of entry leaves very little room between the femur and patella, hence the needle commonly hits the joint surfaces, causing the patient to contract the quadriceps muscle in pain further narrowing the joint space. An alternative route is to insert the needle medial to the patella just superior to the superior margin of the patella on the medial aspect of the knee (this site should be low enough to allow direction of the needle below the quadriceps tendon). The medication is then easily introduced into the suprapatellar pouch, which is contiguous with the synovial cavity and which lies below the quadriceps tendon (thus there is no undue pain or contraction of the quadriceps muscle).

2) **Lateral approach.** It uses similar traditional and alternative routes of entry as that of the medial approach except that the patella is displaced medially to increase the lateral gap between the patella and femur, and the needle is inserted lateral to the patella.

3) **Anterior approach** is used only if the patient cannot extend the knee, if the patient is obese, or if there are osteophytes around the patella.

The knee is flexed to 90 degrees and the needle is inserted just inferior to the inferior patellar pole either from the lateral or medial side of the patellar tendon. The needle is then advanced parallel to the tibial plateau until the joint space is entered. The risk of puncturing the articular cartilage is much higher, as is the risk to the infrapatellar fat pad for necrosis. Moreover, it is hard to obtain synovial fluid from this position because the fluid migrates posteriorly during knee flexion.

   d. Ankle mortise. The foot is positioned at about a 45-degree angle of plantar flexion.

   1) Anteromedial approach. Insert a 22-gauge needle about 1 inch proximal and lateral to the distal end of the medial malleolus with the flexor hallucis longus tendon just lateral to this point. Direct the needle 45 degrees posteriorly, slightly upward, and laterally.

   2) Anterolateral approach. Insert a 22-gauge needle about 0.5 inch proximal and medial to the distal end of the lateral malleolus. Direct the needle 45 degrees posteriorly, slightly upward, and medially.

   e. Subtalar joint. The patient is prone with feet extending over the end of the examination table so that the ankle is in the neutral position. Insert a 22-gauge needle halfway between a line drawn from the most prominent aspect of the lateral malleolus posteriorly to the Achilles tendon and parallel to the plantar aspect of the neutrally positioned foot. Direct the needle toward a point inferior and medial to the medial malleolus.

   f. Intertarsal joint. A 22-gauge needle is used and as with intercarpal bones, fluoroscopic needle guidance is needed.

   g. Metatarsophalangeal (MTP) joints. Insert a 22-gauge needle from the dorsal aspect with the toes plantar flexed and the needle directed distal to the largest palpable part of the joint. The needle should not be inserted laterally or superiorly, but between these two planes to avoid essential structures.

   h. Interphalangeal joints. The technique is similar to those used for IP joint injection of the hands (see section III.A.1.i).

B. Bursal injection techniques. Bursae are synovial-like tissues that form fluid-filled sacs and are usually located adjacent to joints. Their function is to reduce irritation at friction-prone areas between muscles, tendon, skin, and bone. They can get inflamed during repetitive activities as a result of poor body mechanics or from direct trauma. As with joint injections, bursal injections serve both diagnostic and therapeutic roles. A local anesthetic may initially be injected alone for diagnostic purposes (i.e., to determine the source of pain). If the bursa is aspirated, the fluid should be screened for increased leukocytes, gram-negative or positive bacteria, or crystals. When a septic bursa has been ruled out, corticosteroid and anesthetic agents may be injected therapeutically into the inflamed bursa. The lowest effective dose is used and the volume injected is adjusted to the size of the bursa (see Table 4.9-2). Corticosteroid is usually given about 14 to 21 days after bursal injury and should be avoided during the first 7 days as this may theoretically inhibit the healing process. After bursal injection, additional treatment should include ice, nonsteroidal antiinflammatory drugs (NSAIDs), soft tissue mobilization, stretching and strengthening exercises, as well as proper body mechanics. In severe or recurrent bursitis, surgical incision and drainage may be needed.

   1. Upper limb

   a. Subacromial (subdeltoid) bursitis usually coexists with or is secondary to

Table 4.9-2.   Guidelines for bursal injections

BURSAE*	ANESTHETIC VOLUME† (ml)	CORTICOSTEROID VOLUME† (ml)	NEEDLE‡ LENGTH (inch)
Subacromial	4.0-6.0	0.5-1.0	1.5
Trochanteric	4.5-9.0	0.5-1.0	1.5-3.5
Iliopectineal	4.0-4.5	0.5-1.0	3.5
Ischial	2.5-4.0	0.5-1.0	3.5
Anserine	2.5-4.5	0.25-0.5	1.5
Prepatellar	Variable§	0.5-1.0	1.5

* Fluoroscopic guidance may be necessary to increase accuracy of bursa injection. A bursogram may be a useful tool, increasing the diagnostic and therapeutic value of injections.
† The volume refers to the capacity of the bursa, and the clinician should select a corticosteroid or anesthetic concentration appropriate for the bursal volume.
‡ A gauge 20-22 needle is usually used, but the clinician may prefer an 18-gauge needle initially for aspiration if gelatinous fluid is anticipated and then change to a finer gauge for instillation of pharmacologic agents.
§ The prepatellar bursa is often multiloculated, and its capacity may vary.
From Olsen NK, Press JM, Young JL: Bursal injections. In Lennard TA, editor: *Physiatric procedures in clinical practice*, Philadelphia, 1995, Hanley & Belfus, p 42, with permission.

rotator cuff tendinitis or shoulder impingement syndrome. The subacromial bursa rests on the supraspinatus tendon and is covered by the acromion, the coracoacromial ligament, and the deltoid muscle. Although an anterior, posterior, or lateral approach may be used, the posterolateral approach is usually easier to perform. Palpate the tip of the acromion and insert a 25-gauge, 1.5-inch needle approximately 1.5 cm beneath it and superior to the humeral head. Initially inject a total volume of 4 to 6 ml of local anesthetic (e.g., a mixture of 1% lidocaine with 0.5% bupivacaine). If there is a 50% reduction of pain with improved strength (supporting the diagnosis of shoulder impingement, supraspinatus tendinitis, or subdeltoid bursitis), this can be followed by injecting corticosteroid (e.g., 1 ml of betamethasone). If the initial blind injection is unsuccessful or if the diagnosis is unclear, subacromial bursography may be done. If the bursogram is normal, the diagnosis of subacromial impingement is doubtful.

   b. Olecranon bursitis (draftsman's elbow) is commonly seen in rheumatologic disorders (e.g., gout). Insert an 18-gauge needle (because the fluid is usually gelatinous) perpendicular to the central swelling of the enlarged bursa overlying the olecranon process of the ulna. A low-dose corticosteroid injection may be given after aspiration.

2. Lower limb

   a. Greater trochanteric bursitis is common in the elderly and usually manifests as lateral thigh pain (which may radiate down to the leg or up to the buttock) during ambulation. The pain may be elicited by applying deep pressures to the posterior and superior aspect of the greater trochanter in an externally rotated and abducted lower limb. For injection therapy, the patient is placed on sidelying position (the site to be injected is on top) with the hips and knees flexed to about 45 degrees. A 3.5-inch, 22-gauge needle is inserted perpendicularly into the skin at the point of maximal tenderness overlying the greater trochanter. Once the needle has touched bone, it is slightly withdrawn and a mixture of corticosteroid and anesthetic is injected. If pain persists despite injection therapy and comprehensive rehabilitation (including stretching of the long constrictors of the hip, such as tensor fascia lata, hamstring, and rectus femoris muscles), the clinician should consider other sources of pain (e.g., from the lumbar spine, hip joint, and distal joints).

b. **Ischial bursitis (tailor's or weaver's bottom)** is associated with prolonged sitting on a hard surface or may be seen in adolescent runners in conjunction with ischial apophysitis (pain is aggravated during uphill running or with contraction of hamstring muscles). The ischial bursa is located between the inferior part of the ischial tuberosity and the gluteus maximus. If the patient does not respond to rest, ice, NSAIDs, change in sitting duration and surface, or modification in running styles and intensity, then injection therapy may be warranted. The patient is placed in the sidelying position with the knee fully flexed to relax the hamstrings. Palpate the point of maximal tenderness overlying the ischial tuberosity and horizontally insert a 3-inch, 22-gauge needle directed toward it. Fluoroscopic guidance may be needed to do a bursogram and to verify needle placement.

c. **Iliopsoas (or iliopectineal) bursitis,** which is relatively uncommon, manifests as pain referred to the anterior thigh (following the distribution of the femoral nerve). The patient usually externally rotates and flexes the hip to relieve pressure on the inflamed bursa and avoids extension of the lower limb during ambulation. A 20- to 22-gauge, 3.5-inch needle is inserted to the point of maximum tenderness (elicited by passive extension of the patient's hip) usually under fluoroscopic guidance for diagnostic and therapeutic purposes.

d. **Prepatellar bursitis (housemaid's knee)** is often the result of frequent kneeling. Despite the presence of effusion, the patient rarely complains of pain unless direct pressure is applied to the bursa. A 20- to 22-gauge, 1.5-inch needle is inserted to the area of maximal fullness at the middle to superior pole of the patella (either medially or laterally). Repeat injections may be required because the prepatellar bursa is often multiloculated. The patient should be advised to avoid kneeling and to use knee pads when pressure must be applied to the patella.

e. **Tibial collateral ligament (TCL) bursitis** should be considered in any patient with medial joint line tenderness (usually with no evidence of new ligamentous or capsular instability). The TCL is located between the deep and superficial aspects of the tibial collateral ligament. It does not adhere to the medial meniscus, and it appears to reduce friction between the superficial layer of the TCL and the medial meniscus. A 20- to 22-gauge, 1.5-inch needle is inserted perpendicularly to the medial joint line at the point of maximal tenderness where medication (e.g., 2-ml mixture of lidocaine and triamcinolone) is injected.

f. **Anserine bursitis.** The anserine bursa is located approximately 5 cm distal to the tibial joint line on the medial aspect of the tibia and somewhat posterior. It separates the three conjoined tendons of the pes anserinus (i.e., semitendinosus, sartorius, and gracilis muscles) from the medial collateral ligament and the tibia. Anserine bursitis is commonly seen in women with heavy thighs and osteoarthritis of the knees or in athletes (especially soccer players) due to direct knee trauma. Patients usually complain of pain below the anteromedial surface of the knee during stair ascension. This pain can be reproduced by moving the patient's knee in flexion and extension while the leg is internally rotated. In addition to a comprehensive rehabilitation program (including ice, NSAIDs, and exercise), injection therapy may be given. The knee is fully extended, and a 1- to 1.5-inch, 22-gauge needle is inserted perpendicular to the skin over the point of maximal tenderness on the medial tibial flare where the pes anserinus tendon and bursa lie. The tip of the needle is slightly withdrawn once its tip touches bone surface and a 1- to 3-ml combination of anesthetic and corticosteroid is injected. Athletes at risk for repetitive trauma may also benefit from padded protection about the knee.

g. Retrocalcaneal (subtendinous) bursitis. The retrocalcaneal bursa is located between the posterior surface of the calcaneus and the tendon of the triceps surae. It may be inflamed during overstraining (e.g., early assumption of increased mileage in a runner or an ill-fitting shoe resulting in pressure from a restricting heel counter). Pain can be elicited by placing the thumb and index finger on the anterior edges of the Achilles tendon and applying pressure. The first step in treatment is footwear modification combined with ice and NSAIDs. This is followed by daily stretching of the triceps surae. If these measures fail, then a 20- to 22-gauge, 1- to 1.5-inch needle may be inserted with an anterior angle of 15 to 20 degrees to the point of greatest bursal distention, which is often on the lateral aspect of the heel. Care must be taken to avoid instilling corticosteroid into the Achilles tendon because of risk of tendon rupture.

h. Achilles (or subcutaneous) bursitis is common in women who wear high-heeled shoes that apply direct pressure on the bursa that lies subcutaneous to the posterior surface of the Achilles tendon. A midline swelling is usually noted where the upper edge of the heel counter comes in contact with the heel cord. Treatments include changing the patient's shoes and the use of ice and NSAIDs. If these fail, the point of maximal tenderness or distention may be injected with a corticosteroid and anesthetic mixture via a 20- to 22-gauge, 1- to 1.5-inch needle. Care must be taken to avoid instilling corticosteroid into the Achilles tendon because of the risk of tendon rupture.

i. Calcaneal bursitis is common in elderly patients with a calcified heel spur that irritates the bursa during prolonged walking or running. Treatment includes the use of an appropriate walking or running shoe (with good heel cushion) and the use of a heel cup. Athletes are encouraged to change their running shoes every 200 to 300 miles (this amount of mileage usually causes mid-sole breakdown). If these measures fail, a 20- to 22-gauge, 1- to 1.5-inch needle may be inserted to the point of maximal tenderness for diagnostic and therapeutic purposes.

C. Tendon and tendon sheath injections. A tendinitis or tenosynovitis may be caused by either an acute injury or chronic overuse. Injection therapy may be used to facilitate or as part of the overall rehabilitation program (which includes work or environmental modification, proper body mechanics, use of splints, stretching and flexibility exercises, NSAIDs, etc.). Corticosteroid injection for tendinitis or tenosynovitis should be limited to a maximum of three in a given area. It may be injected into the tendon sheath but not directly into the substance of the tendon to avoid tendon rupture. When injecting into the tendon sheath, there is generally no significant resistance felt over the plunger of the syringe. To alleviate the pain of injection, a vapocoolant spray (e.g., ethyl chloride or fluorimethane) or EMLA cream may be used for superficial skin anesthesia.

1. **Upper limb**
   a. **Supraspinatus tendinitis (impingement syndrome, rotator cuff tendinitis).** Palpate the supraspinatus tendon, which is usually located approximately 2.5 cm medial to the most lateral aspect of the spine of the scapula. Insert a 22-gauge needle to the point of maximal tenderness and inject the mixture of corticosteroid and anesthetic in the proximity of the tendon. After the injection, advise the patient to avoid heavy lifting and excessive overhead work for at least 2 days.
   b. **Biceps tendinitis.** The corticosteroid and anesthetic mixture is injected into the immediate proximity of the tendon (not into the tendon substance) through the anterior approach using a 22-gauge needle. After the injection, the patient is advised not to do heavy lifting or vigorous exercises for 48 to 72 hours. In general, steroid injection into the bicipital groove is discouraged because of the possibility of promoting eventual tendon rupture.
      1) **Long head of the biceps tendons.** Insert the needle at the point of maximum tenderness located at the bicipital groove located in the head the humerus.
      2) **Short head of the biceps tendon.** Insert the needle at the point of maximum tenderness, which is usually right on top of the coracoid process.
   c. **Lateral epicondylitis (tennis elbow)** is usually associated with pain when making a fist, doing backhand shots in tennis, lifting objects, using a screwdriver, and when the patient extends the wrist against resistance. Injection therapy may be tried only after conservative treatments (e.g., NSAIDs, tennis-elbow band, exercises, proper body mechanics, and environmental or work modifications) have failed. The elbow is flexed to about 90 degrees and a 22-gauge needle is inserted just below and medial to the lateral epicondyle into the common extensor tendon origin. Deposit about 0.5 ml mixture of local anesthetic into the point of maximal tenderness, and if the symptoms improve, follow this with a corticosteroid preparation (e.g., 10-20 mg of triamcinolone). After injection, the elbow is fully extended and pronated and the wrist is simultaneously flexed to stretch the common extensor tendon. A wrist splint may be beneficial to help immobilize the wrist extensor tendons for a few days.
   d. **De Quervain's syndrome** refers to the stenosing tenosynovitis of the first dorsal wrist compartment, which typically transmits the tendons of both the abductor pollicis longus (APL) and extensor pollicis brevis (EPB). Place the forearm in a neutral position with the wrist in 15 to 20 degrees of ulnar deviation. Insert a 25-gauge needle to the point of maximal tenderness at the level of the distal end of the radius tangential to the skin along the length of the APL and EPB. Inject a small amount of local anesthetic, and note for a small fusiform swelling along the length of the tendons to indicate that the needle is in the tenosynovium. Carefully disconnect the syringe and replace it with a tuberculin syringe containing corticosteroids (e.g., DepoMedrol) and inject about an eighth of 1 ml of the steroid. Other clinicians believe that any attempt to enter a tendon sheath causes more damage than benefit and thus recommend

that the corticosteroid be injected intradermally above the site of tenderness and letting it diffuse into the inflamed tendon sheath.

   e. **Trigger thumb or trigger digit** is a stenosing flexor tenosynovitis for which corticosteroid (mixed with anesthetic) injection is a primary treatment. Insert a 25-gauge needle tangentially and just proximal to the fusiform swelling at about the level of the metacarpal head and inject a small amount of local anesthetic and steroid mixture into the tendon sheath (there should be no resistance felt over the syringe plunger). A more conservative method is to inject intradermally above the site of tenderness and to let the medication diffuse into the inflamed tendon sheath.

2. **Lower limb.** Although quadriceps (infrapatellar) tendinitis and Achilles tendinitis may be treated by injecting corticosteroid and anesthetic, many clinicians avoid injection therapy in these weight-bearing structures because of fear of tendon rupture.

   a. **Hip abductor tendinitis.** The technique for patient positioning and injection is similar to that described for trochanteric bursitis (see section III.B.2.a). A 20- or 22-gauge needle is inserted at the point of maximal tenderness and the mixture of corticosteroid and anesthetic is injected into the proximity of the hip abductor tendon.

   b. **Iliotibial band tendinitis.** The patient lies on the side. Using a 20- or 22-gauge needle, inject a mixture of corticosteroid and anesthetic around the insertion of the iliotibial band at the proximal, lateral tibia, or, depending on the site of symptoms, where it passes over the prominence of the lateral femoral condyle.

   c. **Plantar fasciitis.** Palpate for the exact site of inflammation or point of maximal tenderness (usually at the attachment of the plantar fascia to the calcaneus) and approach it perpendicularly from the plantar aspect of the foot (usually slightly off center, closer to the medial border of the foot). Insert a 22-gauge needle until it touches the underlying bone, then withdraw it slightly by 1 to 2 mm and deposit the mixture of local anesthetic and steroid (e.g., 0.5 ml of DepoMedrol and 1 ml of lidocaine). Steroid injection should be considered only after other measures (e.g., stretching exercises, NSAIDs, and shoe modification) have failed because it can theoretically cause atrophy of the specialized fat pads of the heel leading to a significant disability (especially in athletes).

D. **Other soft tissue injections:**

1. **Carpal tunnel syndrome (CTS)** is an entrapment syndrome of the median nerve at the wrist which manifests as pain and paresthesia at the median nerve distribution. The pain usually occurs at nighttime or after frequent use of hands or fingers. Carpal tunnel syndrome is often caused by overuse of the hand (e.g., forceful gripping or repetitive hand/wrist motions). Corticosteroid injection is considered only after conservative measures (e.g., wearing of wrist splints [in neutral position] during sleeping hours for 4 to 8 weeks, work and activity modification, and NSAIDs) have failed. One method of carpal tunnel injection is to inject 0.5 ml (20 mg) of triamcinolone hexacetonide (Aristopan) without anesthetics (to avoid accidental injection into the median nerve after the area becomes anesthetized). A 25-gauge needle is pointed distally towards the carpal tunnel and inserted at a 35° angle on the ulnar side of the palmaris longus tendon, a few millimeters beyond the distal wrist crease. Another approach is to draw a line connecting the pisiform and trapezoid bones to approximate the position of the transverse carpal ligament. The needle is then inserted through the trans-

verse carpal ligament approximately 6 mm below the surface of the skin. If the patient complains of paresthesias, the needle should be redirected laterally and more superficially.

2. **Morton's neuroma,** which is neither a neuroma nor a neoplasm, is a degenerative process of the nerve characterized by tenderness with distal paresthesia (because of hypertrophic fibrosis of the digital nerve) usually located between the distal metatarsal bones of the second and third or third and fourth digits of the foot. The corticosteroid preparation is injected through the foot dorsum into the point of maximal tenderness via a 22-gauge needle. Morton's neuroma has a tendency to recur.

BIBLIOGRAPHY

Cyriax J, Russell G: *Textbook of orthopedic medicine, vol. 2. Treatment by manipulation, massage, and injection,* ed 9, Baltimore, 1977, Williams & Wilkins.

Gray RG, Gottlieb NL: Intra-articular corticosteroids: an updated assessment. *Clin Orthop* 177:235-236, 1983.

Hasselbacker P: Synovial fluid analysis. In Utsinger PD, Zvaifler JK, Erlich, editors.: *Rheumatoid arthritis.* Philadelphia, 1985, JB Lippincott.

Hollander JL: Intrasynovial corticosteroid therapy in arthritis. *Maryland State Med J* 19:62-66, 1970.

Lennard TA, editor: *Physiatric procedures in clinical practice,* Philadelphia, 1995, Hanley & Belfus.

Nicholas JJ: Joint and soft tissue injection techniques. In Braddom RL, editor: *Physical medicine and rehabilitation,* Philadelphia, 1996, WB Saunders, pp. 503-513.

Pfenninger JL: Injections of joints and soft tissue: Part I: General guidelines. *Am Fam Physician* 44:1196-1202, 1991.

Pfenninger JL: Injections of joints and soft tissue: Part II: Guidelines for specific joints. *Am Fam Physician* 44:1690-1701, 1991.

Sandrock NJG, Warfield CA: Epidural steroids and facet injections. In Warfield CA, editor: *Principles and practice of pain management.* New York, 1993, McGraw-Hill, pp. 401-412.

Stern R: Arthrocentesis and intraarticular injection. In Paget S, Pellicci P, Beary JF III, editors: *Manual of rheumatology and outpatient orthopedic disorders,* ed 3, Boston, 1993, Little, Brown, pp. 33-38.

Zuckerman JD, Meislin RJ, Rothberg M: Injections for joint and soft tissue disorders: when and how to use them. *Geriatrics* 45:45-55, 1990.

CHAPTER 4.10

NERVE BLOCKS

Nerve blocks should only be used as an adjunct in the comprehensive treatment of the patient. It refers to the administration of a local anesthetic agent or neurolytic agent to interrupt the nerve's somatic function (motor, sensory, or both) and/or sympathetic functions. Motor nerve blocks are used to relax specific muscles such as for the treatment of spasticity (see Chapter 5.4, section III.D.2) or trigger points (see Chapter 4.11). Sensory nerve blocks are commonly used for providing anesthesia to facilitate surgical procedures and for pain management. Sympathetic blocks are generally used to dilate blood vessels (e.g., in patients with ischemic rest pain) and for the treatment of sympathetically maintained pain (SMP). This chapter presents an overview of nerve blocks primarily used in pain management for diagnostic, preemptive, prognostic, and therapeutic purposes. Although commonly done by anesthesiologists, nerve blocks are becoming popular among physiatrists who specialize in pain management and who have received additional training in performing these procedures. Clinicians performing nerve blocks should have resuscitation equipment at hand and should be able to perform cardiac/respiratory resuscitation according to the Advanced Cardiac Life Support (ACLS) protocols. For specific injection techniques, the reader is referred to standard anesthesiology textbooks or other standard textbooks on pain management.

I. **Diagnostic nerve blocks** are used to ascertain specific nociceptive pathways, to help determine the possible mechanism of chronic pain syndromes, to aid in the differential diagnosis of the site and cause of pain, and to determine the patient's reaction to pain relief. They use small volumes (2 to 4 ml) of local anesthetics (e.g., lidocaine, bupivacaine, procaine, and tetracaine), which are injected through disposable 21 to 23 gauge, 3.5-inch needles or, for deeper structures (e.g., lumbar sympathetic and celiac plexus blocks), via 5- or 6-inch needles. The different local anesthetic agents used should have different durations which should be correlated with the duration of subjective pain relief (placebo blocks may be included). Neurolytic agents (e.g., chemical agents such as phenol and absolute alcohol) are rarely used for diagnostic nerve blocks due to their destructive effects. Accurate needle placement is recommended by using fluoroscopy or computed tomography (CT) scan with or without prior injection of contrast medium. To avoid contamination of results, patients should be given little or no analgesic medication during diagnostic blocks. Although placebo responses to nerve blocks may suggest pain of psychogenic origin, nerve blocks should never be used to make definitive diagnoses of psychogenic pain. Placebo response (i.e., false-positive result) has been shown to occur in about 30 to 60% of "normal" individuals. Diagnostic nerve blocks should produce consistent results for two or three nerve block sessions before any decisions are made about its effectiveness.

A. **Diagnostic sympathetic and somatic nerve blocks** are used to differentiate between sympathetic and somatic pain for the diagnosis of reflex sympathetic dystrophy (RSD)/causalgia with SMP features and the localization of somatic nerve pain.
  1. **Diagnostic anatomic nerve blocks** utilize the presumed anatomic differences in the sympathetic and somatic nerve pathways to determine the source of pain. One method is to start proximally (i.e., with sympathetic blockade)

and proceed distally (i.e., with somatic blockade). A placebo block is first done by injecting 5 to 10 ml of normal saline into the sympathetic pathway. If pain is relieved, a placebo effect is assumed. If not, then 10 to 15 ml of local anesthetic (e.g., lidocaine and/or bupivacaine) is injected. If pain is relieved, the sympathetic pathway is probably the source of pain, but if pain is persistent, then a somatic block to the painful area is done. Another method of doing anatomic nerve blockade is to start distally with a somatic block then proceed proximally towards a sympathetic blockade.

a. **For head, neck, and upper limb pain,** use the stellate (cervicothoracic) ganglion for sympathetic blockade. For somatic blockade, the nerves used are the trigeminal nerve for the head, the cervical roots for the neck, and the brachial plexus for the upper limb.

b. **For upper chest and thoracic pain,** use the stellate ganglion for sympathetic blockade and the intercostal nerves for somatic blockade.

c. **For upper abdominal pain,** use the intercostal nerves for somatic blockade followed by sympathetic blockade using the celiac plexus.

d. **For lower back and lower limb pain,** use lumbar sympathetic nerves for sympathetic blockade. For somatic blockade, the lumbar paravertebral nerves are used for the lower back pain, and the lumbar paravertebral nerves or the transsacral S1 nerves are used for the lower limb.

2. **Diagnostic pharmacologic (or neurophysiologic) nerve blocks** utilize the differential sensitivity of sympathetic and somatic nerve fibers of different sizes to the blocking effect of local anesthetics. Injection of 0.25% procaine or 0.5% lidocaine selectively blocks the type B, myelinated preganglionic autonomic fibers, while 0.5% procaine or 1% lidocaine blocks the type C, unmyelinated postganglionic fibers and the type A-δ myelinated fibers responsible for touch, pressure, pain, and temperature. A higher dose of procaine (1%) or lidocaine (2%) blocks the type A (α, β, and γ) myelinated fibers responsible for motor function. The following differential blocks are used to distinguish the character of a pain state and to help differentiate somatic sensory from sympathetic, central, or probable pain of psychogenic origin.

a. **Differential spinal blocks** consist of sequential injections of 5 to 10 ml of normal saline followed by 0.25%, 0.5%, and 1% of procaine (or 0.5%, 1%, and 2% of lidocaine) to determine the source of pain. The same volume of local anesthetic (5-10 ml) is used for each injection. The injection may be given via the subarachnoid space **(subarachnoid block)** or the epidural space **(epidural block).** Subarachnoid blocks are generally done in the midthoracic level or caudally because of the cervical origin of the phrenic nerve. Epidural blocks have more limited areas of effect than subarachnoid blocks and these can be done virtually at any point in the spinal cord. However, epidural blocks are seldom used for diagnostic purposes because bilateral effects usually occur and it is more difficult to control its area of action. Relief by normal saline suggests a placebo effect or probably pain of psychogenic origin. If there is no relief, then 0.25%, 0.5%, and 1% procaine (or 0.5%, 1%, and 2% lidocaine) solutions are sequentially injected until patient reports pain relief. Pain relief from 0.25% procaine (or 0.5% lidocaine) suggests sympathetic pain (e.g., RSD/causalgia with SMP features) whereas pain relief from 0.5% procaine (or 1% lidocaine) suggests somatosensory pain. The 1% procaine (or 2% lidocaine) is used to provide motor block. If there is no pain relief after all four injections are completed, an intravenous test for centrally mediated pain (see section I.C) may be done.

   b. Modified differential spinal blocks take advantage of the fact that a complete block wears off in the following sequence: motor, sensory, then sympathetic. A local anesthetic agent (2 ml of 5% procaine, 10-20 ml of 2% lidocaine, or 3% chloroprocaine) is injected into the subarachnoid space to induce a complete motor block. If there is no pain relief, then an intravenous test for centrally mediated pain may be done. If there is pain relief, the origin of pain is identified by assessing which sensation returns during the time when pain returns (as the anesthetic effect wears off). For example, if the pain recurs at the time when pinprick and temperature sensations return, the source of pain is most likely somatosensory (type A-δ or type C fibers). However, if the pain recurs long after the return of pinprick and temperature sensations, then the pain is most likely sympathetic. The modified method is more practical than the original spinal blockade method because it is less time consuming and the patient does not need to stay immobile for long.

B. Diagnostic peripheral nerve blocks

   1. Diagnostic selective nerve root blocks involve the injection of 0.5 to 1 ml of local anesthetic into the lateral margin of a neuroforamen. They are used to determine classic monoradicular pain whose neuroradiologic studies either fail to provide a structural explanation or show an abnormality related only to an adjacent nerve root. In the first case, blocking of the suspected nerve root should abolish pain, while in the second case, blocking of the adjacent nerve root (with neuroradiologic abnormality) should not abolish the pain. They can also be used to distinguish pain whose clinical picture is suggestive of both nerve root and distal nerve origin. If the pain has a distal origin, blockade of a single root should not completely abolish pain because of dermatomal overlap.

   2. Diagnostic motor nerve blocks involve the selective injection of a local anesthetic agent (e.g., lidocaine or bupivacaine) or, in some occasion, a neurolytic agent (e.g., phenol) around a peripheral nerve (identified by electrodiagnostic techniques) to effectively paralyze those muscle innervated by the nerve. They are used to simulate or approximate the clinical outcome of a proposed tenotomy or neurectomy in patients with spasticity so that potential muscle imbalance or voluntary motor control can be assessed. When the blockade is done at the point proximal to or near the terminal innervation within the muscle, it is called a **motor point block** or **intramuscular neurolysis.** The nerves commonly assessed are the median, ulnar, and musculocutaneous nerves for the upper limbs and the obturator, femoral, posterior tibial, common peroneal, and popliteal nerves for the lower limbs.

C. Intravenous (IV) tests for centrally mediated pain are performed if the sequential, differential spinal blockade (original or modified method) fails to provide pain relief. These tests remain controversial.

   1. Intravenous thiopental test (barbiturate test) is based on the assumption that a patient's response to typical pain should be the same during barbiturate sleep as when awake. It is done by slow IV infusion of thiopental until the patient falls into a light sleep. The infusion is then stopped and as the patient awakens slowly, a stimulus other than that which elicits the typical pain (e.g., pressure over the sternum or anterior tibia) is given periodically. If the patient feels the pain, then a stimulus that is known to elicit the typical pain is given. If the patient does not respond to the typical stimulus, then the pain is probably psychogenic.

2. **Intravenous lidocaine test** uses 1.2 to 2 mg/kg of IV lidocaine, injected until patient complains of mild toxicity (tingling or dizziness). Relief of pain (2 minutes after toxicity occurs) suggests pain of central origin. If there is no relief, the pain is probably psychogenic.

3. **Intravenous phentolamine test** is used in the diagnosis and prognosis of RSD/causalgia. Reflex sympathetic dystrophy/causalgia patients with transient relief from IV phentolamine will likely respond to regional IV guanethidine sympathetic blocks.

D. **Diagnostic facet injections** introduce a local anesthetic (e.g., lidocaine or bupivacaine) and a steroid (e.g., methylprednisolone) into the intraarticular facets (most commonly the lumbar facets at two or three levels) under fluoroscopic or CT guidance. If the facet is the source of back pain, there is immediate relief of pain, which may last for about 24 hours.

II. **Prognostic nerve blocks** are used to predict the effects of neurolytic blocks or neurosurgery and allow the patient to experience the sensory changes (e.g., numbness) and other side effects that follow destructive procedures (neuroablative surgical procedures or neurolytic blocks) and help the patient decide whether or not to have it done. As with diagnostic blocks, little or no analgesic medications should be given to the patient during prognostic blocks; and precise needle placement is determined by fluoroscopy or CT scan with or without prior injection of contrast medium. Prognostic blocks can be used to determine any changes in behavior and affect in the absence of pain and analgesic medication; the amount of physical activity tolerated and the degree of physical limitation unrelated to pain; evidence of narcotic dependence and its severity; and the development of new pain in other locations previously unnoticed but now unmasked. Clinical evidence suggests that despite its limitations in predicting long-term effects, prognostic blocks are still useful especially when performed for 2 to 3 days (i.e., using continuous techniques such as indwelling catheters) rather than by just performing a single block.

III. **Preemptive (or prophylactic) nerve blocks** refer to blockade of the proposed site of the operation to prevent or reduce the incidence and intensity of pain and the delay of normal functional activity that follows postoperatively. Clinical evidence has shown regional nerve blocks for several days prior to limb amputation can decrease the incidence of phantom limb pain, RSD/causalgia, and other chronic pain syndromes; thus, resulting in earlier functional rehabilitation, prevention or reduction of complications, and shorter hospitalization.

IV. **Therapeutic nerve blocks (or specific regional blocks)** are done only after the nature and location of the pain is established by diagnostic blocks. They involve the administration of local anesthetic agents or neurolytic agents into the somatic nerves, sympathetic ganglia, or localized pain-sensitive trigger points (see Chapter 4.11 for trigger point injections). In general, they are used in combination with other therapeutic modalities to control severe acute postoperative pain (e.g., postoperative thoracotomy pain) or posttraumatic pain (e.g., fracture of the ribs) or postinfectious pain (e.g., herpes zoster neuralgia); provide pain relief and allow normalization of posture to occur through muscle relaxation by breaking the vicious cycle involved in chronic pain syndromes; and allowing the patient to perform other therapeutic measures (e.g., weight-bearing exercises) during the period of symptomatic pain relief.

Therapeutic blocks using local anesthetics (see Chapter 5.10, section VI.E.2.d) are indicated for providing anesthesia for procedures, treatment of inflammatory compression neuropathies in combination with corticosteroids (see Chapter 4.8 section III), and in the following pain situations: presence of a sympathetic component in a pain state with a positive response to diagnostic sympathetic block (a series of sympathetic blocks are usually needed); presence of somatic pain which is unilateral, well-localized, and confined to a small number of dermatomes; and in patients in whom such blocks are associated with minimal risk and morbidity. Although the mechanism of pain relief from a series of therapeutic nerve blocks using local anesthetic is unknown, a variety of factors may contribute, such as transient increases in tissue blood flow; interruption of abnormal neuronal impulse transmission; isolation or disruption of nociceptive foci, particularly in scar tissue or fascial layers; and an occasionally prolonged placebo response or spontaneous resolution of pain.

Therapeutic blocks using neurolytic agents (i.e., chemical agents such as absolute alcohol and phenol; cold agents such as cryoprobe; and heat agents such as radiofrequency coagulation) are usually confined to patients with cancer pain because of their limited duration of action (the effects of neurolytic nerve blocks range from 8 days to a year and are rarely, if ever, permanent) and potential side effects (e.g., loss of motor, bowel and/or bladder control, small vessel thrombosis and ischemic tissue damage, and chemical neuritis, which may develop into a deafferentation pain syndrome). They are used in relieving spasticity (see Chapter 5.4, section III.D.2.a.2) and in relieving pain in selected patients with noncancer chronic pain due to peripheral vascular disease (particularly elderly patients with lower limb claudication), trigeminal neuralgia, RSD/causalgia, chronic pancreatitis, severe angina pectoris, or other chronic disorders in patients who cannot tolerate a neurosurgical operation. During recent years, the use of the more accurate and selective radiofrequency coagulation (which uses heat) is slowly replacing chemical neurolysis for pain management. As with chemical neurolysis, neuritis may occur with radiofrequency coagulation.

Compared with systemic analgesics, nerve blocks can improve local blood flow and prevent the central effects of sedation, drowsiness, and respiratory depression. Absolute contraindications for therapeutic nerve blocks include anticoagulation, regional infection, and lack of technical expertise. Relative contraindications include pain with documented psychogenic or psychiatric origin, language barrier or inability to grasp the concept of a pain rating scale or questionnaire, uncooperative patients, unstable narcotic addiction, poor stress or pain tolerance, poorly localized pain, episodic pain, lack of proper equipment, and anatomical distortion of injection site.

A. Somatic nerve blocks

1. **Peripheral local blocks** include infiltration of wound margins or incision irrigation with long-acting local anesthetics (e.g., bupivacaine) to decrease incisional or wound pain; local blocks (e.g., upper limb block, lower limb block, trunk block, head block, and penile nerve block) for anesthesia or analgesia for surgical procedures, nerve entrapment syndrome, or other severe painful conditions; trigger point injections (see Chapter 4.11); nerve blocks for controlling spasticity (e.g., peripheral nerve blocks and motor point blocks; both described in Chapter 5.4, section III.D.2.b), and injection of local anesthetic and corticosteroids into joints and soft tissues (see Chapter 4.9). In using local infiltration of wound margins, a more proximal blockade of the same nerve is usually recommended because the wound's acidic milieu limits the amount of anesthetic passing through the neuronal membrane.

2. **Cranial nerve blocks** are useful in managing severe intractable pain of the head and neck region, which is mostly seen in trigeminal neuralgia or in cancer patients (due to local spread of the tumor, neural infiltration of the tumor, or tumor-related nerve injury). Therapeutic cranial nerve blocks commonly performed include blockade of the trigeminal nerve and its branches (e.g., mandibular and maxillary branches), gasserian ganglion blocks (if more than one division of trigeminal nerve is involved), facial nerve blocks, glossopharyngeal nerve blocks, and vagus nerve blocks. All cranial nerve blocks must be done under fluoroscopic or CT guidance and only after prior diagnostic and prognostic blocks with local anesthetics. Side effects include inadvertent injection of or diffusion of the drug to neighboring structures such as motor fibers of the jaw, eye, or the upper cervical sympathetic ganglion or internal jugular vein. Hematoma, permanent neurologic sequelae, and alcoholic neuritis have also been reported.

3. **Spinal nerve blocks**
    a. **Occipital nerve blocks** provide analgesia in the distribution of the posterior division of the C2 spinal nerve for patients who have suffered musculoskeletal trauma or have occipital headaches. There are no side effects other than those that occur with accidental intraarterial injection, which is usually of no consequence because of the small volume of the drug.
    b. **Paravertebral blocks** are used to temporarily provide sensory analgesia of selected spinal nerves for the relief of severe pain (e.g., due to musculoskeletal pathology such as fracture) by the placement of local anesthetic distal to the intervertebral foramen. A successful block is denoted by anesthesia and pain relief in the desired distribution; however, overlapping innervation usually necessitates blocks of one or two neighboring segments. Use of neurolytic agents on the spinal nerves is not recommended for pain of nonmalignant disease because most spinal nerves are mixed nerves and neurolytic blocks affect both motor and sensory modalities to the same extent. Moreover, alcohol and, to a lesser degree, phenol can cause a chemical neuropathy, which in itself may create a pain syndrome. Complications are associated with needle penetration of neighboring structures, for example, accidental injection into the vertebral artery with resultant seizures and/or transient paralysis of vital centers and often unconsciousness. Accidental injection into the subarachnoid space with consequent total spinal anesthesia, concomitant block of the cervical sympathetic chain with development of Horner's syndrome, involvement of the superior aspect of recurrent laryngeal nerves and perhaps even the trunk of vagus, and pneumothorax have all been reported. All of these can be avoided by using proper techniques (with fluoroscopic or CT-scan guidance) and small amounts of solutions.
    c. **Intercostal blocks** are used for the relief of severe acute posttraumatic (e.g., rib or sternal fractures), postoperative (e.g., poststernotomy, postmastectomy, or postthoracotomy), or postinfectious (e.g., acute herpes zoster) pain in the thoracic or abdominal wall. The nerves are blocked as they course along the underside of the ribs. The most important complications of intercostal blocks are pneumothorax and systemic toxic reactions (e.g., sudden hypotension and cardiorespiratory compromise). Disadvantages include the limited duration of action of a single dose of local anesthetic (6-8 hours) and the subsequent need for repeated injections, which are painful for the patient and labor intensive for the physician. An alternative to intercostal block is **intrapleural administration**

of local anesthetic via a catheter placed over the T7 or T8 rib to simulate the effect of multiple intercostal blocks and reduce the labor intensiveness of repeated injections.

d. **Subarachnoid neurolytic blocks** involve segmental injections of small amounts of phenol or alcohol into the subarachnoid space at L2-L5 to produce a chemical posterior rhizotomy (primarily for cancer pain, e.g., pelvic cancer pain). Exact positioning and careful choice of the injection level and volume allow selective sensory anesthesia with sparing of motor fibers. Major complications include permanent weakness and urinary or rectal sphincter dysfunction, chemical meningitis, arachnoiditis, headaches, and neuropathies. Several injections may be necessary, and the duration of action varies from an average of 3 months with alcohol injections to only 3 to 4 weeks with phenol injections.

e. **Epidural blocks,** when compared with subarachnoid blocks, allow for blockade of spinal nerve roots over a more limited area and needle insertion at virtually any point in the spine (including cervical segments) due to less risk of penetrating the spinal cord. Unlike, subarachnoid drugs, epidural fluids do not flow freely or predictably with changes in patient position. Despite the ease of injection to a limited area, epidural blocks usually have bilateral effects. Therapeutic indications of epidural local anesthetics blocks include the management of acute pain in trauma, surgery, and obstetrics.

   In chronic pain patients, epidural blocks may be performed using an opioid (with or without local anesthetic) for relief of chronic cancer pain or using a corticosteroid (e.g., 80 mg of methylprednisolone, which should not be repeated if there is relief of pain but may be repeated up to a maximum of three injections in 3-week intervals if there is no pain relief). Epidural corticosteroid injections reduce acute local edema and nerve root compression and may be beneficial in acute back pain due to diskogenic disease; however, efficacy in patients with spinal stenosis, scoliosis, spondylolysis, or spondylolisthesis or in those who have had laminectomies remains controversial with highly variable success rates. The variable success rates are attributed to variations in technique, ancillary care, patient selection and follow-up period. In patients with nonspecific low back pain, several controlled studies showed that epidural steroid injection showed no significant immediate or long-term improvement. When used for treatment of back pain, the caudal epidural approach may be used instead of the translumbar epidural approach to avoid the higher risk of thecal sac injection. Complications of epidural blocks include dural puncture, intravascular injection (with systemic toxicity such as cardiorespiratory compromise, nausea, and vomiting), hypotension (from sympathetic blockade), motor block, pruritus, bladder dysfunction (e.g., urinary retention), epidural abscess, and meningitis.

f. **Intravenous regional (Bier) somatic block** is a technique for producing anesthesia of a limb using an ischemic isolation with a tourniquet and refilling the vascular system with local anesthetics for surgical anesthesia. With local anesthetics, the duration of action is only minutes longer than the tourniquet time. The therapeutic indication of Bier somatic block is anesthesia of the distal limb for orthopedic or soft tissue surgery. It is contraindicated in patients with infection in the limb, those who do not have an intact venous system, and those who can not tolerate a tourniquet. The complications of Bier blocks involve local anesthetic toxicity if the tourniquet fails or leaks or if the tourniquet is deflated before 30 minutes have elapsed since the primary injection. Tourniquet leak may manifest as tinnitus, circumoral numbness, and dizziness; however, the dose of local anesthetics for the average adult is not usually high enough to cause seizures.

4. **Plexus blocks** include **brachial plexus blocks**, which provide sensory, motor, and sympathetic blockade of the ipsilateral upper limb, depending on the volume and concentration of local anesthetic drug used; **cervical plexus blocks** (superficial and deep), which provide sensory and motor block of the distal C1-C4 nerves prior to surgery in the neck and supraclavicular area; and **lumbar plexus blocks**, which provide sensory and motor block of the anterior thigh and quadriceps muscle (L1-L4). The complications for brachial and cervical plexus blocks include pneumothorax, Horner's syndrome, and phrenic nerve block. For lumbar plexus blocks, complications include accidental injection into the subarachnoid space (causing total spinal anesthesia) and improper needle placement (leading to retroperitoneal hemorrhage and injury to the kidney, ureter, or renal pelvis). Systemic toxicity (e.g., hypotension and cardiorespiratory compromise) can also occur with plexus blocks.

B. Sympathetic nerve blocks

1. **Stellate ganglion (cervicothoracic) sympathetic blocks** are aimed at the sympathetic outflow from the upper four to six thoracic sympathetic ganglia and the lower cervical sympathetic ganglion located in a fascial plane at approximately the C7 level in the neck lateral to the vertebral spine. It is important that at least the upper four thoracic ganglia be blocked to obtain complete sympathetic block of the upper limb because not all sympathetic fibers to the upper limb pass through the stellate ganglion. The procedure is usually carried out with local anesthetics; for prolonged action, an indwelling catheter can be used. The use of neurolytic agents, although rarely performed, may be done using fluoroscopy and contrast solutions. The block is successful if it affects: 1) the ipsilateral upper quadrant of the body (above T8), including the face and head with meiosis, mild ptosis, flushed dry skin, and blocked nasal passage; 2) the upper limb with absence of sweating, measurable skin temperature rise, visible vasodilation (with measurable plethysmographic evidence of increased blood flow), and loss of skin conductance response (or galvanic skin response); and 3) the ipsilateral hemithorax, including visceral pleura and sympathetic supply to the heart.

Therapeutic indications of stellate ganglion sympathetic blocks include chronic conditions such as RSD/causalgia involving the upper limb and the face, central pain, phantom pain, posttraumatic pain syndromes, postamputation pain, shoulder-hand syndrome, chronic obstructive vascular disease, ischemic rest pain, chronic herpetic neuralgia, idiopathic neuralgia, painful invasive lung tumors, collagen vascular diseases (e.g., scleroderma, systemic lupus erythematosus, and Raynaud's disease), atypical facial neuralgias, myofascial syndromes, and whiplash injuries. The advantages of stellate ganglion sympathetic blocks compared with other upper limb blocks include the absence of sensory and motor block and the resultant improved blood flow. The potential complications include spinal or epidural block, toxic reaction to the local anesthetic drug due to vertebral artery injection, bradycardia (with right-sided blocks), pneumothorax, recurrent laryngeal nerve block, which causes temporary hoarseness; brachial plexus block; hematoma formation; and orthostatic hypotension. The presence of temporary meiosis may interfere with the neurologic evaluation of a patient with an elevated intracranial pressure.

2. **Lumbar sympathetic blocks** are aimed at the lumbar sympathetic chain of the ipsilateral lower limb, which lies on the anterolateral surface of the bodies of the L2, L3, and L4 vertebrae adjacent to the aorta and vena cava. A single needle insertion is sufficient for temporary blocks, while multiple insertions are safer if neurolytic agents are used. When prolonged sympathectomy is indicated, continuous epidural infusion of a local anesthetic may be used. The block is successful if there is absence of sweating, measurable skin temperature rise, loss of skin conductance response (or galvanic skin response), and visible vasodilation (with measurable plethysmographic evidence of increased blood flow) in the lower limb.

   Therapeutic indications of lumbar sympathetic block include lower limb RSD/causalgia with SMP features, posttraumatic pain syndromes, compromised peripheral vascular disease, intermittent claudication, circulatory insufficiency (ischemic rest pain), herpes zoster, renal colic, intractable pelvic and urogenital pain, phantom limb pain, amputation or stump pain, and carcinomatous invasion of nerves and plexi. For lower limb RSD/causalgia with SMP features, one of the commonly used protocols is daily blocks for 1 week, followed by every other day, twice a week, and then weekly blocks in combination with early mobilization and aggressive physical and occupational therapy. Complications include spinal or epidural anesthesia; injection into a root sleeve; lumbar plexus block; intravascular injection precipitating a systemic toxicity (e.g., sudden hypotension and cardiorespiratory compromise); L2, L3, or L4 neuralgic pain; neuropathy of the genitofemoral nerve; retroperitoneal hemorrhage; and injury to the kidney, ureter, or renal pelvis.

3. **Celiac plexus sympathetic block** is aimed at the sympathetic ganglia located approximately at the L1 level, anterior to the aorta, anterolateral to the celiac artery, and posterior to the pancreas. Blockade of the celiac plexus provides intraabdominal visceral analgesia. Therapeutic indications include the management of visceral pain associated with abdominal malignancy (e.g., chronic pancreatitis) and postoperative pain selectively after abdominal surgery. Complications include spinal or epidural anesthesia, subarachnoid injection (with paraplegia), intravascular injection, neuralgic pain in the upper lumbar roots, diaphragmatic irritation (with pleuritic and shoulder pain), urinary difficulties or renal trauma, pneumothorax, hematoma, hemorrhage, splanchnic vasodilation (hypotension), and systemic toxicity (e.g., cardiorespiratory compromise and unchecked parasympathetic tone with increased bowel motility and diarrhea).

4. **Intravenous regional (Bier) sympathetic block** is similar to the Bier somatic block using local anesthetics described in section IV.A.3.f. When sympathectomy is the goal, a sympathetically active drug (e.g., bretylium or guanethidine) is added to the local anesthetic. Even without the use of local anesthetics, however, peripheral sympathectomy can last for 1 to 2 weeks. Bier sympathetic block is indicated in patients with sympathetically maintained pain (SMP) syndromes (e.g., RSD/causalgia with SMP features). Complications are similar to that of Bier somatic block except that the addition of a sympathetic blocking drug can further cause orthostatic hypotension and headache.

BIBLIOGRAPHY

Aronoff GM, editor: *Evaluation and treatment of chronic pain,* Baltimore, 1992, Williams & Wilkins.

Bonica JJ, editors: *The management of pain,* ed 2, Philadelphia, 1990, Lea & Febiger,

Hamill RJ, Rowlingson JC, editors: *Handbook of critical care pain management,* New York, 1994, McGraw-Hill.

Lennard TA, editor: *Physiatric procedures in clinical practice,* Philadelphia, 1995, Hanley & Belfus.

Portenoy RK, Kanner RM, editors: *Pain management: theory and practice,* Philadelphia, 1996, FA Davis.

Raj PP, editor: *Practical management of pain,* St. Louis, 1992, Mosby-Year Book.

Sinatra RS, Hord AH, Ginsberg B, et al, editors: *Acute pain: mechanism and management,* St. Louis, 1992, Mosby–Year Book.

Tollison CD, Satterthwaite JR, Tollison JW, editors: *Handbook of pain management,* ed 2, Baltimore, 1994, Williams & Wilkins.

Wall PD, Melzack R, editors: *Textbook of pain,* ed 3, Edinburgh, 1994, Churchill Livingstone.

Warfield CA, editor: *Principles and practice of pain management,* New York, 1993, McGraw-Hill.

CHAPTER 4.11

TRIGGER POINT THERAPY

Trigger points are small, localized tender areas found within skeletal muscles, fascia, tendons, ligaments, periosteum, and pericapsular areas. When "active," they may radiate pain into a specific distant area or a zone of referred pain. The zone of referred pain, which is constant in its distribution for any given muscle (although it does not always follow segmental neurological patterns) can be activated by pressure, by piercing with a needle, during activity, or even spontaneously during rest. If there is no zone of referred pain, then the localized tender area is called a tender spot. Trigger points and tender spots can be caused or perpetuated by local factors (e.g., sports- or work-related injuries, sprains, strains, overuse or repetitive injuries, compressed nerves, disk disease, arthritis, or muscle tension related to nonphysiologic posture or stress) or systemic factors (e.g., hypothyroidism, metabolic electrolyte disorders [such as hypokalemia and hypocalcemia], vitamin deficiencies [such as vitamin B complex or C deficiencies], chronic infections, and, possibly, estrogen deficiency).

The trigger points in the muscles usually involve the fascia and are thus called myofascial trigger points. The symptoms and dysfunctions caused by one or more myofascial trigger points are referred to as myofascial pain syndrome (MPS). In MPS, trigger points are found within palpable taut bands. Taut bands run parallel to the orientation of the muscle fibers and represent constantly contracted group of muscle fibers. When taut bands are snapped by a palpating finger or when it is pierced by a needle, a local twitch response (i.e., transient contraction of the taut band) can be elicited. Electromyographic studies show that although the taut band is electrically silent, the trigger points within the taut band show distinctive spontaneous electrical activity (i.e., motor endplate-like potentials with high frequency and spikes). In chronic cases (6-8 weeks after injury), the taut band usually hardens due to fibrosis. Trigger points within a taut band can be detected by using a dolorimeter or algometer (see Chapter 5.10, section IV.C.1.a), which shows pain thresholds that are 2 kg/cm^2 lower than those of the normal side. The muscles that are commonly involved in MPS include suboccipital muscles, neck muscles (near the transverse processes of the C4-C6), trapezius muscles, levator scapulae muscles, supraspinatus and infraspinatus muscles, rhomboid muscles, extensor communis muscles near the lateral epicondyle, sacrospinous and quadratus lumborum muscles, gluteal muscles, tensor fascia lata, vastus medialis muscles, gastrocnemius muscles, and soleus muscles.

In contrast to myofascial pain syndrome, the tender areas found in patients with fibromyalgia are generalized, diffuse, involving bilateral and symmetrical muscles, typically located in nonmuscular tissues (e.g., suboccipital muscle insertion, C5-C6 intertransverse space, second rib costochondral junction, lateral humeral epicondyle, greater trochanter, and medial knee fat) as well as muscular tissues (e.g., trapezius, supraspinatus, and gluteus muscles), with no zone of referred pain nor taut bands. Patients with fibromyalgia do respond well to medication (e.g., amitriptyline and cyclobenzaprine) but not to trigger point therapy unless they have concomitant myofascial trigger points.

Trigger point therapy encompasses injection therapy as well as noninjection therapy (e.g., spraying with vapocoolants followed by therapeutic exercises; relaxation exercises; electrical stimulation; and other physical modalities). Although there are many variations of trigger point therapy (e.g., Travell and Simon technique and Kraus technique), this chapter deals primarily with the eclectic technique taught by Dr. Andrew Fischer. As with other treatment modalities, trigger point therapy should only be used as one of the components of the overall management of the patient (which includes elimination of perpetuating factors such as bad posture, poor body mechanics, highly stressful lifestyle, hypothyroidism, and vitamin deficiencies). To date, the data about trigger points and trigger point therapy are mostly based on empirical evidence. Randomized controlled studies are still lacking.

I. **Trigger point and tender spot injections** involve needling (i.e., repetitive insertion and withdrawal of the needle), which is theorized to mechanically break up fibrotic pockets that have entrapped the nerve endings along with sensitizing substances, thus allowing blood to enter and wash away the sensitizing substances, leading to interruption of the "vicious cycle" of pain. The primary sites of injections are areas with the most intense pain and most tenderness and which are functionally important. Some of the functionally important muscles are as follows: for walking (quadratus lumborum, gluteus medius, and gastrocnemius), for shoulder movements (supraspinatus), and for normal postures (quadratus lumborum, levator scapulae, and upper trapezius). Depending on the number of trigger points, the size of the taut bands, and on patient tolerance, at least one or two (up to 10) injections per session may be given. The injection sessions are usually two to three sessions per week (with injections in different area) during the acute pain stage and once per week or once every 2 weeks during the recovery stage. To be effective, injection therapy should be combined with noninjection therapy (particularly exercises and proper body mechanics) as well as the elimination of the perpetuating factors. The contraindications for injection therapy include bleeding disorders (e.g., coagulopathies and thrombocytopenia), anticoagulant therapy, local infection, immunosuppression, certain psychiatric conditions (e.g., anxiety, paranoia, and schizophrenia), and inability to avoid heavy activity on the injected body part for 2 to 3 days following the procedure. Depression is not a contraindication for injection therapy (in fact, pain relief from the injection may relieve depression).

A. **Injection techniques.** A 22- to 25-gauge needle is usually large enough for needling. A length of 1.5 inches is usually long enough to reach deeper than the trigger points or tender spots except for the thicker muscles of the lumbar paraspinal and gluteal muscles, which may need about 2- to 3.5-inch needles. The following describes general injection techniques. For injection therapy of specific muscles, refer to the textbooks by Travell and Simons or by Kraus (see bibliography).

1. **Dry needling** is similar to the fluid-injection technique described in section I.A.2 except for the absence of fluid infiltration. It is a painful procedure, which is not well tolerated by patients and is, therefore, not recommended.

2. **Needling combined with fluid infiltration** potentiates the mechanical effects of needling alone and is preferred to dry needling because it is more comfortable. The most commonly used fluid is a local anesthetic (e.g., 1% lidocaine or 0.5% procaine), which blocks the pain and the irritation resulting from tissue damaged by the needling. Although their anesthetic effect usually lasts only for about 45 to 60 minutes, the use of local anesthetics has been reported to reduce the intensity and duration of postinjection soreness as well as postinjection spasm in the surrounding muscles. If the patient is allergic to local anesthetics, however, isotonic saline solution may be used (because ultimately it is the needling, not the infiltrated fluid, that is believed to break up the taut band and trigger points). The use of corticosteroids (alone or in

combination with local anesthetics) are generally not recommended (unless for injection into inflamed passive soft tissues like bursa and tendon sheaths; see Chapter 4.9) because trigger points are usually caused by reflex muscular irritability rather than inflammation. Moreover, corticosteroids are associated with greater potential for side effects including local myopathy.

After explaining the procedure to the patient, the point of maximal tenderness is located by asking the patient to point with one finger, by clinician's palpation, or by using a dolorimeter (see dolorimeter description in Chapter 5.10, section IV.C.1.a). The patient is positioned to allow proper access to the trigger point and the muscle around it is palpated to find the entire taut band (which may span from the origin to the insertion of the muscle). The taut band and trigger point are marked using an indelible felt pen or using fingernail impressions. The skin is then prepared using the technique described in Chapter 4.9, section II. After the skin is decontaminated, the entire taut band area is sprayed with a vapocoolant (e.g., ethyl chloride or fluorimethane). When the skin is slightly frosted, the needle is quickly inserted aiming directly at the point of maximal tenderness. An alternative to vapocoolant anesthesia is to pinch the skin in the area to be injected (to distract the sensory pathways) followed immediately by needle insertion.

Once the needle reaches the taut band, a fibrotic type of resistance (gritty, sandpaper-like) is usually felt. The syringe is aspirated and if it is clear of blood, a small amount (0.1-0.3 ml) of fluid is deposited and the taut band or fibrotic area is mechanically needled. Any time that blood is drawn during syringe aspiration, the injection therapy for that site should be terminated. The needling is continued several times or until normal muscle is reached, i.e., when the pain and fibrotic resistance ceases. Upon reaching normal muscles, deposit 0.1 to 0.3 ml of fluid into the normal muscle and redirect the needle. The redirection of the needle should be done under the skin surface, that is, by gently pulling the needle up to the subcutaneous level (without removing or pulling the needle out of the skin) and redirecting it by either a few millimeters or by 1- to 3-cm increments along the plane of the taut band. As the needle pierces each new area in the taut band, infiltrate 0.1 to 0.3 ml of fluid (making sure no blood is aspirated prior to each fluid deposition). This process is repeated until the entire taut band (including the myotendon junction) is needled and infiltrated (usually up to 10 local infiltrations can be performed in one session depending on the patient's tolerance).

To cover the entire taut bands of large muscles, the needle may need to be pulled out of the skin and reinserted at another site. Otherwise, the remaining parts of the taut band can be injected after a period of about 1 week (to allow for tissue healing). Muscles that are constantly active (e.g., masseters and gluteus medius) should only be given minimum needling per session and may, therefore, need several sessions for complete treatment. The total amount of fluid used per muscle are as follows: 1 to 3 ml for head, neck, hand, or feet muscles; 2 to 5 ml for shoulder muscles; 3 to 4 ml for trunk muscles; 6 to 10 ml for lumbar paraspinals or gluteal muscles; and 3 to 7 ml for leg muscles. If 1% lidocaine is used, the maximum amount per session is 20 ml. When the needle is pulled out, the injected site should be compressed for about 2 minutes to prevent bleeding and then covered with a Band-Aid. After injection, the patient is instructed to perform active full range of motion (ROM) to the injected muscle at least 3 times in positions with gravity eliminated or reduced (e.g., in side lying position for hip flexion and extension).

B. **Postinjection care** is crucial to the success of trigger point injection therapy. For the next 3 consecutive days, the patient should avoid heavy use of the injected muscle (e.g., long walks, long driving, or sports activities). If the muscle soreness is excessive, ibuprofen or acetaminophen may be prescribed for 3 to 5 days. The patient should also receive 3 consecutive days of physical therapy consisting of the following:

1. **Local heat,** for example, hot moist packs for 20 min.

2. **Electrical stimulation** for 15 minutes using sinusoidal surging current to induce muscle squeezing actions, that is, slow, strong contractions of the injected muscles with alternating periods of contraction and rest.

3. **Exercises** that follow a pattern of relaxation, warm-up, limbering/stretching (to be repeated only 3 to 4 times each movement), and cooling off. The exercises include

   a. **Relaxation exercises,** such as controlled breathing with eye movement technique (see Chapter 4.2, section VI.A.1.b), Jacobson's progressive relaxation exercises (see Chapter 4.2, section VI.A.2), or active inhibition techniques (see Chapter 4.2, section I.C). The breathing may be timed so that stretching occurs only when the muscles are relaxed.

   b. **Spray and limbering exercises** (see section II.A.1.a) or **spray and stretch exercise** (see section II.A.1.b); and

   c. **Customized home exercise program,** which consists of limbering exercises and passive stretching to be performed every hour on the first 2 to 3 days after injection, then gradually reduced in frequency until they are done at least 3 times a day. If the patient received an injection to the lower body, he or she is instructed to get up and walk or at least contract and relax the muscles in the sitting position every 2 hours for about 5 minutes to prevent stiffness and to maintain circulation.

II. **Noninjection trigger point therapy** should be included in the comprehensive management of trigger points or tender spots. It may be used solely if injection therapy is contraindicated (see section I) or is refused by the patient. It is useful in complex cases involving many muscles in one or more regions of the body because it permits the release of several closely related muscles at one time.

A. **Therapeutic exercises**

1. **Exercises in combination with vapocoolant spray.** The vapocoolant spray (ethyl chloride or fluorimethane) is used to inactivate the trigger point and facilitate stretching. Its mechanism of action is unclear but probably works indirectly via skin afferent nerves (rather than by direct cooling of the muscles) to inhibit pain and spinal stretch reflexes thus reflexively relaxing the muscle and allow it to be adequately stretched. If ethyl chloride is used, fire hazards must be eliminated, and the patient should not inhale the heavy vapors. In contrast, the same caution is not necessary for fluorimethane, which is nonflammable, nonexplosive, chemically stable, nontoxic, and does not irritate the skin.

   a. **Spray and limber protocol (Kraus).** Ethyl chloride (preferred by Krauss) is sprayed (with very slight frosting) over the area concentrating on the point of maximum tenderness. The patient is then asked to do limbering exercises by actively and slowly moving the joint of the sprayed muscle through its full ROM for 3 to 5 times with minimal effort in a position with gravity eliminated or reduced. This can be combined with deep breathing exercises to induce muscle relaxation. After the exercise, check if the pain is still present or if it has shifted to another location. Repeat the spraying process followed by limbering exercises to full active ROM until pain is relieved completely or no further increase in ROM or relief

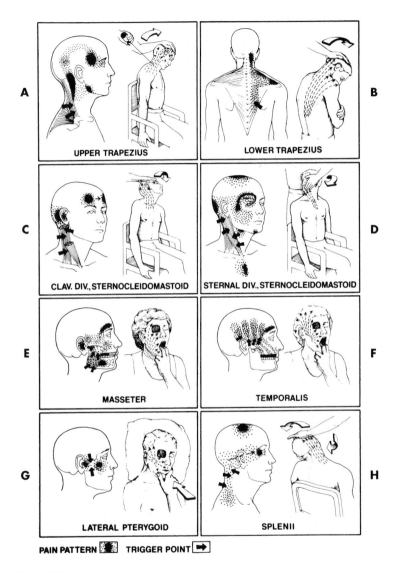

Figure 4.11-1
Location of trigger points (*solid arrows*) and pain patterns (*black stipples*), stretch positions and spray patterns (*dashed arrows*) for muscles that cause head and neck pain. Curved white arrows show the direction of pressure applied to stretch each muscle, and dashed arrows trace the path of parallel sweeps of vapocoolant spray to release tension and permit stretch of each muscle. In **H,** broken arrow in pain pattern deep to ear indicates pain deep in head radiating to back of eye. (From: Simons DG: Myofascial pain syndromes. In Basmajian JV, Kirby RL, eds: *Medical rehabilitation*, Baltimore, 1984, Williams & Wilkins, p. 314, Copyright © 1984 Williams & Wilkins, with permission).

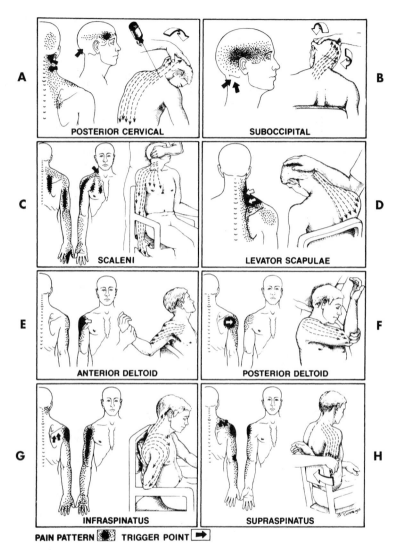

Figure 4.11-2
Location of trigger points (*short, straight black and white arrows*) and pain patterns (*stipples*), stretch positions and spray patterns (*dashed arrows*) for two muscles producing head and neck pain (**A** and **B**) and six muscles causing shoulder and upper limb pain (**C** to **H**). Curved white arrows identify the direction of pressure applied to stretch the muscle. The dashed arrows trace impact of the stream of vapocoolant spray applied to release the muscular tension during stretch. (From: Simons DG: Myofascial pain syndromes. In Basmajian JV, Kirby RL, eds: *Medical rehabilitation*, Baltimore, 1984, Williams & Wilkins, p. 315, Copyright © 1984 Williams & Wilkins, with permission).

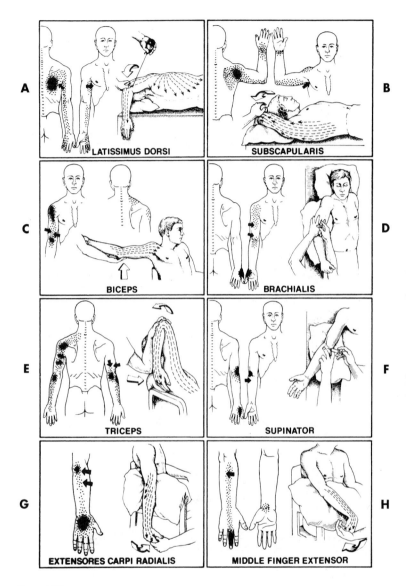

Figure 4.11-3
Location of trigger points (*short, straight black arrows*) and pain patterns (*stipples*), stretch positions and spray patterns (*dashed arrows*) for eight muscles responsible for shoulder and upper limb pain. Curved white arrows identify the direction of pressure applied to stretch the muscle. Dashed arrows trace impact of stream of vapocoolant spray applied to release muscular tension during stretch. (From: Simons DG: Myofascial pain syndromes. In Basmajian JV, Kirby RL, eds: *Medical rehabilitation*, Baltimore, 1984, Williams & Wilkins, p. 316, Copyright © 1984 Williams & Wilkins, with permission).

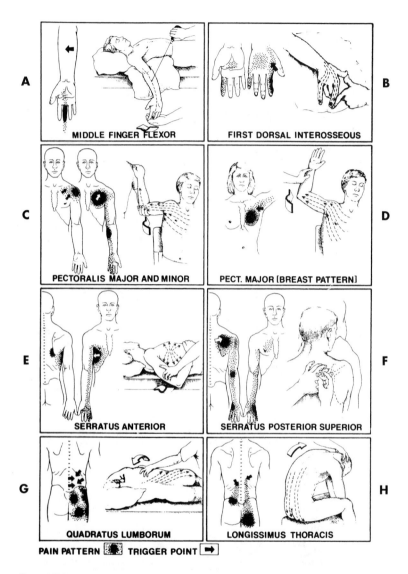

Figure 4.11-4

Location of trigger points (*short, straight white and black arrows*) and pain patterns (*stipples*), stretch positions and spray patterns (*dashed arrows*) for two muscles producing shoulder and upper limb pain (**A** and **B**) and six muscles causing trunk and back pain (**C** to **H**). Curved white arrows identify the direction of pressure applied to stretch the muscle. Dashed arrows trace impact of stream of vapocoolant spray applied to release muscular tension during stretch. (From: Simons DG: Myofascial pain syndromes. In Basmajian JV, Kirby RL, eds: *Medical rehabilitation*, Baltimore, 1984, Williams & Wilkins, p. 317, Copyright © 1984 Williams & Wilkins, with permission).

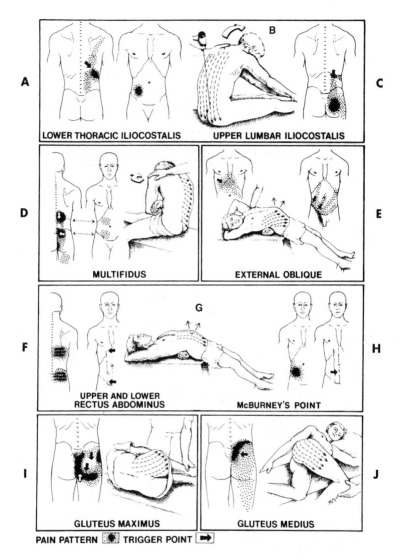

Figure 4.11-5
Location of trigger points (*short, straight black and white arrows*) and pain patterns (*stipples*), stretch positions and spray patterns (*dashed arrows*) for five muscles producing trunk and back pain (**A** to **H**) and two muscles responsible for lower limb pain (**I** and **J**). Curved white arrows identify the directions of pressure applied to stretch the muscle. Dashed arrows trace impact of stream of vapocoolant spray applied to release muscular tension during stretch. (From: Simons DG: Myofascial pain syndromes. In Basmajian JV, Kirby RL, eds: *Medical rehabilitation*, Baltimore, 1984, Williams & Wilkins, p. 318, Copyright © 1984 Williams & Wilkins, with permission).

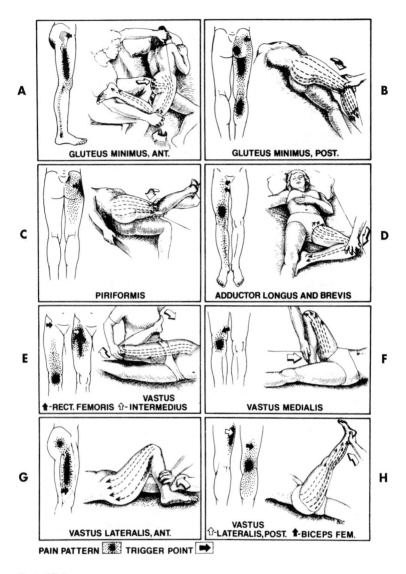

PAIN PATTERN ▓ **TRIGGER POINT** ➡

Figure 4.11-6
Location of trigger points (*short, straight black and white arrows*) and pain patterns (*stipples*), stretch positions and spray patterns (*dashed arrows*) for ten muscles causing lower limb pain. Curved white arrows identify the directions of pressure applied to stretch the muscle. Dashed arrows trace impact of stream of vapocoolant spray applied to release muscular tension during stretch. (From: Simons DG: Myofascial pain syndromes. In Basmajian JV, Kirby RL, eds: *Medical rehabilitation*, Baltimore, 1984, Williams & Wilkins, p. 319, Copyright © 1984 Williams & Wilkins, with permission).

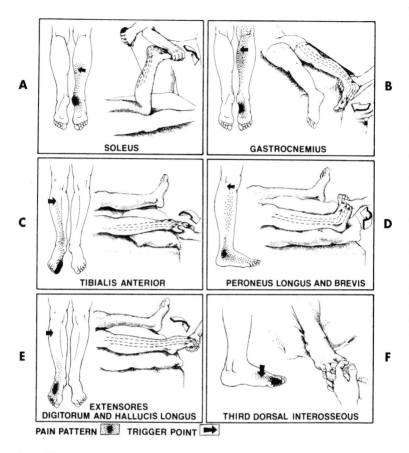

A SOLEUS

B GASTROCNEMIUS

C TIBIALIS ANTERIOR

D PERONEUS LONGUS AND BREVIS

E EXTENSORES DIGITORUM AND HALLUCIS LONGUS

F THIRD DORSAL INTEROSSEOUS

PAIN PATTERN   TRIGGER POINT

Figure 4.11-7
Location of trigger points (*short, straight black arrows*) and pain patterns (*stipples*), stretch positions and spray patterns (*dashed arrows*) for eight muscles producing lower limb pain. Curved white arrows identify the directions of pressure applied to stretch the muscle. Dashed arrows trace impact of stream of vapocoolant spray applied to release muscular tension during stretch. (From: Simons DG: Myofascial pain syndromes. In Basmajian JV, Kirby RL, eds: *Medical rehabilitation*, Baltimore, 1984, Williams & Wilkins, p. 320, Copyright © 1984 Williams & Wilkins, with permission).

of pain can be obtained. In this protocol, all movements are done actively with no passive stretching.
  b. **Spray and stretch protocol (Travell and Simons; see Figures 4.11-1 to 4.11-7).** Fluorimethane (preferred by Travell and Simons) is sprayed until the skin is cool but without frosting; wait until the skin warms before repeating the application. Use a unidirectional sweeping pattern (one or two sweeps) in the direction of the muscle fibers at a slow rate of 10 cm or 4 inches per second from an angle of 30 degrees and a distance of 45 cm (18

inches) over the entire muscle including the zone of referred pain. While spraying, the muscle is passively stretched (for about 30 seconds slowly) using gentle, smooth, steady tension applied by the patient or the clinician's free hand. Then warm the skin using a hot moist pack for a few minutes followed by having the patient perform slow, active, full ROM exercise through both the fully shortened and fully lengthened positions for the muscle group under treatment. This process is repeated 5 times. The stretching may be timed to the exhalation phase of controlled breathing exercise.

2. **Customized home exercise program.** Combine relaxation exercises (see section I.B.3.a) with limbering and stretch exercises.

B. **Physical modalities** (see Chapter 4.1) include electrical stimulation (e.g., transcutaneous electrical nerve stimulation [TENS], high-voltage monophasic pulsed current; see Chapter 4.1, section V), ice application (see Chapter 4.1, section II), ultrasound (see Chapter 4.1, section I.B.1), biofeedback (see Chapter 4.1, section VI), and massage (e.g., deep, kneading or friction massage; see Chapter 4.1, section IX).

C. **Drugs** such as amitriptyline (see Chapter 4.8, section V.A.1.a.1) and cyclobenzaprine (see Chapter 4.8, section II.A.1) may be helpful especially if patient has concomitant fibromyalgia. However, nonsteroidal antiinflammatory drugs (NSAIDs), corticosteroids, and other analgesics are usually ineffective (although NSAIDs or Tylenol may be used to treat postinjection soreness).

D. **Elimination of contributing factors,** such as poor posture, poor body mechanics, leg length discrepancy, vocational and avocational overuse, highly stressful living, poor sleep, and poor physical fitness.

BIBLIOGRAPHY

Fischer AA: Trigger point injection. In Lennard TA, editor: *Physiatric procedures in clinical practice,* Philadelphia, 1995, Hanley & Belfus, pp. 28-35.

Fischer AA: Local injections in pain management: trigger point needling with infiltration and somatic blocks, *Phys Med Rehab Clin Nor Amer* 6(4):851-870, 1995.

Kraus H: *Diagnosis and treatment of muscle pain,* Lombard, IL, 1988, Quintessence Publishing.

Simons DG: Muscular pain syndromes. In Fricton JR, Awad, EA, editors: *Advances in pain research and therapy,* New York, 1990, Raven, pp. 1-41.

Simons DG: Myofascial pain syndromes due to trigger points. In Goodgold J, editor: *Rehabilitation medicine,* St. Louis, 1988, Mosby–Year Book, pp. 686-723.

Simons DG, Simons LS: Chronic myofascial pain syndrome. In Tollison CD, Satterthwaite JR, Tollison JW, editors: *Handbook of pain management,* ed 2, Baltimore, 1994, Williams & Wilkins, pp. 556-577.

Travell JG, Simons DG: *Myofascial pain and dysfunction: the trigger point manual,* vol 1, Baltimore, 1983, Williams & Wilkins.

Travell JG, Simons DG: *Myofascial pain and dysfunction: the trigger point manual. The lower extremities,* vol 2, Baltimore, 1992, Williams & Wilkins.

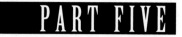

PART FIVE

Basic PM&R Problems

CHAPTER 5.1

DECONDITIONING

Immobilization is the physical restriction of movement involving a body segment or the entire body. Common causes of immobilization in PM&R include neuromusculoskeletal disorders and injuries (e.g., paralysis due to stroke or spinal cord injuries [SCI]; orthopedic casts, body jackets, and splints, usually after trauma or fracture; critical illness requiring bed rest (e.g., after acute myocardial infarction, cardiac dysrhythmia, or septic shock); and prolonged stays in a recumbent position (e.g., chronic low back pain) or sitting position (e.g., wheelchair sitting). Immobilization due to prolonged bed rest results in a clinical entity called *deconditioning*, which is separate from the original process that led to the immobilization. In deconditioning, there is a reduced functional capacity of multiple body systems, especially the musculoskeletal system. The reduced functional capacity of the musculoskeletal system leads to further inactivity and perpetuates the vicious cycle. The severity of deconditioning is dependent on the degree and duration of immobilization. It affects any age and gender, particularly the chronically sick, aged, and disabled population. The adverse clinical manifestations of prolonged immobilization are described below together with the recommended rehabilitation measures to counteract or prevent its deleterious effects. Obviously, prevention is much more cost-effective and is preferable to treatment.

I. Musculoskeletal changes

A. **Contracture** is the lack of full active or passive range of motion (ROM) due to a joint, soft tissue, or muscle limitation. Conditions producing limited joint ROM include pain (e.g., trauma, inflammation, infection, joint degeneration, ischemia, and hemorrhage), muscle imbalance (e.g., paralysis and spasticity), capsular or periarticular tissue fibrosis, primary muscle damage (e.g., polymyositis and muscular dystrophy), or mechanical factors (e.g., improper bed positioning, and casting or splinting in a foreshortened position). The muscle fibers and connective tissues which are maintained in a shortened position (e.g., for 5 to 7 days), adapt to the shortened length by contraction of collagen fibers and a decrease in muscle fiber sarcomeres. In 3 weeks or more, the loose connective tissue in muscles and around joints gradually change into dense connective tissue, causing contracture on the relaxed side of the joint. Contractures occur most commonly at the lower limb with involvement of muscles that cross two joints in the hips, knees, and ankles. In the upper limbs, the shoulders, elbows, wrists, and fingers are most susceptible.

   Contractures are prevented by proper positioning (using pillows, trochanter rolls, hand rolls, or resting splints), active or passive ROM exercises (see Chapter 4.2, section I.A), and early mobilization and ambulation (see Chapter 4.6, section IV). In the supine position, the anterior neck and upper chest should be extended; the trunk and lower limbs should be neutral with the hips extended and slightly abducted; the knees should be extended; and the ankle should be in a neutral position with the toes pointing towards the ceiling (and no pressure at the heels). The shoulders should be in 30 degrees of flexion and 45 to 90 degrees of abduction, the elbows extended, the wrists

425

in 20 to 30 degrees extension, and the hands in the functional position (i.e., the thumb should be abducted and the first web space preserved by using a hand roll or resting splint; and the metacarpophalangeal (MCP) and interphalangeal (IP) joints should be flexed 30 degrees or the MCPs flexed and IPs extended in patients with dorsal hand burns). A prone or sidelying position may also be used. Nurses or family members should be instructed on how to provide ROM for preventing contractures.

Bed treatment of contractures include passive ROM (see Chapter 4.2, section I.A) with terminal stretch at least twice daily; prolonged stretch using low passive tension and heat; sustained stretch using continuous passive mobilization (CPM); progressive, sustained stretching of 2 hours or more (e.g., dynamic splinting or serial casting); treatment of spasticity (see Chapter 5.4, section III); and surgical release (e.g., tendon lengthening, osteotomies, and joint replacements). In spastic patients, a more aggressive ROM exercise 3 to 4 times per day may be necessary, along with medical management of spasticity with medications (see Chapter 5.4, section III.D.1), and nerve or motor point blocks (see Chapter 5.4, section III.D.2.b).

B. **Muscle weakness and atrophy** are usually seen in the antigravity muscles of the lower limbs. With total inactivity there is a 10 to 20% decrease in isometric muscle strength per week, or about 1 to 3% per day. In 3 to 5 weeks, complete immobilization can lead to a 50% decrease in muscle strength. Strength that is lost in 1 week may take 4 weeks to regain even with a maximal strengthening program. To prevent disuse weakness, a muscle must exert 20 to 30% of its maximal capacity for several seconds each day. Muscle exertion at 50% of maximum capacity performed for 1 sec/day is even more effective. Neuromuscular electrical stimulation (NMES) can prevent or retard muscle weakness and atrophy if the muscle is not denervated (see Chapter 4.1, section V). Another technique for maintaining or increasing muscle strength is proprioceptive neuromuscular facilitation (see Chapter 4.2, sections II.A and IV.B.1).

C. **Disuse (immobilization) osteoporosis** is the loss of bone density due to increased resorption caused by lack of stimulus (e.g., weight bearing, gravity, and muscle activity) on bone mass. The adverse effects of prolonged immobilization on the endocrine system cause increased urinary excretion of calcium and hydroxyproline and increased excretion of calcium in the stool which contribute to disuse osteoporosis. Disuse osteoporosis is more marked in the subperiosteal region, in contrast to senile osteoporosis, which develops from the marrow outward. Disuse osteoporosis initially involves the cancellous bone at the metaphysis and epiphysis, and later extends to the entire diaphysis. Bone density is reduced by 40 to 45% after 12 weeks of bed rest. By the thirtieth week, more than 50% of bone density is lost. In patients with disuse osteoporosis, minor trauma or falls may lead to compression fractures of vertebral bodies, or fractures of the hip or other weight-bearing long bones. In patients with neurogenic paralysis (e.g., SCI), disuse osteoporosis is accelerated.

Osteoporosis can only be prevented by weight-bearing standing (see Chapter 4.6, section IV.A). Nonweight-bearing exercise in bed, is in itself not effective in preventing or treating osteoporosis. A standing frame or tilt table may be used in patients who are unable to stand unsupported. As soon as the patient is stable, tilt-table conditioning should begin at a 30-degree tilt for 1 minute. Gradually the tilt may be increased by 10 degrees every 3 to 5 days or earlier as tolerated, until the patient is able to tolerate a 70-

degree tilt for 30 minutes. Then the patient progresses to standing in parallel bars, and finally, to ambulation (see Chapter 4.6, section IV). A general exercise program (see Chapter 4.2), including strengthening, endurance, and coordination exercises, and resumption of activities of daily living (ADL) should be started as early as possible.

II. Cardiovascular changes

A. Orthostatic (postural) hypotension is due to the impaired ability of the circulatory system to adjust to the upright position. As the person stands, blood pools in the lower limbs causing an immediate drop in venous return, which reduces stroke volume and cardiac output. Normally, there is immediate vasoconstriction and increase in heart rate (HR) and systolic blood pressure (SBP). However, prolonged bed rest causes the person to lose this adaptation which is manifested in the following clinical signs and symptoms: tingling, burning in the lower limbs, dizziness, lightheadedness, fainting, vertigo, increased pulse rate (20 or more beats per minute), decreased SBP (20 or more mm Hg), and decreased pulse pressure.

Treatment includes early mobilization (ROM exercises, strengthening exercises, ambulation, and calisthenics); abdominal strengthening and isotonic-isometric exercises of the legs (to reverse venous stasis and pooling); providing the wheelchair with elevating leg rests and a reclining back; use of the tilt table (gradual tilt up to 75 degrees for 20 minutes); use of Ace bandage wraps, full length elastic stockings, and abdominal binders; use of sympathomimetic pressor agents (ephedrine, 10-25 mg slow IV infusion which may be repeated every 5-10 minutes; or phenylephrine [Neo-Synephrine]; 100-200 μg, IV, for severe hypotension or infusion of 20 mg in 250 ml 5% dextrose in water [80 μg/ml] at 40-180 μg/min [35-160 ml/hr]); use of mineralocorticoid (fludrocortisone [Florinef], 0.1 mg, po, qd) to help maintain blood pressure; and maintaining an adequate salt and fluid intake to prevent further blood volume contraction and worsening of hypotension.

B. Changes due to cardiac deconditioning take at least as long or twice as long to recover as it took to deteriorate. Hence early mobilization is important.

1. *At rest,* cardiac changes caused by deconditioning include increased resting HR by one beat per minute every 2 days for the first 3 to 4 weeks of immobilization; decreased resting stroke volume up to 15% after 2 weeks of bed rest, which is related to a decrease in blood volume by 7% after 20 days of bed rest; decreased cardiac size by 11%; and decreased left ventricular end diastolic volume. The cardiac output (CO) remains unchanged or is slightly decreased. Resting systolic and mean blood pressure remains unchanged. Both the oxygen uptake (VO_2) at rest and the arteriovenous oxygen difference remain unchanged.

2. *With exercise,* cardiac changes caused by deconditioning include increased HR response to submaximal exercise (up to 30-40 beats per minute greater than expected after 3 weeks of bedrest), although maximal HR remains unchanged or slightly increased; decreased stroke volume at submaximal and maximal exercise (30%); decreased CO (slightly at submaximal exercise and up to 26% at maximal exercise); decreased maximum oxygen uptake (VO_2 max) by 27%, which indicates reduced aerobic fitness; increased arteriovenous oxygen difference at submaximal exercise but not at maximal exercise.

C. Changes in fluid balance in the recumbent position include increased CO by 24%; increased cardiac work by 30%; shift of 700 ml of blood volume to the thorax; delayed shift of extravascular fluid into the circulation; and compensatory diuresis, which leads to decreased plasma volume with subsequent loss of plasma mineral and protein. By day 4 of bed rest, plasma volume loss is about 13% of the pre-bedrest level. It continues to decline due to a reduced hydrostatic blood pressure and decreased secretion of antidiuretic hormone (ADH) until it plateaus at 70% of normal plasma volume and 60% of normal blood volume. Treatment using isotonic exercise (see Chapter 4.2, section II.B.2) is almost twice as effective as isometric exercises in preventing plasma volume reduction.

D. Venous thromboembolism (see Chapter 5.3) may develop due to venous stasis increased blood viscosity, and hypercoagulability (caused by the decline in plasma volume while red blood cell mass remains unchanged). Preventive measures (see Chapter 5.3, section IV) include active exercise (e.g., calf or ankle pumps and walking; is shown to clear contrast medium injected into the veins 4 times faster than those on bed rest); use of elastic stockings (knee- or thigh-high) or elastic wraps (Ace bandage); use of low molecular-weight heparin (30 mg, SQ, bid) or low-dose unfractionated heparin (5000 to 8000 units, SQ, q8-12h) in patients at high risk for deep venous thrombosis; and proper positioning (legs elevated).

III. Respiratory changes due to bed rest are caused by mechanical restriction of breathing (caused in part by reduced chest excursion due to progressive reduction of ROM in the costovertebral and costochondral joints) which subsequently results in rapid, shallow breathing. Pulmonary function parameters, such as tidal volume, minute volume, vital capacity, and maximum voluntary ventilation, are all reduced. The overall reduction in muscular strength and endurance of deconditioned patients result in reduced movement of the diaphragmatic, intercostal, and abdominal muscles.

In the supine patient, mucus secretions accumulate in the dependent (i.e., posterior) respiratory segments, whereas the non-dependent (i.e., anterior) respiratory segments become dry, rendering the mucociliary mechanism ineffective in clearing secretions. Both the ciliary malfunction and weakness of the abdominal muscles are responsible for the impaired cough. As dependent areas become poorly ventilated and overperfused, there are regional changes in the ventilation-perfusion ratio, and significant arteriovenous shunting with lowered arterial oxygenation. If metabolic demand is increased, hypoxia can occur. Ultimately, the bed-ridden patient may develop atelectasis and hypostatic pneumonia. Preventive measures (see Chapter 5.12, section IV.B) include: early mobilization; frequent change in position; chest physical therapy (deep breathing exercises, incentive spirometry, assisted coughing, and/or chest percussion and vibration may be indicated, depending on the patient's needs); and adequate pulmonary hygiene.

IV. Skin changes

A. Pressure ulcers are fully discussed in Chapter 5.2.

B. Dependent edema can predispose to cellulitis. Preventive measures include adequate mobilization and elevation, use of elastic stockings or gloves, pressure gradient compression, and massage.

C. Subcutaneous bursitis occurs when there is excessive pressure on the bursae (usually prepatellar or elbow bursae). It can be prevented by removal of aggravating pressure on the bursae. Treatment measures include use of nonsteroidal antiinflammatory drugs (see Chapter 4.8, section I.A.3), percutaneous drainage, corticosteroid injections (see Chapter 4.9, section III.B); and surgery in refractory cases.

V. Gastrointestinal changes include decreased appetite, decreased gastric secretion, atrophy of the intestinal mucosa and glands, slower rate of absorption, distaste for protein-rich food (which can lead to nutritional hypoproteinemia), and constipation due to decreased gastric and intestinal motility (caused by increased adrenergic stimulation, which inhibits peristalsis and causes sphincter contraction). The loss of plasma volume and dehydration aggravates constipation. Desire to defecate is also reduced due to embarrassment at using the bedpan. Treatment of constipation (see Chapter 5.8, section VI.B) or fecal impaction (see Chapter 5.8, section VIII.A) include: laxatives, enemas, manual extraction, or in extreme cases, surgical interventions. Preventive measures include adequate fluid intake and fiber-rich diet (raw fruits and vegetables); use of stool softeners and bulk-forming agents; avoidance of narcotics because they produce slowed peristalsis; and limited use of hyperosmotic (e.g., glycerin) or peristalsis-stimulating (e.g., bisacodyl) suppositories combined with a regularly-timed bowel program.

VI. **Genitourinary changes** include increased diuresis and mineral excretion, stone formation, and urinary tract infection. Stones (struvate and carbonate apatite are the most common) are found in 15 to 30% of immobilized patients due to urinary stagnation (incomplete bladder emptying), hypercalciuria (in patients with SCI and fractures), altered ratio of citric acid to calcium, and increased excretion of phosphorus. Bladder stones promote bacterial growth due to irritation and trauma to the bladder mucosa, leading to increased incidence of urinary tract infection (UTI). Long-term immobilization may lead to decreased glomerular filtration rate and decreased ability to concentrate urine. There also appears to be decreased spermatogenesis and androgenesis.

Preventive measures include adequate fluid intake, use of the upright position for voiding, and strict avoidance of bladder contamination during instrumentation. In patients with high post-void residual, an external (condom) catheter (see Chapter 5.7, section IV.B.1) or intermittent catheterization (see Chapter 5.7, section IV.C) may be used. Any UTI should be treated with appropriate antibiotics based on urine culture and sensitivity (see Chapter 5.7, section V.A). Other therapeutic approaches include acidification of the urine through the use of vitamin C (to prevent growth of proteus organisms), use of urinary antiseptics, and, in those patients at highest risk for stone formation, a urease inhibitor. Treatment of stones after they have formed (see Chapter 5.7, section V.B) includes surgical removal or the use of lithotripsy.

VII. **Metabolic and nutritional changes** include decreased lean body mass, increased body fat, disorder of nitrogen balance, and mineral and electrolytes losses (nitrogen loss, calcium loss, phosphorus loss, sulfur loss, and potassium loss). Hypercalcemia due to immobilization is associated with osteoporosis, especially in young adult males with traumatic injuries who were physically active prior to immobilization. As their bones are reabsorbed, serum calcium levels rise. This is associated with hypercalcemic metabolic alkalosis and may lead to renal failure and ectopic calcification. Hypercalcemia manifests clinically as headache, nausea, lethargy, constipation, and weakness. It is treated by achieving adequate calcium excretion through hydration with 0.9% or 0.45% saline and diuresis with furosemide (Lasix, 1 mg/kg up to 20-40 mg IV or 20-80 mg, po, qd/bid). If hypercalcemia is refractory, etidronate disodium (Didronel, 7.5 mg/kg in 250 ml normal saline given IV over 2 hours daily for 3 days) may be used.

VIII. **Endocrine changes** are due to altered responsiveness of hormones and enzymes. They include glucose intolerance; altered circadian rhythm; altered temperature and sweating responses; and altered regulation of parathyroid hormone (PTH), thyroid hormone, adrenal hormones, pituitary hormones, growth hormone, androgens, and plasma renin activity. The glucose intolerance (noted after 8 weeks of immobility) is due to reduced insulin-binding sites which causes decreased sensitivity of the peripheral muscle to circulating insulin. Glucose intolerance induced by bed rest can be improved by isotonic but not isometric exercises of the large muscle groups in the legs. After 2 weeks of bed rest, it takes about 2 weeks of resumed activity before glucose response returns to normal.

IX. **Neurological, emotional, and intellectual changes** include the effects of sensory deprivation (decreased attention span, confusion and disorientation to time and space, decreased hand-to-eye coordination); decreased intellectual capacity; emotional and behavioral disturbances (anxiety, depression, autonomic lability, restlessness, decreased pain tolerance, irritability, hostility, insomnia, and lack of motivation); increased auditory threshold and decreased visual acuity; impaired balance and coordination (probably due to neural factors rather than muscle weakness); and compression neuropathies. Preventive measures include encouraging the patient to interact with staff, other patients, and family members, and recreational therapy for psychosocial integration, resocialization, and adjustment to independent functioning. Nerve compression can be prevented by proper positioning to relieve pressure from the nerve.

BIBLIOGRAPHY

Akeson WH, Amiel D, Abel MF; et al: Effects of immobilization on joints, *Clin Orthop* 219:28-37, 1987.

Baker JH, Matsumoto DE: Adaptation of skeletal muscle to immobilization in a shortened position, *Muscle Nerve* 2:231-244, 1988.

Buschbacher RM: Deconditioning, conditioning, and the benefits of exercise. In Braddom RL, editor: *Physical medicine and rehabilitation,* Philadelphia, 1996, WB Saunders, pp. 687-708.

Dolkas CB, Greenleaf JE: Insulin and glucose responses during bed rest with isotonic and isometric exercise, *J Appl Physiol* 43:1033-1038, 1977.

Downs FS: Bed rest and sensory disturbances, *Am J Nurs* 74:434-438, 1974.

Haines RF: Effect of bed rest and exercise on body balance, *J Appl Physiol* 36:323-327, 1974.

Halar EM, Bell KR: Contracture and other deleterious effects of immobility. In DeLisa JA and Gans BM, editors: *Rehabilitation medicine: principles and practice,* ed 2, Philadelphia, 1993, JB Lippincott, pp. 681-699.

Leadbetter WF, Engster HE: Problems of renal lithiasis in convalescent patients, *J Urol* 53:269, 1957.

Minare P: Immobilization osteoporosis: a review, *Clin Rheumatol* 8:95-103, 1989.

Mueller EZ: Influence of training and of inactivity on muscle strength, *Arch Phys Med Rehabil* 51:449-462, 1970.

Saltin B, Blomquist G, Mitchell JH, et al: Response to exercise after bed rest and after training. a longitudinal study of adaptive changes in oxygen transport and body composition, *Circulation* 38(Suppl VII):1-78, 1968.

Shahzadi S, Vallbona C: Immobilization. In Garrison SJ, editor: *Handbook of physical medicine and rehabilitation basics,* Philadelphia, 1995, JB Lippincott, pp. 185-196.

Spencer WA, Valbona C, Carter RE: Physiologic concepts of immobilization, *Arch Phys Med Rehabil* 46:89-100, 1965.

Taylor HL: The effects of rest in bed and of exercise on cardiovascular function, *Circulation* 38:1016-1017, 1968.

Van Beaumont W, Greenleaf JE, Juhos L: Disproportional changes in hematocrit, plasma volume, and proteins during exercise and bed rest, *J Appl Physiol* 33:55-61, 1972.

CHAPTER 5.2

PRESSURE ULCERS

Pressure ulcers (also called decubitus ulcers, pressure sores, or bedsores) are localized areas of cellular necrosis almost always occurring over bony prominences. They are the results of prolonged, externally applied pressure. In the PM&R setting, they are most frequently seen in the elderly disabled who are bed- or chair-bound in nursing homes or at home; in patients with decreased mobility because of paralysis (e.g., spinal cord injury [SCI], multiple sclerosis [MS], stroke, or traumatic brain injury [TBI]), fractures (e.g., hip fracture), or surgery; and in patients on steroids or chemotherapy. This chapter presents the prevention and treatment of pressure ulcers based on the clinical practice guidelines published by the Agency for Health Care Policy and Research (see bibliography). The prevention of pressure ulcers must be emphasized throughout the care of the disabled because, not only are pressure ulcers preventable, but prevention is more cost-effective than treatment.

I. **Pathophysiology.** Pressure ulcers are caused by unrelieved local external pressure (often over bony prominences). Pressures applied for 30 minutes or less cause hyperemia (skin redness), which disappears 1 hour after pressure is removed. If pressure is applied for 2 to 6 hours, ischemia occurs, and the redness takes 36 hours to disappear after pressure is relieved. If pressure is applied continuously for 6 to 12 hours, a blue demarcation is detected, which does not disappear. Two weeks after necrosis, skin breakdown results in ulceration.

II. **Epidemiology.** In the United States pressure ulcers occur in one million people per year at a cost of $6 billion in hospitalized patients alone for 1991. Every year, 60,000 people die from the complications of pressure ulcers. In hospitalized patients, the incidence ranges from 2.7 to 29.5% with a prevalence of 3.5 to 69%. In chronic or long-term facilities, the incidence is 10.8% with a prevalence of 2.6 to 24%. In critical care units, the incidence is 33% with a prevalence of 41%. In elderly patients admitted for femoral fracture, the incidence is 66%. In patients with SCI, the incidence is 25 to 66% with a prevalence of 60% in tetraplegic patients.

III. **Risk and etiologic factors**

   A. **Biomechanical factors** include pressure, shear, friction, moisture, and temperature. Prolongation of normal activities such as sitting and lying can result in extremely high tissue stresses because small volumes of flesh are compressed between the bony skeleton and an external surface. In the development of pressure ulcers, the duration of pressure is more critical than the intensity of pressure, hence if pressure duration is long enough (even with relatively small loads or small applications of pressure), tissue necrosis results. Other common causes of increased pressure, shear, or friction include use of deteriorated or inappropriate wheelchair cushions, activities involving sitting on uncushioned surfaces (e.g., floor), and continuing to sit after bruising the skin (e.g., from transfer). A slumped sitting posture or the shearing forces created by the posterior pelvic tilt as the patient tends to slide out of the wheelchair, also contribute to the formation of sacral ulcers. Increased skin temperature with resulting perspiration, can increase metabolic demands of cells in a local region, thus predisposing to skin breakdown. Moist skin (e.g., from bowel or bladder incontinence and excessive perspiration) may adhere to clothing and bed linen, causing shearing maceration through direct trauma or exposure to pressure. Fecal and urinary incontinence can also cause chemical irritation of the epidermis, which can lead to infection.

B. Biochemical factors include poor nutrition, which can result in weight loss with loss of fat padding over bony prominences; negative nitrogen balance and poor vitamin intake, which can compromise normal tissue integrity; hypoproteinemia, which can lead to edema causing decreased skin elasticity thus making it more susceptible to inflammation; and anemia with low serum iron and low serum iron binding hence leading to decreased oxygen and nutrients to the tissues. Other biochemical factors include poor collagen metabolism (with increased susceptibility to skin breakdown), heterotopic ossification (possibly because of increased bony areas against which the tissue can be compressed), and poor circulation (decreased tissue oxygen and nutrient supply).

C. Medical factors include any trauma, illness, or disease that decreases mobility, especially if there is associated malnutrition (hypoalbuminemia, vitamin deficiency), anemia, ischemia, infection, severe spasticity, contractures, edema, decreased level of consciousness, decreased or absent sensation (e.g., diabetic neuropathy and SCI), and psychological stress and depression. Elderly patients are particularly susceptible to pressure ulcers because their skin loses elasticity and vascularity, and it becomes more dry and fragile.

IV. Classification. Pressure ulcers are graded or staged according to the degree or extent of tissue damage (see Table 5.2-1). The Shea classification is traditionally used. In this chapter, all references to staging are based on the National Pressure Ulcer Advisory Panel classification.

V. Diagnosis

A. Inspection of skin over bony prominences. The most common sites of pressure ulcers are the ischium (28%), sacrum (17-27%), greater trochanters (12-19%), and the heels (9-18%). Other common sites include the malleoli, tibial crests, patellae, anterior superior iliac spines, elbows, shoulders, scapulae, costal margins, spinous processes, ears, and occiput. Ischial ulcers are most common in paraplegics, and sacral ulcers are most common in tetraplegics. In elderly and diabetic patients, heel ulcers are common. In ambulatory patients, pressure ulcers can occur at the plantar forefoot (the most common site being the metatarsal heads in patients with diabetic neuropathy) and in bodily parts in contact with orthotic or prosthetic devices.

B. Physical examination. Measure the ulcer in centimeters, and determine its depth by inserting a cotton swab to the deepest part of the wound and measuring it in centimeters. Check for signs of infection (redness, induration, exudates, edema, malodor). Probe the ulcer using a sterile cotton swab to rule out communication of ulcers and joint spaces or bony cavities. A polaroid photograph is useful for documenting pressure ulcers and following their progress. Check for predisposing factors such as urinary or fecal incontinence, severe spasticity, contractures, or malnutrition.

C. Laboratory work-up includes complete blood count (CBC), prothrombin time (PT), activated partial thromboplastin time (aPTT), total proteins, albumin/globulin ratio, and blood urea nitrogen (BUN). Erythrocyte sedimentation rate (ESR) may be done to follow progression of osteomyelitis. Iron, folate, vitamins B_6 and B_{12}, and zinc levels may also be checked to determine need for supplementation.

D. Bacteriology reveals that the most common bacteria in pressure ulcers are a

Table 5.2-1.   Comparison of three classification systems for clinically grading or staging pressure ulcers. For accurate classification, eschar or slough must be removed so that the wound base is visible

SHEA* CLASSIFICATION	YARKONY-KIRK† CLASSIFICATION	NATIONAL PRESSURE ULCER ADVISORY PANEL‡ CLASSIFICATION
1. Erythema or induration overlying a bony prominence without ulceration (i.e., an incipient ulcer)	1. Red area (possible sites of future breakdown) 1a. Present >30 min but <24 hrs 1b. Present >24 hrs	Stage I. Nonblanchable erythema of intact skin; the heralding lesion of skin ulceration
2. Shallow full thickness skin ulcer involving dermis extending to junction of subcutaneous fat	2. Epidermis and/or dermis ulcerated, but subcutaneous fat is not seen	Stage II. Partial thickness skin loss involving epidermis and/or dermis; presents as an abrasion, blister, or shallow crater
3. Ulcer extending into subcutaneous tissue, obliterating fat but limited by the deep fascia and does not extend into muscle	3. Subcutaneous fat observed, but muscle is not seen	Stage III. Full-thickness skin loss with damage or necrosis of subcutaneous tissue, which may extend down to, but not through, underlying fascia; presents as a deep crater with or without undermining of adjacent tissue
4. Ulcer extending into or through muscle tissue exposing the underlying bony prominence at its base; "closed pressure sore," i.e., large cavity accessible through a small skin sinus (could be grade 3 or 4)	4. Muscle/fascia observed, but bone is not seen	Stage IV. Full-thickness skin loss with extensive destruction, tissue necrosis or damage to muscle, bone, or supporting structures (e.g., tendon, joint capsule, etc.)
	5. Bone is seen, but joint space is not involved	
	6. Joint space involved; pressure ulcer healed	

Adapted from * Shea JD: Pressures classification and management, *Clin Orthop* 112: 89-100, 1975.
† Yarkony G., Kirk PM, Carlson C, et al: Classification of pressure ulcers, *Arch Dermatol* 126:1218-1219, 1990.
‡ National Pressure Ulcer Advisory Panel: Pressure ulcers—prevalence, cost, and risk assessment: consensus development conference statement, *Decubitus* 2(2):24-28, May 1989.

mix of gram-positive and gram-negative flora, namely *Staphylococcus aureus, Proteus mirabilis, Pseudomonas aeruginosa,* and *Escherichia coli.* Anaerobic cultures often show *Bacteroides* and *Clostridia.*

1. **Qualitative wound culture and sensitivity tests (C/S)** may be done to guide antibiotic choice.
   a. **Swab culture** only indicates what organisms are present in the wound fluid. These organisms are usually microbes that have colonized the wound (without causing tissue infection) from the gastrointestinal (GI) tract or the surrounding skin. They do not always concur with deep tissue culture.
   b. **Irrigation-aspiration** is done immediately after thorough cleansing of the wound. It has 98% concordance for aerobes and 92% concordance for anaerobes compared to tissue biopsy.
2. **Quantitative wound culture (tissue biopsy)** is done by removing 1 g of wound tissue and then counting the microorganisms in it. If the number of bacteria exceeds 10^5 per gram of tissue, infection exists.

E. **Diagnostic tests** include bone radiographs to rule out osteomyelitis and heterotopic calcification. Bone biopsy with trochar needle is the definitive diagnostic procedure for ruling out osteomyelitis. Bone scans and computed tomography (CT) or magnetic resonance imaging (MRI) are not routinely indicated but may be used as an adjunct to rule out osteomyelitis or abscess. Bone scans are nonspecific and have high false-positive results. The sensitivity of bone scan in diagnosing osteomyelitis is increased when a triple phase bone scan is done or in conjunction with a gallium or indium scan. Contrast sinography may evaluate the presence and extent of wound tunneling or sinus tracts.

F. **Pressure ulcer risk assessment scales** can be used to identify at-risk individuals so that risk factors can be reduced through intervention. These individuals should be assessed on admission to the acute- or long-term care facility and reassessed at periodic intervals. Despite their limitations, their use ensures systematic evaluation of individual risk factors.
   1. **Braden scale** assesses the patient's physical activity, mobility, sensory perception, degree to which the skin is exposed to moisture, nutrition status, and friction and shear. This scale has been tested extensively in diverse sites such as medical-surgical units, intensive care units (ICUs), and nursing homes. It has good interrater reliability.
   2. **Norton scale** assesses the patient's physical condition, mental condition, activity, mobility, and continence. A score of 12 or below signifies patients at risk of developing pressure ulcers. This scale has been extensively tested on elderly persons in hospital settings; however, no reliability data is yet available.

VI. **Prevention** of pressure ulcers involves an integrated team management approach with emphasis on good medical and nursing care, proper training and education of patients, family, and caregivers, encouragement of patient compliance, and the proper prescription of support surfaces. It is more cost-effective than treatment of pressure ulcers.

A. **Skin inspection and skin care** as part of the patient's daily routine are the basis of pressure ulcer prevention. The patient's skin must be examined regularly each morning and evening and each time the patient is turned or receives a specific treatment. Potential signs of impending ulcer formation include color variation (redness, skin discoloration), blisters, rashes, swelling, temperature variation, pimples and ingrown hairs, bruises, surface breaks, and dry, flaky skin. If any of these signs are present, all pressure from that area must be removed immediately. The patient and family must be taught the importance of these routine skin checks and care.

The patient's skin should be washed and dried twice daily. Any areas where perspiration, urine, or feces collect should be washed several times daily with mild soap, then rinsed with warm water, and patted dry. Apply a skin moisturizer and massage it well into the skin immediately after washing or bathing the patient. The patient's skin, after a washing or a bath, is well-hydrated so moisturizers applied at this time provide the optimal moisturizing and protective effect. Moisturizing cream and protective ointments are preferred over lotions because they contain a lower proportion of water and offer better barrier protection. Avoid leaving any moist areas as they may cause skin irritation and maceration.

B. **Pressure reduction measures**

   1. **Positioning, turning, and transferring.** Patients at risk for developing pressure ulcers should be turned and repositioned at least every 2 hours around the clock: 2 hours on the side, 2 hours on the back, and 2 hours on the other side regardless of the type of support surface. When lying on the side, the patient should avoid direct pressure on the trochanter by using a 30-degree lateral-inclined position instead. Elevate the head of the bed as little as possible (maximum of 30°) and for as short a time as possible. If able to tolerate it, the patient should sleep in the prone position because the anterior part of the body has larger low-pressure areas and smaller high-pressure areas. Positioning devices such as pillows or foam wedges may be used to keep bony prominences (e.g., knees or ankles) from direct contact with one another. The heels should be raised off the bed by placing a pillow under the calf. Donut-type devices should *not* be used because they create larger areas of ischemia at the center of the donut. Chair-bound patients must be repositioned every hour. If possible, patients must be taught to raise themselves off the seat for 15 seconds every 30 minutes (e.g., pushup exercises or leaning side to side). Sitting uninterrupted for more than 2 hours should *not* be allowed. During transfers, the patient should not be dragged across the bed. Instead the patient should be lifted using a draw sheet under the patient, or the patient can assist by pulling on the bed trapeze.

   2. **Skin protectors** may help prevent skin friction and shear but are usually *not* very helpful in reducing pressure. They include padded dressings, sheepskin mats or pads, silicone gel pads, elbow pads, heel pads, and bunny boots.

   3. **Pressure reducing support surfaces** keep pressures lower than that of the standard hospital bed or standard wheelchair seat, but *not* consistently below capillary closing pressure of 32 mm Hg. They consist of a supporting medium ("the core material") and an enclosing membrane, which separates the patient's skin from the supporting medium. The ideal supporting medium should have high compliance, minimum shearing force, high porosity, and should be light, easy to clean, and durable. Although high compliance is essential for uniform pressure distribution, it makes it difficult for the patient to maintain proper bed positioning that ensures spinal support, prevents contractures, and permits transfer activities. Hence, a firm supporting medium is preferred to a highly compliant medium. Ideally, the enclosing membrane should have low stiffness, a low coefficient of friction, high porosity, and high absorbency so it can prevent

skin friction and shear, and so it can decrease the temperature and moisture at the skin surface. Obviously, no one product fulfills all of these requirements all of the time. In choosing the appropriate product to meet individual patient needs, recognize the advantages, disadvantages, and limitations of the different surfaces.

a. Static overlays attempt to provide pressure reduction by their material and design. They do not eliminate, however, the need for pressure relief by preventive repositioning (see section VI.B.1 above) and do not decrease pressures of the ischium below capillary pressure. Currently no clear evidence supports one static overlay over another.

1) Functional types of static overlays

   a) Mattress overlays are placed directly over a regular mattress. A mattress overlay should be 3 to 4 inches thick with 25% indentation load deflection (ILD) of 30 lb, density of 1.3 lb/ft^3 or more, and modulus of 2.5 or more. A 25% ILD is the force needed to compress a 4-inch piece of foam until it is 3 inches tall. Density measures how much material is in the foam, while the modulus of the foam is the ratio of the 65% ILD to 25% ILD.

   b) Static seat cushions are usually placed over a wheelchair seat. They are used to relieve pressure in vulnerable anatomical areas by providing an additional protective layer between the support surface and the body. They distribute the body's weight away from bony prominences and stabilize the body for balance and functional pelvic positioning. They should be durable and moisture resistant for incontinent persons. Although firmer cushions provide a better base of support, they may be inappropriate in insensate patients.

2) Types of static overlays by materials or contents (see Chapter 4.7, section I.A.3.b for pressure-relief seat cushions used in wheelchairs).

   a) Polyurethane foam overlays are blocks or layers of foam whose compliance, firmness, and density can be varied from supersoft to extra firm. Combinations with soft foam on the top and firm below can provide both high compliance and good support. Foams can be shaped like egg cartons or they can be split in parts (split-foam) so that separate sections support the trunk, the thighs, and the legs. With split-foams, all pressure points from heel to sacrum can be positioned in a space between the mattress sections so that they are free from pressure and air circulates freely by them in any lying position. Foams used as wheelchair cushions can also be contoured to reduce pressure and improve posture and balance. Unlike the gel- or water-filled overlays, compression of foam overlay on one area has little effect on other areas, and the pressure distribution depends on the design and firmness of the foam. Foams are lightweight; can be cut into any size, shape, or thickness; are easy to transfer; and can provide stability and good balance; however, they wear out quickly (average of 6 months), cannot be washed or cleaned, can retain moisture, and can increase temperature of the support surface.

   b) Gel-filled (flotation-gel) overlays are plastic or rubber membranes filled with a plastic-like material that simulates body fat tissue. They adjust to body movements and can act as a shock absorber. They can maintain skin temperature, but cooling of the cushion is necessary every 3 hours to maintain this effect. They can also resist puncture more than water or air-filled overlays; however, they are heavy, difficult to transfer, and expensive.

c) **Air-filled overlays** are inflatable membranes. They are lightweight, easy to clean, can be customized in multiple heights, and can be compartmentalized (with multiple valves). Air-filled overlays with multiple cells (e.g., ROHO overlays, which consist of a series of vertical balloons filled with air) can increase the humidity and temperature of the support surface, but less so than a foam cushion. They are subject to puncture, not easily repaired, require monitoring of the air pressure, and may cause balance or transfer problems.

d) **Water-filled (flotation-water) overlays** are plastic or rubber membranes filled with chemically treated water or other liquid. They adjust to body movements and are easy to clean and can decrease temperature on the support surface; however, they are heavy, may leak if punctured, and are difficult to transfer.

b. **Dynamic overlays or mattresses** are designed to reduce duration of pressure by alternating pressure pads, which provide alternating periods of high and low pressure. They are used if the patient cannot assume a variety of positions without bearing weight on the ulcer, or if the patient fully compress the static support surface, or if the ulcer does not show evidence of healing. They are dependent on an external power source (e.g., battery or wall socket), however, and their use as wheelchair cushions is limited because they can interfere with the patient's functional independence and mobility. They are also noisy and are subject to puncture and breakdown.

1) **Alternating pressure-point mattresses** consist of a series of vinyl tubes or cells, which are connected to a pump in such a way that when one cell or tube is inflated, an adjacent cell or tube is deflated. Its air cells tend to collapse under high local pressure, and lying directly on the plastic can increase discomfort, body heat, and perspiration, hence making the skin prone to maceration.

2) **Rolling mattress (Cloud 9)** consists essentially of two long interconnected sausage-like air sacs. One sac alternately inflates and deflates, so that the other sac responds reciprocally, hence the patient is rolled from side to side while supported on an air cushion. This seems to be more comfortable and more effective in reducing tissue pressure than the alternating pressure-point mattress. It may, however, make some patients nauseous.

c. **Static replacement mattresses** are designed for use on an existing bed frame without an underlying mattress. They reduce staff time and are easy to clean; however, they have a high initial cost, may not control moisture, and lose effectiveness over time. They require at least 4 inches of foam to protect the greater trochanter. Although they may reduce pressures below those of a standard bed mattress, these pressures can be raised by spasm, postural change, and muscle contraction.

4. **Pressure-relieving specialty beds** reduce pressure consistently below capillary closing pressure of 32 mm Hg. They are used to promote healing of pressure ulcers as well as to prevent development of new pressure ulcers in patients with large stage III or stage IV pressure ulcers on multiple turning surfaces. In rehabilitation, they are generally used for short periods of time because they are not practical or are too expensive for home use.

Pressure-relieving specialty beds use air flotation for pressure relief. They are comfortable, keep the skin dry (hence decreasing maceration), and promote healing. They are, however, noisy, heavy, costly, and the sensation of floating can cause motion sickness or disorientation.

a. **Air-fluidized bed (Clinitron)** uses a process in which a high volume of warm compressed air is forced through a diffuser into a medium of silicone beads to simulate a high-density fluid environment. The glass granules are enclosed in a woven polyester filter sheet, which prevents the beads from escaping but permits air to pass easily through it. The patient lying on top of the polyester sheet has the sensation of lying on a water bed, and it is claimed that no point in the body exceeds a pressure of 20 mm Hg. The temperature of the air is usually kept at 31°C for optimal comfort with minimal perspiration. Air-fluidized beds are used for patients with stage III or IV pressure ulcers or in patients with skin grafts. They are also bactericidal by the sequestration and dessication of microorganisms by the silicone beads. To position a patient in a seated or semi-Fowler's position, foam cushions are required.

   The adverse effects of air-fluidized beds are preventable. They include fluid loss, dehydration, and dry, scaly skin caused by the continuous flow of warm, dry air through the filter sheet. This is prevented by extra fluid intake and the use of skin moisturizers. The low relative humidity of the bed environment causes drying of the nasal mucosa, which can potentially result in epistaxis. This is prevented by regular spraying of the nasal mucous with saline nasal spray; but with chronic use, hypernatremia may occur. Moreover, with prolonged periods in a "weightless" environment, hypophosphatemia and hypocalcemia may occur. As much as medically possible, the patient should be placed in the seated, semi-Fowler, or standing position, and laboratory work-ups should be performed regularly. Although turning and repositioning may be difficult in air-fluidized beds, they should be done regularly, otherwise new pressure ulcers may develop, especially at the heels. Due to the lack of a firm back support, the patient's cough mechanism may be rendered ineffective, and thick pulmonary secretions can develop. Pulmonary hygiene is, therefore, essential. Leakage of the silicone beads may cause eye injury to the patient and caregivers; therefore, the filter sheet should be inspected frequently for tears and, if necessary, replaced.

b. **Low-air loss bed (Alamo, Kin-air, Medicus)** consists of air-filled sacs that leak air slowly. A pump keeps the pillows filled to the desired firmess. It uses separate air-permeable sacs that are individually monitored to keep the pressure below 32 mm Hg in the area of bony prominences. Compared to air-fluidized beds, the low-air loss bed requires less volume of air to support the patient, which considerably reduces the noise and size of the blower unit and cost. It needs skilled setup, and, if adjusted properly, its pressures can be equivalent to air-fluidized beds. Its bed temperature can be easily regulated, and it has the additional advantage of allowing the patient to recline, or assume a semi-Fowler's position, thus making it useful for patients requiring both plastic surgery and rehabilitation for skin grafting, pressure ulcers, and burns.

5. **Systemic treatment of predisposing factors** can help prevent pressure ulcers (see treatment under section VII.A).

VII. Treatment
A. Systemic treatment of predisposing factors

1. **Restoration of nutrition** is necessary for wound healing especially in patients with nutritional deficiencies. On a tissue level, the critical local factor that causes skin breakdown is prolonged pressure. On a cellular level, however, the cells break down because they are unable to sustain metabolism because of poor delivery of nutrients and poor elimination of waste products. Fluid containing protein, vitamins, and minerals are lost continuously through the open surface of the pressure ulcer. Patients with pressure ulcers, therefore, should receive supplements of proteins, vitamins and minerals, in addition to their basic nutritional requirements. Adequate calories should also be provided to promote anabolism. Fluid intake must be increased (240 ml every 2 hours or at least 1 L/day) unless medically restricted.

   a. **Protein** must be available for wound granulation to occur. If pressure ulcers are present, the patient's protein requirements may rise to between 1.5 and 2.0 g/kg of ideal body weight to maintain a positive nitrogen balance and promote protein synthesis for healing. Fever, infection, or wound drainage can increase protein demands. The patient's serum protein should be maintained above 6 mg/dl. If the patient's serum albumin drops below 3.1 g/dl, aggressive protein feeding must begin. Protein is given by mouth in the form of nutritionally-complete food, but oral supplements or tube feedings may be used. Total parenteral nutrition is sometimes required. If the patient develops diarrhea because of the high protein and high calorie diet, the diet may be given every third meal to lessen gastrointestinal side effects.

   b. **Vitamin C** promotes collagen synthesis and should be supplemented orally at 1 g/day in divided doses. Excess vitamin C is excreted by the kidneys, and patients may be at risk for stone formation.

   c. **Zinc** is necessary for protein synthesis and repair. Zinc levels should be checked and supplemented only if deficient because excess zinc (more than 400 mg/dl) can interfere with macrophage function. The recommended daily allowance (RDA) for zinc is 15 mg. For zinc deficiencies, give 135 to 150 mg (9-10 times RDA) of elemental zinc daily, e.g., Zinkaps-220, 220 mg (containing 50 mg zinc), one tab, po, tid.

   d. **Vitamin and mineral deficiencies related to anemia** must be treated (see section VII.A.2).

2. **Treatment of anemia** is important because low hemoglobin (hgb) levels cause a lower blood oxygen content and, therefore, a decrease in oxygen delivered to the tissues. Patients with pressure ulcers often have hgb levels of 10g/dl or less because of decreased appetite, loss of serum and electrolytes from the ulcer, infection, and generalized debilitation. Malformation of red blood cells because of various nutritional deficiencies can further aggravate the problem. Nonnutritional-related anemia, such as blood loss through oozing of blood from the wound or from surgical debridement, may be treated with blood transfusion. When laboratory work-up shows anemia caused by the following nutritional deficiencies, they must be treated accordingly:

   a. **Iron deficiency:** Ferrous sulfate, 325 mg, po, tid.

   b. **Folate deficiency:** Folic acid, 1 mg, po, qd.

   c. **Vitamin B$_{12}$ deficiency (nonpernicious anemia).** 30 to 100 μg of cyanocobalamin (vitamin B_{12}), IM/SQ daily for 5 to 10 days depending on the severity of deficiency, followed by 100 to 200 µg/month or prn.

d. Vitamin B_6 deficiency: 10 to 20 mg of vitamin B_6 po or IM or IV daily for 3 weeks, then 2 to 5 mg daily as a supplement to a proper diet.

3. Relief of spasticity or spasm is important because these involuntary movements may cause skin breakdown as the body part rubs against bedsheets, clothing, bedrails, or adaptive equipment. Spasticity can also cause contractures that preclude proper positioning. Treatments include oral medications, positioning, physical modalities (e.g., cold), splints and orthoses, muscle or nerve blocks, and selective rhizotomy. Refer to Chapter 5.4 for details on treatment of spasticity.

4. Systemic antibiotics are only given if there is evidence of systemic infection or in ulcers with surrounding cellulitis. Antibiotic treatment should be combined with surgical debridement in soft-tissue infection or with osteotomy if there is osteomyelitis. Parenteral antibiotics for osteomyelitis are usually given for at least 6 to 8 weeks.

5. Incontinence care (see Chapter 5.7, section IV for bladder care, Chapter 5.8, section VI.A for bowel care) should be provided to prevent wound infection and skin maceration. Skin protection with barrier ointments or thick protective creams should be used. Incontinent patients should be checked frequently and urine or fecal materials should be cleaned immediately. Highly absorbency diapers may be used but should not replace frequent skin checks and cleaning. For male patients, an external (Texas) condom catheter may be used. For stage III or IV ulcers, an indwelling catheter (especially for female patients) or fecal collector may be used. In extreme cases, the patient may need diversion procedures for stool (e.g., colostomy or ileostomy) or urine (e.g., urostomy).

B. Pressure-reduction and pressure-relieving devices as outlined under section VI.B should be used.

C. Conservative wound care

1. Local wound care of pressure ulcers involve proper wound cleaning, debridement of necrotic tissue, and wound dressing. Pressure ulcers in any stage must be kept clean and dry. Any pressure on the wound should be reduced or relieved.

a. Stage I skin erythema heralds skin ulceration. Preventive measures outlined above (see section VI) should be strictly enforced. If there is skin induration, ice may be applied in the first 24 hours to decrease metabolic rate, decrease oxygen demand, and decrease inflammation.

b. Stage II pressure ulcer can either be a blister or an open wound. Blisters should be kept dry and pressure-free. When it breaks, it should be debrided (by sharp or surgical debridement method) and treated as a second-degree burn (e.g., silvadene dressing). If there is a dry superficial scab on the skin, leave it alone and just debride around the periphery.

c. Stage III and Stage IV pressure ulcer. If it is large, an air flotation bed may be needed for pressure relief. Surgery should be considered.

2. Periwound skin care. Periwound skin tissue injury may occur from mechanical stripping, shearing, or maceration of otherwise healthy tissue from prolonged exposure to moisture. Topical management approaches preclude aggressive adhesives on tissue with cutaneous atrophy because removal may result in stripping injuries. An effective approach for wounds with minimal atrophy of periwound skin would be to use a hydrogel in the wound bed with a secondary dressing and a nonadhesive dressing wrap, such as Coban self-adherent wrap. If drainage is significant, however, the periwound skin becomes macerated. A polyurethane foam dressing may be indicated at this point. It is easy to apply and may be secured with a nonadhesive wrap. Selection of a dressing that does not shift or become dislodged from the wound is particularly important for areas of maximum activity and irregular contour. Skin sealants (e.g., Skin Prep), solid form skin barriers (e.g., Stomahesive), or petrolatum ointments protect periwound skin from exudate or solutions used in wound care. These precautions are typically necessary when the wound is being packed with gauze. Maceration of the periwound skin when semipermeable dressings are used is an indication that exudate control is not effective. Absorption products, therefore, can be used in conjunction with hydrocolloids or other dressings.

3. **Growth factors** are currently being investigated for use in pressure ulcer healing. They include epidermal growth factors, fibroblast growth factors, transforming growth factor beta (TGFβ1), extracts of autologous human platelets (platelet-derived growth factors [PDGF]), and others.

4. **Physical modalities** such as electrical stimulation (see Chapter 4.1, section V) have been shown to promote wound healing in animal studies. Their utility and cost-effectiveness for pressure ulcer healing in human beings require further studies.

D. **Surgical care of pressure ulcers** is applicable to stage III or stage IV pressure ulcers. The goals of surgery are to reduce protein loss through the wound, prevent progressive osteomyelitis and sepsis, avoid progressive secondary amyloidosis and renal failure, reduce rehabilitation costs, improve patient hygiene and appearance, and avert future Marjolin's ulcer (a rare malignant degeneration, of a chronic pressure ulcer present for more than 20 years). In general, stage III and IV ulcers heal faster and generate less scar tissue when treated surgically. Although elderly patients are poor candidates for major surgery, they are unable to tolerate large, open pressure ulcers; therefore, simple rhomboid or bilobe flaps may be used in the elderly patient because sensation is intact.

1. **Preoperative care.** Pressure ulcer surgery should not be done until the patient's condition has stabilized, nutritional deficiencies have been corrected, and the pressure ulcer shows signs of improvement (i.e., all necrotic tissues are gone; evidence of healthy granulation tissue is present; and the ulcer is decreasing in size or shows reepithelization). Before surgery, the patient must be well-hydrated and have a hematocrit above 30. If necessary, packed red blood cells (PRBC) may be transfused. Any infections such as urinary tract infections (UTI) should be treated. Immediately before surgery, all patients should be given antibiotics and maintained on them postoperatively until the drains are out (at least 2 weeks in uncomplicated cases).

2. **Surgical closures.** Surgery usually involves total excision of the ulcer, surrounding scar, and underlying bursae and soft tissue calcification. All infected bones should be completely removed, and bony prominences should be recontoured. The wound defect is then closed using one of the following methods:

a. **Primary (direct) closure** consists of excision of the ulcer margin to convert it into an ellipse. The skin margins are then sutured to obliterate the dead space. Direct closure can usually be completed as an outpatient procedure in a day surgery unit. It is inappropriate for large ulcers because paucity of soft tissue coverage can lead to excessive wound tension and poor healing. In this case, tissue expanders may be used to provide more skin surface and to facilitate closure. After direct closure, the patient must keep pressure off the area for 2 weeks. If there is good healing, the patient may be allowed to put short minimal pressure (e.g., sitting) on it after the second week. The sutures are removed on the third week. With this form of treatment, the patient loses a minimum of time and can remain reasonably active.

b. **Skin grafts** are skin segments separated from their blood supply and transplanted from the donor site to the surface of the wound. They provide only skin barrier and when applied directly to granulating bone, they quickly erode, precluding healing. The transplanted skin is never as "tough" as the original skin.

1) **Partial thickness or split-thickness skin graft (STSG)** consists of the epidermis and only a portion of the underlying dermis. The STSG is more likely to survive than full-thickness skin graft (FTSG) because STSG can tolerate a longer phase of plasmatic absorption and, therefore, can survive longer before vascularization occurs. A STSG is the method of choice for shallow defects without exposed bone in sensate patients (e.g., shallow sacral ulcers). It is not indicated for ischial and trochanteric ulcers. The graft site needs to be continually lubricated because it does not contain dermal appendages (i.e., sweat glands and hair follicles).

2) **Full-thickness skin graft** consists of the epidermis and all of the dermis, and is less likely to survive than STSG.

c. **Skin flap** is used when the wound is too extensive for primary closure and loss of tissue mass precludes grafting. It consists of a "tongue" of skin and subcutaneous tissues detached from its surrounding tissue except for a pedicle or base, through which blood supply is maintained. Usually, patients need to be hospitalized for 4 to 6 weeks. Skin flaps are used to cover ischial, trochanteric, or sacral ulcers.

d. **Myocutaneous flaps** consists of a composite of skin, subcutaneous tissue, and underlying muscle, detached from its surrounding tissue with the major blood supply (which enters the proximal undersurface of the muscle) kept intact. It helps eliminate dead space in a deep wound, enhances perfusion and tissue coaptation, and provides a temporary pad for wider dispersion of residual pressure. It can also help heal osteomyelitis, and limit the damage caused by shearing, friction, and pressure. It is the procedure of choice for nonambulatory patients with SCI or when loss of muscle function (of the muscle being flapped) does not contribute to comorbidity. In ambulatory patients, the sacrifice of functional muscle units must be weighted against the need for good wound healing. Myocutaneous flaps can be used for sacral, ischial, and trochanteric ulcers. The most commonly used myocutaneous flaps are tensor fascia lata, posterior hamstring, and gluteal flaps. When the myocutaneous flap is placed over a bony prominence not normally covered by muscle, it eventually atrophies. The pressure ulcer may recur as early as 9.3 months in 61% of pressure ulcers treated.

e. **Free flaps** are muscle-type flaps (usually from latissimus dorsi muscle) in which the vein and artery are disconnected at the donor site and reanastomosed to the vessels at the recipient site by microsurgical techniques. It is used as endstage salvage procedure for recurrent deep ulcers (e.g., ischial ulcers).

f. **Amputation and fillet procedures** are reserved for those patients who have extensive or combined ulcerations, with or without underlying osteomyelitis, and those who cannot be treated successfully with any of the procedures previously described. The amputation (unilateral or bilateral) can be transfemoral (above-knee) with removal (fillet) of the femur and use of the entire thigh for flap coverage. A more extensive procedure comprises amputation at the level of the ankle and fillet of the entire leg to provide the largest possible amount of muscle and subcutaneous tissue to cover the defects. These patients should be referred for psychological counseling when faced with the consequences of amputation.

3. **Surgical procedure selection**

   a. **Sacral pressure ulcers** are best managed with myocutaneous flaps using the gluteus maximus muscle. If the ulcer is shallow (without bone exposure and with good sensation), it can be treated with skin grafting.

   b. **Ischial pressure ulcers** have high rates of recurrence in the seated position and are usually associated with osteomyelitis. Skin graft is not indicated. A local myocutaneous flap using gluteus maximus combined with partial ischiectomy is appropriate for first treatment of deep ischial ulcers. Distant flaps using gracilis muscles, tensor fascia lata (TFL) muscle, or hamstring (biceps femoris) may also be used. As endstage salvage procedure for recurrent deep ischial ulcers, free flaps can be brought from distant sites to provide additional padding.

   c. **Trochanteric ulcers** are best managed with myocutaneous flaps. The local TFL flap is most useful for uncomplicated medium sized ulcers, while the local vastus lateralis muscle flap or the distant gluteal thigh flaps are used for larger, deeper ulcers. Skin grafts should not be used for trochanter ulcers.

   d. **Multiple pressure ulcers or combined pressure ulcers** have large soft tissue defects and are usually associated with osteomyelitis. A myocutaneous flap using the TFL may be used to cover trochanteric and ischial ulcers. If the ulcer is extensive, and all other procedures have failed, then the amputation and fillet procedure may be done.

4. **Postoperative care.** Suction drains (used to prevent hemostasis) are usually left for at least 2 weeks and removed when output is less than 30 ml/24 hours. Drains should be frequently stripped to prevent blockage. After surgery, the patient is usually kept prone for 2 to 4 weeks. If the patient is unable to tolerate the prone position (e.g., due to poor pulmonary reserve), an air-flotation bed (air-fluidized or low-air loss) may be used to allow placement in the supine position. To decrease the need for turning the patient and to prevent soiling and contamination of the surgical site, an indwelling catheter or a fecal incontinence bag is recommended until all drains are removed. Custom padding and scrotal supports, which are prepared preoperatively, are used to help prevent iatrogenic pressure ulcers. Oral feeding and bowel feeding are restarted 3 days postoperatively. Antibiotics given preoperatively are adjusted according to the intraoperative cultures and biopsies. For uncomplicated cases, antibiotics are used for 2 weeks. If there is evidence of osteomyelitis, they are used for 6 to 8 weeks. The dressing from the operating room should be removed on

the third postoperative day, and the wound should be allowed to remain open to the drying effects of the air. Only the drain sites or skin grafts need a protective dressing. Sutures are usually left in place for 3 weeks. Antispasmodic and antispasticity drugs are used to decrease the risk of bleeding and hematoma formation caused by involuntary movements. Patients are usually kept on bedrest 2, 3, or 6 weeks depending on wound healing. Then gradual mobilization is started.

5. **Postsurgical complications**
   a. **Immediate postoperative complications** include hematoma, seroma, infection, and wound separation caused by tension—all of which can lead to flap necrosis. These can be prevented by good surgical techniques, proper hemostasis procedures (e.g., surgical drain for 2 weeks after surgery and fibrin sealant), and adequate antibiotics.
   b. **Long-term postoperative complications** include ulcer recurrence (in 40-50% of cases) caused by persistent osteomyelitis, inadequate osteotomy, a large surgical scar, and a persistent sinus tract. When identified early, these complications can be corrected by appropriate secondary procedures (e.g., more extensive osteotomy and sinus tract resection). Another common cause of recurrence is excessive pressure on the surgical site, which should be prevented by educating the patient and caretaker to strictly comply with the preventive measures outlined in section VI.

BIBLIOGRAPHY

Bergstrom N, Bennett MA, Carlson CE, et al: *Treatment of pressure ulcers*, Clinical Practice Guideline Number 14. AHCPR Publication No. 95-0642, Rockville, MD, 1994, Agency for Health Care Policy and Research, US Dept of Health and Human Services.

Bergstrom N and the Panel for the Prediction and Prevention of Pressure Ulcers in Adults: *Pressure ulcers in adults: prediction and prevention*, Clinical Practice Guideline Number 3. AHCPR Publication No. 92-0047. Rockville, MD, 1992, Agency for Health Care Policy and Research, US Dept of Health and Human Services.

Bryant R: *Acute and chronic wounds: nursing management*, St. Louis, 1992, Mosby–Year Book.

Constantian MB: *Pressure ulcers: principles and techniques of management*, Boston, 1980, Little, Brown.

Donovan WH, Dinh TA, Garber SL, et al: Pressure ulcers. In DeLisa JA Gans BM, editors: *Rehabilitation medicine: principles and practice*, ed 2, Philadelphia, 1993, JB Lippincott, pp. 716-732.

Kosiak M: Etiology of decubitus ulcers, *Arch Phys Med Rehabil*, 42:19-28, 1961.

Krasner D: *Chronic wound care: a clinical source book for health care professionals*, King of Prussia, 1990, Health Management Publications, pp. 74-77, 152-56.

Salcido R, Hart D, Smith AM: The prevention and management of pressure ulcers. In Braddom RL, editor: *Physical medicine and rehabilitation*, Philadelphia, 1996, WB Saunders, pp. 630-647.

Yarkony GM: Pressure ulcers: a review, *Arch Phys Med Rehabil* 75:908-917, 1994.

CHAPTER 5.3

VENOUS THROMBOEMBOLISM

Venous thromboembolism is a frequent occurrence in PM&R in-patients and out-patients. It can involve the superficial or deep veins of the limbs. Superficial thrombophlebitis poses little risk for embolism and is generally controlled by supportive measures (i.e., local heat, elevation of the affected limb, rest, and, if needed, antiinflammatory agents such as aspirin). On the other hand, deep-vein thrombosis (DVT) presents a more difficult diagnostic and therapeutic problem and is associated with a significant risk of pulmonary embolism. This chapter deals mainly with DVT and its major complication, pulmonary embolism (PE).

I. **Pathophysiology.** The calf veins are the earliest and most frequent sites for DVT. The initial lesion begins (intimal lesion is not necessary) as a platelet nidus in the pocket behind a valve cusp of the vein (usually caused by venous stasis). There is activation of thrombin through the coagulation cascade leading to irreversible platelet aggregation and thrombus formation. The subsequent fate of the thrombus depends on the continued formation of fibrin, the degree of local fibrinolytic activity, and blood flow rate. It organizes and becomes adherent to the vein wall in 7 to 10 days then resolves through fibrinolysis. Occasionally the thrombus may dislodge and form a pulmonary embolism. In rehabilitation the following three factors (Virchow's triad) increase the risk of DVT:

A. **Venous stasis** is the principal factor contributing to the DVT formation of the lower limbs. It can be caused by bed rest; immobility (increased risk in paralyzed limbs of patients with stroke or spinal cord injury [SCI]); general anesthesia exceeding 30 minutes (blood flow velocity decreases by 50% in the external iliac and popliteal veins); surgery (possibly due to vein compression during recumbency, use of a tourniquet, or mechanical trauma to femoral or iliac veins); medical problems such as obesity, hypotension, diabetes mellitus, stasis dermatitis, varicosities, circulatory compromise due to congestive heart failure, sepsis, prior DVT (increased risk by 2-3 times if previous DVT is confirmed by objective test); and age (risk to those over 40 years is moderate to high, but for those over 50 years, it increases exponentially).

B. **Endothelial injury to the vessel wall** includes direct trauma, surgery (e.g., during total hip or knee replacement, surgery can cause kinking of vein; scissoring of the femoral vein between the internally rotated femur and pubis; and manipulation and traction of the anterior hip structures especially in anterior dislocation approach), tissue hypoxia, previous venous thrombosis, infection, and labor trauma (this probably accounts for the increased risk in the postpartum period compared to normal risk during pregnancy).

C. **Increased coagulability** plays a limited role. It is caused by altered blood elements; dehydration; increase of platelet aggregation (in SCI); increased fibrinogen during acute inflammatory response; acquired deficiencies including postoperative decrease in antithrombin III; medical problems such as diabetes mellitus, malignancy (particularly adenocarcinoma of the lung, breast, and viscera), and inflammatory bowel disease; and use of oral contraceptives. A rare cause of hypercoagulability is a congenital defect in coagulant inhibitors (e.g., deficiencies in protein C, protein S, and antithrombin III).

Table 5.3-1. Incidence of deep vein thrombosis (DVT) and pulmonary embolism (PE); and successful prophylaxis methods classified by level of risk as recommended by the Fourth American College of Chest Physicians (ACCP) Consensus Conference on Antithrombotic Therapy (1995)

LEVEL OF RISK	CALF DVT (%)	PROXIMAL DVT (%)	CLINICAL PE (%)	FATAL PE (%)	EFFECTIVE DVT/PE PROPHYLAXIS
Low risk (uncomplicated minor surgery in patients under 40 yr with no clinical risk factors)	2	0.4	0.2	0.002	No specific measures
Moderate risk (major surgery in patients over 40 yr with no other risk factors)	10-20	2-4	1-2	0.1-0.4	1. Compressive stockings, 2. LDUH (q12h, SQ), or 3. IPLC
High risk (major surgery in patients over 40 yr who have additional risk factors or myocardial infarction)	20-40	4-8	2-4	0.4-1.0	1. LDUH (q8h, SQ), 2. LMWH, or 3. IPLC
Very high risk (major surgery in patients over 40 yr with previous venous thromboembolism, malignancy, orthopedic surgery, hip fracture, stroke, or spinal cord injury)	40-80	10-20	4-10	1-5	1. LMWH, 2. Warfarin, 3. IPLC (with LDUH or LMWH), or 4. ADUH

Adapted from Salzman EW, Hirsch J: Prevention of venous thromboembolism. In Colman RW, Hirsch J, Marder VJ, et al: *Hemostasis and thrombosis: basic principles and clinical practice*, ed 3, Philadelphia, 1994, JB Lippincott, p. 1332, with permission, and Clagett GP, Anderson FA, Jr, Heit J, et al: Prevention of venous thromboembolism, *Chest Suppl* 108(4):316S, 1995, with permission.
IPLC = intermittent pneumatic leg compression; LDUH = low-dose unfractionated heparin; ADUH = adjusted dose unfractionated heparin; LMWH = low molecular weight heparin.

II. **Epidemiology of DVT** is tabulated in Table 5.3-1.

III. **Diagnosis of DVT**

A. **Clinical evaluation** for the diagnosis of DVT is insensitive and nonspecific. The majority of patients with DVT are clinically silent (probably because the vein is not totally obstructed and because of collateral circulation). Physical examination fails to detect 50 to 90% of DVTs. In more than 50% of patients with a clinical diagnosis of DVT, venography is unable to definitely confirm it. Clinical findings often associated with DVT include pain and tenderness (vague and nonspecific; located at the calf, popliteal fossa, posterior thigh; aggravated by ankle movement); leg swelling (may be localized or pitting; aggravated by prolonged sitting or early ambulation; usually subsides after the leg is elevated); Homan's sign (calf or popliteal pain with forced dorsiflexion of the ankle; an insensitive and nonspecific clinical test for DVT, which is present only with complete occlusion, and even then it is present in only 70% of such cases; Homan's test is discouraged because if a DVT is present, the thrombus may be dislodged and may embolize); palpable cord (in the groin, popliteal fossa, or upper calf); superficial venous distention (around the knee, groin, or anterior abdominal wall; relieved by leg elevation); and fever (usually low-grade). Differential diagnoses for these clinical findings include muscle injury with strain, tear, or hematoma; cellulitis; superficial

thrombophlebitis in a varicose vein; Achilles tendinitis; bursitis; and a ruptured
Baker's cyst. Because the clinical diagnosis of DVT is unreliable, more definitive diagnostic tests (invasive or noninvasive) must be done if DVT (or PE)
is suspected.

B. **Diagnostic tests**

1. **Noninvasive tests** (see Chapter 2.2, section III). Duplex scanning (using
   color-flow doppler scanning [CFDS]) and impedance plethysmography
   (IPG) are considered ideal for monitoring patients who are at risk for DVT
   because they are highly sensitive and are safe to perform serially. The IPG
   test is the most cost-effective in DVT diagnosis especially in symptomatic
   patients. Formal studies on the cost effectiveness of duplex scanning are
   not available; however, there is greater cost with duplex scanning (equipment costs $100,000 to $200,000 vs. about $15,000 for an IPG unit, and
   operating costs are higher for duplex scanning). If the IPG or duplex scan
   study is negative in a symptomatic patient (i.e., patients with clinical features suggestive of DVT), then it is safe to withhold anticoagulant therapy.
   This is because the diagnosis of thrombosis of the proximal vein (i.e.,
   popliteal, femoral, and iliac vein) is virtually excluded if the IPG or duplex
   scan is negative. Even if a calf thrombos remain undetected (because
   IPG and duplex scanning are insensitive for detection of calf thrombi),
   they rarely embolize while confined to the calf. The initial negative IPG
   or duplex scan in a symptomatic patient with high suspicion of DVT should
   either be confirmed by venography or the noninvasive test (either IPG or
   duplex scanning) repeated serially several times during the next 10 to 14
   days. If the results of the noninvasive test are equivocal, venography
   should be done. On the other hand, if IPG or duplex scan becomes positive,
   prompt anticoagulation is warranted. In patients with no DVT symptoms,
   the available noninvasive tests are unsatisfactory for DVT screening due
   to low sensitivity.

   a. **Venous duplex scanning** is a form of vascular ultrasonography (see Chapter
      2.2, section III.E.2.b) that combines pulsed-wave doppler (for detection
      and localization of abnormal blood flow) with high-resolution, real-
      time, B-mode ultrasound imaging (for morphologic confirmation of the
      venous thrombosis). The venous doppler uses the following compressive
      technique for detection of DVT: (1) a doppler sensor is placed over the
      femoral vein with a background signal elicited (the S sound), which
      fluctuates significantly with respiration (i.e., venous flow increased with
      expiration or decreased with inspiration); (2) the thigh vein is then com-
      pressed gently at several distal points (e.g., midthigh) via external pres-
      sure from the hand-held ultrasound transducer, and the normal response
      is an augmented tone (the A sound); and (3) this process is then repeated
      with the sensor placed over the popliteal and posterior tibial veins, and
      the compression is applied distally at the calf and foot respectively. In
      the presence of DVT, the A sound is absent (i.e., there is failure of
      signal augmentation) or the S sound does not fluctuate significantly with
      respiration or the vein is noncompressible (i.e., the vein does not collapse
      under a force sufficient to distort the artery). The thrombus can be visual-
      ized either directly using the B-mode, grey scale or indirectly by the
      lack of color in the lumen using **color-flow duplex scanning (CFDS).** When
      the thrombi are visible, their echo characteristics may help determine
      their age and distinguish acute from chronic venous occlusion.

      Duplex scanning is highly accurate in detecting occluded proximal

DVT but is less accurate in detecting calf DVT (because the calf vein is difficult to compress) or nonobstructing proximal DVTs. In symptomatic patients, the high sensitivity (97%) and specificity (97%) of duplex scanning are slightly better than those of IPG; however, in nonsymptomatic patients, the sensitivity drops to 59%. In symptomatic patients, duplex scanning in itself is sufficient in confirming or disproving suspected cases of DVT, as long as a negative examination is followed by repeated noninvasive testing to detect proximal extension. In patients with clinical suspicion of isolated calf vein thrombosis, a venogram is recommended or the duplex scanning may be repeated every 2 to 3 days for 10 to 14 days to document possible progression of a suspected thrombosis. Duplex scanning is not as convenient as IPG (although some equipment may be transported to the bedside, they are not as easy to handle as an IPG unit).

b. Plethysmography (see Chapter 2.2, section IV.B)

1) Impedance plethysmography (IPG) assesses limb volume by detecting changes in the electrical impedance between two electrodes wrapped around the calf. A thigh cuff is inflated to obstruct venous flow and increase limb volume. Once the cuff is deflated, the limb volume returns to normal size within 3 to 4 seconds. If there is a venous obstruction proximal to the electrodes, the return to baseline is delayed when the cuff is deflated. In symptomatic patients, IPG has high sensitivity (92%) and specificity (95%) comparable to duplex scanning in the diagnosis of proximal DVT. False-negative results occur in patients with distal (calf) thrombi, small nonocclusive proximal thrombi, or when there are sufficient collateral veins. Hence the sensitivity of IPG drops to as low as 22% in nonsymptomatic patients, many of whom have non-occluding thrombi. False-positive IPG tests may occur in patients with congestive cardiac (right heart) failure, excessive leg muscle tension, severe peripheral vascular disease, postoperative lower limb swelling, enlarged pelvic lymph nodes, in patients receiving mechanical ventilation, and in pregnant patients. When these conditions are present, either duplex scanning or venography may be used. In symptomatic patients, if serial IPG is persistently negative, then it is safe to withhold anticoagulation.

2) Phleborheography (PRG) is a sophisticated form of whole leg plethysmography using multiple air-filled cuffs to detect volume changes. Early studies show that its sensitivity and specificity are comparable to those of IPG, however, it is not widely used because it is time consuming and its interpretation is subjective.

2. Invasive tests (see Chapter 2.3, section II.A)

a. Venography (phlebography) of the lower limb is accepted as the final diagnostic test for determining proximal DVT and distal DVT. It is not used routinely nor serially because it is costly, painful, and can cause local venous or skin injury, secondary thrombophlebitis (in 2-3% of patients), and hypersensitivity reactions to the contrast medium. Its use is justified when the diagnosis of DVT requires confirmation in symptomatic patients (e.g., clinical suspicion of isolated calf DVT), when recurrent DVT is suspected, or when patients who have undergone hip operations require screening for postoperative DVT, but less invasive methods lack sensitivity. In such cases, the cost of venography is substantially less than the cost of hospitalization and the treatment for an incorrectly diagnosed illness. A positive venogram warrants prompt anticoagulation. However, a negative venogram does not guarantee that the patient will not develop a late pulmonary embolism even if the chance is extremely small.

   b. Magnetic resonance venography has high sensitivity (87-100%) and specificity (97%) but is generally unavailable because of its cost.

   c. Radionuclide venography can be used to detect proximal DVT. A labeled sample of the patient's platelets, proteins, or red cells is used to highlight the veins of the lower limbs for imaging. The label can either be a radioactive marker or a radiopharmaceutical solution injected into a vein in the foot. Radionuclide venography is still in the developmental stage.

   d. Radioiodine [^{125}I]-labeled fibrinogen, once widely used, has been withdrawn from the U.S. market because it uses blood products and carries the risk of virus transmission (e.g., hepatitis).

C. Laboratory work-ups such as protein S, protein C, fibrinogen, antithrombin III levels, lupus anticoagulant, and anticardiolipin antibodies are indicated (prior to anticoagulation) in young patients with DVT, patients with recurrent DVT without obvious causes, and those with a family history of thrombotic disease.

IV. DVT prophylaxis in patients at risk is highly recommended for the following reasons: (1) The incidence of DVT and PE remains too high for a condition that is preventable (see Table 5.3-1); (2) DVT and PE are clinically silent with few specific clinical manifestations; moreover, clinical diagnosis for DVT is insensitive and unreliable; (3) Use of serial surveillance (e.g., IPG and duplex scanning) is expensive and has only moderate sensitivity and moderate positive predictive value when used in nonsymptomatic high-risk patients; (4) To rely on the diagnosis and treatment of established DVT may expose susceptible patients to unacceptable risk: Although anticoagulant therapy is highly effective in treating DVTs, most patients who die of PE do so within 30 minutes of the acute event, too soon for the anticoagulant to be effective; (5) Unrecognized and untreated DVTs may lead to long-term morbidity from postphlebitic syndrome and predispose patients to future episodes of recurrent DVT; (6) Although there is legitimate concern about bleeding (e.g., hematoma in surgical patients, which can result in wound infection, dehiscence, or infection of the implanted prosthetic device), studies have shown that there is no significant increase in major bleeding with low-dose unfractionated heparin (LDUH) or low-molecular-weight heparin (LMWH): Besides, alternative mechanical methods of effective DVT prophylaxis that carry no bleeding risk (e.g., intermittent pneumatic leg compression) are available; 7) Studies have shown that broad application of DVT prophylaxis is cost-effective.

Effective DVT prophylaxis methods for different levels of DVT risk are summarized in Table 5.3-1. Deep-vein thrombosis prophylaxis for specific conditions commonly encountered in PM&R are shown in Table 5.3-2. Despite prophylaxis, nonsymptomatic DVT and PE may still develop. Although there are sufficient data to make recommendations for the type of DVT prophylaxis, the decision on when to stop DVT prophylaxis remains controversial. For elective total hip replacement (THR) and total knee replacement (TKR), the American College of Chest Physicians (ACCP) recommends at least 7 to 10 days after surgery, regardless of hospital length of stay, although the significant risk of DVT may persist for at least 2 months. For acute nonambulatory SCI patients, the ACCP recommends at least 3 months of DVT prophylaxis. For the other conditions listed in Table 5.3-2, the clinical data are insufficient to make a definite recommendation about duration of prophylaxis. It is very likely that

Table 5.3-2. **DVT prophylaxis in common PM&R conditions as recommended by the Fourth American College of Chest Physicians (ACCP) Consensus Conference on Antithrombotic Therapy (1995)**

PM&R CONDITIONS	ACCP RECOMMENDATION FOR DVT PROPHYLAXIS
Total hip replacement surgery	1. LMWH (postoperative), warfarin (started preoperatively or immediately after surgery), or ADUH (started preoperatively) are most effective for routine use. 2. Adjuvant prophylaxis with CS or IPLC may provide additional efficacy. 3. LDUH, aspirin, dextran, and IPLC are less effective and should not be used routinely.
Total knee replacement surgery	Either LMWH (postoperative) or IPLC is effective for routine prophylaxis.
Hip fracture surgery	1. LMWH (preoperative) or warfarin is most effective for routine prophylaxis 2. IPLC combined with either LMWH or warfarin may provide additional benefit.
Ischemic stroke	1. LDUH or LMWH are effective. 2. IPLC and CS are also probably effective.
Acute spinal cord injury (SCI)	1. ADUH or LMWH is recommended for prophylaxis. 2. Warfarin prophylaxis may also be effective. 3. LDUH, CS, and IPLC when used alone appear ineffective and are not recommended, but these methods may have benefit when used together.
Elective intracranial neurosurgery	1. IPLC with or without CS is recommended. 2. LDUH may be an acceptable alternative (start 2 weeks postoperatively). 3. IPLC and LDUH may be more effective in combination than individually, and should be considered in high-risk patients.
Multiple trauma	1. IPLC, warfarin, or LMWH is recommended. 2. Serial surveillance (with duplex scanning) may be a successful strategy. 3. Prophylactic vena caval filter placement may be used in selected very high risk patients (e.g., lower limb fracture, SCI, indwelling femoral venous catheter).

Data tabulated from Clagett GP, Anderson FA Jr, Heit J, et al: Prevention of venous thromboembolism, *Chest* 108(4) suppl:312S–334S, 1995.
IPLC = intermittent pneumatic leg compression; LDUH = low-dose unfractionated heparin; ADUH = adjusted dose unfractionated heparin; LMWH = low molecular weight heparin CS = compressive stockings.

the risk of DVT is not uniform but varies according to the presence of other risk factors. Most studies report that more severe weakness is associated with a higher risk of DVT, and that more venous thromboembolic events occur in nonambulatory patients. These observations suggest that the risk of late DVT in stroke has a strong relationship to persisting leg weakness and nonambulatory status, and might not be a simple function of time. The evidence supports the value of continuing DVT prophylaxis into the postacute rehabilitation phase until the risk of DVT is low. The best assessment of risk is made on clinical grounds, including consideration of degree of leg weakness and ambulatory status.

A. **Physical or mechanical DVT prophylaxis** has the advantage of being safe, effective, relatively inexpensive, well tolerated by most patients, and not associated with hemorrhagic complications.

1. **Intermittent pneumatic leg compression (IPLC)** provides rhythmic external compression (inflation pressure of 35-40 mm Hg lasting 10 seconds/min for each compression) by intermittent compression of the legs with inflatable leggings. It prevents venous stasis using sequential application of pressure that cyclically increases the venous blood flow velocity from the ankle to the thigh. It also stimulates intrinsic fibrinolysis attributed to the intermittent compression. It is effective in preventing distal DVT formation but has the same effect as placebo in preventing proximal DVT. The duration of daily compression is probably an important factor in determining the effectiveness of IPLC. Hence it may not be as effective in a rehabilitation setting where patients spend considerable time out of bed in therapeutic and recreational activities.

   If IPLC is used at all for DVT prophylaxis in a rehabilitation unit, the leggings should be applied with the compression pump on whenever the patient is in bed. Intermittent pneumatic leg compression is recommended for DVT prophylaxis in moderate-, high-, and very-high-risk patients (see Table 5.3-1). It is effective, by itself, for DVT prophylaxis in patients with total knee replacement; ischemic stroke; intracranial neurosurgery; and multiple trauma. It is effective when combined with other prophylactic agents in THR and SCI. It may also be effectively used in patients in whom anticoagulants are contraindicated because of the risk of hemorrhage, for example, in patients with intracranial hemorrhage or prior history of gastrointestinal bleeding).

2. **Compression stockings (CS) (antiembolic stockings, thromboembolytic disease [TED] hose)** are graded compression elastic stockings, either knee- or thigh-high, available in different standard sizes. They must be applied evenly (without being rolled) so that circulation to the legs is not obstructed. They can control leg edema and reduce the risk of leg DVT, but their effectiveness on proximal DVT prophylaxis remains to be proved. They provide adequate DVT prophylaxis in patients with low-to-moderate risk of DVT. The conditions in which they have been shown to be effective are ischemic stroke (probably effective), total hip replacement (effective as adjuvant prophylaxis), acute SCI (may be beneficial when used with LDUH and IPLC), and intracranial neurosurgery (effective when used with IPLC). In patients who cannot tolerate CS, Ace bandages are an alternative; however, unless the Ace bandage is wrapped properly around the legs (i.e., with adequate pressure to provide decreasing compression from distal to proximal) and maintained throughout the day, they are probably less effective than CS for DVT prophylaxis. Most studies on DVT prophylaxis used CS instead of Ace wrap because CS are more convenient to apply and easier to standardize.

3. **Mobilization (exercises and ambulation)** can help improve peripheral venous flow in the legs and reduce venous stasis; however, they are not adequate in and of themselves for DVT prophylaxis. They include active range-of-motion (ROM) exercises, for example, active contraction of the calf muscle (ankle pumps), passive ROM exercises, use of continuous passive motion

(CPM) machines (their effectiveness in DVT prophylaxis after total knee or hip replacements remains controversial), leg elevation to help reduce leg swelling, and early ambulation (although there is no data available, most physiatrists use ambulation distance as a guide in terminating DVT prophylaxis especially in postsurgical patients).

4. **Functional electrical stimulation (FES)** has been tried for DVT prophylaxis in patients with acute SCI and stroke. It supposedly increases fibrinolytic activity and causes mild to moderate increase in venous flow thus reducing incidence of DVT; however, it has the problem of poor compliance due to discomfort and blister formation. Its effectiveness remains to be proven.

B. **Pharmacological DVT prophylaxis** (see Tables 5.3-1 and 5.3-2)

1. **Anticoagulant drugs**

   a. **Warfarin (Coumadin, Panwarfin)** (see Chapter 4.8, section VII.A.1) are used for DVT prophylaxis in very-high-risk patients, specifically in patients with THR (effective when given preoperatively [on the evening prior to surgery] or immediately postoperatively), hip fracture surgery (may be effective when combined with IPLC), and acute SCI. It may be used in patients with multiple trauma if feasible. Due to hemorrhagic complications, it is not recommended for DVT prophylaxis in patients with TKR, ischemic stroke, hemorrhagic stroke, or intracranial neurosurgery. It must be monitored regularly to maintain international normalized ratio (INR) at 2.0 to 3.0. If the INR is above the therapeutic range, refer to the ACCP guidelines in Table 5.3-3. Unexpected fluctuations in dose response could be attributed to changes in diet (e.g., high vitamin K–diet) or undisclosed drug use (see Table 4.8-10 for drug and food interactions), inaccuracy of prothrombin time testing, poor patient compliance, surreptitious self-medication, or intermittent alcohol consumption.

   b. **Heparin (unfractionated heparin)** (see Chapter 4.8, section VII.A)

      1) **Low-dose unfractionated heparin** can be given subcutaneously in a fixed dose of 5000 U q8-12h for the prevention of DVT in moderate- and high-risk patients. In very-high-risk patients, it may be used effectively with IPLC. Specific conditions include: ischemic stroke, acute SCI (may be effective only when combined with CS and IPLC), neurosurgery (may be an acceptable alternative when given 2 weeks postoperatively and combined with IPLC). It is not recommended in THR, TKR, and hip fracture surgery. Low-dose unfractionated heparin does not require activated partial thromboplastin time (aPTT) monitoring.

      2) **Adjusted-dose unfractionated heparin (ADUH)** can be given by IV (or SQ) route for DVT prophylaxis in very-high-risk patients, specifically patients with THR (start preoperatively) and acute SCI. It is not recommended in patients with TKR, hip fracture surgery, stroke, intracranial neurosurgery, and multiple trauma. It must be monitored regularly to keep aPTT at about 1.5 to 2.5 times normal (see Tables 5.3-4 or 5.3-5 for guidelines on adjusting IV heparin either by using or not using body weight). A commonly used alternative method is to load 5000 U of IV ADUH then infuse 25,000 U in 250 ml 5% dextrose in water (D_5W) or normal saline (NS) (i.e., 100 U/ml) at 800 to 1000 U/hour (8-10 ml/hour) and adjust at the rate 100 U/hour as needed until the therapeutic dose (aPTT of 1.5 to 2.0 × the normal value) is reached. Length of anticoagulation is 5 to 10 days with

Table 5.3-3. **Management of patients with prolonged INR as recommended by the Fourth American College of Chest Physicians (ACCP) Consensus Conference on Antithrombotic Therapy (1995)**

INR	SYMPTOMS	ACCP RECOMMENDATION
Above therapeutic range but less than 6	No bleeding	Withhold warfarin for next few days.*
6-10	No bleeding	Give 1-2 mg of vitamin K_1†; the INR should be reduced in 8 hrs and be in the therapeutic range within 24 hr.* If INR is still too high at 24 hr, give additional 0.5 mg of vitamin K_1.
10-20	No bleeding	Give 3 mg of vitamin K_1; the INR should be reduced in 6 hr,* check INR q6 h and repeat vitamin K_1 as necessary.
Above 20	Serious bleeding	Give 10 mg of vitamin K_1 and supplement with transfusion of fresh frozen plasma (FFP), 2-4 U, or factor concentrates depending on the urgency of the situation; check INR q6 h; repeat vitamin K_1 q12 h if needed.
	Life-threatening bleeding or serious warfarin overdosage	Transfuse factor concentrates (preferably containing factor VII) and supplement with 10 mg of vitamin K_1 (IV route is preferred), which can be repeated as necessary depending on the INR.

Data tabulated from Hirsch J, Dalen JE, Deykin D, et al: Oral anticoagulants: mechanism of action, clinical effectiveness, and optimal therapeutic range, *Chest* 108 (4) suppl: 238S, 1995, with permission.

* When INR returns to the therapeutic range, resume warfarin (if still indicated) at a lower dose.

† Vitamin K_1 or phytonadione (Mephyton, AquaMephyton) is preferably given by SQ route. If given by IV route it should be diluted and infused over 20-30 min. If warfarin therapy needs to be resumed after high doses of vitamin K_1 (e.g., 10-15 mg, which may cause resistance to warfarin for up to a week), then heparin can be given until the effects of vitamin K_1 have been reversed and the patient becomes responsive to warfarin.

warfarin administered jointly with heparin for 4 to 5 days (see Chapter 4.8, section VII.A.2).

    c. Low-molecular-weight heparin (Enoxaparin [Lovenox]) (see Chapter 4.8, section VII.A.3 for details) can be given 30 mg, SQ, bid, for DVT prophylaxis in high and very-high risk patients. It is recommended preoperatively in hip fracture surgery (may be combined with IPLC) and postoperatively (started within 12-24 hrs after surgery provided hemostasis has been established) in patients with THR and TKR. It is also recommended in patients with stroke (within 48 hours), acute SCI, and multiple trauma. It is not recommended for patients with intracranial neurosurgery. Low-molecular weight heparin does not require aPTT monitoring. The duration of treatment (about 7 to 14 days) remains controversial.

  2. Antiplatelet drugs (see Chapter 4.8, section VII.B) are generally *not* recom-

Table 5.3-4. Guidelines for adjusting dose of IV unfractionated heparin using body weight

aPTT	DOSE ADJUSTMENT
<35 s (<1.2 times control)	Rebolus 80 U/kg, then increase rate by 4 U/kg/h
35 to 45 s (1.2-1.5 times control)	Rebolus 40 U/kg, then increase rate 2 U/kg/h
46 to 70 s (1.5-2.3 times control)	Therapeutic range; no change
71 to 90 s (2.3-3 times control)	Decrease rate by 2 U/kg/h
>90 s (>3 times control)	Hold infusion 1 hr then decrease rate by 3 U/kg/h

Adapted from Hyers TM, Hull RD, Weg JG: Antitthrombotic therapy for venous thromboembolic disease, *Chest* suppl 108 (4):339S, 1995, with permission; and Hirsch J, Raschke R, Warkentin TE, et al: Heparin: mechanism of action, pharmacokinetics, dosing considerations, monitoring, efficacy, and safety, *Chest* suppl 108 (4)1:262S, 1995, with permission.
Note: Use full-strength heparin concentration of 25,000 U in 250 ml D_5W (i.e., 100 U/ml). Initial loading dose is 80 U/kg bolus followed by 18 U/kg/h maintenance dose. The aPTT must be checked q6h until therapeutic range is reached (i.e., aPTT of 46-70 s, which should correspond to a plasma heparin level of 0.2-0.4 U/ml by protamine sulfate titration; this should be determined in every laboratory). Once reached, check aPTT q6h for another 24 hr. Thereafter, monitor aPTT once every morning unless it is outside the therapeutic range.

Table 5.3-5. Guidelines for adjusting IV unfractionated heparin dose without using body weight

aPTT	DOSE ADJUSTMENT
≤45	Rebolus 5000 U, then increase rate by 6 ml/hr or 5760 U/24 hr
46-54	Increase rate by 3 ml/hr or 2880 U/24 hr
55-85	Therapeutic range; no change
86-110	Hold infusion 1 hr, then decrease rate by 3 ml/hr or 2880 U/24 hr
>110	Hold infusion 1 hr then decrease rate by 6 ml/hr or 5760 U/24 hr

Adapted from Hull RD, Raskob GE, Lemaire J, et al: Optimal therapeutic level of heparin therapy in patients with venous thrombosis, *Arch Intern Med* 152:1591, 1992; and adapted from Hyers TM, Hull RD, Weg JG: Antithrombotic therapy for venous thromboembolic disease, *Chest* suppl 108 (4):338S, 1995, with permission.
Note: Use half-strength heparin concentration of 20,000 U in 500 ml D_5W (i.e., 40 U/ml). Initial loading dose of 5000-10,000 U is followed by 1300 U/h maintenance dose. The aPTT must be checked q4-6h until a therapeutic range is reached (i.e., aPTT of 55-85 s, which should correspond to a plasma heparin level of 0.2-0.4 U/ml by protamine sulfate titration; this should be determined in every laboratory). Once reached, check aPTT q4-6h for another 24 hr. Thereafter, monitor aPTT once every morning unless it is outside the therapeutic range.

mended for DVT prophylaxis. Aspirin is not as effective as other DVT prophylaxis agents. Dipyridamole is ineffective in DVT prophylaxis. Use of 10% dextran-40 solution for DVT prophylaxis in patients undergoing total hip or knee replacement is controversial, although it has been shown to be ineffective in preventing DVT in stroke patients.

C. **Inferior vena caval filter (IVCF) (e.g., Greenfield filter)** is an umbrella-like filter device that can be inserted percutaneously (with fluoroscopic guidance) through the femoral vein to the inferior vena cava to prevent PE. The IVCF as primary prevention may be used in selected patients with very high risk for developing DVT and PE (e.g., those with multiple lower limb fractures, spinal cord injury, severe head injury, or indwelling femoral venous catheters) but in whom anticoagulation therapy is contraindicated or led to complications. The IVCFs are mainly used as secondary prophylaxis in patients with DVT or recurrent DVT (see section V.C). Complications of IVCF (although infrequent) include misplacement (4%), formation of thrombi on the filter, occlusion of the filter, migration of the filter, or perforation of the caval wall.

D. **DVT surveillance** (duplex scanning or IPG) in high-risk patients is an attractive alternative in DVT prophylaxis; however, both IPG and duplex scanning are expensive and are shown to have only moderate sensitivity and positive predictive value when applied to nonsymptomatic high-risk patients. The DVT surveillance may be used effectively in high-risk patients (e.g., multiple trauma) in whom standard methods of DVT prophylaxis are not feasible or are shown to have uncertain efficacy. The IPG or duplex scanning for screening DVT in high-risk patients admitted to the rehabilitation service may be done (based on the physician's clinical judgment) in those not already on prophylaxis, those with clinical signs of DVT, and those who are nonambulatory because of severe leg weakness. There is insufficient data, however, to indicate whether all patients should be screened on admission to the rehabilitation unit. For patients already on DVT prophylaxis, there is continued risk of developing DVT extension or PE especially in patients with severe leg weakness or with limited or no ability to ambulate (or both). In such cases, serial IPG or duplex scanning may be justified on a case-to-case basis.

V. **Management of DVT** is ultimately aimed at preventing PE by limiting thrombus extension and preventing thrombus recurrence. This is achieved primarily through anticoagulation therapy (ADUH and warfarin). The earliest and most frequent sites for DVT are in the calf. Treatment of isolated calf thrombi has been controversial. Based on recent evidence, the ACCP recommends that symptomatic isolated calf DVTs should be treated with anticoagulation for 3 months (see Table 5.3-6 for the ACCP guidelines for the management of suspected and confirmed DVT or PE). If for any reason anticoagulation cannot be given, serial noninvasive studies of the lower limb (e.g., duplex scanning or IPG) should be performed to assess for proximal extension of thrombus. It is estimated that about 20% of untreated calf DVT eventually extends proximally.

A. **Anticoagulation therapy**

1. **Adjusted-dose unfractionated heparin** should be started (5000 U, IV bolus) in patients with suspected DVT or PE while awaiting diagnostic work-ups (see Table 5.3-6). If DVT or PE is confirmed, the patient should be rebolused with IV heparin (5,000 to 10,000 U) and the aPTT kept at 1.5 to 2.5 times normal (see Table 5.3-6). Heparin should be continued for 5 to 10 days, unless there is a massive pulmonary embolism or ileofemoral thrombosis in which case a longer period of heparin therapy may be considered. On day 1 of heparin treatment, warfarin should be started and should

Table 5.3-6. **Management of suspected and confirmed DVT or PE as recommended by the Fourth American College of Chest Physicians (ACCP) Consensus Conference on Antithrombotic Therapy (1995)**

DVT OR PE	GUIDELINES
Suspected	Obtain baseline prothrombin time, aPTT, CBC. Check for contraindication to heparin therapy. Give heparin, 5000 U IV and order imaging study.
Confirmed	Rebolus with heparin 5000-10,000 U IV and start maintenance infusion at 1300 U/hr (heparin, 20,000 U in 500 ml D_5W, infused at 33 ml/hr). Check aPTT at 6 hr to keep aPTT between 1.5 and 2.5 times control (blood heparin level, 0.2-0.4 U/ml); may use Table 5.3-4 or 5.3-5 for adjusting heparin dose. Check platelet count daily. Start warfarin therapy on day 1 at 5-10 mg and then administer warfarin daily at estimated daily maintenance dose. Stop heparin therapy after 4-7 days of joint therapy when INR is 2.0-3.0 without heparin therapy. Anticoagulate with warfarin for 3 months at an INR of 2.0-3.0 (longer treatment should be given to patients with ongoing risk factors or recurrent thrombosis).

From Hyers TM, Hull RD, Weg JG: Antitthrombotic therapy for venous thromboembolic disease, *Chest* 108 (4) suppl:337S, 1995, with permission.
D_5W = 5% dextrous in water.

overlap with heparin therapy for 4 to 5 days. For many patients, heparin therapy can be discontinued on day 5 or 6 if the INR is 2.0 to 3.0.

2. **Warfarin (Coumadin, Panwarfin)** should be continued for at least 3 months for the treatment of DVT or up to 6 months for PE treatment. The INR should be maintained between 2.0 to 3.0. If INR is above therapeutic range, refer to ACCP guidelines in Table 5.3-3. Reasons for unexpected fluctuations in warfarin dose response are given in section IV.B.1.a. In patients in whom warfarin is either contraindicated (e.g., pregnancy) or inconvenient, long-term ADUH may be considered. Patients with recurrent venous thrombosis or a continuing risk factor, such as antithrombin III deficiency, protein C or S deficiency, lupus anticoagulant, or malignancy, should be anticoagulated with warfarin indefinitely.

3. **Low-molecular-weight heparin** has been used in other countries for treating acute DVT. This particular indication, however, has not been approved by the FDA in the United States.

B. **Thrombolytic therapy (e.g., Streptokinase, Urokinase, tPA)** may accelerate thrombus dissolution, resulting in a reduction in the incidence of postphlebitic syndrome. They may be indicated in selected patients with proximal DVT or pulmonary embolism; however, because of uncertain long-term benefits and the increased risk of hemorrhagic complications, they are not recommended for routine use in patients with acute DVT. Their efficacy still needs further clinical investigation.

C. **Inferior vena caval filter** (e.g., Greenfield filter) (see section IV.C for its description and complications) is recommended when there is a contraindication or complication of anticoagulant therapy in an individual with or at high risk for proximal vein thrombosis or pulmonary embolism. It is also recommended for recurrent thromboembolism that occurs despite adequate anticoagulation, in the presence of a large free-floating vena caval thrombus, in the patient with chronic recurrent embolism with pulmonary hypertension, and during the concurrent performance of surgical pulmonary embolectomy or pulmonary endarterectomy. Whenever possible, anticoagulants should be given following placement of a vena caval filter in a patient with proximal deep vein thrombosis of the lower limb.

D. **Mobilization** of the affected limb and gait training should be restricted in patients with DVT until the patient attains at least 1 to 2 days of therapeutic aPTT range while on IV heparin therapy. During this bedrest regimen, the affected limb is elevated and the patient is prohibited from moving it and from walking; however, other rehabilitation measures (e.g., nursing care measures, upper limb therapy, certain activities of daily living, communication, education, and counseling) may be continued at the bedside. The length of the bedrest regimen may be up to 7 to 10 days for patients with proximal DVTs or a few days for patients with distal DVT, depending on the time it takes for the patient to attain therapeutic aPTT range. Based on its natural history, thrombus resolution by the fibrinolytic system occurs within a few days and organization of the thrombus in 10 to 14 days.

VI. Complications of DVT

A. **Pulmonary embolism** is the most serious and fatal complication of DVT. If the calf thrombus embolizes, it is usually small, and the resulting PE is not likely to be fatal. However, about 20% of calf thrombi progress and extend proximally into the popliteal and thigh veins. Half of these proximal thrombi embolize, and some are large and cause massive PE. In about 20% of cases with clinical features of PE, the event is fatal. (See Table 5.3-1 for incidence of PE.)

1. **Pathophysiology.** PE is caused by the dislodgment of a deep vein thrombus into the pulmonary arterial system causing complete or partial obstruction of the distal lung. This leads to increased intrapulmonary dead space (ventilated without perfusion); air space constriction in the affected lung; atelectasis due to loss of surfactant with decreased alveolar stability; loss of pulmonary vascular capacity with increased resistance to flow (pulmonary hypertension, right ventricular failure); and subsequent development of bronchial collateral arterial circulation. If the PE is massive (i.e., 60% or more of the pulmonary circulation obstructed), the patient can develop right-sided heart failure, which may progress to cardiovascular collapse leading to hypotension, coma, and death.

2. **Diagnosis of PE**

   a. **Clinical diagnosis.** Half of all PEs are clinically silent and are not suspected or diagnosed antemortem. Only 30% of patients with PE have clinical features of DVT, even though in about 70% of these patients DVT can be demonstrated by venography. As with DVT, the clinical diagnosis of PE, is insensitive and nonspecific.

      1) **Submassive PE** can have clinical features that includes tachypnea, tachycardia, and the signs of pulmonary infarction (i.e., pulmonary consolidation, rales, hemoptysis, pleuritic chest pain, pleural friction rub, pleural effusion, and fever). However, only a few of these usually present clinically. Sometimes the patient may only complain of malaise or fever.

      2) **Massive PE** can be fatal within 30 minutes of the acute event. The

typical clinical features consist of an abrupt onset of tachypnea, tachycardia, cyanosis, raised jugular venous pressure, and altered mental status.

  b. **Diagnostic tests** must be done to confirm or disprove a PE suspicion because of the unreliability of the clinical features associated with PE.

   1) **Arterial blood gas (ABG)** values are not helpful diagnostically because up to 15% of patients with PE are not hypoxic, and abnormal gas values occur in many respiratory disorders. Changes in ABG, however, may be used as a simple screening test. If PaO_2 is above 90 mm Hg, significant PE is not likely.

   2) **Chest radiogram** findings may be suggestive of or compatible with a diagnosis of PE, but at least 25% of patients with symptoms of PE have negative chest radiographs. The main value of a routine chest film is to rule out an alternative diagnosis such as a pneumothorax or pulmonary edema.

   3) **Radionuclide ventilation-perfusion lung scan (V/Q scan)** (see Chapter 2.3, section I.D) combines perfusion lung scan (which is very sensitive in detecting PE, but is not specific) with a ventilation scan (which reveals pulmonary disorders in which there is impairment of both ventilation and perfusion). The ability of the lung scan alone to predict pulmonary embolism (as confirmed by angiography) is 88% for high-probability scans, 33% for intermediate-probability scans, 16% for low-probability scans, and 9% for normal or near-normal scans. In a patient with a high clinical suspicion of PE, however, a high-probability lung scan has a 96% likelihood of predicting PE. Patients with high clinical suspicion of PE but low- or intermediate-probability V/Q scan should undergo pulmonary angiography.

   4) **Pulmonary angiography** is the most definitive study for the diagnosis of PE. It may be required in 40 to 60% of patients who have high clinical suspicion of PE but in whom the results of V/Q scan are inconclusive. The need for pulmonary angiography can be reduced by performing leg venograms. Although a venogram is negative in up to 30% of patients with PE, if venography (or IPG or duplex scanning) is positive in a patient with a high clinical suspicion of PE, then pulmonary angiography would not be required, because full anticoagulation would be needed in any case.

 3. **Treatment** for suspected and confirmed PE is similar to that for DVT (see section V and Table 5.3-6). The effectiveness of surgical procedures for PE (e.g., pulmonary embolectomy and transvenous catheter extraction of emboli) are controversial. Because massive PE can be fatal, it is imperative to prevent it through DVT prophylactic measures.

B. **Recurrence of DVT** is high after the initial treatment of DVT with short-term IV heparin, the risk being greatest in the first month and then diminishing over the next 6 months. Hence anticoagulation with warfarin (INR 2.0 to 3.0) for 3 to 6 months (probably indefinitely) is essential for secondary DVT prophylaxis. In patients refractory to warfarin (usually patients with underlying malignancy or other predisposition to thrombosis), chronic anticoagulation with adjusted-dose heparin given subcutaneously may be required.

C. **Postphlebitic syndrome** is a late complication of DVT and is associated with venous insufficiency. There is distal venous hypertension caused by residual obstruction to venous outflow from the limb and incompetent valves in the deep veins. The most frequent clinical feature is leg swelling, which may

Chapter 5.3 Venous Thromboembolism **459**

develop following an acute DVT and then persist to give a chronically swollen limb. In other patients the swelling may not be prominent until later, when patients begin to sit or stand with the limb dependent for long periods of time. The patient with postphlebitic syndrome may also have exercise-induced pain that is relieved with rest and elevation of the leg. About 23% of patients with long-standing venous insufficiency developed pigmentation of the legs, while 5% developed increased ulceration. The early detection and treatment of DVT limits the extent of proximal progression of a thrombus and minimizes the degree of overall venous obstruction that can lead to late postphlebitic syndrome. The use of DVT prophylaxis has decreased the incidence of postphlebitic syndrome, especially in its severe form.

BIBLIOGRAPHY

Brandstater ME, Roth EJ, Siebens HC: Venous thromboembolism in stroke: literature review and implications for clinical practice, *Arch Phys Med Rehabil Suppl* 73:379-391, 1992.

Clagett GP, Anderson FA, Jr., Heit J, et al: Prevention of venous thromboembolism, *Chest Suppl* 108 (4):312-334, 1995.

Ferri FF: *Practical guide to the care of the medical patient*, ed 3, St. Louis, 1995, Mosby–Year Book.

Hyers TM, Hull RD, Weg JG: Antithrombotic therapy for venous thromboembolic disease, *Chest Suppl* 108 (4):335-351, 1995.

Imperiale TF, Speroff T: A meta-analysis of methods to prevent venous thromboembolism following total hip replacement, *JAMA* 271:1780-1785, 1994.

Interchange forum: developments in prophylactic therapy or venous thromboembolic disease, *Orthop Rev Suppl* 23 (3A):1-56, 1994.

Weinmann EA, Salzman EW: Deep vein thrombosis, *New Engl J Med* 331 (24): 1630-1641, 1994.

CHAPTER 5.4

SPASTICITY

Spasticity is a component of the upper motor neuron syndrome characterized by a velocity-dependent increase in muscle tone with exaggerated tendon jerks resulting from hyperexcitability of the stretch reflex. Common PM&R conditions associated with spasticity include spinal cord injury (SCI), demyelinating disease (e.g., multiple sclerosis [MS]), stroke, traumatic brain injury (TBI), and cerebral palsy (CP). Spasticity has to be distinguished from *spasms*, which refer to spontaneous uncontrolled movements, which may be due to spasticity (e.g., painful flexor or extensor spasms) or to other hyperactive spinal reflexes such as cramps, dystonia, rigidity (decerebrate, decorticate, or parkinsonian), stiff-man syndrome, and metabolic contractures (e.g., McArdle's disease). The terms *spasticity* and *spasms* should also be differentiated from *muscle spasms*, which typically refer to focal areas of increased muscle activity associated with tenderness and splinting of the painful part occurring in the setting of nerve or muscle (or myofascial) injury (see also Chapter 4.8, section II).

I. Pathophysiology
  A. Neural mechanism for spasticity can possibly be explained by
   1. Selective increase in motor neuronal excitability due to enhanced excitatory synaptic input, reduced inhibitory synaptic input, and/or changes in intrinsic electrical properties of the neuron.
   2. Increase in stretch-evoked synaptic excitation of motor neurons due to gamma efferent hyperactivity and/or increased sensitivity of excitatory neurons to muscle afferent (e.g., collateral sprouting, denervation hypersensitivity, and decrease in presynaptic inhibition).
  B. Supraspinal mechanism for spasticity can possibly be caused by changes in the balance of the descending pathway activity, that is, increased excitation of the motor neurons innervating antigravity muscles (extensors in the legs and flexors in the arms) or loss of inhibition from the descending tracts.

II. Clinical evaluation of spasticity should include quantification of spasticity and its functional effects so that effective comparisons and justifications can be made following treatment. After treatment, it should be kept in mind that decreasing spasticity in one area may precipitate changes in other unexpected areas.
  A. Physical examination of spasticity: The limb is placed in a relaxed state (as much as possible), then suddenly flexed or extended to check for hypertonia. Spasticity is velocity-dependent whereas spasms, contracture, capsule tightness, or other states of hypertonia are not. Spasticity usually involves the flexors of the upper limbs and extensors of the lower limbs. It occurs at the early range of joint motion and is characterized by a sudden relaxation (as in a clasp-knife release) of the limb when a static force is applied persistently to a spastic limb. Other associated features of spasticity include clonus (a cyclical hyperactivity of antagonistic muscles in response to stretch) and spasms (e.g., painful flexor or extensor spasms). Spasticity is one component in the assessment of upper motor neuron (UMN) lesions (cortical, subcortical, or spinal cord level). Abnormal symptoms of UMN lesions include positive cutaneomuscular reflex (e.g., Babinski's or Chaddock's response of the toes

Table 5.4-1. Modified Ashworth scale for clinical grading of muscle spasticity

SPASTICITY GRADE	DEFINITION
0	No increase in tone
1	Slight increase in muscle tone, manifested by a catch and release or by minimal resistance at the end of the range of motion (ROM) when the affected part(s) is moved in flexion or extension
1+	Slight increase in muscle tone, manifested by a catch, followed by minimal resistance throughout the remainder (<50%) of the ROM
2	More marked increase in muscle tone through most of the ROM; affected part(s) easily moved
3	Considerable increase in muscle tone; passive movement is difficult
4	Affected part(s) rigid in flexion or extension

From: Bohannon RW, Smith MB: Interrater reliability on modified Ashworth scale of muscle spasticity. *Phys Ther* 67:207, 1987, with permission of the American Physical Therapy Association.

and Hoffman's response of the fingers), hyperreflexia, and loss of precise autonomic control below the level of the spinal cord lesion.

B. **Qualitative and quantitative assessment of spasticity:**
1. **Modified Ashworth Spasticity Scale** (see Table 5.4-1) is a qualitative scale which is commonly used in the assessment of spasticity. Assess all involved limbs and use consistent body and joint positions.
2. **Bilateral Adductor Tone Score** is carried out for patients with increased hip adductor tone (0 = no increase in tone; 1 = increased tone; hips are easily abducted to 45 degrees by one person; 2 = hips are abducted to 45 degrees by one person with mild effort; 3 = hips are abducted to 45 degrees by one person with moderate effort; 4 = two people are required to abduct the hips to 45 degrees). Hip adductor spasticity may interfere with sexual function, perineal hygiene, and catheter care for both men and women.
3. **Spasm Frequency Score** is used to assess all muscle groups presenting with spasms (0 = no spasms; 1 = one or fewer spasms; 2 = between 1 and 5 spasms; 3 = between 5 and 9 spasms; 4 = ten or more spasms or continuous contraction).
4. **Visual Analog Scale** for assessment of global pain may be done to assess effects of spasticity. The patient is asked to rate the total amount of pain he or she had in the last 24 hours in the (affected part) using a 10 cm horizontal line with "no pain" written on the left end and "maximal pain" on the other end (see Chapter 5.10, section IV.C.2.a.1).
5. **Other methods** of evaluating or quantifying of spasticity include dynamic multichannel EMG, computerized gait analysis, the pendulum test, temporary anesthetic nerve blocks, and electrophysiologic testing (e.g., H reflex, H/M ratio, F waves, tonic vibration reflex, cutaneomuscular or flexor withdrawal response, and lumbosacral spinal evoked responses). Most of these tests are time-consuming, involve expensive equipment, or are used mainly in research. Electrophysiological studies are not very useful because they study the patient at rest ignoring the biomechanic and neurophysiologic features of movement.

C. **Functional evaluation of spasticity:** Functionally, the performance deficits (negative symptoms) of UMN lesions include decreased dexterity, weakness, paralysis, synergy (i.e., loss of isolated voluntary activation), and increased fatigability. During examination, the adverse functional impact of spasticity must be determined.

1. **Activities of daily living (ADL):** Assess all basic and instrumental ADLs (see Chapter 4.5, sections II.A and II.B). Also note assistive devices used and amount of assistance required.

2. **Transfer abilities:** Assess the type, amount of assistance, and difficulties and safety for all forms of transfers, i.e., tub, chair, bed, toilet, and car.

3. **Resting positions:** Measure the joint resting angles in sitting, standing, and following ambulation. Note any deviations, difficulties, and adaptations with positioning for bed, chair, and wheelchair.

4. **Range of motion (ROM):** Assess active and passive ROMs of the involved limbs.

5. **Balance skills:** Note sitting, standing, and walking balance.

6. **Endurance:** Determine how much endurance is lost because of the energy expended to overcome spasticity.

7. **Orthoses:** Assess existing splints or orthoses by noting fit, function, and joint position.

8. **Sleeping patterns:** Assess the effects of spasticity on sleep, e.g., the number of times per night the patient is awakened by spasms or spasticity, and the remedy or assistance required to resume sleep.

9. **Observational gait analysis** (see Chapter 2.5, section VI.A): Determine gait patterns, compensations, and deviations. Also evaluate how the patient's gait and walking balance are affected by the arm position and swing.

III. **Step-care for spasticity** starts from the most conservative care with the least side effects. If this is unsuccessful, then it progresses to higher steps of care which, although more effective, are more aggressive (invasive), more irreversible, and have more side effects. Before starting any treatment, the functional impairment of spasticity must be carefully assessed. Not all spasticity should be treated because it may help in the patient's function, for example, mild to moderate extensor spasticity of the legs may provide a bracing function and assist in standing and ambulation activities. However, if spasticity is severe (e.g., awakening patient at night) or interferes with function (e.g., hip adductor spasticity, which causes "scissoring" of gait, limit effective ambulation, make catheterization difficult, or makes transfers and positioning difficult), then it must be treated. By limiting the effects of spasticity, deformity and contractures can be prevented, nursing care improved, bracing better tolerated, and function enhanced.

A. **Step 1 care:**

1. **Prevention of noxious stimuli** that can exacerbate spasticity, such as urinary tract infection, bowel impaction, pressure ulcers, fractures, paronychia, and the acute abdomen. The tendency to develop pressure ulcers is increased in spasticity because involuntary spastic movements may rub the body against bedsheets, clothing, bedrails, or adaptive equipment.

2. **Patient education** is geared towards decreasing the adverse effects of spasticity and improving patient function despite spasticity. It includes the use of slow movements and techniques on how to trigger useful extensor or flexor spasms during transfers or bed mobility. Patient should be taught how to use foot protection devices and remove heel-loop bolts from wheelchair footrests to prevent skin breakdown. In severe spasticity, waist or

chest straps or contact guarding from another person may be needed. After giving a treatment that reduces spasticity, the patient should be taught to avoid previous substitutions or patterns that reinforce spasticity (e.g., cradling the upper limb in a flexed position or extending the lower limbs) and to use proper body mechanics for lifting, pushing, and pulling to help prevent future injury.

B. **Step 2 care** includes the following which should be taught to both the patient and the patient's caretaker:

1. **Proper positioning and handling** of the patient in the bed, chair, and wheelchair to prevent or minimize spasticity, contractures, or pressure ulcers;

2. **Daily ROM and stretching exercise program** including static muscle stretch (e.g., standing activities) to prevent contracture and capsule tightness, reduce stretch reflex hyperactivity, and improve motor control.

C. **Step 3 care:**

1. **Physical modalities**

   a. **Muscle cooling** (15 minutes or more) using ice, ice pack, or topical anesthesia reduces phasic stretch reflex activity and clonus. It can also be used with static stretch to overcome hyperactive stretch reflexes.

   b. **Heat (e.g., hot packs or ultrasound)** may be effective in relaxing the spastic muscles in some patients.

   c. **Therapeutic exercises** include techniques to facilitate or strengthen agonist voluntary movement and to inhibit antagonist spasticity. Under-utilized mechano- and proprioceptors may be stimulated with weightbearing, joint compression, tendon vibration, and other techniques (e.g., proprioceptive neuromuscular facilitation) for improving tone and movement control described in Chapter 4.2, section IV.B. Muscle reeducation should be taught to facilitate balance and equilibrium.

   d. **Biofeedback** using either EMG or joint position sensors, and providing auditory or visual feedback have been tried.

   e. **Peripheral electrical stimulation** of muscle or nerve for 15 minutes reduces spasticity and clonus for hours, but functional gains have not been demonstrated. Transcutaneous electrical nerve stimulation (TENS) has also been used.

2. **Splints (static or dynamic), serial casts, or orthoses** are used to provide prolonged static stretching (to reduce spasticity while slowly increasing ROM or flexibility) and to limit further deformities. However, surface electromyography (EMG) has not been able to demonstrate decreased muscle activity when using upper limb splints (e.g., resting splints) or serial casts. Although lower limb resting splints may improve ankle ROM and facilitate motoneuron activity due to cutaneous stimulation, they do not alleviate spasticity. Ankle foot orthoses (AFOs) are used to control spastic equinus deformities at the ankle (e.g., using posterior leaf spring [PLS]). Medial and lateral T-straps or anterior flare can be used to control varus or valgus deformities.

D. **Step 4 care:**

1. **Antispasticity medications** reduce tone, but their dosages have to be titrated so they do not limit the patient's function. Because the drugs act at different sites, they may be combined in dosages low enough to avoid major side effects. The effects of the drugs are nonselective and systemic. They have adverse effects especially in large dosages. Some clinicians believe that drug therapy should only be tried if chemical nerve blockade (section III.D.2), specifically motor point and peripheral nerve blocks, have failed.

a. **Baclofen (Lioresal),** an analog of gamma-aminobutyric acid (GABA), binds to GABA receptors in the spinal cord and is probably the drug of choice in spinal forms of spasticity (e.g., painful flexor spasms in SCI or MS patients). It is less sedating than diazepam and probably plays no role in spasticity of cerebral origin (e.g., stroke or CP). Common side effects are weakness, sedation, dizziness, gastrointestinal symptoms, tremor, insomnia, headache, and hypotension. Hepatic dysfunction may occur. Serious side effects include personality disturbance and hallucinations. Epilepsy is a relative contraindication to its use. Alcohol use should be limited. Baclofen should not be withdrawn suddenly as it may lead to seizures and hallucinations. The half-life of baclofen is 3.5 hrs. It is available in 10- and 20-mg tablets. For adults, start with 5 mg, po, bid, then increase by 5 mg as tolerated every 3 days to 30 to 80 mg daily in divided doses (tid or qid). Although the FDA-recommended maximum dose is 80 mg/day, higher and more therapeutic doses (up to 100-120 mg) have been well-tolerated. For children, start with 2.5 to 5.0 mg, po, qd; then slowly titrate up to 30 mg (for children less than 8 years old) or 60 mg (for those over 8 years old) per day in divided doses. However, in children under 12 years old, it is generally not recommended because its safety has not been established.

b. **Dantrolene sodium (Dantrium)** acts at the level of intra- and extrafusal muscle fibers resulting in decreased release of calcium from the sarcoplasmic reticulum, therefore, reducing the force produced by excitation-contraction coupling. It is preferred for spasticity of cerebral origins (e.g., stroke or CP) and can be a useful adjunct to the treatment of spasticity of spinal origin (especially in wheelchair-bound paraplegics). It produces benefit in proportion to an increasing degree of weakness, but when properly titrated, it usually does not impair motor performance. Its sedative effects are only mild to moderate. Side effects include generalized weakness, fatigue, diarrhea, lethargy, and hepatotoxicity. The hepatotoxic effects may have been overstated because it occurs only in about 1% of patients (usually in women over 30 years old at a dosage of over 300 mg/day for more than 2 months). Liver function tests (aspartate aminotransferase [AST or SGOT] and alanine aminotransferase [ALT or SGPT]) and blood counts must be monitored during treatment. In patients with preexisting liver disease, it is contraindicated. Although dantrolene has little effect on smooth and cardiac muscles, the manufacturer recommends caution when used in patients with severe cardiac or pulmonary disease. The half-life of dantrolene is 8.7 hours. It is available in 25-, 50-, and 100-mg capsules. For adults, start with 0.5 mg/kg/day or 25 mg, po, qd/bid, and titrate up to a maximum of 400 mg daily over a 1 month period. For children, start with 0.5 mg/kg, po, bid, slowly increase by 0.5 mg/kg to tid/qid up to a maximum of 3 mg/kg qid or 100 mg qid. Its long-term safety has not been established in children under 5 years old.

c. **Diazepam (Valium)** acts at both the brainstem reticular activating system and spinal cord. It facilitates postsynaptic effects of GABA although it has no direct GABA-mimetic effect. It is useful for spasticity (e.g., painful flexor spasms) due to SCI and is generally unsuitable in patients with brain injury. It can cause sedation, urinary retention, ataxia, and drug dependence. Long-term side effects include paradoxical insomnia, anxiety, and hostility. Sudden withdrawal may cause seizures. It is contraindicated in patients with narrow-angle glaucoma. It must be used with caution by patients taking alcohol or anticoagulation drugs. The half-life of diazepam is 27 to 37 hours (longer for active metabolites). It is available in 2-, 5-, 10-mg tablets. For adults, start with 2 to 4 mg, po, qd/bid, and titrate up to 60 mg daily in divided doses (there is no absolute maximum dosage). For children, give 0.12 to 0.8 mg/kg, po, daily in divided doses.

   d. **Clonidine (Catapres),** which is an α_2-adrenergic agonist and α_1-adrenergic blocker, has been fairly successful in treating spasticity due to SCI. Side effects include hypotension, syncope, nausea, depression, sedation, and dry mouth. For more details about its ADRs, contraindications, and precautions, see Chapter 4.8, section V.F. The half-life of oral clonidine is 12 to 16 hours. It is available in 0.1-, 0.2-, and 0.3-mg strengths in either tablet or patch (transdermal therapeutic system [TTS]) form. Start with 0.05 mg, po, bid, and increase up to 0.2 to 0.4 mg/day. The adhesive patch form (Catapres-TTS) begins with a 0.1 mg patch and titrates up to a 0.3 mg patch every week. The dose and rate of titration is based on the patient's tolerance of the side effects (especially hypotension).

   e. **Tizanidine (Zanaflex),** is a centrally acting α_2-adrenergic agonist, which is chemically related to clonidine. It has been recently approved by the FDA for use in the acute and intermittent management of spasticity (particularly in patients with MS, SCI, or stroke). Tizanidine presumably acts by increasing presynaptic inhibition of motor neurons. Its antispastic effectiveness in patients with MS or stroke is comparable with baclofen and diazepam. Moreover, it produces less muscle weakness than baclofen, less sedation than diazepam, and less cardiovascular effects (e.g., hypotension) than clonidine. Common adverse effects include dry mouth, sedation, asthenia (tiredness), dizziness, hypotension, bradycardia, and possibly increased muscle tone. Although uncommon, hallucination and psychotic-like symptoms as well as liver injury have been reported. Tizanidine has no specific contraindication except in patients with known hypersensitivity to tizanidine or its ingredients. It must be used with caution in patients receiving concurrent antihypertensives or other sedatives, and in those with impaired liver function. Monitoring of liver function tests is recommended during the first 6 months of treatment (e.g., baseline, 1, 3, and 6 months) and periodically thereafter. Tizanidine is available in 4-mg tablets and may be started at 4 mg then gradually titrated by 2- to 4-mg steps to optimum control of spasticity up to 8 mg, po, tid (or a maximum of 36 mg/day).

   f. **Other oral drugs** used for spasticity when the patient does not respond to the aforementioned drugs include a combination of 300 mg/day of **phenytoin (Dilantin)** and 300 mg/day of **chlorpromazine (Thorazine); ketazomal** (a benzodiazepine which is used in Europe but is not FDA-approved for use in the United States); **cannabinoids; progabide; threonine; vincristine; clonopin;** and **vigabatrin.**

2. **Chemical nerve blockades** reduce localized spasticity with neurochemical agents (e.g., local anesthetics such as lidocaine, or neurolytic agents such as phenol) or neurotoxins (e.g., botulin) on individual nerves. Their potential benefits include: increased ROM; decreased clonus (clonus may interfere with ADL); increased speed and dexterity of movement (due to blockade of inappropriately firing antagonists); improved crawling, sitting, and standing in children; and even diminished spasticity in the contralateral

limbs. They also help prevent joint contractures and deformities; improve function (positioning and/or gait), thus facilitating other therapies; promote better tolerance of orthoses (e.g., serial casting) or positioning devices; buy time to allow rehabilitation to continue while awaiting spontaneous improvement (e.g., in TBI or SCI); allow better timing of surgical procedures in children (e.g., after growth spurt); and evaluate surgical results (by mimicking tendon lengthening).

a. **Chemical agents used for nerve blockade in spasticity**

1) **Local anesthetics** (e.g., lidocaine and marcaine) can block nerve conduction for hours by interfering with the increase in permeability of sodium ions that normally occurs when the membrane is depolarized. It can be used to determine if a decreased ROM is due to contracture or tone and to assess the potential effects of a longer-acting nerve block or surgical procedure.

2) **Chemical neurolytic agents** such as aqueous phenol (2-6% in water, saline, or glycerol) or absolute ethyl alcohol (45-50%) can block spasticity for 6 to 12 months or longer. Usually after 4 to 6 months (less for motor point blocks), the effect is lost due to distal axonal regeneration from the site of injection. Phenol or alcohol may then be repeated once or twice, after which little significant change is seen. Phenol has a higher incidence of skin sloughs and, unlike alcohol, which has no systemic effect when injected intravascularly, phenol can cause severe systemic reactions when injected intravascularly.

3) **Neurotoxin** such as botulinal type-A toxin (available as Botox in the United States) is claimed to be more effective than phenol or alcohol for neurolysis of motor points (i.e., the terminal branches of motor nerves) because Botox diffuses through muscle membranes, causing a ''leaking'' of the neuromuscular effect, thus blocking motor points at multiple sites. Botox inhibits the release of acetylcholine at the neuromuscular junction and interferes with the uptake of cytoplasmic acetylcholine. Botox injections can be carried out with a typical electromyography machine and do not require exact needle placement in the neuromuscular junction as in phenol injections. Unlike phenol motor point blocks, Botox injection is directed toward the muscle belly rather than the nerve in the neuromuscular junction.

   Although the FDA has currently approved Botox use only for blepharospasm and torticollis, Botox has been used in PM&R for spasticity limited to a ''functional unit'' (e.g., thigh adductors, plantar flexors, or neck extensors), movement disorders (e.g., torticollis and focal dystonias), painful conditions due to prolonged muscle spasm and contractures, chronic pain (e.g., postoperative back pain), myofascial pain, thoracic outlet syndrome associated with spasm of the scalene musculature (to improve peripheral blood flow), dystonia, and detrusor sphincter dyssynergia. The FDA statement of efficacy does not include young children (less than 12 years old); however, clinicians have used Botox in children (most common indication being abnormal tone due to CP). Botox is contraindicated in patients receiving aminoglycoside or spectinomycin antibiotics, known sensitivity to botulin, myasthenia gravis, Lambert-Eaton myasthenic syndrome, motor neuron disease, and upper eyelid apraxia. Its safety during pregnancy and lactation has not been established yet.

b. Chemical nerve blockade procedures

1) **Motor point blocks (MPBs)** are applied to distal motor nerve branches to reduce clonus and velocity-dependent increase in the stretch reflex response in a spastic muscle. However, they are less effective for the more incapacitating manifestations of spasticity, that is, nonvelocity-dependent tone, flexor spasms, rigidity, and dystonia. If spasticity is generalized, MPB is generally ineffective; but, if focal muscle groups can be identified as the primary generator of a diffuse spastic reaction or for cases in which individual muscle groups are explicitly involved in function and hygiene, MPB may be helpful. Advantages of MPB include no need for general anesthesia (except when the patient is very young or uncooperative, or when severe spasticity complicates positioning); high acceptance compared to systemic medications; no sensory side effects compared to nerve block; and no apparent tolerance to repeated injections (however, localization in repeat MPB may be more difficult). The use of alcohol and phenol need precise localization of motor points and are not as effective clinically because it is time consuming to locate the multiple number of motor points within a muscle. On the other hand, botulin (as described above) can diffuse into the muscle and is, therefore, less time consuming and does not need as precise localization as alcohol or phenol for MPB.

a) **Botulin preparation:** Botulin for clinical use is marketed by Allergan Pharmaceuticals as Botox. It is supplied in a highly purified, freeze-dried state in vials of 100 units, stored in a styrofoam container at $-5°C$. It is reconstituted by adding 2 ml of preservative-free normal (0.9%) saline to get a final dilution of 5 units per 0.1 ml (if 1 ml of saline is added, the final dilution is 10 units/0.1 ml; if 4 ml of saline is added, the final dilution is 2.5 units/0.1 ml). The saline from the prefilled syringe should be sucked into the vacuum-sealed vial without having to push the plunger. If this does not occur, the unused vial should be returned to the manufacturer. Once reconstituted, the vial should not be agitated and should be stored at 2 to 4°C until use. It remains effective for about 4 hours at room temperature. Due to its high cost (about $280-$300 per vial, which is expected to come down once FDA has approved it for wider use), it is advisable to schedule more than one patient at a time so that any medication left over from one patient can be given to the next.

b) **Selection of patient and muscle for Botox MPB** is crucial for its success. Patients should be informed of possible complications (especially weakness), the variability of outcome, and the possibility of recurrence. If they are on nonsteroidal drugs or are taking anticoagulants, they should be warned of the possibility of increased bruising at the injection site. The joint where the spastic muscle crosses should have no fixed deformity. Botox MPB, which causes weakening of the spastic limb, should not further compromise residual function (including gait). The muscles (e.g., antagonist) to be blocked should be spastic enough that they interfere with normal movement of the opposite (e.g., agonist) muscles. Prior to blocking the spastic muscle (e.g., antagonist), determine if the opposite muscle (e.g., agonist) is capable of hypertrophy and strengthening if allowed to perform through the appropriate ROM. Determine also if induction of partial or complete paralysis (i.e., flaccidity) of one or more muscles improves the overall function of the patient.

c) **Botox MPB injection** can be given with or without EMG guidance. For superficial muscles, a 1.0 ml tuberculin-type syringe with a 25-gauge, 5/8 inch needle may be used. For deeper muscles and for treatment of conditions in which the identity of the hyperactive muscles is difficult, EMG guidance may be necessary. A hypodermic (cannulated) monopolar needle cathode, through which the Botox can be injected, is used. For small muscles (e.g., facial), a 30-gauge, 1-inch needle is used, but for large muscles (e.g., hamstrings), a 26-gauge, 1- or 1.5-inch needle is used. The cannulated needle cathode, insulated with Teflon except at the tip, is inserted into the selected muscle. A surface anode (reference) and ground electrode is then placed near the cathodal needle. The patient should be as relaxed as possible and the joint should be positioned so that the muscles that are contracting are not doing so in a normal postural response to their current positioning. Once the motor point is located, Botox is injected intramuscularly after aspirating to prevent intravascular administration of the drug. If alcohol is used to cleanse the skin, it should be allowed to dry to prevent toxin deactivation.

(1) **For dystonic spastic muscles** associated with hemiplegia or other central nervous system pathology, motor point is located by inserting the needle into the muscle and looking for the classic burst of rhythmic dystonic firing pattern of the muscle group involved on EMG. If dystonic firing is not evident after needle placement, the patient should assume body posture or movements that normally trigger the dystonia. It is frequently helpful to needle muscles that are not obviously involved from the clinical examination alone. If dystonia is demonstrated on EMG, these muscles may also be injected.

(2) **For nondystonic spastic muscles,** the motor point is located by connecting the hub of the cathodal needle to a stimulator that is found in most standard EMG machines. The clinician stimulates the muscle by delivering a square pulse of approximately 0.1 ms once or twice per second at 5 mA intensity through the needle and watches for a brisk visible twitch in the desired muscle. The needle is then gradually moved until only the minimal current (approximately 1 mA) is necessary to obtain a maximal twitch in the desired muscle(s). This site is the motor point.

d) **Dosage of Botox:** Exact dosages of Botox for specific diagnoses have not been clearly established. It is preferable to underdose an individual with botulin during the first treatment (typically, 200 units per session is the starting therapeutic dose). If the desired effect is not achieved, an additional 100 units is given in 30 days. The dosage may be increased proportionately until the desired clinical effect is obtained. About 30 to 75 units of Botox may be injected per muscle site up to a combined limit of approximately 300 units per session per month (which is the FDA-approved maximum dose); however, 500 units have been given in the clinical setting without adverse effect in individual cases. The onset of Botox effect occurs within 24 to 72 hours, peaks at 4 to 6 weeks and lasts 3 to 6 months. Although the effect of Botox on individual nerve terminals is effectively irreversible, recovery of neuromuscular control occurs due to new terminal formation and nerve sprouting.

The average Botox doses in units for the lower limb are hip adductors, 160 to 165; hamstrings, 135 to 175; quadriceps, 200 to 240; triceps surae, 150; tibialis posterior, 50; and anterior tibialis, 50. For the upper limbs, the doses in units are biceps, 150; triceps, 160; wrist flexors, 120; and finger flexors, 80 to 120. For the neck, the doses in units are sternocleidomastoid, 15 to 75; trapezius, 50 to 100; splenius capitis, 50 to 150; levator scapulae, 25 to 100; semispinalis capitis, 50 to 150; and longissimus capitis, 50 to 150. When injecting regional muscles in combination (e.g., wrist flexors, finger flexors, and biceps), the dose per muscle should be reduced so the total is less than 300 units per session. The dose of Botox injected is typically divided between two to four sites per muscle, with higher doses reserved for larger muscles.

e) **Non-response to Botox MPB** can either be primary (i.e., no response to initial injection of Botox) or secondary (i.e., a relative or complete loss of efficacy at subsequent visit). Factors that might contribute to nonresponse include underdosage, poor injection techniques (may require EMG guidance), inappropriate reconstitution or storage of toxin, weakness or atrophy present on examination with no functional benefit, change in pattern of muscle involvement during treatment, and presence of neutralizing antibodies (confirmed by assay). To avoid antibody formation, wait as long as possible between injections (at least 3 months), avoid booster injections (given 1-3 weeks after the initial treatment session), and use the smallest clinically effective dose. A patient should only be classified as unresponsive to Botox therapy if they do not exhibit any reduction in muscle tone 4 to 6 weeks after one or more injections.

f) **Side effects of Botox** are usually temporary and well-tolerated by the patient. Most of them result from diffusion of the toxin into adjacent structures and are site-specific. They include unwanted weakness in injected and neighboring muscles, temporary change in posturing or pain due to realignment of nerve-muscle-bone relationships, and subjective symptoms of weakness and fatigue (''flu-like'' syndrome with headache and nausea), which usually last less than 4 days. No anaphylactic reactions have been reported.

g) **Postinjection care and follow-up:** Pain after Botox MPB is similar to that of a standard EMG examination. Muscle relaxants or acetaminophen may be given to patients after Botox MPB if any discomfort occurs over the next 24 to 48 hours. Stronger analgesics are rarely required. A follow-up appointment in 2 to 3 weeks after the initial treatment is helpful in determining if an adequate dosage was given. Treatments are repeated as necessary based on individual patient needs.

2) **Peripheral nerve blocks** refer to the application of local anesthetics (e.g., lidocaine or marcaine) or neurolytic agents (e.g., phenol or alcohol)

to disrupt peripheral nerve functions. Peripheral nerve blocks may be quite effective and may last 3 to 6 months or more. Compared to oral medications, they are relatively selective and have rare systemic side-effects. They are easier and safer to perform compared to surgery.

a) **Peripheral nerve block procedure** is performed using EMG guidance and a Teflon-coated needle similar to that used for nondystonic spastic muscle MPBs (see section III.D.2.b.1.c). If needed, light general inhalation anesthesia may be given.

b) **Indications for specific peripheral nerve blocks:** In the upper limbs, median and ulnar blocks are generally avoided due to the high risk of sensory complications.

  (1) **Lumbar spinal nerves** may be blocked paravertebrally to reduce hip flexor spasticity. Special caution should be observed due to the proximity of important visceral and vascular structures.

  (2) **Obturator nerves (anterior and posterior branches)** may be blocked to reduce adductor tone, diminish lower limb scissoring during gait, facilitate hip abduction to ease personal hygiene, and promote passive abduction as a means of protecting hip joint integrity.

  (3) **Femoral nerves** may be blocked inferior to inguinal ligament and lateral to femoral pulse to diminish severe spastic genu recurvatum in CP patients, and midstance recurvatum in gait unresponsive to AFO dorsiflexion. Branches to individual component of the quadriceps may be locally blocked.

  (4) **Perineal nerves** may be blocked to significantly reduce postvoid residual volumes when the external urethral sphincter is very spastic.

  (5) **Sciatic nerves (e.g., branch to the medial hamstrings)** may be blocked to diminish crouch gait and internal rotation deformities.

  (6) **Tibial nerves (e.g., tibial branch to the heads of the gastrocnemius)** may be blocked to diminish severe equinovarus ankle posturing (due to increased plantarflexion tone) or painful clawing of the toes thus allowing better tolerance of AFOs.

  (7) **Musculocutaneous nerves** may be blocked at the medial upper arm near insertion of pectoralis tendon to promote elbow extension and facilitate reach. It is helpful in the hemiplegic patient with severe elbow flexion contracture or in the C5 tetraplegic patient with flexor contractures due to loss of triceps function. Elbow flexion is preserved through the action of the brachioradialis muscle which is innervated by the radial nerve.

  (8) **Median nerves** are usually avoided but may be blocked to help relax the tightly flexed wrist and fingers of hemiplegic patients.

c) **Side effects:** Nerve blockade to a major nerve trunk containing a significant number of cutaneous nerve fibers (e.g., tibial, median, and ulnar nerves) can produce 10 to 30% risk of dysesthesia and causalgia (with symptoms of burning sensation and discomfort). Severe persistent dysesthesias may be treated with oral steroids, transcutaneous nerve stimulation, or repetition of the nerve block. To presumably reduce the incidence of dysesthesia, an open procedure may be performed by a surgeon. The selected motor trunk is exposed surgically and phenol or alcohol is injected at the site where the motor nerve enters the muscle bulk, thus leaving the cutaneous sensory fibers unharmed.

Muscle weakness, after nerve blockade is usually temporary, that is, lasting for hours or days. Occassionally permanent weakness may occur, which leads to deformity (e.g., tibial block can cause weakness or paralysis of all posterior compartment muscles resulting in unopposed dorsiflexion and eversion, i.e. calcaneovalgus foot). Overdosage with phenol can cause convulsions, central nervous system depression, and cardiovascular collapse. However, the usual dosages of phenol (e.g., 20 ml of 5 or 6% phenol) are well below its lethal range (at least 8.5 g). Another complication of phenol nerve block is venous thromboses.

3) **Spinal block** is the intrathecal or epidural administration of local anesthetic (e.g., lidocaine or marcaine) or neurolytic agents (e.g., absolute alcohol, which has more permanent effects than phenol) to reduce severe spasticity of the lower limbs. Patients are immobilized to allow layering of the neurolytic material so that damage is limited to the desired spinal roots. However, control over affected fibers is imprecise and complications arise in 1 to 10%, which includes urinary and bowel incontinence, loss of sexual function, paresis, paresthesias, and even death.

E. Step 5 care:

1. Intrathecal medications

a. **Intrathecal baclofen (IT-B)** allows delivery of baclofen directly to the cerebrospinal fluid (CSF) so that higher effective dosages can be attained at the receptor sites in the spinal cord than with oral administration. This is because baclofen has low lipid solubility and does not effectively cross the blood-brain barrier; hence, in some patients, the effective dose cannot be reached with oral baclofen, or side-effects become intolerable at the effective oral dose. A typical intrathecal dose of baclofen is 0.3 to 0.5% of oral dose, because an oral dose of 60 mg baclofen per day gives 24 mcg/L of lumbar concentration of baclofen, while intrathecal infusion of 600 mcg/day gives a lumbar concentration of 1240 mcg/L.

Intrathecal baclofen can be administered via a pump implanted subcutaneously in the abdominal wall, with a catheter surgically placed into the subarachnoid space. The two types of pumps available are Infusaid Pump (a gas-powered bellows device, which is purely mechanical and has no battery, can only infuse drug at a constant rate, and the dosage can only be adjusted at the time of refill) and Medtronic SynchroMed Pump (an electronic battery-operated pump, which can be programmed to deliver precise drug dosage several times daily through an onboard computer so spasticity may be reduced or increased at certain times of the day; its battery lasts about 4 to 5 years). The costs of the pump alone is about $6500 plus another $3000/year for the drug itself plus surgical costs. The IT-B is used if spasticity is multisegmental and diffuse. It may be used in conjunction with Botox MPB. It is effective for spasticity related to spinal cord dysfunction (e.g., SCI or MS) and to CP with some preserved function below the level of the lesion allowing the patient to be ambulatory.

1) **Patient selection for IT-B:** Possible candidates for IT-B should be free of active infection and pressure ulcers, have an anterior abdominal

wall site suitable for pump placement (any abdominal procedures, e.g., colostomies, ileal conduits, and feeding tubes must be separated from the pump site), and have no block in CSF flow (myelography may be needed to ensure communication between the proposed site of infusion and the source of spasticity). Candidates must also live in a place that has access to magnetic resonance imaging (MRI) centers (in case of complications) as well as to clinicians experienced with IT-B maintenance. Prior to implanting the IT-B pump, the patient is admitted to the hospital and injected intrathecally with a trial dose of baclofen (starting at 50 mcg, then increasing to 75-100 mcg) via lumbar puncture or spinal catheter. Effects of baclofen are observed 2 to 8 hrs after each dose. If there is a significant decrease in muscle tone, frequency, or severity of spasms, the patient is scheduled for IT-B.

2) **Surgical phase of IT-B:** The patient is placed under intravenous deep sedation or general anesthesia. The pump is implanted in a subcutaneous abdominal pocket, the site of which is selected with consideration of the patient's belt lines, wheelchair arms, and physical activities. The pump's catheter is tunneled, using a 15- or 16-gauge Tuohy needle, to the midline lumbar area, where it is inserted into the intrathecal space at L3-L4, then advanced up a minimum of 10 cm (with the catheter tip at T10 to T12 level). Intraoperative fluoroscopy is done to confirms catheter placement into the intrathecal sac with no twisting or coiling. This surgical procedure is usually not difficult and takes 1 to 2 hrs.

3) **Drug adjustment of IT-B:** On the first day postimplantation, the pump is programmed to begin continuous infusion of 500 mcg/ml of baclofen at a rate of about 2 times the bolus responsive trial dose (given presurgically) or less if the patient had a prolonged effect (more than 12 hours) from the trial dose. The patient is observed for any untoward effects during the first 24 hours. Then, the dose is increased 10 to 15% every 24 hours. Once clinical response becomes evident, the patient is discharged from the hospital and followed for gradual dose adjustments every 1 to 4 weeks until optimal effect is achieved (i.e., muscle tone as close to normal as possible without weakness; and minimal frequency and severity of spasms without intolerable side effects). If a sudden change in spasticity occurs, causes (e.g., urinary tract infection, or inadequate bowel or bladder regime) should be corrected before changing dosage. Dose is adjusted in the office using a portable computer-based programming device through a telemetry head. Usual infusion rate is 0.004 ml/hr to 0.90 ml/hr or 300 to 800 mcg/day (i.e., average of 600 mcg/day or lumbar concentration of 1240 mcg/L).

Intrathecal baclofen has a half-life of 1.5 hrs in the CSF. The ratio of lumbar to cervical concentration of intrathecal baclofen is about 4 to 1, which is important for patients with spasticity in their lower limbs as it allows relief of spasticity without causing intolerable supraspinal side effects. If the Medtronic SynchroMed pump is used, the drug delivery mode may be changed, during follow-up visits, from continuous to either continuous-complex (drug delivered continuously in a series of 2-10 steps for specified times, e.g., at nighttime for patients who have increased spasms at night) or bolus-delay (drug delivered intermittently at a prescribed dose and at specified intervals, e.g., the flow rate can be programmed to change 2 hours before the time of desired clinical effect).

4) **Maintenance phase of IT-B:** Depending upon the dose, the pump is re-filled percutaneously every 4 to 12 weeks (baclofen is stable in the pump for up to 90 days). The pump alarm should be set to alert the patient of low reservoir. It is important that patients keep their appointment for refill to avoid an empty pump which may lead to withdrawal symptoms (i.e., return of spasticity, agitation, fever, and tachycardia). After the refill procedure, the patient should be moni-tored for any unusual reactions (e.g., swelling around the pump site, which may indicate a pocket infusion due to missed reservoir port).

5) **Side effects and complications of IT-B:** The most common side effects (i.e., drowsiness, dizziness, nausea, hypotension, headache, and weakness) are dose-related and usually subside by reducing the dos-age 10 to 20%. The IT-B can decrease the detrusor reflex, but can also depress the pelvic floor reflex, hence resulting in a bladder with low pressure, which empties less effectively (an undesirable effect in tetraplegic patients). Complications from IT-B include tube dys-function (dislodgment, disconnection, kinkage, and blockage), pump failure, infection, and baclofen overdosage (due to programming error or too rapid increase in dosage). The signs and symptoms of overdose include drowsiness, lightheadedness, nausea, bradycardia, weakness, fatigue, somnolence, seizures, respiratory depression, rostral progres-sion of hypotonia, and loss of consciousness progressing to reversible coma. The anticholinesterase, physostigmine (Antilirium), 2 mg, IV, may be given to reverse the respiratory depression caused by baclofen overdose.

b. **Intrathecal morphine** (1-2 mg) may be used instead of IT-B to reduce spasticity in patients with SCI. Although it can be effective (long-term follow-up shows that patients do not seem to develop drug tolerance), it is currently rarely used.

2. **Rhizotomy,** the sectioning of the spinal roots or rootlets, may be categorized as open (requiring laminectomy) or closed (percutaneous), complete or selective, or anterior or posterior. **Anterior rhizotomy** is associated with severe denervation-type atrophy of all innervated muscles and is seldom done.

a. **Selective dorsal (or posterior) rhizotomy (SDR)** refers to the neurosurgical sectioning of a particular proportion of selected dorsal segmental roots or rootlets to modulate afferent sensory input and reset muscle spindles so that there is less spasticity. Posterior rhizotomy is easier to perform than anterior rhizotomy and does not result in denervation muscle atro-phy. Although SDR disrupts spinal reflex arcs, it does not abolish spas-ticity mediated by suprasegmental pathways. There are reports of im-provement in tone, range, posture, and functional status in about 85% of candidates. Early gait analysis studies show improvement in stride length and hip and knee ROM in children with CP. Objective random-ized studies on gains in the range of functional motor performance defi-cits, however, remain to be seen.

1) **Patient selection for SDR:** Selective dorsal rhizotomy is indicated in young children (3-8 years old) with spastic CP (usually spastic diplegic) and for treatment of spasticity and pain in the hemiplegic upper limb. For CP patients, the favorable selection criteria for SDR

include pure spasticity (absent or very mild dystonia, athetosis, ataxia, rigidity); function limited primarily by spasticity and not significantly affected by primitive reflexes or movement patterns; no severe underlying weakness; selective motor control (e.g., some degree of spontaneous forward locomotion and adequate truncal balance and righting responses); minimal joint contractures or spine deformity; adequate cognitive ability to participate in intensive physical therapy after surgery; no significant motivational or behavioral problems; and a supportive and interactive family. It is contraindicated in neurodegenerative disorders, beneficial pattern of spasticity, and multiple fixed or orthopedic deformities.

2) **Surgical procedure of SDR:** The dorsal aspect of the thecal sac is exposed by multilevel laminectomy (e.g., L1 or L2 to S1) with the facet joints left intact. The dorsal roots are identified and stimulated with an insulated bipolar stimulator at frequencies of 1 to 50 Hz. The responses are recorded on a multichannel EMG (surface or intramuscular) from the ipsilateral and contralateral muscles of various myotomes. The dorsal afferent rootlets that cause reflex "spastic" responses in muscles are chosen for SDR (specific criteria for determining this choice remains controversial). The selected dorsal rootlets are only partially sectioned (25-80%) as complete sectioning may cause complete loss of sensation. Selective dorsal rhizotomy is most frequently performed at L5 and S1 roots. The S2-S4 dorsal roots are avoided to prevent bowel and bladder dysfunction.

3) **Post-SDR care:** Postlaminectomy precautions are observed for 6 weeks (i.e., no passive trunk rotation, no straight leg raising, no hip flexion above 90°, and no hamstring stretching). Intensive physical therapy for up to a year is required to maximize long-term functional changes. These include gentle stretching, neurodevelopmental techniques (NDT), proprioceptive neuromuscular facilitation (PNF) techniques, muscle reeducation prior to controlled ambulation training, use of adaptive equipment (e.g., tricycle), and use of less restrictive hinged AFOs with or without single lateral uprights with pelvic band and free hips and knees to control any residual internal rotation.

4) **Complications of SDR** are most commonly hypotonia (usually temporary) and weakness. Other complications include sensory changes (25% with transient dysesthesias), bladder dysfunction, bronchospasm and pneumonia, hip subluxation and dislocation, ataxia, and recurrence of spasticity. There is also a questionable potential of spinal stenosis in later life due to multilevel laminectomy.

b. **Percutaneous (closed) radiofrequency rhizotomies** are performed under fluoroscopic guidance using a radiofrequency needle to destroy nerve tissue. It is effective in reducing spasticity in the lower limbs with minimal morbidity; however, the effects are not permanent.

F. **Step 6 care:**

1. **Orthopedic surgeries (e.g., tenotomy, tendon lengthening, tendon transfers, myotomy, arthrodesis, and neurectomy)** are done to increase function (e.g., ambulation, grasp, and dressing), to increase ROM (e.g., to facilitate self-care or nursing care), to correct deformity, reduce pain, or for cosmesis. They have been used successfully in spastic patients whose voluntary movements are preserved (e.g., patients with CP, stroke, TBI, spina bifida, and SCI). Surgery should only be done when the recovery has more or less plateaued

(i.e., at least 6 months after a stroke and up to 12-24 months after TBI). Patients must be informed that the original deformity may recur after tenotomies or tendon-lengthening procedures because the number of sarcomeres in the muscle decreases, or an alternate deformity may develop from overcorrection.

A careful physical examination must be done to make sure that the weakness is due to upper motor neuron insult and not undiscovered lower motor neuron injury (e.g., brachial plexopathy or peripheral nerve injury). Static deformities (i.e., fixed contractures that are present both at rest and with movement) must be differentiated from dynamic deformities (i.e., dysfunction that appears with movement) by physical examination or by a diagnostic block with short acting anesthetic (e.g., lidocaine). For example, if after median nerve block at the elbow, deformity of the finger and wrist flexion persists, it is most likely due to a fixed contracture. Preoperative radiograph and bone scans may be done to rule out fractures, dislocations, arthritis, and heterotopic ossification. For the upper limb, sensory input is vital and can be assessed with a variety of tools (e.g., two-point discrimination). To assess the residual motor function in the upper limb, the degree of remaining trunk and shoulder stability must be determined also. For the lower limb, gait analysis with multichannel electromyography is frequently used as an adjunct in planning procedures in the lower limb. The following classification and description of orthopedic surgery for spastic limbs are primarily from Keenan, Kozin, and Berlet's Manual of Orthopedic Surgery for Spasticity (see bibliography).

a. **Orthopedic surgery for the spastic lower limb**
  1) **Static contractures** are corrected to reduce pain; improve perineal hygiene; prevent skin maceration and breakdown; facilitate lower limb dressing, positioning, and transfers; and improve cosmesis. Correcting static contractures also helps increase gait efficiency.
    a) **Hip adduction contracture** is corrected by releasing the adductor longus, adductor brevis, and gracilis muscles. Adductor magnus is not released because it is also a hip extensor. This is followed by 4 weeks of forced abduction with casts (using abduction bar) or an abduction pillow splint.
    b) **Hip flexion contracture** is corrected by releasing the sartorius, rectus femoris, iliopsoas, and pectineus muscles. If involved, tensor fascia lata and the anterior part of the gluteus medius may also be released. The hip joint capsule is left undisturbed. Postoperative care includes the prone position 3 times per day for increasing periods, followed by gentle stretching exercises. Patients may sit in a wheelchair for short periods.
    c) **Hip extension contracture** is corrected by releasing the origins of medial and lateral hamstring muscles. Postoperative care includes gentle hip ROM and sitting activities (e.g., in a wheelchair).
    d) **Knee flexion contracture** is corrected by releasing the distal hamstring (biceps femoris, semitendinosus, and semimembranosus), gracilis, and sartorius muscles. The posterior knee capsule is left undisturbed to prevent posterior tibial subluxation. Transfer of the distal hamstring insertion has also been used. Only 50% of the contracture is corrected during surgery to prevent excessive tension on the contracted neurovascular bundle. Postoperative care includes long leg casting with the knees extended maximally (forced

extension is avoided as it may cause limb ischemia and necrosis). The cast is changed weekly until full extension is achieved. This is followed by 4 weeks of nightly splinting to maintain extension. Transfers and gait training (weight bearing as tolerated) are started once the cast is applied.

e) **Knee extension contracture** is corrected by quadriceps V-Y lengthening, i.e., an inverted-V portion of the distal rectus femoris tendon is harvested, then the knee is flexed to 90 degrees and the rectus tendon is sutured to complete the V-Y lengthening on the flexed knee (V-Y refers to the shapes of the proximal and distal end of the tendon after a V-shaped incision). Postoperative care includes knee casting in 90 degrees of flexion for 3 weeks. Continuous passive motion and gait training (weight bearing as tolerated) are started once the cast is removed.

f) **Fixed equinovarus contracture** is treated similarly as in dynamic equinovarus deformity (see section III.F.1.a.2.e). In addition, a release of the plantar fascia or triple arthrodesis of the ankle, or both may be done.

g) **Fixed equinus contracture** is treated similarly as in dynamic equinus deformity (see section III.F.1.a.2.f).

h) **Fixed toe curling contracture** is treated similarly as in dynamic toe-curling deformity (see section III.F.1.a.2.g).

2) **Dynamic deformities of the lower-limb** are corrected to primarily make gait and transfers more efficient and less energy consuming.

a) **Lower limb scissoring** with narrow-based gait results from spastic hip adductors. A preoperative obturator nerve block is done to rule out static hip adduction contracture, which if present is treated as described in section III.D.2.b.2.b.2 If there is no hip adduction contracture, obturator neurectomy of the anterior branch is done. Complete obturator neurectomy is not done as it may lead to adductor paralysis and inability to walk (because both the anterior and posterior branches of the obturator nerve supply the adductor magnus). Postoperative care includes early gait training with weightbearing as tolerated. No immobilization or abduction splinting is needed.

b) **Crouched gait** results from spastic hip flexors and is associated with compensatory knee flexion and lumbar hyperlordosis. The spastic iliopsoas tendon is released from the lesser trochanter while maintaining its capsular attachments, hence weakening iliopsoas pull and allowing it to recess proximally (i.e., become attached more proximally). Postoperative care includes early hip ROM (active and passive) and gait training (weight bearing as tolerated). There is no need for postoperative immobilization. Knee flexion contracture may also be corrected (see section III.F.1.a.1.d.) to improve the crouched gait.

c) **Stiff-knee (stiff-legged) gait** with inadequate knee flexion during swing phase results from inappropriate firing of the quadriceps muscle (75% involves all four heads whereas 25% involves either rectus femoris or vastus intermedius or both). Lower limb clearance is achieved by hip-hiking gait or by circumduction gait. The spastic heads of the quadriceps are selectively released after they are identified preoperatively by EMG during dynamic gait analysis. Postoperative care includes a posterior knee splint applied for 5 days to control pain. Gait training (weight bearing as tolerated) is allowed on the first postoperative day. ROM and quadriceps strengthening exercises are done on the 5th postoperative day.

d) Dynamic knee flexion deformity results from hamstring spasticity which prevents adequate knee extension during stance phase. Fractional lengthening of the biceps femoris, semimembranosus, and sartorius are done at the myotendinous junction. The semitendinosus and gracilis are transected. The posterior knee capsule is left undisturbed to prevent posterior tibial subluxation. Postoperative care is the same as that for static knee flexion contracture (see section III.F.1.a.1.d).

e) Dynamic equinovarus deformity is the most common deformity in the lower limb. The ankle is plantarflexed (because of spastic gastrocnemius and soleus) and the foot is turned-in and supinated (because of spastic tibialis anterior). Often, the toes are curled (because of spastic extrinsic and intrinsic toe flexors). The spastic muscles are identified preoperatively by EMG during dynamic gait analysis. The split anterior tibialis tendon transfer (SPLATT) procedure is done by splitting the tibialis anterior tendon along its length, then tunneling the distal end of the lateral half of the tibialis anterior into the cuboid and sometimes the third cuneiform bones. This creates an eversion force, which counteracts the varus pull of the remaining medial portion of the tibialis anterior thus rebalancing the forefoot deformity. The SPLATT is usually done in combination with tendo-Achilles lengthening (TAL) and release of the toe flexors. If the posterior tibialis is spastic, it may be transferred through the interosseous membrane to the foot dorsum, or it may be sectioned. Postoperative care includes a short-leg walking cast with the foot in neutral for 6 weeks followed by a rigid molded ankle-foot orthosis for an additional 4.5 months. Transfers and gait training (weight bearing as tolerated) are started once the cast is applied on the first postoperative day.

f) Dynamic equinus deformity due to spastic gastrocnemius and soleus hinders both swing and stance phases of ambulation by making limb clearance difficult and preventing initial heel contact. Tendo-Achilles lengthening (TAL) using a step-cut (Z-plasty) lengthening procedure is done. Postoperative care is similar to that for equinovarus deformity (see section III.F.1.a.2.e).

g) Dynamic toe-curling deformity due to spasticity of the extrinsic and intrinsic toe flexor muscles causes pain, callosities on the dorsum of the toes, and difficulty with shoe wear. Release of all intrinsic and extrinsic toe flexors at the base of each toe (metatarsophalangeal level) is done. Postoperative care includes a soft dressing to maintain toes in the corrected position. If SPLATT, TAL, or both are done, the short-leg walking cast with toe-plate is used (see section III.F.1.a.2.e).

h) Dynamic foot valgus or pronation deformity results from the spastic peroneus longus muscle during stance phase and is usually associated with an equinovarus deformity (i.e., "combination foot deformity") seen during swing phase. It is corrected by the release and transfer of the peroneus longus across the dorsum of the foot into the navicular bone. The equinovarus deformity correction and postoperative care is similar to that for equinovarus deformity (see section III.F.1.a.2.e).

b. **Orthopedic surgery for spastic upper limb**

1) **Static contractures of the upper limbs** are corrected mainly for cosmetic reasons in a nonfunctional spastic upper limb. Correction can also reduce pain, improve axillary hygiene, reduce skin maceration and breakdown, and facilitate upper limb dressing, positioning, and transfers.

a) **Adduction and internal rotation contracture of the shoulder** is corrected by releasing the humeral insertion of the pectoralis major, subscapularis, teres major, and latissimus dorsi muscles. The shoulder capsule is left undisturbed to prevent shoulder instability and capsular adhesion. Postoperative care includes aggressive mobilization and a passive stretching program after wound healing. Recurrence is prevented by positioning (e.g., using sling, splint, or pillows) the shoulder in abduction and external rotation for several months. In the paretic shoulder, inferior subluxation is a frequent problem. When the sling gives inadequate symptomatic or functional relief, the biceps tendon can be looped over the coracoid process of the shoulder to serve as a static sling.

b) **Flexion contracture of the elbow** (usually associated with ulnar nerve compression at the elbow) is corrected by releasing the brachioradialis and biceps tendon at the elbow, and by fractional (or myotendinous) lengthening of the brachialis muscles. Brachialis muscle release is only performed in severe contractures present for several years. The anterior capsule is left undisturbed to prevent postoperative adhesions. Only 50% of the contracture is corrected during surgery to prevent excessive tension on the contracted neurovascular bundle. Postoperative care includes serial casting every week to obtain further extension.

c) **Wrist flexion contracture** (usually associated with median nerve compression at the transverse carpal ligament) is corrected by releasing the wrist flexor tendons (palmaris longus, flexor carpi ulnaris, and radialis). Often there is concomitant finger flexion contractures, which can be corrected by fractional (or myotendinous) lengthening of the finger flexors, or a superficialis to profundus tendon transfer (STP). If carpal tunnel syndrome is present, the medial nerve is decompressed. Postoperative care includes short arm casts for 3 weeks to immobilize the wrist followed by nightly volar splinting for an additional 3 weeks to maintain correction. After the cast is removed, gentle ROM exercise is started. If there is severe wrist flexion contracture, wrist arthrodesis may be done. Postoperative care for wrist arthrodesis includes a long arm splint, which should be elevated until swelling subsides. Then a short arm cast is applied for 6 to 8 weeks until fusion is seen on a radiograph.

d) **Clenched-fist contracture** is corrected by STP, which provide sufficient flexor tendon lengthening with preservation of a passive tether to prevent a hyperextension deformity. Neurectomy of the motor branch of the ulnar nerve in the Guyon's canal is routinely done because intrinsic spasticity, which is always present, may cause intrinsic-plus hand deformity after surgery. Transection of the flexor tendon is not recommended as it may lead to hyperextension deformity due to unopposed extensor muscles. The associated wrist flexion deformity is corrected as described in section III.F.1.b.2.c). Postoperative care includes immobilization for 4 weeks in a short-arm cast extended to the fingertips followed by ROM exercises after the cast is removed.

e) Intrinsic-plus hand contracture results in flexed metacarpophalangeal (MCP) and extended interphalangeal (IP) joints and is often associated with boutonniere or swan-neck deformities of the fingers. It is corrected by releasing the lateral band and oblique fibers of the extensor hood. A concomitant neurectomy of the motor branch of the ulnar nerve in the Guyon's canal is advisable to prevent a recurrence of intrinsic-plus hand deformity. Postoperative care includes hand immobilization in a bulky dressing for 1 week followed by passive ROM exercises.

2) Dynamic deformities of the upper limbs are corrected to improve upper limb function and provide cosmesis. The efficacy of correcting dynamic deformities in hemiplegic patients is unclear because the patient frequently continues to carry out most activities with the uninvolved upper limb.

a) Dynamic elbow flexion deformity due to elbow flexor spasticity is associated with a cog-wheel type of motion during attempted elbow extension, while elbow flexion is relatively normal. It is corrected by myotomy of the proximal brachioradialis, tenotomy of the brachialis tendon, step-cut (Z-plasty) lengthening of the biceps tendon, and fractional (or myotendinous) lengthening of the brachialis muscle. Postoperative care includes a long arm cast with the elbow in 45 degrees of flexion for 4 weeks. After the cast is removed, active ROM exercises are started, and night splints are used for an additional 4 weeks to protect the biceps tendon repair.

b) Dynamic elbow extension deformity due to triceps spasticity rarely occurs. It is corrected by V-Y lengthening of the triceps. In severe cases, triceps release may be done.

c) Dynamic wrist and finger flexion deformity due to wrist and finger flexor spasticity is corrected by fractional (or myotendinous) step-cut (Z-plasty) lengthening of flexor digitorum superficialis (FDS) and flexor digitorum profundus (FDP) combined with step-cut (Z-plasty) lengthening of the flexor pollicis longus and overlengthening of the flexor carpi radialis and flexor carpi ulnaris. The palmaris longus tendon is also released if tight. Postoperative care includes 3 weeks of short arm cast, which includes thumb and fingers with the wrist held in 20 degrees of extension, the MCP joint in 60 degrees of flexion, and the IP joint extended. After the cast is removed, active ROM exercises are started and resting splints are worn at night for an additional 3 weeks to protect the tendon from inadvertent stretching. Because overlengthening of the finger flexors can result in a loss of grip strength, a flexor-pronator origin release may be done for patients with voluntary control but overpowering flexors.

d) Dynamic thumb-in-palm deformity causes the thumb to be flexed and adducted within the palm due to spastic adductor pollicis and thenar muscles. The flexor pollicis longus and the first dorsal interosseous (DI) commonly contributes to the deformity. It is corrected by proximal myotomy at the origin of all thenar muscles. Distal releases are avoided as it may cause hyperextension deformity of the thumb MCP joint. Flexion deformity of the IP thumb joint is corrected by either fractional or Z-plasty lengthening of the flexor pollicis in the forearm. The IP joint can also be stabilized by percutaneous arthrodesis. If the first DI is contracted, it is released. If the web space is contracted, a Z-plasty of the thumb web space is necessary. Postoperative care includes thumb spica cast for 4 weeks followed by active ROM exercises after cast removal.

e) **Dynamic intrinsic-plus hand deformity** results in flexed MCP and extended IP joints and is often associated with boutonniere or swanneck deformities of the fingers. It is corrected by blocking the motor branch of the ulnar nerve in the Guyon's canal either by neurectomy for permanent ablation or by injection of phenol into the exposed nerve under direct vision. Usually, a 5% phenol in glycerine is used because the glycerine allows the phenol to be released more slowly thus prolonging its effects (up to 6 months). Postoperative care includes soft dressing applied to the hand with ROM exercises (active and passive) started on the first day after surgery.

2. **Peripheral neurectomy,** is the sectioning of peripheral nerves to relieve spasticity. For example, anterior obturator neurectomies are used to relieve hip adductor spasticity and improve scissoring of gait in cerebral palsy patients; neurectomy of the motor branch of ulnar nerve is done to prevent intrinsic-plus hand deformity. See section III.D.2.b.2.b for other nerves used in neurectomies.

a. **Complete peripheral neurectomy** abolishes all muscle tone and voluntary movements. It is associated with profound muscular atrophy and sensory loss.

b. **Selective peripheral neurectomy** refers to the partial sectioning of the nerve using microsurgical techniques and intraoperative electrical stimulation, thus preserving some voluntary muscle activity, lessening atrophy, and preserving cutaneous sensory branches.

3. **Central electrical stimulations,** including **epidural (dorsal column) electrical stimulation** and **cerebellar stimulation** have been tried to reduce spasticity, but their long-term objective efficacy and functional gains under blinded conditions have yet to be shown.

G. **Step 7 care: Myelotomy, cordotomy, and cordectomy** are rarely done because they can lead to severe muscle atrophy, loss of bowel and bladder functions, and loss of erectile function. They are contraindicated when useful voluntary motor control is preserved or when motor recovery is possible.

1. **Myelotomy** involves severing of the tracts in the spinal cord.

2. **Cordotomy** involves sectioning and **cordectomy** involves excision of portions of the cord.

BIBLIOGRAPHY

Glen MB. Nerve blocks for treatment of spasticity, *Phys Med Rehabil State Art Rev* 8 (3):481-505, 1994.

Katz RT, Campagnolo. Pharmacological management of spasticity, *Phys Med Rehabil State Art Rev* 8 (3):473-480, 1994.

Katz RT: Management of spasticity. In Braddom RL, editor: *Physical medicine and rehabilitation.* Philadelphia, 1996, WB Saunders, pp. 580-604.

Keenan MA, Kozin S, Berlet A: *Manual of Orthopedic Surgery for Spasticity,* New York, 1993, Raven Press.

Little JW, Massagli TL: Spasticity and associated abnormalities of muscle tone. In DeLisa JA, Gans BM, editors: *Rehabilitation medicine: principles and practice,* ed 2, Philadelphia, 1993, JB Lippincott, pp. 666-680.

MacDonald CM: Selective dorsal rhizotomy: Patient selection, intraoperative electrophysiologic monitoring and clinical outcome, *Phys Med Rehabil State Art Rev* 8 (3):579-604, 1994.

Merritt JL: Management of spasticity in spinal cord injury. *Mayo Clin Proc* 56: 614-622, 1981.

O'Brien C, Yablon S, editors: *Management of spasticity with botulinum toxin: a clinical monograph,* Littleton, 1995, Postgraduate Institute of Medicine.

Schwartz RG: Botulinum toxin injections. In Lennard TA, editor: *Physiatric procedures in clinical practice,* Philadelphia, 1995, Hanley & Belfus, pp. 84-93.

Worldwide Education and Awareness for Movement Disorders (WE MOVE): *Spasticity: diagnosis and treatment.* Mount Sinai Medical Center, New York, 1995, WE MOVE publication.

Young RR, editor: Role of tizanidine in the treatment of spasticity, *Neurology* 44 (suppl 9):S1-S80, 1994.

CHAPTER 5.5

NEUROGENIC COMMUNICATION DISORDERS

This chapter deals only with acquired neurogenic communication disorders in adults encompassing the following dimensions of human communication: language, cognition, attention and perception, speech, voice, fluency, and hearing. It does not include developmental communication problems (e.g., developmental stuttering) or nonneurogenic voice or hearing disorders (e.g., laryngeal cancer and cholesteatoma), as these are beyond the scope of PM&R.

I. **Language impairments** can result from focal injury of the dominant (usually left) hemisphere (e.g., aphasia because of a stroke or neurosurgical procedure) or it may result from a more diffuse axonal injury (e.g., cognitive-communication impairments due to closed head injury). Although mild language impairment may be associated with right hemisphere communication impairments (RHCI), RHCI is discussed separately in section II because its underlying pathomechanism is nonlinguistic in origin (i.e., attentional and perceptual disorders).

A. **Aphasia (dysphasia)** is an acquired focal neurologic disorder (e.g., brain damage due to stroke) resulting in impairment of the processing for receptive language (i.e., auditory and reading comprehension) or expressive language (i.e., expressive speech, intonation, gestures, and written expression) or both receptive and expressive languages. The multimodal loss or reduction in language is disproportional to the impairment of other intellectual functions and cannot be attributed to dementia, sensory loss, or motor dysfunction. Aphasia is characteristically seen in lesions of the dominant hemisphere, which in 85% of all individuals is the left hemisphere. In the United States alone, there are more than a million people who suffer from aphasia, and each day almost 300 new cases are added to the list.

Aphasia must be differentiated from other cortical and subcortical speech and language disorders such as (1) *agnosia* in which, unlike the multimodal aphasia, the disorder tends to be confined to only one input or output modality despite intact end-organ function (e.g., auditory agnosia in which hearing is compromised despite normal hearing threshold, but visual modalities such as reading remain intact); (2) speech disorders (e.g., *apraxia of speech* or *dysarthria*, both described in section III); 3) *dementia*, which is primarily due to cognitive deficits (involving orientation, judgment, memory, and visual-perceptual skills) caused by Alzheimer's disease or multiple infarct dementia, which have a progressively deteriorating course (hence prognosis is less favorable than that for aphasia); and (4) *confusion*, which is characterized by reduced recognition, reduced understanding of and responsiveness to the environment, faulty memory, unclear thinking, and disorientation. Unlike dementia, confusion is often associated with head trauma, is generally not progressive, and has more favorable outcome. Both dementia and confusion have cognitive deficits that extend beyond the communication seen in aphasic patients.

1. **Classification of aphasia:** The algorithm for screening and classifying aphasia

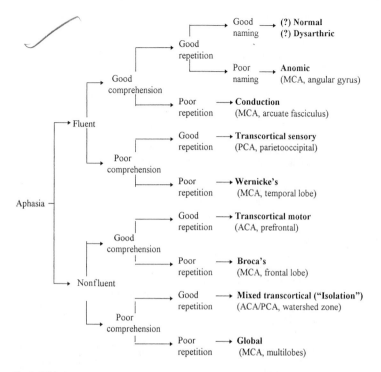

Figure 5.5-1
Algorithm for screening and classifying aphasia (using the Boston classification).
Listed in parentheses are the main sites of pathology and the blood vessels involved,
usually located on the left or dominant hemisphere. See text for explanation of
informal bedside screening of aphasia. MCA = middle cerebral artery; ACA =
anterior cerebral artery; PCA = posterior cerebral artery.

(using the Boston classification) is shown in Fig. 5.5-1. Standardized
screening tests (see section I.A.2) may be used. Informal bedside screening
may be done as follows: (1) Determine the patient's verbal fluency (fluent
vs. nonfluent characteristics are described in sections I.A.1.a and b) by
asking the patient, "What did you have for lunch?" or ask the patient to
say as many words within 1 minute beginning with letter *A* or *S* (most
normal people can list at least 12 words in 1 minute); (2) Check for comprehension by asking the patient to follow one-, two-, or three-step commands
(e.g., "Point your right thumb to your left ear, then to the door, then to
your bed."); (3) Have the patient repeat verbally after you using random
digits (e.g., "two," "eighteen," "twenty-nine," and so on), or words
(e.g., "apple" or "school"), or simple sentences (e.g., "The cat ate the
fish."); sentences can be made progressively more complicated by increasing the length and raising grammatical complexity (e.g., "When the busy
doctor went to the cafeteria he found that all the seats were occupied
by medical students."); and (4) Evaluate confrontation naming ability by

showing the patient a common object (e.g., pencil or tie) and ask for its name. Naming is severely impaired in patients with anomic or global aphasia.

The following subtypes of aphasia (based on the Boston classification) are caused by cortical lesions. Subcortical lesions, however, may also cause aphasias, for example, *anterior subcortical aphasia*, which involves the internal capsule limb and the putamen (aphasia characteristics are sparse verbal output with severely impaired articulation and hypophonic speech) and *posterior subcortical aphasia*, which involves the thalamus or neighboring white matter (aphasia characteristics are fluent aphasia, with intact comprehension and repetition skills but with major difficulty in word-finding and paraphasia [defined in section I.A.1.a]).

a. Fluent aphasia is associated with cerebral lesions posterior to the rolandic fissure, often in the temporoparietal region of the dominant (left) hemisphere. It is relatively normal in the following aspects: word output is 100 to 200 words per minute (wpm); speech production is easy and uneffortful; articulation is good; phrase length is more than 5 to 8 words/phrase; and prosodic quality is at least acceptable. (*Prosody* refers to the speech rate, rhythm, pitch, loudness, and intonation, which can convey additional meaning such as joy, anger, or sadness.) The speech content, however, lacks substance ("empty speech") and is characterized by *circumlocution* (i.e., attempts at word retrieval, which end in descriptions or associations related to the intended word), and frequent *paraphasia* (i.e., substitution of an incorrect or unintended word for a correct one, e.g., pen for pencil). This mostly incomprehensible but well articulated speech output is called *jargon*. Fluent aphasics tend to pause and seem to have word finding difficulty when semantically meaningful and picturable action words are needed. If asked "What did you have for lunch?" The answer might be, "Lunch. Yes, I have great lunches everyday. I love to munch. I would never miss munching for anything in the world. Yum, Yum. I love munching. My lunch I love lunch. I just love it. Everyday of the week is really super." Although verbose, this "fluent" answer lacks substance.

1) Major fluent aphasia

  a) Wernicke's aphasia (also known as "posterior," "receptive," "sensory," "acoustic," or "syntactic" aphasia) is associated with lesions of the posterior region of the superior temporal gyrus (which is supplied by the middle cerebral artery). It is predominantly a "receptive" aphasia, that is, comprehension (auditory and reading) skills are impaired. The well-articulated ("fluent") speech is characterized by paragrammatism (i.e., incorrect use of grammatical words), paraphasia (defined in I.A.1.a), circumlocution (defined in I.A.1.a), and neologism (i.e., partially recognizable, contrived, or "new" fabricated words). Patients with Wernicke's aphasia are unable to monitor their speech, and they seem to have an irrepressible desire to continue in their incomprehensible monologue (i.e., "press for speech"). Their repetition and writing skills are also impaired. Moreover, naming ability is poor (i.e., confrontational naming and word-finding, especially for substantive words). They also tend to show paranoid behaviors probably because of consistent confusion or neglect from their listener.

  b) Conduction aphasia ("afferent-motor" or "central" aphasia) is associated with lesions of the supramarginal gyrus and arcuate fasciculus (which are supplied by the middle cerebral artery). Its most discriminating feature is the significant impairment in repetition (which is more evident on repetition of phrases, short sentences, polysyllabic words, and unfamiliar phrases). While repetition difficulties may also be seen in other aphasias (e.g., Broca's, Wernicke's, or global), patients with conduction aphasia have relatively intact "fluency" and comprehension (auditory comprehension may be slightly impaired but is functional) which are disproportionate to their repetition impairment. Although considered "fluent," their speech (which may be limited to short bursts of fluency) may be interspersed with long pauses and expressive struggles due to naming (i.e., word-finding) difficulties. In addition, writing is impaired while reading skills remain intact.

2) Minor fluent aphasia

a) Transcortical sensory (TCS) aphasia (or "Wernicke's aphasia type II") is a rare syndrome associated with lesions in the parietooccipital area bordering Wernicke's area (which is supplied by the posterior cerebral artery). Like Wernicke's aphasia, the speech is fluent but comprehension (auditory and reading) is poor. Unlike Wernicke's aphasia, however, repetition skill is intact and may be echolalic (i.e., accurate repetition of a preceding utterance when repetition is not required). Naming (including word-finding abilities) and writing skills are also impaired.

b) Anomic aphasia (also known as "semantic," "nominal," or "amnesic" aphasia) is probably associated with lesions in the angular gyrus (which is supplied by the middle cerebral artery). It is a "milder" form of fluent aphasia whose major feature is word-finding difficulty, both orally and in writing. Unlike other fluent aphasias with word-finding difficulties (e.g., Wernicke's, conduction, and TCS aphasias), patients with anomic aphasia have relatively good comprehension (reading and listening skills are at least functional) and good-to-normal repetition skills. Their fluent, grammatically well-formed speech tend to be circumlocutory and may seem empty, as the content words tend to be omitted.

b. Nonfluent aphasia is associated with cerebral lesions anterior to the rolandic fissure, often in the frontal region of the dominant (left) hemisphere. It is characterized by the following: word output is sparse (i.e., less than 50 wpm); speech production is effortful (e.g., slow speech accompanied by facial grimacing and body posturing); articulation is poor; phrase length is short (1-2 words per phrase); and speech is dysprosodic (i.e., unmelodic, dysrhythmic, and incompetently inflected). Paraphasia is rare, however, and speech is packed with substantive words (i.e., nouns, action verbs, or descriptive adjectives) but is significantly lacking in syntactical words. The sparsely worded speech tends to be "telegraphic" and may be characterized by agrammatism (i.e., devoid of any grammatical structure). If asked "What did you have for lunch?" The answer might be, "Uh . . . salad . . . uh . . . chicken . . . fried . . . good." Although the answer is choppy, telegraphic, and agrammatic, it is packed with information.

1) Major nonfluent aphasia

a) Broca's aphasia (also known as "anterior," "nonfluent," "expres-

sive," "motor," "verbal-efferent," "motor-expressive," or "cortical-motor" aphasia) is the most common type of aphasia in patients receiving comprehensive rehabilitation. It is associated with lesions in the third convolution of the frontal lobe. It is predominantly an "expressive" aphasia (featuring all the nonfluent characteristics described above) with relatively intact and often functional auditory and reading comprehension (i.e., patients with Broca's aphasia are able to follow most everyday conversation and communicate through yes and no questions or multiple choices, but they may have trouble following complex grammatical statements). Repetition and naming skills are often moderately to severely impaired. Their writing output also tend to be as "nonfluent" as their speech. Due to their awareness of their inability to express themselves, they tend to show varying degrees of frustration when they make errors (in contrast, patients with Wernicke's aphasia often show little frustration or awareness of error).

b) Global aphasia is associated with lesions involving the frontal, temporal, and parietal lobes (supplied by the middle cerebral artery). It is similar to Broca's aphasia except that comprehension (auditory and reading) is severely impaired. Likewise, naming, repetition, and writing skills are impaired. Global aphasics may be able to utter automatic (stereotyped) words and phrases, but they are rarely able to use them in the appropriate context. They may compensate for their lack of verbal skills by using nonverbal means of communication (e.g., primitive gestures).

2) Minor nonfluent aphasia

a) Transcortical motor (TCM) aphasia is associated with lesions in the prefrontal or supplemental speech area (which is supplied by the anterior cerebral artery). Like Broca's aphasia, the speech is nonfluent (writing is also impaired) and comprehension (auditory and reading) is relatively intact and functional. Unlike Broca's aphasia however, repetition skill is intact (and may be echolalic). Naming ability of TCM aphasics, which is usually fairly good, may be slightly abnormal in some patients, for example during confrontation naming, perseveration may be noted (i.e., patient may continue to give a past answer for a new stimulus). Moreover, unlike Broca's aphasics, patients with TCM aphasia have occasional breakthroughs of grammatical and well-articulated speech with little to no paraphasia. Another feature of TCM aphasia is adynamia (i.e., difficulty in initiating speech or one-word factual responses; marked reduction in initiation and organization; and either akinetic or bradykinetic movements).

b) Mixed transcortical aphasia ("isolation of speech," "mixed nonfluent," or "sensorimotor aphasia") is a rare syndrome associated with lesions similar to those of TCM and TCS aphasias (both anterior and posterior cerebral arteries at the vascular watershed zone may be involved). Like global aphasia, the speech is nonfluent (writing is also impaired) and comprehension (auditory and reading) is poor. Unlike global aphasia, however, repetition skill is intact and may be echolalic. Unlike TCM aphasia, naming skills are impaired.

2. Assessment tools for aphasia can be used clinically to identify the nature and severity of the aphasia and its specific deficits, classify aphasia into subtypes, assess functional communication skills, establish prognosis and determine treatment necessity, guide in the treatment planning, and monitor treatment progress. They are commonly administered by speech-language pathologists (also called speech pathologists or speech therapists). The interpretation of quantitative assessment tools must be done cautiously because they may not always reflect "real-life" communication skills. Likewise, a "mild" impairment rating may be considered "severe" for that individual, especially when one considers occupation.

Screening tests for aphasia may be done informally (using the bedside screening method for classifying aphasia as described in section I.A.1) or formally (using standardized screening tests). Standardized screening tests for aphasia include: Aphasia Language Performance Scale (ALPS), Bedside Evaluation Screening Test (BEST), and Halstead-Wepman Aphasia Screening Test. Most of these can be administered at the bedside within 30 minutes. Another screening test for aphasia, which takes even less time (3-10 minutes) to administer, is the Frenchay Aphasia Screening Test (FAST). The following section describes the more popular aphasia test batteries used to evaluate comprehensive language, functional communication skills, and other related language modalities. Currently, the two most frequently used standardized aphasia examinations are the Boston Diagnostic Aphasia Examination (BDAE) and the Western Aphasia Battery (WAB).

a. Comprehensive language tests

1) **The Boston Diagnostic Aphasia Examination** contains 27 subtests and an additional group of nonlanguage subtests to evaluate parietal lobe dysfunction. It evaluates auditory comprehension, oral expression, understanding of written language, and writing. It is useful in classifying patients into the subtypes of aphasia (based on the Boston classification), assessing therapeutic progress, and in guiding treatment programs. It does not provide, however, prognostic information nor specific treatment plan. It may take several hours to administer. It has good internal validity, but reliability has not been clearly shown.

2) **Western Aphasia Battery** is a modification and expansion of BDAE. It measures oral language abilities (i.e., fluency and information content of spontaneous speech, comprehension, repetition, and naming) and auditory verbal comprehension. Both the auditory and expressive modality yields an aphasia quotient (AQ). An AQ below 93.8 is consistent with aphasia. Like BDAE, it is useful in classifying patients into the subtypes of aphasia (based on the Boston classification). It has high reliability and is highly correlated with Neurosensory Center Comprehensive Examination for Aphasia (NCCEA) scores. It requires 1 to 2 hours to administer (much less than that for the BDAE) and is widely used as a clinical and research tool.

3) **Porch Index of Communicative Ability (PICA)** has 18 subtests and uses 10 common objects to elicit patient responses. Every response is scored by a specially trained tester according to a unique 16-point multidimensional system based on accuracy, completeness, promptness, and responsiveness. Results are reported in percentiles and can be compared with scores of other patients with bilateral and left hemisphere damage. It is useful in determining prognosis, assessing therapeutic progress, and in planning programmed treatment and research. It as-

sesses a narrow range of verbal functions and is not sensitive to patients with mild or severe linguistic deficits. It provides the most detailed qualitative record of response and takes 1 hour to administer and score. It has high reliability and has concurrent validity with BDAE, Functional Communication Profile (FCP), and Communicative Abilities in Daily Living (CADL) tests.

4) **Minnesota Test for Differential Diagnosis of Aphasia (MTDDA)** consists of 47 subtests which focus on five areas of disorders: auditory disturbances, visual and reading disturbances, speech and language disturbances, visuomotor and writing disturbances, and disturbances of numerical relationships and arithmetic processes. It is most useful for recognizing and classifying deficits of auditory comprehension, for classifying patients into aphasia type (on which prognosis for recovery is based), and for treatment planning. The test takes about 3 hours and is given in multiple sessions. Its reliability and validity are not as well documented as for the BDAE or WAB

5) **Neurosensory Center Comprehensive Examination for Aphasia** contains 20 language subtests (to assess level of comprehension and expression, the ability to retain verbally presented material, and the ability to make functional use of reading and writing skills) and four control tests (to assess visual and tactile functions). It compares the patient's specific deficits with the performance of normal adults and has been tested on adult aphasics and on nonaphasic adults with brain damage. It also has norms for children to as young as 6 years old. It can measure severity of aphasia and can distinguish the patient's specific areas of strength and weakness; therefore, it can be used to monitor recovery. However, it does not assess spontaneous speech, does not specify aphasia classification, and does not specify treatment plan. It takes 90 minutes to administer. Its reliability is satisfactory, and has concurrent validity with WAB and FCP tests.

b. **Functional communication tests**

1) **Functional Communication Profile (FCP)** consists of 45 communication behaviors divided into five major groups: movement (gesture), speaking, understanding, reading, and others (e.g., handling of money). Data are collected in a nonstructured, conversational situation as the rater informally interacts with the patient. An overall percentage score reflects the patient's functional communication skills after the injury or disease and compares it to his or her own premorbid norm, which is inferred from the patient's education, personality, etc. It takes 20 to 30 minutes to administer by an experienced clinician. Although rating is subjective, it has high interrater reliability. The FCP can be used to follow recovery and predict outcome.

2) **Communicative Abilities in Daily Living** consists of 68 easily administered items incorporating 10 categories of everyday language activities presented in interview and role-playing situations. It provides information about the functional communication skills of aphasic patients in everyday situations and is used in patients whose PICA score have plateaued. It has high reliability and has high concurrent validity with the PICA, FCP, and BDAE tests.

3) **Communication Effectiveness Index (CETI)** is a more recent functional communication assessment tool that focuses on communicative need and assesses communication for social needs, life skills, basic needs,

and health threats. It is based on direct observation (done by the patient's spouse or significant other) of the patient's ability to perform 16 communicative skills relative to premorbid abilities in those skill areas.

4) **American Speech and Hearing Association–Functional Assessment of Communication Skills (ASHA-FACS)** consists of 43 items, which measure adult functional communication across four assessment domains (i.e., social communication; communication of basic needs; reading, writing, and number concepts; and daily planning) and four qualitative dimensions (i.e., adequacy, appropriateness, promptness, and communication sharing). It has high intra- and intertester reliability and takes about 20 minutes to administer. It has been tested on 131 adult aphasics with left hemisphere stroke (with good correlation with WAB) and 54 adults with cognitive-communication impairments due to traumatic brain injury (TBI) (with good correlation with the Scale of Cognitive Abilities for Traumatic Brain Injury [SCATBI]; see section I.B.2.c).

c. **Specialized aphasia tests** include the Token Test, which measures subtle mild auditory comprehension deficit (in which the patient is asked to manipulate 20 tokens of two sizes [big and small], two shapes [square and round], and five colors through nonredundant language of increasing length and complexity); Reporter's Test, a variation of the Token Test, in which the examiner moves the token and the patient describes the movements to another person who has not seen them; Reading Comprehension Battery, which assesses reading skills in greater detail than most aphasia batteries; Auditory Comprehension Test for Sentences (ACTS), which examines auditory comprehension, may be used in mildly impaired patients; Boston Assessment of Severe Aphasia (BASA), which is used in patients with severe or global aphasia for whom other tests are too difficult; Peabody Picture Vocabulary Test (PPVT), which is used to test naming ability. Multilingual tests of aphasia include the Multilingual Aphasia Examination (MAE) and the Bilingual Aphasia Test (BAT).

3. **Prognosis** for speech recovery in aphasic patients may be determined by using one of the comprehensive language tests (i.e., *WAB, PICA,* or *MTDDA*). In general, the following characteristics of aphasia tend to have poorer prognosis: severe auditory comprehension deficits, the presence of perseveration, the inability to match objects, unreliable yes and no responses, and the use of jargon and empty speech without self-correction. Among the four types of prognostic variables listed below, the medical and speech and language variables are more potent. There is no single variable that exerts such strong negative influence that it precludes a trial of speech therapy.

a. **Medical variables** include

1) **Etiologic factors.** Aphasia of vascular etiology has a poorer outcome than aphasia due to trauma. Aphasia caused by tumor has a variable prognosis (but is often poor).

2) **Site and extent of lesion.** In general, the larger the dominant-hemisphere lesion, the poorer the prognosis; small lesions, if multiple, have a poorer outcome; left-side lesions have a poorer prognosis than right-side lesions; and bilateral lesions, even when small, have a poorer prognosis. However, despite poor prognosis because of the site and

extent of the lesion, there are case reports of good recovery. A trial of speech therapy, therefore, should at least be considered.

3) Coexisting medical problems, if present, contributes to poor outcome.

b. **Speech and language variables**

1) **Severity of disorder.** Middle cerebral artery deficits frequently result in severe aphasia. Patients with severely impaired initial ability to speak or with severe impairment in auditory recognition and comprehension have a poorer prognosis. Likewise, the longer the length of their hospital stay, the poorer the outcome (probably due to coexisting medical problems in addition to severe impairments).

2) **Auditory process.** Patients with peripheral hearing loss or impaired central auditory process have a poorer outcome.

3) **Classification and type of disorder.** Broca's and Wernicke's aphasias have similar prognoses whereas global aphasia has a notably poorer prognosis. The poor auditory comprehension in Wernicke's aphasia makes it less amenable to treatment than other aphasias. Conduction aphasias have the greatest gains. The prognosis for TCM or TCS aphasia is generally good. In mixed transcortical aphasia, the prognosis is relatively good but is generally poorer than that for TCM or TCS aphasia.

4) **Nonlanguage cognitive defects,** for example, major perceptual defects, visual or auditory, or memory and attentional deficits (if any of these are present, the outcome is poorer); coexisting communicative impairment, for example, apraxia (if present, treatment efficacy may be limited).

c. **Patient variables**

1) **Age at onset.** Younger patients possibly have better outcomes (controversial).

2) **Education, premorbid intelligence, and communication skills.** Creative patients with rich vocabularies generally have a better outcome. In illiterates, aphasia is less severe, probably due to more bilateral representation of language.

3) **Handedness.** Reports that left-handed patients have better outcome is controversial (studies seem to indicate that handedness is probably not related to hemispheric dominance, i.e., many left-handed people are left-brain dominant with left-sided language representation).

4) **Multilinguals (polyglots).** Both the Ribot's rule and Pitre's Law are not shown to be consistently true. The Ribot's rule states that in a multilingual aphasic, the language best recovered would be the mother tongue; however, the Pitre's law states that the language that the multilingual aphasic was consistently using at the onset of the aphasia will be the first to be recovered even though it is not the first learned. Currently, there is no simple or steadfast rule of language recovery that can be consistently applied to the multilingual aphasics. There are reports that indicate that probably the language milieu during recovery determines the first language to be recovered. There are also reports of more frequent crossed aphasics in right-handers who are multilingual suggesting greater right-hemisphere participation. Most clinical evidence seems to indicate that the degree of control the left hemisphere has on the first and subsequent languages is probably the same.

5) **Gender** is probably unrelated to prognosis. Data favoring recovery in either sex have been reported.

d. Other variables

   1) Months after onset. The longer the time elapsed, the poorer the prognosis.

   2) Motivation. Poorly motivated patients have poorer outcome.

   3) Environment and attitude of support system. Patients whose family or significant others are supportive have better outcome.

4. **Treatment** of aphasia is a dynamic, organized process tailored to all the personal, neuropsychological, and linguistic factors affecting each patient. Although aphasia therapy is individualized, group therapy with peers can be beneficial in some patients as it can provide a comfortable atmosphere in which patients can vent feelings, meet new friends, gain feedback on their impairment and their progress, and practice functional communication skills. Aphasia therapy mainly uses the language intervention strategies described below. Pharmacological treatment (e.g., bromocriptine, L-dopa, amphetamine, and piracetam) has been reported in a few studies, but their efficacy remains doubtful. The general goals of aphasia treatment are (1) to stimulate the disrupted process and to promote functional reorganization; (2) to teach the use of residual abilities as compensatory strategies for communication; (3) to provide education and counseling and to promote adjustment of the patient and family; (4) to eliminate "bad habits" that interfere with successful communication; (5) to promote a suitable communication environment; and (6) to provide psychological support and improve the patient's attitude, morale, and other significant social factors (i.e., speech therapy can be used to channel attention and energies toward constructive ends, thus reducing depression). The ultimate goal of treatment is to progress toward successful "real-life" communication, outside the professional program, within the limits of the brain damage.

   There are 2 stages of language recovery: (1) an initial spontaneous recovery (reflecting resolution of edema, hemorrhage, and other cellular damage), which starts within a few days of onset and lasts about 1 month (or even further) after onset; and (2) a long-term recovery, which takes place for months or even years (reflecting reorganization of language function in the brain possibly from increased participation of uninjured parts of the brain or from relearning). Ideally, intensive aphasia treatment should be started and maintained as soon as the patient is medically and neurologically stable (even with delay of up to 6 months postonset, therapy has been shown to be beneficial). Speech therapy should be directed to the patient and the patient's family or significant others. It is usually given 3 to 5 times per week for 2 to 3 months during which time the patient is reevaluated on the first month and again after the second or third month. When the treatment progress has plateaued, the treatment may be gradually discontinued (abrupt cessation may be psychologically harmful) by reducing it to 1 to 2 times per week, then every 1 to 2 months with reevaluation at the sixth and tenth months. Strategies commonly used for aphasic therapy are described below. For specific treatment of different types of fluent and nonfluent aphasia, the reader is referred to LaPointe's *Aphasia and related neurogenic language disorders*, and Chapey's *Language intervention strategies in adult aphasia* (see Bibliography).

   Speech therapy (individual or group) for aphasia is generally reported to be beneficial and not harmful in patients with nonprogressive etiologies (e.g., stroke or excised brain tumor). The traditional belief is that significant spontaneous recovery is completed by 3 to 6 months postonset. However, a recent study (Nicholas et al, 1993) on the evolution of severe aphasia in the first 2 years postonset noted significant improvements in communicative functions for up to 18 months, with the greatest improvement occurring in the first 6 months. There is some justification, therefore, for continuing speech therapy longer than 6 months in selected cases.

a. **Language intervention strategies** are based on two schools of thoughts. The first school believes that language in the damaged brain is not "erased," but its access is impaired. The brain, therefore, needs to be retrained to retrieve its individual language units (i.e., use a *retraining approach* to build the lost or inhibited language processes). The second school believes that the language function subserved by the damaged brain is not recoverable; therefore, the patient must compensate for what is lost (i.e., use a *compensatory approach* to learn alternate ways of communicating, which may be nonverbal). Cueing strategies commonly used include varying the speed and means of presentation of an item, providing additional information about an item or providing phonetic or semantic starters. For clinical use, a multimodal (holistic) approach, that is, combining the retraining and compensatory approaches, is probably most effective.

1) **Retraining approach** (or "restorative" approach) attempts to activate any essential verbal behavior and facilitate language recovery through repetitive stimulation, primarily of the auditory system, which is believed to be the primary mode of language acquisition as well as the feedback system that processes and controls the information. Another system frequently stimulated is the visual system. The stimulation is constantly repeated as repetition is essential for organization, storage, and retrieval of information in the brain.

a) **Stimulation techniques** emphasize effective verbal communication through stimulation of input modalities to improve spoken and written language, without putting too much emphasis on personal relevancy of lexicon or grammar. It is exemplified by the Stimulation-Facilitation Therapy, which typically has the following features: the clinician generally assumes the role of stimulator or facilitator and initiates and directs language-based exchanges; auditory stimulations, as well as pictorial and printed stimuli, are used to improve propositional word retrieval and to increase length and completeness of utterances; convergent confrontative strategies are used to increase available vocabulary; and treatments, which are given in an individual clinical setting, are based on the analysis of the individual patient's profiles of language strengths and deficits derived from assessment tools. Other examples include Sentence-Level Auditory Comprehension Treatment Program (SLAC), which is designed to improve auditory comprehension using controlled auditory stimulation, and Language Enrichment Therapy (LET), which uses a pedagogical language training approach (applied by clinicians as well as trained relatives) in an attempt to improve functional communication.

b) **Programmed learning (behavior modification) techniques** involve the use of a methodical framework in which each program contains a defined success criteria, and the course of therapy is planned and conducted in small steps with hierarchy of difficulties. Examples include Respondent-Contingent Small-Step Treatment (RCSST), Audio-Visual Stimulation and Direct-Production Treatment,

Filmed Language Instruction, Sentence Repetition, ''Loose'' training (which facilitates responses by allowing patients to use their
own creative language rather than demanding specific target responses), and group therapy.

c) **Symptom-specific techniques** involve the use of specific types of linguistic deficits as specific communicative goals in therapy (e.g.,
therapy to improve word retrieval or spontaneous speech). Examples include self-cueing, which uses linguistic cues or microcom-
puters to improve word retrieval or improve spontaneous speech;
Treatment of Aphasic Perseveration (TAP), which uses inhibitory
techniques to treat perseveration; and The Preventative Method,
which is used to prevent secondary symptoms, (e.g., telegraphic
speech) from developing.

d) **Language-oriented (psycho- or neurolinguistic) techniques** involve the
use of a programmed instruction approach addressing the actual
deficit and progressing from lower levels of functioning to higher
linguistic levels according to predetermined steps.

   (1) **Structure-based techniques** emphasize the relearning of linguistics
   units through repeated performances (resembling a didactical
   grammar exercise). Examples include Sentence Construction
   Board (SCB), Systematic Therapy for Auditory Comprehension
   Disorders, Training Formal Structure of Language, and Mapping Thematic Relations.

   (2) **Deblocking techniques** systematically pair weak with strong modalities to ''deblock'' impaired performances, for example,
   Helm-elicited Language Program for Syntax Stimulation
   (HELPSS) program used in patients with agrammatism, which
   involves the use of proper cues to remove blocks that interfere
   with the accessing process of syntactic information.

   (3) **Voluntary control of involuntary utterances (VCIU)** is a recently used
   method that attempts to develop a functional vocabulary from
   the spontaneous utterances of patients with global aphasia.

2) **Compensatory approach** (or ''substitutive retraining'') assumes that,
despite a certain amount of neural plasticity in adult brains, other
areas of the brain cannot relearn what the damaged area subserved.
Hence, rather than retraining lost or inhibited language functions,
patients are taught how to compensate using whatever residual function they have (e.g., using gestures or melodic stimulation) to attain
communication, of which language is important but not the only
means.

a) **Functional communication (pragmatic) techniques** focus on effective
verbal communication, stressing the pragmatic approach (i.e., the
context-based use of social rules of communication) rather than on
the grammatical aspects of language. Functional communication
strategies need not replace but instead may be viewed as an extension of language retraining methods. Although patients may benefit
by maximally improving the lexical and syntactic aspects of the
language, the learned language should also be tested and used in
various functional contexts. The pragmatic approach is exemplified
by the Functional Communication Therapy (FCT), which focuses
on the following: (1) the clinician alternates as listener and speaker
by creating situations requiring equal participation from the patient,

(2) patient comprehension and response is maximized by enriching the context of natural conversation with writing, gestures, use of situational cues, and interrogative probes, (3) the environment of the treatment setting (e.g., in a group setting) is made as natural as possible, and (4) when contrived situations are used, the situation should simulate real-life scenes and context and must stress functional communication content (e.g., stimuli such as menus, road maps, calendars may be used in FCT to create role-playing situations).

Other examples of the pragmatic approach are Visual Action Therapy (VAT) in which the patient creates symbolic or representational gestures to represent visually absent objects; Promoting Aphasics' Communicative Effectiveness (PACE) Therapy, which involves getting a message across by any means possible, whether it be via language, drawing, gesture, tone of voice, or any of a variety of other expressive methods; Response Elaboration Training (RET), which is based on the "loose training" concept described in section I.A.4.a.1.b; Visual Communication Therapy (VIC), which was designed for global aphasics and which uses an artificial language consisting of arbitrary symbols representing syntactic and lexical components of language that the patient learns to manipulate; Computer-Aided Visual Communication (C-VIC) System, which is a computerized adaptation of VIC; Communicative Strategies, which includes asking other people to speak slower or to simplify their complicated messages; Conversational Coaching, which involves coaching of the patient by the clinician in different settings as the patient uses a scripted short monologue; and Behavioral Modification to Train Requesting in which the patient is prompted by the clinician to ask for information on chosen topics.

b) **Right hemisphere (or minor hemisphere) mediation techniques** use minor (nondominant, usually right) hemisphere abilities to mediate (facilitate) communication through the use of imagery, contextually rich stimuli, novel stimuli, drawing (e.g., Back to Drawing Board [BDB]), melody (e.g., melodic intonation therapy [MIT], which uses natural melody patterns to facilitate speech in nonfluent aphasics with good comprehension), or humor (e.g., laughter therapy).

c) **Nonverbal communication techniques** substitute spoken words with visual symbols or gestures. It may be augmented or supplemented by Augmentative and Alternative Communication Aids ranging from pointing tools (e.g., communication board, which the patient can use to convey messages by pointing to the board's printed letters, numbers, words, or pictures, using a finger, head pointer, or foot) to computer-based systems (e.g., using a computerized scanning system through which the patient can indicate his or her chosen message displayed on the computer screen by either typing or inputing other signals such as infrared beams transmitted through head nods, eye blink, etc.). Nonverbal techniques differ from previously mentioned methods (e.g., VAT or VIC) in the greater degree of stress they place on nonverbal means of communication. Examples include Blissymbolics, which uses line drawn symbols to represent basic nouns, verbs, adjective, or function words; sign language such as those used by the deaf; Amer-Ind

Code treatment, which uses gestural communication consisting of nearly 250 iconic gestural signals (modified from American Indian sign language) to facilitate oral speech production.

b. Speech therapy aids

1) Social-context aids are used to improve the patient's social interaction abilities and promote understanding of the aphasic syndrome in both the patient and the patient's immediate social support system. Examples include family therapy, which encourages the aphasic patient and their family members to act out the emotional feelings connected with the trauma to improve family communication skills and avoid emotional problems and psychological deterioration, and linguistic role playing to stimulate residual language and develop compensatory communicative abilities.

2) Affective-context aids are aimed at helping the patient cope with the affective aspects such as depression, anxiety, and frustration. Examples include hypnotherapy to sharpen memory and integrate skills learned during therapy; and laughter therapy (see section I.A.4.a.2.b) to relax the patient and improve the mood of the therapy session.

c. Interdisciplinary team approach emphasizes that everyone caring for the aphasic patient (professionals and nonprofessionals) be actively involved in the speech rehabilitation of the patient. Almost all patients with aphasia have some degree of difficulty in comprehending spoken language, and the patient's auditory comprehension varies greatly, depending on the context and complexity of the task at hand. In communicating with aphasic patients, the following guidelines are suggested:

- Use short and simple sentences.
- Speak a little more slowly and give the patient enough time to process the information and formulate a response.
- Ask unequivocal questions that can be answered with ''yes'' or ''no'' or another single word.
- Use physical assistive cues to facilitate the patient's comprehension (e.g., gestures, facial expression, and voice inflection).
- Be aware that aphasic patients often find it easier to respond to whole body or axial commands (e.g., ''stand up'') than distal commands (e.g., ''pick up'').
- Be consistent in giving instructions and, if needed, repeat the instruction or rephrase it and supplement speech with body language or written instructions.
- If the patient becomes visibly frustrated, remain calm and try again later.
- Encourage patients to produce single-word repetitive speech that coincides with physical movements (this supplements the patient's speech practice).
- Do not make demands that are beyond the patient's level of preserved communicative skill (this can be determined by consulting with the speech-language pathologists).

B. Cognitive-communication impairment (CCI) or cognitive-linguistic impairment is a nonaphasic language impairment, which occurs following diffuse brain damage caused by a nonpenetrating TBI, in particular a closed head injury (CHI) in which the primary traumatic force is a sudden acceleration or deceleration of the brain within the skull (e.g., motor vehicular crash, fall, or head blow with a blunt object). Aside from diffuse axonal injury, the pathophysiology of the CHI can also include focal lesions, ischemia, and neurochemical changes, all of which interact with the severity of the CHI and the patient's premorbid status to produce heterogenous patterns of neurobehavioral deficits. The language impairment in CCI is differentiated from aphasia in that its deficit (involving attention, information processing, and cognition) is more discernible on tasks with greater cognitive demands than those discerned in conventional measures used for aphasia. Moreover, the conceptual framework used to explain CCI focuses on how one uses language (e.g., in discourse), not simply on how one performs isolated linguistic measures.

1. Classification of communication deficits associated with CCI.

   a. Aphasic language deficits include anomia (the most common aphasic language deficit in CCI), reduced word fluency, impaired comprehension of complex oral commands, verbal paraphasic errors (especially in complex task, e.g., picture-description task and use of antonyms, synonyms, and metaphor), impairments of reading and writing, impaired sentence repetition, disruption in flow of language (i.e., slowed rate of speech, hesitations, and repetition of words or phrases), and perseveration.

   b. Nonaphasic language deficits, have also been referred to as "subclinical aphasic disorder," "high-level language deficits," "global disorganization of language," "confused thought content," "impaired language processing," and "fragmented and tangential conversation." These deficits, which become evident during discourse, include difficulties in topic management (in both appropriate selection and maintenance of conversational topic); noncoherent topic changes; ambiguous, unrelated, and incomplete ideational units; and unrelated responses. Grammatical or syntactic errors (e.g., omission of the subject or the main verb) occur less frequently but seem to be more than those committed by normal subjects. Although traditional naming ability is commonly disrupted in CCI patients, it does not appear to have a direct association with discourse function.

   c. General cognitive deficits

      1) Attention deficits include impulsivity (in which the patient cannot sustain concentration long enough to monitor the quality of ongoing behavior), inappropriate social judgment, lack of insight, literal interpretations, perseveration, stimulus boundedness, disinhibition, and comprehension difficulties.

      2) Information processing deficits refer to impairments involving areas of language, visual perceptual skills, motor skills, and memory (i.e., analysis and synthesis of information in sequential steps). Specifically, they may include aphasia, alexia (reading disorder), agraphia (writing disorder), acalculia (calculation disorder), agnosia (defined in I.A), apraxia of speech (see section III.A), amnesia, and memory impairments. Perceptual disturbances (e.g., unilateral spatial neglect), associated with CCI can also be considered an information-processing deficit because it reflects failure of the brain to adequately process stimuli to the point of meaningfulness.

      3) Cognition deficits include disorders in perception, discrimination, organization, recall, and problem solving, all of which may be difficult to separate from language disorders or from attention or information-processing deficits.

2. Assessment
   a. Aphasia language batteries (see section I.A.2) may be used to identify certain linguistic deficits in CCI. However, because they measure language primarily at the word and sentence levels, they may be relatively insensitive to the nonaphasic language deficits (e.g., poor discourse and poor cognitive abilities) seen in CCI. One functional communication test that has been validated for CCI is the ASHA-FACS (see section I.A.2.b.4). The ASHA-FACS has a good correlation (0.78) with the Scale of Cognitive Abilities for Traumatic Brain Injury (SCATBI; see I.B.2.c).
   b. Nonaphasia language (discourse) tests focus on narrative, procedural, descriptive, and conversational discourse. They measure informational content, cohesive ties, story and topic production, sequential organization of information, informativity, and semantic coherence at either a global level (i.e., relevance of information to a unifying theme or topic of the conversation) or a local level (i.e., connectivity between sentences as marked by cohesive devices, e.g., reference and connectors).
   c. General cognitive tests for CCI include tests of perception, discrimination, organization, recall, convergent thinking, deductive reasoning, inductive reasoning, divergent thinking, and problem solving. Examples include Scale of Cognitive Abilities for Traumatic Brain Injury (SCATBI), Wechsler Memory Scale, Benton Visual Retention Test, Woodcock-Johnson Test of Cognitive Abilities, Detroit Test of Learning Abilities, Test of Problem Solving, and Ross Information Processing Assessment. Neuropsychologic tests (see Chapter 2.9) may also be used to assess cognitive skills (e.g., Halstead-Reitan Neuropsychological Battery (HRNB) and Luria-Nebraska Neuropsychological Battery (LNNB).
3. Prognosis for CCI recovery is most favorable for younger patients, patients who spend less than 3 months in a coma, and patients who are highly motivated and goal-oriented. While age is important in determining recovery, age alone cannot predict recovery. The severity of diffuse cerebral insult (as reflected by duration of coma) is the major determinant of language competence 1 year after severe head injury. The course of language recovery in CHI is manifested initially by a complete collapse of the language system, followed by gradual recovery (typically within 6 months) until "normal speech" is attained as measured by conventional aphasia language tests. In fact, about two-thirds of CHI patients with aphasia in the acute stage show overall improvement in aphasic linguistic abilities. Certain aspects of language, however, have been reported to remain impaired years after injury, such as, naming or word-finding, word fluency, and comprehension of multistage commands. Nonaphasic linguistic deficits at the discourse level generally have a less favorable prognosis following CHI.
4. Treatment of CCI is ultimately aimed at developing in the patient the ability to practice, to learn from that practice, to use feedback purposely, and to encourage relearning of daily skills, which will then enhance functional living. It may include some of the techniques (and principles) used for aphasia with greater emphasis placed on the cognitive aspects and on discourse. During the earlier stage of recovery the treatment may include environmental intervention, structured activities, and cognitive-communication activities. As recovery progresses, the patient is taught compensatory strategies, memory organization, and problem solving. The interdiscipli-

nary approach must be used to provide consistency, feedback, and reinforcement to the patient. Family involvement at the start of the program cannot be overemphasized.

Treatment program must be individualized although it may be given in a group setting. Group therapy can provide opportunities for the patient to increase social interaction and self-monitoring skills in a communication environment, which is more natural than the individual therapy setting; increase self-esteem and self-motivation; increase ability to develop short- and long-term goals that are meaningful; and allow the patient to share feelings and needs with peers as well as to provide and receive peer review of behaviors. Computers may also be used for CCI rehabilitation to provide a controlled, consistent presentation of task stimuli with objective feedback. However, improvement in computer tasks do not necessarily generalize to other, more meaningful areas of the patient's life. Computerized systems that train attention, visual scanning, and concentration seems to hold the greatest promise for generalizing to "real-life" activities. Neuropharmacologic agents (described below) may also be used to improve attention, memory, and learning. As of present, there are no definitive studies available to suggest what works and doesn't work in CCI rehabilitation.

a. **Aphasic language rehabilitation** include both retraining and compensatory strategies used for aphasia (see section I.A.4.a). Specific strategies used for anomia (the most common aphasic language deficit, which may persist beyond 6 months of recovery) include word retrieval techniques (confrontational naming, confrontational naming with prestimulation, sentence completion, cueing hierarchies, and word focus), generalization (e.g., picture description, prepared monologue, story retelling, story elaboration, referential communication, and role-playing), and compensatory strategies (e.g., develop patient's use of generated cues, gestures, and drawing).

b. **Nonaphasic language rehabilitation,** specifically on discourse, concentrates on the close interaction of cognition and linguistics. Patients are trained through a feedback and cueing system in a different setting to improve sequential organization of information, increase informativity, increase global cohesiveness (i.e., relationship of a response or sentence to the topic of conversation), increase local cohesiveness (i.e., connectivity between adjacent sentences as marked by cohesive devices, e.g., references and connectors), increase cognitive organization of information in the narrative discourse (avoid incomplete episodes), and to decrease use of repetitions and revisions.

c. **Cognitive remediation** is usually administered by neuropsychologists (or specially trained speech-language pathologists). It is quite controversial and seems to be of benefit only to mild or moderate CCI. The treatment has a three-stage hierarchy consisting of arousal and alerting, operant retraining, and a community-oriented, self-reliant treatment program. Computers are usually used in cognitive remediation, although their long-term benefit and generalizability to "real-life" situations remains unproved.

1) **Attention-focusing techniques** include techniques for focusing attention (e.g., using the starter phrase "are you ready?" or waiting for eye contact before initiating a task with the patient); reducing environmental distractions (which can be added gradually as attention im-

proves); techniques to make the session interesting (e.g., varying the treatment concept, time, rates, and sequences); and sensory stimulation to activate any response to a stimulus and to gradually increase the frequency, type, and duration of the response.

2) **Information processing techniques,** specifically on improving memory, which include techniques to facilitate short-term memory storage (e.g., using meaningful verbal information); facilitate short-term to long-term memory storage (by analyzing, organizing, and rehearsing information); decrease reliance on feedback for memory (by gradually weaning the patient from memory cues); and determine the best method of processing information for each patient. The usefulness of rote repetition in improving memory is unclear. Patients with severe deficits can often use external memory aids (e.g., calendars, bulletin boards, message machines, and small notebooks), while patients with more subtle deficits may use internal aids such as mnemonic strategies (e.g., "chunking," i.e., memorizing in smaller segments such as 263-925-424 instead of 263925424, or rhyming).

3) **Cognitive retraining methods** vary from simple low-technology interventions to complex computerized interventions. The selected interventions should match the patient's home and work environment as closely as possible. They include techniques for improving perception (e.g., tracking, sound recognition, shape recognition, and work recognition); discrimination, (e.g., color discrimination, matching objects, pointing to objects, visual matching picture to sentence, and auditory discrimination between words or sentences); organization (e.g., categorization and closure [identification of geometric forms with sections missing], and sequencing); recall (e.g., verbal description, visual imagery, chunking activities, categorization of information, rehearsal, association, temporal spatial ordering, primacy and recency benefits [first and last items are accented visually or auditorily], PQRST approach [preview, question, read, state, and test], and mnemonic devices); and problem solving (e.g., convergent thinking, deductive reasoning, inductive reasoning, divergent thinking, and multiprocess reasoning).

d. **Psychopharmacological interventions** seem to be beneficial in CCI patients with deficits in attention, memory, or learning. They must be used judiciously, however, and their dosages monitored as their "therapeutic windows" are often narrow. The drugs commonly used to improve attention and concentration (which in turn are supposed to improve memory and learning) are central nervous system stimulants (i.e., catecholamine agonists). They include dextroamphetamine (Dexedrine), 2.5 to 5 mg, po, bid (given in the AM and at midday; may be increased to 30-60 mg/day; available in 5- and 10-mg tabs and 5 mg/5 ml elixir); methylphenidate (Ritalin), 0.30 mg/kg, po, bid or 5 to 10 mg, po, bid/tid (available in 5-, 10-, and 20-mg tabs); and Pemoline (Cylert), 37.5 mg, po, every morning (may increase by 18.75 mg at 1-week intervals up to 75-112.5 mg/day; the effective daily dose is 56.25-75 mg; available in 18.75-, 37.5-, and 75-mg tabs). Experimental drugs that are used to improve memory and learning include physostigmine (a cholinergic agonist only available in oral form for experimental use) and pramiracetam (considered a "nootropic" or "cognitive activator"). For details on the drugs, see Chapter 4.8, section V.E.

II. Right hemisphere communication impairment (RHCI) is an acquired disturbance of the attentional and perceptual mechanisms of the right (nondominant) hemisphere (e.g., due to stroke, traumatic brain injury [TBI] or tumor), which results in impaired reception and expression of contextually based communication. Patients with RHCI may appear linguistically adequate (unlike aphasics, they have no apparent difficulty with laboratory language and speech tasks), but they communicate inefficiently because they are neither able to appreciate nor interpret the context of incoming visual and auditory information, e.g., emotion conveyed in another's voice.

A. Classification of communication deficits associated with RHCI

   1. Extralinguistic deficits reflect a failure to adequately interpret cues and organize or express information in an efficient manner. They are actually considered to be the result of processing deficits in the nonlinguistic area.

   a. Receptive deficits may result in difficulty in organizing information due to failure to make use of contextual or emotional cues.

   1) Context-cue interpretation difficulties can lead to failure to recognize the implicit or implied meaning whether in verbal exchange or in pictures and ongoing events. Specifically, the RHCI patient has difficulty in distinguishing relevant from irrelevant information, grasping figurative meaning (i.e., they are literal-minded), and recognizing humor and metaphorical language structures.

   2) Emotional-cue interpretation difficulties include the inability to interpret the tone of voice, prosody, facial expression, and situational context. The emotional impairment is in its superficial expression and comprehension rather than its actual experience.

   b. Expressive deficits can make turn-taking during conversation difficult due to the inability to maintain a conversational topic.

   1) Emotional expression difficulties can result in flat affect and monotonous speech (i.e., lack of facial expression while speaking, failure to maintain eye contact, failure to use gesture, and a lack of vocal inflection or emotional overlay), or it may occasionally manifest inappropriately as hypereuphoric or jocular speech.

   2) Impulsive responses to complex questions are given with no apparent thought or regard for the listener's reaction. The responses given immediately are usually shallow, inaccurate, or inappropriate, and they reflect the RHCI patient's refusal to admit their uncertainty or lack of knowledge.

   3) Interpretive-response difficulties result in a tendency to use more explicit (i.e., excessive irrelevant details due to failure to distinguish significant from insignificant information) rather than interpretive concepts in the response (e.g., ''the young woman in her mid-twenties breastfeeding the baby'' rather than interpreting it as the ''mother breastfeeding the baby.'')

   4) Overpersonalized responses (i.e., excessive reliance on personal or internal associations) are given because it is easier to reminisce than to interact when one is uncertain about the nature of the conversation or unsure of how to organize an opinion or explanation.

   2. Nonlinguistic deficits comprise the underlying pathomechanism of RHCI and are usually manifested in the extralinguistic aspects of communication. In the rehabilitation setting, the nonlinguistic deficits (i.e., attentional and perceptual disorders) can make ambulation and activities of daily living (ADL) training more difficult and can lead to multiple accidents and falls.

a. **Attentional disorders** have recently been shown to involve space in general, rather than being limited only to the contralateral (left) side. Attentional disorders involve the inability to focus attention as well as difficulty deciding which features require attention. Specifically, they include the inability to recognize the boundaries of relevant space, to recognize significant features within that space, and to act upon those features.

1) **Unilateral spatial neglect (USN) (left-sided neglect)** is the inability to register and to integrate stimuli and perceptions from the one side (usually left side) of the body and environment. Patients with pure USN (i.e., without homonymous hemianopsia) have intact vision but seem unaware of the problem and do not attempt to compensate spontaneously by turning their head. In contrast, patients with left homonymous hemianopia have actual loss of vision from the left visual field of both eyes and may be aware of the problem and automatically compensate by turning their head. An extreme case of USN is *anosognosia*, in which the patient not only completely neglects the left paralyzed side (and the left environment), but they may even deny that the left limbs belong to them.

   a) **Sensory neglect** can lead to disrupted input of sensory stimulation from the left side (e.g., failure to read the left side of a book page), hence decreased ability to integrate concrete sensory and perhaps even abstract information. Tests include the visual field cut test to rule out coexisting homonymous hemianopsia and the cortical sensory extinction using simultaneous bilateral stimulation in the visual, auditory, and tactile modalities.

   b) **Motor neglect** can lead to impairment in the interaction with and the exploration or manipulation of the left-sided external space (e.g., impaired use of left-sided margins and punctuation in writing). Constructional abilities and scanning (e.g., visual scanning or tracking) can also be impaired.

2) **Confusion** can result from impaired contextual processing and impaired visual associations. It can lead to an inability to attend adequately to environmental cues resulting in *reduplicative paramnesia* (i.e., geographic disorientation in which the patient is convinced he or she is in another location), *prosopagnosia* (i.e., inability to recognize familiar faces), or topographical disorientation (i.e., inability to get to the destination).

b. **Perceptual disorders (visuospatial perceptual deficits)** can lead to impairment in the rapid recognition and synthesis of features into a form that is more than the sum of its parts (i.e., bits of information are seen but not integrated).

3. **Linguistic deficits** in RHCI, if present, are usually mild. They include problems in word-finding (e.g., confrontation naming, body part naming, and word fluency), auditory comprehension of complex material, oral sentence-reading, and writing (e.g., dysgraphia, which manifests as substitutions, repetitions, and omissions of words). Their speech also tends to be monotonous.

B. **Assessment:** The only formal assessment tool for RHCI is the Rehabilitation Institute of Chicago Evaluation of Communication Problems in Right Hemisphere Dysfunction (RIC-ECPRHD), which provides a check list and rating scale for pragmatic functions (e.g., eye contact and facial gestures), interpretation of metaphorical language, memory skills, writing, visual scanning and tracking, and an analysis of conversation including topic maintenance, verbosity, and reference. The screening battery for assessing cognition in patients with right-sided stroke is an informal tool that screens basic language skills; analyzes single word responses to part-whole tasks, oral opposites, written opposites, oral analogies, and printed analogies; evaluates interpretation of idioms, proverbs, effects of imagery; and evaluates the ability to appreciate humor. Other related tests include tests for visual perception (e.g., Spatial Orientation Memory Test and the Hooper Test of Visual Organization), tests of verbal or nonverbal relationships (e.g., subtests of Detroit Test of Learning Aptitude and Woodcock-Johnson Psycho-Educational Battery, respectively); tests of language function (e.g., standard aphasia battery and "Cookie Theft" picture subtest from Boston Diagnostic Aphasia Examination), and cognitive test batteries (e.g., mathematics subtest to assess mathematics skills, which can be impaired in patients with RHCI).

1. **Extralinguistic tests** assess interpretative skills that measure ability to distinguish relevant from irrelevant information (e.g., "Cookie Theft" picture description and story interpretation; Woodcock-Johnson Psycho-Educational Battery to determine nonverbal ability to see relationship; Detroit Test of Learning Aptitude to assess verbal relationship using analogy tests), organizational skills (e.g., ask patient for opinion on topic of current interest), pragmatic skills (e.g., RIC-ECPRHD to rate pragmatic functions such as facial gestures during conversation), emotional responsiveness (e.g., explain emotional content in pictures and stories), and prosodic skills (e.g., read aloud sentences in a happy, sad, or angry tone).

2. **Nonlinguistic testings** include neuropsychological examinations for motor neglect (e.g., spontaneous drawing and copy drawing of symmetrical objects to determine left versus right details; line bisection tasks to establish sense of midline; and cancellation tests such as uncrossing of lines to determine severity of neglect), sensory neglect (e.g., visual field cuts and cortical extinction), visual perception (e.g., Hooper Test of Visual Organization and the Spatial Orientation Memory Test), attention (i.e., short and immediate memory, e.g., digit span and story retelling), and confusion (e.g., orientation to place and recognition of familiar faces).

3. **Linguistic tests** include the standard aphasia battery or its subtests, the standard reading battery, and the test of writing skills. Even if language appears normal, standardized language tests (to assess visual confrontational naming, word fluency, auditory and written paragraph comprehension, and reading and writing skills) are useful.

C. **Prognosis** for recovery from RHCI, as in aphasia, is affected by the site and size of the lesion, age, and degree of lateralization. Neglect symptoms in stroke patients usually subside 6 months after the stroke onset. If neglect persists beyond the first few months, the prognosis for improvement seems to be poor.

D. **Treatment** for extralinguistic deficits should not only be focused on compensatory strategies but should also incorporate treatments for the underlying nonlinguistic problems. Nonlinguistic deficits can be approached through patient education and through feedback paradigms. The patient is trained to increase awareness of the neglected side by initially presenting stimuli (especially those specialized for the right hemisphere, e.g., shapes or blocks) on the intact side, gradually shifting the stimuli to the midline then to the neglected side. The patient is given training on anchoring visual attention to a certain starting point, systematic scanning (e.g., left-to-right visual scanning), slowing down their performance, recognizing errors and stimulus load via feedback, and manipulating the complexity of the task. He or she is also taught to position the head and eye toward the involved field. During physical therapy, weight bearing (after proper splinting) of the affected side and stimulation of the proprioceptors of the affected joints may provide effective feedback to improve limb perception. Aside from awareness skills, techniques to facilitate recovery of deficits in perception and attention (e.g., "edgness" and "bookness") may also be used. For linguistic deficits, aphasia treatment regimen may be used. The following techniques are used in RHCI patients with nonlinguistic and extralinguistic deficits:

1. **Perception- and attention-recovery techniques**
   a. **"Edgeness" technique** requires the patient to detect (using both visual and tactile tracing methods) the boundaries of relevant space (e.g., a grid) and to explore within the boundaries (e.g., by asking the patient to find colored cubes placed in varying locations on the grid). After practicing with the grid, the patient progresses to the perimeter of any surface (e.g., lapboard or table) on which they are working.
   b. **"Bookness" technique** is an extension of the "edgeness" technique. The patient is asked to use the eyes to trace the outline of the book and to describe what he or she sees. This is done on every reading session, first with the book closed then with the book opened. It also includes reading tasks that involve matching stimuli on the left page with that on the right page. Initial stimuli include shapes that progress to letters, words, and, finally, sentences. In the "bookness" technique, the concept of reading is treated as a whole instead of a left-to-right scanning task.

2. **Compensatory strategies** involve teaching the RHCI patient to use unimpaired language capabilities (e.g., auditory or visual) to compensate for the impaired visuomotor skills. The patient is given tasks that help him or her to pay attention to the contextual and pragmatic cues (e.g., facial expression and tone); to reduce verbosity; to improve the ability to maintain a conversational topic; to retell stories in a fashion that highlights the relevant points; and to produce language that follows a logical sequence. Feedback may be given to the patient in individual (e.g., by cueing from the clinician and playing back taped conversations) or group sessions.

3. **Interdisciplinary team approach** emphasizes active involvement of the entire rehabilitation team. The patient's family or significant others (as well as the rest of the rehabilitation team) are not only counseled on the impact of RHCI on the patient and their own perception of the patient's personality, but they are instructed in a consistent approach for treatment. For example, the whole team should be involved in providing feedback cues on pragmatic skills and in listing step-by-step the approach to accomplishing transfers, ambulation, or other activities of daily living.

III. **Speech disorders**
   A. **Apraxia of speech (AOS)** is a nondysarthric, nonaphasic sensorimotor disorder of articulation and prosody (prosody is defined in section I.A.1.a). Apraxia of speech is similar to other kinds of motor apraxia in that it involves the person's inability to initiate and execute learned voluntary movements (e.g., speech articulation) in the absence of actual paralysis, incoordination, sensory loss, or incomprehension of or inattention to commands. The person hears and understands the requested task, and knows that he is physically capable of performing this task, but when he attempts to do it, he cannot execute the

movements or series of movements needed to complete the task. In patients with AOS, most vegetative and reflexive actions (e.g., coughing or chewing) are intact; however, higher cortical functions are disrupted, specifically the brain's ability to program the positioning of the speech musculature and to sequence the movements for volitional production of speech.

The lesion of AOS is typically in the left frontal lobe adjacent to Broca's area. This has led to controversy as to whether AOS is a separate entity or part of aphasia. Although, AOS can coexist with aphasia and dysarthia, AOS has unique features (e.g., relatively normal pronunciation of serial or automatic speech, absence of significant motor control problems, inconsistent articulatory errors, and rare involvement of the respiratory or phonatory subsystems) that distinguishes it from both disorders. The linguistic hallmarks of AOS include (1) articulatory errors (i.e., omissions, substitution, distortions, additions, and repetition of speech sounds) that are highly inconsistent on repeated productions of the same utterance and that vary with the complexity of the sound patterns and length of target words; moreover, the errors are increased when using less-frequently articulated words and decreased with successive repetition of the word; (2) difficulty with initial consonants and in initiating an utterance; (3) effortful, trial-and-error groping for the proper articulatory position or sequence of positions; although the speaker is often aware of errors, he or she is usually unable to anticipate, modify, or correct them; attempts to monitor and anticipate errors often leads to a slowed speech rate; (4) automatic-spontaneous speech (e.g., counting 1 to 10) is usually intact while volitional-purposeful speech (e.g., counting backwards from 10 to 1) is impaired; and (5) dysprosody unrelieved by extended periods of normal rhythm, stress, and intonation.

1. **Assessment**
   a. **Language screening tests** are similar to those used in aphasia (see section I.A.2) and are done routinely because AOS almost always coexists with aphasia. Aphasia tests for patients with AOS show relatively intact auditory and reading comprehension skills, and better writing than speaking skills.
   b. **Speech production tests** are used to elicit simple and progressively more complex volitional utterances under varying conditions (e.g., by imitation, oral reading, or spontaneous speech).
2. **Treatment** for AOS is usually concomitant with treatment for coexisting aphasia or dysarthria. If accompanied by moderate to severe aphasia, there is poor prognosis for AOS recovery. The treatment goals for AOS are to improve volitional control of the oral musculature for speech purposes and to teach communication strategies that get the message across in the most efficient and effective manner possible. There are some studies that show the beneficial effects of speech therapy even in patients with severe AOS. Long-term recovery of AOS (up to 10 years) has been reported in case studies. As with aphasia treatment, AOS treatment can be categorized into the retraining approach and the compensatory approach.
   a. **Retraining approaches** involve teaching patients with AOS how to program sound patterns to shift from one sound to another and to use preserved melodic and rhythmic patterns to improve their articulation and speech. They are given articulation drills, which start at simple tasks and proceed to exercises of increasing complexity under constant supervision and correction. The drills that are designed to improve phonetic placement accuracy typically use imitation, stress, and progressive approximation.

The cues used for retraining include auditory (i.e., rhythm), visual (i.e., spatial), and kinesthetic (i.e., movement) cues. The AOS patients begin with nonoral imitation, followed by sounds, utterances, words, and finally phrases. They are advanced from limited, automatic reactive speech to appropriate, volitional-purposeful communication to progressively meaningful speech sound sequencing. Based on AOS severity, the following specific strategies are recommended: expanded contrastive stress for mild AOS; inter- and intrasystemic facilitators for moderate AOS; and contrastive stress drills, imitation of contrasts, and segmental/syllabic level imitation for severe AOS.

1) **Rate and melodic (rhythmic) flow training** emphasizes stress and intonation in which patient generates the rhythm to facilitate articulation accuracy. Examples include intersystemic facilitators (e.g., tapping foot, tapping leg, finger-counting, and finger-tapping), intrasystemic facilitators (e.g., pacing board), and expanded contrastive stress drills.

2) **Kinesthetic awareness (movement units) plus rate-and-melody flow training,** for example, contrastive stress drills, which consist of repetitive practice of contrasting words (e.g., pin-bin and day-may) to promote kinesthetic awareness of speech units and facilitate articulation accuracy.

3) **Postural shaping (spatial targeting) plus kinesthetic awareness training,** for example, imitation of contrasts technique.

4) **Postural shaping training,** for example, segmental/syllabic level imitation (with imitation, phonetic placement, phonetic derivation, derivation and placement, and key word techniques).

b. **Compensatory approaches** focus on using residual function (e.g., nonverbal means rather than language-based drills) for communication. Examples include **melodic intonation therapy (MIT),** which uses natural melody patterns (a right hemisphere function) to facilitate speech in nonfluent aphasics with good comprehension; and Amer-Ind code training, which uses gestures modified from the American Indian sign language to facilitate speech; and eight-step task continuum with integral stimulation in which the clinician elicits patient response (utterance) by using cues ranging from spoken words, to mime, written words, and role-playing.

B. **Dysarthria** is strictly a problem with the motor control of speech, affecting articulation (e.g., in stroke patients with upper motor neuron lesions resulting in weakness, spasticity, and slowness of motor speech). Patients with pure dysarthria have intact language function (i.e., they are able to retrieve words and comprehend and express both written and spoken language). The layman's term *slurred speech* is inaccurate as it refers to only one component of dysarthria. The three features of dysarthria that distinguishes it from AOS are: impairment of the automatic (i.e., nonspeech) movements, highly consistent articulatory errors, and involvement of all speech subsystems (including respiration and phonation). In contrast, AOS has intact automatic movements, inconsistent articulatory errors, and rare involvement of respiratory or phonatory subsystems.

1. **Classification of dysarthria (Mayo Clinic classification)**

a. **Flaccid dysarthria** is characterized by a breathy voice (reduced speech volume and audible exhalation), hypenasality (with nasal emission of air during speech), and imprecise articulation of consonants and vowels. It is caused by hypotonia, muscular weakness (e.g., of the tongue and lips), and failure to generate sufficient intraoral breath pressure because of velopharyngeal incompetence. It is seen in patients with bulbar palsy, facial palsy, poliomyelitis, myasthenia gravis, stroke, tumor, trauma, or infection of the lower motor neurons.

b. Spastic dysarthria is characterized by slow and labored speech, imprecise consonant articulation, low and monotonous pitch, a harsh quality to the voice (strained-strangled voice), and hypernasality. It is caused by hypertonia leading to slow, weak movements with reduced range. It is seen in patients with pseudobulbar palsy, spastic cerebral palsy, encephalitis, and stroke, tumor, trauma, or infection involving the upper motor neurons.

c. Ataxic dysarthria is characterized by irregular, imprecise consonant articulation, distorted vowel production, excessive loudness variation, "excess and equal" pattern of syllable stress, and an occasionally harsh voice. It is caused by hypotonia and slow movement with inaccurate range, timing, and direction. It occurs in patients with Friedreich's ataxia, ataxic cerebral palsy, alcohol intoxication, multiple sclerosis, and stroke, tumor, trauma, or infection involving the cerebellar system.

d. Hypokinetic dysarthria is characterized by monotonous pitch and loudness, reduced speech stress, short rushes of speech with illogical and variable silences, reduced speech volume and rate, blurring of consonant articulation, and difficulty in initiating articulation (with repetition of initial sounds). It is caused by slow movements with limited range, rigidity, paucity of movement, loss of automatic aspects of movement, resting tremor, and variable speed of repetitive movements. It is seen in patients with Parkinson's disease or drug-induced (e.g., reserpine or phenothiazine) disorders of the extrapyramidal system.

e. Hyperkinetic dysarthria occurs in patients with excessive motor activity due to extrapyramidal system (EPS) disorders.

1) Predominantly quick pattern is caused by quick, unsustained, random, involuntary movements (e.g., tics and myoclonic jerks) with variable muscle tone. These result in an altered breathing cycle, which causes sudden exhalatory gusts of breath, bursts of loudness, elevations of pitch, imprecise consonants, distorted vowels, abnormally prolonged, variable speaking rate, monopitch, inappropriate silences, harsh voice quality, and overall increase in loudness. It is seen in patients with chorea, myoclonus, Tourette's syndrome, or ballism.

2) Predominantly slow pattern is caused by involuntary body and facial movements (sustained, distorted twisting and writhing movements and postures, slowness, and hypertonus), which leads to unpredictable voice stoppages, imprecise consonant articulation, prolonged and distorted vowels, excessive loudness variation, a harsh voice (strained and strangled quality), monotonous pitch and loudness, and irregular articulatory breakdowns. It is seen in patients with dystonia, dyskinesia (e.g., torticollis and tardive dyskinesia), athetosis (or choreoathetosis), stroke, tumor, infection, or drug-induced (e.g., tranquilizers) disorders of the EPS.

f. Mixed dysarthria pattern has components of different dysarthric types and occurs in patients with extensive neurologic involvement. It can be spastic-flaccid (amyotrophic lateral sclerosis, stroke, head trauma), spastic ataxic hypokinetic (Wilson's disease), or spastic-ataxic-flaccid or variable (multiple sclerosis).

2. Dysarthria assessment

a. Speech impairment assessment techniques includes perceptual tools (which rely on the trained eyes and ears of the clinician) and the use of instruments (to measure acoustic, aerodynamic movement, or myoelectric aspects of speech). They systematically evaluate the different subsystems along the vocal tract where speech activities occur. The following have rating scales that indicate the severity of the impairment of each subsystem:

1) **Respiratory subsystem measurements** include perceptual tools (i.e., ratings of the number of words per breath, loudness of samples of connected speech, and visual observation of clavicular breathing) and instrumental tools (i.e., respiratory inductive plethysmography to measure movement of the rib cage and abdomen during breathing and speech; acoustic measure of vocal intensity and utterance durations; and aerodynamic measurement of subglottal air pressure).

2) **Phonatory or laryngeal subsystem measurements** include perceptual tools that rate pitch characteristics (pitch level, pitch breaks, monopitch, voice tremor), loudness (monoloudness, excess loudness, variation of volume), and voice quality (harsh voice, hoarseness, wet voice, breathiness, strained and strangled voice). It also includes instrumental tools, that is, acoustic measures of frequency and intensity, and aerodynamic measures of laryngeal resistance.

3) **Velopharyngeal subsystem measurements** include perceptual tools (i.e., judgment of hypernasality or occurrence of nasal air emission) and instrumental tools (i.e., acoustic measurement of nasalization; aerodynamic measures of air pressure and air flow during selected speech samples; and cineradiographic techniques to measure velopharyngeal movement).

4) **Oral articulation subsystem measurements** include perceptual tools (i.e., rating of consonant and vowel precision) and instrumental tools (i.e., the use of cineradiographic and EMG recordings).

b. **Speech functional disability assessment techniques** include measurements of speech intelligibility, rate, and naturalness to determine severity of disability, monitor progress over time, and measure the effectiveness of specific interventional techniques. Among these, intelligibility tests (e.g., standardized tools to measure single word and sentence intelligibility) are most commonly used to assess the index of overall speech adequacy.

3. **Treatment** of dysarthria in nonprogressive disorders focuses mainly on maximizing speech intelligibility. Unfortunately, this is not always a realistic goal, especially in patients who are unable to communicate verbally due to severe impairment in intelligibility; therefore, alternate means of communication and augmentative communication devices may be used. In patients with progressive disorders (e.g., Parkinson's disease, multiple sclerosis, and amyotrophic lateral sclerosis), the patients are initially encouraged to maximize the functional communication level by paying special attention to the clarity and precision of their speech. Subsequently the patients need to modify speaking patterns by controlling rate, consonant emphasis, and reducing the number of words per breath. In severe cases, a communication augmentation system may be considered.

a. **Techniques that maximize speech intelligibility** can be enhanced through breathing exercises (to facilitate control of pitch, phonation, and volume), or exercises of the tongue, mouth, and facial muscles (to help improve control of oral musculature), or exercises that strengthen the soft palate and adjacent muscles (to counteract hypernasality).

1) **Rate control,** that is, slowing the rate of speech, is often used in patients with coordination problems (e.g., ataxic dysarthria) and patients with Parkinson's disease. Techniques include pacing boards, alphabet supplementation, rhythmic cueing (computerized or clinician-controlled), delayed auditory feedback, and the use of an oscilloscope (for visual feedback).

  2) Precision training involves techniques that emphasize speech sounds in the final position of words, controls the number of words per breath, and stresses important words in a sentence. Techniques used include articulatory drills and natural stress patterning. Exercises of the tongue, mouth, and facial muscles help improve control of oral musculature.

  3) Palatal lift fitting uses a dental retainer to elevate the soft palate to the height necessary to reduce hypernasality and nasal emission. When fitted properly, it allows certain dysarthric speakers to better produce speech sounds that require the build up of oral air pressure (e.g., /p/, /t/, and /d/).

  b. Functional speech training includes exercises in production of sounds, melodic flow of speech, or coordination of respiration and speaking.

  c. Augmentative communication systems are used in patients who are unable to communicate verbally to augment, supplement, or replace verbal and/or written communication. They include communication boards, books, or computer-based systems, which employ speech synthesis and printed output.

IV. Voice disorders exist when the quality, pitch, or loudness of the voice differs from that of other persons of similar age, sex, cultural background, and geographic location. A common defining feature of a voice disorder is when a given voice draws attention to the speaker. Disorders range from aphonia (no voice) to various dysphonias (disorders of sound quality). In PM&R, voice disorders of neurological origins are commonly encountered. They may be due to unilateral or bilateral vocal cord paralysis (e.g., after intubation or in tracheostomized patients). Patients with cords fixed in an adducted position usually require a tracheostomy (see Chapter 5.12, section V.A.2) to maintain a functional airway. Voice disorders of psychosocial origin may require psychological intervention in concert with the speech-therapy voice regimen.

A. Assessment. Voice disorders must be referred to an otolaryngologist (ear, nose, and throat [ENT] specialist) to rule out organic (e.g., laryngitis; laryngeal ulcers, nodules, polyps, or cancer; and laryngeal paralysis) or functional (e.g., psychogenic or hysterical) causes. If there is no need for further medical or surgical intervention, the patient is referred to a speech-language pathologist for voice assessment, which typically includes an extensive interview, oral peripheral examination, voice analysis (including respiration, phonation, resonance, and prosody), as well as an objective voice analysis using instrumentation. The purpose is to uncover the factors contributing to the vocal problem (e.g., voice misuse or abuse, smoking, and alcohol use); to determine the patient's stimulability to achieve an improved vocal cord approximation; to gauge the degree of the patient's understanding of the disorder; and, finally, to assess willingness to participate in a remediation program.

B. Treatment for dysphonia typically involves a systematic step-by-step patient education and implementation regimen attempting to identify misuse or abuse, describe the effects of the patterns of misuse or abuse, define the specific instances or circumstances of abuse or misuse, modify the behavior, and monitor vocal change. The regimen may include periods of voice rest and often includes counseling to reduce or eliminate substance abuse. Management of the vocal components basically involves reestablishing the proper coordination of respiration, phonation, resonance, and prosody and determining appropriate pitch, quality, and intensity.

1. **Speaking options**
   a. **Nontracheostomized patients.** Speaking options include the use of electrolarynx prosthesis (e.g., a neck type or intraoral type, which must be coordinated in placement and timing with articulated speech), artificial larynx (to generate sound for speech production purposes), esophageal voice (produced by oral injection of air into the esophagus followed by a rapid vibrating expulsion), and tracheoesophageal shunt (a one-way valve prosthesis, which permits air to pass from the trachea into the esophagus, producing an ''esophageal sound'' within the esophagus).
   b. **Tracheostomized patients.** Speaking options include the use of specialized tracheostomy tubes (e.g., a talking tracheostomy tube, a one-way speaking valve attached to the tracheostomy tube adapter, and a tracheal button or plug) or cuff deflation or downsizing of nonspecialized tracheostomy tubes. These are discussed in Chapter 5.12, section V.A.2.b.4.
2. **Nonspeaking options** include the use of writing, complex and simple gestures, communication boards, or portable personal computers.

V. **Fluency disorders (stuttering)** is defined as the phenomenon of gaps, prolongations, or involuntary repetitions of a sound or syllable that occur during speech production. The most common type of stuttering is developmental and is beyond the scope of physiatry. The acquired type is fairly rare (only 2% of cases estimated after the age of 10 years) but is occasionally encountered by the physiatrist; therefore, only this type is discussed. Acquired stuttering is primarily due to brain injury and is thus also called neurogenic or cortical stuttering. Nonneurogenic stuttering (i.e., psychogenic and malingering) are extremely rare.

A. **Classification** of neurogenic stuttering can be subdivided into dysarthric (poor motor speech control), dyspraxic (poor volitional vocal control due to impaired motor programming), and dysnomic (word-finding problem).

B. **Assessment** of neurogenic stuttering should include a detailed history relating to its onset; an oral peripheral examination; a voice, speech, language, and cognitive screen; and an extensive speech sample that includes imitation, oral reading, narrative discourse, conversation, and singing. Differential diagnoses of neurogenic stuttering include palalalia (a paroxysmal speech characterized by sudden involuntary vocalizations such as rhythmic repetitions of syllables, words, and phrases; the words or phrase repetition gets faster and faster with each repetition and may or may not become more unintelligible); multiple self-corrections (may be seen in fluent aphasics); psychogenic stuttering (caused by emotional trauma); or malingering stuttering (faked for some secondary gain).

C. **Treatment** of neurogenic stuttering has been reported to be effective for all three subtypes. This includes patient education and counseling; breathing exercises to control phonation; the use of masking noise to distract speakers from their own speech; the use of delayed auditory feedback forcing the speaker to reduce speech rate; and use of pacing strategies such as finger- or foot-tapping.

VI. **Hearing impairment** interferes with the patient's quality of life by hampering free and easy communication. It most commonly leads to depression and social isolation. In patients with severe hearing loss, paranoid behaviors have been reported. In the United States, 20 million Americans, or 1 out of 10, have some degree of hearing loss. About 12 million Americans have serious hearing impairment, and 2 million are either totally deaf or lack sufficient hearing to understand speech. Any PM&R patients with hearing loss should be referred to an otologist (for diagnosis and management of medical and surgical hearing problems) and to an audiologist (for audiologic testing and management). The physiatrist should be able to detect basic hearing problems and know the available tests and treatment options.

A. **Classification.** Hearing impairment can be categorized as temporary, progressive, or permanent; unilateral or bilateral; and partial (i.e., hard of hearing) or complete (i.e., deaf).

The following classification of hearing impairment is by site of structural damage (using audiograms):

1. **Conductive hearing impairment** results from involvement of the outer and middle ear systems. Possible causes include external blockage, perforated ear drum, otitis media, and otosclerosis.

2. **Sensorineural hearing impairment** stems from damage to the inner ear or neural fibers of the eighth cranial nerve. Possible causes include presbycusis, hereditary hearing loss, trauma, tumors, noise, viral and bacterial illness, or Meniere's disease.

3. **Mixed hearing impairment** comprises both conductive and sensorineural components. Possible causes are the same as for sensorineural hearing impairment.

4. **Central hearing impairment** influences one's ability to comprehend spoken language and is related to damage in the auditory pathways of the brain. Possible causes include trauma, tumors, and vascular damage.

B. **Assessment**

1. **Pure tone audiometry** is used to classify hearing impairment.

   a. **Air conduction audiometry** provides information on the degree of hearing impairment as well as the configuration of the hearing loss. It measures each ear separately using earphones. A hearing impairment can be due to a disorder anywhere in the auditory system from external auditory canal to the brain.

   b. **Bone conduction audiometry** uses a small vibrator placed on the mastoid process to bypass the outer and middle ear, thus reflecting only the sensitivity of the sensorineural system. A masking noise in the nontest ear ensures that bone conduction is not perceived by the nontest ear.

2. **Speech audiometry** tests the patient's ability to discriminate (i.e., recognize or understand) speech. It augments the findings of pure tone audiometry and helps determine the extent of a patient's hearing loss and tolerance. They are used in hearing aid evaluations. Speech audiometry tests are usually presented through earphones in either ear (monoaurally) or in both ears simultaneously (biaurally). Other less common modes of testing are through a bone-conduction vibrator or in the sound field through a loudspeaker. The patient is then asked to repeat back each word heard.

   a. **Speech threshold testing** measures the speech reception threshold (SRT), which is the softest intensity level at which 50% of spondees (i.e., familiar two-syllable words pronounced with equal stress and effort such as "hotdog" or "baseball") are correctly repeated. Normally, the SRT should agree within +10 dB of the pure tone average (PTA) threshold levels at 500, 1000, and 2000 Hz. Otherwise, hearing loss is suspected.

   b. **Word discrimination (WD) test (or speech discrimination test)** analyzes the patient's ability to understand words and is not a threshold nor sensitivity test. It measures the word discrimination score (WDS), which is the percentage of words correctly repeated. The words, which are phonetically-balanced (e.g., darn or art), are presented at comfortably loud levels to the patient from a standardized list of 25 or 50 single-syllable words. The WDS interpretations are as follows: 90 to 100% (normal limits); 75 to 90% (slight difficulty in discrimination); 60 to 75% (moderate difficulty in discrimination); 50 to 60% (poor discrimination, i.e., marked difficulty in following conversation); and less than 50% (very poor discrimination, probably unable to follow running speech).

3. **Auditory tests for site-of-lesion** are special tests indicated for patients with asymmetric sensorineural or clinical suspicion of eighth nerve or central auditory involvement. They include the loudness recruitment tests (to measure the growth of loudness in the pathological ear as compared to normals); differential intensity discrimination tests (to determine the smallest change in intensity that can be recognized as a change in loudness); threshold tone decay tests (to determine the rates at which tones fade away from audibility); Bekesy audiometry (to determine the ability to detect the presence of transient changes in intensity); measurements of impedance (static and dynamic impedance tests) and compliance in the plane of the tympanic membrane (tympanometry); BAEP audiometry (the electrophysiologic analysis of brainstem auditory evoked potentials [BAEP], which is sensitive for diagnosing cochlear tumors); and electrocochleography (which measures electrophysiologic signals from the cochlea).

C. Treatment

1. **Hearing aid** is a miniature amplifier that amplifies sound intensity for the hearing-impaired ear. It is indicated for patients with hearing loss above 40 dB due to difficulty in understanding normal speech. For its successful use, patients must accept their hearing difficulties and express their desire to improve, be motivated, have positive attitudes, and have a good support system. Aside from being easy to use, affordable, and cosmetically appealing, the ideal hearing aid should provide the lowest SRT, the highest WDS, a most comfortable loudness level close to the level of normal conversation, a broad range of comfortable loudness, and the least amount of noise and background interference.

   a. **Body- or pocket-hearing aids** are housed in a case worn at chest level. Although powerful and durable, they are larger than other hearing aids and are uncosmetic. They are indicated for patients who have severe or profound hearing loss, as well as those with poor manual dexterity who are unable to manipulate smaller hearing aids.

   b. **Eyeglass hearing aids** are housed in an eyeglass frame. They are seldom used because wearers find them annoying.

   c. **Behind-the-ear (BTE) aids** fit into a curved base that rests behind the ear. They are indicated for severe as well as mild and moderate hearing loss patients. They have power equivalent to most body-hearing aids.

   d. **In-the-ear (ITE) hearing aids** are custom-fitted into the ear concha. They are cosmetically appealing and easier to use than BTE.

   e. **In-the-canal (ITC) or custom-canal hearing aids** are custom-molded to fit within the ear canal. Because of their extremely small size, they can only provide adequate amplification for patients with mild-to-moderate hearing loss. They are highly appealing cosmetically and are expensive.

   f. **Contralateral routing of signals (CROS) hearing aids** are indicated for patients with unilateral severe or profound hearing loss but with a normal contralateral ear. A microphone on the hearing-impaired ear transmits radio waves to a receiver unit attached to the normal ear. This permits the wearer to "hear" people speaking on their hearing-impaired ear side. A variation is the **bi-CROS hearing aid**, which is used in patients with bilateral hearing loss but whose poorer ear is not suitable for amplification.

2. **Assistive listening devices (ALDs)** are designed to reduce the level of noise and background interferences in adverse listening situations. One form of ALD transmits sound directly from the source to the hearing-impaired listener through infrared, audio loop, FM radio system, or direct audio input to the hearing aid. Other forms of ALDs include amplified telephones, low-frequency doorbells and telephone ringers, and closed-caption TV decoders. Visual cues (e.g., flashing alarm clocks, flashing smoke detectors, and use of typed messages via telephone modem) and vibration cues (e.g., alarm bed vibrators) may be used instead of sound to alert the hearing-impaired person.

3. **Speechreading and auditory training** combines visual input and auditory input for understanding speech. Speechreading teaches the patient how to interpret visual cues (e.g., facial expression, body movements, or gestures); however, only about one-third of English speech sounds are clearly visible. Hence, auditory training needs to be supplemented to teach the patient how to make the most effective use of the minimal auditory cues imposed by the hearing loss.

4. **Cochlear implants** are internal electrode wires surgically placed into the cochlea. They are connected to an external microphone and signal converter. Sound waves are converted into electrical impulses and are delivered directly to the cochlea. Cochlear implants are indicated for patients with profound sensorineural hearing loss. Although sound or speech can be detected (hence increasing patient's environmental awareness), the patient is unable to understand or discriminate the speech.

5. **Tactile aids** convert sound into vibrations to provide the patient with awareness of sound. It is indicated in profoundly deaf patients who are not candidates for any of the aforementioned treatments.

BIBLIOGRAPHY

Adamovich BB, Henderson JA, Auerbach S: *Cognitive rehabilitation of closed head injury patients,* San Diego, 1985, College-Hill Press.

Benson DF, Ardila A: *Aphasia: a clinical perspective,* New York, 1996, Oxford University.

Cardenas DD, McLean A, Jr.: Psychopharmacologic management of traumatic brain injury, *Phys Med Rehabil Clin North Am,* 3(2):273-290, 1992.

Chapey R, editor: *Language intervention strategies in adult aphasia,* ed 3, Baltimore, 1994, Williams & Wilkins.

Chapman SB, Levin HS, Culhane KA: Language impairment in closed head injury. In Kirshner JS, editor: *Handbook of neurological speech and language disorders,* New York, 1995, Marcel Dekker, pp 387-414.

Damasio AR: Aphasia, *New Engl J Med,* 326(8):531-539, 1992.

Frattali CM, Thompson CK, Holland AL, et al: *American Speech and Hearing Association (ASHA): Functional assessment of communication skills for adults,* Rockville, MD, 1995, ASHA.

Kerman-Lerner P: Communication disorders. In Goodgold J, editor: *Rehabilitation medicine,* St. Louis, 1988, Mosby–Year Book, pp 787-814.

Kirk A, Kertesz: Assessment of aphasia, *Phys Med Rehabil State Art Rev* 6(3): 433-450, 1992.

LaPointe L, editor: *Aphasia and related neurogenic language disorders*, New York, 1990, Thieme Medical Publisher.

Miller RM, Groher ME, Yorkston KM, et al: Speech, language, swallowing, and auditory rehabilitation. In DeLisa JA, Gans BM, editors: *Rehabilitation medicine: principles and practice*, ed 2, Philadelphia, 1993, JB Lippincott, pp 201-226.

Methe S, Huber W, Paradis M: Inventory and classification of rehabilitation methods. In Paradis M, editor: *Foundations of aphasia rehabilitation*, Oxford, 1993, Pergamon Press, pp 3-60.

Porcelli J: Aphasia assessment and treatment, *Phys Med Rehabil Clin North Am*, 2(3):487-500, 1991.

Rao PR: Adult communication disorders. In Braddom R, editor: *Physical medicine and rehabilitation*, Philadelphia, 1996, WB Saunders, pp 49-65.

Sarno MT, editor: *Acquired aphasia*, ed 2, New York, 1991, Academic Press.

Sarno MT: Neurogenic disorders of speech and language. In O'Sullivan SB, Schmitz TJ, editors: *Physical rehabilitation: assessment and treatment*, Philadelphia, 1994, FA Davis, pp 633-653.

Yorkston KM, Beukelman DR: Speech and language disorders. In Kottke FJ, Stillwell G, Lehmann JF, editors: *Krusen's handbook of physical medicine and rehabilitation*, ed 4, Philadelphia, 1990, WB Saunders, pp 126-152.

Wertz RT, LaPointe LL, Rosenbeck JC: *Apraxia of speech in adults*, New York, 1984, Grune & Stratton.

CHAPTER 5.6

DYSPHAGIA

Swallowing disorders of neurologic origin (which usually involve the oral or pharyngeal stage or both) are commonly managed by physiatrists in a multidisciplinary inpatient setting (involving the patient, family or significant others, occupational therapist, speech-language pathologist, nutritionist or dietitian, rehabilitation nurse, home health attendant, respiratory therapist, radiologist, etc.). In addition to neurogenic dysphagia, physiatrists also deal with nonneurogenic dysphagias such as those due to rheumatologic conditions (e.g., scleroderma, Sjogren's syndrome, systemic lupus erythematosus, mixed connective tissue disease, and rheumatoid arthritis) or foreign devices (e.g., tracheostomy tube). Although this chapter deals specifically with neurogenic dysphagia, most of the diagnostic and treatment strategies presented here can also be applied to dysphagia of nonneurogenic origin. For a discussion on assistive and adaptive equipment and strategies for oral feeding (i.e., food preparation and mechanisms for bringing food to the mouth), refer to Chapter 4.5, section II.A.3.a.

I. **Pathophysiology** of swallowing can arbitrarily be divided into 3 overlapping stages:

A. **Oral stage** is concerned with bolus preparation and transportation. As the food is placed in the mouth and the lips come together, food is chewed (if necessary) and mixed with saliva into a bolus. The bolus is moved around by the muscles of the tongue and cheeks and transported to the anterior faucial arch where the pharyngeal swallow reflex is triggered. Oral stage pathologies include decreased labial seal (leading to anterior spillage; inability to remove food from utensil), jaw weakness (resulting in chewing difficulty), tongue and buccal weakness (causing difficulty in forming the bolus resulting in pooling or pocketing of food between the cheeks and teeth; difficulty in retaining the bolus resulting in drooling; difficulty in moving food to the back of the mouth), poor tongue coordination (i.e., slow diodochokinetic rate; multiple anterior-posterior tongue movements or tongue pumping before swallow), and problems with oral sequencing, which results in aspiration before the swallow.

B. **Pharyngeal stage** is the reflex phase of swallowing. As the bolus reaches the anterior faucial arch and is propelled by the tongue into the pharynx, it is sealed by the tongue within the pharynx by forceful apposition to the soft palate (velum) and posterior pharyngeal wall. Peripheral sensory input from the taste, fluid, or pressure sensory receptors (located mainly in the fauces, pharynx, and posterior larynx) travel through cranial nerves V, VII, IX, and X to the central nervous system. Cortical and subcortical pathways modulate the swallowing threshold (the exact mechanism is as yet unclear) and the input is passed to the brainstem "swallowing center" (where either swallowing or a gag reflex is triggered). When the swallowing reflex is triggered, output is passed from the brainstem to the nuclei of cranial nerves V, VII, IX, X, and XII and subsequently to the muscles they innervate. This results in the following reflex responses: soft palate elevation and velopharyngeal port closure (to close off the nasal cavity and prevent regurgitation into the nasopharynx), laryngeal elevation with folding (i.e., tilting down) of the epiglottis and vocal cord adduction (to protect the trachea from food contamination), and coordinated pharyngeal constriction and cricopharyngeal relaxation (to facilitate bolus transport into the esophagus). During the pharyngeal phase, inspiration and expiration are inhibited to prevent aspiration. Pharyngeal stage pathologies include difficulty in initiating the swallowing reflex, nasal regurgitation, mid-throat sticking of the bolus, choking and coughing, aspiration during or after the swallow, and aspiration pneumonia.

C. **Esophageal stage** begins as the bolus travels beyond the cricopharyngeus and is propelled by peristalsis from the esophagus through the gastroesophageal (GE) junction into the stomach. Between swallows, the cricopharyngeus contracts continuously to prevent aerophagia and GE reflux. Esophageal stage pathologies include esophageal pain and obstruction (e.g., stricture, tumor, web, spasms, and dysmotility) and GE reflux.

II. **Epidemiology.** The overall incidence and prevalence of dysphagia is difficult to quantify as they vary according to the patient's stage of recovery from the underlying cause. Some of the reported incidence for dysphagia caused by specific neurologic disorders are stroke (up to 30-45%; 28% of all left hemispheric strokes; 21% of all right hemispheric strokes; up to 67% of brainstem strokes), traumatic brain injury [TBI] (up to 27%), cerebral palsy (40%), parkinsonism (50-70%), myasthenia gravis (15-63%), and postpolio syndrome (18%).

III. **Dysphagia evaluation** is performed to screen for the presence or absence of a swallowing impairment; establish a possible local anatomic and physiologic cause for the dysphagia; assess the patient's ability to protect the airway (i.e., aspiration risk); determine the practicality of oral feeding and/or recommend alternative methods for nutritional management; determine the need for additional specific diagnostic tests, studies, or referrals; and collect baseline clinical data, which can be used to chart changes in swallowing function of patients. Clinical (bedside) evaluation tends to underestimate aspiration occurrence in patients who are elderly, have expressive aphasia, and in whom more than 30 days have elapsed since the onset of injury. In most cases, because of the patient's altered mental status or severely impaired speech, information may be obtained from a health care attendant, family member, or medical records. The swallowing evaluation is usually performed by the speech-language pathologist or occupational therapist with the radiologist, if necessary.

A. **History**

1. **History of present illness**

   a. **Dysphagia symptoms** including duration, frequency (intermittent vs. constant), factors exacerbating or relieving the symptoms, influence of food texture (solids, semisolids, and liquids; influence of hot and cold foods), and course of symptoms.

   b. **Associated symptoms** including sensation of obstruction while swallowing, a "globus sensation" or foreign body feeling, intermittent obstruction, mouth or throat pain (odynophagia), nasal regurgitation, foul mouth odor, choking or coughing while swallowing, change in speech and voice (e.g., wet voice), history of pneumonia, other respiratory symptoms (chronic cough, dyspnea, asthmatic episodes), GE reflux (sensation of heartburn, globus sensation, hiccups, a sour taste, dry throat, or pain in the throat or tongue), and chest pain (can be related to diffuse esophageal spasm).

   c. **Ancillary symptoms** including weight loss, change in eating habits (e.g., avoidance of certain foods, such as lettuce, because of pharyngeal weakness; increase in eating time; decrease in usual meal size; increase fluid intake with meals), decrease in appetite, change in taste, dry mouth, thickening of saliva consistency (e.g., due to chronic dehydration from impaired swallowing of liquids or related to mouth breathing, salivary gland dysfunction, or medications), change in speech or voice (hoarseness or temporary loss of voice, slurred or clumsy speech), and sleep disturbance (e.g., due to GE reflux).

2. **Past history** including neurologic conditions (e.g., stroke, TBI, central nervous system infection, demyelinating disease, and motor neuron disease), previous swallowing examinations, neck problems (e.g., cervical spondylosis or ankylosis), dental disorders, presence of dentures, radiation therapy to the head and neck or mediastinum, cardiopulmonary disease (e.g., chronic obstructive pulmonary disease [COPD], congestive heart failure, and recurrent pneumonia), psychiatric and psychologic history (e.g., dementia), and surgery of the head, neck, or gastrointestinal tract.

3. **Family history,** for example, muscular dystrophy or myopathy.

4. **Current medications** that may contribute to dysphagia including sedatives (can cause disorientation and confusion), antispastics (can cause oropharyngeal muscle weakness), anticholinergics (can cause mucosal drying), antidepressants with anticholinergic effects, diuretics (can cause dehydration with drying of the mouth), antipsychotics or neuroleptics (can cause extrapyramidal symptoms, which may affect feeding and swallowing, such as tardive dyskinesia, dystonia, and pseudoparkinsonism), topical mouth anesthetics or denture powders with anesthetics, and any drugs that may decrease appetite. In addition, β-adrenergic drugs, theophylline, alcohol, and tobacco have been reported to lower or overcome esophageal sphincter tone and promote GE reflux.

B. **Physical examination**

1. **General inspection** including current feeding methods (e.g., oral route vs. extraoral route, such as through nasogastric tube [NGT], surgically placed gastrostomy, percutaneous endoscopic gastrostomy [PEG], or percutaneous endoscopic jejunostomy [PEJ]), presence of tracheostomy (note the type and size of tube and the status of the cuff, i.e., inflated, partially inflated, or deflated), nutrition and hydration status, and presence or absence of drooling.

2. **Oropharyngeal status** including lip protrusion or closure, lip and mandibular tone, range of motion (ROM), strength, and sensation of the lips, tongue, and mandible; abnormal oropharyngeal reflexes; teeth condition (e.g., dental plates, false dentures, and malocclusion); and oropharyngeal mucosa condition (e.g., dryness, tenacious mucus, sores, odor, and presence of pocketed food).

3. **Pulmonary system** including rate and depth of breathing (too rapid and shallow breathing can affect timing of swallowing), cough reflex (voluntary and involuntary cough, cough strength, measurement of vital capacity to predict cough effectiveness), and chest auscultation to rule out pneumonia or COPD.

4. **Musculoskeletal system** including posture, deformity, muscle tone (spasticity, flaccidity, rigidity, dystonia), and ROM, strength, and coordination of the neck and limbs.

5. **Neurologic system**

   a. **Mental status** including level of consciousness, cognition (i.e., alertness, orientation, attention, judgment, memory, ability to cooperate and follow instructions), behavioral characteristics (e.g., agitation and impulsivity), and perception (e.g., unilateral neglect).

b. **Language ability,** such as receptive and expressive aphasia, to determine the ability to communicate and follow instructions.

c. **Speech and voice** including quality and strength of voice (e.g., a hoarse voice may indicate reduced laryngeal closure; a wet or gurgly voice, extreme breathiness, or loss of voice may indicate pooling of saliva or secretions at the laryngeal level and possible acute aspiration); phonation (e.g., hypernasality may suggest impaired palatopharyngeal function; hyponasality may imply filling of the nasopharynx or occlusion of the nasal passages); and speed and precision of articulation (e.g., oral diadochokinetic tasks, i.e., forced rapid alternating movements using consonant-vowel combinations to determine the integrity of the oral motor system). If the dysphagic patient has unimpaired voice and speech, the swallowing problem is probably related to the late pharyngeal stage (cricopharyngeal function) or to esophageal function.

d. **Cranial nerves (CN)** including CN V (biting, side to side jaw grinding, sensation of forehead, face, and jaw), CN VII (facial expression, cheek puffing, lip sealing, taste in the anterior two thirds of the tongue), CNs IX and X (phonation, position of uvula, palatal elevation, gag reflex, swallowing, taste in the posterior third of the tongue), CN XI (head movement), and CN XII (tongue movement).

e. **Reflexes**
   1) **Swallowing reflex,** which can be palpated by placing a finger on the thyroid notch between the hyoid bone and the larynx and feeling the larynx move up and forward during swallowing. Failure to detect laryngeal elevation may indicate weak swallowing muscles or an inadequate swallowing reflex, which leaves the airway unprotected. The swallowing reflex can be clinically tested on the right and left sides by:
      a) **Pressure stimulation,** for example, applying an empty spoon to the anterior third of the tongue to stimulate a dry pharyngeal swallow.
      b) **Tactile and taste stimulation,** for example, rubbing a lemon glycerin swab (that has been squeezed out) to the lips, teeth, gums, and tongue to stimulate a pharyngeal swallow and to determine the ability to taste (which in turn can stimulate salivary flow and, eventually, swallowing).
      c) **Thermal stimulation,** for example, tapping an ice-cold laryngoscopic mirror (size 00) or small metal spoon to the base of the anterior fauces to facilitate a pharyngeal swallow (either with or without verbal cueing).
   2) **Gag reflex,** which is highly variable even among healthy persons, should be elicited from both sides (the right and left sides should also be compared). A diminished or absent gag does not automatically mean that the patient is unable to swallow or protect the airway although it may give information about both cranial nerve function and the ability to achieve laryngeal closure. A diminished gag reflex is probably significant only when found in patients who have evidence of weakened or paralyzed pharyngeal palatine musculature, an asymmetric gag reflex, or other signs of cranial nerve dysfunction.
   3) **Cough reflex,** which is the final protective mechanism to prevent aspiration, is in itself not an indication that the patient is experiencing

tracheal aspiration. In fact, oral feeding should not be started unless the patient has an adequate cough reflex (as patients with inadequate cough reflex may silently aspirate without this protective mechanism). The cough reflex can be assessed by having the patient swallow 3 oz of water. Coughing during the swallow may indicate reduced vocal cord closure while coughing elicited within 1 minute after the pharyngeal swallow may indicate decreased laryngeal elevation, reduced pharyngeal peristalsis, or upper esophageal sphincter deficits. Likewise, if the patient develops a wet, hoarse voice or cough after the swallow, or if the patient experiences some choking or respiratory distress that is not immediately relieved by coughing, then probably some aspiration has taken place.

    4) Pathological reflexes including suck, bite, tongue thrust, suck-swallow, asymmetric tonic neck, and tonic labyrinthine reflexes.

  f. Motor control including coordination (e.g., finger-to-nose test, rapid alternating hand movements, tongue wiggling, and finger wiggling), involuntary movements (e.g., tremors, chorea, athetosis, ballismus, dystonia, myoclonus, asterixis, tics, and tardive dyskinesia), and motor planning ability (e.g., feeding apraxia).

C. Diagnostic tests

  1. Swallowing tests

    a. Clinical (or bedside) swallowing studies (CSS) are not as reliable as videofluoroscopic swallowing studies (VFSS) (see section III.C.1.b), which remains the "gold standard" in determining the safety of oral feeding. Unlike VFSS, CSS is incapable of detecting "silent" (or coughless) aspiration and can only provide limited information about either structure or function of the swallowing mechanism. However, CSSs are still done because patients who are able to swallow safely during VFSS may have different functional skills at the bedside because of problems with endurance, insight, judgment, and planning during mealtime. Also, CSS may be used to screen for the need of VFSS except in patients with high risk for aspiration (in which case, VFSS should be done prior to CSS). Patients undergoing CSS must have an intact cough reflex to protect the airway in case of aspiration. They should also have adequate hydration and moist mucosa. Any CSS should be done during mealtime (if possible) with the patient in an upright position (i.e., seated at 90° or reclining backward at a 45° angle or more) and the head tilted slightly forward. If the patient is hemiplegic, the weaker side should be elevated above the stronger side. During CSS, the following feeding behaviors are observed: impulsivity (which can affect the rate and size of the bolus), attention and distractibility during the meal, abnormal head and body positions, rate of intake, bolus size, and drooling or oral spillage of liquids or the bolus.

      For each food consistency, laryngeal elevation is determined by observing the elevation of the hyoid and thyroid cartilages. The time delay should be about 1 second from the initiation of lingual movement after bolus formation to the elevation of the larynx, indicating triggering of the pharyngeal swallow and laryngeal protection of the airway. A stethoscope may be placed against the patient's neck during the swallow to listen for the occurrence of the swallow and also to detect possible aspiration. For each food presentation, the following are noted: the average number of swallow required per bolus (i.e., repeated swallows, which may indicate possible pooling in the pharyngeal area or reduced pharyngeal peristalsis); chewing difficulties (for solid or semisolid foods); fatigue during chewing or swallowing (swallowing or chewing can be performed successively to elicit fatigue if the patient has subjective complaints suggestive of fatigue); the location of any discomfort/pain during swallowing; occurrence of the cough reflex (see section III.B.5.e.3) during or after the swallow; presence of excessive secretions; and nasal regurgitation (especially when testing with liquids).

After each swallow, the following are noted: any changes in the patient's color (a possible sign of choking), any changes in phonation and vocal quality (see section III.B.5.c), and presence of food pocketing, i.e., retention of food in the oral cavity, which may indicate reduced bolus formation and/or sensory loss (e.g., pocketing of food on the neglected side of parietal stroke patients). To reduce the risk of aspiration of any residual food in the oropharynx, the patient must be seated upright for at least 30 minutes after the CSS. Also, monitor the patient for any changes in his or her respiratory or medical status over a 24-hour period (e.g., increased temperature or increased amount of secretions). If the patient does not exhibit any signs of aspiration, a trial oral feeding program may be initiated. If needed, a VFSS can be used to confirm the results of the CSS and to help determine appropriate compensatory head postures and swallowing techniques that may be necessary for safe swallowing.

1) Nontracheostomized patients are initially evaluated by presenting them with a small ice chip from a spoon and observing lip function, tongue propulsion, any chewing ability, and the initiation of the pharyngeal swallow (by palpating for laryngeal elevation). Ice chips are initially used because they are relatively safe if partially aspirated; they provide a good medium for eliciting the chewing reflex (because of their solid texture and stimulatory effect on the cold receptors in the gums); and they help facilitate a pharyngeal swallowing reflex (probably due to cold stimulation). If the patient appears to have difficulty with ice chips, there must be extra caution in completing the swallowing evaluation. If there is adequate laryngeal elevation and a cough reflex, the patient may be tested with food of different textures and consistencies (e.g., pureed foods, thick liquids, ground solids, chopped solids, regular solids, and thin liquids; see section V.A.2.b.1 for description and examples of different food textures) unless contraindicated due to medical or behavioral problems.

The sequence of presentation of different food consistencies is based on the patient's history, his or her medical status, prior observations of the patient, and suspected areas of difficulty. If a delayed pharyngeal swallow is suspected during ice-chip testing, then pureed foods and thick liquids should be presented before thin liquids to reduce the possibility of aspiration. However, if upper esophageal sphincter dysfunction or esophageal stricture is suspected (e.g., complaints of discomfort), then thin liquids should be presented first because they can easily pass through the esophagus. If the patient does not voluntarily initiate chewing, the lateral side of the tongue may be rubbed with a soft solid food to facilitate a chewing response. It is safest to begin with small amounts (e.g., $\frac{1}{4}$ teaspoon) and gradually increase the amount of each presentation up to 1 to 2 teaspoons of each consistency. In a patient with NGT, the tube should be removed prior to testing as it may potentially interfere with normal swallowing because of altered pharyngeal sensations and deflection of the bolus. Patients with NGT may need to be properly hydrated because they tend to mouth breathe, thus causing dry oral mucosa, which can interfere with swallowing.

2) **Tracheostomized patients** rarely have dysphagia that can be directly attributed to the tracheostomy tube itself. However, the presence of the tracheostomy tube may predispose these patients to tracheal aspiration for the following reasons: (1) the tracheostomy cannula has a tendency to tether the larynx anteriorly (to the trachea) thus restricting normal laryngeal elevation and resulting in reduced glottal closure and increased laryngeal penetration; (2) the lack of movement of the laryngeal muscles, together with restricted movement of the pretracheal strap muscles, can interfere with laryngeal elevation and cricopharyngeal relaxation; and (3) the cannula in the trachea may desensitize the airway, thus raising the threshold for coughing and throat-clearing activities, which are necessary to expel any material from the airway.

To test swallowing in tracheostomized patients, a blue food coloring (e.g., Evans blue or methylene blue dye) is used so the aspirated material can be distinguished from other possible tracheal secretions. The blue dye is initially applied to the tongue, and the trachea is suctioned to detect the dye's presence. If the test is negative (i.e., dye is absent in the trachea), the patient is presented with small amounts (e.g., $\frac{1}{4}$ teaspoon) of food or liquid colored by the blue dye. The tracheostomy is momentarily occluded with a finger to establish near-normal tracheal pressure. Laryngeal elevation is observed as well as signs of swallowing difficulties such as coughing, gurgling, or leakage of blue substance around the tracheostomy site. If difficulty is noted, the patient is suctioned immediately to see if any blue-tinged solution shows up in the trachea. If not, the amount of food or liquid is increased to 1 to 2 teaspoons, followed by tracheal suctioning to detect any blue-tinged secretions. Before proceeding to a new consistency, the patient is suctioned thoroughly to help differentiate the specific consistencies with which the patient is having difficulty. If a very small amount of blue-tinged secretion is detected in the tracheostoma several minutes after a test swallow, it does not necessarily indicate impaired swallowing (as this is a common finding due to the tendency of the color-contrast solutions to coat the entire oropharyngeal mucosa). In tracheostomized patients with negative dye tests, a trial oral feeding program may be initiated.

a) **Occluded versus unoccluded tracheostomy.** Before testing the swallow, the tracheostomy tube should be plugged for several seconds to assess the patient's ability to breathe through the larynx, and the voluntary laryngeal cough. When the tracheostomy tube is not occluded, the risk of aspiration may increase due to the patient's inability to expel air to clear the larynx of foreign materials.

b) **Inflated versus deflated tracheostomy cuffs.** Inflated tracheostomy cuffs do not guarantee safety as they can cause swallowing difficulties because of increased compression of the bolus material around the cuff into the tracheal area, tracheal irritation, restriction of laryngeal elevation, and prevention of the exhalation of pulmonary air that normally clears the larynx. Cuff deflation, therefore, is usually recommended during the CSS (a deflated cuff also makes it easier to immediately detect any signs of aspiration). If the cuff cannot be deflated for medical reasons (e.g., in ventilator-dependent patients, who need the cuff inflated to maintain adequate ventilation), then oral feeding may be premature. Prior to cuff deflation, the trachea above the cuff should be suctioned to prevent aspiration of any residual food above the inflated cuff. The cuff is then deflated slowly and the patient suctioned again. If the patient has been given blue-tinged food, the amount and quality of the secretion is observed for any traces of food coloring.

b. **Videofluoroscopic swallowing study** is the ''gold standard'' for evaluating swallowing disorders. For most patients, it is done after the CSS to confirm the results of the CSS and to help determine appropriate compensatory head postures and swallowing maneuvers that may be necessary for safe swallowing. If the patient is at high risk for aspiration, however, VFSS is recommended prior to CSS. In VFSS, the patient is tested in an upright position to reflect normal eating and drinking (this is unlike an esophagram, i.e., a contrast study of the esophagus, which is conducted in the horizontal position to eliminate the effect of gravity on esophageal contraction). Controlled amounts (e.g., using a teaspoon, tablespoon, cup, or straw) of barium-impregnated food and liquid substances of different textures (e.g., thin liquid, thick liquid, pureed food, mechanical soft food, or solid food such as cookies; see section V.A.2.b.1 for description and examples of different food textures) are administered to the patient by an occupational therapist or speech-language pathologist. As the patient chews (if necessary) and swallows the bolus, a video recording is made of the fluoroscopic radiogram (usually a lateral view; see Fig. 5.6-1) of the oral, pharyngeal, and esophageal stages of swallowing. The videotape can then be subsequently played at a slow speed for swallowing analysis.

Qualitative swallowing pathologies (e.g., ''silent'' or coughless aspiration, laryngeal penetration, pharyngeal pooling, and delayed oral stage) and quantitative swallowing pathologies (e.g., abnormal pharyngeal transit time over 2 second) can be identified from the VFSS to determine the quantity and texture of food or liquid that the patient can tolerate safely. By trying various swallowing techniques (e.g., dry swallowing and chin tucking during swallowing), feeding and swallowing strategies can also be recommended based on the VFSS. The clinician must be aware, however, that patients who are able to swallow safely during VFSS may have poor functional skills at the bedside due to problems with endurance, insight, judgment, and planning during mealtime. A VFSS is contraindicated if the patient has a low level of consciousness or is unable to cooperate or follow commands. Although the radiation exposure to the patient is generally small (especially in a well-planned VFSS session), the patient or family must be informed about it and, if the patient is a female of child-bearing age, the patient should be screened for pregnancy.

c. **Swallowing ultrasound** is useful in studying the oral stage of swallowing, in particular tongue motions. In itself, it is not useful in studying the

Oral palate

Pharyngeal palate

Uvula

Genioglossal muscles

Vallecula

Hyoid bones

Epiglottis

Vocal cord

Thyroid cartilage

Cricoid cartilage

Trachea

Esophagus

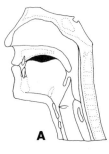

A

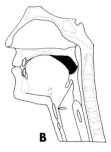

B

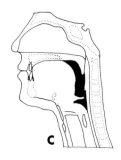

C

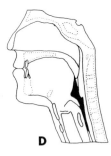

D

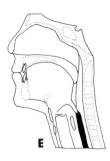

E

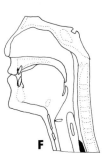

F

pharyngeal stage of swallowing. When combined with VFSS, however, it may be used to document aspiration and to further evaluate esophageal function.

d. **Swallowing surface electromyography** can be used to screen the risk for aspiration and serve as a bedside biofeedback tool for teaching compensatory swallowing maneuvers. It uses surface electrodes to determine laryngeal movement during swallowing (normal age-specific amplitude is 50-100 mV; duration is 1-2 seconds; wave pattern has two peaks; swallowing rate is 1-5 per minute; and swallowing rhythm is stable). It can also indirectly determine the swallowing duration in the oral phase (about 1 second) and in the esophageal phase (about 7 seconds between successive laryngeal movements). For both oral and esophageal phases, the laryngeal electromyographic amplitude should be close to 0 mV.

e. **Swallowing scintigraphy,** that is, radionuclide imaging of the swallowed bolus mixed with radioisotopes (e.g., technetium-99 sulfur colloid), can be used to quantify aspiration and to evaluate esophageal motility disorders and GE reflux.

f. **Fiberoptic videoendoscopy** may be used to directly visualize the upper aerodigestive structures to rule out aspiration and to determine appropriate compensatory head postures and swallowing maneuvers that may be necessary for safe swallowing.

2. **Laryngoscopy (mirror or fiberoptic),** done by an otolaryngologist, can detect premature spillage, laryngeal penetration, tracheal aspiration, and pharyngeal residue in patients who are too ill to undergo VFSS or unable to tolerate any risk of aspiration, or in patients with a weak or absent cough or with an altered vocal quality (e.g., hoarse or breathy).

3. **Imaging studies** include chest radiograph to determine pulmonary infiltrates (this may raise the suspicion but is not pathognomonic of aspiration pneumonia) and computed tomography or magnetic resonance imaging (MRI) scan to identify and stage masses in the upper digestive tract or diagnose a central or peripheral nervous system mass, which could explain the swallowing disorder. An MRI scan is superior to CT scan for this purpose.

Figure 5.6-1
Lateral videofluoroscopic view of oropharyngeal swallow of large liquid bolus in an adult. **A.** Bolus preparation in the oral cavity (the velum is approximated with the tongue; nasal respiration can continue). **B.** Bolus is transported by the tongue to the anterior faucial arch where the pharyngeal swallow reflex is triggered (the velum is displaced upward and backward and is approximated by a protrusion on the posterior pharyngeal wall). **C.** The bolus is propelled to the laryngopharnyx (the epiglottis is folded downward; the hyoid and larynx are fully displaced upward and forward; the vocal cord adducts to protect the trachea from food aspiration; peristaltic waves descend in the constrictor wall). **D.** The bolus penetrates the opened pharyngoesophageal segment (peristaltic waves descend further; the upper part of the palatopharyngeal isthmus reopens). **E.** The bolus has nearly traversed the pharynx (peristaltic waves reach the hypopharynx; the oropharynx is beginning to reopen). **F.** The mouth (now empty) and the pharynx return to their usual position. (From: Donner MW, Bosma JF, Robertson D: Anatomy and physiology of the pharynx. *Gastrointestinal Radiology* 10: 196, 205, 1985, copyright © 1985, Springer-Verlag, with permission)

4. **Esophageal manometry** uses a multilumen catheter system to evaluate esophageal motor disorders; however, it is time consuming and uncomfortable.
5. **Nutritional work-up** includes serum total protein, prealbumin (a better indicator than serum albumin for determining the patient's current visceral protein stores and protein status change over time), cholesterol, triglycerides, creatinine, blood urea nitrogen (to determine protein catabolism), electrolytes, and glucose; caloric counting; and serial weighing.

IV. **Classification by causative factors**
  A. **Neurogenic disorders**
    1. **Upper motor neuron (UMN) and cortical disorders**
      a. **Vascular:** stroke, intracranial hemorrhage, cerebral palsy.
      b. **Degenerative and extrapyramidal:** parkinsonism, spinocerebellar degeneration, olivopontocerebellar atrophy, progressive supranuclear palsy, Huntington's disease, Alzheimer's disease, adrenoleukodystrophy, dystonia, tardive dyskinesia, dementia.
      c. **Demyelinating:** multiple sclerosis.
      d. **Infectious:** encephalitis, meningitis, Creutzfeldt-Jakob disease, AIDS.
      e. **Structural:** neoplasm, Arnold-Chiari malformation, syringomyelia, and syringobulbia.
      f. **Exogenous:** TBI, cervical spinal cord injuries, drug-induced causes.
      g. **Other cortical etiologies:** mental retardation.
    2. **Combined upper and lower motor neuron disorders:** amyotrophic lateral sclerosis, progressive muscular atrophy, progressive bulbar palsy, primary lateral sclerosis.
    3. **Lower motor neuron (LMN) disorders**
      a. **Motor neuron:** spinal muscular atrophy, poliomyelitis, postpolio syndrome.
      b. **Peripheral nervous system:** Guillain-Barre syndrome, sarcoidosis, porphyria.
      c. **Neuromuscular junction:** myasthenia gravis, Eaton-Lambert syndrome, botulism.
      d. **Muscles:** inflammatory myopathies (e.g., polymyositis and dermatomyositis), metabolic myopathies (e.g., mitochondrial and thyroid myopathies), myotonic dystrophy, oculopharyngeal dystrophy, Duchenne's muscular dystrophy (late phase).
  B. **Nonneurogenic disorders: rheumatologic disorders** (e.g., scleroderma, Sjogren's syndrome, systemic lupus erythematosus, mixed connective tissue disease, and rheumatoid arthritis); **metabolic disorders** (e.g., hypercalcemia and diabetes mellitus); **structural disorders** (e.g., cervical osteophytes, goiters, neoplasm, scarring [especially due to tuberculosis]; tracheoesophageal fistula, foreign bodies, congenital anomalies [such as cleft palate]; vascular aneurysm or anomalies; hypertonic cricopharyngeus muscle; fixation of larynx; Zenker's diverticulum; esophageal stricture, tumor, or web; Schatzki's ring; and severe dental anomalies); **esophageal dysmotility disorders** (e.g., GE reflux, achalasia, diffuse esophageal spasm, and "Nutcracker" esophagus); **gastrointestinal diseases** (e.g., Crohn's disease, ulcerative colitis, and amyloidosis); **infectious disease** (e.g., caused by *Candida*, cytomegalovirus, herpesvirus, and human immunodeficiency virus); **psychiatric disorders** (e.g., globus hystericus); **skin diseases** (e.g., mucus membrane pemphigoid, epidermolysis bullosa dystrophica, lichen planus, psoriasis, Stevens-Johnson syndrome, and chronic graft-vs.-host disease); **treatment-related etiologies** (e.g., postoperative head and neck radiation, foreign devices [such as tracheostomy and nasogastric tubes], and postchemotherapy mucositis).

V. Nonsurgical management of dysphagia has the following general goals: to minimize the risk of aspiration and to advance the difficulty and variety of oral intake, both for the nutrition and the enjoyment of the patient. Short-term goals address the immediate needs of the patient and are attainable within a short period of time (e.g., 2-4 weeks). These include indirect therapy (e.g., appropriate bolus volumes and feeding rates), direct swallowing therapy (e.g., prefeeding exercises and compensatory swallowing maneuvers), and appropriate professional referrals for further evaluation or management of dysphagia. Long-term goals include using prescribed feeding techniques (e.g., consistent oral ingestion of a pureed diet) that meets the daily nutritional needs with constant supervision or independent self-feeding on a regular diet.

In severe dysphagia, an NGT may be temporarily used to provide full or supplemental nutrition to the patient. An NGT should not be used for more than 2 to 3 weeks as it is uncomfortable, may cause erosion of the nasopharynx, and does not prevent aspiration. If a prolonged extra-oral feeding route is required, a gastrostomy tube (e.g., percutaneous endoscopic gastrostomy [PEG]; see section VI.D) or jejunostomy tube (e.g., percutaneous endoscopic jejunostomy [PEJ]; see section VI.D) is indicated as it is more comfortable and provides lesser (but not absent) aspiration risk than an NGT. In addition to specific swallowing treatment, oral hygiene (e.g., cleaning the dentition and mucosa after meals and removing pocketed food particles) as well as prefeeding and feeding activities can be used to provide stimulation to the oral cavity and reinforce normal patterning. Therapeutic interventions focusing on postural and limb control as well as cognitive, behavioral, and perceptual remediation, if necessary, can enhance dysphagia interventions. Progression of treatment should be made based on individual performance with appropriate grading to ensure safety. Swallowing can be assessed by using sophisticated techniques (e.g., VFSS) or by quantifying clinical outcomes (e.g., decreases in pharyngeal swallow time, increases in the frequency of spontaneous swallows, advancements to oral feedings, upgrades in food or liquid textures, reductions in the degree of required supervision, improved nutritional status, and decreases in the time required to eat a meal safely). Nonsurgical treatment options for common swallowing problems are shown in Table 5.6-1.

A. Indirect management does not involve direct hands-on patient contact but involves giving feeding recommendations and education to the caregivers and interdisciplinary team members. In indirect management, other interdisciplinary team members (e.g., dietitian, nutrition support team, speech-language pathologist, occupational therapist, respiratory therapist) are actively involved. It is the sole treatment approach in patients who suffer from end-stage progressive disease or who have severe cognitive impairments that preclude the ability to follow even simple commands.

1. Cognitive stimulation

    a. Dysphagia education including the nature of the swallowing disorder, safety precautions, nutritional requirements, diet modifications, and the rationale for treatment methods, are given not only to the patient but also to the family or caregiver(s) and other interdisciplinary team members.

    b. Verbal cueing, such as telling the patient with cognitive deficits to close the lips, move the tongue, and "think" swallow, are more effective than simply telling the patient to "swallow" after placing the bolus in the mouth.

2. Feeding modification

    a. Food placement alteration involves food placement in the part of the oral cavity that enhances the patient's ability to feel the location of the bolus

Table 5.6-1. Nonsurgical treatment options for common swallowing problems

SWALLOWING PROBLEMS	NONSURGICAL TREATMENT OPTIONS
I. Cognitive status	
A. Impulsivity	Supervise feeding; place utensils on table after each bite; and present one food item at a time
B. Poor judgment	Use small-bowled utensils or covered cups with small openings or pinch the straw
C. Poor attention	Feed in a quiet, distraction-free environment
II. Oral phase	
A. Facial weakness	Modify diet texture (e.g., pureed, thick liquids); place food toward back of mouth or on stronger side of mouth; tilt head toward stronger side; assist lip closure
	Tactile stimulation of face; facial exercises (with mirror); EMG biofeedback; sucking or blowing exercises
B. Poor lingual control	Modify diet texture (foods that need little oral manipulation); place food toward the back of the mouth; tilt head toward the stronger side; forward and backward head movement to assist with bolus propulsion; oral inspection after mealtime to check for residue
	Tongue AROM and strengthening exercises; encourage precise articulation
III. Pharyngeal phase	
A. Delayed swallow reflex (aspiration)	Diet with no thin liquids; chin tuck; head rotation to the weaker side; supraglottic swallow
	Cold stimulation
B. Unilateral decrease in pharyngeal peristalsis (with unilateral pharyngeal pooling)	Turning of head to weaker side; tilting of head to stronger side
C. Decreased bilateral pharyngeal peristalsis (with pharyngeal pooling)	Effortful swallow; double (or dry) swallow; alternating liquids and swallows
D. Reduced laryngeal closure	Chin tuck; supraglottic swallow
E. Incomplete relaxation or premature closing of the cricopharyngeus (with pooling in pyriform sinus)	Mendelsohn's maneuver; turning of head to weaker side

EMG = electromyogram; AROM = active range of motion.

and to facilitate optimum bolus hold and transport. This can improve swallowing efficiency and safety, not only in patients with partial or complete oral, labial, or facial sensory deficits, but also in cases of impaired facial and lingual muscle strength.

    b. Bolus characteristic modifications are individually determined for each patient during CSS or VFSS.

        1) Bolus texture (consistency) modifications involve the gradual progression of the patient's diet through food of different texture or consistency with the goal of returning to a regular diet. In general, food of thinner consistencies (e.g., thin liquids) are more difficult to control and have a higher risk for aspiration because they can leak into the pharynx before swallowing is triggered. Hence, thickened liquids and soft cohesive solids are generally the safest consistencies. By increasing the viscosity or thickness of the food or liquid bolus in patients with oral sensory or motor deficits, there is reduced tendency for the material to escape from the oral cavity, fall into the laryngeal inlet, or penetrate the incompletely sealed larynx during the delay before pharyngeal swallow initiation. Also, more viscous materials may increase tongue movements and enhance mechanoreceptor displacement thus facilitating more timely initiation of the pharyngeal swallow. However, if the patient has a delayed pharyngeal swallow and is unable to significantly clear the pharynx of viscous materials, then the use of thick or viscous materials will not improve swallowing safety. Moreover, liquid thickening can adversely affect the patient's hydration (if necessary, these patients should be hydrated intravenously or through the feeding tube).

a) **Dysphagia NPO (*non per os* or nothing by mouth)** is indicated in patients with high risk for aspiration because of reduced alertness, reduced responsiveness to stimulation, absent swallow, absent protective cough, and difficulty handling secretions as evidenced by excessive coughing and choking, copious secretions, and a wet gurgly voice quality; or significant reductions in the range and strength of oral pharyngeal and laryngeal movements. Even if indicated for aspiration prevention, NPO is disadvantageous to treating dysphagia because swallowing itself is the best exercise for its recovery. Hence, although a patient may remain NPO, treatment may be recommended to improve prefeeding skills such as oral-pharyngeal sensorimotor functioning or alertness and responsiveness. If indicated, single food items may be used in NPO patients for trial feeding purposes. Patients on NPO can be given intravenous (IV) hydration, total parenteral nutrition (central or peripheral), or can be fed through a nasogastric tube or gastrostomy tube.

b) **Dysphagia pureed diets** are smooth, soft, moist, blenderized foods that do not require chewing (e.g., applesauce and whipped potatoes). They are indicated for patients with chewing difficulty or who are unable to form a cohesive bolus because of decreased tongue function. In these patients, liquids are not allowed.

c) **Dysphagia mechanical soft (semisolid) diets** require little chewing and are easy to control in the mouth. Examples include minced food (e.g., ground meats with gravy and meatloaf) and soft foods (e.g., bananas). In these patients, liquids are not allowed.

d) **Thick liquids,** which are liquids that have body, are easier to control in the mouth than thin liquids because they have less tendency to leak from the base of the tongue before swallowing is triggered. They should be introduced gradually under supervision in conjunction with the dysphagia pureed or dysphagia mechanical soft diet.

   (1) **Full-thick (or spoon-thick) liquids** include thickened cream soups, applesauce, mashed potatoes with gravy, and cooked cereal.

   (2) **Medium-thick liquids** are used as a transition from full-thick to

thin liquids. They include eggnogs, milkshakes, regular or strained cream soups, tomato juice, sherbet, and nectars (e.g., peach or apricot).

e) **Thin liquids** are clear with little or no body (e.g., water, tea, fruit juice, coffee, and milk). Ice cream and Jello are also considered thin liquids because they melt in the mouth. Thin liquids are only recommended when medium-thick liquids are tolerated and should be introduced gradually under supervision in conjunction with the dysphagia pureed or dysphagia mechanical soft diet.

f) **Regular diets** have no texture restrictions and are allowed if the patient can safely tolerate pureed or semisolid foods as well as thick or thin liquids. Solid foods used in the regular diet may be chopped or cut to the size of a fingernail or smaller.

2) **Bolus volume modifications** involve the use of smaller volumes to prevent or minimize the degree of aspiration that may occur. Recommended bolus volumes, as determined during the VFSS are 2 ml ($\frac{1}{2}$ teaspoon), 5 ml (1 teaspoon), 10 ml (small sip or by straw), and 20 ml (average bolus in normal adults; by filled tablespoon or by cup). The timing of food presentation is also important in controlling bolus volume. There should be at least a 30-second delay between bolus presentations to avoid overloading the mouth in patients with problems in oral preparation and oral transit.

3) **Bolus temperature modification** involves the use of a cold stimulus to facilitate more rapid posteriorward tongue movement and pharyngeal swallow elicitation. It is recommended in patients with oral sensory deficits or poor initiation of oral bolus transport. In some dysphagic patients with chronic respiratory problems, however, cold may be perceived as a noxious stimulus, hence a tepid or warm bolus should be used instead.

4) **Modification of bolus taste, aroma, and appearance** is quite variable as it is dependent on the patient's premorbid preferences as well as alterations in taste after the neurologic, surgical, or medical insult. Anecdotally, carbonated beverages have been used in dysphagic patients because the carbon dioxide bubbles stimulate pain fibers, which may enhance patient awareness of the liquid during pharyngeal swallowing.

5) **Salivary enhancement** includes the use of swabs, humidified air, or drugs (e.g., pilocarpine or artificial saliva) to moisturize the bolus and facilitate swallowing.

c. **Feeding adaptations** include the use of adapted feeding utensils (e.g., small-bowled utensils to decrease bolus size and covered cups with small openings or pinching the straw to limit amount of liquids) and the use of feeding adaptations for patients with decreased upper–limb function (such as limited grasp, incoordination, decreased ROM, hemiparesis, and hemiplegia), which are described in Chapter 4.5, section II.A.3.a. Feeding strategies for different pulmonary-related symptoms (e.g., dyspnea) in patients with chronic obstructive pulmonary diseases are shown in Table 5.12-3 in Chapter 5.12.

d. **Feeding environment adaptations** include feeding in a quiet, distraction-free environment for patients with problems in judgment, attention, or motor planning.

e. **Feeding route,** oral versus extra-oral, can be determined by the swallowing tests. If oral intake is inadequate, it may be supplemented by extra-oral (e.g., NGT, PEG, or PEJ) feedings. Patients with extra-oral feeding sources can be progressed as follows: as the patient recovers swallowing abilities or learns compensatory strategies (as indicated by changes in VFSS findings or increased ability to manage secretions), he or she receives therapeutic feedings by an allied health personnel. When the amount of intake increases and safe feeding behaviors are noted, the patient is permitted to eat under the supervision of other health care-givers or trained family members. As intake improves and calories are consistently sufficient, the extra-oral feeding source may be used only for hydration and medication intake. Eventually, if the patient continues to improve, he or she will become able to drink enough fluid and take medication so that the extra-oral feeding source can be removed. It is important that throughout this process that patient be weighed at regular intervals and be monitored for signs of dehydration or malnutrition.

f. **Degree of feeding supervision** depends on the patient's cognitive status.
g. **Feeding positions or postures** should be combined with other measures such as controlling bolus volumes, modifying bolus textures, slowing feeding rates, cognitive stimulation techniques, and compensatory airway protective maneuvers (see section V.B.4). Their effectiveness can be objectively tested using the VFSS. Ideally, they should serve only as temporary measures during the recovery period (although they may be needed permanently in some severe dysphagia cases). After feeding, patients should remain upright for at least 30 minutes to decrease the risk of aspiration and GE reflux.

1) **Sitting position**
   a) **A 90-degree-angle sitting position** with the trunk erect, the head in the midline, and the neck slightly flexed forward, is the optimal feeding position that achieves maximum airway protection in most patients with neurogenic dysphagia.
   b) **A 45-degree-angle sitting (i.e., reclining) position** can facilitate drainage of the residue from the valleculae down the posterior pharynx and into the pyriform sinuses, thus preventing laryngeal penetration and aspiration. This position may be beneficial for patients with a moderate degree of vallecular or pyriform sinus residue and who have poor cognitive ability to follow each wet swallow with a dry swallow (i.e., double swallow; see section V.B.4.a), and for patients with a poor prognosis for significant recovery of neuromuscular dysphagia who express a strong desire for some oral intake. Feeding in this position is typically used only to supplement the extra-oral route of feeding. Bolus volumes must be kept to a minimum (2-5ml) with appropriate texture as specified during the VFSS.

2) **Head position**
   a) **Chin-tuck (chin-down)** can reduce the opening to the airway, draw the tongue forward, and widen the vallecular space, thus preventing or minimizing premature entry of the bolus into the pharynx and open larynx. The open laryngeal vestibule is also drawn forward and is somewhat channeled under the tongue base, thereby making it less vulnerable to penetration due to the additional protection from the tongue. Chin-tuck is an effective airway protective position in appropriate patients who present with delayed initiation of

the pharyngeal swallow; however, it must not be used for all types of dysphagia as it can promote aspiration in some cases. For example, in patients whose pharyngeal swallow is so delayed that it is not initiated until the bolus reaches the pyriform sinuses and in whom there is also delay in laryngeal elevation and closure, the chin-tuck posture may facilitate the anterior diversion of the hesitated bolus in the pyriform sinus into the airway during laryngeal elevation. In patients with sensorimotor impairment of the lips and tongue, the chin-tuck may also cause inefficient oral bolus containment, control, and transport. Also, if the chin-tuck is not combined with bolus volume control, the large thin liquid bolus can fill the valleculae causing an overflow into the pharynx and into the laryngeal inlet.

  b) **Head-rotation position** toward the weaker pharyngeal side can increase pharyngeal clearance by directing the bolus to the stronger side.

  c) **Head-tilt position** toward the stronger pharyngeal side can increase pharyngeal clearance by directing the bolus towards the stronger side.

 3) **Side-lying position** can reduce hypopharyngeal pooling in selected patients.

3. **Secretion management** includes pulmonary toileting, i.e., oral or tracheal suctioning.

4. **Calorie counts,** which are done by nutritionists or dietitians, are used to determine the patient's nutritional status especially when diet modifications (e.g., purees and thickened liquids) or rather laborious feeding methods (e.g., controlled bolus volumes and double swallows) are initiated (as these may influence the patient's motivation and potential for sufficient oral intake).

B. **Direct management** involves direct hands-on patient contact and should be done only if it is likely to improve the patient's quality of life, nutritional status, or safety. The patient must be alert, have adequate communicative and cognitive abilities, be medically stable, and have good endurance and pulmonary function. If the patient is unable to tolerate oral intake safely, direct management without liquid or food substances may be done. In direct management, a treatment applied to one structure can usually facilitate improvement in other areas of the upper aerodigestive tract. For example, ROM and strengthening exercises of the tongue, which are aimed at improving the tongue's propulsive mechanism for more efficient oral bolus transport can also facilitate pharyngeal clearance (by tongue base retraction) and enhance speech production and articulation. Likewise, increasing the frequency of dry swallows, which is aimed at reducing accumulated oral secretions may also simultaneously strengthen pharyngeal muscle contraction.

1. **Sensory stimulation** remains controversial especially in its long-term efficacy.

  a. **Cold stimulation** is a sensory facilitative technique based on the hypothesis that mechanical and thermal sensory receptors in the anterior oropharynx are the most reflexogenic for swallow elicitation and, when mechanically stimulated with a blunt cold object, will heighten the sensitivity and increase the speed at which the pharyngeal swallow occurs. A laryngeal mirror (size 00) or a metal rod of similar size is placed in ice for approximately 10 seconds and then placed along the area of the anterior faucial arch (bilaterally or alternating between the right and left sides) and rubbed or tapped 5 to 8 times. After this icing procedure, the patient is asked to swallow food or, if oral feeding is not allowed, to perform a dry swallow. Cold stimulation is performed for short periods (i.e., stop after 5 minutes, or if fatigue occurs as evidenced by increased time before initiation or coughing) and several times throughout the day as well as before mealtimes. Patients with delayed initiation of the pharyngeal swallow have reported an easier time in initiating the swallow when cold stimulation is done immediately before mealtime.

    b. Tactile and pressure stimulation includes the application of an empty spoon or a tongue depressor to the anterior third of the tongue or rubbing a squeezed-out lemon glycerin swab to the lips, teeth, gums, and tongue to stimulate a dry pharyngeal swallow; and tapping or applying a quick stretch of the facial muscles in patients with facial weakness or sensory loss.

2. Swallowing reflex modulation

    a. Gag reflex modulation to normalize gag is recommended although a gag reflex per se is not required for safe swallowing.

        1) Facilitation of an hypoactive gag can be done by applying a tongue depressor, cotton-tipped swab, or quick tap or stretch to the arch of the soft palate in an upward and outward direction.

        2) Desensitization of hyperactive gag can be done by using firm pressure with a tongue depressor to slowly "walk" back on the tongue. As the gag reflex becomes less sensitive, the tongue depressor can be advanced farther back in the mouth.

    b. Bite reflex inhibition can be done by applying sustained pressure to the tongue with a padded stick and positioning the head in an upright position with the chin tucked.

    c. Tongue-thrust reflex inhibition can be done by a sequence of techniques, including pressure under the chin applied to the tongue retraction musculature, manual vibration under the tongue, and quick stretch of the tongue into protrusion to facilitate retrusion.

3. Therapeutic exercises are used to facilitate oral motor strength, range of motion, and coordination. They are best done 5 to 10 times per day. Patients must be able to follow instructions (one-step or more) and be able to imitate isolated orofacial movements. Their anecdotal efficacy remains to be proved scientifically.

    a. Active range of motion exercises for patients with oropharyngeal swallowing impairments are preferred over passive ROM exercises.

        1) Jaw AROM exercises are used to facilitate jaw opening and closure as well as rotary and lateral movements to help maintain any bolus within the oral cavity. Exercises include opening the mouth as wide as possible; moving the jaw from side to side; alternating left to right jaw extensions; chewing a soft piece of chewing gum wrapped in gauze and tied to a string that is held by the clinician; chewing lightly against the tip of a soft-sponged toothette held firmly by the clinician; and biting against a block made of soft material of different widths applied interdentally between the central incisors to facilitate a gradual increase in the distance between the upper and lower teeth (using a mirror, the patient later attempts to match the opening width without the use of the bite block device). In patients with an exaggerated bite response, systematic desensitization techniques should be used (i.e., the jaw is pushed closed and held firmly for a few seconds, then the pressure is released and the jaw is allowed to relax) rather than trying to pry the mouth open.

2) Lip AROM exercises can help prevent food or liquid from leaking out of the oral cavity. These include opening the mouth wide; smiling, grinning, or sneering; repeating "pa, pa, pa, ba, ba, ba"; and blowing through a straw or blowing bubbles. Any exercise that is directed toward increasing mandibular elevation can also improve the approximation of the upper and lower lips. Patients can also be taught to imitate lateral and medial labial movements to prevent lip stiffening and enhance mobility for speech, swallowing, and better physical appearance. On each trial, the patient should be instructed to maintain the targeted lip posture for a few seconds before returning to the rest position.

3) Tongue AROM exercises are used to facilitate control of the bolus and its propulsion through the oral cavity or to aid pharyngeal swallowing ability by improving retraction of the tongue base. They include exercises to improve tongue lateralization (e.g., alternating lateral movements of the tongue tip with the main objective of sustaining the isolated posture), tongue elevation (e.g., approximation of the tongue tip toward the front teeth or repeating "la, la, la, ta, ta, ta"), tongue protrusion, and posterior retraction of the tongue base (e.g., hard swallow; see section V.B.4.b).

b. Strengthening exercises are indicated for nonprogressive or recovering dysphagic patients with weakness of the striated muscles of the oral cavity (e.g., lips and tongue), pharynx, and larynx. They are not indicated for patients with progressive neurologic diseases. Any AROM exercises for the lips, tongue, or jaw can be modified into strengthening exercise by applying manual resistance.

1) Lip strengthening exercises are used to improve the integrity of the lip seal to maintain foods and liquids in the oral cavity. The patient is asked to purse the lips tightly holding them tightly together for about 5 seconds, followed by a slow release. To further increase lip strength, an intervening tongue blade or soft-sponged swab may be pulled by the clinician from the patient's lips as the patient purses his or her lips against it.

2) Tongue strengthening exercises can help control the bolus and propel it to the pharynx. Exercises include manual depression of the top, side, and back of the tongue with a tongue blade and asking the patient to displace the tongue against the blade. The patient may also be asked to use the tongue to cup an oral stimulus or a controlled bolus to the hard palate while the clinician attempts to remove it. Examples of oral stimuli include a moistened, soft-sponged toothette, flavored suckers, or rolled pieces of flavored gauze held at one end by the clinician.

3) Palate strengthening exercises can help seal the back of the tongue and prevent premature spillage of bolus into the pharynx. The elevation and retraction of the soft palate (i.e., contraction of the levator veli palatini muscles) are also required during swallowing to effect velopharyngeal closure and prevent misdirection of foods or liquids into the nasal cavity. Exercises include tongue cupping of an oral stimulus or a controlled bolus to the hard palate while the clinician attempts to remove it (see section V.B.3.b.2). The application of resistive activities that promote increased strength of the levator muscle is difficult. Hence patients with flaccid or surgically altered soft palates are typically managed by fitting them with palatal augmentation prostheses (see section V.B.6).

4) Respiratory strengthening exercises are needed so that the patient can hold respiration to swallow and can clear penetrated or aspirated material from the airway. They include inhaling deeply and exhaling slowly; repeating "ah, ah, ah" as long as possible; blowing through a straw or onto a windmill; and reading poems or singing songs. Patients with a weak cough should also be taught assisted-coughing (see Chapter 5.12, section IV.B.1.b.1.c), which involves having the supine patient take a deep breath, followed by coughing effort done in synchrony with the clinician (or assisting person) pushing on the patient's abdomen and lower ribs. This can help achieve normal cough airflow velocity despite paralysis and can also help clear the tracheobronchial tree of secretions and aspirated materials.

5) Vocal cord adduction exercises are performed as an attempt to strengthen weak cords and approximate them to prevent aspiration. Examples include repeating "ah, ah, ah," or saying "ah" for 5 seconds while pushing down on a chair or pushing the hands together. These exercises can create a Valsalva effect and should be used cautiously in patients with cardiac disorders.

c. Coordination exercises can be done by increasing the speed of AROM or using strengthening exercises. Patients may also be taught motor planning skills.

4. Compensatory swallowing maneuvers are used to improve airway protection and the efficiency of bolus passage through the aerodigestive tract. The patient must be able to understand the rationale for the maneuver, follow two- to three-step instructions, concentrate on the execution of the maneuver, and retain instructions over time. The efficacy of the compensatory swallowing maneuvers can be confirmed by VFSS or by fiberoptic endoscopy.

a. Double (or dry) swallowing involves having the patient swallow twice (or more if needed) per bolus (e.g., after wet swallows with subsequent dry swallows). This technique may be used in patients with incomplete pharyngeal clearance during the initial swallow or in patients with oral residue related to slow and inefficient lingual motility. It can also help improve pharyngeal muscle strength.

b. Hard (or effortful) swallow involves having the patient swallow with forceful backward motion of the tongue in an attempt to help propel the bolus through the pharyngeal cavity in a timely manner. It can improve the strength of the tongue base retraction and the pharyngeal wall contraction, which are both needed to complete pharyngeal clearance.

c. Supraglottic swallow is designed to voluntarily close the airway before and during the swallow to clear potential residue, primarily from the laryngeal vestibule and pyriform sinuses. It is indicated in patients with reduced laryngeal closure, delayed initiation of the pharyngeal swallow, incomplete supraglottic valving, and incomplete pharyngeal clearance. The patient is instructed to take a deep breath and hold it (more effective if patient bears down on a table or presses the hands together to create a Valsalva effect); place food or liquid in the mouth; swallow (once or twice, depending on the efficiency of pharyngeal clearance); clear the throat "out" (rather than cough because most patients will attempt to inhale before a coughing); and swallow again. Patient should only reestablish breathing after the sequence to prevent inhalation of pharyngeal stasis or residue.

   d. Mendelsohn maneuver is designed to voluntarily prolong cricopharyngeal relaxation in patients with incomplete relaxation or premature closing of the cricopharyngeus (as shown by VFSS). During dry swallows or 1-ml water swallows, the patient is instructed to "hold" the swallow for 3 to 5 seconds (i.e., voluntarily hold the larynx in its involuntarily initiated, elevated, and anteriorly displaced position), and then to complete the swallow and relax. This increases the strength and range of the hyolaryngeal complex and prolongs the retraction of the tongue base, both of which help in laryngeal vestibular closure and in prolongation of cricopharyngeal relaxation for more complete pharyngeal clearance.

   e. Alternating liquid and solid swallowing is effective in cases of decreased pharyngeal peristalsis. The liquid swallows help to clear any solid material remaining in the pharyngeal recesses.

5. **Biofeedback techniques** using taped VFSS or ultrasonography can be used to promote lingual bolus control and coordinated tongue movement during the oral stage of swallowing. Electromyography and esophageal manometry may be repeated over the course of treatment and used to demonstrate progress towards the goals of increasing strength and pressure exerted by the tongue and the pharynx during swallowing. For teaching laryngeal valving maneuvers, fiberoptic videoendoscopy may be used as a biofeedback tool by allowing visualization of laryngeal valving during compensatory breath-holding strategies.

6. **Prosthetic devices,** e.g., palatal augmentation prostheses, can be used to lower the palatal vault to enhance tongue-to-palate contact and to potentially improve the pharyngeal phase of swallow (i.e., by improving pharyngeal transit time). Use of palatal augmentation prostheses requires training regarding optimum oral bolus positioning and compensatory tongue placements for articulation; therefore, the patient must be motivated to tolerate and adapt to the prosthesis during speech and swallowing. Palatal augmentation prostheses have been used in dysphagic patients who suffer from surgical ablation or neuromuscular impairment of the oral structures.

VI. Surgical procedures

A. **Tracheostomy** (see Chapter 5.12, section V.A.2) can be used for short-term protection of the airway from aspiration. However, tracheostomy can also possibly increase aspiration risk due to impaired laryngeal elevation caused by tethering of the tracheostomy tube to the larynx and trachea. If an inflated tracheostomy cuff is used (see section III.C.1.a.2.b), careful suctioning is needed prior to deflation because food that accumulates above the cuff may be aspirated on cuff deflation. The treatment of dysphagia in patients with tracheostomy tubes is controversial. Oral intake for either evaluation or treatment should probably be postponed if the patient's tracheostomy tube is a Jackson size 5 or larger or if the patient's respiratory status necessitates an inflated cuff.

   In tracheostomized patients, treatment should be directed toward decannulation, which can be accomplished by gradual reduction in the size of the tracheostomy tube; removal of the cuff; introduction of a fenestrated tube; gradually increasing the period of time that the patient tolerates occlusion for uncuffed or fenestrated tubes; and the use of a one-way valve (e.g., Passy-Muir Speaking Valve and Olympic Trach-talk; see Chapter 5.12, section V.A.2.b.4.b). A one-way valve opens on inhalation and closes on exhalation thus forcing expired air through the larynx and upper glottis. This helps blow out any food residue in the trachea (which might otherwise penetrate more deeply into the airway) and restore-phonation. Swallowing evaluation and treatment may proceed in conjunction with decannulation for patients who demonstrate limited success with oral intake as swallowing treatment may improve the patient's ability to handle his or her secretions (thus facilitating decannulation). A patient with a cuffed tracheostomy tube can be decannulated by drinking 4 oz of blue-dyed water (e.g., with methylene blue) at intervals of 15 minutes for an hour and thoroughly suctioning the trachea to note any blue-tinged secretions. If this test is negative, the cuff is deflated for meals and at other times, with close supervision for 24 hours. Although a positive test result suggests aspiration, decannulation may still proceed if the patient shows adequate swallowing during meals with the cuff deflated.

B. **Cricopharyngeal myotomy,** which is used in patients with Zenker's diverticulum and cricopharyngeal achalasia, can also be effectively performed in patients with generalized dysphagia because of neuromuscular disease.

C. **Laryngeal protection procedures,** for example, vocal cord augmentation for mild aspiration and laryngeal diversion for more severe and chronic aspirations, may be used.

D. **Surgical feeding tube insertion** (e.g., surgically placed gastrostomy, PEG, or PEJ) may be used for nutritional purposes in patients with high risk for aspiration (NGT may initially be used temporarily for less than 2-3 weeks). Surgically placed gastrostomy or PEG do not necessarily protect the patient from aspiration as the patient may aspirate his or her saliva or gastric contents, which reach the pharynx by reflux. However, PEJ (wherein a thin tube is deposited in the distal duodenum or proximal jejunum through a mature PEG tract) may possibly reduce the risk of aspiration.

VII. **Complications**

A. **Aspiration pneumonia** usually occurs at the time of eating although it may occur even during sleep. It can be prevented by elevating the head of the bed, using H_2-blockers or antacids to increase the gastric pH above 2.5, and decreasing food intake before sleep. In patients with recurrent aspiration, a PEG or PEJ tube may be inserted.

1. **Chemical pneumonitis** is caused by gastric reflux and aspiration of a sufficient quantity of stomach acid with pH below 2.5. Clinical features include acute dyspnea, hypoxemia, tachypnea, tachycardia with or without cyanosis, bronchospasm, and fever. Sputum may be pink and frothy. Radiographs may show infiltrates in one or both lower lobes. The clinical course is variable, ranging from rapid improvement within 5 days to a fulminant course, which may lead to death. Treatment is supportive and includes positive-pressure breathing, IV fluids, and tracheal suction as needed. The benefit of corticosteroids and antibiotics remain controversial.

2. **Bacterial infection** is usually caused by aspiration of oropharyngeal bacteria (usually anaerobes in community-acquired pneumonias and *Staphylococcus aureus* in hospital-acquired pneumonias). Onset is usually insidious. Symptoms include cough, fever, and purulent sputum. The radiograph

shows infiltrates involving the dependent pulmonary segments or lobes with or without cavitation. Treatment is antibiotics given empirically or based on sputum culture.

3. **Mechanical airway obstruction** results from aspiration of particulate matters (e.g., food) or inert fluids and usually involve the right mainstem bronchus territory. Symptoms include wheezing, coughing, choking, and respiratory distress (e.g., acute dyspnea and cyanosis with or without apnea). Depending on the level of obstruction and the size of the particle aspirated, the patient may develop an irritating chronic cough (with or without recurrent infections) or develop acute apnea leading to rapid death. Treatment is extraction of the particulate matter (e.g., by the Heimlich maneuver) or, if inert fluids are present, tracheal suction and intermittent positive pressure breathing (IPPB) with oxygen and isoproterenol as needed. If there is a superimposed bacterial infection (due to obstruction of normal pulmonary drainage), antibiotics may be given.

B. **Malnutrition** is an imbalance between nutrient intake and bodily requirements. It is significant if the patient has a recent weight loss of more than 10 to 15%; weight below 90% of ideal body weight (IBW) (see Table 5.6-2 for IBW computation); or serum albumin below 3.5 g/dL. In malnutrition, the daily caloric needs can be determined by the Harris-Benedict formula for basal energy expenditure (BEE):

- Male: BEE in Kcal/day $= 66 + (13.7 \times$ wt in kg) $+ (5 \times$ ht in cm) $- (6.8 \times$ age in years)
- Female: BEE in Kcal/day $= 655 + (9.6 \times$ wt in kg) $+ (1.8 \times$ ht in cm) $- (4.7 \times$ age in years)

Table 5.6-2. Quick calculation for ideal body weights (IBW)

BODY CONDITION	MALE IBW	FEMALE IBW
Medium build	Allow 106 lb for the first 5 feet, plus 6 lb for each additional inch	Allow 100 lb for the first 5 feet, plus 5 lb for each additional inch
Small build	Subtract 10% of IBW	Subtract 10% of IBW
Large build	Add 10% of IBW	Add 10% of IBW
Para- or tetraplegia	Subtract 5-10% of IBW	Subtract 5-10% of IBW
Amputations		
Foot	Subtract 1.8% of IBW	Subtract 1.8% of IBW
Below knee	Subtract 6.0% of IBW	Subtract 6.0% of IBW
Above knee	Subtract 15.0% of IBW	Subtract 15.0% of IBW
Entire unilateral lower limbs	Subtract 18.5% of IBW	Subtract 18.5% of IBW
Hand	Subtract 1.0% of IBW	Subtract 1.0% of IBW
Below elbow	Subtract 3.0% of IBW	Subtract 3.0% of IBW
Entire unilateral upper limb	Subtract 6.5% of IBW	Subtract 6.5% of IBW

Tabulated from the IBW formulas used by the nutrition departments of the New York University Medical Center, New York, NY and Goldwater Memorial Hospital, Roosevelt Island NY; Data adapted from Peiffer SC, Blust P, Leyson JFJ: Nutritional assessment of the spinal cord injured patient, *J Amer Dietetics Assoc* 78:501-505, 1981; and LeVeau B: *Williams and Lissner: biomechanics of human motion*, ed 2, Philadelphia, 1977, WB Saunders, pp 205-215.

The caloric needs of general hospital patients are about 120% of BEE, but if there is a major medical stress, caloric requirements can be as high as 150 to 200% of BEE. Caloric need (i.e., Kcal per kg) for sedentary activity is 20 to 30 × IBW; for light activity, 25 to 35 × IBW; for moderate activity, 30 to 40 × IBW; and for heavy activity, 45 to 50 × IBW. The protein requirement for healthy adults is 0.8 g/kg/day, but for hospitalized patients, it is about 1.0 to 1.5 g/kg/day (higher in catabolic state and lower in renal or liver disease). Fluid requirement is approximately 30 to 35 ml/kg. Enteral feeding (e.g., nasogastric tube feeding) may be used if nutritional needs are not met by oral feeding (e.g., due to recurrent aspiration). For prolonged enteral feeding, a PEG or PEJ is preferred over NG tubes. In the PM&R setting, intermittent or bolus feeding in the daytime is preferred so the patient can participate in rehabilitation activities.

In patients with chronic pulmonary disease (especially COPD), there is increased energy cost of breathing even at rest; therefore, the result of the above BEE computation needs to be adjusted by multiplying it with a correction factor of 1.2 to 1.5 (the higher factor is used for emaciated patients). If the patient is not confined in bed, the adjusted BEE is further adjusted by multiplying it by a factor of 1.06. In using IBW to determine the status of patients with chronic pulmonary disease, cutoff values of less than 90% or as low as less than 70 to 85% IBW may be justifiable (as discussed in Chapter 5.12, section IV.A.1.b). For further discussion about the pulmonary relationship, effects, and management of malnutrition in patients with chronic pulmonary problems, refer to Chapter 5.12, section IV.A.1.b.

BIBLIOGRAPHY

Bartlett JG: Aspiration pneumonia. In Baum GL, Wolinsky E, editors: *Textbook of pulmonary diseases*, ed 5, vol 1, Boston, 1994, Little, Brown, p 593.

Cherney LR: *Rehabilitation Institute of Chicago: clinical management of dysphagia in adults and children*, ed 2, Gaithersburg, MD, 1994, Aspen.

Greenbaum DM: Decannulation of the tracheostomized patient, *Heart Lung* 5:119-123, 1976.

Groher M, editor: *Dysphagia: diagnosis and management*, ed 2, Boston, 1992, Buttersworth-Heinemann.

Johnson R, McKenzie S, Rosenquist C, et al: Dysphagia following stroke: quantitative evaluation of pharyngeal transit times, *Arch Phys Med Rehabil* 73:419-423, 1992.

Langmore SE, Miller RM: Behavioral treatment for adults with oropharyngeal dysphagia, *Arch Phys Med Rehabil* 75:1154-1160, 1994.

Logemann J: *Evaluation and treatment of swallowing disorders*, San Diego, 1983, College-Hill Press.

Miller RM, Langmore SE: Treatment efficacy for adults with oropharyngeal dysphagia, *Arch Phys Med Rehabil* 75:1256-1262, 1994.

Noll SF, Bender CE, Nelson MC: Rehabilitation of patients with swallowing disorders. In Braddom RL, editor: *Physical medicine and rehabilitation*, Philadelphia, 1996, WB Saunders, pp 533-554.

Nutrition and Food Service: *Goldwater Memorial Hospital pocketbook of diet manual*, New York, 1993, Goldwater Memorial Hospital.

Stefans V, Gray RP, Sowell T: Pediatric and adult swallowing videofluoroscopy. In Lennard TA, editor: *Physiatric procedures in clinical practice*, Philadelphia, 1995, Hanley & Belfus, pp 105-113.

CHAPTER 5.7

VOIDING DYSFUNCTIONS

Aside from urinary tract infections, voiding disorder is the most common urinary problem managed by physiatrists in the inpatient rehabilitation setting. This chapter concentrates mainly on voiding dysfunctions of neurourologic origin.

I. **Neuroanatomy and neurophysiology of voiding**
  A. **Peripheral pathways**
    1. **Efferent fibers**
      a. **Autonomic efferents**
        1) **Parasympathetic efferents** from **S2-S4** travel through the pelvic nerves (also called pelvic splanchnic nerves or nervi erigentes) to the parasympathetic (cholinergic muscarinic M2) receptors distributed throughout the detrusor muscle (more in the body of the bladder than at the base). Its stimulation results in bladder contraction (i.e., emptying).
        2) **Sympathetic efferents** from **T11-L2** travel through the hypogastric plexi to sympathetic (α and β-2 adrenergic) receptors. Stimulation of β-2 receptors located primarily in the body of the bladder causes bladder relaxation (urine storage). Stimulation of α (mainly α-1) receptors, which are located primarily at the base of the bladder cause constriction (i.e., closing) of the internal urethral sphincter (IUS) at the detrusor outlet (smooth muscles circling the bladder outlet) promoting urine storage.
      b. **Somatic efferents** from **S2-S4** travel through the pudendal nerves to innervate the striated muscles of the external urethral sphincter (EUS). The EUS is marginally closed with its normal tone (thus preventing urine emptying or leakage) and is opened passively by forceful urinary flow with contraction of the detrusor and of the abdominal muscles. Voluntary contraction can hold the urine in the bladder for a limited period of time.
    2. **Afferent fiber** signals travel through the pudendal and pelvic nerves to the conus medullaris and through the hypogastric plexi to the thoracolumbar spinal cord. They originate from the detrusor muscle stretch receptors, external anal and urethral sphincters, perineum, and genitalia. Filling of the bladder up to a threshold level activates the stretch receptors in the bladder, which send impulses through the afferent nerves (probably through pudendal and/or pelvic nerve; exact physiology is unknown) to the sacral micturition center to stimulate the parasympathetic efferents, hence resulting in a reflex detrusor contraction, opening of the sphincters, and emptying of the bladder.
  B. **Central pathways ("voiding centers")**
    1. **Loop I (corticopontine-mesencephalic nuclei)** originates from the frontal lobe and exerts inhibitory influence on parasympathetic sacral micturition center (loop III) thus allowing bladder storage. Loop I lesions above the pontine micturition center (e.g., stroke, traumatic brain injury [TBI], hydrocephalus, multiple sclerosis [MS], brain tumor, and Parkinson's disease,)

cause lack of inhibitory effect of the cerebral cortex on the sacral (parasympathetic) micturition center; therefore, a low threshold detrusor reflex (hyperreflexic detrusor) and small bladder capacity results. Because the pontine micturition center remains intact, there would be no sphincter dyssynergia.

2. **Loop II (pontine-mesencephalic-sacral nuclei or "pontine micturition center")** coordinates efficient sphincter and detrusor interaction (i.e., during voiding, it coordinates bladder contraction and opening of the sphincter). Lesions at or below the pontine micturition center and above the sacral cord (e.g., traumatic spinal cord injury [SCI], transverse myelitis, MS involving the cord, syringomyelia, and primary or metastatic spinal cord tumor) would have both detrusor hyperreflexia and sphincter detrusor dyssynergia hence inefficient voiding pattern (e.g., bladder contraction on a closed sphincter may lead to vesicoureteral reflux or hydronephrosis).

3. **Loop III (pelvic and pudendal nuclei or "sacral micturition center")** is responsible for integrating stimuli from cephalic centers and for sorting out, passing on, and initiating sensation, inhibition, and excitation of the end organs. It also mediates the parasympathetic S2-S4 sacral micturition reflex (i.e., stretching of the detrusor stimulates the parasympathetic efferents resulting in a reflex detrusor contraction and emptying of bladder). Lesions involving the sacral micturition center (e.g., conus and cauda equina injuries, L4-L5 or L5-S1 disc herniation, primary or metastatic tumors, myelodysplasias, arteriovenous [AV] malformation, lumbar stenosis, and inflammatory process such as arachnoiditis) or peripheral nerves (e.g., diabetic neuropathy and pelvic trauma) cause dyssynergia of detrusor and external sphincter interaction as well as loss of the sacral micturition reflex resulting in urinary retention (areflexic or atonic bladder).

4. **Loop IV (motor cortex to pudendal nucleus)** is responsible for the voluntary control (contraction or inhibition) of the external urethral sphincter.

II. Evaluation

A. **Urologic history** includes voiding complaints (urgency, frequency, hesitancy, dysuria, and incontinence), previous voiding history, previous surgery (abdominal, pelvic, transurethral, and lower limb), medications (sedatives, hypnotics, anticholinergics, antidepressants, antipsychotics, antihistamines, antispasmodics, opiates, adrenergic, and calcium channel blockers), other medical problems (stroke, cognitive disorders, endocrine disorders such as diabetes mellitus, recurrent urinary tract infections [UTIs], restricted mobility, and stool impaction or incontinence), fluid intake and output over several 24-hour periods, activities of daily living (ADL) (hand function, ability to perform transfers, and ability to dress and undress), availability of support system (e.g., family and home health aides), lifestyle, and sexuality. The mnemonic for the reversible (transient) causes of incontinence in the elderly that must be ruled out in history taking is **DIAPPERS—D**elirium or confusional state, **I**nfection (urinary, symptomatic), **A**trophic vaginitis and/or urethritis, **P**harmaceuticals (sedatives or hypnotics, especially long-acting agents; anticholinergic agents; loop diuretics; alpha-adrenergic agonists and antagonists; calcium channel blockers), **P**sychological disorders (depression), **E**ndocrine disorders (hyperglycemia or hypercalcemia), **R**educed mobility, and **S**tool impaction.

B. **Physical examination** includes assessment of motor level, sensory level (sacral sensation), deep tendon reflexes, pathological reflexes (e.g., Babinski), anal wink (S1-S4), bulbocavernosus reflex (S2-S4), ice water test (instill 50-100 ml of ice water into the bladder through a catheter; if the bladder contracts and expels the catheter, it signifies that patients with upper motor lesions are out of spinal shock stage), prostate examination in men, and degree of vaginal support and estrogenization in women.

C. Diagnostic tests

1. Upper urinary tract studies

a. **Intravenous pyelogram (IVP) or excretory urogram** is used to visualize the size, shape, and function of the whole urinary tract (kidney, ureters, and bladder) to detect hydronephrosis, pyelonephritis, calculi, tumor, and renovascular hypertension. A radiopaque substance is injected intravenously, and a series of radiographs are taken 3, 5, 10, 15, and 20 minutes after dye injection. At the end of the test, the patient voids and another radiograph is taken to visualize the residual dye in the bladder. The major disadvantage of IVP is patient's potential allergic reactions to the dye, radiation exposure, and patient inconvenience (patient should be *non per os* [NPO] and take laxatives). It can cause contrast nephropathy in patients with compromised renal function (especially in patients with insulin-dependent diabetes mellitus or creatinine greater than 1.5 mg/dl).

b. **Renal ultrasound (US)** is useful for detecting hydronephrosis and kidney stones. Unlike IVP, it does not subject the patient to radiation; however, it is operator-dependent, and it does not give information on kidney function.

c. **Plain radiogram of kidneys, ureter, and bladder (KUB)** is used with renal US to identify possible radiopaque calculi missed by US.

d. **Quantitative renal scan** monitors renal function and drainage.

1) **Technetium-99m (^{99m}Tc) scan** using ^{99m}Tc-dimercaptosuccinic acid (DMSA) is used for both differential function and evaluation of the functioning areas of the renal cortex. ^{99m}Tc-mercaptoacetyltriglycine (MAG3) is used to also assess urinary tract drainage as well as differential function.

2) **Hippuran I-131 scan** is used to monitor renal perfusion and determine glomerular filtration rate (GFR) and excretory renal plasma flow (ERPF).

e. **Twenty-four hour urine creatinine clearance** may be used to follow quantitative renal function; however, it may remain normal despite moderate to severe renal deterioration.

2. Lower urinary tract studies

a. **Urinalysis and urine culture and sensitivity** are used to detect urinary tract infection (UTI). Pyuria accompanied by a bacterial colony count of 100,000 or more organisms of a single microbial species per ml indicates UTI. The antibiotic sensitivity of the cultured bacteria is used to guide the choice of antibiotic therapy.

b. **Postvoid residual (PVR)** involves transurethral catheterization to measure residual urine volume in the bladder immediately after voiding to determine the ability of the bladder to empty and to gauge the effectiveness of any therapeutic interventions for the bladder. A "balanced bladder" has less than 100 ml PVR with reflex voiding frequency greater than every 2 hours (e.g., in men with SCI). A large PVR must be interpreted with caution because it may not have been taken immediately after voiding or the patient may not have understood the instruction to void completely. Consistently low PVR may rule out outlet obstruction, but incontinence does not rule out urinary retention.

c. **Voiding cystourethrography** is a radiologic study that provides structural and dynamic measures of bladder function. Contrast dye is introduced into the bladder via catheter and a cystography radiograph is taken. The patient is then asked to void and the radiographs taken during micturition display the bladder size and shape, sphincter function, urinary flow, and presence of reflux. This can help detect neurogenic bladder, fistulas, tumors, and a rupture in the bladder.

d. **Cystoscopy** is the direct visualization of the bladder wall and urethra. It is also used to obtain tissue biopsy and to remove stones and debris from the distal ureter, bladder, or urethra. Clinical indications include hematuria, recurrent symptomatic UTI, an episode of genitourinary (GU) sepsis, urinary retention or incontinence, small calculi, and long-term use of indwelling catheter (to rule out carcinoma).

e. **Urodynamics or cystometrogram (CMG)** documents the bladder pressure (via an intravesical pressure transducer), the electrical activity of the urinary sphincter (via surface electromyograph [EMG] electrodes), and the patient's subjective sensation of voiding as the bladder is progressively filled transurethrally with either water or carbon dioxide. Although water is more physiologic, it takes a long time to fill the bladder. In the office or bedside setting, carbon dioxide is commonly used because it fills the bladder fast; however, the voiding phase of micturition cannot be evaluated with carbon dioxide. The bladder and the urethra can also be visualized using fluoroscopic (e.g., **video urodynamics**) or sonographic technique. Common indications for urodynamic studies include recurrent UTIs in a patient with voiding dysfunction, urinary incontinence, frequency, large PVRs (i.e., retention), deterioration of the upper tracts, monitoring of voiding pressures, and evaluation and monitoring of neurourologic drugs.

1) **Filling-phase study.** As the bladder volume increases, there is a slow rise in intravesical pressure due to the viscoelasticity of the bladder. The urethral sphincter shows EMG activity, which gradually increases to prevent urine leakage. At around 100 to 200 ml, the first sensation of bladder filling normally occurs. At around 300 to 400 ml, a mild desire to void usually occurs. As the bladder fills to around 400 to 500 ml, there is a strong desire to void (urgency). A full normal bladder during the filling phase (maximum capacity of 400 to 750 ml in adults) has intravesical pressures of 0 to 6 cm H_2O, which should not rise above 15 cm H_2O. In patients with bladder (detrusor) hyperreflexia caused by upper motor neuron lesions, the bladder contracts and empties at low volumes. Patients with atonic (areflexic) bladders due to lower motor neuron (i.e., loop III and below) lesions, however, have large capacity and do not show increase in intravesical pressure despite the introduction of large volumes of fluid.

2) **Voiding-phase study** is used to determine the coordination of bladder and urinary sphincter during micturition. During voiding, there is normally a sudden silence of EMG activity and drop in proximal urethral pressure (due to inhibition of the sympathetic α-adrenergic receptors). The bladder (detrusor) then contracts and voiding occurs. The detrusor contraction results from the sacral parasympathetic outflow to the bladder via the pelvic nerve in addition to the suppression of sympathetic beta-2 adrenergic influence on the detrusor muscle. The bladder contraction and sphincter relaxation is coordinated by the ''pontine micturition center.'' After voiding, the EMG becomes

active again to keep the sphincter closed. This coordination is lost in patients with detrusor-sphincter dyssynergia. The detrusor pressure is below 30 cm H_2O in women and between 30 to 50 cm H_2O in men during voiding. The flow rate is between 15 to 20 ml H_2O for men if there is at least 150 ml of urine in bladder. The urethral sphincter EMG should remain silent throughout voiding.

III. **Classifications of voiding dysfunctions** have been based on neurologic lesions (e.g., Bors-Comarr or Bradley), functional classification (Wein), urodynamic findings (e.g., Lapides or Krane-Siroky), combination of bladder and urethral function based on urodynamics (e.g., International Continence Society). In the PM&R setting, the functional classification by Wein (determined by urodynamics) is useful for deciding on treatment options (see Table 5.7-1). Classification terms such as *neurogenic bladder* should not be used when referring to non–bladder (e.g., outlet or sphincter) dysfunction.

IV. **Treatment** goals are to decrease or prevent lower tract complications (e.g., by maintaining continence), preserve the upper tracts (e.g., by avoiding high intravesicular pressures, which may cause vesicoureteral reflux), and implement a realistic bladder management program.

A. **Behavioral management**

1. **Timed (scheduled) voiding** before the bladder reaches full capacity to prevent urine leakage due to high intravesical pressure. Demented persons need constant reminding.

2. **Bladder training** is done by progressively increasing the time between voiding by 10 to 15 minutes every 2 to 5 days until a reasonable interval between voiding is attained (regular voiding of at least every 3 hours). The patient is made fully responsible for adhering to a drinking, voiding, and catheterization schedule. The drinking schedule usually consists of a well-timed fluid intake of 1,800 ml per day (400 ml at meal times and 200 ml at 10 AM, 2 PM, and 4 PM). The patient attempts to void at least every 3 hours while awake by using specific techniques that gave the best response during urodynamics. Intermittent catheterization schedule is adjusted in accordance with the residual urine volume. The following records are made by the patient: fluid intake, intentional voiding (amount in milliliters), unintentional voiding (in relative degrees), and the amount of residual urine volume obtained by intermittent catheterization after attempted voiding. These day-to-day data are then represented in graph form and kept on a clipboard at the bedside to determine the efficiency of voiding. Bladder training is most effective in the patient who has recovered or is recovering from a neurologic lesion (e.g., stroke or TBI) but is voiding frequently due to fear of incontinence or out of habit, SCI, in selected brain-injured patients, and in patients who have atonic myogenic detrusor insufficiency (underactive bladder and normoactive outlet) associated with habitual contraction of the external urethral sphincter. Bladder retraining may be contraindicated in patients with decompensating renal function, especially when accompanied by incompetent vesicoureteral junctions. It is also contraindicated in patients with severe cystitis, bladder calculi, or major structural changes of either the bladder or the urethra; in patients who cannot adhere to the necessary training procedures and record keeping; in the very young; in debilitated elderly patients; in unmotivated or undisciplined patients; and in patients who are unable to do the necessary

Table 5.7-1. Functional classification of voiding dysfunctions and their treatment options

FUNCTIONAL CLASSIFICATION	TREATMENT OPTIONS
I. Incontinence (failure to store)	
A. Due to bladder hyperreflexia (e.g., suprapontine lesions such as stroke, TBI, MS, neoplasm, hydrocephalus, PD)	1. Behavioral: timed voids, fluid restrictions 2. Collecting devices: diaper, catheter (condom or indwelling) 3. Clean intermittent catheterization 4. Drugs: anticholinergics, musculotropics, tricyclic antidepressant, intrathecal baclofen*, prostaglandin inhibitors* 5. Surgery: augmentation, continent diversion, denervation procedures,* neurostimulation*
B. Due to the outlet or sphincter incompetence (e.g., children with myelodysplasia; stress incontinence in women with infrasacral lesion and denervated pelvic floor; or rarely, men with complete denervation)	1. Behavioral: timed voids, pelvic floor exercises, biofeedback, fluid restrictions 2. Collecting devices: diaper, catheter (condom or indwelling) 3. Drugs: α-adrenergic agonists, imipramine, estrogen cream 4. Surgery: collagen injection, fascial sling, artificial sphincter, Teflon injection,* neurostimulation*
II. Retention (failure to empty)	
A. Due to bladder areflexia (e.g., spinal shock in SCI; MS; peripheral neuropathies; sacral lesions such as spinal trauma, herniated lumbar disc, spinal tumors, myelodysplasia, AV malformation, lumbar stenosis, arachnoiditis)	1. Behavioral: timed voids, bladder stimulation (suprapubic jabbing, transurethral electrical bladder stimulation), Valsalva's and Crede's maneuvers 2. Collecting devices: indwelling catheter 3. Clean intermittent catheterization 4. Drugs: cholinergic agonists, intravesical prostaglandins,* narcotic antagonists* 5. Surgery: neurostimulation*
B. Due to outlet or sphincter dyssynergia (e.g., suprasacral traumatic SCI)	1. Behavioral: anal stretch void, suprapubic tapping, biofeedback 2. Collecting devices: indwelling catheters 3. Clean intermittent catheterization 4. Drugs: α-adrenergic blockers, oral striated muscle relaxant (baclofen, diazepam, dantrolene), intrathecal baclofen* 5. Surgery: sphincterotomy incision, bladder neck incision, prostate resection, pudendal neurectomy,* stent, sphincterotomy*
III. Failure of storage and emptying with nonusable urethra	Surgery: suprapubic catheter with or without bladder neck closure, ileal conduit

Adapted from: Linsenmeyer TA, Stone JM: Neurogenic bladder and bowel. In DeLisa JA Gans BM, editors: *Rehabilitation medicine: principles and practice*, ed 2, Philadelphia, 1993, JB Lippincott, p 744; Cardenas DD, Mayo ME, King KC: Urinary tract and bowel management in the rehabilitation setting. In Braddom RL, editor: *Physical medicine and rehabilitation*, Philadelphia, 1996, WB Saunders, p 561, with permission.

* Experimental or nonstandard treatment.

TBI = traumatic brain injury; MS = multiple sclerosis; PD = Parkinson's disease; SCI = spinal cord injury; AV = arteriovenous.

activities for voiding, such as transferring to the toilet or dressing and undressing.

3. **Bladder stimulation**
   a. **Suprapubic jabbing,** that is, by pressing deep over the bladder to mechanically stretch its wall, is more effective than suprapubic tapping (rapid, yet light tapping at a place where the highest degree of reflex response is obtained) or stroking or pinching of the perineal skin.
   b. **Transurethral electrical bladder stimulation** has recently been used experimentally to supposedly activate mechanoreceptor afferents, which restore the sensation of bladder filling, and in turn, activate efferent nerves, resulting in detrusor contraction and bladder contraction.

4. **Valsalva's maneuver** increases intravesical pressure by increasing intraabdominal pressure. It involves sitting and resting the abdomen forward on the thighs for both men and women. During straining in this position, hugging of the knees and legs may prevent any bulging of the abdomen. In this manner, all of the increase in intraabdominal pressure is transferred to the bladder and the pelvic floor. Adverse effects include exacerbation of hemorrhoids, rectal prolapse, or hernia. In patient with vesicoureteral reflux, they are contraindicated.

5. **Crede's maneuvers** increase intravesical pressure by manually pushing down on the bladder. They have the same adverse effects and contraindications as Valsalva's maneuver.
   a. **The open-hand Crede's method** involves placing the thumb of each hand over the area of the left and right anterosuperior iliac spine and the digits over the suprapubic area with slight overlapping of the tips. The slightly overlapped digits are then pressed into the abdomen. When they have gotten well behind the symphysis, the pressure is directed downward to compress the fundus of the bladder. Both hands are then pressed as deeply as possible downward into the pelvic cavity.
   b. **Closed-hand Crede's method** compresses the bladder by using the closed fist of one hand or a rolled-up towel.

6. **Anal stretch voiding** involves relaxation of the pelvic floor by first stretching the anal sphincter and then evacuating by Valsalva's maneuver. It can be used in paraplegic patients who have no anal sensation and are able to transfer to a toilet and do Valsalva's maneuver.

7. **Pelvic floor exercises or Kegel exercises** (see also Chapter 5.8, section VI.A.6.b.1) are effective only in women with mild to moderate stress incontinence because of a hypotonic sphincter. Patients need to be highly motivated as it may take 4 to 8 weeks before any effect is seen.

8. **Biofeedback** (see also Chapter 4.1, section VI) may be used in conjunction with Kegel exercise. It may also be used in patients (often children) who voluntarily tighten their sphincters during voiding.

B. **Urine collection devices**
   1. **External condom catheters** are used in men with detrusor hyperreflexia or normal unobstructed bladder function with incontinence because of immobility (e.g., tetraplegia) or dementia. Unlike diapers, it can only be changed once a day; however, the patient must wear a leg bag, and there is a slight increased risk for UTI and potential for penile skin breakdown and urethral damage. The condom catheter can also get dislodged.
   2. **Indwelling urethral or suprapubic catheters** are used when other treatment options have failed or for the patient's convenience. Complications include bladder stones, hematuria, bacteremia (especially when catheter is ob-

structed), metal erosions, penile and scrotal fistulas, vesicovaginal fistula, epididymo-orchitis, urethral stricture, urethral diverticulum, and bladder carcinoma (with long-term use). To prevent or reduce complications, indwelling catheters must be changed every 2 to 4 weeks; patient must orally take at least 2 L/day of fluids; catheters must be taped up to the abdomen in men to prevent traction and risk for penile and scrotal fistula; urethral meatus must be cleaned with soap and water; collecting bags must be sterilized with bleach; detrusor hyperreflexia must be controlled with anticholinergics; and collecting bag must never be raised above the bladder level to prevent reflux of urine into bladder.

3. **Adult diapers and other protective garments** are a combination of high-absorbent gel-impregnated material that allows the lining against the patient's skin to stay dry. They are used in incontinent demented patients with adequate bladder emptying. They tend to be expensive, may be difficult to put on and take off, and can potentially cause skin maceration if not changed within 2 to 4 hours after getting wet.

C. **Intermittent catheterization (IC)** requires a bladder that is sufficiently areflexic and compliant (i.e., low pressure bladder with a greater than 300 ml capacity and enough outflow resistance to maintain continence with normal daily activities). Anticholinergics or musculotropics may be used in patients with detrusor hyperreflexia and incontinence. In an acute care setting (e.g., acute SCI centers), the sterile technique is recommended to prevent UTI; however, in outpatient or chronic care facility settings, a nonsterile but "clean" technique (called **clean intermittent catheterization [CIC]**) may be used. To keep the catheter "clean," patients may wash it with soap and water, or if there is recurrent bacteriuria, they should either soak it in Cidex solution or boil it. The use of concomitant bacteriostatic medications for UTI prophylaxis remains controversial (e.g., trimethoprim-sulfamethoxazole [Bactrim, Septra], one single-strength tablet, po, qhs; or methenamine salts such as Mandelamine, 1 g, po, qid, or Hiprex, 1 g, po, bid).

Patients should be restricted to about 600 ml in the time interval between catheterization or to a total of 1.8 to 2 L per day. The IC schedule may be on demand if the patient has a sensation of voiding, or it may be timed to keep the residual urine below 400 to 450 ml. For a timed IC schedule, an easy mnemonics is the "1-2-3-4" system, i.e., for residual volume of 100 (± 50) ml, catheterize once a day; 200 (± 50) ml, twice a day; 300 (± 50) ml, thrice a day; 400 (± 50) ml, four times a day). If the patient's residual volume is consistently below 100 ml, IC is not necessary.

Relative contraindications to a self-IC program include significant leg adductor spasticity, PMH of urethral false passage, poor hand-eye coordination, poor cognition, and poor motivation. Complications of IC are symptomatic bacteriuria, urethral trauma, and bladder stone formations (hair or lint introduced during catheterization has been found to be the nidus for stone formation). If there is sphincter spasm, extra lubrication and local anesthetic urethral gel (lidocaine 2%) or a curved-tip (coude) catheter may be used. Repeated bleeding during IC may warrant use of indwelling catheter until the traumatic source (e.g., urethral mucosa trauma or urethral false passage) is resolved.

D. **Drugs**

1. **Drugs used in incontinence caused by hyperreflexic bladder** act by relaxing the detrusor hence increasing bladder capacity.

   a. **Anticholinergic drugs** are used to relax hyperreflexic bladder by blocking acetylcholine receptors competitively at the postganglionic cholinergic receptor sites. Adverse drug reactions (ADRs) include decreased secretion of tears, saliva, sweat, and milk; mydriasis, blurred vision, and increased intraocular pressure; tachycardia and palpitations; mental confusion, headache, dizziness, nervousness, drowsiness, insomnia, and weakness; nausea, vomiting, and decreased GI mobility (i.e., paralytic ileus and constipation); impotence; and allergic reactions. Contraindications include glaucoma, urinary outlet obstruction (e.g., hypertrophic prostate), acute paralytic ileus, GI obstruction (e.g., pyloroduodenal stenosis), severe colitis, and myasthenia gravis.

1) **Propantheline bromide (Pro-Banthine)** is a muscarinic receptor antagonist that decreases the frequency and amplitude of uninhibited bladder contractions and, therefore, increases total bladder capacity.

2) **Oxybutynin (Ditropan)** exerts direct antispasmodic effect on smooth muscle cell membrane (musculotropic effect) and, to a lesser extent, inhibits the muscarinic action of acetylchonine on smooth muscles. It increases bladder capacity; decreases the frequency of uninhibited bladder contractions; and decreases urgency, frequency, and urge incontinence. It can also decrease dysuria because of its local anesthetic effects on the bladder. Aside from the oral route, it may be instilled intravesically during IC by dissolving a 5-mg tablet in sterile water. This reportedly has less ADRs than when given orally.

3) **Hyoscyamine (Levsin)** inhibits acetylcholine receptors at the postganglionic cholinergic nerves hence relaxing hyperreflexic bladder. It is available in an extended-release (Levsin Timecaps) preparation.

b. **Tricyclic antidepressants (TCAs)** are known to cause urinary retention because of their anticholinergic effects. They are also theorized to cause sphincter contraction by potentiating adrenergic responses (via inhibition of norepinephrine reuptake). The TCAs may be used alone or in combination with anticholinergics (e.g., oxybutinin or propantheline). For details about the mechanism of action, ADRs, contraindications and precautions, and drug administration guidelines of TCAs, see Chapter 4.8, section V.A.1.

1) **Imipramine (Tofranil)** is mainly indicated for children with nocturnal enuresis (nonorganic etiology).

2) **Amitriptyline (Elavil, Endep)** causes urinary retention due to its anticholinergic effects. Its effects are potentiated by cimetidine and other anticholinergic drugs.

c. **Experimental drugs** include **terodilene** (a calcium channel blocker that relaxes the detrusor; has been withdrawn due to cardiac arrhythmias), **prostaglandins (PG) inhibitors** (e.g., nonsteroidal antiinflammatory drugs such as **flurbiprofen**), and **intrathecal baclofen.** Intrathecal baclofen decreases detrusor reflex but also depresses pelvic floor reflex with the net result of a bladder with low pressure, which empties less effectively; therefore, it is not desirable in tetraplegic patients in whom intrathecal baclofen is used to control spasticity.

2. **Drugs used in incontinence caused by outlet or sphincter incompetence** act primarily by stimulating alpha-adrenergic receptors or potentiating adrenergic effects via inhibition of norepinephrine reuptake, hence enhancing the closure of the internal urethral sphincter (IUS) at the detrusor outlet and promoting urine storage. Beta agonists and antagonists are not used because they have little effect on bladder functions. To prevent vesicoureteral

reflux due to increased intravesical pressure (caused by increased outlet resistance), urodynamics must be done to rule out detrusor hyperreflexia or poor bladder compliance.

    a. Alpha-adrenergic agonists are useful for improving mild to moderate stress incontinence due to the sphincter. For severe stress incontinence, surgery is needed. Potential side effects include anxiety, insomnia, headache, increased blood pressure, respiratory difficulty, cardiac arrhythmias, and palpitations. Contraindications include hypertension, cardiovascular disease, and hyperthyroidism. Their oral forms are usually available in combination with decongestants, bronchodilators, antitussive, and/or antihistamine.

        1) Ephedrine directly stimulates the alpha and beta adrenoceptors and causes release of norepinephrine. It has anecdotally been used in enuretic children with myelodysplasia at 25 to 50 mg, po, qhs. It is rarely used in adults.

        2) Phenylpropanolamine is similar to ephedrine but has less CNS side effects. It may be given at 25 mg, po, q4h.

        3) Pseudoephedrine (e.g., Sudafed) works well with oxybutinin.

    b. Premarin (conjugated estrogen) vaginal cream is helpful in postmenopausal women with stress incontinence caused by atrophy of the urethral epithelium or irritative symptoms from atrophic urethritis. It probably increases the sensitivity or increases the number of α-adrenergic receptors. To be effective, the pelvic floor has to be at least partially innervated. Dosage is 2 to 4 g (0.625 mg/g) applied intravaginally daily. If used for short duration (4-6 weeks), the risk for endometrial carcinoma, thrombosis, or withdrawal bleeding is negligible. It is contraindicated in women with breast cancer, pregnancy, genital bleeding, or thromboembolic disease.

    c. Tricyclic antidepressants (see section IV.D.1.b)

3. Drugs used in retention caused by bladder areflexia (see Table 5.7-2)

    a. Bethanechol (Urecholine) is a cholinergic agent that stimulates release of acetylcholine. It is also resistant to rapid hydrolysis by acetylcholinesterase. It increases detrusor tension but probably does not stimulate physiologic bladder contraction. At oral dose tolerated by patients, its effectiveness has been controversial; however, it may be used to augment mechanical stimulation of the detrusor by giving it 45 minutes before voiding maneuvers (e.g., Crede's). Contraindications include bowel or bladder outlet obstruction, sphincter detrusor dyssnergia, asthma, peptic ulcer, cardiac arrhythmia, coronary artery disease, and hyperthyroidism. Adverse drug reactions include flushing, salivation, nausea, vomiting, diarrhea, GI cramps, bronchospasms, sweating, lacrimation, miosis, difficulty with visual accommodation, headache, malaise, and hypotension with reflex tachycardia.

    b. Experimental drugs include narcotic antagonists (to block enkephalins, which are thought to inhibit sacral micturition reflex) and intravesical prostaglandin $F_{2\alpha}$ to increase detrusor pressure.

4. Drugs used in retention caused by sphincter contraction (see Table 5.7-2)

    a. Alpha-adrenergic blockers improves bladder emptying in patients with sphincter-detrusor dyssynergia (e.g., in SCI) or prostate outlet obstruction (because prostate smooth muscle is also mediated by α–adrenoceptors). They are also useful in decreasing the frequency of autonomic dysreflexia (AD) associated with bladder distention and in controlling

Table 5.7-2. Drugs commonly used in treating voiding dysfunction

GENERIC	BRANDNAME (PARTIAL LIST)	AVAILABLE PREPARATIONS (mg)	DOSAGE (mg), ROUTE, FREQUENCY	MDD (mg)
I. Anticholinergics				
Oxybutinin	Ditropan	*tab* 5; *elixir* 5/5ml	5 po bid/tid/qid	20
Propantheline	ProBanthine	*tab* 7.5, 15	7.5-15 po 30 min ac tid & 30 mg qhs	75
Hyoscyamine	Levsin	*tab* 0.125; *elixir/drops* 0.125/5ml; *timecaps* 0.375	0.125-0.25 po/sl tid/qid; *timecaps*: 0.375 po bid	1.5
Imipramine	Tofranil	*tab* 10, 25, 50	50-150 po qhs	100-150
Amitriptyline	Elavil, Endep	*tab* 10, 25, 50, 75, 100, 150	10-25 po tid; or 20-75 po qhs	150
II. Cholinergics				
Bethanechol	Urecholine	*tab* 5, 10, 25, 50	10-50 po bid/qid	50
III. α-adrenergic agonists*				
Pseudoephedrine*	Sudafed*	*tab* 30, 60; *elixir* 30/5ml	60 po q4-6h	360
IV. α-adrenergic blockers				
Prazosin	Minipress	*cap* 1, 2, 5	start 1 po bid/tid up to 40/day	40
Terazosin	Hytrin	*tab* 1, 2, 5, 10	1 po qhs; ↑ stepwise to 2, 5, 10, 20 qhs	20
Doxazosin	Cardura	*tab* 1, 2, 4, 8	1-16 po qd	16

* Available in combination with antitussive, bronchodilators, nasal decongestant, or antihistamines.
MDD = maximum daily dose.

of the vascular manifestations of AD. They are contraindicated in situations in which hypotension is undesirable. Common ADRs include dizziness, headache, orthostatic hypotension, palpitation, fatigue or malaise, weakness, nausea, edema, dyspnea, and nasal congestion. Less common ADRs include vertigo, rash, arthralgia, myalgia, paresthesia, ataxia, dry mouth, flushing, abnormal vision, eye pain, tinnitus, somnolence, nervousness, depression, insomnia, sexual dysfunction, diarrhea, constipation, polyuria, and chest pain.

1) **Doxazosin (Cardura)** is a selective blocker of α-1 adrenoceptor. It is available in once-a-day doses.
2) **Terazosin (Hytrin)** is a selective blocker of α-1 adrenoceptor. In 70% of patients with urinary retention due to benign prostatic hyperplasia, there is an increase in urinary flow.
3) **Prazosin (Minipress)** is a postsynaptic blocker of α–adrenoceptors.
b. **Oral striated muscle relaxants (baclofen, diazepam, and dantrolene)** may be used to promote relaxation of the striated muscles of the external urethral sphincter muscles. They are discussed in Chapter 5.4, section III.D.1.
E. **Invasive procedures (injections or surgery)** to improve voiding are used only if conservative treatment methods have failed.
1. **Bladder augmentation (augmentation cystoplasty)** is used to increase bladder capacity and reduce intravesical pressure. It is indicated in patients with

detrusor hyperreflexia or with reduced bladder compliance that failed non-surgical treatment options. Distal ileum is usually used for augmentation. Patients may require long-term IC due to inefficient bladder emptying. Immediate postoperative complications include autonomic dysreflexia, prolonged intestinal ileus or obstruction, anastomotic leak with peritonitis, wound infection, and pulmonary complications (pneumonia and emboli). Increased mucus secretion, which can be annoying in the first 3 postoperative months may be controlled with good CIC and bladder irrigation. Long-term sequelae include chronic bacteriuria, theoretical risk of neoplastic change, possible diarrhea or malabsorption from a shortened gut or decreased intestinal transit time, and hyperchloremic acidosis due to absorption of urine with secondary mobilization of skeletal calcium as a buffer.

2. **Continent diversion** uses bowel not just to increase bladder capacity but also to form a continent catheterizable channel, which opens into the abdominal wall. It is useful in women who have difficulty with IC through the urethra (e.g., leg adductor spasticity, severe urethral incontinence, and obesity) or men who are unable to do IC because of strictures, false passages, or fistulas. Patient must be compliant with IC, otherwise an overdistended bowel may rupture internally.

3. **Denervation procedures,** used in patients with bladder hyperreflexia, can be done at either root (e.g., sacral rhizotomies), peripheral nerve (e.g., unilateral pudendal nerve block or neurectomy), or at the perivesical area (gangliectomy). It is not widely accepted because of bladder areflexia.

4. **Surgically implanted electrical neurostimulation** can selectively stimulate detrusor contraction without stimulating the EUS or can cause relaxation of hyperreflexic bladder. It uses electrodes implanted on the bladder wall, pelvic nerves, sacral roots (most common site), and conus. Its use remains experimental and controversial.

5. **Bladder outlet procedures** are indicated for severe stress incontinence, which does not respond to α-adrenergic agonists.

    a. **Injection therapy** into the urethra using Teflon is currently not used because of the danger of particle migration. Injections of autologous fat and bovine collagen have low potential side effects and are especially suitable for elderly and poor surgical-risk patients. Botulin (Botox) may be injected into the striated sphincter in patients with detrusor dyssynergia. Pudendal block may also be done.

    b. **External compressive surgical procedures**

      1) **Fascial sling procedure** uses a fascial strip taken from the anterior abdominal rectus or tensor fascia lata and wrapped around the bladder neck. Patients must have compliant low-pressure bladder and must agree to do self-IC indefinitely as they will be unable to void using Valsalva's maneuver.

      2) **Artificial urinary sphincter (AUS) implant** consists of a cuff implanted around the bladder neck, a pressure regulating balloon, and a control pump (implanted in the labia or scrotum to allow the patient to open the cuff for voiding). Problems of AUS include mechanical failure, cuff erosions, and infection. Advantage is that patients can do Valsalva's maneuver to void and do not need an IC program; however, there may be uncontrolled hyperreflexia in 10% of patients with myelodysplasia in the first year after implantation (and they may probably need bladder augmentation). An AUS is rarely used in SCI patients because of potential damage to the upper tract in those with detrusor

hyperreflexia and high intravesical pressure. There is also increased risk of prosthesis infection or erosion of the cuff because of frequent bacteriuria. It is better tolerated in children with myelodysplasia or SCI with detrusor areflexia. It is wise to delay the AUS implantation at least 6 to 12 months to make sure there is no return of function.

c. **Sphincterotomy** is the ablation (usually by incision) of the striated sphincter up to the bladder neck. It is used to decrease outflow resistance in patients with low volume bladder (less than 200 ml) and adequate detrusor contraction (less than 20 seconds rise time of contraction with more than 50 cm H_2O amplitude, and duration of at least 2 minutes); male SCI patients unable or unwilling to do self-IC; and patients with selective injury to the sphincter mechanism (e.g., postprostatectomy or pelvic fracture). Other indications include vesicoureteral reflux, high residuals with severe AD or recurrent UTI, upper tract changes with sustained high intravesical pressures, and poor compliance or side effects from drugs used to relax the outlet. It has relatively high immediate postoperative morbidity because of bleeding, clot retention, and infection. Long-term complications include recurrent obstruction from stricture or recurrent dyssynergia. The procedure is irreversible, and the patient must wear a leg bag for life. Its main advantages are less need for attendant care and no need for fluid restriction.

d. **Stainless inert stent** can be implanted to maintain the sphincter mechanism open. This procedure is still considered experimental.

6. **Urinary diversion** are restricted to patients with severe urethral problems such as stricture, fistula, periurethral abscess, and intractable incontinence with perineal skin breakdown. The simplest method is suprapubic catheterization and closure of bladder neck.

V. Complications of voiding dysfunctions

A. **Urinary tract infection** is the most common complication of voiding dysfunctions. Prophylactic antibiotics for those on ICP or for asymptomatic bacteriuria remain controversial (because of the possibility of developing antibiotic resistant organisms). Indwelling Foley catheter by itself (short-term use) is not associated with renal deterioration and generally does not need prophylactic antibiotics. Bacteriuria should only be treated if patient is symptomatic (e.g., fever, urine leakage around the Foley, increased spasticity, and AD). Common urine pathogens in uncomplicated UTI is *Escherichia coli;* and in patients with catheter-associated UTI there is usually a mixture of organisms (especially in indwelling catheters) including *Proteus, Klebsiella, Pseudomonas, Serratia, Providencia,* enterococci and staphylococci.

Antibiotic treatment is based on urine culture and sensitivity. If unavailable, empirical treatment should be started immediately. Amoxicillin, ampicillin, nitrofurantoin, and sulfa drugs are generally poor choices for empirical treatment due to high prevalence of resistance in hospitalized patients. **Trimethoprim-sulfamethoxazole (Bactrim, Septra)**, one tab, po, bid (double strength 160/800 mg or single strength 80/400 mg), is a better choice but does not cover *Pseudomonas aeruginosa.* Oral fluoroquinolones are generally good choices for most mild to moderate UTIs because they also cover *P. aeruginosa.* Examples are **ciprofloxacin (Cipro)**, 250 to 750 mg, po, bid; **ofloxacin (Floxin)**, 200 to 400 mg, po, q12h; or **norfloxacin (Noroxin)**, 400 mg, po, bid. For more seriously ill patients, IV antibiotics may be needed. Antibiotics should be given for at least 7 to 14 days depending on the severity of UTI.

In recurrent UTIs or severe UTIs, urodynamic evaluation, excretory urogram, and cystogram should be done to rule out treatable causes.

B. Stones

1. **Bladder stones** are usually associated with an indwelling Foley catheter or prolonged urinary retention. It can occasionally be caused by foreign body introduction (pubic hair or retained portion of the Foley balloon). It predisposes the patient to hematuria, persistent UTI infection, autonomic dysreflexia or occasionally obstruction; however, it is not associated with renal deterioration. Treatment of choice is electrohydraulic lithotripsy.

2. **Kidney stones** are seen in 8% of SCI patients in a period of 10 years of SCI, more commonly in young men within the first 3 years of injury, and in those with bladder stones. If left untreated, there is a 50% chance of losing the kidney. In 98% of urinary calculi, the stone is made up of magnesium ammonium phosphate (struvite) and calcium phosphate because of alkaline urine from urease producing bacteria. Treatment of choice is extracorporeal shock wave lithotripsy (ESWL) for stones less than 3 cm in diameter and the percutaneous approach for stones above 3 cm in diameter.

C. Vesicoureteral reflux (VUR) is often associated with detrusor-sphincter dyssynergia (i.e., hyperreflexic detrusor and spastic external urinary sphincter) and high pressure voiding, or it could be congenital. It can lead to renal deterioration, especially in the presence of bacteria. Patients with bilateral reflux have creatinine clearance, which is 30% less than those without reflux.

D. Pyelonephritis, often associated with VUR, kidney stones and obstruction, can lead to renal deterioration. Upper urinary tract studies (e.g., IVP or excretory urogram, renal US, KUB, quantitative renal scan, or 24-hour urine creatinine clearance) should be done to rule out correctable causes.

E. Bladder cancer (usually squamous cell carcinoma) is more prevalent in SCI patients who have had an indwelling Foley catheter for more than 10 years. These patients should be monitored with cystoscopy, cell cytology, and bladder biopsy of suspicious areas.

F. Autonomic dysreflexia, which can occur in patients with SCI at or above T6, is characterized by exaggerated autonomic response to stimuli, which are innocuous in normal individuals (e.g., bladder distension). The AD symptoms include headache (pounding), hyperhydrosis (especially of the forehead), cutaneous vasodilation (i.e., flushing above level of lesion), nasal obstruction, piloerection, paresthesia, or anxiety. Clinical signs include hypertension, reflex bradycardia (tachycardia or normal sinus rhythm are often seen) or nonspecific ST-T changes. If untreated it may cause mental status changes, seizure, intracerebral hemorrhage, or even death. It is usually precipitated by noxious stimuli from the bladder distention (e.g., blocked urinary catheter), urinary tract infection, bladder stones, or from other sources (e.g., bowel distention, pressure sores, tight leg bag, tight clothing, ingrown toenail, orgasm, labor and delivery, spasticity, fractures, hemorrhoids, or abdominal emergencies such as appendicitis). In the acute phase, immediate management includes

1. Sitting up the patient.

2. Finding and removing the noxious stimuli causes (e.g., catheterizing the patient if bladder is distended).

3. If there is no resolution, any of the following drugs may be used (listed according to rapidity of onset in lowering blood pressure):

a. **Nitrates (peripheral vasodilator):** amyl nitrate, 1 ampule, inhaled for 30 seconds; or nitroglycerin (Nitrostat), 0.4 mg, SL.

b. **Direct arterial vasodilator:** hydralazine (Apresoline), 10 mg, IM or slow IV push (over 30 seconds).

c. **Calcium-channel blocker:** nifedipine (Procardia, Adalat), 10 mg, SL (puncture capsule first); may repeat in 30 minutes if hypertension persists (for details about calcium-channel blockers, see Chapter 4.8, section IX.B).

d. **Central alpha$_2$-adrenergic agonist:** clonidine (Catapres), 0.1 to 0.2 mg, po. For details about clonidine, see Chapter 4.8, section IX.A.1.

BIBLIOGRAPHY

Bradley WE: Innervation of the male urinary bladder, *Urol Clin North Am* 5(2): 279-293, 1978.

Cardenas DD, Mayo ME, King KC: Urinary tract and bowel management in the rehabilitation setting. In Braddom RL, editor: *Physical medicine and rehabilitation*, Philadelphia, 1996, WB Saunders, pp 555-579.

Chancellor MB. Urodynamic evaluation after spinal cord injury, *Phys Med Rehabil Clin North Am* 4(2):273-298, 1993.

Doughty DB, editor: *Urinary and fecal incontinence: nursing management*, St. Louis, 1991, Mosby–Year Book.

Linsenmeyer TA, Stone JM: Neurogenic bladder and bowel. In DeLisa JA, Gans BM, editors: *Rehabilitation medicine: principles and practice*, ed 2, Philadelphia, 1993, JB Lippincott, pp 733-762.

Perkash I: Urologic diagnostic testing. In Lennard TA, editor: *Physiatric procedures in clinical practice*, Philadelphia, 1995, Hanley & Belfus, pp 114-122.

Resnick NM, Yalla SV: Management of urinary incontinence in the elderly, *New Engl Med J* 313:800-805, 1985.

Wein AJ: Lower urinary tract function and pharmacologic management of lower urinary tract dysfunction, *Urol Clin North Am.* 14 (2):273-296, 1987.

CHAPTER 5.8

BOWEL DYSFUNCTION

This chapter deals with bowel dysfunction commonly encountered in PM&R, with special emphasis on neurogenic bowel dysfunction. Neurogenic bowel dysfunction is the loss of voluntary control of defecation caused by impairment of the extrinsic (sympathetic, parasympathetic, or somatic) nervous control of the bowel and anorectal mechanisms, resulting in fecal incontinence (FI) or difficulty with evacuation (DWE). In neurogenic bowel dysfunction (e.g., caused by spinal cord injury [SCI], stroke, traumatic brain injury [TBI], multiple sclerosis [MS], diabetic neuropathy, or myelomeningocele), the rehabilitation goal is not necessarily to restore normal defecation (as this may not always be feasible) but rather to attain ''social continence,'' i.e., predictable scheduled adequate defecation without incontinence at socially unacceptable times.

I. Neuroanatomy and neurophysiology

A. Efferent fibers

1. **Autonomic efferents** modulate the enteric nervous system (ENS) rather than directly control the smooth muscles of the gastrointestinal (GI) tract. The intrinsic **enteric nervous system** (ENS) of the GI tract is a collection of highly organized neurons in two primary layers, i.e., the submucosal (Meissner's) and myenteric (Auerbach's) plexi. The ENS is located along the bowel wall from esophagus to internal anal sphincter (IAS) and forms the final common pathway to control the bowel wall smooth muscle. The autonomic efferents inhibit the ENS, which in turn directly inhibits the GI tract peristalsis (i.e., the continuous, distal-moving phasic contractions produced by the inherent electromechanical automaticity of the GI tract smooth muscles). Ablation of all ENS activity by neurotoxin (e.g., tetrodotoxin) causes uninhibited GI tract contraction (from esophagus to IAS).

   a. **Parasympathetic efferents** inhibit the inhibitory influences of the ENS hence increasing GI tract motility. The upper or right colon (i.e., ascending and proximal transverse colons) is innervated by the **vagus nerve (cranial nerve X)** from the medulla, while the lower (or left) GI tract, i.e., distal transverse colon, descending colon, rectum, and IAS, is supplied by the pelvic nerves (also called pelvic splanchnic nerves or nervi erigentes) from **S2-S4**. Injury to the S2-S4 (e.g., conus medullaris or cauda equina lesion) or the pelvic nerves can lead to flaccidity of the lower GI tract, which often leads to DWE, including fecal impactions and functional obstructions. In impacted patients, liquid stool (which accumulates due to decreased absorption capacity of the lower colon) may flow past a bolus of solid feces and may erroneously be diagnosed as fecal incontinence.

   b. **Sympathetic efferents** promote the storage function by enhancing anal tone and inhibiting colonic contractions. Sympathetic stimulation leads to adynamic ileus and decreased bowel activity. But bilateral sympathectomy only causes minor clinical deficits. Sympathetic efferents from **T11-L2** travel through the pelvic ganglion and hypogastric plexi to increase contraction of the IAS. In the resting state, the tonic contraction of the IAS, which accounts for about 80% of resting sphincter pressure, maintains fecal continence. Sympathetic efferents from **L1-L2** travel through the inferior mesenteric ganglion to inhibit contractions of the lower (or left) GI tract.

2. **Somatic efferents** are not affected by the ENS or the parasympathetic efferents but are under sympathetic efferent and voluntary (cortical) control. They consist of α-motor neurons, which directly innervate the external anal sphincter (EAS) and puborectalis muscles. Both of these voluntary striated skeletal muscles are normally in continuous tonic contraction (even during sleep) hence maintaining continence. Tonic contraction of the circular EAS (which surround the IAS and extends distally to the subcutaneous tissue surrounding the anus) closes the anal canal while tonic contraction of the puborectalis (which extends from the pubic arch and loops around the posterior part of the rectum and back to the pubic arch) draws the rectum forward, producing an angulation between the axis of the rectum and the axis of the anal canal of about 90 degrees, which is most crucial for maintaining solid continence. This 90-degree anorectal angle maintains solid continence by: occluding the lumen; providing a sharp curve, which makes it difficult for the stool bolus to pass through; and making it likely that increases in intraabdominal pressure result in compression of the anterior wall of the rectum against the posterior wall, further occluding the lumen.

The EAS is innervated by the **S2-S4 roots** through the pudendal nerves, and the puborectalis is innervated by **direct sacral root branches from S1-S5 roots** (mainly S3-S4). In an isolated pudendal injury (e.g., "stretch neuropathy" during childbirth, injury caused by anorectal surgery, and chronic straining), fecal transit time is normal, but there is predominant fecal incontinence because of EAS flaccid paralysis. Likewise, injury to the sacral roots innervating the puborectalis muscle (e.g., polyneuropathy or cauda equina lesions), causes a predominant fecal incontinence with normal fecal transit time. In women over 50 years old, there is a significant decline in EAS function (thus predisposing to incontinence) compared with that of younger women. This decline is not seen in men and is probably because of previous childbirth or hormonal changes affecting the pelvic floor muscles after menopause.

B. **Afferent fibers** originate from the sensory receptors of the GI tract. The intestine and rectal mucosa are sensitive only to distention (most people can differentiate distention caused by solid, liquid, or gas in the rectum), while the epithelium of the anal canal is sensitive to pain, touch, and temperature. Afferent impulses are processed in three centers: the central nervous system (CNS) (through the vagus nerve through cell bodies in the nodose ganglia or through the sympathetic nerves through cell bodies in the dorsal root ganglia); the prevertebral sympathetic ganglia; and the interneurons within the GI tract wall. Afferent impulses to the CNS and the prevertebral sympathetic ganglia interact with each other and influence the GI tract interneurons; however, afferent impulses going to the GI tract interneurons can interact directly with the efferent fibers. All these afferent impulses ultimately modulate the autonomic efferents (which also control the ENS) but not the somatic efferents. Loss of afferent (sensory) input results in a lack of awareness of rectal filling and may contribute to constipation and eventually to fecal impaction.

II. Phases of bowel evacuation

A. **Colonic phase** is a continuous process of phasic colonic contractions, which propels the feces into the rectum but is not sufficient to overcome EAS tonic contraction. Colonic contents of the ascending and transverse colon are constantly stirred and mixed so they can be exposed to the colon wall for further reabsorption. Typically, the colonic walls reabsorb up to 30 L of fluids per day (with only 100 ml water loss in feces) and up to 90% of the 7 to 10 L of gas produced by bacterial fermentation. Stool transit time in the colon is also affected by the time of day, and even the person's surroundings. Normally, the fecal transit time from cecum to anus is 12 to 48 hrs with giant migratory contractions (GMCs) of the colon occurring up to 2 times per day in a normal colon or approximately 4 times per day in a fasting colon. The GMCs are associated with mass movement of the feces (to as far as one-third the length of the colon) and can increase in the first 30 to 60 minutes after a meal (because of the gastrocolic reflex) leading to shortened fecal transit time. The fecal transit time can also be shortened or decreased (i.e., GMCs and defecation frequency are increased) by the type of diet (e.g., fiber supplements, which increase stool bulk) and by physical exercise. Patients with SCI have prolonged fecal transit time, reduced frequency of GMCs, and less GMC facilitation by defecation, exercise, or food ingestion, all of which predispose them to chronic constipation and fecal impaction. Specifically, the fecal transit time for patients with upper motor neuron (UMN) lesions is more than 72 hours while for patients with lower motor neuron (LMN) lesions, it is more than 6 days (especially of the left colon).

B. **Voluntary defecation phase** (see Fig. 5.8-1)

1. **Holding phase** starts upon the delivery of feces of an appropriate consistency into the rectum. The amount, consistency and rate at which feces enters the rectum, is controlled by the proximal bowel. The feces are initially retained in the sigmoid colon and are intermittently propelled to the rectum at about 100 g of solid stool per day through rectorectal reflex (i.e., bowel proximal to the stool contracts as the distal bowel relaxes; exact mechanism underlying this process is unclear). As the feces enter the rectum, there is a decrease in intraluminal pressure proportional to the distending volume because of rectal accomodation and partial relaxation of the IAS; therefore, the rectum, which does not actively contract, serves as an accommodating and compliant reservoir of feces. Continence in the holding phase is maintained by the tonic contraction of the puborectalis and EAS muscles (see above discussion under section I.A.2), which are normally reinforced by cortical control until defecation is socially acceptable. Moreover, as the feces comes in contact with the upper anal canal, there is reflex contraction of the EAS. Continence can be maintained for both solid and liquid stools, unless there is voluminous phasic flows of liquid stool, which overwhelms the continence mechanism leading to urgency and incontinence. In patients with supraconus disease processes, from SCI (i.e., UMN lesions) to dementia, the cortical modulation is lost and spontaneous defecation may occur reflexively even in socially unacceptable situations. In patients with combination UMN lesions with posterior rhizotomy or in patients with LMN lesions, reflex defecation is absent.

2. **Initiation phase** starts with the sensation of rectal distention (which is perceived at volumes as low as 10 ml). When the rectal volume reaches at

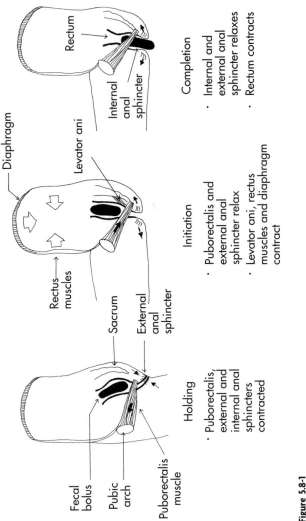

Figure 5.8-1
Voluntary defecation phases. (Adapted from Schiller LR: Fecal incontinence. In Sleisenger MH, Fordtran JS, editors: *Gastrointestinal disease: pathophysiology, diagnosis, management,* ed 4, Philadelphia, 1989, WB Saunders, p 322.)

least 100 to 150 ml (i.e., intrarectal pressure reaches at least 100 cm H_2O), the urge to defecate becomes strongly felt, but the urge may dissipate as accommodation occurs (i.e., the initial rise in intrarectal pressure soon drops back to its original level as the compliant rectum relaxes and accommodates the fecal mass) or the urge may be cortically suppressed. The ability to sense the urge to defecate is decreased in patients with UMN lesions caused by impaired spinal-cortical pathways (although in 43% of these patients, there is a vague sense of abdominal distention or discomfort probably mediated by afferent fibers bypassing the zone of cord injury in sympathetic nerves). Compared to normals, the rectal distention studies of patients with UMN lesions show elevated rectosigmoid pressures especially when higher or continuous filling rates are used. The elevated rectosigmoid pressure is probably associated with increased EAS pressure because of sacral reflexes (rather than associated with true decreased colonic compliance as seen in patients with ischemic or postinflammatory rectal bowel wall caused by fibrosis).

When the person decides to defecate, he or she voluntarily contracts the levator ani (to reflexively open the proximal anal canal) and voluntarily relaxes the EAS and puborectalis muscles. Puborectalis relaxation in combination with the sitting or squatting position make the anorectal angle more straight thus facilitating stool passage. Stool passage is propelled distally with the aid of Valsalva's maneuver, that is, closure of glottis and contraction of the abdominal muscles to increase intraabdominal pressure (IAP) by at least 100 cm H_2O. The inability to do Valsalva's maneuver because of paralyzed abdominal muscles (e.g., patients with C5-C6 level SCI who can rarely generate more than 10 cm H_2O of IAP) contributes significantly to DWE. During Valsalva's maneuver (see section VI.B.1.c.2), the EAS pressure increases (so-called protective vesicoanal reflex) to prevent incontinence; however, this protective vesicoanal reflex can be overcame by coordinated voluntary relaxation of the EAS during defecation. In patients with UMN lesions, the protective vesicoanal reflex is present (because of intact or increased anal sphincter tone), but in patients with denervation and atrophy of the EAS (e.g., in patients with LMN lesions or in patients with a combination of UMN lesion and posterior rhizotomy), the protective vesicoanal reflex is absent. The loss of the protective vesicoanal reflex can result in fecal incontinence (caused by increased abdominal pressures associated with daily activities) and in excessive perineal descent and even rectal prolapse during Valsalva's maneuver.

3. **Completion phase** occurs as the IAS and EAS continues to relax, and the rectal propulsive contractions (in conjunction with the forces described in the initiation phase) expel the bolus through the open canal. Once evacuation is initiated, the entire left colon may empty by mass peristaltic action, or the fecal bolus may be passed bit by bit. In the American norm, approximately 100 g of solid feces is expelled daily or less frequently. The major factor in determining the pattern of defecation is probably the consistency of the stool. In SCI patients, IAS and EAS relaxation occurs upon rectal distention (resulting in expulsion of the fecal bolus) as in normals.

III. **Epidemiology:** The prevalence of fecal incontinence (FI) and fecal impaction range from 0.3 to 5.0% in the general population. Fecal incontinence in the elderly is often caused by local factors (most commonly undetected fecal impaction) rather than from cerebral deterioration, and it decreases the return-to-home rates for stroke patients. The 1983 cost for the care of fecally incontinent institutionalized patients in the United States was 8 billion dollars. The prevalence of DWE ranges from 10 to 50% among hospitalized or institutionalized elderly. In SCI patients, 43% have chronic complaints of vague abdominal distention and discomfort, which eases with bowel evacuation. In outpatient SCI patients, the prevalence of bowel disturbances is 29%, especially in those with more than 5 years of complete SCI.

IV. Diagnosis

A. History

1. **History of present illness:** A bowel function diary for 1 to 2 weeks may be needed to determine current bowel patterns.

   a. **Current and premorbid bowel function,** such as defecation frequency and duration; typical time(s) of the day for defecation; associated predefecatory activities (e.g., effect of body position, eating, trigger foods, bowel care medications and techniques, and urinary function); presence of GI sensations or pain, warning sensations for defecation, sense of urgency, and ability to prevent stool loss during Valsalva activities (e.g., laughing, sneezing, coughing, or transfers); stool consistency; onset of bowel symptoms and the events that occur around that time (e.g., change in living situation); and functional impact of bowel function on ability to work, travel, interact with others, and carry out activities of daily living (ADLs).

   b. **Associated symptoms,** such as autonomic dysreflexia, abdominal wall spasticity, fever, weight change, and rectal bleeding.

2. **Past medical history,** such as number of pregnancies or deliveries, history of traumatic deliveries, history of anorectal surgery or GI surgery, trauma to the perineum, trauma to the spinal cord, neurologic disease, diabetes, radiation therapy, neurogenic bladder, impotence, and other illness (premorbid GI disease).

3. **Medication history:** Past and present use of medications that can cause diarrhea (see section V.A.2.c) or constipation (see section V.B.2.c).

4. **Diet history,** such as, intake of fluids, dietary bulks and fibers, and dietary irritants.

5. **Personal history,** such as physical activity and emotional status.

B. Physical examination

1. **Anal inspection:** Anal-buttock contour (normal in patients with UMN lesions or combination UMN lesions with posterior rhizotomy; flattened, fanned-out, or "scalloped" in patients with LMN lesions because of loss of EAS muscle bulk), perianal soiling or excoriations (caused by fecal incontinence), anal opening (e.g., patulous gaping orifice because of overdistention or trauma), and perineal descent during Valsalva's maneuver (i.e., bulging of the anus below the ischial tuberosities in excessive descent or prolapse of the perineum).

2. **Digital examination of the anus and rectum:** Assess rectal vault for fecal impaction; sphincter tone (which should normally be in a state of contraction at rest); length of anus (i.e., 2.5-4.5 cm long from anal opening to anorectal junction where finger senses a decrease in rectal pressure; a shortened length of anal pressure zone suggests EAS muscle atrophy, e.g., in LMN lesions); puborectalis muscular sling (palpated as a ridge along the posterior wall, 1.5-2.5 cm from the anal verge; absence of the ridge suggests puborectalis atrophy or dysfunction such as in LMN le-

sions); volitional EAS and puborectalis tone and control (by asking the patient to volitionally squeeze the anus; patients with SCI are unable to do this); bulbocavernosus (BC) reflex, that is, anal contraction elicited by rapid tapping or squeezing of the clitoris or glans penis, and anocutaneous (AC) reflex or "anal wink," that is, visible anal sphincter contraction elicited by sharp stimulation to the perianal skin (both BC and AC reflexes are present or increased in UMN lesions; and absent or decreased in LMN lesions or in combination UMN lesion with posterior rhizotomy); and anal closing reflex (which is normally brisk when the finger is withdrawn).

3. **Transabdominal palpation** to detect hard stool in the colon (this should not be present in the ascending colon at the right side of the abdomen).

4. **Musculoskeletal system:** Assess patient's gait, the time required for position change and ambulation, use of assistive devices, and the patient's ability to manipulate clothing rapidly in preparation for toileting.

C. **Diagnostic tests** may be helpful when the cause of FI or DWE is obscure, conservative interventions have failed, or surgical intervention is contemplated.

1. **Laboratory studies** may be needed if disease or disorder of the intestinal tract is suspected, for example, acute diarrhea of undetermined origin. They include complete blood count (CBC), serum electrolytes and biochemistry, stool culture and sensitivity tests, stool analysis for ova and parasites, and stool assay for *Clostridium difficile* toxin.

2. **Morphological studies** are used to identify anatomical lesions or causes of GI obstruction; however, they have limited benefit in assessing bowel function.

   a. **Endoscopy,** for example, colonoscopy, rectosigmoidoscopy, and anoscopy are used to directly visualize the lower GI tract.

   b. **Anatomical radiologic studies,** that is, radiographs (e.g., barium enema studies), computed tomography (CT) scans, or magnetic resonance imaging (MRI) studies, may be used for further anatomical investigation of diseases or disorders of the GI tract.

   c. **Biopsy,** for instance, rectal biopsy, may be used for histopathologic diagnosis.

3. **Functional studies**

   a. **Sensory function studies**

      1) **Sensory electromyography (EMG)** is used to assess sensory pelvic afferents (by nerve conduction studies), or somatosensory evoked potentials. It can also be used to assess the bulbocavernosus reflex (e.g., **sacral evoked response study** described in Chapter 5.9, section III.D.1.a).

      2) **Intra-rectal balloon distention test** is used to determine the rectal sensory threshold (i.e., normally the smallest volume of rectal distention sensed by the patient is 15 ml within less than 2 seconds).

   b. **Motor function studies**

      1) **Motor EMG** using needle or wire electrodes can be used to assess volitional motor control of the puborectalis, anococcygeus, levator ani, and EAS; however, abnormal potentials may be difficult to detect because the EAS is an atypical striated muscle (i.e., it maintains tonus even when it is not voluntarily contracted). Motor EMG may help identify the location of the EAS when the normal anatomy has been disrupted (e.g., because of congenital anomaly or trauma).

Single-fiber EMG may be used to identify muscle denervation and give an estimate of its degree.

2) **Anorectal pressure and sphincter function studies**

   a) **Anorectal catheter manometry** uses an intraanal pressure-sensitive catheter balloon probe, which is connected to a transducer and a recorder or computer. It measures the pressures and resting tone of the IAS, the contractility of the EAS, and the functional length of the anal canal. The parameters measured are anal canal pressures (both resting pressure and maximum squeeze pressure) and the rectoanal or rectosphincteric reflex (i.e., relaxation of the internal sphincter and contraction of the external sphincter in response to balloon distention of the rectum). Manometric resting and contractile pressures are decreased in cases of sphincter laceration or denervation and during a reflex reaction to rectal distention (e.g., because of fecal impaction). These pressures are increased in cases of anal fissure and in some patients with hemorrhoids.

   b) **Balloon sphincterography or kymography** is a simpler method than manometry and is used to evaluate the EAS mechanism of anal canal closure and the production of the anorectal angle by the puborectalis. It uses an intrarectal cylindrical balloon connected by tubing to a bag of radiopaque dye (the pressure in the balloon corresponds to the height of the fluid in the bag and can be measured or controlled by raising or lowering the bag). Plain radiograph, fluoroscopy, or ultrasound is used to visualize the shape of the dye-filled balloon within the anal canal and rectum during voluntary contraction and relaxation of the external sphincter and puborectalis. The parameters measured include the resting and maximum squeeze pressures, the length of the anal canal, and the degree of perineal descent. The accuracy and reliability of this method have been questioned recently.

3) **Rectodynamics** is a combination of anorectal pressure studies and motor EMG. A concentric EMG needle is placed in the EAS to measure resistive forces of bowel evacuation and a triple-lumen balloon catheter is inserted through the anus to measure expulsive forces of bowel evacuation (i.e., intraabdominal pressure, colorectal contraction, and rectal compliance). The catheter is positioned so that the first lumen measures the rectal pressure and the second lumen measures the pressure of the anal canal. The third lumen is used to fill a balloon located in the rectum. Rectal and anal pressures, as well as EMG of EAS, are measured at rest and during stimulation of the anorectum by digital stimulation, Valsalva's maneuver, rapid rectal distention (i.e., rapid injection and removal of air from the rectal balloon to elicit the rectoanal inhibitory reflex), and slow, continuous filling of the rectal balloon at a constant rate of 20 ml/min. Rectodynamics can help in the management of patients with neurogenic bowel by identifying the following patterns of bowel evacuation: anorectal dyssynergia (i.e., loss of coordination between the rectal pressure and anal relaxation) versus insufficient expulsive forces to overcome normal anal sphincter tone (i.e., rectal volumes over 500 ml, instead of the normal 100 to 150 ml, are needed to

trigger anal relaxation; seen in patients with long-standing cervical cord injuries, often with associated megacolon and megarectum).

4) Functional radiographic studies may be used to examine anal continence mechanisms, colonic transit time, and defecation mechanism.

   a) Defecography is used to visualize the kinesiology of defecation and evaluate the pelvic floor muscles. The rectum is filled with a barium suspension and the patient is placed on a radiolucent chair and asked to alternately defecate and contract the sphincter while sequential lateral radiographic films are taken. The anorectal angle, the length of the anal canal, and perineal descent (if present) can be demonstrated.

   b) Serial radiographs of tiny radiopaque plastic beads ingested with food are used to evaluate colonic transit time. This is useful in confirming constipation history and in identifying dysfunctional bowel segments (for planning colostomy level).

5) Anal continence studies

   a) Saline continence test is used to objectively assess the degree or severity of fecal incontinence. A saline solution is run into the rectum through a length of polyethylene tubing at the rate of 60 ml/min for 25 minutes. In normal continent individuals, 1500 ml can be retained before the first leakage of over 10 ml occurs (as measured via a funnel connected to a graduated cylinder placed beneath the seat of a toilet). In patients with incontinence, however, the first leakage almost invariably occurs when approximately 500 ml have been instilled. The result varies with the strength of the EAS, degree of rectal compliance, and the patient's motivation.

   b) Solid-sphere continence test measures maximal anal resistance to the active and passive passage of solid spheres of standard sizes, which are attached to a string and inserted into the rectum.

   c) Functional radiographic studies (see section IV.C.3.b.4) may be used to examine anal continence.

c. Rectal accommodation (i.e., reservoir function) studies

   1) Rectal capacity and compliance test uses a large capacity balloon (or condom) inserted into the rectum. The balloon is tied to a polyethylene tubing, which is connected to a three-way stopcock and a 50 ml syringe. Rectal accommodation is determined by inflating the balloon in 50 ml increments.

   2) Colon capacity and motility test, for example, using colonoscopy, barium enema, or both.

V. Classification by causative factors

A. Failure to store (fecal incontinence and diarrhea)

1. Neurogenic causes

a. Upper motor neuron and/or cortical lesions that cause constipation (see section V.B.1.a) can lead to unrecognized fecal impaction with overflow incontinence (i.e., seepage of watery stool around the obstructing fecal mass; or stool leakage because of loss of normal rectal tone caused by chronic constipation thus resulting in loss of sensation of rectal fullness and loss of voluntary contraction of the external sphincter). Also, patients who are demented, sedated, mentally retarded, or with cognitive deficits may be fecally incontinent (although not diarrheic).

b. **Lower motor neuron lesions,** such as isolated pudendal nerve injury with EAS denervation (e.g., because of childbirth, anorectal surgery, or chronic straining), injury to the sacral roots with puborectalis denervation (e.g., polyneuropathy or cauda equina lesions), LMN myelomeningocele, or Guillain-Barre syndrome (GBS) (may have occasional transient FI).

2. **Nonneurogenic causes**

a. **Medical diseases**

   1) **Gastroenteritis,** which can be caused by viruses, bacteria (e.g., Clostridium difficile, Shigella, Salmonella, Mycobacterium avium intracellulare, or invasive Escherichia coli), parasites (e.g., Giardia or amoeba), or fungus (e.g., intestinal candidiasis caused by aggressive antibiotic therapy that destroys normal intestinal flora). Patients prone to gastroenteritis are immunocompromised patients (e.g., patients receiving cancer treatment or steroids, malnourished patients, or patients with the human immunodeficiency virus) and patients who are receiving organ and bone marrow transplants (because of graft-versus-host disease or immunosuppresive drugs).

   2) **Bowel diseases,** such as celiac disease, malabsorption conditions, inflammatory bowel disease, or chronic intestinal conditions that result in motility change (e.g., radiation injury to the bowel).

b. **Dietary factors,** such as caffeine, alcohol (in large quantities), artificial sweeteners or additives (e.g., fructose, sorbitol, mannitol, and nutmeg), any food to which the person is intolerant (e.g., milk products, meat, potatoes, or wheat), fruit juices, cruciferous vegetables, fatty food, or enteral feedings (especially if the patient is severely malnourished or has received nothing by mouth for several days).

c. **Medications causing diarrhea,** such as antacids (e.g., those containing magnesium), antibiotics, cardiac medications (e.g., digitalis or quinidine), antihypertensives (e.g., hydralazine, methyldopa, propranolol, or guanethidine), potassium supplements, cholinergic agents (e.g., bethanechol), diuretics, anticoagulants, sulfasalazine, indomethacin, colchicine, theophylline, cholestyramine, chenodeoxycholic acid, stool softeners, or laxatives (see section VI.B.3.a).

d. **Others causes,** such as, women over 50 years old (men are not affected) because of significant decline in EAS function probably caused by previous childbirths or hormonal changes affecting the pelvic floor muscles after menopause; and any unrecognized fecal impaction (e.g., because of poor bowel hygiene or other nonneurogenic causes), which can lead to overflow incontinence.

B. **Failure to eliminate (i.e., constipation or DWE)**

1. **Neurogenic causes**

a. **Upper motor neuron or cortical lesions,** which causes constipation because of loss (complete or partial) of voluntary control of defecation, loss or decrease in the ability to sense the urge to defecate, prolonged colonic transit time, reduced frequency of GMC, or increased EAS tone. Their causes can be vascular (e.g., stroke or intracranial hemorrhage); degenerative and/or extrapyramidal (e.g., parkinsonism, Alzheimer's disease, or dementia); demyelinating (e.g., MS); structural (e.g., neoplasm or UMN myelomeningocele); exogenous (e.g., TBI, supraconus SCI, or drug-induced lesions), or others (e.g., mental retardation).

b. **Lower motor neuron lesions,** for example, neuropathy involving the parasympathetic nerves (which can lead to constipation due to prolonged colonic transit time) caused by diabetes, tumor, trauma (e.g., from childbirth, pelvic surgery, or chronic straining), or lesions of the conus medullaris, cauda equina, or nervi erigentes.

2. Nonneurogenic causes

a. Medical diseases

1) Metabolic causes, such as, diabetic acidosis or neuropathy, porphyria, uremia, amyloidosis, or electrolyte abnormalities (e.g., hypokalemia).

2) Endocrine causes, such as, hypercalcemia, hyperparathyroidism, hypothyroidism, pheochromocytoma, or panhypopituitarism.

3) Large intestinal causes, such as, obstruction to flow in the ileal and colonic area (e.g., malignant carcinoma or benign conditions such as polyp, abscess, adhesion, diverticular stricture, or ischemic stricture), anal abnormalities (e.g., paradoxical puborectalis contraction, rectoanal intussusception, rectocele, fibrosis, or abscess), Hirschprung disease (or aganglionic megacolon), pelvic floor abnormalities, or muscular diseases (e.g., scleroderma or dermatomyositis).

4) Other disorders that cause pain on defecation, such as, thrombosed external hemorrhoids, anal fissures, or anal strictures.

b. Dietary factors, such as, inadequate intake of fluids and dietary bulk.

c. Medications causing constipation, such as, analgesics (e.g., opiates or nonsteroidal antiinflammatory drugs), anesthetic agents, antacids (e.g., cimetidine, ranitidine, or aluminum compounds), anticholinergics (e.g., oxybutinin or propantheline), anticonvulsants (e.g., carbamazepine, phenytoin, or valproic acid), antidepressants (e.g., amitriptyline, desipramine, doxepin, imipramine, or nortriptyline), barium sulfate, bismuth, ganglionic blockers, hematinics (especially dietary iron supplements), hypotensives (e.g., diltiazem, nifedipine, or verapamil), laxative or enema abuse, loop-diuretics (producing electrolyte abnormalities such as hypokalemia), monoamine oxidase (MAO) inhibitors, metallic intoxication (e.g., arsenic, lead, mercury, or phosphorus), muscle paralyzers, parkinsonism medications (e.g., amantadine, benztropine, biperiden, or procyclidine), psychotherapeutic drugs, smooth-muscle relaxants, or tranquilizers.

d. Others, such as, reduced peristaltic activity because of aging or inactivity (e.g., chronically ill, immobilized, or postoperative patients), poor bowel hygiene (e.g., prolonged failure to defecate), or impaired diaphragmatic and abdominal wall function.

VI. Nonsurgical management involves the determination and correction of the underlying reasons for diarrhea or constipation, as well the use of general symptomatic control measures. The treatment of nonneurogenic medical bowel diseases (except for diarrhea caused by *Clostridium difficile*) is beyond the scope of this book.

A. Failure to store (fecal incontinence and diarrhea)

1. Dietary measures that help thicken stool consistency by absorbing fluid from the stool or by forming stool bulk.

a. Constipating diet, which increases fluid absorption from the colon, such as, rice, bananas, apples or unfiltered apple juice, yogurt, cheese, marshmallows, or some wheat products.

b. High-fiber (bulk-forming) diet: See section VI.B.2.

c. Avoidance of diarrheic diet, as partially listed in section V.A.2.b.

d. **Fluid and electrolyte replacement,** given orally or intravenously, may be needed to prevent fluid volume deficit caused by diarrhea. Oral fluid replacements include electrolyte drinks (developed for athletes and ostomy patients) or a homemade electrolyte solution (e.g., mix 1 tbsp salt, 1 tbsp baking soda, 1 tbsp corn syrup, 6 oz of orange juice concentrate, and add water to make one quart of liquid). If possible, replace fluid volume lost through diarrhea with an equivalent volume of solution or if unable to estimate fluid loss, replace with 8 oz of solution every bowel movement. If unable to tolerate oral fluids, the patient may be temporarily placed on nothing by mouth (NPO) and intravenous (IV) fluids may be given if needed.

e. **Modification of enteral feeding:** Although the diarrhea during enteral feeding is usually attributed to the formula itself, it is more commonly caused by an underlying malnutrition (i.e., albumin level of less than 2.8/100 ml) that results in edema of the gut wall and malabsorption (may be associated with intestinal villi atrophy). Enteral feeding modification includes the use of isotonic formula with bulk agents and with antidiarrheals, and gradual increase in feeding rate (starting at 50 ml/hr). Short-term use of antiperistaltic drugs (e.g., loperamide [Imodium] or diphenoylate with atrophine [Lomotil]) may be warranted in refractory cases.

f. **Bacterial cultures** may be ingested to normalize intestinal flora for cases of diarrhea caused by antibiotics. Examples are *Lactobacillus* products (Lactinex) or dairy products that contain bacterial cultures (e.g., buttermilk or yogurt). These should not be used by patients with high fever or by children under 3 years old.

2. **Drug therapy**

a. **Antidiarrheal drugs** are used either to achieve appropriate stool consistency or to reduce intestinal peristalsis and stool frequency. They are nonspecific and tend to be overused. In most acute diarrhea they are not necessary, and in chronic cases, they must not be used as a substitute for treatment of the underlying illnesses. Prior to giving antidiarrheal drugs, any drug causing diarrhea (see section V.A.2.c) should be discontinued if possible.

1) **Antiperistaltic drugs** should only be used after fecal impaction is ruled out. They may precipitate toxic megacolon in patients with invasive bacterial infection. Most of them contain opium or its derivative and have potential for abuse. They should be used with caution by patients with asthma, chronic lung disease, benign prostatic hypertrophy, and acute angle-closure glaucoma. Of the following drugs, only loperamide (Imodium) and Lomotil have been scientifically assessed for effectiveness in controlling diarrhea:

a) **Loperamide (Imodium),** a synthetic opioid, is the drug of choice for antiperistalsis because it acts directly on the smooth and circular muscles to decrease peristalsis and prolong transit time. It also increases the basal anal sphincter tone. It must be used with caution in patients with acute ulcerative colitis, antibiotic-induced pseudomembranous colitis, hepatic dysfunction, and dehydration with electrolyte imbalance. It is contraindicated in acute dysentery. Adverse drug reactions (ADRs) include nausea, vomiting, skin rash, dry mouth, drowsiness, bloating, and GI distress. It is available in 2 mg capsules or 1 mg/5 ml elixir. Oral dosage is 4 mg initially, then 2 mg, prn (after each loose bowel movement), to a maximum of 16 mg/day. If ineffective, discontinue after 48 hours.

b) **Diphenoxylate with atropine (Lomotil)** is a combination of opioid (meperidine congener) and anticholinergic agents, which act on smooth muscle to inhibit motility and propulsion. The ADRs are uncommon although nausea, vomiting, sedation, paralytic ileus, and headache have been reported. Its use is contraindicated in pseudomembranous enterocolitis, obstructive jaundice, electrolyte imbalance, and glaucoma. It must be used with caution by patients with dehydration, acute ulcerative colitis, and advanced hepatic or renal disease, and drug abusers. It is available in tablet or liquid forms (i.e., 2.5 mg of diphenoxylate with 0.025 mg of atropine per tablet or per 5 ml). Oral dosage is 2 tablets or 10 ml, qid, until initial control of diarrhea is achieved, followed by the lowest effective dose.

c) **Cholinergic blockers** act locally on the gut to inhibit intestinal secretions and motility and reduce GI tract spasms. The ADRs include dry mouth; blurred vision; dizziness; headache; dry, flushed skin; drowsiness; tinnitus; vertigo; changes in affect and behavior; and vitamin B deficiency. Its use is contraindicated in patients with glaucoma, unstable cardiovascular status, paralytic ileus, chronic lung disease, asthma, pyloric stenosis, liver damage, pregnancy, renal insufficiency, and convulsive disorders. Examples are atropine (see Lomotil described above) and belladonna (e.g., combination of 25 mg powdered opium and 15 mg belladona, one capsule, po, tid or qid, prn).

d) **Other opium derivatives,** which act on the smooth muscle of the large bowel to increase tone and decrease motility. The ADRs include addiction as well as sodium and potassium loss. Examples include paregoric (camphorated tincture of opium), 4 to 8 ml, po (diluted in 3 oz of water to ensure stomach absorption), qid or after each liquid stool, not to exceed 32 ml/day; or deodorized tincture of opium, 0.3 to 1.0 ml, po, qid, prn up to a maximum of 6 ml/day; or codeine, 30 to 60 mg, po, bid to qid, prn.

2) **Absorption agents**
   a) **Kaolin and pectin (Kaopectate)** act as protectants and demulcents. They are contraindicated in pseudomembranous colitis. Oral dosage is 60 to 120 ml of regular strength or 45 to 90 ml of concentrate after each loose bowel movement.

   b) **Attapulgite (Parepectolin; Donnagel)** acts as an absorbent. It is available in 600 mg/15 ml and 600 mg/chewable tablet. The oral dosage is 30 ml or 2 chewable tablets after each loose bowel movement for a maximum of 7 liquid doses or 14 tablets per 24 hrs for 2 days.

   c) **Activated charcoal** may be used to absorb water to firm stool. No adverse effects have been reported. For treating diarrhea, combination agents may be used, e.g., Flatulex, which has 250 mg of activated charcoal with 80 mg of simethicone, given 1 tab, po, qid (after meals and at bedtime) for a maximum of 6 tabs/day.

3) **Astringent and coating agents**
   a) **Bismuth subsalicylate (Pepto-Bismol)** acts by coating and astringent

effects. It may decrease the effects of anticoagulants and interfere with abdominal radiographs. It is useful in cases of traveler's diarrhea. It is available in tablets (262 mg) and suspension (262 and 524 mg/5 ml). Oral dosage is 2 tabs or 30 ml, every hour for each loose bowel movement up to 8 doses/day.

  b) Aluminum hydroxide (Alternagel; Amphojel) produces a barrier coating between the intestinal contents and intestinal wall. The ADRs include constipation, nausea, vomiting, and phosphate deficiency with prolonged use. It is contraindicated in patients on low-sodium diets, tetracycline, or anticoagulants. It is available in tablets (300 and 600 mg) and suspension (320 and 600 mg/5 ml). Oral dosage is 500 to 1500 mg up to 6 times daily.

b. **Antibacterials** for *Clostridium difficile* diarrhea are commonly prescribed in the rehabilitation ward because of frequent use of broad-spectrum antibiotic therapy (e.g., for treatment of infections of the urinary tract and wound), which can alter the normal intestinal flora and cause proliferation of the anaerobic *C. difficile*. If untreated, the toxin of *C. difficile* can cause psudomembranous colitis. *C. difficile* diarrhea is clinically presumed in patients who develop watery diarrhea during or after an antibiotic (for as long as 1-3 weeks after cessation of antibiotics). This can be confirmed by assaying of *C. difficile* toxin. Treatment consists of discontinuation of the antimicrobial therapy (if possible), avoidance of antiperistaltic drugs, and use of oral metronidazole or vancomycin.

  1) Metronidazole (Flagyl) is available as capsules (250 and 500 mg). Oral dosage is 500 mg, bid or tid, for 7 to 10 days.

  2) Vancomycin (Vancocin) is available as capsules (125 and 250 mg) or as powder for oral solution (1 and 10 g). Oral dosage is 125 mg, qid, for 7 to 10 days.

3. **Stool containment measures** provide skin protection, improve patient comfort, reduce nursing time, and provide an accurate measurement of fluid losses.

  a. **External collection devices** consist of a drainable pouch attached to a synthetic, adhesive skin barrier, which conforms to the perianal area and buttocks. These devices adhere to the skin for an average of 24 hours. They are most effective when applied to clean, dry skin that is free of skin breakdown (any skin breakdown must be treated, e.g., with a skin barrier powder, before the pouch is applied).

  b. **Internal drainage systems** may be used on a short-term basis if external devices are not feasible (e.g., because of skin breakdown or lack of adherence). They consist of a large-bore catheter (e.g., French size 30 catheter) inserted into the anorectal junction and connected to a bedside drainage bag. The catheter balloon may be inflated to prevent catheter slippage, but this carries the risk of bowel wall necrosis (unless the balloon is regularly deflated). Internal drainage systems are contraindicated in patients with rectal disease or neutropenia, or those who are immunocompromised.

  c. **Incontinence pants** may be used by patients with severe diarrhea that cannot be managed with external collection devices; however, contact dermatitis and odor may limit the use of incontinence pants.

4. **Skin care**

  a. **Routine skin care** includes gentle cleansing of the perianal area after each bowel movement or incontinent episode followed by protection of intact skin with a moisture barrier cream or ointment (most with petrolatum base) or a skin sealant (e.g., copolymer film product). Tepid water, pH-balanced soaps, commercial formulas designed for incontinence care, or mineral oil may be used for cleansing.

b. **Skin-breakdown care** (see Chapter 5.2 for details) includes application of a skin barrier powder (above which a moisture barrier may be applied), premixed ointments and pastes, or hydrocolloid wafer dressings.

c. **Fungal rash care** includes nystatin (Mycostatin) applied bid or tid for *Candida albicans* and the more broad-spectrum antifungal imidazole, for example, clotrimazole (Lotrimin, Mycelex), econazole (Spectazole), ketoconazole (Nizoral), miconazole (Monistat), or oxiconazole (Oxistat), each applied bid. If available, the powder form (over which a sealant or moisture barrier cream may be applied) is preferred over the ointment or cream forms, which appear to lengthen the time required for healing because of the retention of moisture at the skin surface.

5. **Odor control,** such as, pouch deodorants (if perianal pouch is used), deodorizing skin cleansers, and effective room-deodorizing sprays.

6. **Behavioral management** for patients with fecal incontinence because of cognitive dysfunction and alterations in sensory awareness or sphincter control.

a. **Timed (scheduled) bowel movements** can decrease incontinence between bowel movements (because of less stool accumulation between desired defecation times) and can enhance stool elimination (the establishment of regular, soft, bulky stools is discussed in section VI.B.2).

b. **Anal sphincter retraining** involves training the patient to voluntarily contract the EAS when the rectal vault fills to prevent stool leakage. It is indicated if the patient has a weak but contractable EAS and if anatomic defects are minimal or absent, that is, no large amount of scar tissue (from episiotomy or surgical procedure) nor severe congenital defects.

1) **Pelvic floor exercises** involve repeated tightening of the pelvic floor muscles to increase their muscle tone to help prevent stool leakage. The correct muscle is identified by squeezing as tightly as possible around a finger placed in the anal canal or vagina, or by instructing the patient to stop urine flow in midstream and concentrate on the muscle used. Once identified, the muscle squeezed for 10 seconds followed by a 10-second relaxation, for a total of 20 to 25 times, 3 times per day. This exercise can be done while standing, sitting, or lying down, and even incorporated into the patient's daily lifestyle. When done in combination with biofeedback techniques, this exercise seems to be more effective in reducing incontinence.

2) **Anorectal biofeedback (BF) therapy** (see Chapter 4.1, section VI) can help restore not just social continence but normal defecatory control. It is indicated in motivated individuals with incomplete neurogenic bowel deficits (i.e., with some residual degree of anorectal sensation and volitional EAS activation). It involves the use of a sensing device inserted into the rectum to record the baseline resting pressure as well as the squeeze pressure. Two common anorectal BF methods include (1) the use of a manometric device with three balloons to provide feedback on a recording apparatus, and (2) the use of a rectal plug to provide feedback from an EMG or a computer monitor. The patient is then taught how to squeeze the EAS around the balloon

or plug. A video monitor or a strip recording provides immediate visual or auditory (or both) feedback on any changes in the squeeze pressure. Additional EMG readings may also be taken from the abdominal and puborectalis muscle to prevent any inappropriate contractions of the abdominal muscles and to provide visual correlation between contractions of the EAS and the puborectalis. All these feedback signals are used to reinforce the patient's anorectal squeeze sensation as well as squeeze efforts. The BF sessions last from 30 minutes to 2 hours and take an average of one to three sessions to learn.

B. **Failure to eliminate (constipation, DWE)** is difficult to objectively define because the patient's perception of ''normal'' bowel habits varies widely. In 94% of unimpaired persons, the average bowel movement is at least 3 times per week. Frequent bowel evacuation (e.g., every other day or more frequently) can decrease stool accumulation and hardening. The general treatment goal is to prevent long-term complications by minimizing anorectal overdistention, anal trauma, and chronic use of oral laxative stimulants. The key to success in any bowel program is consistency, adequate follow-up, modifications as necessary, and ongoing support. A step-care system for sequential nonsurgical management of constipation or DWE in nonneurogenic and neurogenic patients is provided in Table 5.8-1.

1. **Behavioral management** is indicated if the patient is willing to alter prior bowel habits.

   a. **Timed (scheduled) bowel movements** must be done at a consistent time that is convenient for the patient (or caregiver) at a frequency of every other day or more frequently. An adequate time for evacuation (10-15 minutes for nonneurogenic patients and longer for neurogenic patients) should be set aside for evacuation at periods of high colonic motility (e.g., after waking up in the morning or 20-40 minutes after regularly-scheduled meals). Failure to produce a bowel movement at that specific time should not discourage the patient as evacuation can be attempted again at another time in the day. It may take several weeks of training to establish a consistent time for bowel movements.

   b. **Exercises** include getting out of bed, exercises in the upright position, walking (e.g., shortly after breakfast), abdominal training (e.g., pelvic tilt or modified sit-ups), and aerobic exercises, if appropriate. For patients with rectal sensory deficits, rectal sensory reeducation may be done. This technique involves the inflation of a rectal balloon catheter to an initial sensory threshold level (i.e., when pressure sensation is first felt) followed by patient training (with or without biofeedback) to sense progressively less degree of inflation (until sensory threshold is within normal limits of 15-30 ml). For patients with anal sphincter motor deficits, anal sphincter training (i.e., Kegel exercise and biofeedback training, described in sections VI.A.6.b.1 and VI.A.6.b.2) may be used to improve defecation.

   c. **Defecation techniques** include

      1) **Proper defecation position,** that is, approximation of squatting position to achieve the proper angle between the rectum and the anal canal (if needed, a footstool may be used), or if unable to sit, a left side-lying position is best.

      2) **Valsalva's maneuver** involves having the patient ''bear down,'' that is, lean forward, close the glottis, hold the breath, and contract the

Table 5.8-1.   Step-care system for sequential nonsurgical management of constipation

STEP	SEQUENTIAL RECOMMENDATIONS FOR CONSTIPATION*
I	Behavioral training, e.g., time schedule, diet modification (i.e., high-fiber diet), regular exercise, Valsalva's maneuver, proper defecation position, digital-rectal stimulation
II	Bulk forming agents or high-fiber supplements
III	For nonneurogenic bowel (with refractory constipation)

> III (continued)
>
> For nonneurogenic bowel (with refractory constipation)
> 1. Oral stool softeners (i.e., docusates; avoid those combined with stimulant laxatives) or, if with high colonic constipation, oral mineral oil lubricants (unless contraindicated).
> 2. a. Oral hyperosmotic agents (e.g., lactulose or sorbitol); or
>   b. Sparing use of hyperosmotic suppositories (e.g., glycerin, which may be combined with digital stimulation 20 min after suppository insertion).
> 3. Sparing use of mini-enemas (e.g., Therevac) or enemas (e.g., tap-water enemas, mineral oil retention enemas, or sodium phosphate enemas).
> 4. Intermittent and sparing use of rectal stimulant laxatives or enemas (e.g., bisacodyl suppository or enema) for refractory constipation. Avoid oral stimulant laxatives.
>
> For neurogenic bowel (bowel habituation program)
> 1. Bowel clean-out at the start of the bowel training program (e.g., using multiple saline or bisacodyl enemas if stool is present at the rectal vault; or using oral mineral oil if stool is palpable proximal to the descending colon).
> 2. Hyperosmotic suppository (e.g., glycerin) 20-30 min after meal and 10 min later on toilet. Suppositories must be placed against rectal wall and not into fecal mass.
>   a. If no defecation 20 minutes after suppository insertion, digital stimulation is done and repeated once every 5 minutes up to three times.
>   b. If defecation occurs in less than 10 minutes after suppository insertion, wean off suppository and only use digital stimulation to trigger defecations at desired time. If liquid glycerin with docusate is used (e.g., Therevac mini-enema), a faster response time is anticipated as it does not have to wait for the solid suppository to melt.
> 3. Same as 2 but stimulant suppository (e.g., bisacodyl) is used instead of glycerin.
> 4. Oral stimulant laxatives, e.g., casanthranol-docusate sodium combination (e.g., Peri-Colace), senna (e.g., Senokot), bisacodyl (e.g., Dulcolax) given 6-10 hrs before anticipated bowel movement schedule (time can be adjusted so that defecation would otherwise result 30 min to 1 hr after the scheduled bowel triggering with suppository and/or digital stimulation).

* Note: Steps I and II should be implemented vigorously in younger patients (below 50 yrs old). Each new step or substep should only be implemented if the previous step or sub-step has failed after a consistent trial for a reasonable period (e.g., 2 weeks). Details are described in the text.

diaphragm and the abdominal muscles to increase intraabdominal pressures (IAP) and pelvic muscle tone. The increase in IAP is transferred to the pelvic floor and rectum to facilitate defecation. This should not be done in patients with rectal prolapse, hernias, hemorrhoids, or vesicoureteral reflux.

   d. **Manual bowel stimulation** is most effective when the patient is sitting or squatting.

1) **Digital bowel (or digital-rectal) stimulation** is favored over manual disimpaction. It is done by inserting a gloved, lubricated finger into the anal canal and gently moving the finger in a circular motion (with the finger continually maintaining contact with the mucosa) until the IAS relaxes and the rectum dilates. It is performed for 30 seconds to 2 minutes and repeated every 5 minutes up to 3 times or it may be done continuously without interruption until defecation occurs or for a maximum period of 20 minutes. A suppository or enema is usually applied prior to digital bowel stimulation.

2) **Manual disimpaction** of feces should be done only if digital stimulation has failed. It is performed gently to prevent inadvertent overstretching of the anal sphincter (especially in insensate patients) or traumatic anorectal injury (e.g., ulceration or perforation, which can lead to bacterial sepsis). In patients predisposed to autonomic dysreflexia because of fecal impaction (e.g., patients with T6 or higher SCI), lubrication with lidocaine gel (see section VI.B.3.e) may help decrease nociceptive sensory input.

2. Dietary measures

a. High-fiber (bulk-forming) diet is the cornerstone in the prevention and treatment of constipation. It has hydrophilic properties that increase the stool's weight, bulk and fluidity; decrease the colonic transit time (hence increasing stool frequency); and enhance colonic bacterial load (hence increasing colonic fecal mass). For the high-fiber diet to be effective (and prevent further constipation), the person must have adequate oral fluid intake (i.e., 2.0-3.5 liters per day of any fluid except those containing alcohol, caffeine, or other diuretic agents). Costs can be minimized by promoting dietary changes (i.e., increasing intake of fruits, vegetables, and cereals) rather than by addition of dietary fiber supplements. Dietary fiber should be increased gradually, as rapid and sudden increases can result in flatulence, eructation (belching), diarrhea, and abdominal bloating.

Daily recommended dietary fiber varies from 14.4 g to 20 to 35 g. The ingestion of water-soluble fibers (i.e., mucilages and pectin such as those found in oats, barley, peas, dried beans, potatoes, seeds, apples, oranges, and grapefruits) has the additional benefit of decreasing levels of serum cholesterol and lipids. The effect of a high-fiber diet in decreasing bowel malignancy is controversial. The use of a high-fiber diet and bulk-forming agents are contraindicated in patients with intestinal obstruction (as documented by radiologic or endoscopic procedures), with allergic reactions (e.g., urticaria and bronchial asthma) either to the bulk-forming agent or to substances contained in the preparations, and who are under strict fluid restriction for medical reasons (e.g., hyponatremia).

1) **Natural high-fiber foods**

a) **Cereals,** such as, bran, shredded wheat, wheatgerm, oats, and barley. The recommended dosage for bran is 1 to 2 tbsp taken 1 or 2 times a day with subsequent doses titrated based on individual response. Although an increase in stool frequency and flatus may occur during the first 2 to 3 weeks of bran therapy, bowel regularity is usually established within 1 month.

b) **Vegetables,** such as, brussel sprouts, peas, artichokes, pumpkins, lima beans, and potatoes.

c) Fruits, such as, dates, avocadoes, raisins, blackberries, blueberries, apples, oranges, and grapefruits.

2) Commercial fiber supplements (see section VI.B.3.a.1). The bulk-forming laxative with the highest fiber content is psyllium.

b. Fruit juices, such as, 4 oz of prune, fig, or pear juices can provide mild defecation stimulus when given 30 minutes to 1 hour before established time of defecation.

3. Drug therapy

a. Laxatives are used either to achieve appropriate stool consistency or to increase intestinal peristalsis and stool frequency. They are available for oral or rectal use (enemas are also discussed in section VI.B.3.b), and most of them can be obtained over the counter. When suppositories are used, they must be applied against the rectal wall and not into the fecal mass. They are contraindicated in patients with intestinal obstruction (partial or complete).

1) Bulk-forming agents thicken stool by absorbing fluid in the bowel and forming stool bulk. They also provide dietary fiber (especially psyllium seed derivatives which can also lower serum cholesterol with chronic use) and as with fiber intake, fluid intake of 2.0 to 3.5 liters per day are necessary (otherwise, further constipation and dehydration may ensue). Their effectiveness generally occurs within 12 to 24 hours (or may take several days depending upon transit times). The dosage is based upon individual patient response (usually 1-2 doses every 12-24 hours is sufficient).

The ADRs of bulk-forming agents (e.g., diarrhea, bloating, abdominal distress, and possible appetite reduction) can be decreased by reducing their doses or by using gradual dose titration. Bulk-forming agents must be used with caution by patients taking loop diuretics (as hypokalemia may occur) and by patients taking cardiac glycosides, nitrofurantoin, salicylates, and coumadin (because intestinal absorption of these drugs may be decreased). The adverse effect on serum electrolyte or blood urea levels in dialysis patients remains controversial. For diabetic patients, a sugar substitute may be used (nonabsorbable sugar substitutes may also help promote catharsis by an osmotic mechanism). Contraindications to the use of bulk-forming agents are similar to those noted previously for high-fiber diets (see section V.B.2.a).

Commercial preparations are supplied as individual packets, bulk packages, capsules, pills, or wafers. The manufacturer's recommended dosage is usually one teaspoon, tablespoon, pill, capsule or wafer to be taken 1 to 3 times daily with water or juice. Examples include psyllium or plantago seed derivatives (Konsyl, Metamucil, Modane-Bulk, Mucilose, Fiberall, Effersyllium, Hydrocil instant, Sarake, Syllact, Siblin, Naturacil, Nuggets), methylcellulose (Cologel, Citrucel, Hydrolose), polycarbophil (Mitrolan, Fibercon, Equalactin), malt soup extract (Maltsupex), plant gum, and guar. They are also available in combination with other laxatives, for example, psyllium with senna (Perdiem), plant gums with mineral oil (Kondremul), or plant gums with docusate sodium (Gentlax-B). Isphagula husk, a natural nonwheat source of fiber, is not indicated as it may cause serious allergic reactions.

2) Emollient (or surfactant) laxatives soften the stool without adding bulk, increasing peristalsis, or causing any sense of urgency. They act primarily as surfactants that facilitate the mixture of aqueous and fatty substances in the fecal mass to soften it. The prototype is docusate (active ingredient is dioctyl sodium sulfosuccinate), which is supplied as either a sodium or calcium salt. They are non-habit-forming and are indicated for hard stools or for short-term use when straining at stools is to be avoided (e.g., postmyocardial infarct and postanorectal surgery). They are primarily not absorbed, but they may increase the absorption of other agents administered concurrently. In fact, this is suspected to be the mechanism of hepatotoxicity when combined with danthron (see section VI.B.3.a.5.b.3) and the mechanism of foreign body reactions in lymphoid tissues when combined with mineral oil (see section VI.B.3.a.3). They may be safe, however, when used concomitantly with bulk-forming agents. Docusate sodium has been reported to be associated with periportal hepatitis but not with chronic active hepatitis.

The oral daily dose for docusate sodium and calcium is 50 to 360 mg with adequate fluid intake. Docusate sodium is available as either 50 mg or 100 mg tablets or as an elixir containing 20 mg per 5 ml, while docusate calcium is available as 240 mg capsules. Examples include docusate sodium (Afko-lube, Colace, Coloctyl, Comfolax, Dio-Medicone, Dialose, Diosate, Diosul, Doctate, Doxinate, Kasof, Modane-Soft, Regul-Aid, Regutol, Softenex) and docusate calcium (Surfak). Both are also available in combination with other laxatives, for example, docusate sodium with phenolphthalein (Correctol, Dialose-plus, Modane-plus) or with casanthranol (Peri-Colace, Constiban) or with cascara (Stimulax) or with danthron (Doctate, Dorbantyl, Unilax) or with senna (Senokot-S, Gentlax-S), and docusate calcium with phenolphthalein (Doxidan). Docusate sodium is also available for rectal use, for example, as one of the ingredients in the Therevac mini-enema (see section VI.B.3.b). Oral docusate is indicated in situations in which straining must be avoided, for example, in patients with angina, painful hemorrhoids, or who are prone to autonomic dysreflexia.

3) **Lubricant laxatives** promote defecation by facilitating the movement of stool. The prototype for lubricant laxatives is mineral oil, which consists of aliphatic hydrocarbons, which coat and penetrate the fecal material thus decreasing colonic absorption of water and allowing easier passage of oil-coated feces. It is given in doses of 5 to 45 ml either orally or as enemas (see Enemas in section VI.B.3.c) for short-term management of constipation (especially if there are formed stools in the transverse colon or higher as detected by radiographs). The ADRs include pruritus ani, leakage of mineral oil from the anus (in some patients with poor sphincter tone), lipoid aspiration pneumonia, foreign body reactions in lymphoid tissues (especially when combined with docusates), inhibition of absorption of fat-soluble vitamins (i.e., A, D, E and K) in chronic use, and anal stenosis in long-term use. It is contraindicated in elderly patients and in patients prone to gastroesophageal reflux or aspiration (e.g., poststroke). Also, it should not be ingested at bedtime or when lying down (because of aspiration risk) nor should it be combined with docusates. Commercial preparations of mineral oil include Milkinol, Neo-Cul-

trol, Petrogalar, Fleet Mineral Oil Retention Enema, and Saf-tip Oil Retention Enema. It is also available in combination with other laxatives, such as mineral oil with magnesium hydroxide (Haley's M-O, Milk of Magnesia-Mineral Oil Emulsion), or with bulk-forming agents (Agoral Plain, Kondremul). Other lubricant laxatives include liquid paraffin and seed oils, such as croton and arachis oils.

4) Osmotic laxatives are relatively nonabsorbable salts or carbohydrates that osmotically retain water in the lumen of the colon. They are indicated for immediate evacuation of bowel contents (e.g., at the start of bowel training program or for preparing the bowel for endoscopy, surgery, or radiologic studies) and should not be used chronically.

a) Saline laxatives: Magnesium (Mg) salts and sodium phosphates must be used with caution in patients with renal impairment, heart disease, or preexisting electrolyte imbalance.

(1) Magnesium salt usually has an effect within 3 to 4 hours and is most effective when given on an empty stomach. It can cause hypermagnesesemia (which may manifest as hypotension and muscle weakness) in patients with renal failure. Examples include Mg citrate (Citrate of Magnesia, Citroma, Citronesia, Evac-Q-Mag), 200 ml or 11 to 18 g in 10 oz, po; Mg hydroxide (Milk of Magnesia), 15 to 30 ml or 2.4 to 4.8 g, po; and Mg sulfate (Phillip's Milk of Magnesia), 10 to 30 gm, po.

(2) Sodium phosphates can be given orally (e.g., Fleet Phosphosoda, 20-45 ml, po) or as enemas (e.g., Fleet Phosphate Enema or Saf-Tip Phosphate Enema). They should not be used in patients with congestive heart failure as they may cause hypernatrenic dehydration.

(3) Polyethylene glycol with salts in colonic lavage solutions (Colyte, GoLytely, Nulytely) are effective for rapid bowel cleansing (dose of 4 to 6 L, po, over 3-4 hours which may be ingested at 8 oz every 10 minutes) or for chronic constipation (oral dose of 224-448 g or 8-16 oz per day). Polyethylene glycol does not cause either electrolyte imbalance or mucosal irritation, although some patients may be allergic to it.

b) Hyperosmotic laxatives

(1) Glycerin should be applied rectally as it is well-absorbed when given orally. It softens the fecal material and lubricates the anus and rectum, causing bowel evacuation within 30 minutes. Recommended rectal dose is 3 g. Chronic or daily use is not recommended as it may cause rectal irritation. It is available as Fleet Glycerin, Fleet Babylax, or generically as glycerin suppository. It is also one of the ingredients in *Therevac minienema* (see section VI.B.3.b).

(2) Lactulose is a nonabsorbable synthetic disaccharide, which exerts an osmotic effect when unmetabolized. When metabolized by colonic bacteria into lactate, it has both an osmotic and a stimulant effect. It is commonly used in the elderly patients with constipation. The ADRs include GI complaints (e.g., flatulence, cramps, diarrhea, nausea, and vomiting) and electrolyte imbalance. Serum electrolytes need to be monitored in long-term use. It is contraindicated in patients on galactose-

restricted diets and should be avoided when concomitant ant-
acid is taken. Daily oral dose is 15 to 30 ml (maximum of 60
ml/day), qd or bid. To prevent ADRs, it may be started at
5 ml, po, qid and increased as necessary. Examples include
Constulose, Enulose, Cephulac, Cholac, Chronulac, Constilac,
and Duphalac.

(3) Other carbohydrates, such as sorbitol and lactilol may be used
as hyperosmotic laxatives. Sorbitol (30-70%, 30 ml, po, qd)
is shown to be as effective as lactulose but is not widely used
because of its limited commercial availability. Yogurt modified with lactilol, wheat bran, and guar may be given as snacks
to elderly patients with chronic constipation.

5) Stimulant (irritant or contact) laxatives stimulate peristalsis by promoting water and electrolyte movement into the gut and inhibiting their
absorption. They should be used sparingly and intermittently only
if other laxative methods have failed. Local rectal stimulant suppositories and enemas carry less risk than oral stimulant medications
and do not appear to lead to chronic inflammatory changes of the
rectal mucosa. The chronic abuse of oral laxative stimulants can
lead to atonic "cathartic bowel" syndrome caused by dysfunction
or damage to the enteric neuron system (ENS). This is specially true
for the chronic use of anthroquinone stimulant laxatives in patients
with nonneurogenic bowel dysfunction (however, it remains unes-
tablished for patients with neurogenic bowel dysfunction, e.g., because of SCI). Stimulant laxatives can cause autonomic dysreflexia
due to hyperperistalsis in SCI patients with T6 lesions or higher (in
these patients, senna, which is a mild stimulant, may be used if
necessary). In nauseous patients, stimulant laxatives may cause vomiting because of reverse peristalsis.

a) Diphenylmethane derivatives

(1) Phenolphthalein stimulates colon motility and inhibits absorption of sodium and glucose (which causes accumulation of
intraluminal fluid). It is best taken at night because the laxative
effect occurs 6 to 10 hours after administration (this lag time
occurs because it needs to be metabolized by colonic bacteria).
Prolonged action (3-4 days) of phenolphthalein may occur
because of enterohepatic circulation. The ADRs include dermatologic reactions (e.g., erythema multiforme and erythema
nodosum), Stevens-Johnson syndrome, osteomalacia and pro-
tein-losing enteropathy, hypokalemia, hyperaldosteronism,
and laxative dependence. Daily oral dose varies from 30 to
270 mg for adults and from 15 to 60 mg for children. It is
available as tablets or as a liquid. Examples include Alophen,
Espotabs, Evac-U-Gen, Ex-Lax, Feen-A-Mint, Modane, and
Phenolax. It is also available in combination with other laxatives such as with docusate sodium (Correctol, Dialose-plus,
Modane-plus), docusate calcium (Doxidan), or mineral oil
(Agoral).

(2) Bisacodyl, a congener of phenolphthalein, stimulates the mucosal nerve plexus of the colon, producing contractions of the
entire colon and inhibiting water absorption in the small and
large bowel. Unlike phenolphthalein, it does not require ab-

sorption and subsequent metabolism before being effective. Rather, it is readily converted to its active desactyl metabolite by intestinal enzymes, both bacterial and mucosal. Its laxative effect occurs within 6 to 12 hours after oral administration or 15 to 60 minutes after rectal administration. It must be taken at least 1 hour before milk or antacids are given. The usual dose is 10 to 15 mg (0.3 mg/kg), po or pr, as needed. It is available in 5 mg enteric-coated tablets, 10 mg suppositories, or 10 mg/30 ml rectal enemas. The ADRs include abdominal cramps and laxative dependence. Examples are Dulcolax, Fleet Bisacodyl Enema, Carter's Little Pills, and Theralax.

(3) Oxyphenisatin is no longer available due to its association with chronic active hepatitis.

b) **Anthraquinone derivatives** stimulates colonic motility via Auerbach's plexus. It needs to be metabolized by colonic bacteria when orally administered and needs approximately 6 to 10 hours for the laxative effect to occur. The ADRs include melanosis coli (when used in large amounts over long periods; reversible upon cessation; benign) and acute nephritis (when ingested in large doses). Because metabolites of the anthraquinones are found in breastmilk, urine, and saliva, toxic quantities of these secretions can have laxative effects in the infants of nursing mothers.

(1) Senna is the mildest of the anthraquinone derivatives and may be used safely even in tetraplegic patients. Oral administration of senna results in poor initial absorption from the small intestine. More significant absorption occurs after metabolism by colonic bacteria. These agents produce primarily a colonic effect, which accounts for the 6 to 10 hours usually required for its laxative action to occur. It is available in 8.6-mg tablets, 15-mg granules, and in 8.8-mg/5 ml syrup. Daily oral dose is 1 to 2 tablets, 1 tsp granules, or 10 to 15 ml, po, qhs or bid. Examples include Senokot, Dosaflex, Fletcher's Castoria, and Nytilax. It is also available in combination with docusate sodium (Gentlax-S).

(2) Cascara usually requires 6 to 10 hours for its laxative action to occur. Dosage varies from 2 to 6 ml, po, qhs because of variable amounts of cascara in commercial preparations. Examples include Cas-Evac and Extract of Cascara. It is also available in combination forms, for example, cascara with milk of magnesia (also called "black and white," an effective laxative after barium swallow) or with docusate sodium (Stimulax).

(3) Danthron is given at a dose of 75 to 150 mg orally. Examples include Dorbane and Tonelax. It is also available in combination with emollient laxatives, for example, danthron with docusate sodium (Doctate, Dorbantyl, Unilax). This combination, however, has been shown to cause hepatotoxicity similar to chronic active hepatitis.

(4) Casanthranol is given at a dose of 30 mg orally. Examples include Black Draught and Lanes Pills. It is also available in combination with emollient laxatives, such as, casanthranol with docusate sodium (Constiban, D-S-S plus, Peri-Colace).

(5) Other anthraquinones include *Cassia alata* from Thailand and mulberry extract used primarily in China. Their effectiveness and mechanism of action have not been well studied in the West.

c) Castor oil is metabolized into ricinoleic acid, which promotes intestinal peristalsis and reduces the absorption of fluid and electrolytes. It acts within 2 to 6 hours and can result in a complete bowel evacuation. It is given at 15 to 45 ml, po, qhs or up to 60 ml if used for bowel preparation for radiologic or endoscopic procedures. However, it has a disagreeable odor and taste and is seldom prescribed for constipation as it can cause painful cramps, watery bowel movements, malabsorption, electrolyte abnormalities, and dehydration. Examples include Fleet Flavored Castor Oil Emulsion, Neoloid, and Purge Evacuant.

6) Carbon dioxide suppository (e.g., Ceo-Two) releases carbon dioxide as it melts into the rectum causing rectal distention, a reflex colonic peristalsis, and subsequent mechanical expulsion of stool. It may be used during bowel training for low-level SCI patients with loss of anorectal reflex; however, it is expensive and may cause autonomic dysreflexia in SCI patients with T6 lesions or higher.

b. Mini-enemas, so named because they contain a small volume of fluid (4 ml), can help improve rectal evacuation by increasing the response time. They produce a bowel movement within 15 minutes because, unlike a solid suppository, they do not need a waiting period for melting. An example is Therevac mini-enema, which contains docusate sodium in a soap base of glycerin and polyethylene glycol. Some variants also contain benzocaine, an anesthetic. Therevac mini-enema triggers reflex-mediated colonic peristalsis by acting as a mucosal stimulus, and provide lubrication by penetrating stool and softening it by the action of the docusate. It is commonly used in SCI patients, especially those with T6 or higher lesions because it reduces nociceptive stimuli that might precipitate autonomic dysreflexia. It is packaged in a single-use, ready-to-squeeze container with applicator tip. The tip should be punctured and *not* cut (to prevent sharp edges which could injure the anal sphincter, especially in insensate SCI patients).

c. Enemas are usually used as purgatives for bowel cleansing in preparing the patient for surgery or x-ray or endoscopic procedures. They may also be used in selected patients to help maintain regular bowel function and prevent skin breakdown (e.g., elderly patients with chronic constipation in whom rehabilitation is not feasible and who do not respond well to lesser stimuli, such as suppositories). Enemas must be used sparingly and intermittently because of their potential to cause enema-dependency bowel, rectoanal trauma, bowel perforation, electrolyte disturbances, bacteremia, colonic infections, and autonomic dysreflexia. They should only be used when more conservative bowel-care procedures (e.g., use of suppositories and digital bowel stimulation) failed. In the elderly or insensate patients, enemas should be administered using a cone tip (such as the tip used for colostomy irrigations) or using the nipple of a baby bottle fitted around the tip of the catheter to prevent backflow. If the enema is prepackaged in ready-to-use plastic squeeze bottles with applicator tips, the tip should not be cut to prevent sharp edges.

1) **Enemas containing laxative drugs** include saline osmotic enemas (see sodium phosphates described in section VI.B.3.a.4.a), mineral oil enemas (see section VI.B.3.a.3), stimulant enemas (see bisacodyl described in section VI.B.3.a.5), and lactulose enemas (which generate the release of carbon dioxide and hydrogen to break up impacted feces).

2) **Tap-water enema** is benign and may be used to break up impacted stool. It is safer than **soap-suds enema,** which can also be used to break up fat in the stool. Soap-suds enema is popular among the elderly but has been reported to cause acute colitis (mechanisms of action are unknown; probably caused by long-chain fatty acid toxicity). Although the colitis is usually benign, there have been reports of anaphylaxis, rectal gangrene, excessive fluid loss, and death attributed to the use of soap-suds enemas.

3) **Nontraditional enemas** containing coffee, herbal laxative additives, wheat grass, or hydrogen peroxide have been used not just for relief of constipation but as part of alternative medicine (e.g., for cancer treatment, increasing sexual potency, or total-body cleansing). These claims, however, have little scientific basis.

d. **Other peristaltic drugs**

1) **Prokinetic agents**

a) **Cisapride (Propulsid)** is a new prokinetic and noncholinergic agent that stimulates colonic smooth muscle through muscarinic receptors, thus accelerating colonic transit and increasing the frequency of stools with normal consistency. It is available in 10- and 20-mg tablets. If given in doses of 5 to 10 mg, po, tid for 8 to 12 weeks, it appears to be beneficial in SCI patients with chronic or refractory constipation. The ADRs include GI distress (i.e., cramping, diarrhea, and borborygmi), headache, rhinitis, infections, abnormal vision, and cardiac arrhythmias (rare). It is contraindicated when GI motility may be dangerous (e.g., mechanical obstruction, perforation, and hemorrhage) and should not be used concomitantly with oral ketoconazole, fluconazole, itraconazole, erythromycin, clarithromycin, or IV miconazole.

b) **Metoclopramide (Reglan)** is an antiemetic agent that also promotes gastric emptying probably by sensitizing tissues to acetylcholine. Although it has no direct effect on the colon, it can help resolve ileus after SCI. In high-dose or long-term use, it can cause dystonic reactions and other extrapyramidal side effects. It can be given at a dosage of 5 to 20 mg, po, tid or qid.

2) **Erythromycin** is a macrolide antibiotic that stimulates gastric, small bowel, and colon motor activity, thus accelerating colonic transit and increasing stool frequency. It has been effective at a dosage of 500 mg, po, qid in selective SCI patients with refractory constipation because of ileus.

e. **Viscous 2% lidocaine,** applied topically, may be beneficial if rectodynamic studies show anorectal dyssynergia. It may also be used during manual disimpaction (see section VI.B.1.d.2) in SCI patients with T6 or higher lesions who are predisposed to autonomic dysreflexia.

VII. Surgery to improve defecation is used only if conservative treatment methods have failed.

A. **Surgery for FI patients** to improve sphincter mechanism

1. **Anal sphincter repair** involves direct apposition or the overlapping of the EAS muscle. It is indicated for patients who have a deficient EAS with no neurologic damage (e.g., aging).
2. **Muscle transplant** involves the transposition of innervated muscles (e.g., gracilis, adductor longus, or gluteus maximus) or free muscle graft (e.g., palmaris longus) to replace puborectalis, levator ani, or EAS functions in patients with sacral nerve deficits. Chronic electrical stimulation may be used with these transplants.
3. **Artificial anal sphincters** involve the use of a subcutaneous pump mechanism that controls defecation by manually deflating a cuff placed around the EAS, which automatically reinflates over a period of 10 minutes to provide continence. It is indicated only for patients who have failed other surgery because of high complication rates and poor outcomes.

B. **Surgery for patients with DWE**
   1. **Myotomy** involves IAS or partial EAS incision to improve incomplete EAS relaxation during defecation (e.g., in anorectal dyssynergia). Although it relieves constipation in 62% of patients, it causes FI in 16%.
   2. **Transrectal (Brindley) stimulation** of anterior (parasympathetic) roots of S2-S4 is used in complete SCI patients to stimulate the distal colon and increase defecation frequency; however, electrodefecation results are unpredictable.

C. **Surgery for patients with FI or DWE**
   1. **Fecal diversion (e.g., colostomy or ileostomy)** can be used in patients with fecal incontinence (to attain social continence in intractable FI), chronic DWE or impaction (for reducing bowel care time and relieving abdominal distention), intrinsic bowel deficits (e.g., Hirschsprung's disease or atonic ''cathartic colon''), pressure ulcers or other skin lesions that cannot be effectively healed because of frequent soiling, or frequent urinary tract infections caused by seeding from frequent fecal impactions. Aside from the surgical risks, problems include cosmetic difficulties and embarrassing leakage of stool (e.g., loosening of ostomy bag). Due to the improvement in quality of life it provides (i.e., simplification of bowel care), however, many patients with neurogenic bowel have refused to have their fecal diversion reversed (e.g., after healing of pressure ulcers).
   2. **Bowel resection** may be done on diseased bowel that contributes to FI or DWE.

VIII. **Bowel complications**
   A. **Fecal impaction** has a morbidity range between 0% and 6% in the normal population (being higher in the cognitively impaired elderly). It is the most common bowel complication of chronic SCI patients (i.e., seen in at least 80% of the 27% of SCI patients who 5 years after injury develop significant bowel complications despite previous satisfactory bowel management). It is a common and potentially dangerous cause of autonomic dysreflexia in SCI patients with lesions at or above T6 because of the substantial time that may be required for its clearance. It can also lead to perforation or even death. Treatments include manual disimpaction (see section VI.B.1.d.2) in conjunction with laxatives or enemas, disimpaction by hydraulic lithotripsy, or by surgical decompression. Preventive measures are described previously (see step-care system in Table 5.8-1).
   B. **Hemorrhoids** are frequently (i.e., in over 90% of Americans or over 70% of SCI cases) caused by high pressures in the anorectal marginal veins associated with DWE. They can cause pain as well as rectal bleeding. They can

be prevented by adequate softening of stool (see under diet in section VI.B.2 and medications in section VI.B.3) without causing incontinence. Hemorrhoids surgery (e.g., by rubber band ligation or operative hemorrhoidectomy) may be done if there is bleeding (i.e., blood dripping into the commode or passage of clots), mucus soilage, or difficulty with anal hygiene.

C. **Rectal prolapse** can be associated with an overstretched patulous noncompetent sphincter because of the passage of very large hard stools through a weakened or atonic anorectal mechanism (e.g., because of lower motor neurogenic bowel). Treatment includes avoidance of straining and stretching of atonic bowel (e.g., softening of stool by diet or medications and avoidance of Valsalva's maneuver). If manual disimpaction is used, it must be done gently to avoid trauma to the denervated structures. A temporary colostomy (see section VII.C for indication) may allow the overdistended bowel to regain tone.

D. **Rectal bleeding** (i.e., streaks of blood on the glove or stool) after SCI is most commonly caused by traumatic superficial circumferential mucosal erosion (which can be treated conservatively). In patients over 45 years old, a flexible sigmoidoscopy may be done followed by a full colonoscopy if polyps or tumors are seen.

E. **Bloating, abdominal distention, and flatulence** can be especially severe in those with anorectal dyssynergia (i.e., hyperactive EAS in response to rectal distention). Treatment includes increasing the frequency of the bowel program, avoidance of foods that produce excessive gas (e.g., beans), digital release of flatus, and antiflatulent medications (e.g., those containing simethicone).

BIBLIOGRAPHY

Banwell JG, Creaswey GH, Aggarwal AM, et al: Management of the neurogenic bowel in patients with spinal cord injury, *Urol Clin North Am* 20:517-526, 1993.

Cardenas DD, Mayo ME, King KC: Urinary tract and bowel management in the rehabilitation setting. In Braddom RL, editor: *Physical medicine and rehabilitation,* Philadelphia, 1996, WB Saunders, pp 555-579.

Christensen J: The motor function of the colon. In Yamada T, editor: *Textbook of gastroenterology,* Philadelphia, 1991, JB Lippincott, pp 180-196.

Devroede G: Constipation. In Sleisenger MH, Fordtran JS, editors: *Gastrointestinal disease: pathophysiology, diagnosis, management,* ed 4, Philadelphia, 1989, WB Saunders, pp 331-368.

Doughty DB, editor: *Urinary and fecal incontinence: nursing management,* St. Louis, 1991, Mosby-Year Book.

Linsenmeyer TA, Stone JM: Neurogenic bladder and bowel. In DeLisa JA, Gans BMW, editors: *Rehabilitation medicine: principles and practice,* ed 2, Philadelphia, 1993, JB Lippincott, pp 733-762.

Schiller LR: Fecal incontinence. In Sleisenger MH, Fordtran JS, editors: *Gastrointestinal disease: pathophysiology, diagnosis, management,* ed 4, Philadelphia, 1989, WB Saunders, pp 317-330.

Stiens SA, Bergman SB, Goetz LL: Neurogenic bowel dysfunction after spinal cord injury: clinical evaluation and rehabilitative management, *Arch Phys Med Rehabil* 78 (3-S):S86-S102, 1997.

Tedesco FJ, Di Piro JT: American College of Gastroenterology's committee on FDA-related matters: laxative use in constipation,. *Am J Gastroenterology* 80: 303, 1985.

Wexner SD, Bartolo DCC: *Constipation: etiology, evaluation and management,* Oxford, 1995, Butterworth-Heinemann.

CHAPTER 5.9

PROBLEMS IN HUMAN SEXUALITY

The impact of disability on the patient's sexuality and sexual function is a common concern of PM&R patients. Although sex is considered one of the basic activities of daily living (ADLs), it is often neglected because the sex drive does not have immediate consequences for survival and most health care providers are uncomfortable with the subject. As experts in the rehabilitation of the whole patient, physiatrists must be knowledgeable in dealing with sexual issues considering that 80% of sexual complaints can be successfully managed in the office setting. This chapter deals with the physiological, mechanical, and psychosocial issues of sexual dysfunction and related sexual issues, such as fertility, contraception, pregnancy, labor, and lactation. For other important issues, such as sexually transmitted diseases, the reader is referred to any standard medical textbook.

I. Definitions

    A. Sex drive (libido) is a primary drive similar to hunger, thirst, and avoidance of pain. The conscious or unconscious decline in sexual drive or desire (e.g., because of anxiety, pain, malaise, stress, or fatigue) is referred to as *decreased libido*. Sex drive is not abolished by physical disability.

    B. Sex acts (or "sex") are human behaviors that result in pleasurable sensations through contact with one's own or another person's body, usually, but not necessarily, involving erogenous zones. *Sexual intercourse,* which is an example of a sex act, should not be limited to *coitus* (penetration of erect penis into the vagina). In PM&R, *sexual intercourse* refers to communication involving sexual self-expression and associated pleasuring, with or without genital involvement.

    C. Sexuality refers to the expression of one's sex drive through learned sex acts within the context of the sexual identity of the person. It integrates the physical, emotional, intellectual, and social aspects of an individual's personality, and expresses maleness or femaleness. It is a dynamic process grounded in developmental learning experiences involving the individual's self-concept, relationships with others, and specific repertoire of sexual behaviors. Interactions with others, personal hygiene, dress, speech, and expressions of affection are all important parts of sexuality. Sexuality is not determined by physical characteristics, and persons with physical disabilities do not lose their sexuality.

    D. Intimacy should not be equated with sexuality as it does not always involve sexuality. Intimacy is a special state of mutual understanding, trust, and acceptance. The need and capacity for intimacy remains although physical disability may interfere with sex drive and sex acts.

    E. Sexual dysfunction refers to any sexual behavioral problem that makes sexual expression consistently unsatisfying for the individual or partner. It is affected by physical, mechanical, and psychological factors as well as by aging and various medications (see Table 5.9-2). Sexual dysfunction can be classified into four types based on disability type (Cole & Cole, 1990).

        1. Type I disabilities are nonprogressive and occur at birth or before puberty. Examples include congenital loss of sight or hearing, spina bifida, and mental retardation. People with type I disabilities often fail to encounter the social learning opportunities associated with adolescent sexual development for various reasons, such as overprotective parents and societal ambivalence about sexuality training for developmentally disabled persons.

2. **Type II disabilities** also begin before puberty but are progressive. Examples include cystic fibrosis, muscular dystrophy, diabetes mellitus, and juvenile rheumatoid arthritis. Persons with these disabilities find it difficult to establish a stable body image and constantly face the uncertainty of further physical deterioration. As in the case of persons with type I disabilities, these persons frequently miss important socializing opportunities of a psychosexual nature.

3. **Type III disabilities** occur after adolescence and are nonprogressive. These stable, late-onset disabilities include stroke, spinal cord injury (SCI), traumatic brain injury (TBI), and physical disfigurement (e.g., amputation, burns). Affected persons have gone through the socializing experiences connected with adolescence and often developed the interpersonal skills required to initiate and maintain intimate social relationships, particularly of a sexual nature. After injury, they are taught to adapt their already developed skills to maximize their sexual lifestyle.

4. **Type IV disabilities** include progressive degenerative diseases and are usually found in older adults. In fact, 60% of all male sexual dysfunction at a performance level is physical in origin, and this dysfunction increases with age. Type IV disabilities can be caused by arthritis, Alzheimer's disease, heart disease, pulmonary disease (e.g., chronic obstructive pulmonary disease [COPD]), renal disease, circulatory changes, autonomic nervous disorders, venous leakages or arteriovenous shunting, peripheral neuropathies (diabetic or alcoholic), amyotrophic lateral sclerosis (ALS), multiple sclerosis (MS), or terminal illness, such as cancer or AIDS. Affected patients usually have a long history of intimate relationships. They face the problem of coping with either a discrete event or slow deterioration, which may impair their intellectual and physical ability to communicate sexually. Others face negligible impairments but may harbor fear of further losses should they engage in strenuous physical activity. These fears coupled with the necessity of frequent medical interventions often result in marked changes in sexual behavior.

F. **Sexual adjustment** refers to the intimate communication involving a mutually pleasurable and practical repertoire of behavior, which may or may not emphasize genital behavior. Its adequacy is solely determined by the patient and partner.

II. **Neurophysiology of sexual response** presented below is classified in four phases (based on the Masters and Johnson's classification of sexual response).

A. **Excitement or arousal phase,** which lasts several minutes to hours, occurs in response to sexual stimulation either because of touch (reflexogenic) or imagination (psychogenic). In men, the penis becomes erect, the scrotum contracts, and the testes are brought close to the body. In women, there is vaginal lubrication (with vasocongestion leading to a transudate of fluid), swelling of the labia, clitoral erection, expansion of the inner two thirds of the vagina and elevation of the uterine body, cervix, and labia majora. The vascular mechanism of erection occurs because of vasocongestion of the erectile tissues of the genitals resulting from arteriolar and sinusoidal dilation, which passively occludes venous outflow. Both sexes have increased muscle tension, blood pressure, and heart rate. In elderly men, the following changes may be noted: erections occur 2 to 3 times slower than with younger men; tactile stimulation may be necessary; erection which is not as firm approaches full rigidity only seconds before ejaculation. In elderly women, the arousal phase is also delayed and there is less voluminous vaginal secretion with delayed and reduced vaginal expansion.

1. **Reflexogenic excitement** can be elicited by direct genital stimulation (e.g., stroking, oral stimulation, vibration, pulling pubic hair, or a full bladder) independent of erotic stimuli or thoughts. The sensory impulse travels through the dorsal afferent nerve to the sacral cord through the pudendal nerve. From the sacral cord, **parasympathetic efferents** originate from the anterior division of **S2-S4** and travel via the cauda equina through the pelvic nerves (also called pelvic splanchnic nerves or nervi erigentes) to the cavernosal nerves and into the corporal trabeculae. The parasympathetic efferent stimuli causes vasodilation, which leads to vasocongestion of the genitalia. Hence, interruption of the S2-S4 parasympathetic reflex arc (e.g., in complete lower motor neuron lesions) leads to loss of reflexogenic excitement; but, if the sacral reflex activity (i.e., bulbocavernosus reflex) is intact (e.g., in upper motor neuron lesion), reflexogenic excitement can occur.

2. **Psychogenic excitement** is believed to originate in the cerebral cortex through the different senses, such as audio-visual stimuli (e.g., erotic movies or pictures) or through erotic fantasies. The stimulating psychogenic impulses travel through the hypothalamic and thalamic centers to the thoracolumbar (sympathetic) cord and the sacral (parasympathetic) cord. Hence, even if reflexogenic excitement is lost because of abolished S2-S4 parasympathetic reflex arc (e.g., in patients with complete lower motor neuron lesions), psychogenic excitement may still occur (although rarely) as long as the thoracolumbar (sympathetic) cord is intact. In SCI patients with incomplete upper motor neuron lesion above T10 (i.e., intact sympathetic cord), psychogenic as well as reflexogenic excitement is possible. The **sympathetic efferents** originate from **T11-L2** and travel to the genitalia through the hypogastric plexi. In the nonexcited state, tonic sympathetic discharge (probably through postsynaptic α-receptors) causes contraction of the genital arterioles and sinusoids thus keeping the blood from entering the erectile tissues of the genitals. During excitement, it is theorized that norepinephrine acts on the postsynaptic β-receptors resulting in smooth muscle relaxation and vasodilation of the genital arterioles and sinusoids, which leads to vasocongestion of the genitalia.

B. **Plateau phase,** which can last from seconds to minutes, consists of the high levels of sexual arousal that precede the threshold levels required to trigger orgasm. It involves maximal vasocongestion of the sexual organs with additional increases in heart rate and blood pressure. In men, vasocongestion continues; the penis enlarges further and can deepen in color. The testes elevate and rotate anteriorly, coming to rest against the perineum. In women, the processes of vaginal expansion and clitoral and nipple engorgement continue. A "sex flush" may spread over the abdomen, breasts, and chest wall. In both sexes, there is tachypnea, tachycardia, elevated blood pressure, and generalized myotonia. In elderly men, the plateau phase is prolonged, and there is a poorly defined sense of impending orgasm whereas in elderly women, there is less discernible nipple swelling and erection. Patients who have anorgasmy do not progress further than the plateau stage.

C. **Orgasm phase** involves rhythmic contractions of the penis and prostrate in men (i.e., ejaculation). In women, there is rhythmic contractions of the uterus and outer one-third of the vagina. In both sexes, there is also rhythmic contraction of the perineal muscles and other more diffuse responses (e.g., peripheral muscular contractions and changes in electroencephalographic activity). Orgasm has been described as a cortical experience of "supreme pleasure," which is generally followed by a feeling of "well-being and satisfaction." It is theorized to occur in the limbic system and to be triggered by a neural reflex under **sympathetic** control once the orgasmic threshold is reached.

Although orgasm in men is usually associated with ejaculation, it is not a prerequisite (likewise, erection is not a prerequisite of ejaculation, which is reflexive). Men with transurethral prostatectomy (TURP) may still experience orgasm despite 90% incidence of ejaculatory failure (with 50 to 60% incidence of retrograde ejaculation). In elderly men, there is reduced volume of the seminal fluid, and the ejaculatory event is shorter with fewer and less forceful expulsive contractions of the urethra (i.e., seepage may occur instead of forceful ejaculation). In women, ejaculation is not an easily quantifiable response as in the men. The nature of female ejaculate remains controversial (it has been reported to consist of vaginal transudate, which accumulates throughout the arousal process). Women who have had a hysterectomy or clitoridectomy may still experience orgasm. During menopause, there is a decrease in the frequency of vaginal and uterine contraction during orgasm because of a relative estrogen deficit.

In both sexes, orgasms are rare in complete upper motor neuron (UMN) lesions (a recent study by Sipsky et al, 1995, reported that women with complete UMN lesions did experience orgasm described as "throbbing in the vaginal area" or as sensation "all over"). In general, the higher the spinal cord lesion (i.e., the further away from the sacral parasympathetic reflex arc), the more likely the patient is to have a reflexogenic excitement, but the less likely to have ejaculation or orgasm. Ejaculation is more common with lower motor neuron lesions and with more caudal lesions (supporting the theory that ejaculation or orgasm is under sympathetic control). Orgasm in patients with complete lower motor neuron lesions may occasionally be perceived as a pleasurable sensation in the abdomen, pelvis, or thighs.

D. Resolution phase, which usually occurs over a period of 5 to 15 minutes, involves the return of the body to its normal resting state. Sympathetic tonic discharge resumes in the genitals, resulting in contraction of the smooth muscles around the sinusoids and arterioles. Arterial blood flow is decreased and venous channels are reopened. In men, there is a refractory period immediately after ejaculation in which further ejaculation cannot occur (although erection may occur). In contrast, women do not experience a refractory period and have the potential to experience several successive orgasms. In elderly men, detumescence is more rapid and the refractory period is longer (i.e., about 12-24 hours in those over 55 years old).

III. Sexual assessment should be initiated by the physiatrist and, ideally, it should be performed in a multidisciplinary fashion (to identify psychological factors). History and physical examination can be incorporated with sexual counselling by using the ENIGMA model (i.e., **E**ngage, **N**ormalize, **I**nform, **G**uide, **M**aximize, and **A**ssess) described in section V.B.

A. History should be open-ended and nonjudgmental (see Table 5.9-1 for sample format). It should include general and specific current and premorbid sexual functioning (e.g., ability to obtain reflex and psychogenic erections, ability to lubricate, and sexual positioning difficulties), current medications (see

Table 5.9-1.   Sample interview format

CATEGORY	QUESTION OR STATEMENT
Introduction	• I'd like to discuss with you your present sexual functioning. (Assure patient of confidentiality)
Current sexual functioning (general)	• Are your sexually active at present? Have you ever been sexually active? • Are you satisfied with your current sexual relationship(s)? With your current sexual adjustment? • How has your illness or injury affected your enjoyment of or ability to engage in sexual relations? (Frequency, quality, course of adjustment) • What is your sexual repertoire? Or what type of sexual and affectionate behavior do you engage in? Is self-stimulation or masturbation one of the options that you choose? • Do you have any concerns or questions about your sexual functioning? [Stop interview here if no questions or concerns]
Current sexual functioning (specific)	• (Men) Are you able to have and maintain an erection sufficient for coitus? Is this a problem for you or your partner? Under what circumstances do you have difficulty? • (Women) Are you able to reach orgasm? From intercourse or by means of other stimulation? In what situations do you have difficulty?
Partner satisfaction and relationship history	• Are you able to have sexual relations without pain or discomfort? Are you sufficiently lubricating? Under what circumstances? • Are you able to stimulate and satisfy your partner? Does your partner know what pleases you? Are you able to communicate effectively about sex? About other aspects of the relationship? • How long have you been in your present relationship? Have you been able to work out a compatible adjustment? What difficulties have you encountered, and how did you resolve them successfully? How has having children/not having children affected your relationship?
Other effects on the relationship	• How stable is your health at present? What is expected in the future? • Do you take any prescription medication? • What method of contraception do you use? Are you satisfied with it? • Do you use alcohol or other drugs? How often? How does this affect your relationship? Your sexual relationship? • Have you had any negative or traumatic sexual experiences?
Follow-up	• Would you be interested in speaking with a specialist in sexual functioning about the questions or problems that you've raised in this interview?

From Ducharme S, Gill KM, Biener-Bergman S, et al: Sexual functioning: medical and psychologica aspects. In DeLisa JA and Gans BM, editors: *Rehabilitation medicine: principles and practice*, ed 2, Philadelphia, 1993, JB Lippincott, p. 767, with permission.

Table 5.9-2. **Partial list of prescription medications that can cause sexual dysfunction**

DRUG CLASSIFICATION	DECREASED LIBIDO (M/F)	ERECTILE DYSFUNCTION (M)	IMPAIRED EJACULATION (M)	COMMENTS
Anticholinergics		+	(+)	Decrease vaginal lubrication; dry mouth may affect oral sex
Antihypertensives	(+)	+	(+)	Decreased penile perfusion due to decreased blood pressure
Antiseizure	(+)	(+)		Can lower testosterone and estrogen; sedation
Antispasmodics				
Baclofen		+	+	
Dantrolene		+		
Diazepam	+	(+)		Sedation; menses changes
Diuretics	(+)	+	(+)	Menstrual changes
Estrogen	+	(+)		Menstrual changes
H2-blockers	(+)	+		Dry mouth may affect oral sex
Psychotherapeutics (TCA, MAOI, SSRI)	(+)	+	(+)	Sedation, anticholinergic
Recreational drugs (alcohol, cocaine, heroin, marijuana, tobacco)		(+)		Relationship problems; alcohol may suppress libido
Steroids (anabolic)	(+)	(+)		High dose can suppress hypothalamic-pituitary-adrenal axis and spermatogenesis; menses changes.

Note: + indicates that the sexual dysfunction is listed for that drug or most of the drugs in that classification in the *Physicians' Desk Reference*; (+) indicates that the sexual dysfunction has been reported for that drug or most of the drugs in that classification in the medical literature (but not in the *Physicians' Desk Reference*).
TCA = tricyclic antidepressants; MAOI = monoamine oxidase inhibitor; SSRI = selective serotonin reuptake inhibitors; M = male; F = female.

Table 5.9-2), recreational drugs (e.g., alcohol, heroin, marijuana, and tobacco can all cause erectile dysfunction and probably decrease libido), associated injuries (e.g., pelvic fracture or prior pelvic surgery), the patient's and the partner's psychological adjustment to injury, and the patient's need for additional services concerning sexuality.

B. **Physical examination** sessions should be used as an opportunity to check the patient's knowledge of sexually transmitted diseases (STDs). All patients who are sexually active in nonexclusive relationships without STD precautions (i.e., condoms used consistently) should be screened for infection. Most patients, female and male, are neither aware of the signs or symptoms of STDs, nor are they aware of the fact that a significant portion of the infected population is without signs or symptoms.

1. **General.** Demeanor, posture, clothing, and grooming.
2. **Skin.** Scars, rashes, open wounds, pressure ulcers, and skin lesions.
3. **Mental health**
   a. **Cognition.** Competence in consenting to sexual activity; judgment to make safe decisions about high-risk sexual activity and contraception.

      b. Mood. Depressed, abusive.
  4. Neurologic. Educate about possible new erotic areas (insensate-sensate border); instruct patient and partner to concentrate on sensate skin; if patient has dysesthesia, teach techniques for desensitization or position to avoid stimulating dysesthetic areas.

      a. Sensation. Sensory distribution; potential for touching, caressing, receiving touch; erogenous zones (identified by patient or believed to be important by physician, e.g., dermatomal levels just above anesthetic area); areas of dysesthesia.

      b. Strength. Paralysis or paresis (special attention to S1-S3 motor segments of the lower limbs).

      c. Communication. Aphasia, dysarthria, visual and hearing disorders.

  5. Breast. Gynecomastia; teach female patients how to do breast self-examination (or arrange to have their breasts examined at least every 3 months).

  6. Musculoskeletal

      a. Contractures. Arthritic deformities, patient's knowledge of stretching, need for surgery.

      b. Spasticity. Adductor spasticity in females (may interfere with coitus).

  7. Genitalia

      a. Hygiene. Odors or yeast infection, need for attendant care.

      b. Sensation. Perineal sensation (in men with intact pinprick sensation in the penile, scrotal, and perianal dermatomes can expect a return of normal psychogenic erections, ejaculation, and orgasm; women with sensation of the clitoris and labia have better chances of attaining orgasm); evidence of reflexogenic erection or lubrication.

      c. General. Genital anatomy; open lesions; STDs (condyloma, herpes); in females, pelvic examination (may need to be done in a modified position)

  8. Urologic. Continence (if incontinent, check for skin breakdown; if with indwelling catheter, check for scrotal fistula; if with external catheter, check if there is a good seal); epididymitis

  9. Gastrointestinal examination provides an opportunity to instruct patients about reflexogenic erection or lubrication.

      a. General. Check for any ostomy sites or equipment.

      b. Rectal. Anal wink, sphincter tone, voluntary control, bulbocavernosus reflex (in both male and female), open lesions.

  10. Vascular. Diabetes mellitus and peripheral vascular disease (both may contribute to erectile or lubrication problems because of vascular sclerosis).

  11. Cardiac. Blood pressure (prolonged hypertension may lead to vascular sclerosis), pulse rate, arrhythmias, heaves, rubs, murmur.

  12. Pulmonary. Cough, rales, shortness of breath, consolidation, signs of COPD.

C. Laboratories. Electrolytes and glucose, hormonal assays (e.g., prolactin, luteinizing hormone, follicle-stimulating hormone, testosterone, and estrogen), thyroid work-up, diabetes work-up.

D. Diagnostic tests can be used to determine organic versus psychogenic sexual dysfunctions.

  1. Neurophysiological studies are used in patients with sexual dysfunction to confirm the presence, location, and nature of a previously diagnosed neurological lesion (e.g., early polysensory neuropathies).

      a. Sacral evoked response (SER) study determines the integrity of the bulbocavernosus reflex, i.e., the afferent dorsal nerve pathway, the S2-S4 cord, and the efferent pudendal nerve pathway. It confirms the presence, the anatomical location (peripheral, sacral, and suprasacral lesions), the side (left or right), and the nature (motor or sensory) of the neurological lesion associated with the sexual dysfunction (e.g., erectile dysfunction). A stimulus is applied to the skin pudendal sensory nerve through electrodes applied to the penis or clitoris. The motor response is recorded through an electromyography (EMG) needle electrode from the bulbocavernosus muscle, from the external urethral sphincter, or from the external anal sphincter. Normal SER has a stable mean latency of 35 (± 5) msec. The SER is prolonged if patients with abnormal bulbocavernosus reflex (e.g., sacral cord or cauda equina lesions).

b. **Dorsal nerve somatosensory evoked potential (DN-SEP or genitocerebral SEP) study** is used to assess the entire peripheral and central nerve afferent pudendal pathways. It is analogous to the SER test except that instead of recording the motor EMG response, it records only the sensory evoked potential from the sacral cord and cerebral cortex through surface electrodes applied to the sacrum or scalp, respectively. It is most useful in confirming the presence and the anatomical location (peripheral, sacral, and suprasacral lesions) of the afferent pudendal sensory dysfunction in patients with subtle abnormalities determined by screening tests (e.g., penile biothesiometry).

c. **Penile biothesiometry** is a quantitative vibratory somatosensory evaluation. A portable hand-held electromagnetic vibration device with a fixed frequency, but variable amplitude, is applied to the lateral aspects of the penile shaft as well as the glans penis. The patient is then asked to tell the examiner when the vibratory stimulus is first felt. This test is an inexpensive, noninvasive screening method to assess for an abnormality within the dorsal nerve afferent pathway. Abnormal biothesiometry and abnormal DN-SEP suggest an underlying sensory neuropathy, which is usually related to diabetes or alcoholism. A normal biothesiometry and abnormal DN-SEP, however, suggest a somatosensory receptor cell damage or collagen infiltration of the penile shaft.

d. **Cavernous efferent neurointegrity evaluation**
   1) **Indirect tests**
      a) **Nocturnal penile tumescence (NPT) studies** can be performed in a sleep laboratory with monitoring of sleep electroencephalogram (EEG), electrooculogram, or EMG. A normal NPT done in a sleep laboratory shows erections lasting 15 to 30 minutes and occurring 3 to 5 times per night during rapid eye movement sleep. The NPT can also be done at home (without formal sleep monitoring) using a portable unit (e.g., RigiScan). A normal NPT using RigiScan shows erections lasting an average of 10 to 15 minutes and occurring 3 to 6 times per 8-hour sleep session. In addition to NPT, the RigiScan also determines penile compressibility by measuring the tightening of the loops placed around the penis and determining the penile resistance to compression. Compressibility should not be confused, however, with rigidity, which can be determined by awakening the patient during maximal tumescence and measuring the force sufficient to buckle the penile shaft. The minimum buckling resistance required for coital penetration is 500 to 550 g.

      b) **Cystometrogram (CMG)** may be obtained as the bladder is served by many of the same nerve roots serving sexual function (see Chapter 5.7, section II.C.2.e).

      c) **Diagnostic intracavernosal injection of vasoactive agents** (e.g., papaverine and prostaglandin E_1) is done to determine the integrity of the autonomic pelvic-cavernous nerve. Patients with denervation of the pelvic-cavernous nerve (e.g., complete cauda equina lesion) shows a supersensitive response, that is a significantly lower dose is needed to achieve a rapid and sustained pharmacological erection. Erection can be measured using doppler ultrasonography (also known as pharmacopenile duplex ultrasonography [PPDU]) to determine penile-brachial indices (PBI).

    2) **Direct tests,** including the corpus cavernosum smooth muscle EMG (needle and surface electrodes) and the single potential analysis of cavernous electric activity (SPACE) do not ''directly'' evaluate the cavernous efferent nerves in a manner analogous to DN-SEP or SER.

  2. Tests of penile vasculature include PPDU, corporal cavernosometry and sonography, external vacuum diagnosis, penile angiography, and radionuclear scintigraphy.

E. Questionnaire assessments may be used to determines psychological factors affecting sexuality and relationships. They include the Psychological Adjustment to Illness Scale (PAIS), which focuses on sexuality and relationships; Dyadic Adjustment Inventory (DAI), which determines relationship satisfaction or quality of a marital relationship; Sexual Interaction Inventory (SII), which measures sexual adjustment and satisfaction in couples; Derogatis Sexual Functioning Inventory (DSFI), which measures current sexual functioning; Sex-role Inventory (SRI), which measures gender role definition; Sexual Knowledge and Attitude Test (SKAT), which measures sexual attitudes, knowledge, demography, and experiences; Mosher Forced-Choice Guilt (FCGI), which measures sex guilt; and sex history form (SHF). Standardized personality tests such as Minnesota Multiphasic Personality Inventory (MMPI) or Millon Clinical Multiaxial Inventory II (MCMI-II) may be used to detect underlying psychological problems.

IV. Classification and management of sexual dysfunction in PM&R

A. Physiologic dysfunction is usually caused by a lesion in the neural pathways.

  1. Erectile dysfunction (ED) (preferred term instead of impotence) is defined as the inability to achieve an erect penis as part of the overall multifaceted process of male sexual function (not necessarily for coitus). Organic causes are vasculogenic (most common), neurogenic, endocrine, and iatrogenic (medications are estimated to cause 25% of ED; sphincterotomy or TURP can also cause ED). Psychogenic causes are discussed under section IV.C. In PM&R, the most commonly encountered organic ED are neurogenic in origin, such as SCI, MS, diabetic neuropathy, or, rarely, stroke. In general, erection may be achieved by reflexogenic means (e.g., manual stimulation of the genital area or by rubbing the genital on clothing or bed linen) or by psychogenic means (e.g., fantasizing, videos, magazines, or books). However, it is usually difficult to maintain erection for successful coitus (i.e., intromission and intravaginally sustained erection long enough to satisfy the partner) because once stimulation has been removed, the erection may subside. The following are mainly used for neurogenic-based ED:

    a. Noninvasive techniques

      1) **Education.** Patients should be counseled that they could satisfy their sexual partners even without penile erection (e.g., using a vibrator, or through oral or digital sex). Likewise they could satisfy themselves through masturbation using manual or vibratory techniques. In many patients, it may be sufficient just to be aware that there are treatment options for their erectile dysfunction. In SCI patients, erectile functioning may not return for 6 to 12 months postinjury, hence aggressive intervention should be limited initially. There is no evidence to support the belief that patients will interpret sexuality education as an endorsement and thus increase the frequency of sexual behavior.

2) **Vibrator stimulation** at a frequency of 80 Hz can induce erection when, applied to the glans, frenulum, shaft, or base of the penis; however, the erection may not be sufficient for coitus.

3) **"Stuffing"** refers to the insertion of the semierect penis into the vagina and through the "milking activity" of the vaginal muscles, blood flow into the penis may be improved long enough for successful coitus.

4) **Artificial penis (dildo)** can be strapped on the groin to simulate a natural erection.

5) **Vacuum tumescence constriction therapy (VTCT)** has been reported to achieve an erection rigid enough for coitus in up to 90% of men. Although it can maintain the erection for up to 30 minutes, it does not change the patient's ability to ejaculate or achieve orgasm. The sequence of VTCT is the flaccid penis is inserted in a rigid plastic cylinder; a manual or battery-operated pump is operated to create negative pressure (i.e., vacuum) in the cylinder, which draws blood into the penile corpora causing it to become erect; and finally, a constricting band (made of rubber) is guided through the cylinder and placed at the base of the penis to maintain the erection, after which the cylinder is removed. When erection is not desired, the band is removed and detumescence follows rapidly. Common side effects include pain; penile hematoma, ecchymosis, or petechiae; penile numbness; "cold" penis; pulling of scrotal tissue into the cylinder; pivoting of penis (because of lack of erection at the band); and blocked antegrade ejaculation (may be painful). In patients with upper-limb dysfunction and poor hand function, their partners can be trained in its use or a battery-operated unit may be used. Patients must remove the constricting band after 30 minutes to prevent penile ischemia and necrosis. The VTCT is contraindicated in patients receiving anticoagulant medications or with bleeding disorders.

6) **Oral or topical erectogenic medications** should ideally be effective, useful "on demand," free of toxicity and side effects, and affordable; however, there is currently no such universal drug. Many erectogenic drugs (e.g., cantharidin or Spanish fly) are based on anecdotal information or poorly designed studies. The following are some promising erectogenic drugs reported in the medical literature. They probably act on the central mechanism of erection and have very limited peripheral activities. They are given orally unless stated otherwise.

   a) **Adrenergic receptor antagonists.** Yohimbine (controversial "aphrodisiac" available as Yocon, Yohimex, Aphrodyne, Erex, or Yovital; some studies did not show it to be more effective than a placebo; others show it to be effective in psychogenic ED; it can be given at 5.4 mg, po, tid (up to 20-30 mg/day) in patients without coronary disease or moderate-to-severe hypertension, who are unwilling to try other treatment options. Major side effects include angina exacerbation, central nervous system [CNS] excitation with increased pulse rate and blood pressure, anxiety, fine tremors, dizziness, or nausea); buccal phentolamine (20-40 mg applied through a strip of filter paper to the oral mucosa 15 minutes before coitus; further studies needed); and delquamine (new selective α-2 adrenergic antagonist).

b) **Serotoninergic receptors.** Trazodone (Desyrel) 100 to 200 mg, po, qhs; probably acts by inhibiting serotonin reuptake; may be tried with yohimbine for 1 month for synergistic effects (widely accepted belief but no scientific proof).

c) **Dopamine receptor agonists.** Levodopa (55-60% of patients reported to achieve rigid erection; needs further confirmation); apomorphine (buccal tablets; experimental); bromocriptine (see under Hormones).

d) **Nitric oxide (NO) vasodilators.** Nitroglycerine paste (2 cm of 2% paste applied directly to the penis or to the perineum in an attempt to avoid partner contamination; erection rigid enough for coitus in only 25% of patients; frequent side effects include hypotension and headaches, which may manifest in contaminated partner; and L-arginine (precursor of NO; given at 2800 mg, po, daily; no side effects reported; further studies needed).

e) **Other vasodilators.** Minoxidil (Rogaine topical solution used for treating baldness; probably not effective as a single agent; minoxidil combined with capsaicin, a topical analgesic, which acts by depleting substance P, has been reported but needs confirmation); prostaglandin E_1 (popular injectable single intracavernosal agent; new delivery system through topical intraurethral use has been tried but needs further studies; large doses of 500 μg needed compared to 1-40 μg when injected intracavernosally; prominent side effects are pain and hypotension); papaverine (a formerly popular single intracavernosal agent; has been tried transdermally but with disappointing results).

f) **Hormones.** Testosterone (for patients with hypogonadism) and bromocriptine (for patients with hyperprolactinemia).

b. **Invasive techniques**

1) **Intracavernous injection of vasoactive substances** can produce an erection in patients with neurogenic-based erectile dysfunction but whose vasculature is intact. Although partner satisfaction is high, these medications do not affect the man's ability to ejaculate or have orgasm. The vasoactive agents are injected (by the patient or his partner, using a 26- to 30-gauge needle and a 1-ml insulin syringe) with a sterile technique without aspiration into the posterolateral aspect of the base of the penile shaft (3 or 9 o'clock position), avoiding midline neurovascular structures. The dose is carefully titrated by a urologist because of the risk of priapism (prolonged painful erection [over 4 hours] because of lack of drainage of the corpus cavernosum). Men with neurogenic-based erectile dysfunction are more prone to sustain erections lasting more than 6 hours and can develop priapism even with small doses. The dose is typically titrated upward until an erec-

tion adequate for coitus lasting 30 to 60 minutes (or less than 4 hours) is attained.

Complications of intracavernous injection of vasoactive agents include pain (common at the injection site); minor hematoma or ecchymosis at the injection site (which can be prevented by compressing the injection site for 2-5 minutes); liver function abnormalities (common but clinically insignificant); vasovagal episodes (e.g., dizziness and hypotension, usually self-limited, rare); infection (rare); corporal fibrosis or penile plaque formation, rarely with subsequent penile angulation, occurs in 2 to 5% of patients after at least 1 year of use (chance of plaque formation can be reduced by injecting alternate sides of the penis and by limiting injections to twice a week); and priaprism in 3 to 10% of patients.

Patients with priaprism can take oral terbutaline (Bricanyl or Brethine tablets), 5 mg, which can be repeated every 15 minutes until detumescence occurs (for a maximum of 15 mg or three doses). If priaprism persists (over 4 hours), the old blood may be aspirated from the side of the corpus cavernosum using a 19-gauge scalp vein needle. This is followed by slow intracavernosal injection of an α-adrenergic drug, such as phenylephrine solution, 0.5 to 1.0 ml (made by mixing 0.5 ml from a 10 mg/ml phenylephrine vial with 9.5 ml of saline to make a total of 10 ml phenylephrine solution), which may be reinjected after 15 to 20 minutes if erection persists, or Neo-Synephrine, 200 μg, given every 5 minutes until detumescence occurs. After the intracavernosal injection, the penis is wrapped in a compression bandage for several hours.

The following vasoactive agents are commonly used for intracavernosal injections in patients with ED (except for alprostadil, these agents are not FDA approved and, therefore, the patient must sign an informed consent form):

a) Single therapy agents

   (1) Papaverine is a nonspecific smooth muscle relaxant, which decreases resistance to arterial inflow and increases resistance to venous outflow. As the sinusoids fill up, venous outflow is also passively obstructed. In neurogenic ED, a starting dose of 3 mg (0.1 ml of 30 mg/ml vial) is used, which can be increased at 3-mg increments. Typically, less than 12 mg is required to attain an adequate erection, although doses as high as 80 to 120 mg have been used with erections lasting up to 18 hours. Because repeated injections can cause corporal fibrotic nodules, papaverine use as monotherapy has declined. Instead it is usually combined with other agents.

   (2) Prostaglandin E$_1$ (PGE$_1$), also called alprostadil (Prostin; Caverject), is currently the most commonly used monotherapy agent because of its superior pharmacologic profile (i.e., a powerful smooth muscle relaxant with very low incidence of fibrosis). It is also the only injectable drug that is FDA-approved for the treatment of neurogenic ED. It is used in doses ranging from 1 to 40 μg (patients with SCI may respond to as little as 1-2 μg). Adverse effects include penile pain at injection site (a common complaint) and development of hypotension. One way of alleviating the penile pain is to add 20 mg of procaine to the PGE_1.

b) Combination therapy agents

(1) Duo-mix (papaverine + phentolamine) is made by aspirating 1 ml of papaverine solution from 300-mg/10-ml vial and injecting it into a 5-mg vial of phentolamine (Regitine) powder. The powder is shaken until dissolved, then the mixture is aspirated and reinjected into the original papaverine vial to create a 10 ml solution containing 30 mg/ml of papaverine and 0.5 mg/ml of phentolamine. In patients with neurogenic impotence (e.g., SCI), a low dose of 0.1 to 0.2 ml of duo-mix is injected into one of the corpora cavernosa. If no erection occurs within 20 minutes, another injection is given which can be repeated up to a total of 1 ml of the duo-mix. The erection usually lasts 1 to 2 hrs and should subside in 4 hours. Phentolamine produces an alpha-adrenergic blockade, which reduces arterial resistance; however, it does not increase resistance to venous outflow and is less effective than papaverine.

(2) Tri-mix (papaverine + phentolamine + prostaglandin E_1) is made as follows: 0.2 ml (100 μg) of prostaglandin E_1 is added to a vial of papaverine (300 mg/10 ml); two 5-mg vials of phentolamine are reconstituted as described above for duo-mix; both solutions are then added to 6.8 ml of injectable normal saline to yield a total volume of 17 ml consisting of 17.6 mg/ml of papaverine, 0.58 mg/ml of phentolamine, and 5.9 μg/ml of PGE_1. The protocol and dose for injection is similar to that of the duo-mix. The use of low dose of PGE_1 in tri-mix reduces penile pain at the injection site.

2) Implantable penile prostheses can either be semirigid (hinged, malleable, or articulating) or inflatable (self-contained or multicomponent). Semirigid prostheses consist of two flexible silicone or polyurethane rods implanted into both corpora cavernosa to provide a permanent partial erection, which may not be noticeable if patient is sitting in a wheelchair but may be embarrassing in ambulatory patients. Inflatable prostheses consist of a pair of inflatable tubes, which are implanted adjacent to the corpora cavernosa, and which can be inflated to full erection using fluid from an abdominal wall reservoir by means of a pump located in the scrotum or deflated by opening a valve. Some of the manufacturers of penile prostheses include: American Medical System (AMS), Mentor, Dacomed, Jonas, and Small-Carrion. Penile prostheses must only be considered when other options have failed because patients with implants are often not able to benefit from other options because of the disruption of the normal anatomy. There is recent decline in the use of penile prostheses because of its complications (e.g., postoperative infection, urethral or corporal erosion and perforation, extrusion of the device, mechanical failure, and cosmetic deformity because of inadequate sizing) and the availability of other simpler, safer, cost-effective, nonsurgical methods of attaining erection (see above). The best results with penile prostheses have been obtained when they are used for maintenance of external catheters (i.e., semirigid hinged penile prostheses to keep condom catheters from falling off the penis) rather than for correction of sexual dysfunction due to erectile dysfunction.

2. **Ejaculation or emission failures** are seen in 30% of men with incomplete lower motor neuron lesions, 99% of men with complete upper motor neuron lesions, and 90% of men with TURP. Psychological reasons may also contribute to this problem. Emission, or secretion of seminal fluid into the posterior urethra, should be distinguished from actual ejaculation, that is, expulsion of fluid from the urethra to the outside (antegrade ejaculation) or back towards to the bladder (retrograde ejaculation). Retrograde ejaculation can be caused by failure of closure of the internal sphincter or the use of a constriction band in VTCT techniques. There is no known physiologic cure for both ejaculation or emission failure. Vibroejaculation and electroejaculation have been tried to induce ejaculation for procreative purposes (see section VI.A). Patients with ejaculation or emission dysfunction need counseling. They should also be told that orgasm or other pleasurable feelings are not always associated with ejaculation or emission. Awareness of mind and of other bodily changes can enhance their sensation of pleasure. Oral drugs reported to be beneficial for ejaculatory disturbances include propranolol (Inderal; see Chapter 4.8, section IX.A.5), clomipramine (Anafranil; see Chapter 4.8, section V.A.1.a.4), and fluoxetine (Prozac; see Chapter 4.8, section V.A.2). It is likely that their effect is secondary to their anxiolytic properties.

3. **Lubrication dysfunction** in women may be caused by similar events, which cause erectile dysfunction in men. In SCI women, vaginal lubrication may occur reflexively with lesions at T9 but not at all with lesions between T10 and T12, and psychogenic lubrication may occur in lesions below T12. Inadequate lubrication can lead to dyspareunea (i.e., painful coitus) or difficulty with attainment of orgasm. Its psychological ramifications (e.g., doubting of one's attractiveness or femininity) may affect relationships or potential relationships. As with male erection, similar reflexogenic and psychogenic means can be used to elicit lubrication. If needed, vaginal lubricants such as saliva, Astroglide, Aqualube, Replens, or K-Y jelly may be used. Patients should also be counseled that they could satisfy their sexual partners even without coitus (e.g., using a vibrator or through oral or digital sex). Likewise they could satisfy themselves through masturbation using manual or vibratory techniques.

4. **Difficulty in attaining orgasm** may be caused by physical dysfunction (e.g., sensory deficits, lubrication dysfunction, or SCI) or psychological reasons. In able-bodied females, approximately 10% have never achieved orgasm and up to 75% do not routinely achieve orgasm with penile thrusting alone. In men, orgasm may be attained without ejaculation or emission. Patients must be counseled that the brain can work independent of genitalia in the generation of erotic experience and that orgasm may be experienced differently than in premorbid states (e.g., in SCI patients it may be experienced as sudden enhancement of spasticity followed by prolonged relaxation; or it may just be a pleasurable sensation in the abdomen, pelvis, or thighs). Although pleasurable sensations are practically nonexistent below the level of complete upper motor neuron lesions, these patients may experience pleasure at the cutoff sensory level (especially common at the T4 or T5 level) or at nongenital erogenous zones (e.g., neck or ears).

B. **Mechanical dysfunctions** that interfere with sexual activity may result from problems related to bladder or bowel care or problems in positioning (e.g., because of pain, weakness, limited range of motion, or spasticity). If a comfortable position for coitus cannot be attained, masturbation or mutual masturbation may be considered.

1. **Positioning difficulties due to**

   a. **Spasticity** can be reduced by movements that inhibit spasticity (e.g., performing sexual motions slowly, slow rocking motions; gentle shaking, or slow stroking); by using heat or cold modalities; by using antispasticity agents (see Chapter 5.4 section III.D.1); or by experimenting with different sexual positioning that lessens spasticity (e.g., positioning a bolster between the knees may decrease adduction spasticity or scissoring of the hips).

   b. **Weakness** can be alleviated by using physical support (e.g., pillows, towels, or even bolsters) to prop up body parts, or if pelvic thrusting is difficult (e.g., in patients with poor arm or leg function), the down position with the partner on top may be tried.

   c. **Decreased range of motion (ROM)** can be accommodated with rear entry or side-lying sexual positions (e.g., in patients with arthritis or hip flexion contractures).

   d. **Pain** can be reduced with side-lying or partner-on-top positions (to reduce stress on the joints), scheduling sexual activities when pain is diminished (e.g., after taking pain medications), or taking a warm bath.

   e. **Low endurance** can be accommodated by assuming positions in which sexual performance takes less energy (usual positions with the same partner are least stressful; positions that do not restrict breathing; consider masturbation as it requires less energy than coitus) and timing of sex when there is most energy or after resting (e.g., upon waking up).

2. **Bladder and bowel problems,** especially incontinence during sex is of high concern in both disabled men and women. To avoid embarrassing reflex loss of urine during intercourse, patients are advised to limit fluid intake during the hours preceding sexual activity and to empty their bladder prior to having intercourse (e.g., self-catheterization or suprapubic tapping to elicit a bladder contraction). Likewise, patients with bowel incontinence should avoid heavy meals and should empty their bowels (e.g., using enema) prior to sexual activities. In men with indwelling catheters, the catheter may be folded on itself (if needed, taped to the side of the penis) and covered with a condom. In the disabled woman, the indwelling catheter tube may be taped to the abdomen and ignored. If so desired, the catheter may be removed just prior to intercourse and then replaced afterward. Patients with SCI lesions above T6 should be counseled on how to recognize and acutely manage autonomic dysreflexia (see Chapter 5.7, section V.F) as it may be triggered by a distended bladder or orgasm. After sexual activities, patients are advised to void or to catheterize themselves to lessen the chances of urinary tract infection.

C. **Psychosocial dysfunctions** that may play a role in sexual dysfunction, include social isolation (e.g., from poor sexual-social skills to attract a partner), altered body image and self-concept, inability of the disabled person or partner to accept changes in sexual functioning because of the disability (e.g., role changes of patient and partner), unhealthy attitudes and perceptions of the patient by others, poor judgment, egocentricity, emotional lability, disinhibition, low tolerance for delayed gratification, and poor memory. They may result in sexual desire disorders (hypoactive or hyperactive sexual desires), sexual aversion disorders, sexual arousal disorders (female sexual arousal disorder, male erectile disorder), orgasm disorder (inhibited female orgasm, inhibited male orgasm, premature ejaculation), sexual pain disorder (dyspareunias and vaginismus), and sexual dysfunction not otherwise specified.

Treatment of sexual problems because of psychosocial dysfunction is more intensive than the sexual rehabilitation counseling given by clinicians within the context of the patient's other rehabilitation problems. It involves sex therapy in which sex is assumed to be the highest priority at the time of treatment. Sex therapy may be in the form of prolonged and intensive psychotherapy (integrating psychodynamic, systems, behavioral, and cognitive approaches), which often involves intrapersonal and psychological issues and relationship counseling. It may also include behavioral modification and intensive symptom-oriented sex therapy. It may be done in an individual setting or it may involve family or couple therapy. Group therapy settings may also be used. For a free list of a specially trained professional or professional sexual therapists in each state, the clinician should send a self-addressed, self-stamped business envelope to the American Association of Sex Educators, Counselors, and Therapists, P.O. Box 238, Mount Vernon, Iowa 52314.

V. Sexual rehabilitation counseling can be approached using the following models:

A. PLISSIT (or P-LI-SS-IT) counseling model, which was developed by Annon (1980), refers to three levels of brief counseling (i.e., **P**ermission, **L**imited **I**nformation, and **S**pecific **S**uggestions) and a fourth level of **I**ntensive **T**herapy. All physiatrists should be skilled in the first two levels of counseling, permission and limited information. Some may have further training and develop the skills needed to intervene at the third level, specific suggestions. Patients needing intensive therapy because of psychosocial dysfunction should be referred to appropriate sources (see section IV.C). General information about sex may be obtained from Sex Information and Education Council of the United States (SIECUS), 130 W. 42nd St., Suite 2500, New York, NY 10036, tel. (212) 819-9770; Through the Looking Glass, 2198 6th St., Suite 100, Berkeley, CA 94710, tel. (510) 848-1112; and United Cerebral Palsy Associates, 1660 L St., NW, #770, Washington, DC 20036-5682, tel. (800) USA-5UCP.

1. **P—permission** is the first and most basic level of sexual counseling. The clinician generates an attitude in which the patient with sexual concerns senses permission and feels comfortable to ask questions, seek advice, and experiment about sexual issues. This can be done by asking leading questions, initiating talk about sensitive subjects (do not expect the patient to initiate the discussion), or simply by listening to the spoken or body language of the patient or making observations about physical manifestations such as reflex erections in SCI men. The mere taking of a sexual history usually produces a therapeutic effect by giving the patient permission to be sexual, filling knowledge gaps, and providing reality-based feedback. Patients are reassured that their sexual concerns are neither unique nor unusual and that sexuality is a legitimate concern in the rehabilitation process. Permission is directed toward their thoughts, fantasies, feelings, and sexual activities that do not carry the risk of being dangerous or illegal. To develop proficiency on this level, the clinician should read general textbooks and review articles about sexuality (see examples under Supplemental Reading).

2. **LI—limited information** entails provision of specific limited information for general problem solving of a specific sexual concern, either by the clini-

cian or by way of educational materials. This limited information is typically educational and nonpersonal and deals with the disability and its implications on sexual health in a general sense (for cardiac patients, see Table 5.13-2). It gives factual information, which serves to dispel general sexual myths relating to breast and genital size, masturbation, oral-genital contact, anal intercourse, sexual frequency, etc. The disabled persons may also be given information about alternative methods of giving and receiving sexual pleasure (e.g., to seek out new areas of hypersensitivity or erogenous zones), changes in sexual response secondary to disease or medications, and fertility. The overall goal is to change relevant attitudes and behavior. The limited information can be provided during physical examination (see section III.B). Limited information should be provided to family and significant others as well (see examples of pamphlets or educational handouts listed under supplemental reading).

3. **SS—specific suggestions** is the third and final level of brief counseling. It involves providing specific suggestions about sexual concerns and dysfunctions, e.g., sensate focus exercises. The clinician takes a limited history about the sexual problem, including a description of the problem, its onset and course, the patient's concept of cause and maintenance of the problem, past treatment, and current expectations and goals of treatment. Specific suggestions tailored to the patient's sexual concerns and dysfunctions are then provided. These interventions are usually simple, have a behavioral focus, and need to be practiced either alone or with a partner at home. Specific techniques (see also section IV.A.1.a) include sexual positioning for comfortable lovemaking, sensual ways of undressing, exploration of erogenous zones, foreplay techniques, the use of erotic fantasy, use of available sexual mechanical devices, and ways of dealing with urinary or bowel problems. Peer counseling may also be helpful. Examples of books with specific suggestions (e.g., different lovemaking options) for patients with sexual dysfunction are listed under Supplemental Reading.

4. **IT—intensive therapy** is indicated for patients whose sexual dysfunction is caused by deep-seated psychosocial dysfunctions (see section IV.C).

B. **ENIGMA counseling model** is part of the process of assessment and recommendation for sexual satisfaction (PARSS), the main goal being to minimize sexual dysfunction and maximize sexual satisfaction by enabling patients to express their concerns openly and to offer them counseling and education, whenever possible. It encompasses the first three levels of brief counseling in the PLISSIT model (i.e., P-LI-SS) and includes specific strategies for the physician to initiate discussions related to sexual concerns (e.g., incorporating sexual counseling and education to physical examination; see section III.B). The ENIGMA model is open-ended and allows the patient to make sexual issues an ongoing subject for subsequent doctor's visits.

1. **E—engage** the patient in conversation, which provides opportunities to discuss topics that may not be directly sexual, such as, history of surgery or other significant medical conditions. In this step, the clinician can determine the patient's interpersonal skills for expression of need, as well as the status of the patient's current relationships. Although the first contact may be solely with the patient, the patient's partner should be included as soon as the patient gives permission.

2. **N—normalize** and legitimize the patient's sexual interest and activity. In a matter-of-fact open discussion, acknowledge individual variations; clarify

sexual concerns, preferences, interests, experiences, values; and clarify satisfaction with sexual functioning and the existence and nature of any problem with sexual functioning. The goal is to help patients gain self-acceptance and to validate their sexual interests.

3. I—inform the patient and partner about sexual physiology and anatomy thus answering their questions in a more natural fashion. This step includes a thorough, frank but sensitive education of function and response, both physical and emotional, of the disabling condition and its effects on motor and sensory function, communication, cognition, and fertility, a discussion on health issues relevant to patient's sexual behavior (e.g., risk factors for HIV), reeducation about masturbation, and discussion about health issues relevant to the patient's medications.

4. G—guide the patient and his or her partner by responding in the same language the patient uses (may be vernacular) and metaphors, rather than in medical terminology (e.g., ''hard-on'' for erection and ''come'' for experiencing orgasm). Problems such as pain, spasticity, decreased endurance, and bowel and bladder function may also be introduced by the clinician.

5. M—maximize their problem-solving ability by encouraging experimentation, reading, and peer counseling. This step includes discussion on experimentation of masturbation, sexual aids (e.g., vibrators), or couple-play and provision of a list of reading materials (medical and lay) or educational videos about sexual issues (see examples of reading materials listed under the PLISSIT section).

6. A—assess and reassess the sexual issues at subsequent visits and make it an ongoing subject, not a one-time thing. At each visit, briefly review a checklist through the ENIGMA model to monitor progress, hang-ups or anxiety, and acceptance of each area. This step may include patient reassurance about their anxieties and misconceptions (e.g., on issues about sex after heart attack [see Table 5.13-2], hysterectomy, stroke, or life-altering medical conditions), discussion about the patient's sexual experience since the onset of the disability, and assessment of interpersonal and psychosocial factors that may enhance or interfere with sexual relationships.

VI. Related sexual issues including fertility, contraception, pregnancy, delivery, and lactation may not be the primary domain of physiatry; however, if proper sexual counseling and education is to be given to the patient, the physiatrist should at least be knowledgeable about these issues. An excellent resource is Haseltine FP, Cole SS, Gray DB: *Reproductive issues for persons with physical disabilities*, Baltimore, 1993, Paul H. Brooks.

A. Male fertility is retained in most types of physical disabilities; however, in men with SCI, infertility may occur. The spontaneous fertility rate in men with complete and incomplete SCI is less than 10%. In general, men with incomplete lesions are more likely to be fertile than those with complete lesions. Among patients with incomplete SCI, lower motor neuron lesions are more likely to be fertile than are those with upper motor neuron lesions. Possible reasons for infertility causing poor semen quality include stasis of prostatic fluid, testicular hyperthermia (which can be caused by the lifestyle of sitting in wheelchair with thighs together or crossed, not shifting position frequently, or wearing tight clothes; some studies have shown that lowering the testicular temperature can reverse the maturation arrest caused by the increased temperature), repeated urinary tract infections (UTIs), abnormal testicular histology (decreased spermatogenesis and interstitial sclerosis; testicular atrophy, which is commonly associated with weakness and marked debility), sperm contact with urine (e.g., in retrograde ejaculation), possible changes in the hypothalamic-pituitary-testicular axis (although most studies seem to indicate close to normal levels of testosterone and gonadotropin with an intact hypothalamus-pituitary-testicular axis), possible antisperm antibodies (because of blockage of ductal tracts and UTIs), and long-term use of various medications (e.g., nitrofurantoin can cause temporary spermatogenesis arrest in rats). Other reasons for male infertility may arise from ejaculatory failure, obstruction of genital passages, impairment of spermatogenesis, or a combination of the above. Methods of collecting sperm (which can be kept in a sperm bank and used for in-vivo or in-vitro fertilization) include the following:

1. **Electroejaculation (EEJ)** is currently the most common method used in the United States. It involves transrectal electrical stimulation (using 5-30 V, 200-500 mA, 60 Hz current) of the myelinated preganglionic efferent sympathetic fibers of the hypogastric plexi to obtain seminal emission into the posterior urethra, from where the semen can be obtained by milking the urethral bulb and by catheterization. Its effectiveness is unrelated to the duration of injury (may be used successfully within the first 6 months postinjury) or to the level of injury as long as T10-L1 spinal segments are intact. It may be successful even in patients with conus or caudal lesions. The sperm collected by EEJ appears to have decreased motility, with normal fertility seen in only 25% (probably because of the use of electric current and aqueous jelly and changes in semen osmolarity). The semen quality, however, seems to improve by repeated ejaculation. Electroejaculation must be done in an office or hospital setting because of the need to monitor for autonomic dysreflexia (AD) and to do anoscopy to evaluate the rectal mucosa. Pretreatment with sublingual nifedipine (10 mg) for patients with lesion above T6 has decreased the risk of AD. Patients with incomplete lesions may need anesthesia because of pain.

2. **Vibroejaculation (VEJ)** involves the use of a vibrator (e.g., Ling vibrator or Relax vibrator) applied to glans, frenulum, shaft, or base of the penis of patients with lesions above T10 or intact conus and cauda equina (i.e., intact lumbosacral reflexes, e.g., reflex hip flexion after stroking the bottom of the foot and positive bulbocavernosus reflex). Suggested vibratory parameters are 2.5 mm peak-to-peak amplitude at a frequency of 100 Hz applied for 3 minutes (may be repeated for 6 consecutive times after 1 to 2 minutes of rest in between stimulation). Its advantages include noninvasiveness, home use, possibility of "natural" fertilization, less likely occurrence of retrograde ejaculation, and overall better quality semen (fertility rate is about 50% of SCI males). With weekly use of the VEJ, the quantity and quality of sperm seems to improve. The main disadvantage of VEJ is the unpredictability of response in many patients and the high risk of AD in patients with lesions above T6 (may give pretreatment of 10 mg of sublingual nifedipine). Moreover, unlike EEJ, it does not work during the spinal shock period (which may occur within the first 6 months up to a year postinjury). Adjunctive use of neostigmine (Prostigmine) is not recommended as it can lead to greater risk of AD and even death.

3. **Chemical ejaculation** involves the use drugs or chemical agents to improve ejaculation and the quality of the sperm. Oral alpha-adrenergic agonists (pseudoephrine, 60 mg, qid; or imipramine, 25 mg, bid; or ephedrine, 50

mg, qid; or phenylpropanolamine, 75 mg, bid) have been used to convert retrograde to anterograde ejaculation. If this is unsuccessful, the retrograde ejaculation may be harvested either by having the patient void (almost completely) prior to masturbation and then collecting the postejaculatory voided urine. To ensure optimal sperm survival, the bladder may be washed with a sperm-processing buffer after which 30 ml of the buffer is left in the bladder and the patient masturbates and collects the postejaculate fluid. The collected ejaculate is then processed carefully to obtain a concentrated healthy sample of sperm. The use of such drugs as physostigmine or neostigmine has lost favor because of complications, mainly autonomic dysreflexia.

4. **Direct extraction of sperm** can be attempted through cannulation of the vas deferens when the other methods have failed.

5. **Surgery** may be done to release obstructed passages of the vas deferens, epididymis, and seminiferous tubules, all of which can be the result of repeated UTIs.

B. **Female fertility** is usually not affected by most disabilities. In SCI women, menses may continue without interruption or they may temporarily cease, returning to normal within about 6 months or up to a year. Once their menstrual periods return, fertility returns to preinjury levels. Because their first few ovulation cycles may be unpredictable, SCI women engaging in sexual activities must consider contraception (see next section) from the beginning.

C. **Contraception methods** with the lowest failure rates in able-bodied women are oral progestin-estrogen contraceptives, subdermal Norplant, intrauterine devices (IUDs), and sterilization. Failure rates are commonly reported as either optimal failure (i.e., failure of the method despite correct use) or typical failure (i.e., failure caused by incorrect use).

1. **Barrier methods** either kill spermatozoa or block their entry into the cervix. They are reversible and are among the safest methods (if properly used); however, patients need to be highly motivated to use it with each coitus. In patients with poor hand dexterity, adaptive applicators may be used or the partner may help in putting it on.

a. **Condom** for men consists of a cylindrical sheath (usually made of latex) applied to the erect penis; while the condom for women consists of a polyurethane pouch which lines the vagina and partially covers the perineum. Both male and female condoms are readily available, do not need a prescription, are relatively inexpensive, and have the additional advantage of being the only contraceptive method that offers protection against STDs, including HIV. They must be reapplied for each act of coitus. Female condoms have recently been available commercially (e.g., Reality) but are not as popular as male condoms because they are relatively more expensive and more cumbersome to use.

The following discussions are about male condoms. The tip of the penile condom should extend beyond the end of the erect penis by about one half inch to collect the ejaculate. They are available as nonlubricated or lubricated (may contain spermicides). If the condom needs to be lubricated (e.g., to protect indwelling catheter), a water-based lubricant (e.g., Aqua-Lube, Astroglide, and K-Y jelly) should be used to preserve the integrity of the condom latex. Oil-based lubricants, e.g., Vaseline, should not be used as they weaken the latex. For patients with allergy to latex, nonlatex condoms (e.g., lamb's intestine) are available, although they may not offer the same protection against STDs as latex condoms. The taste of the condom may be offensive for oral sex. The optimal failure rate of the penile condom is 2%, but its typical failure rate is 12%.

b. Spermicides (nonoxynol-9), which must be applied within 30 minutes before coitus, are available as an intravaginal sponge, foam, jelly, cream, gel, suppository, or film. Among the vehicles of spermicide application, the sponge (i.e., cervical sponge) is the most popular because it is effective for 24 hours and does not have to be reinserted into the vagina before each coitus. Spermicides are readily available and do not require prescription. Side effects include toxic shock syndrome (incidence is slightly higher in users of the sponge) and allergy to the spermicide. Its optimal failure rate is 3 to 9%, and typical failure rate is as high as 21 to 28%.

c. Diaphragm is a shallow, dome-shaped rubber cup with flexible rim, which is inserted between the posterior vaginal wall and the recess behind the pubic arch. It must be initially fitted by a health care professional, after which the user must be taught how to insert and remove it. Patients with weakened pelvic muscles may not be able to hold the diaphragm in place. Spermicide cream or jelly must be applied to the diaphragm and added intravaginally each time coitus is repeated, especially more than 8 hours after diaphragm insertion. After coitus, the diaphragm must be left in place for at least 8 hours but not more than 24 hours. Using it more than 24 hours increases the risks for UTI (because of mechanical obstruction of urine outflow) and for vaginal ulceration. Its optimal failure rate is 6%, and its typical failure rate is as high as 18%.

d. Cervical cap is a deep, soft rubber cup with a firm round rim. It is commonly used in Europe and is available in the United States as Prentif cavity-rim cervical cap. As with the diaphragm, it is initially fitted onto the cervix by a health professional, after which the patient is taught how to insert and remove it and to place spermicide inside the cap before each use. It can be left in place for up to 48 hours (longer use may cause ulceration, unpleasant odor, or infection). Users are advised to have a Pap smear done every 3 months to detect any abnormal cervical cytology. Its optimal failure rate is 6%, and typical failure rate is as high as 18%.

2. Intrauterine device consists of a flexible, usually plastic device inserted by a physician into the patient's uterus. To increase its contraceptive effectiveness, metal or hormones (e.g., progesterone) may be added. The most commonly used metal is copper (e.g., copper T-380A), which interferes with the effects of estrogen or progesterone on the endometrium. The IUD produces a local sterile inflammatory response caused by the presence of a foreign body in the uterus, which causes lysis of the blastocyst and sperm and the prevention of implantation. It also has deleterious effects on spermatozoa as they pass through the uterus. Adverse effects of the IUD include pelvic inflammatory disease (PID) and abnormal uterine bleeding patterns. Contraindications include cervicitis, vaginitis, endometritis, PID, a nonmonogamous sexual relationship, history of STD, or ectopic pregnancy. Manual dexterity is needed to regularly check for its placement. In SCI patients, IUD may be easier to insert; however, because of sensory deficit, there is a higher incidence of bleeding, cramping, perforation of the uterus, or PID. Hence, IUD is not the best choice for contraception in SCI women. But if it is used at all, SCI women must be taught how to look for spotting, irregular periods, increased spasticity, fever, and increased or unusual vaginal discharge. The optimal failure rate is 2% (progesterone IUD) or 0.8% (copper T-380A), and the typical failure rate is less than 2% for the progesterone IUD and less than 1% for the copper T-380A.

3. **Hormonal contraception** works by altering cervical mucus, thus inhibiting sperm transport; by inhibiting ovulation; and by causing atrophy of the endometrium, thus inhibiting implantation. Contraindications include active thromboembolic disease, undiagnosed vaginal bleeding, breast cancer, and acute liver disease.

   a. Oral steroid contraceptives

   1) Progestin-estrogen contraceptives (the "pill") are the most effective type of oral contraceptives because they consistently inhibit the mid-cycle gonadotrophin surge and thus prevent ovulation. However, they carry the risk of venous thromboembolism (especially in SCI patients) and are associated with cardiovascular, cerebrovascular, and thrombophlebitic disease. They are strongly contraindicated in women with severe headaches, hypertension, diabetes, smokers over age 35, long leg casts or with major surgery to the legs, anticipated elective surgery within 4 weeks, and sickle cell disease. There are multiple brands available. The brand name contains the number of the dose of both progestin and estrogen. Triphasic pills change the dosing of the components throughout the cycle and can be identified by "tri-" in the name or by the use of three numbers instead of two.

   The FDA recommends using the least amount of estrogen (e.g., 35 μg or less of ethinyl estradiol) and progestin (1 mg or less of norethindrone) that is compatible with a low failure rate and the need of the individual patient, such as Ortho-Novum 1/35, Ovcon 35, Norinyl 1 + 35, Loestrin 1.5/30, or Tri-Norinyl. The combination pill is given daily 3 out of every 4 weeks (e.g., started on the Sunday after period begins). If estrogen-related or progesterone-related side effects occur with one formulation, a different agent with less estrogenic or progesterogenic activity can be given. For example, if symptoms of estrogen excess occurs (e.g., weight gain or breast tenderness), change to a lower estrogen concentration (e.g., 30 μg) or instead of using norethindrone, change to a progestin with less estrogenic effect such as norgestrel (Lo/Ovral), norgestimate (Ortho-Tri-Cyclen), or levonorgestrel (Levlen, Tri-Levlen, or Triphasil); if symptoms of androgen excess occurs (e.g., nausea, dizziness, acne, hirsutism, and pruritus), change to a progestin with fewer androgenic effects such as ethynodiol diacetate (Demulen); if menses are missed and patient is not pregnant, it is probably because of estrogen deficiency, which can be treated by increasing the estrogen (e.g., 50 μg). The optimal failure rate for combination progestin-estrogen is 0.1%, but its typical failure rate is 3%.

   2) Progestin-only pills (POPs) or "minipill" may be used by women who must avoid estrogens. Although POPs (e.g., norethindrone [Micronol, NorQD], 0.35 mg, given daily, every day of the year, starting on the first day of menstruation) have a lower incidence of adverse metabolic effects, they cause high frequency of abnormal uterine bleeding patterns. The optimal failure rate for POPs is 0.5%, but its typical failure rate is 3%.

3) Estrogen compounds ("morning after pills") may be used as postcoital oral contraception or as emergency contraception (e.g., when condom breaks). They have good effectiveness if used within 72 hours after coitus and if taken for 5 days. They include diethylstilbestrol (DES), 25 to 50 mg/day; ethynyl estradiol, 5 mg/day; and conjugated estrogens, 30 mg/day. The higher dose estrogens are most effective with an overall failure rate of 0.7%.

b. **Injectable long-acting steroid contraceptives** include the commonly used depo-medroxyprogesterone (DMPA) (Depo-Provera), given at 150 mg, IM, every 3 months, and other agents such as norethindrone enanthate given at 200 mg, IM, every 2 months, and other once-a-month injections of combinations of different progestins and estrogens. The DMPA is highly efficacious and requires no motivation after injection; however, users may experience intermittent spotting, and 50% become amenorrheic at the end of 1 year of use. There are variable rates of return of fertility, controversy over carcinogenicity, and occurrence of progesterone side effects (e.g., headache, weight gain, and depression). Its optimal failure rate is 0.3%, and its typical failure rate is likewise 0.3%.

c. **Levonorgestrel (Norplant)** consists of six Silastic capsules, each containing 36 mg of levonorgestrel, which are implanted into the forearm (for 5 years). Once inserted, it requires no motivation for use. When removed, there is rapid return of fertility. Side effects include frequent irregular menstrual bleeding and progesterone-related side effects (e.g., headaches, weight gain, depression, and psychic symptoms similar to menopause or premenstrual syndrome). Its optimal failure rate is 0.2%, and its typical failure rate is likewise 0.2%. It is a good option for women who do not desire children for a period of years and has the added benefit of reducing or totally eliminating menstrual bleeding, which can facilitate hygiene. Unlike estrogenic agents, it has not been shown to produce thromboembolic, cerebrovascular, or cardiovascular disease; however, patients need to be monitored for hypertension and thrombophlebitis. Its effectiveness in SCI women needs to be studied.

4. **Natural family planning** involves periodic abstinence during the days of the menstrual cycle when the ovum can be fertilized. It includes the calendar rhythm method, basal body temperature method, cervical mucus methods, and symptothermal method (combination of the calendar, temperature, and cervical mucus methods; more effective but more difficult to learn). It requires training, strong motivation, and can only be used in woman with regular cycles. It has relatively high failure rates (optimal failure rate of 1-9% and typical failure rate of 20%). In SCI women, the basal body temperature method is extremely unreliable because of poor temperature control.

5. **Sterilization** includes bilateral tubal ligation in women or vasectomy in men. The optimal failure rate is 0.1% (for men) and 0.2% (for women), but the typical failure rate is 0.15% (for men) and 0.4% (for women). Sterilization is generally not reversible.

6. **Induced abortion** is controversial. The patient (preferably with the patient's partner) should receive proper counseling.

7. **Experimental methods** for women include the vaginal contraceptive pill,

contraceptive vaccine, and pills to terminate early pregnancy, e.g., RU-486. For men, they include the contraceptive pill, contraceptive implant system, injectable contraception, contraceptive vaccine, and percutaneous vasectomy (via small puncture hole of scrotal skin).

D. Pregnancy once attained usually progresses without difficulty in a disabled woman. Possible problems include UTIs (acidification of urine and hydration may help; see Chapter 5.7, section V.A), anemia (the hematocrit should be monitored; iron supplements should be given and, if needed, blood transfusion), constipation (suppositories and stool softeners may be used; see Chapter 5.8, section VI.B.3), altered balance due the expanding uterus (wheelchair-bound patients may need seating system modifications [see Chapter 4.7]; ambulatory patients may need assistive devices to prevent falls and possible fractures [see Chapter 4.6]), thrombophlebitis (see Chapter 5.3), pressure ulcers (see Chapter 5.2), deconditioning (see Chapter 5.1), osteoporosis (may be due to immobility; treat with calcium-rich diet), premature labor, small-for-date infants, and toxemia of pregnancy (especially in patients with repeated UTIs). However, there is no increase in the number of spontaneous abortions. As with able-bodied women, disabled women should receive regular prenatal care with an obstetrician-gynecologist who is knowledgeable about disabled women. The role of the physiatrist is to educate both the patient and other physicians concerning disability-related issues, e.g., on the recognition and management of AD in women with lesion above T6 (see Chapter 5.7, section V.F).

E. Labor takes place normally in most disabled patients because the uterus retains its ability to contract, despite denervation, due to hormonal influences. Due to paralysis of the abdominal muscles, however, the expulsive force may be ineffective, hence forceps delivery or episiotomy (because patient may not sense tears during delivery due to perineal insensitivity) may be necessary. In most SCI women, the discomfort of labor is felt as in able-bodied women, and the onset of labor is typically detected as a different sensation. Labor contractions may be stronger, more prolonged, and more frequent, but the duration of labor is shorter than for the able-bodied women. Women with complete SCI lesions above T10 will not appreciate uterine contractions or fetal movement; therefore, they need to be admitted to the maternity ward about 10 days before their estimated date of birth to prevent a precipitous, unsupervised birth due to the inability to feel the onset of labor. Spinal cord injury per se is not an indication for caesarean section (except in women with lesions at T10-T11 as the uterus is deprived of all reflex function), and it should only be performed when indicated (as with able-bodied women).

In women with lesions above T6, autonomic dysreflexia occurring during labor should be distinguished from eclampsia or preeclampsia. In AD, blood pressure rises with contractions, and falls between contractions; there is headache, piloerection, and tachycardia or reflex bradycardia; and it does not respond to magnesium sulfate. While in toxemia of pregnancy, there is hypertension, proteinuria, edema, and the blood pressure increase is not episodic and is not associated with uterine contractions or bowel or bladder distension. Treatment of choice for AD during labor is epidural anesthesia, which can be administered continuously. Other alternatives include oral antihypertensives (e.g., premedication with Arfonad) or immediate delivery if the blood pressure cannot be controlled by any other means. Post partum, there is a high incidence of UTI and venous thrombosis.

F. Lactation (breast-feeding) can be successfully administered by disabled mothers (although it may require adaptation of wheelchairs or assistance from others). As in all nursing mothers, any medication that is not absolutely necessary for the mother's health should be discontinued. Women with lesions above T6 usually experience a decrease in milk production after 6 weeks (possibly due to lack of nipple sensation). For contraception in lactating women, the following "rule of 3s" applies: for women giving full breastfeeding, a contraceptive method should be used at the beginning of the third postpartum *month*; however, for women giving partial breastfeeding or no breastfeeding, a contraceptive method should begin during the third postpartum *week*.

BIBLIOGRAPHY

Annon JS, Robinson CH: Treatment of common male and female sexual concerns. In Ferguson JM, Taylor CB, editors: *The comprehensive handbook of behavioral medicine*, vol 1, New York, 1980, SP Medical & Scientific Books, pp 273-296.

Baum N, Rhodes D: A practical approach to the evaluation and treatment of erectile dysfunction: a private practitioner's viewpoint, *Urol Clin North Am* 22(4):865-878, 1995.

Berard EJJ: The sexuality of spinal cord injured women: physiology and pathophysiology: a review, *Paraplegia* 27:99-112, 1989.

Boone TB: Evaluation and management of impotence in physically disabled men, *Phys Med Rehabil State Art Rev* 9(2):523-537, 1995.

Cheadle MJ: The screening sexual history: getting to the problem, *Clin GeriatrMed* 7:9-13, 1991.

Cole TM, Cole SS. Rehabilitation of problems of sexuality in physical disability. In Kottke FJ, Stillwell G, Lehmann JF, editors: *Krusen's handbook of physical medicine and rehabilitation*, ed 4, Philadelphia, 1990, WB Saunders, pp 988-1008.

Derogatis LR: Psychological assessment of psychosexual functions, *Psych Clin North Am* 3(1):113-131, 1980.

Ducharme S, Gill KM, Biener-Bergman S, et al: Sexual functioning: medical and psychological aspects. In DeLisa JA, Gans BM, editors: *Rehabilitation medicine: principles and practice*, ed 2, Philadelphia, 1993, JB Lippincott, pp. 763-782.

Gilbert DM: Sexuality issues in persons with disabilities. In Braddom RL, editor: *Physical medicine and rehabilitation*, Philadelphia, 1996, WB Saunders, pp 605-629.

Hatcher RA, Trussel J, Stewart F, et al: *Contraceptive technology*, ed 16, New York, 1994, Irvington.

Hirshkowitz M, Ware JC: Studies of nocturnal penile tumescence and rigidity. In Singer C, Weiner WJ, editors: *Sexual dysfunction: a neuro-medical approach*, Armonk, NY, 1994, Futura, pp 77-99.

Masters WH, Johnson VE, Kolodny RC: *Human sexuality*, Boston, 1982, Little, Brown.

Mishell DR: Overview of contraception. In Wallach EE, Zacur HA, editors: *Reproductive medicine and surgery*. St. Louis, 1995, Mosby–Year Book, pp 289-316.

Morales A, Heaton JPW, Johnston B, et al: Oral and topical treatment of erectile dysfunction: present and future. *Urol Clin North Amer* 22(4):879-886, 1995.

Ohl DA, Menge AC, Sonksen J: Penile vibratory stimulation in spinal cord injured men: optimized vibration parameters and prognostic factors. *Arch Phys Med Rehabil* 77:903-905, 1996.

O'Keefe M, Hunt DK: Assessment and treatment of impotence. *Med Clin North Am* 79(2):415-434, 1995.

Padma-Nathan H: Neurophysiological studies of sexual dysfunction. In Singer C, Weiner WJ, editors: *Sexual dysfunction: a neuro-medical approach*, Armonk, NY, 1994, Futura, pp 101-115.

Physicians' desk reference, ed 51, Montvale, NJ, 1997, Medical Economics.

Rohe DE: Sexuality and disability. In Sinaki M, editor: *Basic clinical rehabilitation medicine*, St. Louis, 1994, Mosby–Year Book, pp 425-432.

Sipsky ML, Alexander CJ, Rosen RC: Orgasm in women with spinal cord injuries: a laboratory-based assessment, *Arch Phys Med Rehabil* 76:1097-1102, 1995.

Smith EM, Bodner DR: Sexual dysfunction after spinal cord injury. *Urol Clin of North Am* 20(3):535-541, 1993.

Speroff L, Darney P: *A clinical guide for contraception*, ed 2, Baltimore, 1996, Williams & Wilkins.

Yarkony GM, Chen D: Sexuality in patients with spinal cord–injury. *Phys Med Rehabil State Art Rev* 9(2):325-344, 1995.

Supplemental reading

General references about sexuality

Brecher EM, and the Editors of Consumer Report Books: *Love, sex, and aging*, Boston, 1984, Little, Brown.

Butler RN, Lewis MI: *Love and sex after sixty: a guide for men and women for their later years*, New York, 1976, Perennial Publications.

Comfort A: *Sexual consequences of disability*, Philadelphia, 1978, GF Stickley.

Croft LH: *Sexuality in later life: a counseling guide for physicians*, Boston, 1982, John Wright.

Hite S: *The Hite report*, New York, 1976, Macmillan.

Kaplan HS: *The evaluation of sexual disorders: psychological and medical aspects*, New York, 1983, Brunner-Mazel.

Kennedy E: *Sexual counseling: a practical guide for those who help others*, New York, 1989, Continuum Publishing Co.

Klein E, Kroll K: *Enabling romance: a guide to love, sex, and relationships for the disabled*, New York, 1992, Harmony Books (Crown).

Lief HI, editor: *Sexual problems in medical practice*, Monroe, Wisconsin, 1981, American Medical Association.

Masters WH, Johnson VE, Kolodny RC: *Human sexuality*, Boston, 1982, Little, Brown.

Munjack DJ, Oziel LJ: *Sexual medicine and counseling in office practice: a comprehensive treatment guide*, Boston, 1980, Little, Brown.

Neidstadt ME, Feida M: *Choices: a guide to sex counseling with physically disabled adults*, Malabar, FL, 1987, Krieger.

Sandowski C: *Sexual concern when illness or disability strikes*, Springfield, 1989, Charles C. Thomas.

Schover LR, Jensen JB: *Sexuality and chronic illness: a comprehensive approach*, New York, 1988, Guilford Press.

Yoselle H: *Sexuality in later years*, Rockville, MD, 1981, Aspen Systems.

Pamphlets and educational handouts about sexuality for the disabled

Sexuality after spinal cord injury: fact sheet No. 3, 1987, National Spinal Cord Injury Association.

Male reproductive function after spinal cord injury: fact sheet No. 10, 1988, National Spinal Cord Injury Association.

Boggs J: *Living and loving with arthritis: information on sex and arthritis*, 1978, Honolulu, Honolulu Arthritis Center of Hawaii.

Books or articles with specific suggestions for patients with sexual dysfunction

Bregman S: *Sexuality and the spinal cord injured woman*, Minneapolis, 1975, Sister Kenny Foundation.

Cole SS, Hossler CJ: Intimacy and chronic lung disease. In Fishman AP, editor: *Pulmonary rehabilitation*. New York, 1996, Marcel Dekker, pp 251-287.

Comfort A, editor: *The joy of sex: a gourmet guide to lovemaking*, New York, 1972, Simon & Schuster.

Gregory MF: *Sexual adjustment: a guide for the spinal cord injured*, Bloomington, Illinois, 1993, Accent on Living.

Griffith ER, Lemberg S: *Sexuality and the person with traumatic brain injury: a guide for families*, Philadelphia, 1993, FA Davis.

Herbert L: *Sex and back pain*, Bloomington, MN, 1987, Educational Opportunities.

Leyson JF: *Sexual rehabilitation of the spinal-cord-injured patient*, Totowa, 1991, Humana Press.

McCormick GP, Riffer DJ, Thompson MM: Coital positioning for stroke afflicted couples, *Rehabil Nurs* 11:17-19, 1986.

Mooney TO, Cole TM, Chilgren RA: *Sexual options for paraplegics and quadriplegics*, Boston, 1975, Little, Brown.

Rabin BJ: *The sensuous wheeler*, Long Beach, CA, 1980, Barry J. Rabin.

CHAPTER 5.10

ACUTE AND CHRONIC PAIN

Pain is defined by the International Association for the Study of Pain as "an unpleasant sensory and emotional experience usually associated with actual or potential tissue damage, or described in terms of such damage." It is one of the most common reasons patients seek care in the medical, as well as PM&R, settings. This chapter deals with acute and chronic pain affecting the neuromuscular and musculoskeletal systems.

I. **Neuroanatomy and neurophysiology.** Peripheral pain receptors (i.e., free-nerve endings called nociceptors) are found in virtually every cutaneous, deep somatic, or visceral structure of the body (including skin, fat pads, muscles, ligaments, fascia, joint capsules, periosteum, subchondral bone, and blood vessel walls). In the presence of noxious or potentially noxious stimuli, the nociceptors release endogenous chemicals, which peripherally transduce these stimuli to pain (or nociceptive) impulses via unknown mechanisms. The three types of endogenous chemical mediators of pain include: (1) those that produce direct local pain (e.g., bradykinin, histamine, acetylcholine, and potassium); (2) those that facilitate pain by sensitization of nociceptors without stimulating it (e.g., prostaglandins, leukotrienes, interleukins, and thromboxanes); and (3) those that produce extravasation of neuropeptides (e.g., substance P and calcitonin gene-related peptide [CGRP]). The excessive release of substance P and other neuropeptides may exert proinflammatory effects in tissues (i.e., "wheal and flare" type reaction mediated, in part, by mast cells) and may lead to "neurogenic inflammation," which can contribute to chronic pain syndromes (see section V.B).

The pain impulses are then transmitted to the dorsal horn of the spinal cord via the following afferent fibers: (1) the large (1-4 μm diameter), fast (velocity of 12-30 m/sec), myelinated A-δ fibers, which transmit sharp, localized pain; (2) the small (0.1-1.0 μm diameter), slow (velocity of 1-2 m/sec), unmyelinated C fibers, which transmit diffuse, burning, throbbing, and aching pain; and (3) the A-α (diameter of 12-20 μm; velocity of 70-120 m/sec) and A-β (diameter of 5-12 μm; velocity of 30-70 m/sec) fibers, both of which transmit episodic, sharp, and stabbing pain, which are difficult to control (because they can become involved through recruitment and plasticity in the injured nervous system, and their input does not undergo the same checks and balances as does that of the A-δ and C fibers in the central nervous system [CNS]). Different function-specific cell layers for A-δ, C, A-α, or A-β fibers are found in the substantia gelatinosa of the dorsal horn, and they serve as relay stations for the pain impulses.

From the spinal cord, pain impulses ascend through the contralateral spinothalamic tracts to the lateral and medial thalamic nuclei and via the spinoreticular tracts to the brainstem. The myelinated (A-δ) fibers relay painful stimuli to the neothalamus and somatosensory cortex where the pain quality can be discriminated and its position localized so the person can promptly withdraw from the noxious stimulus. On the other hand, the unmyelinated C fibers establish numerous synaptic contacts within the brainstem, midbrain nuclei, and cortical limbic system. Because of its persistent nature, the C fibers are primarily responsible for conditioned behavior and learned avoidance. On a teleological level such behavior serves to avoid further injury and promote wound healing; however, other less desirable affective responses can also be produced such as profound suffering, increased anxiety, and release of stress hormones and catecholamines.

Pain impulses also stimulate the sympathetic nervous system, which in turn can contribute to pain (e.g., in sympathetically maintained pain [SMP], reflex sympathetic dystrophy [RSD] with SMP features). The increase in sympathetic tone produces peripheral vasoconstriction (which causes peripheral ischemia, which in turn can aggravate pain) presumably by repeated incoming afferent C-fiber nociceptive impulses causing hypersensitivity in the dorsal horn of the spinal cord. It has been hypothesized that following trauma (e.g., peripheral nerve injuries, fractures, soft tissue traumas, myocardial infarctions, or strokes), norepinephrine is released from peripheral sympathetic terminals to activate nociceptors and that there is a change in the residual (and intact) sensory nerves so that nerves previously unresponsive to sympathetic stimulation can be excited by sympathetic stimulation. It remains unclear whether sympathetic-adrenergic interactions are mediated via the α_1- or α_2-adrenoceptor; however, it is clear that drugs or procedures that cause sympathetic blockade at either receptor can relieve pain under the correct circumstances. Persistent peripheral pain input (e.g., if pain is left untreated) may induce changes in the spinal cord neurons that enhance responsiveness to the same stimuli and increase the receptive field thus possibly contributing to chronic pain syndromes (see section V.B).

Pain impulses can be inhibited by both pre- and postsynaptic stimulation of the opioid receptors (see Chapter 4.8, section I.B), e.g., through exogenous sources such as opioid or nonopioid analgesics or through endogenous sources such as β-endorphins and enkephalins. Pain impulses can also be modulated by many substances including serotonin (5-hydroxytryptamine [5-HT]) and norepinephrine, which inhibit the response of dorsal horn neurons to noxious stimuli. Substance P, which is one of the endogenous chemical mediators of pain, can be inhibited by endogenous opioid peptides (e.g., β-endorphin, enkephalins, and dynorphins) in the CNS and periphery. In addition, descending circuits from many levels of the CNS can also modify the transmission and processing of pain impulses. These descending modulation systems can be triggered by drugs or by hypnosis and can be modified by behavioral mechanisms (e.g., operant conditioning in which good consequences produce increased frequency of the behavior and bad consequences produce decreased frequency of the behavior). Examples of behavioral modifiers that can possibly reinforce loss of function in chronic pain patients include worker's compensation or social security paying the patient for not working, significant others giving attention in response to illness behavior, and pain occurring in association with physical activity.

II. **Physiologic effects.** As the pain input reaches the CNS, it triggers the following reflex responses: (1) segmental spinal reflexes, which result in muscle spasm and vasoconstriction; (2) suprasegmental reflex responses, which are the result of noxious input from a number of spinal segments accumulating to cause the release of catecholamines, steroids, and renin-angiotensin, all of which result in metabolic and physiologic effects; and (3) cortical reaction to the seemingly inescapable pain (i.e., what the patient thinks and believes about the pain can strongly influence the effectiveness of the other therapy provided). The physiologic effects resulting from the summation of the spinal, suprasegmental, and cortical responses can either be beneficial (e.g., maintenance of BP, maintenance of cerebral perfusion, maintenance of cardiac output, maintenance of intravenous [IV] volume, enhanced hemostasis, substrate mobilization, enhanced energy production, immobilization [to minimize further tissue injury], and learned avoidance) or it can be detrimental to the body (e.g., overstressing of one physiologic system in an already compromised, critically ill patient can result in multisystem organ failure).

A. Physical effects include cardiovascular (tachycardia, hypertension, increased cardiac work, increased myocardial oxygen demand), pulmonary (hypoxia, hypercarbia, atelectasis, perfusion/ventilation [V/Q] mismatch, decreased cough, decreased vital capacity, decreased functional residual capacity), gastrointestinal (nausea, vomiting, ileus, intolerance for oral intake), renal (oliguria, urinary retention), musculoskeletal (spasm, limited mobility), vascular (thromboembolism), endocrine (excessive adrenergic activity, vagal inhibition, catabolic metabolism, increased oxygen consumption, negative nitrogen balance, hyperglycemia), CNS (sedation, fatigue) and immunologic (inhibited cellular immunity, possible increased risk of infection and impaired wound healing).

B. Psychophysiologic effects include general arousal (mediated by the sympathetic nervous system); sleep disturbance; reduced activity (including overall level of work, social and recreational activity, as well as activities of daily living [ADL]), which lead to a vicious pain cycle (i.e., inactivity, fatigue, and muscle weakness further increase pain, which promotes inactivity, fatigue, and muscle weakness); impaired behavioral and cognitive responses (including concentration, problem solving, memory, and ability to make decisions); negative emotional reactions (e.g., fear, anxiety, depression, anger, and frustration); and negative family and social responses (e.g., fear, confusion, and helplessness or overprotectiveness).

III. Psychosocial factors have recently been found to affect pain in addition to traditionally known factors, such as the type, location, and extent of tissue involvement, and the physical state of the patient. Factors that lower pain threshold (and increase pain perception) include discomfort, insomnia, fatigue, anxiety, fear, anger, sadness, depression, mental isolation, introversion, and past experience. Factors that raise pain threshold (and decrease pain perception) include relief of symptoms (e.g., analgesics), anxiolytics, sleep, rest, sympathy, understanding, diversion, and elevation of mood (e.g., antidepressants).

A. Internal (i.e., individual difference) factors

1. The **specific meaning attributed to pain** varies according to the one's personal history (e.g., in a patient with a history of physical or sexual abuse, the current pain may reactivate disruptive but previously repressed memories), prior learning about pain (i.e., early childhood pain experiences and observation of how parents or role models respond to pain), environmental factors (e.g., secondary gain, dysfunctional family support of pain behavior, or interpersonal conflict with the caregivers), cultural factors (i.e., racial, religious, and ethnic groups), and the character of the illness or injury and the circumstances surrounding them.

2. **Preexisting levels of problem-solving skills,** i.e., patients with positive problem solving skills in the major arenas of life (e.g., education, work, family, and social interaction) tend to have more productive problem-solving behaviors and positive attitudes toward pain.

3. **Coping style,** which is an internalized way of balancing personal emotional reactions with externally oriented, problem-solving behavior.

   a. **Coping strategies,** that is, use of active coping or problem-focused coping (e.g., by seeking out information and taking specific action) tends to decrease pain perception especially in a situation in which one's own efforts can reduce pain. The use of avoidant coping or emotion-focused coping (e.g., efforts toward suppressing or dealing with emotional reactions such as by relaxation, denial, or avoidance) can also be effective under certain circumstances (e.g., in dealing with short-term situations especially if there is little ability to control aspects of the situation).

   b. Locus of control refers to whether one perceives that control over one's environment and over the outcome of events (such as pain) lies within oneself (internal locus of control) or with powerful others (external locus of control). In general, patients with an internal locus of control are more likely to cope actively and report less severe pain than those with an external locus of control.

   c. Negative thinking and catastrophizing are consistently ineffective in helping cope with pain.

4. **Emotional age** reflects the emotional fluctuations (i.e., regression) often generated by the stress of acute pain. Pervasive regression may represent a character-disordered patient.

5. **Hypnotic capacity** reflects the capacity to assume a natural state of focused attention similar to that of daydreaming. This can be an asset or a liability depending on whether these states occur spontaneously and unwittingly or are purposefully elicited. For example, patients with hypnotic capacity who are prone to negativity and catastrophizing can unwittingly aggravate their pain experience through negative self-suggestion. If hypnotic capacity is purposefully elicited and directed (e.g., by training), however, it can help alleviate pain.

B. **Process factors**

1. **Affective and cognitive principles** governing the awareness of pain include pain beliefs and "meaning" attributed to pain (e.g., childbirth pain is generally perceived as more tolerable than is cancer pain) and emotional arousal (i.e., negative emotional arousal caused by anxiety, fear, depression, anger, irritability, and frustration can lead to increased awareness of pain). The meaning of pain can be altered by primary and secondary gain factors.

2. **Perceived control,** i.e., patients with an increase in perceived control, are more likely to exhibit self-initiated pain management and increased cooperation with treatment. Situational factors such as predictability and familiarity of events also increases one's perceived control and may increase pain tolerance. Patients who actually have a degree of control (e.g., use of patient-controlled analgesic pumps) typically report adequate pain management and actually use less pain medications than patients receiving conventional methods of postoperative injections.

3. **"Recovery" status** of patient, that is for pain treatment to be successful, patients must progress from "victim of injury" to "manager of recovery" and must move through the grieving process (i.e., from shock to denial to anger to bargaining to mourning, and finally, to acceptance) and not be arrested in one grief stage.

IV. **Assessment** of pain is difficult to objectify because its perception is subjective. Despite its subjectivity, however, all pain complaints must be assumed to be real.

A. **History** includes pain description (i.e., quality; location, extension or radiation, intensity, onset, duration, frequency, pattern of involvement, progression, aggravating or relieving factors, previous tests results and treatment effects, and other associated manifestations), mechanism of the injury (if present), presence of chronic medical problems (including chronic pain syndromes and other preexisting conditions that may affect the physical consequences or physiologic reserve of the patient), personal and psychosocial history (i.e., current and past social situation, including vocational, family, and interpersonal stresses), current medications, functional limitations in ADL, dependence on adaptive equipment, litigation status, and other aspects of potential secondary gain which may impede recovery.

B. **Physical examination** is generally directed to neuromuscular and joint examination. Observe the patient walking, sitting, and moving in situations when being directed and when patient is unaware of being observed. Identify the painful structures and document variations from the normal, which may interfere with function. Seek alterations in muscle strength, sensation, and deep tendon reflexes. Search carefully for dermatomal or root level dysfunction of sensory and reflex systems. Examine joint structures for effusion, decreased range of motion, and deformity. Palpate tendons and ligamentous structures. Palpate muscles to evaluate for trigger areas or tight bands of muscle that, when deeply palpated, cause referred pain. Instruct the patient to perform specific maneuvers such as a straight leg raising test (patient supine, leg raised from horizontal), Tinel's sign (tap over median nerves of wrist), or the Finkelstein test (thumb wrapped up in fist, wrist ulnar deviated) to aid in the clinical confirmation of the suspected diagnosis. Vital signs do not necessarily correlate with the intensity or the seriousness of the pain. Observation for signs of distress, body posturing, and the cooperation with verbal responses is important. In addition, the area of injury and the associated physiologic systems must also be evaluated.

C. **Pain measurement tools** attempt to measure pain "objectively." In patients with chronic pain, psychosocial factors play an important role.

1. **Physical and psychophysiologic assessment**

   a. **Pressure algometry (dolorimetry)** uses hand-held mechanical instruments (Pressure Threshold Meter, Tissue Compliance Meter) to measure the amount of force (pressure), which induces pain or discomfort. These devices consist of a rubber disk tip (with 1 cm^2 surface) attached to an analog force gauge, which measures pressure ranging from 0.1 kg to 5 or 10 kg). They can be used to quantify pain because of trigger point (taut and fibrotic bands), tender spots, muscle spasm, edema, hematomas, and other soft tissue pathologies. They have good reliability (intratester is higher than intertester reliability) in trained examiners. They are valid in terms of pressure measurement, but they must be used with caution because pain perception varies in different persons under various conditions, psychological states, and levels of motivation.

   b. **Surface EMG biofeedback** records muscular electrical activities, which are assumed to correlate with the patient's underlying pain syndrome; however, this area remains controversial.

2. **Pain scales**

   a. **Unidimensional pain scales** are simple subjective pain measurements designed to assess a single dimension of pain such as intensity, location, or degree of relief. It is clear and simple and can be used with children and elderly populations of various cognitive levels. Administration and scoring are simple and straightforward. Although it supposedly measures only a single dimension such as pain intensity, it is actually influenced by other factors such as the emotional state of the patient.

      1) **Visual analog scale (VAS)** (see Fig. 5.10-1) is the most commonly used

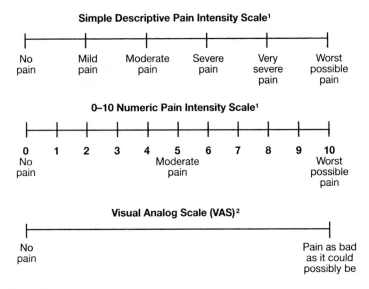

Figure 5.10-1
Three commonly used self-report pain intensity scales.[1] If used as a graphic rating scale, a 10-cm baseline is recommended.[2] A 10-cm baseline is recommended for VAS scale. (From Jacox A, Carr PR, Payne R, et al.: *Management of Cancer Pain: Clinical practical guideline No. 9.* AHCPR Publication No. 94-0592, Rockville, MD, March 1994, Agency for Health Care Policy and Research, U.S. Department of Health and Human Services, p. 26, with permission.)

pain scale. It consists of a 10 cm (100 mm) unmarked line, either vertical or horizontal with verbal or pictorial anchors indicating a continuum from ''no pain'' to severe pain (''pain as bad as it could be'') at each end. There is no descriptor along the length of the line. The patient is asked to mark on the line the pain he or she is experiencing (e.g., how bad is your pain?). This mark is then measured with a ruler and expressed in cm (or mm), with 10 cm (100 mm) representing severe pain. The advantages of VAS include: simple to use, information is quickly obtained, sensitive (i.e., a high number of response options, so that it is sensitive to changes in pain intensity; also with good sensitivity to treatment effects), reproducible results, positive association with other self-report measures, and useful in a wide range of clinical and research conditions. Also, it can be used to reassess pain in the same patient at different times. The disadvantages of VAS include a lack of quantification of pain between the end points; the need for a certain level of cognitive functioning to cooperate with it; patients must be at least 8 years old; and the linear measurement of the patient's response, which adds time and a potential source of error.

2) **Numerical rating system (NRS)** (see Fig. 5.10-1) uses a number span (e.g., 0-5, 0-10, 1-100, or 0-100%) to reflect increasing degrees of

pain. Some patients find it easier to assign a monetary value to their pain, perhaps because it offers a slightly more concrete image of the 0 to 100 scale. The patient is asked, ''If 0 = no pain and $1.00 = the worst pain imaginable, how much is your pain worth?'' The numerical scale is discrete and not continuous. Although simple it is not as sensitive as the VAS. The advantages of numerical scales include their being easy to score and administer, the high number of response categories possible, good patient cooperation, and support of their validity. The disadvantages relate to the weak statistical basis of the data and the low treatment sensitivity. Additionally, like the VAS, numerical scales demand a requisite level of mental functioning and abstract thinking to be usable.

3) **Verbal scales** involve asking the patient to pick a descriptive word that reflects the intensity of his or her pain from a list of words or from words spaced along a horizontal or vertical line (see Fig. 5.10-1). A patient's self-report is probably the best verbal test, but this option may be severely limited in the intensive care unit (ICU) patient. Verbal scales can be used to assess not only the intensity of pain or symptom but also the relief of pain or symptom after treatment, depending on the grouping of words chosen. The advantages of verbal scales are that they are easy to administer and score and that there is good evidence of their validity. The disadvantages include the demand on the patient to choose a word that may not be exactly descriptive of the pain, the need for education to understand the words and the concept, there being only as many response categories as there are words, and the fact that the data are only somewhat amenable to statistical review. Example is the *Patient Assessment Inventory and Narrative* from the University of Virginia, which became the basis for the *McGill-Melzack Pain Questionnaire* (see section IV.C.2.b.1; Fig. 5.10-2).

4) **Pain drawings** (Fig. 5.10-3) on body figures is a technique that provides more data about the location of pain than other pain scales. In general, the more widespread the drawing of the pain, the more intense, frequent, and disruptive the pain is. This pain scale requires coordination, visual integrity, and, depending on the task given, a variable level of cognitive functioning.

5) **Category rating scale (CRS) or graphic rating scale (GRS)** consists of a series of words along a continuum of increasing values (absent, mild, moderate, severe pain). In children, pictures of faces expressing varying amounts of distress (e.g., **Face Scale, Oucher Scale**) or colors, and poker chips representing ''pieces of hurt'' **(Poker Chip Tool)** may be used. Category rating scales are nonspecific, not very sensitive, and not consistently reproducible. A variation is the pain relief scale with the following descriptors of pain relief: none, slight, moderate, good relief.

b. **Multidimensional or complex pain scales** measure not only the intensity but also the quality of pain and its resultant effects on other psychological and social variables. They are not practical for most acutely injured or critically ill patients.

1) **McGill-Melzack Pain Questionnaire (MPQ)** is the most thoroughly researched multidimensional pain scale (see Fig. 5.10-2). It consists of 20 category scales of pain adjective descriptors, which can be

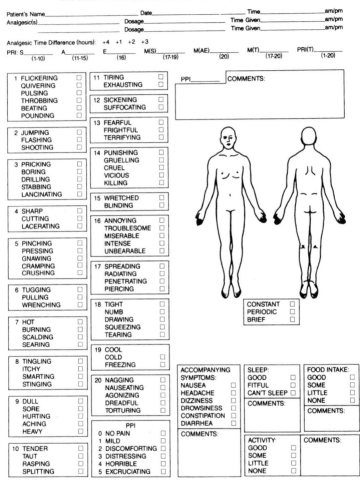

Figure 5.10-2
McGill-Melzack Pain Questionnaire (MPQ). (Used with permission of Ronald Melzack, M.D., McGill University.)

grouped into four major dimensions of the pain experience: sensory (scales 1-11), affective (scales 12-15), evaluative or intensity (scale 16), and miscellaneous (scales 17-20). It provides three measures: pain rating index (PRI), which is the sum of the rank value for each descriptor based on its position in the word set; present pain intensity (PPI), which is based on a scale of 0 (no pain) to 5 (excruciating pain); and number of words chosen. The MPQ is a consistent, useful, easy, and rapid way of measuring pain; however, it takes

Mark the areas on your body where you feel the described sensations. Use the appropriate symbol. Mark areas of radiation. Include all affected areas.

Numbness	—	INC Sensitivity	0000
Constant	xxx	Sharp Twinge	////
Throbbing Ache	xxx		

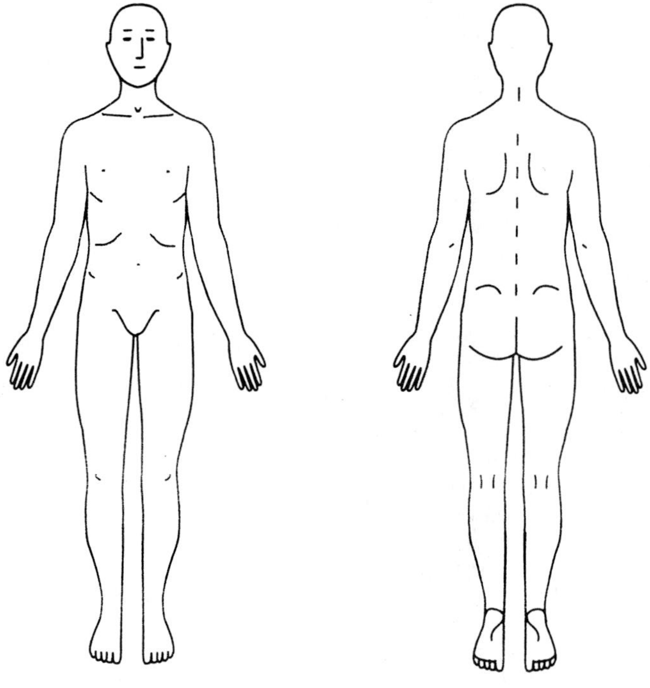

Figure 5.10-3
Pain drawing. (From Bigos SJ, Bowyer OR, Braen GR, et al.: Acute low back problems in adults: Clinical practice guideline No. 14. AHCPR Publication No. 95-0642, Rockville, MD, December 1994, Agency for Health Care Policy and Research, U.S. Department of Health and Human Services, p. 146, with permission.)

both time and education (i.e., greater vocabulary base to understand the pain adjective descriptors) and can be influenced by repeat testing, past experience, and unrelated events. The reported ability of the MPQ to differentiate among various pain syndromes (e.g., neuralgia, arthritis, RSD, and radiculopathy) as well as its reliability remain controversial.

2) **West Haven–Yale Multidimensional Pain Inventory (WHYMPI)** is a 52-item inventory that is divided into three parts: (1) general dimensions of the experience of pain and suffering, interference with normal family and work functioning, and social support; (2) patient's perceptions of the responses of others to displays of pain and suffering; and (3) frequency of engagement in common daily activities. It can be completed in 10 to 15 minutes and has a broader approach than the MPQ in that it includes assessment of the impact of the pain problem on the patient's general functioning.

3) **Emory University Pain Estimate Chart** evaluates four pain factors: overall physical findings, neurologic examination, radiological findings, and laboratory results. Each factor is assigned a numerical value from 0 (normal) to 2.5 (maximum pathology). Other specific measures of pain behavior (verbalization, activity, drug use, and psychological dysfunctions) are also scaled. A score below 5 is low and a score above 5 is high for any given category. Patients are divided into four classes, which aids in quantifying impairment, choosing treatment, and in prognostication of pain. Class I is low in pain pathology but high in pain behavior. Class II is low in both categories, and class III is high in both categories. Class IV is high in pain pathology but low in pain behavior.

D. **Behavioral assessment** includes the psychosocial ramifications (i.e., impact on patient's attitudes, behavior, lifestyle, and functional abilities, be they physical or psychological); perceived consequences of the pain; patient's understanding and degree of acceptance of his or her situation, attitudes, and the premorbid emotional status of the patient; signs of depression (e.g., irritability, decreased energy, poor concentration, and decreased appetite); and issues of loss of control due to hospitalization. Some of the common psychological tests used for chronic pain patients are

1. **Functional status (life-style impact) scales**

   a. **Sickness impact profile (SIP)** is a 136-item self report or interviewer-administered measure yielding 12 subscale scores reflecting mobility, social functions, and elements of self-management. Its scores (range of 0-100%) discriminate between psychosocial and physical dysfunction. It has satisfactory internal consistency, good test-retest reliability, and construct validity.

   b. **Activity diaries** are self reports of hourly activities in sitting, standing, walking, and reclining positions, as well as type and amount of medications taken and pain ratings on a 0 to 10 scale of severity, recorded in 1 to 2 weeks. Weekly total sitting and standing times of under 80 hours (normal is about 112 hours) suggests considerable functional impairment. The validity and reliability of activity diaries remain to be established.

2. **Tests of general psychopathology** involving structured tests and questionnaires, such as the Minnesota Multiphasic Personality Inventory (MMPI), Millon Clinical Multiaxial Inventory II (MCMI-II), Beck Depression Inventory (BDI), and Zung Depression Scale, all of which are described in Chapter 2.9, section VII.B. Other psychological tests commonly used in chronic pain patients are

   a. **Symptom Checklist 90-revised (SCL-90R)** is a 90-item problem checklist that allows the patient to rate symptoms of physical and emotional distress on a 5-point scale. It scores nine symptom dimensions (e.g., depression, anxiety, and hostility) and three global indices of distress.

It takes 15 to 30 minutes to complete and is reliable. Its generalizability to pain patients is questionable because it was standardized using psychiatric patients. It can be used as a screening device and should be correlated with the MMPI.

- **b. Millon Behavioral Health Inventory (MBHI)** is a self-reported inventory consisting of 150 true-false items based on 20 clinical scales that measure personality styles, physical concerns, and behavioral reactions to disease or illness. It takes 30 to 45 minutes to complete. It also contains a prognostic index that attempts to predict one's response to pain treatment. Its reliability is good, but its validity remains to be proved.

E. Diagnostic tests include radiographs or computed tomography (CT) scans to identify fractures and other bone and joint pathologies; magnetic resonance imaging (MRI) to identify muscle, tendon, and ligament abnormalities; electrodiagnostic testing to evaluate the neuromuscular system and nerve entrapments; radiculopathies, myopathies, or CNS reactivation; measures of specific organ system function (e.g., vital capacity, functional residual capacity, and liver function tests); physical quantitative testing (e.g., exercise stress test); laboratory tests (e.g., diagnosis-specific tests, such as rheumatoid factor, antinuclear antibodies [ANA], and creatine phosphokinase [CPK], or stress-response tests, such as corticosteroid levels, renin-angiotensin-aldosterone release, negative nitrogen balance, and sodium/water retention); in addition to diagnostic blocks (see Chapter 4.10, section I). It must be emphasized, however, that negative diagnostic results do not always mean that there is no ''real'' pain or that psychopathology is dominant.

V. Pain classification by duration

A. Acute pain is usually linked to a precipitating event (e.g., trauma or surgery). The pain symptom is physiologically useful as it can provoke an escape or protection reaction to potentially dangerous tissue damage. Acute pain may be accompanied by anxiety, anger, and temporary lifestyle adjustments. Its evaluation and treatment usually takes less time because of its short, self-limiting course (usually less than 3 months) and its high rate of successful cure. Acute pain may be superimposed on a chronic pain (e.g., surgery in a cancer patient) or an acute exacerbation may occur in a chronic pain patient (e.g., pathological fracture of long bones in a cancer patient or acute exacerbation of rheumatoid arthritis during cold weather). The differential diagnosis of acute pain is discussed in Chapter 3.1.

B. Chronic pain can be caused by persistence of organic pathology (e.g., cancer) or it can be caused by persistence of pain despite the resolution of the original tissue damage with excessive loss of function (i.e., noncancer chronic pain, also referred to as ''nonmalignant chronic pain,'' ''benign chronic pain,'' or ''chronic pain syndrome''). In noncancer chronic pain (NCP), the pain has lost its physiologic adaptive value, and the persistent pain has become a disease in itself (with morphologic changes in the nervous system, the exact mechanism of which is unknown; see section I). Noncancer chronic pain is accompanied by physical deconditioning (due to inactivity), frustration and depression, and major changes in behavior, productivity, lifestyle, and attitudes toward becoming healthy. Its course is prolonged (over 3-6 months), and its evaluation and treatment is time-consuming. The treatment goal is aimed at helping the patient control or cope with the residual pain (rather than in curing it as in acute pain). Examples of NCP include chronic neuropathic pain (e.g., painful polyneuropathy, painful mononeuropathy, phantom pain, central pain, postherpetic neuralgia, avulsion of nerve plexus, sympathetic mediated pain syndromes, and RSD/causalgia), and chronic musculoskeletal pain (e.g., fibromyalgia, myofascial pain syndrome, chronic low back pain, and chronic arthritic and bone pain). The differential diagnosis for acute and chronic pain is discussed in Chapter 3.1, section I.A. Treatment options for musculoskeletal pain are shown in Table 5.10-1, while Tables 5.10-2 and 5.10-3 show the treatment options for neuropathic pain.

VI. **Management** of pain begins with the assumptions that all pain complaints are real until proved otherwise and that almost all pain has a psychosocial component (see psychosocial factors affecting pain in section III). Pain is best approached by treating its underlying etiology, although this is not always present or easy to identify. Timely treatment of pain is not only humane but can also help in increasing the patient's cooperation with his or her rehabilitative program, restoring the patient's normal activity, shortening the patient's hospital stay, and reducing health care costs. In postoperative patients, additional benefits of adequate analgesia include improvement in postoperative pulmonary function; decreased length of postoperative ventilation and ICU stay; decreased mortality in patients with traumatic thoracic injuries; attenuation of the stress response to surgery; associated improvement in the metabolic response to injury; maintenance of immunocompetence; earlier mobilization, which may lead to a decreased incidence of thrombotic sequelae; and overall hastening of recovery. Hence, delay in pain treatment and undermedication of pain (especially acute pain) are medically unacceptable.

Because of marked individual variations in pain response, pain treatment protocols should be individualized and flexible. There should also be favorable interaction between the patient and physician (which has been demonstrated to enhance patient compliance). Treatment principles for acute pain include discontinuing the source of tissue damage, resting of the damaged part, pain-relieving physical modalities, informal (or minor) use of behavioral management, and short-term use of nonnarcotic analgesics (acetaminophen, nonsteroidal antiinflammatory drugs [NSAIDs]) or adjuvant analgesics (e.g., "skeletal muscle relaxants" or diazepam) or, if indicated (i.e., in severe pain), the limited use of opioid analgesics. The use of the PRICE treatment approach (i.e., protection, relative rest, ice, compression, and elevation) can be initially helpful in acute injuries. The three stages of recovery in acute pain are: stage one—pain relief through modalities; stage two—regaining of normal resting muscle length through range of motion (ROM) and flexibility exercises, and stage three—gradual muscle strengthening and aerobic exercises. All throughout treatment, the patient must be educated on preventive and ergonomic measures. It is imperative to prevent chronicity of pain because the longer pain persists (over 3-6 months), the less likely complete resolution becomes and the less likely the patient will return to a productive life. Patients with a tendency of developing chronic pain are those with significant psychosocial issues, secondary gain motives, or lack of insight. In patients with chronic pain, the principles of treatment emphasize mobilization of underused affected areas, the use of formal behavioral management (usually in an interdisciplinary setting), and avoidance of addicting medications (e.g., opioids).

A. **Patient education** should be an integral part of the comprehensive clinical care of patients with acute or chronic musculoskeletal and neuropathic pain. It consists of a combination of planned learning experiences to empower the patients and make them active participants in their own treatment program by facilitating them to voluntarily adopt and maintain good health-conducive behaviors and to prevent relapse of disease-related behavior. Clinical evidence shows that patient education can enhance compliance to the therapeutic

Table 5.10-1. Pain treatment options for acute and chronic musculoskeletal pain. These treatments have been tried but have not been definitely proved

MUSCULOSKELETAL PAIN	PAIN TREATMENT OPTIONS
I. Acute*	**PM&R:** PRICE (protection, relative rest, ice, compression, elevation); sensory modulation (e.g., TENS, acupuncture); patient education†. **Drugs:** NSAIDs, opioids, muscle relaxants, and possibly benzodiazepines
II. Chronic*	
1. Chronic low back pain	**PM&R:** sensory modulation (e.g., TENS, acupuncture); exercise (e.g., conditioning, strengthening, aerobic); patient education†; short-term bracing, manipulation, or passive modalities (heat, cold, and massage) in conjunction with active exercises; trigger point injections. **Drugs:** NSAIDs; opioids on selected patients; adjuvants (e.g., tricyclic antidepressants, anticonvulsants, baclofen); pain cocktails. **Nerve blocks:** epidural steroid injections in selected patients. **Surgery:** spinal fusion
2. ''Noninflammatory'' arthritis (e.g., osteoarthritis)	**PM&R:** reduce the stress on the joints (e.g., rest, cane, strengthening exercises, weight reduction); sensory modulation (e.g., TENS, acupuncture); helium-neon laser (?); patient education†. **Drugs:** acetaminophen; judicious and short-term use of NSAIDs and topical analgesics (e.g., capsaicin); antidepressants, anticonvulsants, intra- and periarticular injections (corticosteroids); opioids for severe pain. **Surgery:** total joint replacement; synovectomy; arthrodesis
3. Inflammatory arthritis (e.g., rheumatoid arthritis)	**PM&R:** rest, splinting, exercise, orthotics; heat/cold; sensory modulation (e.g., TENS); cold laser (?); patient education†. **Drugs:** NSAIDS (with acetaminophen); antidepressants; anticonvulsants; corticosteroids; disease-modifying antirheumatic drugs (e.g., gold, D-penicillamine, methotrexate); opioids for severe pain. **Surgery:** total joint replacement; synovectomy; arthrodesis
4. Fibromyalgia	**PM&R:** exercise (especially aerobic); patient education†; biofeedback; short-term manipulation; sensory modulation (e.g., TENS). **Drugs:** amitriptyline; cyclobenzapine, alprazolam, NSAIDs in selected cases; corticosteroids are ineffective
5. Myofascial pain syndrome	**PM&R:** stretch and spray; cold; trigger point injection (with or without steroids); exercise (especially aerobic); patient education†; sensory modulation (e.g., TENS, acupuncture); cold laser (?). **Drugs:** short-term NSAIDs or opioids; antispastics (e.g., baclofen); antidepressants

* Psychosocial interventions (e.g., cognitive behavioral modification, psychotherapy, hypnotherapy, relaxation) and vocational counseling (if appropriate) should be included especially in chronic cases.
† Patient education including joint conservation, lifting techniques, and other biomechanic and ergonomic principles.

Table 5.10-2. **Pain treatment options for neuropathic pain of predominantly "central" process. These treatments have been tried but have not been definitely proved**

"CENTRAL" PAIN	PAIN TREATMENT OPTIONS
I. Deafferentation	
1. Phantom pain	**PM&R:** prosthesis; sensory modulation (e.g., TENS); exercise; biofeedback. **Drugs:** adjuvant analgesics (e.g., calcitonin, antidepressants, anticonvulsants, propranolol); opioids. **Anesthetic:** local anesthetic injection into stump or into hyperalgesic *contralateral* limb; sympathetic blockade. **Surgery:** dorsal root entry zone (DREZ) lesion; ''preemptive analgesia'' prior to amputation; cordotomy; neurectomy; rhizotomy. **Psychosocial interventions***
2. Avulsion of nerve plexus	**PM&R:** splinting; exercise; TENS; vocational retraining. **Drugs:** adjuvant analgesics (e.g., anticonvulsants); opioids; nonopioid analgesics. **Anesthetic:** sympathetic blockade. **Surgery:** DREZ lesion. **Psychosocial interventions***
3. Postherpetic neuralgia	**PM&R:** sensory modulation (e.g., TENS); exercise; helium-neon laser. **Drugs:** adjuvant analgesics including topical agents (e.g., lidocaine, EMLA, capsaicin); antidepressants (e.g., amitriptyline, desipramine, maprotiline); combination of tricyclic antidepressants with neuroleptics (e.g., phenothiazines); anticonvulsants (e.g., carbamazepine, clonazepam, phenytoin, valproate); clonidine; NSAIDs; opioids. **Anesthetic:** skin infiltration with local anesthetic, or local anesthetic and steroids; IV local anesthetic; temporary or permanent blocks of peripheral nerves or nerve roots; sympathetic blocks; epidural steroid, use of cryoprobe to painful scar. **Surgery:** DREZ lesion (neurectomy, rhizotomy, sympathectomy, trigeminal tractotomy, cordotomy, thalamotomy, mesencephalotomy, mesencephalothalamotomy). **Psychosocial interventions***
4. Central pain	**PM&R:** sensory modulation (e.g., TENS); exercise. **Drugs:** adjuvant analgesics (e.g., tricyclic antidepressants [especially amitriptyline], anticonvulsants [e.g., carbamazepine], naloxone infusion, local anesthetics [e.g., mexiletene], antihistamines, neuroleptics, propranolol); nonopioid analgesic; opioids. **Anesthetic:** temporary somatic nerve block with local anesthetic; sympathetic block. **Surgery:** dorsal column stimulation; deep brain stimulation; DREZ lesion. **Psychosocial interventions***
II. Sympathetic maintained pain (e.g., reflex sympathetic dystrophy/causalgia subtype)	**PM&R:** sensory modulation (e.g., TENS, acupuncture); exercise; biofeedback; contrast baths. **Drugs:** adjuvant analgesics (e.g., calcitonin, nifedipine, prazosin, propranolol, clonidine, phenoxybenzamine, antidepressant, anticonvulsants, oral local anesthetics, pulsed oral corticosteroid); opioids. **Anesthetic:** sympathetic blockade. **Surgery:** sympathectomy; percutaneuous electrical stimulation; dorsal column stimulation; deep brain stimulation. **Psychosocial interventions***

* Psychosocial interventions include cognitive behavioral modification, psychotherapy, hypnotherapy, relaxation, etc. If appropriate, vocational counseling should also be included.

Table 5.10-3.   Pain treatment options for neuropathic pain of predominantly "peripheral" process. These treatments have been tried but have not been definitely proved

"PERIPHERAL" PAIN	PAIN TREATMENT OPTIONS
I. Painful polyneuropathies	**PM&R:** orthotics (e.g., shoe lift); bedsheet cradle at night; sensory modulation (e.g., TENS); exercise. **Drugs:** replacement of missing compounds; primary treatment of diabetes with hypoglycemics; use of aldose reductase inhibitors; adjuvant analgesics (e.g., tricyclic antidepressantrs, oral local anesthetics, topical capsaicin, anticonvulsants, propranolol); NSAIDs; opioids. **Anesthetic:** sympathetic blockade. **Surgery:** surgical interruption of afferent neural pathways (no evidence of efficacy). **Psychosocial interventions***
II. Painful mononeuropathies	
1. Lancinating neuralgia	**PM&R:** sensory modulation (e.g., TENS); helium-neon laser. **Drugs:** adjuvant drugs (e.g., anticonvulsants [carbamazepine is first choice, phenytoin, valproate, clonazepam], baclofen, oral local anesthetics [mexiletine], tricyclic antidepressants, propranolol, pimozide, if refractory). **Anesthetic:** temporary or prolonged nerve blocks with local anesthetics; chemical neurolysis/rhizotomy. **Surgery:** neurectomy; microvascular decompression; percutaneous radiofrequency lesioning; rhizotomy; cryotherapy; gangliolysis; peripheral nerve avulsion. **Psychosocial interventions***
2. Nerve trauma, compression, inflammation, or neoplasm	**PM&R:** sensory modulation (e.g., TENS); exercise. **Drugs:** adjuvant drugs (e.g., antidepressants, anticonvulsants, topical analgesics [e.g., capsaicin], clonidine, others); nonopioid analgesics; opioids; short-term systemic steroids or epidural steroid (both controversial). **Anesthetic:** temporary or prolonged nerve blocks with local anesthetics; chemical neurolysis; cryoblock. **Surgical:** nerve decompression; excision of neuroma; neurectomy, rhizotomy, cordotomy, DREZ lesion; **Psychosocial interventions***

* Psychosocial interventions include cognitive behavioral modification, psychotherapy, hypnotherapy, relaxation, etc. If appropriate, vocational counseling should also be included.

regimen, produce physiologic and immunologic changes in response to behavioral change, and result in clinically significant improvement in health outcomes. Contrary to popular beliefs, informing patients about possible side effects of therapy does not increase the occurrence of side effects or have other adverse effects.

To ensure successful patient education, the clinician should deal with the following patient issues: specific behaviors (e.g., appointment keeping, taking medications, performing exercises, changing diet, and managing stress), belief systems about the disease and efficacy of treatment, motivation and perceived self-efficacy, locus of control, skills and resources necessary to make behavioral changes (e.g., communication skills and skills to perform specific disease-related management tasks, such as exercises and self-medication), and reinforcing factors (e.g., from family members, members of the health care team, and even fellow patients). Patient education can be classified into preoperative education, medication self-administration, outpatient education programs, discharge planning education, family education, peer education, cooperative care, early discharge education, home health education programs, and mutual aid and self-help groups. It may be given individually or in small groups (e.g., Back School, Neck School, or Stress School) (see Chapter 5.11, section VI.A.2). Educational techniques include

- Using direct instruction during clinical visits with repetition and reinforcement of the instructions during subsequent visits
- Encouraging patients to take notes
- Having patients clarify instructions and repeating the instructions back
- Having patients set short-term goals
- Encouraging patients to self-monitor (e.g., checklists or diaries)
- Having patients sign a written contract specifying the duration, frequency, and quality of required behaviors (e.g., exercise)
- Using a variety of audiovisual aids when teaching (e.g., slides, audio- or videotapes, films, charts, and model skeletons);
- Providing the patient with tip sheets, pamphlets, newsletters, and other written instructions to supplement oral instructions
- Providing language translations and large-type versions of instructions when appropriate
- Including family members or significant others during patient education
- Telephoning patients a few days following office visits to follow up, clarify, and reinforce instructions

The emphasis of patient education should be focused not only on improving knowledge but also on changing attitudes, beliefs, and behaviors. The information should be presented more than once, and in more than one way because patients seek information from multiple sources. The general content of patient education includes

1. **General overview,** that is, definition of pain (acute vs. chronic), anatomy and pathophysiology of pain, pain assessment scales, preventive approaches to pain control, the importance of reporting pain to doctors and nurses as active participants in their own care, emphasizing that almost all pain can be effectively managed, and the important role that the patient needs to play in pain control.

2. **Pharmacological management,** that is, overview of drug management of pain, overcoming fears of addiction (i.e., use of opioid analgesics will not in itself lead to addiction), understanding drug tolerance (i.e., tolerance to opioid analgesics can be dealt with by upward dosage adjustment), understanding respiratory depression and the methods of controlling common side effects of drugs, and emphasizing the importance of pain prevention by the use of regularly scheduled analgesics. It should also address fears that the pain cannot be effectively controlled without unacceptable consequences or that choices might have to be made between treating the disease or treating the pain and other misconceptions (e.g., pain medication should be saved for when pain is severe or else it might not be effective).

3. **Nonpharmacological management,** that is, its importance; the use of nonpharmacologic modalities as adjuncts to analgesics, review of previous experience with nonpharmacologic modalities, peer support groups and pastoral

counseling, and demonstration of heat, cold, massage, relaxation, imagery, and distraction. For patients with musculoskeletal pain, it should also include joint and energy conservation techniques (see Chapter 4.5, section I.B.3), lifting and carrying techniques (see Chapter 5.11, section VI.A.2.c.2), sitting and standing techniques (see Chapter 5.11, section VI.A.2.c.1), environmental or workplace modifications (see Chapter 4.5 section VI.A.2.d.1 and Chapter 5.11, section VI.A.2.d), and other biomechanic and ergonomic principles (see Chapter 5.11, section VI.A.2.c).

B. **Physical modalities** for pain relief are discussed in Chapter 4.1. (All cross referenced sections are in Chapter 4.1.) They include therapeutic heat (i.e., superficial and deep heating agents; see section I), therapeutic cold (e.g., cold packs and vapocoolant sprays; see section II), hydrotheraphy (including pool therapy; see section III), electrotherapy (e.g., transcutaneous nerve stimulation [TENS] and high-voltage monophasic pulsed current; see section V); iontophoresis (see section V.A.1.a) or phonophoresis (see section I.B.1), low-power cold laser (see section IV.B), biofeedback (see section VI), traction (see section VII), mobilization and manipulation (see section VIII), massage (see section IX), and acupuncture (see section X). Because of their passive nature, these physical modalities must only be used in the acute phase in combination with more active exercises. The use of some of these physical modalities, which are considered sensory modulation modalities (e.g., TENS, acupuncture, alternating use of hot and cold, and massage including vibration and percussion), are based on the hypothesis that hyperstimulation of the nervous system will "drown out" pain messages to the CNS and, thereby, prevent the cascade of adverse physiologic consequences.

C. **Orthoses** (e.g., casts, splints, or braces), **gait aids** (e.g., cane, crutches, or walker), and **adaptive devices** for ADLs may be used temporarily if a specific joint or limb must be rested or protected due to pain. See Chapter 4.3 for details about orthoses, Chapter 4.6 for details about gait aids, and Chapter 4.5 for details about adaptive devices for ADLs.

D. **Therapeutic exercises** (discussed in Chapter 4.2) are an important adjunct in pain therapy. In acute pain, rest (for 2-3 days or up to a week) may initially be necessary to allow healing of the acutely inflamed muscle or joint (e.g., in rheumatoid arthritis); however, complete immobility can rapidly lead to muscle weakness and joint contracture. Isometric exercise (in combination with heating or cold modalities), therefore, may be initiated even in the presence of acute joint inflammation, and, if the patient can tolerate, gentle ROM and flexibility exercises should be started as soon as the inflammation subsides. As the pain improves, strengthening and aerobic exercises can be started to prevent recurrences of the painful episodes. In the acute phase, ROM exercise may be done up to, but not past, the point of pain. Causing pain during the ROM of the joint may only restart the vicious cycle of pain and may delay tissue healing. In contrast, pain is not necessarily a good guideline for exercise in chronic pain patients (as the original tissue has already healed in most cases, and the pain is usually caused by immobilization and deconditioning). In fact, the quota system is more effective in the chronic pain patient (i.e., a goal is set within the patient's capability, and the patient is encouraged to attain that goal regardless of pain complaints). Aside from mobility, strengthening, and aerobic exercises (e.g., walking and swimming), the use of relaxation exercises are beneficial, especially in chronic pain patients.

E. **Oral and parenteral medications**

1. **Analgesics** should only be considered as one component of a multimodality approach to pain treatment (including physical and psychosocial measures

and adjuvant drugs). The general principles in initiating and monitoring analgesic therapy are

- Individualize analgesic therapy based on the severity and nature of the pain as well as underlying condition(s).
- Begin with a simple, single-entity agent, which is appropriate for the patient's pain and which produces the most benefit with the least adverse effect.
- If a single-entity analgesic agent is ineffective or produces intolerable adverse effects, combination therapy should be tried.
- If possible, give the analgesic on a scheduled basis with constant adjustment of doses (depending on pain control) rather than the traditional 'prn' dosing, which is frequently ineffective for adequate pain control.
- Use the analgesic for an adequate period of time (avoiding long-term use if possible).
- Warn the patient about the drug's potential adverse effects and inform him or her that these adverse effects may gradually subside with time or that measures can be taken to reduce the severity of or eliminate a particular adverse effect.
- When using centrally acting analgesics (e.g., opioids), be aware of tolerance and dependence tendencies (especially in chronic pain patients with prior history of substance abuse or in patients with severe personality disorders).
- Monitor all patients for impending tolerance to centrally acting analgesics by slowly titrating the doses of these analgesics, spreading the interval of administration, avoiding excessive renewal of prescriptions, or switching to an alternative drug if dependence becomes apparent. If addiction is suspected, the drug should be slowly withdrawn or the patient should be referred to an addiction specialist.

a. Nonnarcotic analgesics

1) Acetaminophen is a centrally acting analgesic with similar effectiveness to aspirin but unlike aspirin, it does not have antiinflammatory or antiplatelet properties and does not cause gastric toxicity. Because of its low side-effect profile, it is the first-line drug for the relief of mild to moderate pain. It is available in an oral form either singly or in combination with NSAIDs or opioids. It is also available singly in suppository forms. For details, see Chapter 4.8, section I.A.1.

2) Tramadol (Ultram) is an oral synthetic nonopioid drug, which probably causes analgesia by binding to the mu-opioid receptors and by inhibiting reuptake of norepinephrine and serotonin. It is used as an alternative to opioids for the relief of mild to moderate pain. For details, see Chapter 4.8, section I.A.2.

3) Nonsteroidal antiinflammatory drugs reduce inflammation by inhibiting the synthesis and release of prostaglandins (specifically E_2), but they are not prostaglandin antagonists. This implies that the previously existing prostaglandins (PGs) need to be depleted before the NSAID can take effect. Thus, in patients with preexisting tissue trauma (e.g., rheumatoid arthritis), the antiinflammatory (and, indirectly, the analgesic) effect of the NSAID may not be felt until after several days of regular, repeated dosing. In fact, it has been reported that, in certain situations (e.g., patients with low risk for gastrointestinal [GI] bleeding), starting NSAIDs preoperatively is more effective than starting them postoperatively.

The antiinflammatory effect of NSAIDs is not the most important factor in producing NSAID analgesia. This is shown in dental pain studies in which NSAIDs achieve analgesia exceeding that produced by corticosteroids even though the antiinflammatory effect of corticosteroids is greater. Aside from reducing peripheral inflammation, therefore, NSAIDs probably produce analgesia by decreasing painful responses to peripheral chemical mediators as well as by acting centrally. The analgesic effect of NSAIDs (present even without a peripheral focus of inflammation) has a more rapid onset of less than 1 hour (i.e., 10 minutes for the injectable ketorolac [Toradol] and, generally, 30-60 minutes for most oral NSAIDs). For the oral NSAIDs, the limiting factor for onset is the rate of GI absorption of the drug. Even for pro-drug NSAIDs, which must be metabolized in the liver to the active form (e.g., nabumetone [Relafen] and sulindac [Clinoril]), the onset is not significantly delayed because hepatic metabolism is rapid. The NSAID dosage needed to produce analgesia is 2 to 4 times lower than that required for the antiinflammatory effect. The mechanism of action (MOA), indications, contraindications, adverse drug reactions (ADRs), chemical classification, and dosages of NSAIDs are described in Chapter 4.8, section I.A.3.

The NSAIDs have the following advantages over opioid analgesics: low abuse potential; fewer respiratory, cardiovascular, and CNS adverse effects; and ease of prescription and administration (i.e., absence of controlled substance restrictions and availability of multiple over-the-counter oral preparations such as aspirin, ibuprofen, and naproxen). The NSAIDs are indicated in the management of mild to moderate pain. For severe acute pain, NSAIDs are used to supplement a primary analgesic agent (e.g., morphine) to decrease the need for the opioid and to minimize the opioid side effects. For mild to moderate pain, one of the first-line NSAIDs are the nonacetylated salicylates (e.g., choline magnesium salicylate), which have less GI ulcer potential than other NSAIDs. Topical nonsteroidal antiinflammatory preparations are also available (see section VI.E.2.e.3).

b. Opioid (or narcotic) analgesics are discussed in detail in Chapter 4.8, section I.B. They inhibit afferent nociceptive impulses at the dorsal horn of the spinal cord and at supraspinal sites by interacting with opioid receptors (i.e., μ, κ, δ, and σ–receptors). Opioids are relatively safe and effective in the short-term management of moderate to severe acute pain (e.g., postoperative or posttraumatic pain) and in the long-term management of chronic cancer pain. All pain, however, is not responsive to opioid analgesics alone. Opioid-resistant pain can be classified into 1) *pseudoresistant,* for example, underdosing, poor alimentary absorption (rare), poor alimentary intake because of vomiting, and ignoring of psychosocial aspects of care; 2) *semiresistant,* that is, pain that is relieved by the concurrent use of an opioid, an adjuvant drug and/or nondrug measures (examples of opioid semiresistant pain include bone metastasis, activity-related pain, and some cases of neuropathic pain); and 3) *resistant,* that is, pain that is not relieved by opioids but is relieved by other drugs and/or nondrug measures (examples of opioid-resistant pain include muscle spasm and some cases of neuropathic pain).

The use of opioids in NCP remains controversial although it is no longer uniformly rejected by pain specialists. The available data suggests that the population with NCP is extremely heterogenous and that some patients benefit while others deteriorate during opioid treatment. After all other reasonable analgesic therapies have failed, therefore, opioid therapy may be tried in selected NCP patients using clinically derived guidelines (see Table 5.10-4), which stress a structured approach and ongoing monitoring of efficacy, adverse effects, functional outcomes, and the occurrence of aberrant drug-related behaviors. It must be clearly emphasized that opioid therapy would not be useful if it augmented pain-related disability or undermined the efficacy of rehabilitation efforts, regardless of its effects on the pain. Thus, opioid therapy should only be used as a complement to, not as a substitute for, a comprehensive pain management approach, which incorporates psychosocial and rehabilitative therapies. The patient must agree in a contractual arrangement (which can be in the form of a written document) that opioids will be supplied for a limited term (i.e., time-contingent rather than pain-contingent) in exchange for meeting agreed goals such as increased mobilization, return to work, no unauthorized use of other opioids, and changes in unacceptable or nonproductive behaviors. The patient must also understand that there will be regular and random blood samples collected to ensure compliance with dosing schedule and that other opioid drugs are not being used.

Even for acute pain, many clinicians are reluctant to use opioid analgesics because of concerns about life-threatening side effects and the potential for iatrogenic addiction. These concerns, while legitimate, are not supported by current scientific data and hence do not justify a delay in the initiation of opioid therapy, if otherwise indicated, or the withholding of therapy from those with long life expectancies (e.g., noncancer patients). Clinical evidence shows that life-threatening side effects of opioids (e.g., respiratory depression) are extremely uncommon in patients who undergo gradual dose escalation. Even if it occurs, it can promptly be reversed by administering an opioid antagonist (naloxone). Likewise, studies have shown that mere exposure to an opioid, even for prolonged periods, does not produce the aberrant behaviors consistent with addiction disorders. Other factors such as underlying personality, social environment and availability of money are more strongly correlated with drug abuse. Unless the patient has a prior history of drug abuse, addiction appears to be extremely low (less than 0.1%) during chronic opioid therapy for cancer and noncancer pain. In addition to the opioid, nonopioid analgesics and adjuvant drugs should be used concurrently if indicated.

Addiction should not be equated with drug tolerance or physical dependence. Tolerance is a process defined by the occurrence of decreasing effects at a constant dose or the need for a higher dose to maintain an effect. With the exception of constipation and meiosis, tolerance to the nonanalgesic adverse effects of opioids (e.g., nausea, somnolence, mental clouding, and respiratory depression) occurs more readily than tolerance to analgesia in patients whose pain is stable. This is clinically beneficial because it increases the likelihood that a favorable balance between analgesia and side effects will be attained during dose escalation. Tolerance should not be assumed in patients

---

Table 5.10-4. Proposed guidelines for the use of opioid therapy in noncancer chronic pain

---

I. Pretreatment considerations
1. Consider opioid only after all other reasonable analgesic therapies have failed.
2. A single practitioner should take primary responsibility for treatment.
3. A history of substance abuse, severe character pathology, or chaotic home environment should be viewed as relative contraindications.
4. Informed consent (a written contract may be used) should include (a) Recognition of the low risk of true addiction as an outcome; (b) Potential for cognitive impairment from the drug alone or from the combination of the drug with other centrally acting drugs; (c) Potential for other side effects; (d) Likelihood that physical dependence will occur (abstinence syndrome possible with acute discontinuation); (e) Need for responsible drug-taking behavior (e.g., no unsanctioned dose escalation, no prescriptions from other physicians, etc.)

II. Drug administration
1. Oral route must be used (except in rare circumstances).
2. Long-acting opioids (e.g., controlled-release morphine or methadone) are preferred.
3. "Around the clock" dosing is preferable if with continuous or frequently recurring pain.
4. Allow patient to escalate dose transiently on days of increased pain by either method
   a) Prescription of an additional 4-6 "rescue doses" to be taken as needed during the month; or
   b) Instruction that one or two extra doses may be taken on any day but must be followed by an equal reduction of dose on subsequent days.
5. Initial dose titration should be done after the agreed period of several weeks.
6. Failure to achieve at least partial analgesia at relatively low initial doses in the patient with limited prior opioid consumption should raise questions about the potential treatability of the pain syndrome with opioids and lead to reassessment.
7. Exacerbations of pain not effectively treated by transient and small increases in dose are best managed in the hospital, where dose escalation, if appropriate, can be observed closely and return to baseline doses can be accomplished in a controlled environment.

III. Follow-up
1. Initially, patients must be seen and drugs prescribed at least monthly; when patient is stable, less frequent visits may be acceptable.
2. Follow-up visits should specifically address and document (a) Comfort or degree of analgesia (may use self-report instruments); (b) Functional status (physical and psychosocial; may use self-report instruments); (c) Opioid-related side effects; and (d) Existence of persistent aberrant drug-related behaviors during the course of therapy (see Table 5.10-5).
3. Determine if opioid therapy should be continued with rigid guidelines, be tapered and discontinued, or if the patient needs to consult an addiction specialist.

Adapted from Portenoy RK: Opioid therapy for chronic nonmalignant pain: current status. In Fields HL, Liebeskind IC editors: *Progress in pain research and management; vol 1; pharmacological approaches to the treatment of chronic pain: new concepts and critical issues,* Seattle, 1994, IASP Press, pp 274-275, with permission.

with chronic diseases who experience diminishing analgesia after a period of stable dosing. Studies have shown that the main reason for increasing the dose is not tolerance but progression or recurrence of the disease or the development of new pathology. Should tolerance to analgesia develop, an upward adjustment of dose is all that is necessary to regain pain control.

Physical dependence, which refers to a physiologic phenomenon characterized by the development of an abstinence syndrome, does not indicate the presence nor absence of the behaviors that define addiction. While addicted patients can be physically dependent, physically dependent patients are not necessarily addicted. Physical dependence can develop after as little as a few days of opioid therapy. When the opioid is suddenly withdrawn or when an opioid antagonist is administered in a physically dependent patient, abstinence syndromes (which are rarely life-threatening) can develop. Prevention and treatment of abstinence syndromes are discussed in Chapter 4.8, section I.B.

If the patient engages in aberrant drug-related behaviors (listed in Table 5.10-5), the clinician must assess whether the problem is transitory and impulsive (perhaps related to a flare of unrelieved symptoms)

Table 5.10-5. Aberrant drug-related behaviors that raise concern about addiction potential

I. Behaviors more suggestive of an addiction disorder
- Selling prescription drugs
- Prescription forgery
- Stealing or "borrowing" drugs from others
- Injecting oral formulations
- Obtaining prescription drugs from nonmedical sources
- Concurrent abuse of alcohol or illicit drugs
- Multiple dose escalations or other noncompliance with therapy despite warnings
- Multiple episodes of prescription "loss"
- Repeatedly seeking prescriptions from other clinicians or from emergency rooms without informing prescriber or after warnings to desist
- Evidence of deterioration in the ability to function at work, in the family, or socially that appears to be related to drug use
- Repeated resistance to changes in therapy despite clear evidence of adverse physical or psychological effects from the drug

II. Behaviors less suggestive of an addiction disorder
- Aggressive complaining about the need for more drug
- Drug hoarding during periods of reduced symptoms
- Requesting specific drugs
- Openly acquiring similar drugs from other medical sources
- Unsanctioned dose escalation or other noncompliance with therapy on one or two occassions
- Unapproved use of the drug to treat another symptom
- Reporting psychic effects not intended by the clinician
- Resistance to a change in therapy associated with "tolerable" adverse effects, with expressions of anxiety related to the return of severe symptoms

---

From Portenoy RK: Opioid therapy for chronic nonmalignant pain: current status. In Fields HL, Lieberskind JC, editors: *Progress in pain research and management, vol 1: Pharmacological approaches to the treatment of chronic pain: new concepts and critical issues,* Seattle, 1994, IASP Press, p 267; with permission.

or more serious and abiding. Patients with drug-seeking behavior because of uncontrolled pain ("pseudoaddiction") must be distinguished from true addicts who compulsively seek the drug to experience its psychological effects and who continue drug use despite harm. In patients with pseudoaddiction, the aberrant behaviors can be eliminated by improving pain control, which is often achieved by escalation of the opioid dose. If opioid addiction is suspected, tapering and discontinuation of opioid therapy may be necessary or the patient should be referred to an addiction specialist.

General guidelines for opioid administration are discussed in Chapter 4.8, section I.B. For patients with cancer pain, the following additional guidelines must be considered: opioids should be given "by the mouth," "by the clock" (i.e., fixed intervals), "for the individual," "with an adjuvant medication," and "by the ladder" (i.e., analgesic ladder). Adjuvant medications are discussed in section VI.E.2. The analgesic ladder approach, which was developed by a committee of the World Health Organization, is as follows:

Step 1. For mild to moderate cancer pain, use nonopioid drugs (e.g., NSAIDs, acetaminophen; see sections VI.E.1.a.1 and VI.E.1.a.3). If indicated, adjuvant drugs (see section VI.E.2) may be added for additional analgesia or for the treatment of a different symptom (either a side effect of the analgesic or a coexisting symptom other than pain).

Step 2. If mild to moderate pain persists despite step one, add a "weak" pure-agonist opioid drug to the nonopioid analgesic (see Table 4.8-4 for classification and initial dose of "weak" opioids). If indicated, add adjuvant drugs (as in step one). The pure-agonist opioid drugs, which are operationally (rather than pharmacologically) classified as "weak," include codeine, hydrocodone, dihydrocodeine, oxycodone (combined with aspirin or acetaminophen), propoxyphene, and, occasionally, meperidine. Although these opioids do not have a "ceiling" effect for analgesia, they are not indicated in the management of more severe pain because of relatively increased toxicity at higher doses (particularly propoxyphene, meperidine, and codeine). Oxycodone, hydrocodone, and dihydrocodeine (all of which are given in combination with aspirin or acetaminophen) cannot be given in quantities that exceed the maximal safe amount of the nonopioid coanalgesics (e.g., 4-6 gm of acetaminophen per day). Another nonopioid alternative for "weak" opioids is tramadol.

Step 3. If pain is moderate to severe, or if pain persists despite step 2, then replace the "weak" pure-agonist opioids with "strong" pure-agonist opioids (see Table 4.8-4 for classification and initial dosing of "strong" opioids). Depending on indication, the patient may or may not need nonopioid analgesics or adjuvant drugs. The pure-agonist opioid drugs, which are operationally classified as "strong," include morphine (first-line drug), hydromorphone, methadone, fentanyl, and levorphanol. Hydromorphone is used in cases of morphine toxicity in patients with renal disease.

2. **Adjuvant analgesics** are drugs primarily approved for the treatment of conditions other than pain but act as analgesics in selected circumstances. They have large interindividual and intraindividual variability, hence sequential trials (i.e., multiple series of trial and error) are usually needed before a therapeutic regimen is attained. Some groups of adjuvant drugs (e.g.,

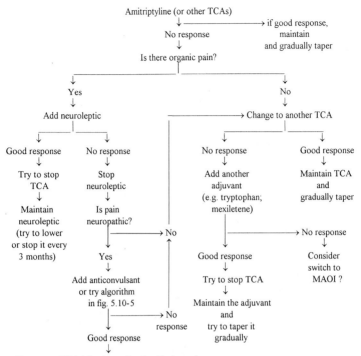

Figure 5.10-4.
Suggested algorithm for sequential trial of adjuvant analgesics in patients with chronic pain syndrome. Each drug must be given adequate dose and period of trial (see text). Monitor ECG and laboratory test as needed (see text). If neuropathic pain is lancinating, may start with anticonvulsant (e.g., carbamazepine). TCA = tricyclic antidepressant; MAOI = monoamine oxidase inhibitor. Adapted from Monks R: Psychotropic drugs. In Wall PD, Melzack R, editor: *Textbook of pain,* ed 3, Edinburgh, 1994, Churchill Livingstone, pp 977-978.

antidepressants, neuroleptics, α_2-adrenergic agonists) are considered multipurpose adjuvant analgesics (i.e., they have established utility in different pain syndromes) and are potentially useful in the management of any chronic pain patients. Figures 5.10-4 and 5.10-5 show the algorithm for the sequential trial of adjuvant drugs in patients with chronic pain syndrome.
  a. Antidepressants (see Chapter 4.8, section V.A) enhance the availability of neurotransmitters (e.g., serotonin and norepinephrine) probably by inhibiting their reuptake at the neuronal membrane. Their multifactorial mechanism of analgesia probably includes raising the pain threshold, allowing improved sleep, altering the perception of pain, and possibly improving mood (although analgesia can occur independent of mood elevation since it is usually given at a dose lower than that needed for

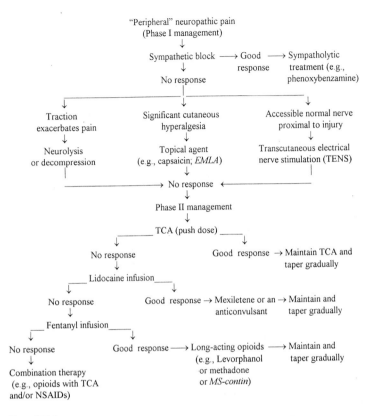

Figure 5.10-5

Suggested algorhithm for management of neuropathic pain with predominating "peripheral" pain generator. Phase I outlines the steps to be taken prior to starting long-term medical management. Phase II outlines one systemic approach to pharmacological treatment. TCA = tricyclic antidepressant; NSAIDs = nonsteroidal anti-inflammatory drugs. Adapted from Fields HL: Peripheral neuropathic pain: an approach to management. In Wall PD, Melzack R, editors: *Textbook of pain*, ed 3, Edinburgh, 1994, Churchill Livingstone, pp 994.

antidepression). Antidepressants also potentiate the analgesic effectiveness of concomitant use of opioids, NSAIDs, or both.

Antidepressants are multipurpose adjuvant analgesics used in patients with chronic neuropathic pain (except possibly pure lancinating neuropathic pain such as trigeminal neuralgia, which responds better to anticonvulsant therapy), chronic musculoskeletal pain (e.g., rheumatoid arthritis, osteoarthritis, fibromyalgia, or myofascial pain), chronic headache, chronic facial pain, cancer pain, posttraumatic encephalopathies, and psychogenic pain. They are rarely indicated in patients with acute pain (except when used in patients expected to have long-term pain problems) because it takes them 2 to 4 weeks to achieve effective analgesia. The average analgesic response rate to antidepressant medications is reported to be 62% (range of 44-70%). In general, antidepressants classified as tricyclics (see Table 4.8-6 for side-effect profiles) should not be used by patients with recent myocardial infarction or cardiac conduction problems and by those who cannot tolerate anticholinergic effects such as symptomatic prostatic hypertrophy or narrow angle glaucoma (tricyclics with secondary amines, such as desipramine and nortriptyline, or non tricyclic antidepressants may be tried because of lesser anticholinergic effects). It is advisable to check the electrocardiogram (ECG) (especially when using tricyclic antidepressants) and laboratory tests (e.g., complete blood count, differential count, and liver and renal function tests) before starting treatment and periodically thereafter. For details about the pharmacology of antidepressants, see Chapter 4.8, section V.A).

Tricyclic antidepressants (TCAs), in particular **amitriptyline (Elavil),** are the most common nonanalgesic medications used in the treatment of chronic pain. Cardiovascular monitoring in TCA use is discussed in Chapter 4.8, section V.A. For chronic pain treatment, a trial of amitriptyline should be considered as first-line therapy, unless relatively contraindicated by its side-effect profile or if another antidepressant has been shown to be more clinically effective for that particular diagnosis. The usual starting dose for amitriptyline is 10 mg in the elderly or 25 mg in younger patients. The dose is then titrated every 2 to 4 days or weekly (with the initial dosing increments being usually the same size as the starting dose) in accordance to individual patient response. The dose needed for pain relief ranges from 25 to 100 mg per day (with occasional patients benefiting from a dose higher or lower than this range). It can be given as a single dose at bedtime to take advantage of its sedating effect and minimize daytime drowsiness (in some patients with late afternoon pain, the dose may need to be divided). Although sedation and other side effects may occur within a week, the analgesic effect may require an average of 2 to 4 weeks to occur. Once the effective dosing level is achieved, the dose should be maintained for a week since analgesic effects usually occur within the next 4 to 7 days. To ensure drug compliance, the patient must be educated about this delay in clinical benefit (and the fact that side effects may decrease after a few weeks as the patient develops tolerance).

If within the 2 to 4 week period (or more), the patient fails to achieve the analgesic benefit and has no limiting side effects, the amitriptyline dose may be escalated beyond the usual analgesic dose range (even if the patient has no evidence of clinical depression). Plasma drug concentration, if available, can help guide dose titration for analgesia. If the plasma concentration is relatively low compared to established antidepressant range, the drug can be increased (as long as there are no intolerable side effects). However, if the plasma concentration is relatively high compared to the established antidepressant range, the drug should be stopped (despite absence of adverse effects) because the likelihood of benefit is probably low and the risks of toxicity are increased. The duration of amitriptyline therapy for pain management is controversial. Once sustained analgesia is achieved for a period of months, the dose can be gradually reduced until the drug is discontinued if neither pain nor any other rebound effects occur.

If treatment with amitriptyline has failed or is not indicated because of concerns about side effects, **desipramine (Norpramine)** or **nortriptyline (Pamelor, Aventyl)** are appropriate alternatives, given their good evidence of analgesia and favorable side-effect profiles (see Chapter 4.8, section V.A and Table 4.8-6). Among the TCAs, it is generally considered that desipramine has the least sedating effect while nortriptyline probably has lesser orthostatic hypotensive effect than desipramine. In refractory cases, another tricyclic (e.g., **imipramine [Tofranil]** or **doxepin [Sinequan, Adapin]**) may be tried sequentially because of variations in individual response. Although the selective serotonin reuptake inhibitors (SSRIs) have very low sedative effects, only **paroxetine (Paxil)** (see Chapter 4.8, section V.A.2) has been shown to have analgesic benefit (i.e., in painful polyneuropathy). If SSRIs are used, they should be given in the morning as they may cause insomnia.

b. **Neuroleptic drugs** (see Chapter 4.8, section V.B) are multipurpose adjuvant analgesics with potential usefulness as second-line agents in the management of chronic neuropathic pain (e.g., continuous dysesthesias) or arthritic pain that is refractory to sequential trials of antidepressants, oral local anesthetics, and other drugs (e.g., anticonvulsants and baclofen). They are also useful in treating acute delirium and can occasionally be used for their sedative and anxiolytic effects. Some of their adverse effects include postural hypotension, excessive sedation, anticholinergic effects, and extrapyramidal reactions (e.g., tardive dyskinesia in long-term use). The use of lower initial doses, which can then be increased to these levels, is particularly important in the elderly. A trial of several weeks is reasonable, given experience with other adjuvant analgesics, and the failure to obtain a clear-cut analgesic response should be followed by discontinuation of the drug.

Only one neuroleptic drug, **methotrimeprazine (Levoprome)**, has been shown to have an unequivocal analgesic effect (mechanism of action is unknown; probably involving the dopaminergic pathways or through alpha-adrenergic blockade). Methotrimeprazine is a phenothiazine, which also has antiemetic and anxiolytic effects. It is often considered for intermittent, short-term use in patients with refractory chronic pain (e.g., because of advanced cancer) who have some other indication for a neuroleptic (e.g., delirium), are largely bedridden, or in whom GI disease (e.g., acute bowel obstruction) or pulmonary disease is sufficient to impede opioid use. Fifteen mg of intramuscular (IM) methotrimeprazine is equianalgesic to 10 mg of IM morphine. Methotrimeprazine is initially given at 5 mg, IM, and titrated up to 10 to 20 mg, IM, q6h. It has prominent sedative side effects and is not available in oral form.

Fluphenazine (Prolixin), a phenothiazine, has mild analgesic properties and can be used in combination with a tricyclic antidepressant (e.g., amitriptyline) to treat refractory neuropathic pain (e.g., postherpetic neuralgia). Evidence of efficacy is controversial. The doses recommended are between 1 and 3 mg a day (given po or IM), starting with a low dose and slowly escalating to 3 mg in combination with 50 to 100 mg of amitriptyline. Because the antihistamines, such as hydroxyzine (Vistaril, Atarax; see section VI.E.2.g.2), often seem to be as effective as the phenothiazines when used by chronic pain patients, the long-term use of phenothiazines must be weighed against the potential risk of tardive dyskinesia.

The other nonphenothiazine neuroleptic drugs with potential usefulness in chronic pain management are haloperidol (a butyrophenone) and
pimozide. **Haloperidol (Haldol)** has been suggested to have coanalgesic
properties at low doses (0.5-1 mg titrated to no higher than 2-5 mg,
po, bid/tid). **Pimozide (Orap)** at high dose (4-12 mg per day) has been
shown to be effective for patients with refractory neuropathic pain characterized by lancinating or paroxysmal dysesthesia. However, pimozide
also has high incidence of physical and mental slowing, tremors, and
slight parkinsonian symptoms.

c. **Anticonvulsants** (see Chapter 4.8, section IV) produce analgesia by an
unknown mechanism, which probably involves stabilization of neuronal
membranes in both the peripheral and central nervous systems. Moreover, sodium valproate has also been reported to increase central levels
of gamma amino butyric acid (GABA). Anticonvulsants should be considered early in the treatment of neuropathic pain characterized by lancinating or paroxysmal pain (e.g., trigeminal neuralgia or other cranial
neuralgias). However, they are second-line or third-line agents (i.e.,
they are appropriate only after failure of other adjuvant analgesics,
including antidepressants and oral local anesthetics) in patients with
neuropathic pain characterized by predominating continuous dysesthesias such as painful polyneuropathies (including diabetic neuropathies),
painful mononeuropathies (e.g., nerve inflammation or trauma, including surgical trauma as well as brachial and lumbosacral plexus pain
syndromes caused by either tumor infiltration or traumatic neuroma),
deafferentation pain (e.g., central pain due to spinal cord injury, phantom limb pain, postherpetic neuralgia, or nerve root avulsion) and SMP
(e.g., RSD with sympathetic features).

The usefulness of anticonvulsants is often limited by their ADRs
(including bone marrow depression, hepatic dysfunction, nystagmus,
diplopia, ataxia, nausea, lymphadenopathy, confusion, and vertigo). All
anticonvulsant drugs used for chronic pain treatment should be initiated
at low doses, except possibly for phenytoin which is usually well tolerated during a cautious oral or intravenous loading regimen. Low dose
titration also minimizes side effects. The minimal effective anticonvulsant dose for analgesia is unknown. To date, no studies have compared
the relative efficacy of the anticonvulsant drugs in various types of
neuropathic pain. Guidelines on drug administration and laboratory
monitoring (including complete blood count, differential count, liver
function tests, and drug levels) are discussed in Chapter 4.8, section
IV.

There is great individual variation in the response to anticonvulsants,
hence, trials with alternative drugs should be considered if the patient
fails to respond or is unable to tolerate any particular anticonvulsant.
In the absence of a contraindication, most clinicians begin with **carbamazepine (Tegretol)** due to the abundant data supporting its efficacy for
neuropathic pain. The other commonly used anticonvulsant for pain
control is **phenytoin (Dilantin).** The effectiveness of phenytoin has been
reported to be approximately 20 to 40% in patients with neuralgic pain.
A favorable response to **clonazepam (Klonopin)** has been reported in patients with trigeminal neuralgia, paroxysmal postlaminectomy pain, and
posttraumatic neuralgia. Patients with chronic pain associated with anxiety or insomnia may benefit from an early trial of clonazepam, which

may also be effective for these symptoms. **Valproic acid (Depakene)** has been reported to be effective in patients with trigeminal neuralgia and postherpetic neuralgia.

The newer anticonvulsants, **felbamate (Felbatol)** and **gabapentin (Neurontin),** have not been fully evaluated in the management of chronic pain. Felbamate interacts with the N-methyl-D-aspartate (NMDA) receptor, which has been associated with painful nerve injuries. However, felbamate is *not* recommended because of its increased potential for aplastic anemia. Gabapentin, a GABA analog, has anecdotally been reported to be effective in certain types of neuropathic pain (e.g., RSD/causalgia nerve trauma, and brachial and lumbosacral plexus pain syndromes) but further controlled studies are needed to confirm this. The mechanism of analgesic action of gabapentin is theorized to be due to increased CNS serotonergic-like activities, which reciprocally block catecholamine outflow, resulting in a gradual reduction of the noradrenergic-induced hyperalgesia. Gabapentin (Neurontin) is available orally at 100-, 300-, or 400-mg capsules. It can be given at 300 mg, po, qhs, on day one; 300 mg, po, bid, on day two; and 300 mg, po, tid, on day three. The effective dose range is 300 to 600 mg, po, tid, which can be titrated as needed up 2400 mg (or even as high as 3600 mg) per day.

d. **Local anesthetics** produce analgesia probably by stabilizing the neuronal membrane, blocking depolarization of the action potential, and suppressing aberrant electrical activity generated by central neurons, damaged peripheral axons, or both. They are third-line drugs, which should be considered in the treatment of patients with continuous dysesthesias (e.g., diabetic peripheral neuropathy) refractory to antidepressants and patients with lancinating pains (e.g., trigeminal neuralgia) refractory to anticonvulsant drugs and baclofen. The ADRs, which are dose-dependent, include CNS effects (e.g., dizziness, sedation, perioral numbness and other paresthesias, tremor, progressive encephalopathy, and seizures), cardiovascular effects (e.g., bradycardia, hypotension, and cardiac arrest), allergic effects, and other effects (e.g., respiratory depression and vomiting). All local anesthetic should be avoided in patients with severe heart failure or cardiac rhythm disturbances and in those on antiarrhythmic drugs. Patients with other significant cardiac disease should be monitored with repeated electrocardiograms or consultation with a cardiologist prior to treatment. A trial of IV infusion of local anesthetic may be implemented prior to starting oral local anesthetic or vice versa. There is no data to support the belief that the patient's response to IV local anesthetics is predictive of the response to oral local anesthetics and vice-versa. Hence oral local anesthetics are justified even if there is no response to the IV local anesthetic and vice versa.

1) **IV local anesthetics** (e.g., **lidocaine [Xylocaine], procaine [Procan]**) can occasionally produce durable effects after a brief infusion but analgesia is usually not prolonged. An IV local anesthetic commonly used for pain management is **lidocaine (Xylocaine)**, given at 2 to 5 mg/kg infused over a period of 20 to 30 minutes.

2) **Oral local anesthetics** (e.g., **mexiletene [Mexitil], tocainamide [Tonacard],** and **flecainide [Tambocor]**) provide an opportunity for long-term pain management. The preferred agent is **mexiletine (Mexitil)** started at 150 mg per day, then gradually titrated up every 2 to 3 days to a maxi-

mum of 300 mg, po, tid. Additional ADRs of mexiletene include nausea and vomiting (which can be diminished by ingesting the drug with food) and rare but serious side effects, including liver damage and blood dyscrasias. Hence, complete blood count and liver function tests should be done periodically.

   3) Topical local anesthetic preparations (e.g., EMLA; see section VI.E.2.e.2).

e. **Topical analgesic agents** have generally been applied to neuropathic pain characterized by both a predominating peripheral mechanism and continuous dysesthesia. Their systemic absorption is minimal hence making them useful for patients who are predisposed to side effects from systemically administered drugs, such as the elderly or those with comorbid conditions such as dementia.

   1) Capsaicin (Zostrix) is an alkaloid neurotoxin (found in hot peppers), which renders the skin and joints insensitive to pain by depleting and preventing reaccumulation of the principal chemical pain mediator, substance P, in peripheral sensory neurons (nociceptors). It is indicated for treating pain due to rheumatoid arthritis and osteoarthritis, as well as for treating allodynia (i.e., pain produced by a normally nonpainful stimulus such as light touch, wind, and mild temperature changes), which occurs in postherpetic neuralgia, RSD/causalgia, painful diabetic neuropathy, traumatic mononeuropathies (e.g., in postmastectomy scar), and other painful mono- and polyneuropathies. It has no known systemic side effects or drug interactions, hence making it especially helpful for older patients taking systemic medications for concomitant diseases. Some patients complain of a local burning sensation, which is not related to tissue damage and appears to pose no risk to the patient. This is usually transitory, that is, disappearing with repeated administrations over days to weeks. If it is persistent, it may be preceded by application of a local anesthetic, ingestion of an analgesic, or the capsaicin may be discontinued. Capsaicin (Zostrix) is available in 0.025 and 0.075% creams. It is applied to the affected area 3 to 4 times daily. Before deciding on its ineffectiveness, the 0.075% cream given 4 times daily should be tried for 4 weeks.

   2) Topical local anesthetics (e.g., EMLA cream) produce an area of dense cutaneous anesthesia presumably by blocking local nerve conduction or activation of receptor organs at a peripheral level. EMLA cream consists of 2.5% lidocaine and 2.5% prilocaine. It is indicated as a local analgesic on normal intact skin and has been used in patients with neuropathic pain (e.g., postherpetic neuralgia). Although systemic effects are unlikely, it should not be used in patients with congenital methemoglobinemia (because of rare reports of methemoglobinemia caused by the metabolites of the prilocaine). To produce an area of dense cutaneous anesthesia, a relatively thick application must remain in contact with the skin under an occlusive dressing for at least 1 hour. The occlusive dressing can be an ordinary plastic wrap for large areas or a synthetic occlusive dressing (e.g., Tegaderm) for smaller areas. This mode of administration, however, may be difficult if the area of pain is on the face on a mobile area of the body.

   3) Topical NSAID preparations probably reduce tissue levels of PGs, thereby diminishing the impact of PGs on the peripheral activation of nociceptive primary afferent neurons. Various NSAIDs (e.g., aspirin, indomethacin, and diclofenac) have been investigated for topical use in neuropathic pain (e.g., postherpetic neuralgia). Although, they appear to be safe (with minimal systemic absorption), the efficacy of topical NSAIDs remain questionable.

f. **Skeletal muscle relaxants** (see Chapter 4.8, section II) produce nonspecific analgesia whose precise mechanism of action remains unknown although it probably is related to their central depressant effects. The name ''skeletal muscle relaxants'' is misleading because (except perhaps for diazepam) they have little or no direct relaxation effect on the skeletal muscles of man. ''Skeletal muscle relaxants'' are indicated for short-term relief of acute musculoskeletal pains (with or without muscle spasm). They should be viewed as alternatives to the nonopioid and opioid analgesics or, in more severe cases, potentially useful drugs to combine with these other analgesics (and help lessen the need for high doses of these other agents). Available data have shown that their analgesic efficacy in treating common acute musculoskeletal pains is superior to placebo, acetaminophen, or aspirin; however, there are no controlled studies comparing them to NSAIDs or opioids. Also, there is no data on the relative efficacy or side effect profiles of different ''skeletal muscle relaxants.'' Except for the use of **cyclobenzaprine (Flexeril)** (see Chapter 4.8, section II.A.1) in fibromyalgia, their use in the treatment of chronic pain is probably limited (there is report of abuse of these drugs in some patients with NCP). Also their sedative effects can hamper rehabilitative efforts. ''Skeletal muscle relaxants'' are available orally in single formulations and in combination with other compounds (usually with aspirin or codeine). In some types of skeletal muscle relaxants, parenteral forms are also available. For details, see Chapter 4.8, section II.

g. **Anxiolytics and sedatives**

   1) **Benzodiazepines** (see Chapter 4.8, section V.C.1) are CNS depressants whose exact mechanism of action is unknown (probably act by potentiating the inhibitory effects of GABA). By themselves, they generally don't have specific analgesic properties (except possibly for clonazepam) and do not produce additive effects when combined with another analgesic (e.g., opioids). Their roles as analgesics are probably limited to the following: **diazepam (Valium)**, 2 to 10 mg, po, tid/qid (see Chapter 4.8, section V.C.1.b.1), for use as a short-term ''skeletal muscle relaxant'' in patients with acute musculoskeletal pain; **clonazepam (Klonopin)**, 0.5 mg, po, tid, titrated up by 0.5 to 1 mg q3d to a maximum of 20 mg/day (see Chapter 4.8, section IV.D) for use in patients with refractory lancinating or paroxysmal neuropathic pain; and **alprazolam (Xanax),** 0.25 to 0.5, po, bid/tid, maximum of 4 mg/day (see Chapter 4.8, section V.C.1.a.3), for use in cancer patients with neuropathic pain or in patients with fibromyalgia. The benzodiazepines, however, play a significant role in the total management of acute or chronic pain patients with anxiety as the overriding clinical symptom (e.g., anxiety that is acute, severe, disabling, or lasting longer than 2 weeks).

   Some pain specialists believe that benzodiazepines should not be used at all in chronic pain patients (except for very short-term

treatment). Aside from their abuse potential (especially after prolonged use) and the possibility of hampering functional restoration,
benzodiazepines (especially in prolonged use) are believed to be
antianalgesic, that is, they may increase pain perception probably
by inhibiting serotonin release and inducing benzodiazepine receptor
subsensitivity. Benzodiazepines may also cause an increase in anger
and hostility when given over a period of 8 weeks.

2) **Hydroxyzine (Atarax, Vistaril)** is discussed in Chapter 4.8, section VI.A.
   It is an antihistaminic agent, which has anxiolytic and sedative effects as well as an analgesic effect (i.e., 100 mg of parenteral hydroxyzine is equianalgesic to that of 8 mg of morphine). When
   combined with morphine, it has additive analgesic effects, while the
   sedative effect is only slightly greater than that of morphine alone.

h. **Antispasticity drugs**, including **baclofen (Lioresal)** and **diazepam (Valium)** act
   as agonists of the inhibitory neurotransmitter GABA. Baclofen (see
   Chapter 5.4, section III.D.1.a) acts presynaptically, and diazepam (see
   above section VI.E.2.g.1; also Chapter 4.8, section V.C.1.b.1; Chapter
   5.4, section III.D.1.c) acts postsynaptically. In addition, baclofen may
   also reduce the release of excitatory transmitters (possibly including
   substance P) from nociceptive afferent nerve endings. The analgesic
   efficacy of baclofen in trigeminal neuralgia has been established. Baclofen can also be used empirically in treating myofascial pain syndromes
   and other types of lancinating or paroxysmal neuropathic pains in which
   muscle spasm is contributing to the pain. It can be started at a dose of
   5 mg, po, tid, which can be gradually titrated up until favorable effects
   occur or side effects supervene. Common side effects include nausea,
   confusion, drowsiness, dizziness, and hypotension. Baclofen should not
   be abruptly withdrawn as this may produce seizures and hallucinations.

i. **Antihypertensive drugs**

1) **Clonidine (Catapres)**, an α_2-adrenergic agonist and α_1-adrenergic
   blocker, is a multipurpose adjuvant analgesic, which is beneficial
   in various neuropathic pain syndromes, including migraine, postoperative pain, painful diabetic neuropathy, postherpetic neuralgia,
   nocturnal leg pains, sympathetically maintained pain, and cancer
   pain. It is considered a second-line adjuvant analgesic in chronic
   pain patients refractory to trials of NSAIDs, antidepressants, and
   other drugs. The MOA of its analgesic effect is probably related to
   its effects on norepinephrine as well as its inhibition of firing of
   dorsal horn nociceptors. Clonidine can be administered through the
   oral or transdermal route (choice of either route is based on patient
   preference). To avoid adverse effects (especially hypotension), it
   should be started at 0.1 mg/day, po, and gradually titrated up until
   side effects occur or a significant effect on blood pressure is noted
   (usual analgesic dose is 0.1 to 0.4 mg/day; maximum of 2.4 mg/day).
   See Chapter 4.8, section IX.A.1 and Chapter 5.4, section III.D.1.d
   for details about its ADRs, contraindications and precautions, and
   dosing administration guidelines.

2) **Prazosin (Minipress)** is a selective α_1-adrenergic blocker, which has
   anecdotally been reported to be effective for neuropathic pain, possibly from up-regulation of α_1-adrenergic receptors in injured nerves.
   Its ADRs include hypotension, syncope, dizziness, headache, drowsiness, lack of energy, weakness, palpitations, and nausea. It can be

started at 1 mg, po, qhs, then gradually titrated up to 4 to 12 mg/day (maximum daily dose is 20 mg in divided doses). It is available in 1-, 2-, and 5-mg capsule forms. See also Chapter 4.8, section IX.A.3.

3) **Phenoxybenzamine (Dibenzyline)**, an α_1- and α_2-adrenergic blocker primarily used in the management of hypertension in patients with pheochromocytoma, has been anecdotally reported to be effective in relieving pain by producing and maintaining "chemical sympathectomy" in selected cases of RSD/causalgia and possibly painful plexopathies. Because of unopposed β-adrenergic activity, there is exaggerated hypotension and tachycardia. If these side effects are intolerable, a β-blocker (e.g., propranolol) may be used concomitantly. Phenoxybenzamine is available in 10-mg capsules and can be given at 10 mg, po, q8h, gradually titrated up to 120 mg over a 6-week period.

4) **Propranolol (Inderal)**, a nonselective β-blocker, has been used in patients with RSD/causalgia, trigeminal neuralgia, phantom pain, and diabetic neuropathy. It is described in Chapter 4.8, sections IX.A.5 and V.F.

5) **Nifedipine (Procardia, Adalat)**, a calcium channel-blocker (see Chapter 4.8, section IX.B), which induces vasodilation, can be used in patients with RSD/causalgia, and Raynaud's phenomenon. The major ADRs include headache, hypotension, dizziness, flushing, weakness, nausea, muscle cramps, tremor, peripheral edema, nervousness, palpitation, dyspnea, and nasal congestion. It can be given at 10 mg, po, tid, and, if needed, increased weekly up to 30 mg, po, tid. If there is partial or complete improvement, the effective dose is continued for 2 weeks after which the dose is tapered and discontinued over several days.

6) **Peripherally acting adrenergic blockers**, e.g., **guanethidine** and **reserpine**, can be used as ganglionic-blocking agents for IV regional sympathetic blocks in patients with RSD/causalgia. They appear to act on the sympathetic nervous tissue, displacing norepinephrine from presynaptic vesicles and preventing reuptake. Their ADRs include a burning pain upon injection, prolonged postural hypotension, vertigo, nausea, vomiting, somnolence, and facial flushing. Clinical trials have shown that IV regional guanethidine block appears to yield more consistent and more reliable response than blocks performed with reserpine. At present, the parenteral forms of guanethidine and reserpine are only available for experimental use.

j. **Corticosteroids** (see Chapter 4.8, section III) have been shown to have analgesic effects probably due to their antiinflammatory effects, antiedema effects, and possibly due to a direct influence on the electrical activity of injured nerves. Steroids have been used as an adjuvant analgesic in cancer patients, specifically in patients with metastatic bone pain, neuropathic pain (e.g., plexopathy) because of infiltration or compression by the tumor, acute spinal cord compression, superior vena cava syndrome, raised intracranial pressure, symptomatic lymphedema, and hepatic capsular distension. They have also been used in NCP, such as postherpetic neuralgia, RSD/causalgia, and lumbar disk disease, although patient response has been variable. For chronic pain treatment, dexamethasone is usually used due to its relatively low mineralocorticoid effects. The dose varies from 4 to 16 mg/day or higher (initial dose may be as high as 100 mg IV) depending on the clinical situation. The use of corticosteroids has to be balanced with the potentially serious side effects (see Chapter 4.8, section III) especially in long-term use.

The analgesic benefit of corticosteroids in rheumatic and collagen disorders is probably related to their ability to modify the specific disease. Their analgesic role in acute neuropathy is controversial. High-dose oral steroids (e.g., prednisone, 60-80 mg, every morning) given for a short period (e.g., 5 days) has anecdotally been reported to have analgesic effects in patients with acute radiculopathy because inflammation in the nerve root is believed to cause the pain. Corticosteroid use for less than 1 week helps minimize adverse effects (e.g., there is no suppression of hypothalamic-pituitary-adrenal axis).

  k. L-**Tryptophan** is the amino-acid precursor of serotonin, which may be used singly or in combination with antidepressants (e.g., tricyclics or MAOIs) in treating patients with refractory neuropathic pain. Although the use of L-tryptophan is theoretically sensible, its analgesic efficacy has not yet been confirmed clinically; however, its use in refractory neuropathic pain may be justified because it is a relatively safe and well-tolerated drug. The alleged causal relationship of tryptophan supplements to eosinophilia-myalgia syndrome (EMS) has recently been shown to be caused by a contaminant originating from supplements provided by a single Japanese manufacturer. L-tryptophan can be started at a low dose (e.g., 1 g, po, bid) and then titrated up to 3 to 5 g per day. Side effects, which appear to be dose-related, include sedation and nausea. The effect of L-tryptophan may be potentiated by adding a low-protein/high-carbohydrate diet with vitamin supplements (e.g., niacin and B_6) which probably ensures adequate entry of L-tryptophan into the brain for conversion to serotonin.

  l. **Psychostimulants**, such as **dextroamphetamine (Dexedrine)** and **methylphenidate (Ritalin)**, may be used to counteract the unwanted sedative effects caused by other analgesics (e.g., opioids); however, they should be used with caution by patients receiving opioids with long half-lives (e.g., methadone). Moreover, sedation and respiratory depression masked during the day may manifest when the effect of the amphetamine has worn off and the patient goes to sleep. Caffeine is another psychostimulant, which is used in combination forms with opioids, NSAIDs, or "skeletal muscle relaxants" (see Chapter 4.8, section I.A.4; I.B.2). For details about psychostimulant drugs, see Chapter 4.8, section V.E.

  m. **Bone-pain drugs** used in cancer patients include calcitonin **(Calcimar, Miacalcin)** (see Chapter 4.8, section VIII.A.2), biphosphonates such as pamidronate (**Aredia;** see Chapter 4.8, section VIII.A.3), and bone-seeking radionuclides such as **strontium-99.** Calcitonin given at a starting dose of 25 IU daily titrated up to 100 to 150 IU once or twice daily may be used as a last resort in the treatment of refractory neuropathic pain including sympathetically maintained pain and phantom limb pain.

3. **Pain cocktail program** is a patient-blinded detoxification protocol used in chronic pain patients for reducing and eliminating excessive or abusive use of opioids, tranquilizers, and sedative-hypnotics medications. All parenteral medications are first switched into oral forms. The oral medications are then given on an as-needed ("prn") basis for 24 to 48 hours to obtain the typical 24-hour baseline requirement. No new or additional opioid, tranquilizer, or sedative-hypnotics are added during the entire program.

For patients with opioid abuse, the pain cocktail can be made up of a long-acting opioid (e.g., methadone), in an equivalent dose equal to the currently used opioid, mixed in a masking vehicle (e.g., cherry syrup). The pain cocktail is given orally around the clock at an interval established for the patient. Over a 3 to 6 week period, the active ingredient (e.g., opioid) is gradually reduced (e.g., 5-20% reduction per day) with an equal increase in the masking vehicle. The decrements are made slowly so as not to elicit withdrawal syndromes. When the patient is receiving the masking vehicle only, the vehicle is maintained for 2 to 10 days prior to discontinuation. Before starting the pain cocktail program, the entire procedure is explained to the patient, except the time when the active ingredient will be reduced. This approach used for opioids can also be used for tranquilizer or sedative-hypnotic drugs. To ensure compliance, pain cocktail programs are usually incorporated as part of a structured in-hospital or day-hospital program. (Chronic pain center treatment program is described in Chapter 5.11, section VI.B.4.) The pain cocktail is usually mixed and prepared by the pharmacist.

F. **Psychosocial and self-regulation techniques** give the patient a sense of control over postoperative and posttraumatic pain and its consequences, as well as demonstrating to the patient that his or her opinions and beliefs are important.

1. **Psychosocial support** refers to reassurance supplied through social and professional interactions with trained personnel as well as through individual psychotherapy and peer support groups.

2. **Procedural and sensory information** can be provided to the patient and the patient's family or support system. Procedural information is the specifics of the surgery or medical procedure, such as the time of the procedure, the risks associated with the anesthetic or surgery, and the sequence of events. Sensory information describes the sensory experiences the patient may confront such as aching, cramping, or burning pain at the incision. The methods of transmitting information include booklets, verbal presentations by staff, and audiotaped or videotaped presentations. The patient must have a good memory to remember information (or it may be repeated or given in written form). The clinician must be aware that for patients who use denial as a means to cope, the information may increase their anxiety.

3. **Coping-skills training** refers to teaching patients specific behaviors and strategies that may be used to cope with pain during the postoperative period or during the actual procedure (e.g., procedures in which the patient is awake).

   a. **Cognitive coping skills** include distraction, calming self-statements, pleasant imagery, humor, music, reading, stress-inoculation training, brief psychotherapy, reinterpreting pain stimuli, and cognitive reappraisal of the event.

   b. **Relaxation training** (see Chapter 4.2, section VI) are alternative forms of self-regulation that are based on modifying a chosen physiologic parameter, such as heart rate, breathing, or muscle spasm, with progressive training. Relaxation training activity takes time and practice, so the patient must be alert, responsive, and interactive. Relaxation may be incorporated with **biofeedback** training (see chapter 4.1, section VI).

   c. **Systemic desensitization** includes procedures in which the steps or parts of an experience such as a painful procedure are enumerated in a hierarchical order from the least distressful or painful for the patient to the most distressful or painful. The patient is then gradually exposed (either in imagination or in vivo) to each step, while applying relaxation or cognitive coping strategies and given positive reinforcement for mastering each step.

   d. **Modeling and exposure** involves the patient watching a videotape of another person who serves as a role model by showing successful techniques of coping with pain and anxiety in a situation similar to that experienced or to be experienced by the patient (e.g., preparation for surgery or other specific procedures).

   e. **Hypnosis** is a general term for states of focused attention, which can be achieved by many individuals under various circumstances. Hypnosis involves training and practice and can be an effective analgesic and anxiolytic tool in patients with long-term problems. It includes hetero- and autohypnoses and may use complex hypnotic phenomena (e.g., dissociation, sensory alteration, and time distortion).

4. **Intervention with family members** who were trained to help the patient cope with painful procedure (e.g., by coaching the patient to use paced breathing and distraction techniques).

G. **Vocational counseling** should be included as part of pain management if indicated.

H. **Invasive techniques** should only be used if noninvasive techniques have failed, except in rare cases where the invasive procedure can correct the underlying pathology (e.g., surgical decompression of the nerve).

1. **Joint and soft tissue injections** using corticosteroid or mixtures of corticosteroid and local anesthetic agents are considered as adjunct treatments for the relief of pain and inflammation of the joint (e.g., synovitis) and soft tissues (e.g., bursitis, tendinitis, or tenosynovitis). They are described in detail in Chapter 4.9. Facet joint blocks, which may be indicated in patients with deep, dull, aching back pain without neurological abnormalities, have variable success rates.

2. **Nerve blocks** involve the administration of local anesthetics or a neurolytic agent (e.g., chemical agents such as phenol and absolute alcohol, cold agents such as cryoprobe, and heat agents such as radiofrequency coagulation) into a somatic nerve (see Chapter 4.9 section IV.A), a sympathetic ganglia (see Chapter 4.9 section IV.B), or a localized pain-sensitive trigger point or tender spot (see Chapter 4.11). Epidural blocks using steroids are discussed in Chapter 4.9 section IV.A.3.e.

3. **Surgical interventions**

   a. **Neurosurgical procedures** for pain relief are generally reserved for refractory cases of chronic pain only after conservative measures fail. They have been associated with high morbidity and mortality in the past, but recent improvements in the understanding of the pathophysiology of pain and in the neurosurgical techniques have resulted in a high rate of success and a low incidence of complications. If patients are carefully selected, surgery performed by a skilled surgeon may provide dramatic relief. A significant number of patients, however, may have recurrence of some symptoms as early as 3 to 6 months after the procedure (probably due to nerve regeneration or scar formation). Procedures that are used to arrest nociceptive transmission include

      1) **Nondestructive techniques,** which attempt to correct the disordered physiology of nerves without creating a lesion, such as carpal tunnel

release, thoracic outlet decompression, root decompression, and cranial nerve decompression.

2) Destructive or interruptive techniques (neuroablation)

 a) Primary afferent procedures transect the primary afferent fibers at the level of the peripheral nerve, root, or ganglion. Examples include peripheral neurectomy, excision or relocation of neuromas, rhizotomy (cranial nerve or spinal), glycerol injection, gangliolysis, and ganglionectomy.

 b) Spinal cord procedures interrupt ascending sensory tracts in the spinal cord or brain stem. Cordotomy is the most effective and widely used, e.g., anterolateral cordotomy (spinal tractotomy), which may be done percutaneously by radiofrequency under fluoroscopic guidance or by open laminectomy at the low cervical or upper thoracic spine. Other procedures include commissural myelotomy (which disrupts pain conducting fibers as well as polysynaptic pain pathways that run through the center of the spinal cord) and dorsal root entry zone (DREZ) lesions (using radiofrequency).

 c) Deep brain procedures include stereotactically placed lesions of deep brain structures, such as stereotactic tractotomy (pons, thalamus, hypothalamus, or spinal thalamic or spinal reticular tracts) and psychosurgery (e.g., cingulotomy).

 d) Pituitary destruction (hypophysectomy), that is, anterior pituitary ablation.

 e) Sympathetic nerve procedures include thoracic or lumbar sympathectomy (in selected cases of sympathetically-maintained pain) and cortical and subcortical ablation.

3) Modulatory techniques

 a) Implantation of drug infusion systems (e.g., morphine infusion). Epidural, spinal intrathecal, intraventricular.

 b) Chronic stimulation (neuroaugmentation) of deep brain structures or the spinal cord to stimulate an analgesia mechanism in the central nervous system (e.g., to alter the gate-control mechanism or to increase secretion of endogenous opioids). Examples include stimulation of the dorsal columns, lemniscal pathway in brain, nerve (especially fifth nerve), periventricular-periaqueductal gray (PVG-PAG), internal capsule, and thalamus.

 b. Musculoskeletal procedures include total joint replacement, synovectomy, and curative excision or palliative debulking of a tumor.

4. Radiation therapy can be used for cancer patients to relieve metastatic pain as well as symptoms from local extension of the primary disease. Radiation therapy includes localized radiation therapy, wide-field radiation therapy, and radiopharmaceuticals (e.g., iodine-131 and strontium-99).

BIBLIOGRAPHY

Acute Pain Management Guideline Panel: *Clinical practice guideline: acute pain management,* AHCPR Publication No. 92-0032, Rockville, MD, Feb, 1992, Agency for Health Care Policy and Research.

Allegrante JP: Patient education. In Paget S, Pellicci P, Beary JF, III, editors: *Manual of rheumatology and outpatient orthopedic disorders,* ed 3, Boston, 1993, Little, Brown, pp 49-53.

Aronoff GM, editor: *Evaluation and treatment of chronic pain,* Baltimore, 1992, Williams & Wilkins.

Bartlett EE: Which patient education strategies will pay off under prospective pricing? *Patient Educ Couns* 12:51, 1988.

Bonica JJ, editor: *The management of pain,* ed 2, Philadelphia, 1990, Lea & Febiger.

Dean BZ, Williams FH, King JC, et al: Pain rehabilitation. 4. Therapeutic options in pain management, *Arch Phys Med Rehabil* Suppl 75:21-30, 1994.

Fordyce WE: *Behavioral methods for chronic pain and illness,* St. Louis, 1978 Mosby–Year Book.

Grabois M, VanDeventer J: Chronic pain. In Garrison SJ, editor: *Handbook of physical medicine and rehabilitation basics,* Philadelphia, 1995, JB Lippincott.

Hamill RJ, Rowlingson JC, editor: *Handbook of critical care pain management,* New York, 1994, McGraw-Hill.

Katz WA: Approach to the management of nonmalignant pain, *Am J Med* 101 (suppl 1A):54S–63S, 1996.

Markenson JA: Mechanism of chronic pain, *Am J Med* 101 (suppl 1A):7S–18S, 1996.

Management of Cancer Pain Guideline Panel: *Clinical practice guideline: management of cancer pain.* AHCPR Publication No. 94-0592, Rockville, MD, March, 1992, Agency for Health Care Policy and Research.

Physicians' desk reference, ed 51, Montvale, NJ, 1997, Medical Economics.

Portenoy RK, Kanner RM, editors: *Pain management: theory and practice,* Philadelphia, 1996, FA Davis.

Sinatra RS, Hord AH, Ginsberg B, et al. editors: *Acute pain: mechanism and management,* St. Louis, 1992, Mosby–Year Book.

Tollison CD, Satterthwaite JR, Tollison JW, editors: *Handbook of pain management,* ed 2, Baltimore, 1994, Williams & Wilkins.

Turk DC, Michenbaum DM, Gemest M: *Pain and behavioral medicine: a cognitive-behavioral perspective.* New York, 1983, Guilford.

Wall PD, Melzack R, editors: *Textbook of pain,* ed 3, Edinburgh, 1994, Churchill Livingstone.

Warfield CA, editor: *Principles and practice of pain management,* New York, 1993, McGraw-Hill.

World Health Organization: *Cancer pain relief and palliative care,* Geneva, 1990, World Health Organization.

CHAPTER 5.11

WORK-RELATED MUSCULOSKELETAL PROBLEMS

At present, work still poses considerable risk of musculoskeletal injury despite major advances in industrial safety and technology. This is costly to both the worker (because of lost wages) and to the industry (because of lost productivity and lost revenues). The two most important factors contributing to musculoskeletal injuries are: (1) increasing worker specialization, which has lead to an increase in task repetitiveness (hence boredom and greater chance for musculoskeletal overexertion), and (2) the combination of open hiring policies and workers' compensation insurance, which promotes hiring of any and all job applicants, resulting in greater likelihood that a worker will apply for and obtain employment that may not be physically suitable for him or her.

Physiatrists, because of their extensive training in neuromusculoskeletal disorders as well as their interdisciplinary team approach, play an important role in the evaluation, treatment, and rehabilitation of workers to help them recover and return to work. The goals of PM&R in work-related musculoskeletal injuries include pain reduction; enhancement of functional capabilities, work tolerance, and job safety; instruction in proper body mechanics and posture; prevention and reduction of work-related injuries and disabilities; and return of workers to significant gainful employment in an expedient and cost-effective manner. Information resources on the manufacturers and suppliers of musculoskeletal and work-related testing devices as well as on work-related organizations, associations, and government agencies, are listed in Appendices G-7 and G-12.

I. **Epidemiology** Studies indicate that work injuries are certainly not unique to the United States but are universal. In 1990, the U.S. Department of Labor's Bureau of Labor Statistics reported that the U.S. workforce experienced approximately 6.8 million job-related injuries and illnesses, which occurred at a rate of 8.8 per 100 full-time workers with resulting loss of approximately 60 million workdays. Nearly half (i.e., more than 3 million) of the reported cases were serious enough to require restricted work duties or lost workdays. Among occupational injuries, more than 2 million cases every year are associated with musculoskeletal injuries.

II. **Costs** resulting from work-related injury are reflected by direct costs (e.g., expenditures for medical care and compensation for lost wages) and the less tangible indirect costs (e.g., lost production, consumer cost increases, expenses of employee retraining or replacement, and litigation). Approximately two-thirds of the direct costs are payments for partial or permanent disability and one-third for medical expenses. The average cost to employers for an injury resulting in lost workdays was $14,000 in 1978. The Rand Corporation estimated that the direct costs of work-related injuries were $83 billion in 1989 and that worker's compensation premiums cost America industry more than $60 billion annually. In 1988, the amount paid in Workers' Compensation benefits was $30.8 billion. This figure was projected to increase at a rate of more than 12% per year. The percentage of compensation awards based on body parts affected are 24% for back, 20% for lower limbs, 14% for upper limbs excluding fingers, 12% for fingers, 11% for trunk excluding back, 8% for multiple parts, and 11% for all other body parts. The costs of medical care and disability benefits are greatest for persons with prolonged disability (in fact 10% of claims account for approximately 80% of costs because of disability). In addition to the monetary costs, work-related disability results in inestimable human pain, suffering, and decreased quality of life for the individual and the worker's family. Often, workers with long-term, work-related disabilities become exceedingly depressed, have limited activity levels, and undergo interpersonal disruptions (e.g., divorce).

III. **The Americans with Disabilities Act (ADA) of 1990** provides persons with disabilities civil rights protection in five areas: employment, public services, transportation, public accommodation, and telecommunication. Title I of the ADA (implemented in July 26, 1994 for employers with 15 to 24 employees) pertains to protection of the "qualified individuals with a disability" against discrimination from employers or labor organizations. A "qualified individual with a disability" is a disabled person who, with or without reasonable accommodation (see section III.B), can perform the essential functions of the job being sought. Aside from physical disability, a person with psychiatric disorder can also qualify as being disabled; however, a person who is currently engaged in the illegal use of drugs is not considered a "qualified individual with a disability." The employer will decide essential job functions and is advised to develop a written detailed job description. Discrimination against disabled persons is outlawed in every aspect of the employment process, including preemployment examination inquiries related to the disability, medical examinations to screen out workers, and the limiting or classifying of job applicants to adversely affect job opportunity. Ability to perform job-specific functions (as opposed to generic inquiries about physical, sense organ, or cognitive limitations) may, however, be considered in the hiring decision. Also, an employer may require a posthiring testing (i.e., preplacement testing), and may make the employment offer contingent on the results of that testing.

A. **Preplacement testing** may be done only after a job offer has been made to the prospective employee. All new employees for the same job must be examined with the same tests. The test must be job-specific (or related to "essential" job functions; factors determining job or task "essentiality" are described in section V.D.2.a) with the goal of ensuring that the employee is physically and emotionally capable of performing the job so as to not endanger himself or herself or other employees. If the employee is unable to successfully perform the testing due to some functional limitation, the industry is obliged to determine if reasonable accommodations (see below) could be implemented that would allow the successful performance of the required job tasks. All information obtained is collected confidentially.

B. **"Reasonable accommodation"** may include making physical facilities accessible (see Chapter 4.5, section II.B.2.e) for persons with disabilities; job restructuring; modifying work schedules; reassigning to a vacant position; modifying or acquiring equipment or devices; modifying or adjusting examinations, training materials, or policies; providing reserved parking; and providing a person (e.g., an interpreter) to help an employee. The ADA, however, does not require "reasonable accommodation" if it causes "undue hardship" on the employer as determined on a case-by-case basis.

IV. **Return to work (RTW) issues.** The interdisciplinary rehabilitation team plays significant roles in determining the patient's capability to return to work, in task-analysis of the patient's job, as well as in adaptations of work tools and work environment (e.g., barrier-free architectural designs). First, the health status of the patient is determined by medical, physical, and psychosocial testing. The health status or restriction is then matched to the job profile, which includes an analysis of both the physical abilities required for performing the job and the working conditions at the worksite. Job profiles compiled from one workplace cannot be used at another place because job titles of the same name may not involve the same tasks. If the patient is able to match all the critical tasks identified in the job profile, then he or she can be recommended to return to full duty with no limitation. However, this is not always feasible. Most of the time, the patient may either return to work with some limitations (e.g., light duty with limitations or part time) or the employer may modify the job or workplace to suit the impairment. Returning a worker to modified duty has been shown to be cost-effective. If this is not possible, an alternative job may be found in the same company making use of the worker's residual skills; however, if alternative jobs cannot be found or if the patient has severe injuries, then retraining for a different vocation may be considered. Usually, this is the last resort because retraining is costly. In making legal determinations of disability and fitness to work, the classification of jobs in the United States based on levels of exertion (Table 5.11-1) is commonly used. The following variables are associated with poor RTW:

A. **Occupational variables** including increased time off work (likelihood of RTW is about 50% if off 6 months, 25% if off 1 year, and less than 5% if off 2 years), poor job satisfaction (which also contributes to increased risk of injury, lost time, and delayed recovery), mismatch between the patient's physical capacities and demands of the job, and unavailability of job or unwillingness

Table 5.11-1. **Physical demand characteristics of work for any jobs in the United States based on the U.S. Department of Labor's *Dictionary of Occupational Titles*.***

PHYSICAL DEMAND LEVEL OF WORK	OCCASIONAL LOAD (1/3 OF THE TIME)	FREQUENT LOAD (1/3-2/3 OF THE TIME)	CONSTANT LOAD (>2/3 OF THE TIME)	TYPICAL ENERGY REQUIRED (METS)
Sedentary†	≤10 lb	Negligible	Negligible	1-2
Light	10-20 lb	≤10 lb‡	Negligible§	2-4
Medium	20-50 lb	10-25 lb	≤10 lb.	4-6
Heavy	50-100 lb	25-50 lb	10-20 lb.	7-8
Very heavy	>100 lb	>50 lb	>20 lb.	>8

Data adapted from US Department of Labor Employment and Training Administration: *Dictionary of Occupational Titles,* vol II, ed 4, revised, Washington, DC, 1991, US Government Printing Office, p 1013.
* (See also Table 2.7-5 in Chapter 2.7 for correlation with the New York Heart Association Functional and Therapeutic Classification of cardiac or cardiopulmonary impairment/disability).
† Sedentary work involves sitting most of the time but may require occasional walking or standing or lifting/carrying (of papers, small tools, or file folders).
‡ Even though the load is less than 10 lb, the job is classified as light if it requires a great deal of walking, standing, pushing, or pulling of arm or leg controls.
§ Even though the load is negligible, the job is classified as light if it requires a great deal of pushing or pulling of arm or leg controls while seated.

of the employer to make reasonable accommodations or to modify the job or consider temporary light-duty work for the employee.

B. **Psychosocial variables** including poor language proficiency, a disabled spouse, anger or excessive fault finding at the system or employer (i.e., adversarial relationship between the employer and employee), pending litigation, and secondary gain (e.g., financial compensation, increased attention and support from family and friends, and use of the illness as a tool of control in the family and against the employer).

C. **Medical variables** including history of previous injury, history of substance abuse (including prescription medication), poor cardiovascular fitness, and physical and psychological deconditioning.

V. **Work assessment** consists of an interview (to determine subjective information), direct measures of physical capacities (to objectively measure strength, range of motion [ROM], sensation, coordination, balance, functional mobility, and cardiovascular fitness and endurance), diagnostic tests, and functional capacity evaluation (including physical and work capacity evaluation). The duration of work assessment can range from 2 hours to 1 week. It is used to determine the worker's existing physical capacities following injury (based on the medical conditions, the individual's transferable skills, vocational interest, and aptitudes, interpersonal skills, and psychological and motivational status) and to compare them against given criteria to predict the worker's potential to engage in work. The criteria used for comparison may be job-specific (to determine if the injured worker may eventually return to that specific job) or it may be general (i.e., based on general classification of work levels as defined by the U.S. Department of Labor in Table 5.11-1). Work assessment can also be used to formulate recommendations for intervention (e.g., work hardening programs) with the ultimate goal of returning the injured patient to work.

Medical evaluation of the injured worker is important for determining the stability of the patient's medical condition. The physiatric evaluation may be in the form of preemployment exam, postinjury assessment, recovery assessment after injury, physical impairment rating (or anatomic incapacity rating), Social Security disability evaluation, independent medical evaluation, and evaluation on compliance with regulations of the ADA. The insurance company (e.g., Worker's Compensation Board) may request the physiatrist to determine if the illness or injury is work-related, if the history of the illness or injury is consistent with the clinical findings and diagnosis, if there are any preexisting conditions or nonoccupational factors that could account for the clinical problem, and if there is a clear cause-and-effect relationship between the work activities and the clinical presentation. In some states, the physiatrist may be asked to determine compensation awards by "rating" the physical impairment (e.g., limitation of ROM or muscle weakness) of the worker based on a standardized system (e.g., using the *American Medical Association's Guides to the Evaluation of Permanent Impairment*) and by determining if the patient has reached maximal medical improvement (MMI) (i.e., patient's progress has reached a plateau and is not expected to change further). Physiatrists may also be asked to provide medical testimony as a factual or expert witness in ongoing work-related litigation.

A. **History**

1. **History of present illness**

    a. **Pain description,** for example, pain quality, location, radiation, intensity, and timing; aggravating and alleviating factors; other associated manifestations; previous tests results; effects of previous treatments such as active physical therapy, work conditioning, or work hardening.

    b. Accident history, for example, position, posture, and footing at the time of the accident; time of day and day of week the accident occurred; nature of the job (i.e., is it a new task? or how long has the worker been on this specific job?); occurrence of similar incidents with other workers on that job; problems with the equipment used on the job; initial medical examination and treatment; and initial response of the employer to the injury.

  2. Past history including general physical fitness; preexisting problems that could have contributed to the accident or injury or will affect the recovery process (e.g., diabetes, arthritis, heart disease, pulmonary disease, and obesity); prior hospitalizations; past traumas and accidents; past surgeries and treatments (and their effectiveness); past minor and major psychiatric illnesses.

  3. Current medications including all current prescription and nonprescription drugs.

  4. Personal history including life styles (e.g., a description of the patient's typical day; time spent in bed, in watching television, in getting out of the house, in hobbies and recreation, and in performing exercises), habits (e.g., use of recreational drugs, alcohol, and tobacco), and premorbid personality and emotional response to previous illnesses and injuries (e.g., is the worker passive and inactive or is there any attempt to stay active and productive or to return to work? Is there a positive or negative outlook for the future?)

  5. Social history including marriage status and history, home situation, and available support systems.

  6. Vocational and economic history including educational and training history, work history (e.g., previous jobs and attempts to return to work), work environment (see Chapter 4.5, section II.B.2.e); current relationship with the employer (e.g., does the worker have a job to return to? Is the employer willing to accept the worker back on the job?), financial situation, insurance, and pending litigation (which often slows down recovery and limits response to treatment).

B. Physical examination should include all the pertinent systems (see Chapter 1.1, section II) with special emphasis on the neuromuscular and musculoskeletal systems as well as on nonorganic signs (seen in patients with symptom magnification syndromes). Pain measurement scales (e.g., Visual Analog Scale) and dolorimetry (see Chapter 5.10, section IV.C.2.a.1) may be used to assess pain.

  1. Musculoskeletal system. ROM, joint stability, strength, pain behavior (e.g., marked grimacing, groans, and limping), tenderness (focal or widespread, trigger and/or tender points), muscle tightness and guarding, deformities, muscle atrophy (focal and localized or generalized), and deep pain (for the upper limb, hyperextend the small finger; for the lower limb, firmly compress the calf muscle or Achilles tendon).

    a. Spine. Posture, straight leg raising, Spurling's test.

    b. Upper limb. ROM (include cervical ROM), grip strength, tests that provoke symptoms (e.g., Tinel's, Phalen's wrist flexion test, and Finkelstein's test), tests for thoracic outlet syndrome, scapular winging, and pain pattern (is it produced at any point in the arc of motion?).

    c. Lower limb. Patrick's test, Gaenslen test, Drawer's test, Lachman's test, pivot shift test, and leg-length inequalities.

  2. Neuromuscular system. Motor functions, sensation (e.g., superficial and deep sensation, vibratory sensation, joint position or proprioception, and sensory distribution), reflexes (including hamstring and gastrocsoleus reflexes because more than 90% of lumbosacral radiculopathies involve S-1 or L-5 nerve roots), gait (e.g., assistive device used and type of gait), and functional activities (e.g., toe-walk, heel-walk, squat, touch toes, hop on one foot, and run in place).

3. **Nonorganic findings** are seen in patients with symptom magnification syndrome (usually with excessive complaints of pain with disproportionately low objective findings). In these patients, a psychologically or behaviorally based intervention may be warranted. Examples of nonorganic findings include "ratchety" (instead of smooth) quality of the "give-way" during muscle testing; right-to-left difference in vibratory sensation in a midline bone, such as the skull or sternum; a pain drawing chart showing extracorporeal pain markings, additional writings or comments, demarcating lines, and nonanatomic drawings; Waddell signs for nonorganic back pain (i.e., tenderness of the skin to light pinch over a widespread area; deep tenderness in a nonanatomical distribution; reproduction of back pain with axial loading by pressing down on the worker's head while he or she is standing; reproduction of back pain when the shoulders and pelvis are rotated together as a unit; inconsistent responses to straight-leg raising in the seated versus the supine position; widespread, inconsistent, and/or nonanatomic weakness or sensory loss; and overreaction during examination (e.g., disproportionate verbalization, facial expression, slow exaggerated movements, muscle tension and tremor, collapsing, or sweating).

C. **Diagnostic tests** should not be used in "shotgun" fashion but should be used for specific indications. They include noninvasive imaging studies (see Chapter 2.2), invasive imaging studies (see Chapter 2.3), laboratory testing (see Chapter 2.1), electrodiagnostic testing (see Chapter 2.4), and diagnostic injections (see Chapter 4.10). Diagnostic tests are useless unless they are closely correlated with clinical findings.

D. **Functional capacity evaluation (FCE),** in the context of RTW programs, usually refers to a physical and work capacity evaluation. The FCE is typically performed by physical or occupational therapists. The information obtained from FCE can be used to establish maximal permissible limits for nonrepetitive activities and to delineate safe parameters for repetitive activities. Examples of commercially available FCEs are the Blankenship system and the EPIC system (which provides six modules that evaluate lift capacity: motor coordination, finger and hand dexterity, standing whole body ROM, balance while walking, carrying and climbing, and industrial pushing and pulling).

1. **Physical capacity evaluation (PCE)** typically assesses isolated parts of the body or functional units, such as lumbar region or upper limbs. Physical tests include gross physical capabilities (e.g., ROM, strength, endurance, lifting capacity, walking balance, carrying, and climbing), finger and hand dexterity skills (e.g., Purdue Pegboard, Crawford Small Parts, Minnesota Rate of Manipulation, Stromberg Dexterity, Bennet Hand Tool tests, and using equipment available from Baltimore Therapeutic Equipment (BTE), EPIC Functional Capacity Evaluation System, Isernhagen Work Systems, Key Functional Assessment, Lafayette Instruments, Valpar, Work Evaluation Systems Technology (WEST), and Work Recovery System), and movement accuracy (e.g., Employee Aptitude Survey #9, EPIC 2 Motor Coordination test, and the ERGOS Work Simulator). An example of a commer-

cially available PCE is the Smith Physical Capacity Evaluation (which measures 154 performance items) and the Blankenship system.

2. **Work capacity evaluation (WCE)** is a comprehensive process that systematically uses work (real or simulated) to assess and measure an individual's capacity to work safely and efficiently in specific job tasks. In persons with disabilities, WCE can help determine if the person needs to change his type of employment (i.e., undergo vocational or prevocational rehabilitation) or to resume previous employment using adapted tools or methods. Primary factors measured by WCE include work feasibility (e.g., using the Feasibility Evaluation Checklist, which consists of 21 behavior-anchored rating scales for items such as the ability to accept supervision and work with others, safety in the workplace, and the quantity and quality of the patient's productivity), which is determined prior to assessing work tolerance (e.g., strength, energy reserve, flexibility, and the effect of pain and other limiting factors on task performance such as sitting and standing tolerance). Secondary factors measured by WCE include aptitudes, interests, and vocational skills. The WCE results are then compared with the demands of the job as listed by the U.S. Department of Labor in the *Dictionary of Occupational Titles*. If there is a deficit that affects performance of the job, intervention (such as modified work hardening or a work conditioning program) may be recommended. During performance of the WCE it is helpful to learn from the worker the amount of energy and effort being expended by using the Rating of Perceived Exertion Scale (Borg Scale) described in Chapter 4.2, section III.A.3. The following discussion provides an overview of the four common categories of WCE tools that can be used independently or as part of a FCE:

a. **Job analyses (on-the-job or worksite evaluations)** are done to determine whether the abilities and physical status of a person with a disability can match the physical demand characteristics of the job so that the worker can return to his or her old job or apply for a particular new job. Under the ADA, a "formal job analysis" is not required because it may not be job specific and may not adequately identify the essential functions of a particular job. To meet the ADA criteria, a job analysis must focus on the purpose of the job and how essential the actual job function is in achieving this purpose. Factors determining the essentiality of a task or function include its frequency, the amount of time required to perform the task, and the consequences if it is not performed (i.e., does removal of that task or function fundamentally change the job or make the position nonexistent?). Job analysis should preferably be done at the worksite or, if that is not feasible, it may be simulated (e.g., in work hardening centers). Data collection for job analysis in the workplace and the clinic can either be expert-based (i.e., rated by expert observers) or incumbent-based (i.e., rated by the workers themselves).

1) **Surveys** are screening methods used to determine whether the workplace, job, individual worker, or working situation contributes significantly to the job stress. Once these problems are identified, surveys can be used to recommend work interventions to reduce the problem or further objective studies (e.g., quantifying a worker's performance on the job and the physiological cost of that performance). Survey questionnaires may include objects handled (weight, size, shape, surface texture, presence or absence of handles); amount and fre-

quency of physical tasks such as lifting, pushing, pulling, climbing, stooping, and squatting; positions and postures that must be utilized to successfully perform the job; tools used (handle size, weight, vibration, position of use); layout of work site (e.g., a desk or table with appropriate height, width, length, and presence of space underneath; height of workbench; and arrangement of tools utilized); amount of lighting present (type and intensity of lighting, windows); temperature of the facility; amount of noise present (e.g., are hearing protectors available and used if excess noise is present?); cleanliness of floor surface (e.g., spills, greasy spots, clutter, and obstacles present on floor that could lead to stumbles and falls); and general ambiance of the facility (e.g., pleasant, relaxed, clean, organized, and orderly or hurried, hostile, and hectic jobs).

2) **Time activity analyses**
   a) **Job activity analysis** is similar to a job description. It is used to estimate the whole job and define its overall physical workload demands to establish the need for recovery time that will bring the job demands within the worker's capacities.
   b) **Work task analysis** consists of a detailed recording of the pattern of activities over the shift, the distribution of heavy and light physical work, the time required to perform a task (used to assess time pressure), and the frequency of occurrence for more demanding activities. It is used to identify the tasks that are most likely to exceed worker capacities.
   c) **Work cycle analysis** measures the time to complete a task and is expressed in minutes. It is used to identify the variability in performance of a task and the potential fatigue factors (i.e., time to complete a task usually increases during a shift when fatigue is occurring).
   d) **Methods-time measurement (MTM)** is a technique in which work is broken down into elemental tasks such as "move, grasp, turn." It is used for evaluating individual efficiency of motion, especially on highly repetitive jobs (e.g., how long a highly repetitive task should take or how it can be modified to reduce the time required). It can also be used for setting production standards in some plants and for identifying where new methods can increase productivity. Because it is too finely divided, it is unable to make an accurate estimate of the energy demands and physiological stresses on the worker; therefore, it is less useful than work task or work cycle analysis for characterizing job demands.

3) **Motion analyses** are used to analyze complex, repetitive motions in industry (i.e., the frequency, degrees of rotation, duration, positions or postures, and dexterity or coordination requirements of a task); to determine the efficiency of motion and the effectiveness of training; and to investigate movements that might contribute to joint irritation. They include goniometry (e.g., electrogoniometers; see Chapter 2.8, section I.B.4) and photometric or video-based motion analysis systems (see Chapter 2.8, section I.E).

4) **Biomechanical analyses** include the use of force transducers (dynamometers and cable tensiometers; see Chapter 2.8, section II.D), force plates (to study ground reaction force that resists the feet during standing, walking, and running, and which can be used to study

the dynamic aspects of industrial tasks when a worker is standing, walking, or lifting), electromyography (EMG), accelerometers (to help determine limb vibration), and motion analysis systems. These devices can be used to follow the motion of the limb during task performance; to identify the maximum torque in the most active muscles; to determine the time of contraction for each muscle group and derive the recovery time (to assess work endurance); to define resistance force and the direction of force; to determine the exact position of the joint around which the muscles are active; and to determine if there are any postural changes. Some applications of biomechanical analyses include assessment of back stress during manual lifting activities (e.g., by measuring reach, forces and torques, and load weight and dimensions; see Chapter 2.8, section III); evaluation of the effects of different body postures during seated and standing work; determination of the effects of vibration or cumulative stress on the joints; and for setting work speed according to the time of contraction and the derived recovery time.

5) **Cardiovascular and metabolic measurements of job demands**

   a) **Heart or pulse rate** is the most convenient measure of the physiological cost of work, for example, the time required for the heart rate to return to a preexercise level can be used to evaluate work stress and individual fitness levels. Heart or pulse rate can be measured by palpation (radial pulse, carotid pulse), radiotelemetry, or continuous electrocardiogram.

   b) **Blood pressure (BP)** is not commonly used because BP measurement requires that the work be stopped during the measurement period. The BP can be used to evaluate the stress of postural static-work, which may show very high BP changes with minimal heart rate changes.

   c) **Minute ventilation** measures the volume of gas breathed out per minute to determine the respiratory demand of work. The expired volume is measured by breathing through a spirometer, which mechanically determines the volume per breath (tidal volume) and accumulates the volume measurement over several breaths (respiratory rate) for a fixed time period, such as 1 minute. To collect the expired air, the worker must wear a partial face mask or a mouthpiece and nose clip, which can become a problem when communication and good visual control are needed on the job. Minute ventilation is usually done in conjunction with measurement of oxygen consumption and carbon dioxide production. During sample taking, the worker must be in a steady state (i.e., the ventilation rate is not changing frequently) to reflect an average of all of the activities performed during the time of the sample.

      (1) **Oxygen consumption** in the lungs is determined by measuring the amount of air exchanged per minute (minute ventilation) and determining the amount of oxygen in the inspired and expired air. The difference between the amount of oxygen breathed in and the amount breathed out is the measure of the amount consumed. In reporting the oxygen consumption values for a job or task, one should include the average demands over the shift, the working demands over the shift

weighted for the amount of time spent in each activity, and the peak demands.

(2) **Carbon dioxide production** is estimated by measuring the minute ventilation and the amount of carbon dioxide in the expired air. It is very reliable if the work sustains a steady state for at least 5 minutes so adequate amounts of expired air sample can be collected.

b. **Situational assessments** involve placing a worker into a realistic work situation and systematically altering variables, such as physical demands or stress factors, to ascertain the worker's performance under each circumtance (e.g., how will a worker's performance be affected by increasing the distance a load must be transported?).

c. **Psychometric instruments** include numerous pencil-and-paper as well as apparatus instruments used for measuring vocational interests, general intelligence, achievement, aptitude, personality, and other related psychological issues. These tests are commonly used in chronic pain patients who are unable to return to their former job duties. They can be used to delineate the individual's response to pain and stress (e.g., depression, coping strategies, and self-image of pain and disability), to identify the patient's interpersonal and vocational strengths and weaknesses, and to determine the best method to motivate the patient to succeed in the rehabilitation program. Most of these tests are described in Chapter 2.9 and in Chapter 5.10, section IV).

1) **Vocational interest tests** are designed to identify broad categories of work with characteristics that an individual would find suitable. Examples include the Wide Range Interest-Opinion Test (WRIOT), the California Occupational Preference Survey (COPS), the Strong-Campbell test, the Work Values Inventory, and the Kuder Occupational Interest Survey.

2) **General aptitude tests** are useful in vocational counseling for placement in work settings or training programs. Examples include the Differential Aptitude Tests (DAT), the General Aptitude Test Battery (GATB), and the Oral Directions Test (ODT). The GATB has been standardized for more than 450 different occupations, especially in unskilled and semiskilled areas, and it is useful for individuals with limited transferable skills.

3) **Specific aptitude tests** are used for further evaluation of specific aptitudes recognized to be important in particular vocations. Examples include the Bennett Mechanical Comprehension Test, the Revised Minnesota Paper Form Board Test, the Minnesota Clerical Test, Computer Operator Aptitude Battery, the Computer Programmer Aptitude Battery, the MacQuarrie Test for Mechanical Ability, the General Clerical Test, and the SRA Tests of Clerical Aptitude.

4) **General intelligence tests** (see Chapter 2.9, section II) include the Wechsler Adult Intelligence Scale-Revised (WAIS-R), the Standford-Binet test, the Peabody Picture Vocabulary, and the California Test of Mental Maturity. In some cases, memory assessments may be used to provide a memory quotient.

5) **Achievement tests** (see Chapter 2.9, section III) are used to determine past learning performance. Examples include the Wide Range Achievement Test (WRAT), the Adult Basic Learning (ABLE), and the Peabody Individual Achievement Test.

6) **Personality inventories** (see Chapter 2.9, section I) that assess major personality characteristics related to personal and social adjustment can help determine an individual's suitability for adapting to particular work environments. Examples include the Minnesota Multiphasic Personality Inventory (MMPI), Millon Clinical Multiaxial Inventory II (MCMI-II), Strong Interest Inventory (SII), Sixteen Personality Factors Questionnaire (16PF), and the Edwards Personal Preference Schedule (EPPS).

7) **Tests for depression** (see Chapter 2.9, section VII) include the Beck Depression Inventory (BDI) and the Zung Self-Rating Depression Scale.

8) **Multidimensional pain questionnaires** (see Chapter 5.10, section IV.C.2.b) include the McGill-Melzack Pain Questionnaire (MPQ), the West Haven-Yale Multidimensional Pain Inventory (WHYMPI), and the Emory University Pain Estimate Chart.

9) **Functional status or life-style impact scales** (see Chapter 5.10, section IV.D.1) include the Sickness Impact Profile (SIP) and Activity Diaries.

10) **Test of general psychopathology in chronic pain patients** (see Chapter 5.10, section IV.D.2) include the Symptom Checklist 90-revised (SCL-90R) and the Millon Behavioral Health Inventory (MBHI).

11) **Other psychological tests** include the Back Stress Indices Determination and the Symptom Magnification Testing.

d. **Work samples** are the primary technique of work evaluation used to assess an individual's vocational aptitude, worker characteristics, and vocational interests. They consist of a well-defined work activity involving tasks, materials, and tools that are identical or similar to those in an actual job or cluster of jobs. In addition to the systems described below, other work sample series include Singer Vocational Evaluation System, the Philadelphia Jewish Employment and Vocational Service Work Sample Battery, the Talent Assessment Program, the Key Functions Assessment, the Work Recovery Systems, the Isernhagen work Systems, Blankenships, and ARCON, ERGASYS.

1) **Testing, Orientation, and Work Evaluation in Rehabilitation (TOWER) system** is the oldest complete work evaluation system originally developed and normed for people with physical disabilities. It is useful for thorough evaluation in limited areas and may take up to 3 weeks to complete. It is not commonly used because it has not been normed for the industry, and its applications are limited to jobs that relate to the TOWER work samples and do not relate to *Dictionary of Occupational Titles* classifications.

2) **Work Evaluation Systems Technology (WEST)** series of work samples commonly used in RTW programs include the WEST 2A-Whole Body Range of Motion Work Sample, the WEST 3-Comprehensive Weight System, WEST 4A-Upper Extremity Strength and Fatigue Tolerance Work Sample, and WEST 7-Bus Bench. They all include norms for healthy male college students or MTMs identified by the *Dictionary of Occupational Titles.*

3) **Valpar Component Work Samples (VCWS)** consists of subtests to measure those worker characteristics that have been found to be basic indicators of success within numerous job families. They are keyed to the worker traits listed in *Dictionary of Occupational Titles* and include

MTMs and norms derived from various groups of employed workers and special disability groups. There are at least 18 VCWS, the most popular of which include Small Tools (measures the person's ability to understand and work with small mechanical tools for repair of small appliances or for jewelry making), Upper Extremity Range of Motion (measures upper torso work tolerance), Multilevel Sorting (measures a person's ability to make decisions while performing tasks requiring physical manipulation and visual discrimination of colors, numbers, letters, and a combination of these), Simulated Assembly (measures a person's ability to do a task requiring repetitive physical manipulation and bilateral use of the upper limbs), Whole Body Range of Motion (measures the agility of a person's gross body movements as they relate to the functional ability to perform job tasks), and Dynamic Physical Capacities (composed of 28 individual tasks, such as, lifting, climbing, stooping, and balancing, which are similar to those of a shipping and receiving clerk or parts order clerk).

4) **Baltimore Therapeutic Equipment (BTE) Work Simulator** is a computerized system that quantifies work output by measuring repetitive upper limb motions against measurable resistance over a specified amount of time. The BTE system consists of interchangeable handles, which simulate the physical demands of most jobs, such as gripping, pinching, lifting, carrying, and reaching. It can be used to estimate work tolerance, cardiac stress, and pulmonary stress and to provide feedback for work hardening tasks.

VI. **Work rehabilitation** benefits the workers by making them learn ways to safely and productively do their job; by building their strength, flexibility and endurance; by hastening their return to gainful employment; by returning them to productive roles with family and coworkers; by helping them gain confidence in their physical ability to do the job; and by lessening their chances of repeat or new injury. For the employer, work rehabilitation has the following benefits: reduction in direct costs, facilitation of claim settlement, increase in successful RTW attempts, improvement in employee job satisfaction, and regaining productive use of an injured employee. Case managers should ideally be involved in work rehabilitation (especially in chronic cases) to ensure that the worker does not get "lost in the system." Specifically, the case manager assesses job availability with the current employer or in another company and investigates the existence of light-duty alternatives or other jobs to which the patient's skills can be transferred and communicates with the insurer to be sure that prompt coverage is provided for the necessary diagnostic, therapeutic, and rehabilitative efforts and to be certain that the insurer fully understands the proposed program, expected outcome, and time frames. It also helps to communicate with the worker thereby preventing any misunderstandings about diagnosis, treatment plans, and RTW options; monitors attendance by the injured worker at appropriate therapy sessions; and helps ensure compliance if nonattendance occurs. Return-to-work options should preferably be the same job with the same employer or even with a different employer. If this is not possible, then a more extensive vocational training program may be needed for a different job preferably with the same employer.

A. **Acute (early) interventions** include first aid measures, as well as appropriate acute and postacute care. The goals of acute intervention are accurate diagnosis and appropriate treatment to facilitate the worker's safe return to work as soon as possible. The worker should be seen promptly after the injury and followed up closely at short intervals (daily if necessary) so he or she does not "get lost in the system." In the acute stage, about 80 to 85% of workers generally experience improvement and return to productive work. If symptoms (e.g., pain, stiffness, or weakness) persist longer than expected into the subacute phase, the treatment effort should be intensified to prevent chronicity (see section VI.A.2). In the subacute phase, the patient may need a structured and regularly scheduled therapy program focused around reconditioning (similar to the work conditioning program in section VI.B.1).

1. **Acute management** is generally directed towards the symptomatic treatment of pain (which is a major complaint in the acute phase) and other accompanying symptoms (e.g., sleep disorders). The acute management is described in Chapter 5.10. Often the PRICE (i.e., protection, relative rest, ice, compression, and elevation) treatment approach can be initially helpful. Studies have shown that rest should be limited in duration (e.g., 1-2 days of complete bedrest with bathroom privileges for patients with acute back pain). When resting, patients with acute back pain should lie in the supine or sidelying position with bent hips and knees, and if they need to be upright they should avoid full sitting, which is 40% more stressful on the back than standing (instead, the patient should stand or semi-sit on the back of a chair or on a high stool). Appropriate physical modalities (see Chapter 4.1) such as heat, cold, transcutaneous electrical nerve stimulation units, massage, and gentle stretching may be used with or without nonnarcotic analgesics and/or antiinflammatory agents (e.g., NSAIDs or steroids; all described in Chapter 4.8, sections I.A.3 and III). Muscle relaxants and narcotics are generally less helpful in the acute phase. Tricyclic antidepressants (see Chapter 4.8, section V.A) may be used to improve the accompanying sleep disorder and may also help reduce pain (probably by increasing pain threshold). Active exercises (e.g., flexibility, strengthening, or aerobic exercises—all described in Chapter 4.2, sections I to III) may be started as early as the third day postinjury to prevent deconditioning. Splints (e.g., wrist splints for patients with carpal tunnel syndrome, lumbosacral corsets for back pain patients, or cervical orthosis for neck pain patients) may be used temporarily. As acute symptoms subside, use of medications, physical modalities, and splints should be decreased, but active exercises should increase.

2. **Preventive measures** must be initiated in the acute or subacute phase to prevent future recurrences. Instead of symptomatic treatment, preventive measures should be directed towards the underlying factors (e.g., poor physical conditioning, unhealthy lifestyle, poor posture and body mechanics, and poor working conditions), which lead to the injury in the first place. Patient must be taught about the underlying causes as well as anatomy and pathomechanics of musculoskeletal injuries. Patient education may be given individually or in groups (e.g., Back School or Neck School). See Chapter 5.10, section VI.A for discussion of patient education techniques.

   a. **Early return to work** (e.g., "light duty" or a modified job) is encouraged as long as the medical outcome is not compromised and no further tissue damage occurs. This helps prevent both physical and mental deconditioning.

   b. **Healthy lifestyle** includes appropriate treatment for drug and alcohol abuse, cessation of smoking, proper nutrition (for weight loss if needed), regular conditioning exercises (i.e., flexibility, strength, and aerobic exercises—all described in Chapter 4.2), and relaxation exercises (described in Chapter 4.2, section VI).

c. **Proper body mechanics**

1) **Postural awareness** can be trained through exercises (e.g., using McKenzie's "slouch-overcorrect" procedure or nontraditional techniques such as the Alexander technique or the Feldenkrais method) and patient education. The neck or back should be maintained either in a neutral (normal lordosis) or slightly extended position. A lumbar roll is useful in maintaining normal lumbar lordosis. Excessive forward bending and rotation of the neck or back should be avoided (because they increase spinal load and can overstretch the ligaments making them prone to injury). Workers who sit and do repetitive, monotonous, or static workload should be taught to take a stand-and-stretch moment (also called mini-break or pause gymnastics) every 20 to 30 minutes. This is not a break or rest period but simply a means of getting the worker out of the chair to perform 2 to 3 minutes of gentle movements (see sample exercise program in Table 5.11-2) designed to loosen the muscles, break up the constrained posture, and improve blood flow and tendon lubrication in the affected areas.

2) **Proper lifting and carrying techniques** include the following practical points:

Table 5.11-2. An example of a stand-and-stretch (or mini-break) program for people who sit

The following program takes 3 minutes to complete (each exercise is performed for 20 seconds).

1. Inhale slowly through your nose and gently exhale through your lips.
2. Drop your ear toward your shoulder and repeat on the other side.
3. Make circles with your shoulders by shrugging them up to your ears, pulling them back, and dropping them down.
4. Rotate your ankles in a circle to pump blood back up to your heart.
5. Place your hands on your pelvis and practice increasing and reducing the curve of your low back.
6. Drop your head down to your knees and rub the muscles on your back.
7. Place hands on your seat on either side of your hips. Push down and attempt to lift your weight off the chair.
8. When standing, support your low back with your hands and gently arch backwards.
9. Stand with your back flat against a wall and gently slide down the wall, 4 or 5 inches, bending your knees. Count to 3 and stand tall. If no wall is available, walk on site.
10. Sit up straight! Pull your head back while tucking your chin.

Reprinted with permission of the Back School and Neck School programs of the Occupational and Industrial Orthopedic Center, Hospital for Joint Diseases-Orthopedic Institute, New York, NY.

- Avoid excessive forward bending (because forward bending, even slightly, increases the back stress by 50%) by standing close to object and bending the knees even to pick up light objects or to reach for objects close to the ground (e.g., garage door handle located near the ground).
- Avoid trunk twisting, instead use the feet to pivot.
- Use the strong lower limb muscles for lifting (i.e., knee and hip extensors).
- Maintain normal lumbar lordosis.
- Use wide stance for balance and support.
- Use low loads. If heavy (e.g., 25 pounds is considered heavy), get help from another person or use a mechanical lifting device.
- Pace the lift so it is sufficiently slow and deliberate to allow for the use of good body mechanics.
- Mentally lift (i.e., mentally plan and review the lifting or carrying techniques prior to carrying it out).
- Emphasize the lowering of carried object as well as its lifting.
- Get a firm grasp on the object.
- Keep the load close to the body (especially moving objects such as babies or pets).
- Use symmetrical upper body motions to carry or move objects (e.g., use knapsack or two grocery bags instead of one).
- Put the shoulder strap of the bag on the opposite shoulder to even out the load.
- Push instead of pull (use firm grasp on load; keep a wide stance by putting one foot in front of the other; stay down low; and shift weight in the legs as needed).
- Use a wheeled cart (with wheels sufficiently maintained and large enough to allow smooth movement and to easily clear obstacles such as irregularities in the workplace floor).

d. **Ergonomic intervention** refers to human factors designed to fit or accommodate the work place to the individual and to enhance worker comfort, safety, and productivity.

  1) **Workplace redesign** includes modification in the work space design (see Chapter 4.5, section II.B.2.e for barrier-free architectural design) or tools and equipment. The traditional workplace in the United States is based on anthropometric measurements of selected men or women in the Air Force and is inappropriate for the increasing number of women in the workforce today (especially minority women with different anthropometric measurements). Ideally, the furniture should be fully adjustable for use in multiple tasks. If the company cannot afford new furniture, modifications may be done, such as elevating the chair and providing footstools if the work surface is too high; elevating the work surface with blocks if it is too low; using pillows or lumbar rolls if chairs are too deep; or wrapping arm rests in foam if they are too short or too widely separated.

    a) **Visibility distance,** which is the distance needed between the eye and the work object (e.g., computer screen or book), should be about 12 inches or adjusted to the worker's focal distance (if wearing glasses) to prevent leaning forward to see. While holding the head upright and looking straight ahead, the eye should focus a little below the horizontal top of the book or screen to prevent head extension. Workers are discouraged from wearing bifocals to prevent the backward tilting of the head.

b) Lighting must be sufficient to see well, and there should be no blinding reflections.

c) Work surface should have the same height as the level of the elbow. The traditional work surface height of 29 to 31 inches for a 5'10'' man is inappropriate for a 5'1'' female who needs a surface height of 23 to 25 inches. Everything on the work surface should be arranged so that it is within easy reach and, if tilt is needed, the surface (not the person's head) should be tilted.

d) Keyboards and peripherals (e.g., mouse and trackball) should be positioned so that the worker can type with shoulders relaxed, elbows comfortably at the side of the body, and bent at a 90-degree angle or slightly more open. The worker should also be provided with a wrist rest for the keyboard and a separate one for the mouse or trackball. Ideally, the wrist rest should have a foam core, a smooth surface (e.g., felt, or, for multiusers, vinyl) and rounded edges. It should extend under the keyboards so that it is weighted down, and it should be about 4 inches deep by 1 to 1.5 inches thick (i.e., deep enough to comfortably support the wrist during use of all keys including the space bar and thick enough so that the wrist of the user is not extended or flexed in use). It should also be placed at the edge of the work surface to eliminate ulnar pressure from the sharp edge of the desk. Adjustable forearm support (clamped on the work surface edge and articulated for full movement of the forearms) may also be used.

e) Chairs should have a back support below the shoulder blades, a well-designed lumbar support (detachable or adjustable lumbar rolls or pillows may be used), swivel and rollers (to avoid twisting the spine), arm rests for support, and adjustable seat height. The seat height should allow the feet to rest comfortably flat on the floor or footrest with hips and knees bent at about 90 degrees. The seat edge should be rounded and the seat depth should be three-quarters of leg length. A high sit-stand stool on which the worker can lean back against a semi-sit surface is useful if the worker has a high work surface and needs to frequently stand.

f) Phone adaptations are described in Chapter 4.5, section II.A.4.d. For those involved in heavy phone work, a headset is effective in preventing neck and upper back problems associated with trying to hold the phone between the neck and shoulder while using the hands for a different task.

g) Tool adaptations include grip modification (e.g., covering tool handles with caulking or thermophylic plastic to make them larger, softer, and rougher to reduce the force of grip and wrist deviation or covering mouse or trackballs with a piece of sponge to provide a custom grip and to reduce the finger flexion needed to depress the buttons) and toolweight modification to increase functional efficiency.

2) Administrative changes include rotation of job assignments (e.g., by cross-training), staggered breaks, encouraging breaks away from work area, regular supervised stand-and-stretch mini-breaks (see

Table 5.11-2), varying of work tasks (to reduce repetitiveness), lowering production rates (e.g., slow down typing rates), allowing only limited overtime, training employees on safe and efficient use of equipment (e.g., keying with forearms and wrists relaxed), and proper preemployment selection.

B. **Chronic intervention** is indicated in a small percentage of workers (about 10%) who still have pain complaints and physical disabilities that prevent return to work after the completion of acute and subacute care. It is well recognized that the longer workers are off the job (whether measured as time since date of injury or last date worked), the more difficult it becomes to return them to work (regardless of the type of impairment). In chronic cases (i.e., more than 3 to 6 months consecutively out of work), the initial injury is often resolved, but because of prolonged inactivity and sedentary lifestyle, the worker may develop chronic weakness and deconditioning as well as inflexibility and poor endurance. In addition, the worker may also be psychologically deconditioned. They also tend to smoke more, drink more, and take more medications than they were taking prior to the injury. Other characteristics of chronicity include patient's negative perception of disability, disability claims for compensation, subjective complaints that are disproportionate to objective signs, symptom magnification (see section V.B.3), lack of motivation to recover, and negative attitude to work return.

1. **Work conditioning** is a RTW program consisting of progressive structured reconditioning, which is recommended for a patient with an uncomplicated injury but whose physical limitations preclude return to work. It is typically provided as a unidisciplinary or bidisciplinary (i.e., occupational or physical therapy, or both) program that uses exercise, aerobic conditioning, education, and limited work tasks to restore an individual's systemic and neuromusculoskeletal function (strength, endurance, movement, flexibility, and motor control). The treatment focus is on active rehabilitation and physical restoration rather than passive modalities and medications. Work conditioning is usually tailored to the specific needs of the job (determined by worksite visit, if possible; see section V.D.2.a), e.g, emphasizing upper torso exercises for jobs requiring upper torso functions. It can usually be made acceptable to the worker if it is presented as a sports medicine model of treatment (e.g., using the analogy of an injured athlete who initially requires a period of rest after an acute injury, after which the athlete has to return to the training room to restore fitness before returning to competition). The work conditioning program usually consist of half-day sessions given 3 to 5 times per week for a relatively short period of time (e.g., 3-6 weeks) with periodic reassessment of the worker's fitness level and work capacity. When the worker is sufficiently conditioned to perform light duties, the worker is usually returned to the job, and arrangements are made to continue the conditioning program until the worker has maximally improved or has met the requirements for returning to the original job.

2. **Work hardening** (also called work simulation, work readiness training, or work rehabilitation) is a work-oriented, highly structured, individualized program that uses the interdisciplinary approach to provide a transition for the deconditioned, disabled worker to return him or her to work-ready status through progressively strenuous work (real or simulated) or work-related activities. It is more comprehensive than work conditioning and is recommended for workers who have been off work for protracted periods of time (e.g., longer than 3-6 months) and whose injury and physical limita-

tions are complicated by more severe deconditioning as well as by psychosocial factors that interfere with ability to return to work. The interdisciplinary team members (i.e., physician, physical therapist, occupational therapist, psychologist, vocational specialist, social worker, ergonomist, and industrial engineer) must have a complete understanding of the worker's job and work conditions. Since 1988, the guidelines from the Commission of Accreditation for Rehabilitation Facilities (CARF) have ensured the quality of work hardening programs for structure and content.

The work hardening process includes job analysis (see section V.D.2.a), establishing a work tolerance baseline (e.g., medical history, worker interview, job description with critical work demands, pain assessment, physical assessment, lifting and carrying ability, pushing and pulling, stooping and bending, kneeling and crawling, sitting and standing, and work task simulation), and an individualized work hardening plan with the goal of maximizing the patient's functional improvement while simultaneously providing it in a safe environment. Other goals are increasing physical tolerance identified as deficient for critical work demands, attaining optimal work tolerance and ability, increasing proficiency with work adaptations or assistive devices, reducing fear and increasing confidence for resumption of productive work, developing problem-solving skills for self-management at the work site, facilitating appropriate worker behaviors (e.g., timeliness, attendance, and dress), maximizing cognitive and psychosocial functioning, and identifying problems that may require placement in an alternative job.

Although physical modalities and medications may be used to help reduce pain perception and increase work tolerance, active exercise remains the single most important approach for the greatest number of patients. Aside from continuing to emphasize generalized conditioning (similar to that provided by the work conditioning program), work hardening also incorporates job-specific worktask simulation activities (e.g., if the job requires the patient to lift boxes, then box lifting is incorporated into the program), which can be graded in difficulty or length of time involved. A typical program initially trains the patient to develop endurance for remaining in static positions, including sitting and standing postures, while performing activities. As the patient's tolerance improves, additional work-type activities (e.g., lifting, carrying, bending, kneeling, or climbing—depending on the patient's work requirements) are added. Examples of work hardening modalities include a balance monitor that provides feedback on weight bearing and symmetry of posture; a multiworkstation, which simulates construction jobs; a truck or a car simulator with a computerized video road screen to simulate and measure the driving process; a computerized pneumatic lift to simulate the lifting process; an upper-limb work simulator (e.g., BTE) to simulate various upper-limb work tasks (including reaching overhead and manipulating tools); and a lower-limb simulator (e.g., foot controls). Most of these modalities are homemade, although many are commercially available.

Work hardening programs also try to simulate actual working conditions (e.g., the worker is required to clock in and out daily; breaks are scheduled; and warehouse or other "work-like" settings are used, instead of a medical clinic or hospital, to minimize the worker's perception of illness and sickness). Patients also maintain an activity log to develop a sense of responsibility for their own rehabilitation and pain control. Another integral part of the program is education in proper use of the body to avoid reinjury, proper pacing on the job, relaxation (e.g., biofeedback, hypnosis, and progressive muscle relaxation techniques), stress management skills, assertiveness, interpersonal skills to facilitate conflict avoidance and resolution, and maintaining a healthy lifestyle. Education can be provided through discussion, demonstration, active participation, and audiovisual aids. It may be given individually or in a group setting (e.g., back or neck school).

A typical schedule for work hardening is usually 5 days per week (4 or 8 hours per day) for up to 6 to 12 weeks. Treatment time is gradually increased to equal the person's premorbid work schedule. The cost of these programs is relatively high, but well-organized programs often have favorable success rates. Work hardening is most effective in patients who are motivated to return to work, have jobs available, and are free of overwhelming psychological or secondary gain issues, which can undermine progress. Return-to-work rates, obtained from individual programs that carefully select their clients, range from 50 to 60% to 85 to 88%. The RTW rate decreases as the length of disability (whether measured as time since date of injury or last date worked) increases. The chance of returning to work after 6 months of disability is about 50%. By 1 year, it decreases to about 25%; and by 2 years, almost no patient returns to work even with exhaustive rehabilitation measures.

3. **Vocational training** is considered if the injured worker does not have the option of returning to his or her former job because of inability to physically meet the job demands despite work conditioning or work hardening; poor worker-job match, which would increase the risk of reinjury; lack of desire on the worker's part to return to the former job; or lack of willingness on the former employer's part to accept the worker back on the job. Vocational training refers to the actual training program the worker has to undergo to learn the chosen trade or profession. It involves an interdisciplinary team effort coordinated by the vocational counselor.

The vocational counselor should be familiar with job options in the geographic area and be able to assist the individual with formulating a reasonable plan in finding a suitable vocation and training program. After medical clearance by a physician, the patient is given vocational testing (e.g., vocational interest inventories, achievement testing, aptitude testing, and assessment of the ability to perform work activities) and psychological testing to determine aptitude for specific vocations and for various levels of vocational or educational training (e.g., vocational school, junior college, and college). If the patient does not have a job after training, the vocational counselor can assist with job or volunteer work placements. The vocational counselor may also coach the prospective worker on filling out a job application, preparing a resume, dressing for and conducting oneself at a job interview as well as on the job, dealing with authority figures and coworkers effectively, dealing with stress or conflict in the work situation, and managing finances. For prospective workers with physical impairments (e.g., head injuries or spinal cord injuries), the physical and occupational therapists as well as the ergonomist, industrial engineer, or employer can help formulate specific job and workplace adaptations or modifications.

4. **Chronic pain center treatment program** is an interdisciplinary team approach that focuses on behavioral modification, exercise for reactivation, stress

reduction, and pain management. It is recommended as the last resort for workers with chronic pain whose primary nociceptive insult may no longer account for the greater part of the patient's disability and who are resistant to the above methods. Drug (e.g., narcotic) detoxification (e.g., using "pain cocktail" described in Chapter 5.10, section VI.E.3) may be necessary and antidepressant medications may be used for sleep and for pain modification. Psychologic counseling may be needed for the patient and family (to help them understand and adjust to the patient's behavior). Because most of these patients will not return to their previous employment, alternative vocational strategies (e.g., vocational training as in section VI.B.3) should be incorporated in the program.

BIBLIOGRAPHY

Burt CM, Smith P: Work evaluation and work hardening. In Pedretti LW, editor: *Occupational therapy practice skills for physical dysfunction,* ed 4, St. Louis, 1996, Mosby–Year Book, pp 553-563.

Chaffin DB, Andersson GBJ: *Occupational biomechanics,* ed 2, New York, 1991, John Wiley.

Commission on Accreditation of Rehabilitation Facilities (CARF): *Guidelines for work hardening programs,* Chicago, 1988, CARF.

Demeter SL, Andersson GBJ, Smith GM, editors: *American Medical Association: disability evaluation,* St. Louis, 1996, Mosby–Year Book.

Doege TC, editor: *American Medical Association: guides to the evaluation of permanent impairment,* ed 4, Chicago, 1993, American Medical Association.

Eastman Kodak Company: *Ergonomic design for people at work,* vol 2, New York, 1986, Van Nostrand Reinhold.

Herrington TM, Morse LH, editors: *Occupational injuries: evaluation, management, and prevention,* St. Louis, 1995, Mosby–Year Book.

Jacobs K: Preparing for return to work. In Trombly CA, editor: *Occupational therapy for physical dysfunction,* ed 4, Baltimore, 1995, Williams & Wilkins, pp 329-349.

Matheson LN, Ogden L, Violette K, et al: Work hardening: occupational therapy in industrial rehabilitation, *Am J Occup Ther,* 39(5):314-321, 1985.

National Institute for Occupational Safety and Health: *Application manual for the revised NIOSH lifting equations* (NTIS Publication No PB 94-176930 OSM), Springfield, VA, 1991, U.S. Department of Commerce.

Scheer SJ, Weinstein SM: Industrial rehabilitation medicine. 1. An overview, *Arch Phys Med Rehabil* 73:S-356-S-359, 1992.

Schuchmann JA: Occupational rehabilitation. In Braddom RL, editor: *Physical medicine and rehabilitation,* Philadelphia, 1996, WB Saunders, pp 938-954.

Smith P: American with Disabilities Act: accommodating persons with disabilities. In Pedretti LW, editor: *Occupational therapy practice skills for physical dysfunction,* ed 4, St. Louis, 1996, Mosby–Year Book, pp 541-551.

United States Department of Labor Employment and Training Administration: *Dictionary of occupational titles,* vol II, ed 4, revised, Washington, DC, 1991, US Government Printing Office.

Waddell G, McCulloch JA, Kummel E, Verner RM: Nonorganic physical signs in low-back pain, *Spine* 5:117-125, 1980.

Weinstein SM, Scheer SJ: Industrial rehabilitation medicine. 2. Assessment of the problem, pathology, and risk factors for disability, *Arch Phys Med Rehabil* 73: S-360-S-365, 1992.

CHAPTER 5.12

CHRONIC PULMONARY PROBLEMS

Chronic pulmonary diseases can be classified into those primarily causing oxygenation impairment (e.g., chronic obstructive pulmonary disease [COPD]) or ventilatory impairment (e.g., chronic restrictive pulmonary disease) or both. Patients with chronic pulmonary diseases tend to avoid activities for fear of causing pulmonary discomfort (e.g., dyspnea). This sedentariness leads to deconditioning, which makes physical exertion even more unpleasant, hence leading to a slow and insidious but steady downward spiral in physical capability. The purpose of pulmonary rehabilitation is to halt this downward spiral. Ideally, the pulmonary rehabilitation program should involve an interdisciplinary team, which, aside from the patient and the patient's support system, consists of the physician, physical therapist, occupational therapist, nurse, respiratory therapist, cardiopulmonary technologist, exercise physiologist, nutritionist, speech-language pathologist, social worker, psychologist, vocational counselor, durable medical equipment supplier, and other allied health professionals.

The general goals of pulmonary rehabilitation are to at least stabilize or possibly reverse both the physical and psychopathological aspects of the pulmonary disease, and to help the patient return to the highest possible functional capacity despite the pulmonary disease. Specific goals include measures to support or improve cardiopulmonary function as well as prevent and treat complications; foster compliance with medical regimens; reduce the number of exacerbations, emergency room visits, and hospitalizations; educate the patient to confront the disease realistically; prepare the patient to take responsibility for his or her rehabilitation and well-being; optimize psychosocial functioning and coping mechanisms; and return the patient to a more active, productive, and emotionally satisfying life.

Documented benefits of pulmonary rehabilitation include a reduction in the average number of hospitalization days per year and subjective improvement in symptoms and quality of life. Patients with chronic pulmonary diseases may have a superimposed acute pulmonary disease (e.g., upper respiratory tract infection, common cold, or pneumonia). In general, acute pulmonary care includes appropriate medications (e.g., antibiotics and bronchodilators) and a program of breathing exercises (to expand the lungs and increase breathing efficiency), secretion removal techniques (to enhance gas exchange), and general conditioning exercises (to maintain functional capacity). This chapter gives an overview of pulmonary rehabilitation as it pertains only to chronic pulmonary problems encountered in the PM&R setting.

I. **Epidemiology.** In the United States, COPD and allied conditions are the fifth leading cause of death and the fourth largest cause of major activity limitation (including loss of work days and premature retirement due to disability). The incidence of COPD has doubled since 1970, and the prevalence has been increasing. In patients with traumatic tetraplegia and neuromuscular disorders, the most common cause of premature death is respiratory insufficiency.

II. **Pulmonary evaluation**

  A. **History**

    1. **Chief complaint.** Dyspnea (see functional classification of dyspnea in Table 5.12-1), cough, sputum production, wheezing, fatigue, orthopnea, de-

Table 5.12-1. Impairment or disability rating secondary to respiratory diseases based on the American Medical Association (AMA) and American Thoracic Society (ATS) rating systems

PARAMETERS	RATING SYSTEM	CLASS 1 (0% IMPAIRMENT)	CLASS 2 (10-25% MILD IMPAIRMENT)	CLASS 3 (30-45% MODERATE IMPAIRMENT)	CLASS 4 (50-100% SEVERE IMPAIRMENT)
FVC	AMA‡ (ATS§)	≥80% Pr (≥80% Pr)	60-79% Pr (60-79% Pr)	51-59% Pr (51-59% Pr)	≤50% Pr (≤50% Pr)
FEV_1	AMA‡ (ATS§)	≥80% Pr (≥80% Pr)	60-79% Pr (60-79% Pr)	51-59% Pr (41-59% Pr)	≤50% Pr (≤40% Pr)
FEV_1/FVC*	AMA‡ (ATS§)	≥0.70 (≥0.75)	(0.60-0.74)	0.41-0.59 0.41-0.59)	(≤0.40 (≤0.40)
D_{LCO}	AMA‡ (ATS§)	≥70% Pr (≥80% Pr)	60-69% Pr (60-79%)	41-59% Pr (41-59% Pr)	≤40% Pr (≤40% Pr)
VO_2 max†	AMA‡	>25	20-25	15-20	<15
METs†	AMA‡	>7.1	5.7-7.1	4.3-5.7	<4.3
Dyspnea	AMA‖	No dyspnea; if present it is due to nonrespiratory reasons or is consistent with the circumstances of the activity	Dyspnea on fast walking on level ground or when walking uphill; person can keep pace with persons of same age and body build on level ground but not on hills or stairs	Dyspnea while walking on level ground with person of same age or walking up one flight of stairs; can walk a mile at own pace without dyspnea but cannot keep pace on level ground with others of same age and body built.	Dyspnea after walking >100 m at own pace on level ground; sometimes dyspneic with less exertion or even at rest.
Comment		Must meet all the PFT criteria	Must meet only one PFT criterion	Must meet only one PFT criterion	Must meet only one PFT criterion

Data compiled from ‡ Harber P, Chen-Yeung M: Assessment of respiratory impairment and disability. In Doege TC, editor: *American Medical Association: guides to the evaluation of permanent impairment,* ed 4, Chicago, 1993, American Medical Association, p. 162.‖ Engelberg AL, editor: *American Medical Association: guides to the evaluation of permanent impairment,* ed 3, Chicago, 1988, American Medical Association, p. 108; and § American Thoracic Society: Evaluation of impairment/disability secondary to respiratory disease, *Am Rev Respir Dis* 133:1206, 1986.
% Pr = percent of predicted value; FVC = forced vital capacity; FEV_1 = forced expiratory volume in 1 second; D_{LCO} = diffusing capacity of carbon monoxide.
* The ratio FEV_1/FVC is expressed as an absolute number (rather than as % Pr, which can be confusing).
† VO_2 max = maximum volume of oxygen consumption (expressed in ml O_2/min/kg; can be converted into metabolic equivalents [METs] by dividing VO_2max with 3.5, because 1 MET = 3.5 ml of O_2 consumed/kg/min).

creased exercise tolerance, morning headache, excessive drowsiness (with particular attention to symptom frequency), precipitating factors (such as, cold, infection, allergy, and humidity), relieving factors, complicating factors, rate of progression, and past treatments.

2. **Past and present occupational history.** Exposures to toxins and irritants.
3. **Functional history.** Effect of pulmonary disease on self care, vocational, and avocational activities.
4. **Allergy and medication history.** Prolonged use of corticosteroids can potentially cause osteoporosis.

5. **Personal history.** Smoking, alcohol consumption, and recreational or habitual drug use.

6. **Social history.** Home situation and architectural barriers, psychosocial history, and support system.

7. **Family history.** Alpha-antitrypsin deficiency, which predisposes one to emphysema.

B. **Physical examination** is generally directed to the pulmonary (and cardiac) systems. Observe the patient's breathing rate (e.g., tachypnea), breathing pattern (e.g., shallow; abdominal; chest; pursed lip; paradoxical, i.e., inward motion of abdomen with inspiration; and respiratory alternans, i.e., alternating movements of the rib cage and abdomen and pathognomonic of diaphragmatic fatigue), chest shape (e.g., barrel-chested), posture (e.g., kyphosis, scoliosis, or forward-leaning posture described in section IV.B.4), respiratory muscle aids (e.g., ventilators), signs of advanced lung disease (e.g., use of accessory muscle activity during quiet breathing, jugular venous distention because of cor pulmonale, cyanosis [e.g., perioral and periorbital sites], clubbing, and dependent edema); and capacity to clear secretions (e.g., cough). Auscultate the lungs (for decreased breath sounds [BS], crackles or rales, wheezing, ronchi) and heart (for tachycardia, arrhythmia, increased intensity of the pulmonic second sound). Check vital signs including temperature, blood pressure, height (which has a direct relationship with lung volumes), weight (increase may be due to dependent edema; unexplained loss may be due to carcinoma or other systemic diseases), and nutritional status.

C. **Diagnostic and monitoring tests**

1. **Radiographic tests** include chest radiographs (described in Chapter 5.13, section III.C.1), computed tomography (CT) scans, and magnetic resonance imaging (MRI) scans to image the chest and the intrathoracic structures (to help identify tumors, infections, cardiovascular changes, lung parenchymal changes, etc.). They must be correlated with the clinical findings and may need to be done serially for follow-up.

2. **Cardiac tests** include electrocardiogram (ECG) (described in Chapter 5.13, section III.C.2a) and echocardiogram (described in Chapter 5.13, section III.C.2.b) to rule out cardiac dysfunctions, which may contribute to pulmonary problems.

3. **Laboratory tests**

   a. **Blood tests,** such as complete blood count (hemoglobin and hematocrit), serum electrolytes, serum protein electrophoresis (for alpha-1-antitrypsin), and serum prealbumin or albumin (to determine nutritional status).

   b. **Sputum examination** (microscopy, Gram's stain, culture and sensitivity, cytology) to help diagnose specific infections and malignant conditions.

   c. **Blood gas monitoring** includes arterial blood gas (ABG) (see Chapter 2.6, section IV.A), capillary blood gas monitoring, transcutaneous or pulse oximetry (see Chapter 2.6, section IV.B), and capnography (end-tidal CO_2 monitoring). Although ABG testing is more accurate than other methods, obtaining the arterial sample may be difficult in about 25% of patients (if the patient either hyperventilates or hypoventilates during ABG sampling [because of anxiety or pain], the ABG result may not reflect the patient's actual pulmonary condition). The invasive ABG sampling is usually unnecessary in stable patients without intrinsic pulmonary disease. Daytime ABG for confirming suspicions of nocturnal hypoventilation may be misleading (as it may be normal) in patients with severe paralytic respiratory insufficiency (but no intrinsic lung disease). In these patients, pulse oximetry and capnography, both of which are noninvasive methods, are useful for continuous overnight monitoring of their blood gases. Pulse oximetry and capnography are also useful for monitoring the patient's blood gases during exercise.

d. **Pulmonary function tests** (PFTs) are fully described in Chapter 2.6. They include tests of ventilation (i.e., lung volumes and flow rate), pulmonary mechanics (airway resistance and lung compliance), lung diffusion capacity, and blood gases (see section II.C.3.c). In the PM&R setting, they are primarily used to differentiate between obstructive and restrictive pulmonary disorders and to estimate the severity and progression of a disease. They are usually done with the patient seated; however, in patients with chronic alveolar hypoventilation (CAH), PFTs should also be done in the supine position. For functional classification of pulmonary impairment or disability based on PFT, see Table 5.12-1.

e. **Integrated cardiopulmonary (CP) exercise tolerance tests** are fully described in Chapter 2.7, section II. They are used to assess cardiovascular and pulmonary parameters during exercise in patients with an established pulmonary diagnosis to determine a safe and individualized prescription of exercise or activity (e.g., intensity of exercise or activity or need for O_2 supplementation during exercise or activity). They include the **cardiopulmonary graded exercise tolerance tests (CP-GXTT)** (see Chapter 2.7, section II.A) using treadmill or bicycle ergometers for 6 to 12 minutes and the **timed-walking test** (see Chapter 2.7, section II.C), which involves the patient walking as far as possible in 12 minutes (may be modified to 6 or even 2 minutes for some patients).

f. **Special pulmonary studies** may occasionally be done. They include
   1) **Comprehensive sleep study,** which uses oral and nasal masks to detect airflow; chest wall monitoring to detect respiratory efforts; pulse oximetry to document desaturation; electroencephalogram (EEG) and electrooculogram (EOG) to monitor the stages of sleep; ECG to detect hypoxia-induced arrhythmias; and chin electromyography (EMG). This is indicated only in COPD patients suspected of having sleep apnea/hypopnea syndrome (SAHS) or in those who have cor pulmonale or polycythemia and whose daytime arterial oxygen tension (PaO_2) is above 60 mm Hg. In these patients (who are already hypoxemic when awake), overnight monitoring using only oximetry and capnography may be difficult to interpret.
   2) **Airway reactivity tests** such as the bronchoprovocation test using methacholine inhalation to detect asthma.

III. **Classification by etiology**
   A. **Chronic obstructive pulmonary disease,** including emphysema, chronic bronchitis, bronchiectasis, asthma, and cystic fibrosis, is characterized by air trapping, increased flow work or energy expended in moving air, and normal or increased compliance. Pulmonary function test patterns (summarized in Table 2.6-2) generally show decreased FEV_1/FVC ratio (i.e., ratio of forced expiratory volume in 1 second to forced vital capacity) as well as low $FEF_{25-75\%}$, (i.e., forced expiratory flow rate at 25-75% of the FVC). During maximal voluntary ventilation (MVV), the respiratory baseline gradually rises (due to air trapping) as ventilation progresses. The FEV_1 in COPD decreases by 45 to 75 ml per year, which is 3 times normal rate of decline due to aging. When the FEV_1 is less than 1500 ml, exertional dyspnea often occurs. In COPD patients with FEV_1 less than 750 ml, 30% die within 1 year and 50% within 3 years.

B. **Chronic restrictive pulmonary diseases** are characterized by reduction in the following PFT parameters (summarized in Table 2.6-2): total lung capacity (TLC), vital capacity (VC), residual volume (RV), expiratory reserve volume (ERV), functional residual capacity (FRC), minute ventilation, and compliance. Because air flow rates remain normal, however, the FEV_1/FVC ratio remains normal or may be increased. There is also increased elastic workload (i.e., energy consumed in stretching the elastic tissues of the lung) for which the patient compensates by producing rapid, shallow breathing. Unless the lungs are expanded by effective deep insufflations, these shallow breaths can eventually lead to atelectasis and hypoxia.

In addition, chronic restrictive pulmonary diseases often progress to chronic alveolar hypoventilation (CAH), which may be defined by the presence of chronic hypercapnia. Common symptoms of CAH include fatigue, dyspnea, headaches (morning or continuous), loss of concentration and memory, anxiety, personality changes (e.g., depression and irritability), sleep disturbances (e.g., daytime drowsiness, difficulty falling asleep, frequent awakening at night with shortness of breath, violent nightmares, difficulty awaking in the morning), and difficulty in managing airway secretions (especially with weak oropharyngeal and abdominal muscles). Sequelae of CAH includes pulmonary problems (e.g., atelectasis, pneumonia, pulmonary scarring, decreased lung compliance, impaired ventilation/perfusion ratio, and pulmonary hypertension); cardiovascular problems (e.g., cor pulmonale, arrhythmia, systemic hypertension, and polycythemia,); psychosocial problems (e.g., due to hypersomnolence, loss of concentration, anxiety, and irritability); and muscle aches and stiffness. The greater the severity of the CAH, the greater the risk of acute respiratory failure (which can be triggered by innocuous respiratory tract insults, fatigue, or stress). Chronic restrictive pulmonary diseases that can cause CAH can be classified into the following five categories:

1. **Neuromuscular causes** (the most common cause of neuromuscular respiratory failure in the United States is Guillain-Barre Syndrome [GBS]).

   a. **Upper motor neuron disease** causing central alveolar hypoventilation syndrome because of idiopathic causes (Ondine's curse), brain disorders (Arnold-Chiari malformation, stroke, extrapyramidal disorders), spinal cord disorders (e.g., cervical or upper thoracic spinal cord injury, thoracic myelomeningocele, and syringomyelia), or both brain and spinal cord disorder (e.g., multiple sclerosis).

   b. **Combined upper and lower motor neuron disease,** such as amyotrophic lateral sclerosis and progressive bulbar palsy.

   c. **Lower motor neuron disease** involving the anterior horn cells (e.g., poliomyelitis, postpolio syndrome, and spinal muscular atrophies), peripheral nerves (e.g., GBS, phrenic neuropathies, idiopathic or postsurgical diaphragm paralysis, polyneuropathies [because of toxic, metabolic, or infectious causes]), or neuromuscular junction (e.g., myasthenia gravis, Lambert-Eaton myasthenic syndrome, botulism, and organophosphate poisoning).

2. **Myopathic etiologies,** such as muscular dystrophies with dystrophinopathies (i.e., Duchenne's or Becker's), other muscular dystrophies (i.e., fascioscapulohumeral, limb-girdle, and myotonic dystrophy), polymyositis, and congenital and metabolic myopathies.

3. **Chest wall and diaphragmatic defects,** such as kyphoscoliosis, ankylosing spondylitis, postthoracotomy, and diaphragmatic hernia.

4. **Sleep disordered breathing,** which may be caused by SAHS or obesity.

Table 5.12-2. **Management options of chronic obstructive and restrictive pulmonary diseases**

CLASSIFICATION	MANAGEMENT OPTIONS
Obstructive	**Medical:** Medications (e.g., bronchodilator, pulmonary vaccines); nutrition therapy; hydration, cessation of smoking; patient education (avoid extremes of humidity and temperature, excessive fatigue, crowded areas) **Respiratory:** O_2 supplement to maintain SaO_2 >90% (include home or long-term use); may consider nocturnal noninvasive intermittent positive pressure ventilation (IPPV) **PT/OT:** Controlled breathing techniques CBT (e.g., diaphragmatic breathing; incentive spirometry; pursed lip breathing; paced breathing; ventilatory muscle training such as inspiratory resistive loading); secretion mobilization and airway clearance techniques; postural-relief techniques; abdominal strengthening exercises; general conditioning exercises (aerobic; limb range-of-motion [ROM] and strengthening; avoid excessive fatigue); energy and work conservation (including assistive and adaptive devices, and home modification); may combine CBT with biofeedback and relaxation techniques **Invasive:** Tracheal intubation **Others:** Psychosocial interventions; vocational counseling
Restrictive	**Medical:** Medications (e.g., vaccines [flu and bacterial]; judicious use of antiviral agents [e.g., amantadine] or antibiotics; avoid sedatives and other drugs); hydration; patient education (avoid obesity, heavy meals, extremes of humidity and temperature, excessive fatigue, crowded areas), cessation of smoking **Respiratory:** Mechanical ventilation (e.g., home ventilator; noninvasive IPPV; body ventilators); airway clearance management (consider Mechanical InExsufflator); use O_2 with caution; management of sleep disordered breathing **PT/OT:** CBT (e.g., diaphragmatic breathing; glossopharyngeal breathing; incentive spirometer; paced breathing; ventilatory muscle training such as inspiratory resistive loading); secretion mobilization and airway clearance techniques; abdominal strengthening exercises; may use abdominal binder; general conditioning exercises (e.g., limb ROM and strengthening; avoid fatigue); postural relief techniques; energy and work conservation (including assistive and adaptive devices, and home modification); may combine CBT with biofeedback and relaxation techniques **Invasive:** Tracheal intubation; diaphragmatic pacing **Others:** Psychosocial interventions, vocational counseling

5. **Primary pulmonary disorders,** for example tracheomalacia, bronchiectasis, chronic bronchitis, bronchopulmonary dysplasia, emphysema, cystic fibrosis, interstitial lung disease, adult respiratory distress syndrome, and chronic aspiration.
IV. **Noninvasive management** (see Table 5.12-2)
  A. **Medical modalities**
    1. **General medical care**
      a. **Cessation of smoking** is the most important preventive component in the care of patients with chronic pulmonary diseases. Studies showed that cessation of smoking can decrease the excessive rate of decline in lung

function associated with smoking. Smoke-cessation techniques include cognitive approach (e.g., information, books, articles, and physician's orders), propaganda (e.g., posters, brochures, and mass media messages), drugs (e.g., nicotine gum, patch, or nasal spray; lobeline; dextroampheta- mine; and imipramine), aversion-satiation (e.g., rapid smoking, imagina- tion, smoky air in face or mouth, or electric shock), affective approach (e.g., fear), therapy programs (e.g., hypnosis, psychotherapy, smoking cessation clinics, and individual or group therapy), behavior modifica- tion (e.g., desensitization, role-playing, self-monitoring, sensory depri- vation, and gradual reduction), and others (e.g., acupuncture, meditation, relaxation, and exercise). Resources on cessation of smoking are avail- able from the American Lung Association (1740 Broadway, New York, NY 10019; tel [212] 315-8700) and the American Cancer Society (1599 Clifton Rd, Atlanta, GA 30329; tel. [404] 320-3333). Self-help materials based on empirical research are also available at low cost from the Office of Cancer Communications ("Quit for Good" kit), National Cancer Institute, Bldg. 31, Room 10A18, Bethesda, MD 20205, and the Stanford Health Promotion Resource Center, 1000 Welch Road, Palo Alto, CA 94304-1885, tel. (415) 723-1000.

b. **Nutritional therapy** is essential for patients with chronic pulmonary dis- ease whose body weight is low (especially those with COPD or on mechanical ventilation) because low body weight is associated with in- creased morbidity and mortality in COPD patients. Improving nutritional status increases endurance for activities of daily living (ADLs) and am- bulation, reduces dyspnea, and increases subjective well-being; how- ever, the resting arterial blood gases (ABGs) usually remain unchanged. Also, the role of nutritional therapy in improving long-term outcomes out- side the controlled hospital environment remains unclear. Nonetheless, nutritional support for patients with low body weight is recommended because of the above benefits in addition to improvement in respiratory function, immune function, skeletal muscle mass, and strength.

The two main reasons for weight loss in patients with chronic pulmo- nary disease are increased energy expenditure for breathing even at rest (thus increasing daily caloric need) and decreased caloric intake because of dyspnea while eating (especially large meals) caused by the need to breath-hold during swallowing. Other reasons for weight loss include the side effects of prescribed medications (e.g., bronchodilators); the limitations of diaphragmatic excursion as a result of a full stomach (thus further causing dyspnea); and concomitant depression and a reduced sense of taste and smell (thus causing loss of appetite and further weight loss). The vicious cycle whereby weight loss in COPD patients lead to hypoxemia and hypercapnia is shown in Fig. 5.12-1. Table 5.12-3 shows the general recommendations on feeding strategies to improve caloric intake for different pulmonary-related complaints of COPD patients.

Energy expenditure should be determined by indirect calorimetry. If this is unavailable, a practical method of calculating for the basal energy expenditure (BEE) is using the Harris-Benedict formula and then applying the correction factors for patients with COPD (see Chapter 5.6, section VII.B). Based on the BEE, the caloric needs for the patient can be calculated and the patient given appropriate nutritional supplements to attain ideal body weight (IBW). The cutoff weight for determining undernutrition in patients with chronic pulmonary disease is less than

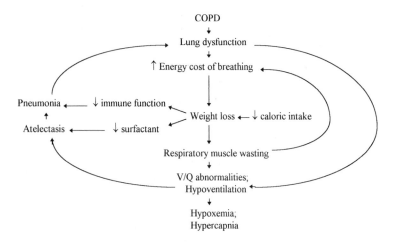

Figure 5.12-1
The vicious cycle whereby weight loss in patients with chronic obstructive pulmonary disease (COPD) lead to hypoxemia and hypercapnia. ↑, increased; ↓, decreased; V/Q, ventilation/perfusion. (Adapted from: Axen KV: Nutrition in chronic obstructive pulmonary disease. In Haas F, Axen K, eds: *Pulmonary Therapy and Rehabilitation. Principles and Practice,* ed 2. Baltimore, 1991, Williams & Wilkins, p. 97, Copyright © 1991 Williams & Wilkins, with permission.)

90% IBW although values as low as below 70 to 85% IBW may be justifiable because: (1) the percentage IBW does not give information about body composition (i.e., lean vs. adipose tissue), hence a weight of 90% IBW may reflect athletic fitness if the low weight is due to loss of adipose tissue; (2) there is generally no associated biochemical or clinical signs of undernutrition at 90% IBW; and (3) the value used for calculating % IBW (i.e., the midpoint of the weight range for a given category) tends to overestimate the lower end of the weight range.

As with other patients, protein usually makes up 20% of the total caloric requirement. Protein supplementation can also be given at 1.7 g/kg of body weight to promote nitrogen retention and physiologic improvement. The distribution of calories among fat and carbohydrate remains controversial. Dietary fat has a respiratory quotient (RQ) of 0.7 compared to 1.0 for carbohydrates. The RQ (see Chapter 2.7, section II.A) is the ratio of the carbon dioxide produced to the oxygen consumed, thus dietary fat produces lower levels of carbon dioxide per kilocalorie of energy expended than carbohydrate, making it more efficient as a source of fuel than carbohydrate. Studies have shown that the intake of relatively higher dietary fat is preferred in hypercapnic patients (e.g., severe COPD or acute respiratory failure requiring mechanical ventilator support) in whom high carbohydrate diet (particularly those providing an excess of calories to promote weight gain) may lead to further retention of carbon dioxide. However, this does not connote excessively high fatty intake, but rather the intermediate caloric distribution of about 45% carbohydrate and 35% fat (in addition to 20% protein and recommended

Table 5.12-3. **General recommendations on feeding strategies to improve caloric intake for different pulmonary-related complaints of COPD patients**

COMPLAINT	ESTIMATED FREQUENCY*	GENERAL RECOMMENDATIONS ON FEEDING STRATEGIES
Early satiety	87%	1. Eat high-calorie foods first. 2. Limit liquid consumption during meal; sip liquids 1 hr after meals. 3. Eat cold food first as this can give less of a sense of fullness than hot foods.
Bloating	80%	1. Treat shortness of breath early to prevent air swallowing. 2. Eat smaller, more frequent meals. 3. Avoid rushed meals. 4. Avoid gas-forming foods (individual to patient).
Dyspnea	73%	1. Rest before meals. 2. Use bronchodilators before meals. 3. Use secretion clearance strategies if indicated. 4. Eat more slowly. 5. Use pursed-lip breathing between bites. 6. Use tripod position for meals. 7. Have readily prepared meals available for periods of increased shortness of breath. 8. Evaluate for meal desaturation; refer for O_2 evaluation if needed.
Anorexia	73%	1. Eat high-calorie food first. 2. Have favorite foods available. 3. Try more frequent meals and snacks throughout the day. 4. Instruct patients to push themselves to eat. 5. Add margarine, butter, mayonnaise, sauces, and gravies to diet to add calories.
Fatigue	60%	1. Rest before meals. 2. Have readily prepared meals available for periods of increased fatigue or illness. 3. Have patient try to eat larger meals when less tired.
Constipation	50%	1. Incorporate exercise as tolerated. 2. Instruct patient in high-fiber foods and adequate fluids. 3. Refer to Chapter 5.8, section VI.B for constipation management.
Dental problems	30%	1. Instruct patient to eat soft, high-calorie foods. 2. Refer to dental services as appropriate.

Adapted from Donahoe M, Rogers RM: Nutritional assessment and support in chronic obstructive pulmonary disease. *Clin Chest Med* 11:499, 1990, with permission.
* Estimated frequency based on a survey of 19 malnourished COPD patients.

daily allowances of vitamins and minerals). In acute respiratory failure, a fat emulsion (e.g., Pulmocare) may be used not only to reduce carbon dioxide production but to provide a volume concentrated source of calories in the fluid-restricted patient.

c. **Education.** Both the patient and family or support system should be educated about the underlying pulmonary disorder, the goal of treatment (as well as side effects), the use and cleaning of respiratory therapy equipment, techniques of pulmonary rehabilitation modalities for home use (including exercise conditioning programs), avoidance of exposure to irritants (e.g., dust and chemicals) at home and at the workplace, and safe techniques for intimacy (see Supplemental References; see also Table 5.13-2 for sexual counseling of patients with concomitant cardiac problems). For discussion on patient education techniques, see Chapter 5.10, section VI.A.

2. **Pharmacotherapy.** Because pulmonary drugs are primarily prescribed by pulmonologists, this section provides only an overview of the pulmonary drug as it relates to patients undergoing pulmonary rehabilitation. The administration routes of some pulmonary drugs include inhalation routes (e.g., through nebulizers, metered-dose inhalers [MDIs] or dry powder inhalers [DPIs]) and oral and parenteral routes. The advantages of the inhalation route over the oral and parenteral routes include a lower dose requirement and fewer side effects; however, drugs given via the inhalation route have a shorter duration of action and must be given more frequently.

The most commonly used inhalation method is the MDI (e.g., for delivery of β-adrenergic, anticholinergic, steroid, and mast cell stabilizing drugs) because of its portability, relatively high lung deposition (10-15%), and low cost. The formerly recommended MDI technique (which can still be found in some package inserts) in which the mouth is closed over the MDI mouthpiece has been shown to be ineffective as it results in greater deposition of aerosols in the mouth and throat rather than in the lung parenchyma; therefore, the following open-mouth technique is currently recommended by the American College of Chest Physicians:

- Shake the inhaler to mix the medication with the propellant (e.g., freon).
- Breathe out completely to end of a normal breath (i.e., to functional residual capacity).
- Open the mouth wide and hold canister in the upright position 2 to 4 cm from mouth, aiming the inhaler towards the mouth. In some patients (e.g., elderly or neurologic patients) spacers or aerosol reservoirs (which hold the MDI) may be used to decrease the proximal deposition of large particles.
- Depress the top of the MDI canister while breathing in deeply and slowly over a period of 5 to 6 seconds (to total lung capacity).
- Close the mouth and hold the breath for about 10 seconds.
- For each additional puff ordered, wait for at least 1 to 2 minutes between actuations.

The DPI, which appears to be equivalent to a properly used MDI, may cause heavy oropharyngeal deposition and clumping of particles in high-humidity environments. There are only a limited number of medications available through DPI (e.g., spin-inhaler for delivery of cromolyn sodium [Intal] and rotacaps for delivery of Ventolin). Nebulizers (e.g., jet nebulizer and ultrasonic nebulizer) can deliver larger volumes and higher doses than MDIs; however, they are bulky, expensive, and subject to bacterial contamination. The nebulizer, therefore, is only used for patients who cannot use inhalers (e.g., because of cognitive or motor deficits) or who do not obtain relief of bronchospasm with inhalers (e.g., advanced COPD).

a. **Bronchodilators** are considered first-line treatment for COPD.

1) **Sympathomimetic drugs,** in particular β_2-**adrenergic agonists,** causes the activation of adenyl cyclase, which catalyzes the conversion of adenosine triphosphate (ATP) to cyclic adenosine monophosphate(cAMP). Increased intracellular level of cAMP, in turn, causes bronchodilation, increased mucus clearance, pulmonary artery dilation, and a decrease in antigen-induced release of mediators from basophils and mast cells. There are also nonpulmonary effects such as skeletal muscle tremors and some direct cardiac stimulation. Sympathomimetics are indicated for the relief of acute or chronic bronchospasm and in the prevention of exercise-induced bronchospasm. They are contraindicated in patients with hypersensitivity to any component of the drug or cardiac arrhythmias associated with tachycardia.

   a) **Cathecholamines** are first generation β_2-adrenergic agonists; however, they are nonspecific as they also stimulate α-adrenergic and β_1-adrenergic receptors, thus causing unwanted effects because of positive chronotropy and inotropy of the heart (e.g., palpitations, tachycardia, and hypertension) and hyperglycemia and hypokalemia. They generally have a short duration of action (only 1-2 hours) and can lead to the development of tolerance in some patients. Examples include **epinephrine, isoproterenol (Isuprel, Medihaler-Iso), isoetharine (Bronkosol),** and **bitolterol (Tornalate).** Epinephrine is a potent stimulator of α- and β-adrenergic receptors. Isoproterenol has mostly β-adrenergic effect but is equally potent on both β_1 and β_2 receptors. Isoetharine has more selective β_2 effect but is a less potent bronchodilator than isoproterenol. Bitolterol is a pro-drug that is inactive until it is cleaved in the lung by esterase to produce its active form, colterol. Because esterase levels are higher in the lung than in the heart, bitolterol has fewer cardiac side effects. Bitolterol is also slowly hydrolyzed and has a sustained duration of up to 8 hours.

   b) **Resorcinols** are second generation β_2-adrenergic agonists. They are more selective β_2-adrenergic agonists, more active orally, and have a longer duration of action (about 4-6 hours) than that of catecholamines. They include **metaproterenol (Alupent)** and **terbutaline (Brethaire, Brethine, Bricanyl).** Terbutaline is more β_2-specific than metaproterenol.

   c) **Saligenins** are third generation β_2-adrenergic agonists. They show more β_2-specificity than the other sympathomimetic drugs, are active orally, and have a duration of action of 4 to 6 hours or longer. They include **albuterol (Proventil, Ventolin, Volmax), pirbuterol (Maxair),** and **salmeterol (Serevent).** Pirbuterol has less potent bronchodilator effects than albuterol. Salmeterol, which was approved by the FDA in 1994, has a duration of action of up to 12 hours and is more potent than albuterol. Its only drawback is its slower onset of action than albuterol; hence, salbuterol is not indicated for rapid relief of acute bronchospasm.

2) **Anticholinergic bronchodilators** compete with acetylcholine for receptors at the parasympathetic postganglionic effector cell junctions. Acetylcholine, which stimulates guanyl cyclase to produce cyclic

guanosine monophosphate (cGMP), can cause both bronchial smooth muscle contraction and mast cell degranulation; therefore, anticholinergic agents, which decrease the intracellular level of cGMP, result in bronchodilation (this effect is independent from the actions of sympathomimetic drugs). In contrast to sympathomimetic drugs, which primarily affect the smaller distal airways, the anticholinergics primarily affect the larger central airways. Anticholinergics, which do not cause drug resistance, may be more effective when used on a long-term basis than β-adrenergic drugs.

The preferred anticholinergic bronchodilator is an inhaled form of **ipratropium bromide (Atrovent)**, which is a derivative of atropine. Ipratropium acts locally as it is poorly absorbed from the bronchial mucosa and generally has less side effects than atropine (common side effects of atropine include dry mouth, tachycardia, blurred vision, and urinary retention). It reaches its peak effect in 1 to 2 hours and is thus not indicated for the initial treatment of acute bronchospasm. It is contraindicated in patients with allergy to atropine or other components of Atrovent (e.g., soya lecithin found in peanuts and soybeans) and is to be used with caution in patients with narrow-angle glaucoma, prostatic hypertrophy, tachycardia, and unstable cardiovascular status (e.g., myocardial ischemia and acute hemorrhage).

3) **Methylxanthines** are traditionally believed to cause bronchodilation through phosphodiesterase inhibition, thus leading to increased intracellular levels of cAMP. Other proposed mechanisms include competitive antagonism at adenosine receptors, reduction in the uptake or metabolism of catecholamines, interference with the uptake and storage of calcium, and inhibition of prostaglandin synthesis. Aside from bronchodilation, they also stimulate breathing, enhance ciliary function, inhibit the release of histamine, vasodilate pulmonary vessels and decrease pulmonary hypertension, improve diaphragmatic contractility, and cause other nonpulmonary effects (e.g., vasodilate coronary artery blood vessels, vasoconstrict cerebral blood vessels, promote diuresis, stimulate the central nervous system and skeletal muscles, increase secretion of gastric acid, and relax uterine smooth muscle).

The methylxanthines most selective in their smooth muscle activity are **theophylline (Theo-Dur, Theolair, Theoclear, Throchron, Uni-Dur, Aerolate, Elixophyllin, Slo-phyllin, Quibron, Respbid)** and its salts, **aminophylline (Mudrane)**, and **dyphylline (Lufyllin, Dilor, Dyline)**. Aminophylline is 75 to 85% less active than theophylline. A blood level of 10 to 20 mg/dl of theophylline is considered therapeutic, although many patients show mild bronchodilation with subtherapeutic levels of 5 to 10 mg/dl. Theophylline blood levels can be increased by many drugs (e.g., erythromycin, ciprofloxacin, flu vaccine, cimetidine, calcium channel blockers, nonselective β-blockers, corticosteroids, isoniazid, allopurinol, and oral contraceptives) and conditions (e.g., pneumonia, congestive heart failure, liver disease, renal disease, shock, and diets high in caffeine). Some drugs that may decrease theophylline blood levels include β-adrenergic agonists, rifampin, phenytoin, and barbiturates. Loop diuretics and isoniazid may either increase or decrease theophylline blood levels. Due to its absorption characteristics and potential side effects, theophylline is contraindicated in patients with unstable blood pressure, gastrointestinal bleeding, hepatic failure, hyperthyroidism, nausea, history of seizures, tachyarhythmias, extreme tremulousness, peptic ulcer, or vomiting.

Other methylxanthines such as caffeine (a central nervous system stimulant found in coffee, tea, cola, and cocoa) and theobromine (found in chocolates) are not approved for use as bronchodilators.

b. Glucocorticoids (discussed in Chapter 4.8, section III), which have bronchodilatory as well as potent antiinflammatory effects, are used in pulmonary patients to treat primarily asthma and other pulmonary diseases (e.g., COPD, sarcoidosis). Steroids may be given intravenously (e.g., **hydrocortisone [Solu-Cortef], methylprednisolone [Solu-Medrol]**), orally (e.g., **prednisone**), via a respiratory inhalant (e.g., **beclomethasone [Beclovent; Vanceril], dexamethasone [Decadron Phosphate Respihaler], triamcinolone [Azmacort], flunisolide [AeroBid]**), or through intranasal sprays (e.g., **beclomethasone [Vancenase Nasal Inhaler, Beconase Inhalation], dexamethasone [Decadron Phosphate Turbinaire], triamcinolone [Nasacort], flunisolide [Nasalide], and budesonide [Rhinocort]**).

c. Prophylactic antiasthmatic agents act by stabilizing mast cells or by inhibiting the release of inflammatory mediators. They include **cromolyn sodium** (also called **disodium cromoglycate**, e.g., **Intal, Gastrocrom, Nasalcrom**), **nedocromil sodium (Tilade)**, and the experimental drug, **ketotifen (Zaditen)**. These drugs are used to decrease the frequency and intensity of asthmatic attacks in both allergic and nonallergic asthma, to treat and prevent allergic rhinitis, and to prevent exercise-induced bronchospasm. Because they are not bronchodilators and have delayed onsets of action (4-6 weeks), they should not be used to reverse acute bronchospasm.

d. Mucokinetic agents alter the composition and volume of airway secretions to promote mobilization and removal of these airway secretions. The most important mucolytic agent is water. Adequate hydration (2-4 L/day) is essential for easier expectoration of mucus; however, patients should not be overhydrated as it may cause pulmonary edema in those with congestive heart failure or renal failure. Other mucokinetic agents (mostly in inhaled form) include **acetylcysteine (Mucomyst, Mucosal), sodium bicarbonate, hydrating agents** (iso-, hyper-, or hypotonic saline), **recombinant human deoxyribonuclease (Pulmozyne)**, and **propylene glycol**. The effectiveness of acetylcysteine in patients with COPD or asthma is controversial as it may also cause bronchospasm. If used at all, acetylcysteine should be limited to only a few doses and should be accompanied by bronchodilators.

e. Cough and cold preparations do not cure the cold nor lessen its duration, but are used to modify or relieve the symptoms (e.g., nasal congestion, headache, fever, general malaise, cough, and rhinorrhea) of cold or allergy. They can be given singly or in combination with each other or with other chemicals (e.g., analgesics, anticholinergic agents, preservatives, caffeine, and alcohol). When using combination preparations, the benefits of each ingredient must be considered. Many cough and cold preparations are available over-the-counter and have high potential for abuse.

1) Antitussives are used to suppress an ineffective, dry, hacking, nonproductive cough or in patients who cannot get enough rest because of excessive coughing. They can be given locally (e.g., topical anesthetics such as **lidocaine**) through an endotracheal or tracheostomy tube, or they can be given systemically using either narcotic (primar-

ily **codeine;** see Chapter 4.8, section I.B.1.a.2) or nonnarcotic preparations **(dextromethorphan** [e.g., **Robitussin DM, Drixoral, Vicks Formula 44],**
diphenhydramine [e.g., **Tusstat, Benylin Cough]**, and benzonatate [e.g.,
Tessalon Perles]). Systemic antitussives act centrally by suppressing
the cough reflex located at the medullary cough center.

2) **Expectorants** are used to relieve dry, nonproductive coughs by increasing the amount of fluid (i.e., mucus production) in the respiratory
tract, therefore, making the cough more productive. These include
guaifenesin (e.g., **Robitussin, Humibid), iodine products** (e.g., **potassium
iodide, SSKI), iodinated glycerol** (e.g., **Organidin),** and **terpin hydrate**. Patients must be adequately hydrated for the expectorant to have maximal efficacy.

3) **Nasal decongestants** are sympathomimetic amines with primary α-adrenergic actions used to relieve nasal congestion and edema via local
vasoconstriction of blood vessels in patients with upper respiratory
allergies and the common cold. Nasal decongestants are to be used
only on a limited basis (3-5 days) as prolonged use may result in
rebound congestion upon drug discontinuation. Examples include
pseudoephedrine (e.g., **Sudafed, Actifed), phenylephrine** (e.g., **Neo-Synephrine), ephedrine** (e.g., **Vicks Vatronol),** and **oxymetazoline** (e.g., **Allerest
12-hour Nasal).**

4) **Antihistamines** reduce inflammation and allergic reactions by competitively antagonizing histamine at the H_1 receptor rather than binding
to histamine to deactivate it. Most antihistamines also have anticholinergic, antipruritic, sedative, and antiemetic effects. The first generation antihistamines include **alkylamines (chlorpheniramine** [e.g., **Chlor-
Trimeton], dexchlorpheniramine** [e.g., **Poladex]), brompheniramine** [e.g.,
**Bromfed, Dimetane, Dallergy, Rondec, Lodrane, Poly-Histine CS, and Respa-
hist], triprolidine** [e.g., **Actifed Cold]), ethanolamines** (i.e., **diphendydram-
ine** [e.g., **Benadryl], clemastine** [e.g., **Tavist],** and **doxylamine** [e.g., **Ny-
quil, Unisom]), ethylenediamines** (i.e., **tripelennamine** [e.g., **PBZ]** and **pyril-
amine** [e.g., **Triaminic, Codimal, Poly-Histine Elixir, Atrohist]), phenothiazines** (i.e., **prometazine** [e.g., **Phenergan, Prometh],** and **piperidine** (i.e.,
cyproheptadine [e.g., **Periactin], azatadine** [e.g., **Trinalin],** and **phenindam-
ine** [e.g., **Nolahist]**. They are short-acting and sedating. In contrast,
the second-generation antihistamines, which include **fexofenadine [Al-
legra], terfenadine [Seldane], astemizole [Hismanal],** and **loratadine [Clari-
tin]**, are long-acting and are nonsedating. Terfenadine can cause QT
interval prolongation and ventricular arrhythmias and has been replaced by the safer fexofenadine.

f. **Pulmonary vaccines** are generally recommended for patients with chronic
pulmonary diseases to prevent major respiratory tract infections, which
can trigger respiratory failure.

1) **Pneumococcal vaccines (Pneumovax 23; Pnu-Imune 23)** contain purified
capsular polysaccharide antigen of up to 23 of the most prevalent
types of *Streptococcus pneumoniae* (pneumococci) which are responsible for approximately 90% of serious pneumococcal diseases. The
vaccine's popular name, ''pneumonia vaccine,'' is misleading because pneumococci are responsible not only for pneumonia but other
infections such as meningitis and otitis media. The vaccine is effective only against the named types of pneumococci and is generally
given once in a lifetime (with no booster dose) to individuals over

2 years old. It is injected intramuscularly (or subcutaneously) at a single dose of 0.5 ml and may be given concomitantly with the influenza virus vaccine (see below) injected at a different site. Aside from local muscle soreness, some patients may develop a low-grade fever and mild myalgia for about 24 hours. Although rare, there are reports of high fever, arthralgia, and anaphylaxis.

2) **Influenza virus vaccines** or **"flu shots"** (e.g., **FluShield, Fluvirin, Fluzone**) are prepared from extraembryonic fluids of chicken eggs infected with influenza virus. The infected fluid is then inactivated (hence it becomes noninfectious and cannot cause influenza), concentrated, and highly purified to create a surface antigen vaccine against types A and B strains of influenza. The formula is updated yearly to contain new strains from the previous year. It is contraindicated in patients with (a) allergy to egg, chicken, or egg products; (b) allergy to any components of the vaccine, including thimerosal; (c) any signs of active infection; and (d) past history of GBS. The vaccine is administered intramuscularly every year, ideally in the fall (before December) when influenza activity sharply increases, to individuals over 6 months old. The recommended dose for individuals over 3 years is 0.5 ml. Aside from local muscle soreness, the major but inconsequential side effects of the influenza vaccine are fever, malaise, and myalgia, especially in patients who have not taken the flu vaccine previously. These symptoms usually appear in 6 to 12 hours and persist for 1 or 2 days.

g. **Others pulmonary drugs** include **diuretics** to reduce fluid overload (e.g., cor pulmonale) and **antiinfective agents** to reduce mucus and improve arterial blood gases in patients with pulmonary infection, especially in those with limited respiratory reserve. Ideally, antiinfective therapy should be directed by cultures. In pulmonary patients with viral infection, antibiotics are frequently prescribed due to the patient's increased susceptibility to secondary bacterial invasion resulting from altered immunity.

3. **Home oxygen therapy.** Based on medical consensus and the guidelines established by Medicare for its reimbursement in the United States, home oxygen is indicated for

- Exercise or activity use if the hemoglobin saturation (SaO_2) is equal to or less than 88%, or the arterial oxygen tension (PaO_2) is equal to or less than 55 mm Hg with the exercise or activity for which oxygen is prescribed, or if there is demonstration of increased exercise tolerance or endurance with oxygen in conjunction with a rehabilitation program.
- Nocturnal use if SaO_2 is less than or equal to 88% or PaO_2 is less than or equal to 55 mm Hg during sleep with evidence of cor pulmonale, erythrocytosis, or other physical or mental impairment attributable to nocturnal hypoxemia, or if sleep-related hypoxemia is corrected or improved by oxygen supplementation.
- Intermittent or stand-by oxygen if SaO_2 is less than or equal to 88% or PaO_2 is less than or equal to 55 mm Hg in association with acute bronchospasm, heart failure, or other cardiopulmonary disease in a patient who is subject to frequent changes in clinical stability.
- Long-term oxygen therapy (LTOT) for continuous (24 hours a day) use if SaO_2 is less than or equal to 88% or PaO_2 is less than or equal to 55 mm Hg when breathing room air as documented by two ABGs drawn

at rest in the seated position in outpatients in stable condition receiving optimal medical therapy (if home oxygen is prescribed for an inpatient, the ABGs must be repeated 1-3 months after discharge when the patient has recovered from the acute illness and is receiving optimum therapy for any remaining chronic respiratory disease). However, because some patients with PaO_2 above 55 mm Hg can have evidence of hypoxic organ dysfunction, the following criteria may also be used: PaO_2 less than or equal to 59 mm Hg and evidence of at least one of the following: pulmonary hypertension (P wave greater than 3 mm in leads II, III, or aVF), cor pulmonale (dependent edema), or erythrocytosis (hematocrit above 56%).

When home oxygen is prescribed, the FiO_2 (fraction of inspired O_2) and oxygen flow rate should be titrated to the minimum needed to achieve adequate tissue oxygenation as confirmed by ABG to determine an increase in PaO_2 by 5 mm Hg or to above 60 mm Hg, or by using pulse oximetry to determine increase in SaO_2 above 90%. To reduce the incidence of pulmonary oxygen toxicity (e.g., diffuse alveolar damage), an oxygen concentration of below 40 to 50% and oxygen pressure of 90 to 110 mm Hg should be used. The oxygen flow should be increased over the resting requirement by 1 L/min during sleep or by 0.5 L/min during air travel. The advantages and disadvantages of different modes of oxygen supply and delivery are shown in Tables 5.12-4 and 5.12.5, respectively.

Table 5.12-4. Advantages and disadvantages of common modes of O_2 supply

OXYGEN SUPPLY	ADVANTAGES	DISADVANTAGES
1. Compressed gas cylinders	100% O_2 up to high flow rates; inexpensive; reliable; relatively portable; no power needed; for intermittent use (e.g., for sleep or exercise)	High pressure; unsafe to transfill at home; bulky; needs frequent deliveries from vendors
2. Liquid O_2 systems	100% O_2 at all flow rates; excellent portability; smaller storage volume; generally lighter; no power needed; for active patients or those who need high liter flows	Low pressure; can transfill from larger tanks; can freeze (may cause frostbite at connections and if spilled); settings can be inaccurate; evaporates if not used; expensive except for patients on >3L/min rate
3. Molecular sieve O_2 concentrators	90-93% O_2 up to flow rates of about 3L/min; least expensive for patients who stay home	Not portable; needs power from wall electrical outlet; needs back-up system; high maintenance; provides only flow rate of <2-3 L/min
4. Membrane-separator O_2 enrichers	Low maintenance (only filter needs to be changed); well humidified; ideal for transtracheal O_2 therapy	Low O_2 concentration (45%)

Table 5.12-5. Advantages and disadvantages of common modes of O_2 delivery

OXYGEN DELIVERY	ADVANTAGES	DISADVANTAGES
Continuous mode		
1. Nasal cannulas or prongs	Inexpensive; relatively comfortable; patient can eat, talk, sleep, expectorate; no CO_2 rebreathing; FiO_2 independent of nose or mouth breathers; FiO_2 delivered is 22-40% at 0.5-6.0 L/min	Less efficient than face mask; FiO_2 elevation is modest even at high flow rates; may cause mucosal drying and dermatitis unless well-humidified
2. Face mask	Efficient delivery of air (if mask is tight) at wide range of FiO_2; air is humidified (except in the venturi mask, where gas is not completely humidified)	Less comfortable; awkward eating, talking, expectorating; not reliable when FiO_2 of <35% is needed; partial rebreathing of CO_2
3. Transtracheal	Cosmetic; lighter equipment; improved mobility; better oxygenation; reduced O_2 flow requirement; reduced inspiratory work; better sense of taste; good patient compliance	Invasive (needs mini-tracheostomy, e.g., with 16-gauge angiocatheter); needs humidification; causes complications (e.g., mucus balls; subcutaneous emphysema; cough; local infection; dislodged catheter; reinsertion failure)
Noncontinuous mode*		
1. Reservoir O_2-conserving device†	Can be used with nasal cannulas; least expensive; simple; reliable	Unsightly; obtrusive; needs frequent replacement of filter; low compliance; decreased effectiveness in mouth breathers
2. Pulsed delivery‡	Most efficacious	Subject to mechanical failure

* Maximizes O_2 delivery at the beginning of inspiration (because at the latter phase of inspiration, the O_2 enters the dead space and is wasted). The reduced O_2 flow requirement can reduce size and weight of O_2 equipment as well as potentially reduce cost of long-term oxygen therapy (LTOT).

† Uses a storage bag (e.g., in nonrebreathing or partial-rebreathing reservoir mask) with an internal diaphragm and a reservoir of about 20 ml, which fills with O_2 during expiration. On inspiration, the diaphragm collapses, thus providing a volume of O_2 at the beginning of inspiration.

‡ Can deliver fixed or variable volume of O_2 at the end of expiration and the beginning of inspiration; uses thermistor detectors or pressure sensors to detect chest wall motion; rapid, shallow breathing can cause continuous activation without O_2 conservation.

The use of home oxygen in COPD patients, when indicated, decreases reactive pulmonary hypertension, polycythemia, perception of effort during exercise, and hospitalizations, as well as improves cognitive function and prolongs life. In hypoxemic COPD patients, these potential benefits of home oxygen outweigh the risks of pulmonary oxygen toxicity (seen in 50% of COPD patients receiving LTOT for 7-60 months). In normoxemic COPD patients, the use of LTOT (to improve exercise performance or to treat dyspnea) remains controversial. In general oxygen should not be prescribed for prophylactic use or for "as needed" use at home (unless the patient meets the criteria described above).

The use of home oxygen may also be beneficial in patients with other chronic pulmonary diseases such as severe restrictive lung disease (e.g., kyphoscoliosis), cystic fibrosis, or pulmonary fibrosis (e.g., interstitial pneumonitis); however, the benefit is not as well documented as for COPD patients. In general, home oxygen is more harmful than beneficial in patients with chronic respiratory failure especially those who are chronic carbon dioxide retainers (e.g., due to paralytic restrictive pulmonary diseases). These hypercapneic patients rely on the central hypoxic ventilatory drive; and oxygen supplementation may suppress ventilatory drive thus leading to more carbon dioxide retention and to respiratory arrest. In these patients, mechanical ventilation (see below) is recommended instead of oxygen supplementation.

4. **Mechanical ventilation** (whether daytime or nighttime) is mainly used in patients with CAH (due to various chronic restrictive pulmonary diseases; see section III.B) either as a life support system (e.g., high-cervical spinal cord injury [SCI] patients with respiratory muscle paralysis and patients with respiratory failure) or as an elective therapy (e.g., patients with progressive chronic respiratory insufficiency in an attempt to prevent acute respiratory failure, to preserve function, and possibly to increase survival). In general, the decision to initiate mechanical ventilation is based on the clinical assessment, that is, presence of apnea, tachypnea of over 40 breaths/min, and respiratory failure that cannot be adequately corrected by any other means. Other less reliable parameters (because they cannot distinguish between acute and chronic respiratory insufficiency) include ABG parameters, that is, PaO_2 less than 55 mm Hg despite high-flow oxygen or $PaCO_2$ above 50 mm Hg and PFT parameters (if patient is able to perform PFT) of, vital capacity less than 15 ml/kg, inspiratory force less than -25 cm H_2O, and FEV_1 less than 10 ml/kg.

Indications for the elective use of chronic nocturnal mechanical ventilation in patients with CAH have not been clearly established. Factors to be considered include the rate of progression of the primary disease process, age, PFT results, ABG level (especially decreased PaO_2 and increased PCO_2) taken when awake and when asleep, sleep disordered breathing, acute respiratory compromise, or "fatigue" from intercurrent respiratory tract infections, and cognitive function, motivation, and cooperation. Noninvasive monitoring of nocturnal sleep blood gases (e.g., pulse oximetry or capnography) should be done at least once a year in patients whose supine VC is below 40 to 50% of predicted normal, especially those with rapidly evolving conditions and loss of VC. More frequent nocturnal monitoring (every 3-12 months unless VC has increased) should be done in the presence of progressive paralytic restrictive pulmonary disease with a sudden drop in VC, a VC of less than 1000 ml or below 25 to 35% of predicted normal; a VC significantly lower in supine than sitting; or in any patients with symptoms or signs of CAH. Nocturnal ventilatory support is indicated in symptomatic patients with a VC less than 50% of predicted normal, mean SaO_2 below 95% for at least 1 hour during sleep, and maximum PCO_2 over 50 mm Hg, and in nonsymptomatic patients with PCO_2 above 50 mm Hg and mean SaO_2 below 95% during much of the night.

Mechanical ventilation (e.g., using oral or nasal intermittent positive-pressure airway ventilators, or using negative pressure body ventilators; see descriptions below) have been used at night in hypercapnic COPD patients to provide "rest" of "fatigued" respiratory muscles. However, this is controversial. Recent evidence suggests that the principal cause of hypercapnia in COPD patients with respiratory failure is weakness, not fatigue. The nocturnal use of mechanical ventilation in these patients, therefore, is actually to support weak respiratory muscles rather than to provide "rest" therapy as previously postulated. Reports on the benefits of nocturnal mechanical ventilation in COPD patients have been unpredictable and inconsistent. They include improvement in daytime blood gases, increased vital capacity, increased respiratory muscle strength and endurance (with increased 12-minute walking distance, functional activities, and quality of life), as well as decreased dyspnea and decreased need for hospitalizations. These potential benefits outweigh the potential adverse effects (e.g., air trapping) of nocturnal mechanical ventilation in COPD patients with any combination of the following: maximal inspiratory force below 50 cm H_2O, FEV_1 less than 25% of predicted normal, $PaCO_2$ over 45 mm Hg, chronic tachypnea (over 30/min), or chest and abdomen dyssynchrony (i.e., paradoxical breathing).

When mechanical ventilation is applied to the body, a positive pressure pushes the diaphragm cephalad to cause expiration, while a negative extrathoracic pressure on the chest wall and abdomen causes inspiration. The opposite occurs when mechanical ventilation is directly applied to the airway, that is, positive airway pressure causes inspiration by pushing air into the lungs, and negative airway pressure causes expiration. The following sections discuss both positive- and negative-pressure mechanical ventilations applied to the body as well as positive-pressure airway mechanical ventilation. Negative-pressure airway mechanical ventilation, which is mainly used for exsufflation in airway clearance, is discussed in section IV.B.1.b.3. Major complications of mechanical ventilation include pulmonary barotrauma (e.g., pneumomediastinum, pneumothorax, and emphysema), pulmonary thromboemboli, gastrointestinal bleeding, dysrhythmias, accumulation of large amounts of secretions, and others (e.g., nosocomial infections, laryngotracheal injury, malnutrition, hypophosphatemia, and oxygen toxicity).

a. **Positive-pressure airway ventilation** can either be intermittent, continuous, or bilevel. In the PM&R setting, the intermittent positive-pressure (airway) ventilation (IPPV) is the most common method used for noninvasive ventilatory support. Occasionally, a continuous positive-pressure mechanical ventilation (i.e., using continuous positive airway pressure [CPAP] may be used to provide a "pneumatic splint" to maintain airway patency in patients with sleep disordered breathing (e.g., obstructive sleep apneas) or to provide positive pressure ventilation for 24 to 48 hours to treat nonintubated patients with rapidly reversible respiratory failure. Noninvasive CPAP can be provided via a tight-fitting CPAP mask. The CPAP is inadequate and poorly tolerated in patients with restricted pulmonary volumes and CAH. Instead, a bilevel positive airway pressure (BiPAP), which is more effective and comfortable, or an IPPV is preferred in treating the sleep disordered breathing in these patients. A BiPAP has independently varying inspiratory positive airway pressures (IPAP) and expiratory positive airway pressures (EPAP). The greater the IPAP/EPAP difference (i.e., span), the greater the inspiratory muscle support. To ensure adequate ventilation, BiPAP spans of at least 20 cm H_2O are often needed. The BiPAP can be applied via a face or nasal mask through a home ventilator unit (e.g., Respironic BiPAP unit).

1) **Types**
   a) **Volume-preset airway ventilators** deliver a preset volume of air with each breath; thus, maintaining constant ventilation by the minute despite changes in compliance or resistance (e.g., due to secretions) of the respiratory system. Volume-preset ventilators are the initial ventilators used in emergency situations (e.g., acute respiratory failure) and are the ventilator of choice for home use in adults. Examples of popular home-care ventilator units used for IPPV include Aequitron LP-6 and LP-10, Lifecare PLV-100 and 102, and Puritan-Bennett Companion 2800 or 2801 and Intermed Bear 33. The manufacturers of ventilators are listed in Appendix G-11. Most home-care airway ventilators are powered by 12-volt, direct current, automotive-type batteries, are portable, and have alarm, monitors, and oxygen-enrichment capability). They are usually prescribed with a battery-powered suction machine, a manual resuscitator, and a back-up ventilator and power generator. For comparative evaluation of home-ventilator units, refer to the latest report of *Health Devices* (e.g., issue 21(8):1-289, 1992) or to the standards published by the American Society of Testing and Materials (ASTM), e.g., ASTM: *Minimum standard specifications for electrically powered home care portable ventilators. Part I: positive pressure ventilators,* Philadelphia, 1991, ASTM, D1246-91.
   b) **Pressure-preset airway ventilators** deliver air until a preset amount of pressure is reached (to prevent excessive airway pressures); thus, the tidal volume varies with airway resistance. They are seldom indicated for home use by adults but may be used by children who have large or variable leak around the tracheostomy tube or who need tidal volumes below 200 ml (because most volume-preset ventilators are not reliable in delivering less than 200 ml of tidal volume). All of the above examples of volume-preset, home-care airway ventilators (except the Intermed Bear 33) have pressure-preset capabilities.

2) **Routes**
   a) **Invasive routes** include intubation and tracheostomy (see section V).
   b) **Noninvasive routes** are usually used for IPPV for elective long-term ventilatory support in patients with CAH. They are generally more convenient and provide good alternatives to invasive IPPV routes. Noninvasive IPPV is also more convenient and often more effective than the noninvasive negative-pressure body ventilators

(NPBVs) (discussed in section IV.A.4.b.3 below) because, in at least 30% of patients, NPBV may cause significant nocturnal oxygen desaturation due to upper airway collapse. Noninvasive IPPV for long-term care can be provided using portable home-care ventilator units with pressure limits (the criteria for prescription of home ventilator units are given in section IV.A.4.a.4.b). An IPPV is contraindicated in patients with pneumothorax, bullous lung disease, asthma, recent esophageal or gastric surgery, cardiac dysfunction, or in an uncooperative patient.

(1) **Nasal IPPV (NIPPV)** is the most popular and practical route for elective long-term nocturnal ventilatory support. It can also be used for elective long-term daytime ventilatory support in patients who cannot use oral IPPV (OIPPV) due to inability to turn the neck and grab the mouthpiece for OIPPV or in patients with no significant ventilator-free time (i.e., the maximum period of time tolerated off ventilator support without resorting to glossopharyngeal breathing [GPB]). A commercially available CPAP mask is generally used for NIPPV because it is simple to use, inexpensive, and durable. However, if the CPAP mask is not comfortable or produces air leaks (especially at NIPPV airflow pressures above 15 cm H_2O), a custom-molded nasal interface may be constructed (e.g., using acrylic materials or using the Lifecare SEFAM Mask assembly kit consisting of silicone putties, elastic straps, and small plastic housings) to increase comfort and decrease insulation leakage.

(2) **Oral IPPV** is ideal for elective long-term daytime ventilatory support and can be as effective as a tracheostomy IPPV. It may also be used for elective long-term nocturnal ventilatory support if NIPPV is inadequate. Because OIPPV is safe, effective, and associated with few complications, it can also be used to convert patients from a tracheostomy to a noninvasive aid and can also be used in weaning a patient from ventilatory support. For daytime OIPPV, a mouthpiece is either kept in the patient's mouth or fixed near the mouth, adjacent to the powered-wheelchair controls (e.g., Sip-and-Puff, tongue, or chin controls; see Chapter 4.7, section III.B.2), so the patient can easily grab it up to 6 to 8 times a minute for full ventilatory support. The commercially available mouthpiece is simple, inexpensive, and permits the patient to use a mouthstick, to eat, and, if the patient can do GPB (see section IV.B.2.a), to talk with a more normal rate, rhythm, and volume. For nocturnal OIPPV, a lip-seal retention flange (or bite-plate retention) is recommended to retain the mouthpiece in the mouth. For additional comfort and relief of orthodontic pressure, a soft, flexible scuba mouthpiece or a custom-molded acrylic mouthpiece may be used. In patients with excessive nasal leakage, cotton pledgets (for plugging the nose) or a nose clip may be used.

(3) **Strapless oral-nasal interface IPPV (SONI-IPPV)** is indicated for the patient who can not use a strap-retained interface or if NIPPV and OIPPV are inadequate or uncomfortable. A SONI consists

of a custom-molded acrylic bite-plate with metal clasps for retention to the teeth. The bite plate is then fixed to an extraoral mask shell, which is connected through a hose to the ventilator. The air-tight extraoral mask may be open to both the nose and mouth, allowing concurrent nasal and mouth IPPV. If not needed, the SONI can be thrusted out by tongue movement alone. Because the bite-plate is crucial to its construction, a SONI cannot be fitted in patients with inadequate or unstable dentition.

3) Modes of assisted ventilation

a) Assist/control ventilation or assisted mechanical ventilation (AMV) allows the patient to trigger a ventilator-delivered breath (at a preset tidal volume) by initiating a minimal inspiratory effort. If the patient's inspiratory effort falls below a preset rate, the ventilator ensures a minimal minute ventilation at a preselected rate and tidal volume. The AMV is the recommended mode for home ventilator units because it allows the patient to interact with the ventilator thus minimizing discomfort and allowing for an increase in minute ventilation in response to changes in physiologic demands. The sensitivity of the patient-triggering mechanism should be set (usually at an inspiratory effort of 2-3 cm) so as to avoid unintentional machine ventilation (which can lead to hyperventilation, hypocapnia, and respiratory alkalosis) but should allow for patient-triggered breaths without excessive effort (or without "fighting the ventilator") especially during sleep to assure adequate support of the ventilatory muscles.

b) Intermittent mandatory ventilation (IMV) delivers a preset rate and tidal volume of air to guarantee a minimum ventilator-delivered minute ventilation, but also allows the patient to breathe spontaneously without triggering the ventilator. It should be tried in patients who are "fighting the ventilator" in the AMV mode or in patients whose cardiac output is reduced during positive pressure ventilation (e.g., because of hypovolemia) because it results in less reduction of cardiac output. It is also useful for treating patients with some capacity for spontaneous breathing (e.g., those with COPD or sleep apnea) because it helps maintain respiratory muscle tone. It can be used for expediting weaning (i.e., by reducing the IMV rate, the patient gradually assumes the bulk of the breathing work). In IMV, the work of breathing as well as oxygen consumption are increased (when compared to AMV), thus making it deleterious to patients with myocardial insufficiency. Moreover, IMV should not be used by patients with depressed respiratory drive or impaired neurologic status. A form of IMV that is synchronized with the patient's spontaneous inspiratory effort is called the **synchronized IMV (SIMV)**. The SIMV prevents the stacking of mandatory breaths on spontaneous breaths. In home ventilator units (unlike the bedside consoles) there is no demand- or continuous-flow of gas, hence IMV/SIMV is not recommended because of the marked increase in breathing workload.

c) Controlled mechanical ventilation (CMV) has a preset tidal volume and rate and does not allow the patient to breathe spontaneously (this can be uncomfortable). It is seldom used except in unconscious and apneic patients.

4) Prescription guidelines

   a) Ventilator setting: Initially a volume-preset ventilator is used with the following parameters: tidal volume of 10 to 15 ml/kg (ideal body weight is preferred); respiratory rate of 12 machine-delivered breaths per minute (depending on the desired $PaCO_2$ or pH; i.e., to decrease $PaCO_2$, the rate should be increased); and an oxygen concentration (FiO_2) of 100% (unless with evidence that lower FiO_2 will provide adequate oxygenation; the goal is to reduce the FiO_2 to a nontoxic level of below 40-50%). The choice for mode of assist is discussed above. The ABGs should be obtained 15 to 30 minutes after initiating mechanical ventilation and periodically thereafter to adjust the ventilator settings. If arterial oxygenation is inadequate (e.g., PaO_2 less than 60 mm Hg; SaO_2 below 90%) despite FiO_2 above 50%, use positive end-expiratory pressure (PEEP) to prevent the closure of edematous small airways. The initial PEEP setting is 5 cm of H_2O, which can be increased by 2 to 5 cm to maintain PaO_2 above 60 mm Hg or SaO_2 above 90%. Subsequent ventilator settings are adjusted so that the lowest FiO_2 is used to maintain of PaO_2 over 60 mm Hg (SaO_2 over 90% in patients with normal pH) and the optimal minute ventilation (tidal volume $\times$ rate) is used to normalize the pH and $PaCO_2$.

   b) Criteria for home ventilation

     (1) Clinical stability, that is, no significant sustained dyspnea or severe dyspnea or tachypnea; acceptable ABG with PaO_2 at least 60 mm Hg using FiO_2 less than or equal to 40%; psychosocial stability; no life-threatening cardiac dysfunction or arrhythmias; no anticipated readmission to hospital for more than 1 month; able to clear secretions; presence of gag or cough reflex; no significant aspiration, and no endotracheal tube (tracheostomy is acceptable for home ventilator).

     (2) Physiological stability, that is, no acute infections; optimal acid-base and metabolic status; other organs are stable; stable time on and off the ventilator; stable lung impedance (i.e., resistance and compliance); and the following ventilator parameters: FiO_2 stable and below 40%, PEEP less than 10 cm H_2O, and IMV not in use.

     (3) Commitment from the patient as well as the caregiver (who must ensure that the ventilator unit as well as the IPPV route are properly adjusted especially during the night).

5) Weaning guidelines

   a) Criteria for ventilator weaning include improved clinical status (i.e., the patient is alert and is hemodynamically stable); adequate oxygenation (PaO_2 over 60 mm Hg on FiO_2 below 40-50%); pH 7.33 to 7.48, with acceptable $PaCO_2$; respiratory rate at or below 25/min (may be at or below 30 for COPD patients); vital capacity at least 10 ml/kg; tidal volume at least 5 ml/kg; resting minute ventilation less than 10 L/min, with ability to double the resting minute ventilation by maximum voluntary effort; maximum inspiratory pressure more negative than -25 cm H_2O; PEEP less than 5 cm H_2O; and spontaneous ventilation via T tube (or other continuous airflow circuit tube, with or without CPAP) for 1 to 4 hours with acceptable blood gases and without marked increases in respiratory rate, heart rate, or change in general status. The above criteria are only guidelines. Some patients (e.g., those with COPD) can be weaned despite failure to meet these criteria.

b) **Ventilator-weaning techniques** involve the progressive withdrawal of ventilator support, that is a progressive increase in ventilator-free time. Various ventilator-weaning protocols have been described, such as those that use or gradually reduce IMV, SIMV, AMV, positive-pressure support ventilation (PSV), CPAP, or PEEP. Following strict protocols (with strict time-schedules), however, may cause unnecessary anxiety in the patient. A simple and effective method that decreases patient anxiety by allowing the patient to follow his or her own weaning schedule is by using the OIPPV, that is, the patient is given access to a mouthpiece so that he or she may take an assisted breath only when needed to prevent dyspnea and to maintain SaO_2 above 90% (e.g., monitored via pulse oximetry). In this method, other modes of ventilator assistance (e.g., IMV, SIMV, PEEP, and PSV) can be turned off, and as the patient becomes more capable of independent ventilation, he or she takes fewer assisted breaths; thus, effectively weaning without an imposed schedule or any complicated protocols.

c) **Criteria for termination of weaning** include a rise or fall in systolic blood pressure of at least 20 mm Hg or a rise or fall in diastolic blood pressure of at least 10 mm Hg; an increase in respiratory rate of at least 10 /min, or a respiratory rate above 30/min; change in pulse rate of at least 20/min, or a pulse rate of at least 120/min or 20% greater than baseline; or when any of the following occur: onset of cardiac arrhythmias, a decrease in tidal volume, an increase in $PaCO_2$, and signs of increased work of breathing such as labored breathing, use of accessory muscles, or fatigue.

d) **Reasons for failure to wean** include excessive airway secretions, incompletely treated pulmonary infection, bronchospasm, depressed cardiac output, respiratory muscle weakness, hypophosphatemia and nutritional deficiency, drug toxicity (e.g., excessive CNS depression from sedatives), significant acid-base disturbances, and hypothyroidism. All these problems are reversible and must be treated before reattempting weaning.

b. **Body ventilation** is another noninvasive technique used for ventilatory support in patients with CAH. It can be administered through either positive- or negative-pressure body ventilators.

1) **Positive-pressure body ventilators** promote expiration by assisting the cephalad movement of the diaphragm through positive pressure on the abdomen. As the pressure is removed and the diaphragm returns to its resting position, passive inspiration occurs (to which the patient can add his or her own tidal volume).

a) **Intermittent abdominal-pressure ventilator (IAPV) (e.g., Pneumobelt, Exsufflation Belt)** consists of a battery-operated rubber air sac contained in an abdominal corset, which can be intermittently inflated to move the diaphragm cephalad, causing a forced expiration. The IAPV may be worn beneath the patient's outer clothing (for better cosmesis), but it must fit snugly over the abdomen from the xiphoid process to just above the pelvic arch. When the IAPV sac is deflated, the abdominal contents and diaphragm fall to the resting position, and inspiration occurs passively (which can be supplemented by active forms of inspiration). The usual IAPV cycle is 40% inspiration and 60% expiration.

The IAPV is the most cosmetic and convenient mode of assisted ventilation in wheelchair bound patients with no significant ventilator-free time (i.e., less than 1 hour). It can be used as an elective long-term noninvasive alternative to ventilatory aids if NIPPV, OIPPV, and SONI-IPPV are inadequate or uncomfortable. Its use is only effective, however, in the daytime because the patient must be in a sitting position (a trunk angle of 75 degrees from horizontal is optimal, although 45 degrees may be adequate in most cases). The patient also should not have significant scoliosis or be extremely obese. The IAPV can deliver from 250 to 500 ml (with reports of up to 1200 ml) of tidal volume and these volumes can be augmented by diaphragm action (when present) as well as by the use of GPB (see section IV.B.2.a). Although the IAPV has been used for daytime support by patients who receive tracheostomy IPPV overnight, its greatest benefit is derived when it is used in conjunction with the noninvasive nocturnal NIPPV or OIPPV. IAPV frees the mouth for mouthstick and other activities and its use may also prevent the development of significant scoliosis.

b) **Rocking bed with head down** (see section IV.A.4.b.2.a).

c) **External oscillation ventilator set at *positive* pressure** (see section IV.A.4.b.2.b).

2) **Negative- and positive-pressure body ventilator**

a) **Rocking bed** tilts the patient through a 15-degree, head-down position to a 30-degree, head-up position at an adjustable rate of 8 to 34 per minute and is usually used in conjunction with other approaches to ventilatory support. When the head of the bed is up, negative pressure is produced to assist inspiration by using gravity to pull the diaphragm caudad; however, when the head is down, positive pressure is produced to assist expiration by the cephalad movement of the abdominal viscera, which pushes the diaphragm cephalad. In patients of relatively normal body weight and with some abdominal girth, the rocking motion of the bed assists in establishing tidal volumes of 250 to 400 ml. It is best for patients who have diaphragm paralysis and some accessory muscle use and who do not have primary pulmonary disease (i.e., those with good pulmonary compliance). The rocking motion produces a more physiologic type of breathing, aids circulation (thus preventing venous stasis and pressure ulcers), and assists in bowel motility and in the clearance of bronchial secretions. It is easy to use without the need for any restricting appliances, and it allows free access to the patient; however, it is one of the least effective ventilatory aids and is heavy, bulky, not portable, and rarely helpful in ventilating patients with poor chest wall or lung compliance.

Although the bed has a break at the knee to prevent sliding, there are reports of patients falling from the bed. Moreover, although movement occurs only in one plane, some patients may complain of motion sickness.

b) **External oscillation ventilator (Hayek Oscillator)** is a new type of ventilator, which consists of a lightweight flexible chest enclosure (cuirass) and an external computerized oscillating ventilator. The oscillating ventilator uses negative and positive pressures to generate a pressure change between the cuirass and the chest wall. The negative pressure causes the chest wall to expand and pulls air into the lungs thus producing inspiration. Positive pressure compresses the chest wall and forces air out to produce expiration. The oscillating ventilator provides full control over the whole respiratory cycle, because both inspiratory and expiratory phases are active and not reliant on passive recoil of the chest. While inspiratory pressure is always negative, expiratory pressure can be made positive, zero (atmospheric), or negative. This means that the ventilation cycle can commence above, at, or below functional residual capacity (FRC). The oscillating ventilator can also be used for secretion clearance by increasing the frequency of the oscillations (up to 999) per minute. It can be used for normal and abnormal lungs (including lungs with poor compliance) and has the same disadvantage as cuirass (see section IV.A.4.b.3.b).

3) **Negative-pressure body ventilators (NPBV)** promote inspiration by creating an intermittent negative-extrathoracic (subatmospheric) pressure in the chest wall and abdomen. These are mainly used for nocturnal ventilatory support (except for the cuirass ventilators, which can also be used in the daytime in a sitting position), because they are not as convenient nor as effective in providing long-term ventilation as the other noninvasive methods (e.g., NIPPV or OIPPV). Most NPBVs are not flexible in that they do not have mechanisms for aborting the development of negative pressure once the unit activates the inspiratory phase, regardless of what the patient desires (thus causing patient discomfort). In general, they are cumbersome and require the assistance of another person to apply or assemble the external device. Patients using NPBV also have difficulty in getting out of bed in the middle of the night or sleeping in any position but supine, are unable to sleep with their significant other, are unable to travel, and frequently complain of being cold during therapy because the negative pressure causes air to be drawn across the patient's chest during inspiration.

The NPBVs are contraindicated in patients with upper airway obstruction because they enhance the development of negative intrathoracic pressure (because the assisted breaths are not initiated by the patient), which increases the frequency and severity of upper airway collapse and obstruction to airflow during sleep (in these patients concurrent CPAP may be required). There are reports that associate NPBV with significant obstructive apneas and oxyhemoglobin desaturations during sleep (thus causing fatigue and other symptoms of ventilatory insufficiency, especially in patients using little or no daytime ventilatory aids) and with recurrent aspiration. The NPBVs should also not be used when there are excessive airway secretions (due to difficulty in the use of mechanical exsufflation or manually assisted airway secretion clearance techniques) or in other cases in which lung compliance or airway resistance is expected to vary extensively throughout the period of assisted ventilation.

a) **Tank or "Drinker" ventilators (e.g., Emerson Iron Lung, Lifecare Porta-lung)** enclose the entire body of the patient (sealed from neck down) in a chamber that produces intermittent subatmospheric pressure by a motor-driven bellow (Iron Lung) or by a separate negative-pressure generator (Porta-lung). They are reliable NPBVs with 100% efficiency and are indicated for the management of patients with acute respiratory failure; for ventilatory support in otherwise hard to ventilate patients with decreased pulmonary compliance or significant scoliosis; and for temporary ventilatory aid in patients with acute upper respiratory tract infections who otherwise use NIPPV or OIPPV (because they free the nose and mouth for clearing secretions). General disadvantages of tank ventilators include difficulty in comfortable fitting of some patients with severe skeletal deformities or with an indwelling tracheostomy; claustrophobic reactions in some patients; and, although patients may be turned while inside the tank, other routine nursing or medical care requires that the patient be pulled out (or the chamber opened) and be given alternative ventilatory supports (preferably OIPPV or GPB). The Iron Lung is heavy (over 300 lb or 136 kg), immobile, requires assistance to enter or exit, and costly; while the Porta-lung also requires assistance to enter or exit but is lighter (about 110 lb or 50 kg) and can be portable.

b) **Cuirass (or chest-shell) ventilators (e.g., Thompson Huxley Shell, Turtle Shell)** consist of an easy-to-don firm shell (which covers the anterior chest and abdomen) and a negative-pressure ventilator unit (which creates the subatmospheric pressure under the shell). They have only 45% efficiency compared to tank ventilators but are adequate for most patients provided that there is no complete respiratory paralysis or impairment of pulmonary compliance, apnea, intrinsic lung disease, severe back deformity, or morbid obesity. The cuirass ventilators are the only NPBV that can also be used for daytime ventilatory support in the seated position (although the IAPV, OIPPV, or NIPPV are invariably preferred). Because of their simplicity and convenience (patient can enter and exit without assistance), the cuirass ventilators are the method of choice for providing temporary ventilatory support when converting a patient from tracheostomy- or intubation-IPPV to OIPPV or NIPPV (e.g., while waiting for the tracheostomy sites to close, which usually takes 2 or more days; or during extubation for patients being converted from IPPV through endotracheal intubation). The customized chest cuirass is better tolerated and provides less air leak than those mass-produced. In insensate patients, the cuirass ventilator may cause pressure ulcers especially at the area anterior to the axilla.

c) **Wrap ventilators (e.g., Poncho; Pneumosuit)** consist of a firm plastic grid or frame (covering the thorax and abdomen) and are covered by a wind-proof wrap made of various materials (e.g., Gortex which is cooler, more flexible, and more comfortable but more expensive than plastic or cloth) in several styles (e.g., Poncho, which covers chest, part of arms, and torso to midhip, or a one-piece Pneumosuit). The wrap is sealed around the patient's wrists, neck, and abdomen or lower limbs depending on the style. As with cuirass ventilators, a negative-pressure ventilator unit is used to create the subatmospheric pressure under the grid and wrap; however, they provide greater volumes and are more efficient than cuirass ventilators. Wrap ventilators have about 60% efficiency compared to tank ventilators when carefully placed and correctly used. They are excellent for patients with difficult fit (e.g., patients with scoliosis but not for markedly obese patients) or with sensory deficits; however they are time-consuming to don, are difficult to access for nursing or medical care of the body, and also make patient turning difficult. As with other NPBVs, they are only used for nocturnal assisted ventilation.

d) Rocking bed with head *up* (see section IV.A.4.b.2.a).

e) External oscillation ventilator set at *negative* pressure (see section IV.A.4.b.2.b).

B. Pulmonary rehabilitation modalities

1. Secretion removal techniques consist of secretion mobilization followed by airway clearance techniques. Their benefits include reduced work of breathing, increased ventilation and gas exchange capabilities, prevention of infection and atelectasis, and improved performance of exercise and ADL.

a. Secretion mobilization techniques usually involve the use of percussion, shaking, or vibration to loosen and mobilize secretions in a patient placed in specific positions for postural drainage. To be effective, they must be followed by airway clearance techniques. An inhaled bronchodilator may be used 10 to 20 minutes prior to secretion mobilization techniques to facilitate secretion movement. The patient should also be adequately hydrated by daily fluid intake. The use of inhaled moisture from a nebulizer or humidifier is mainly beneficial to patients with a tracheostomy due to loss of upper respiratory tract humidification. Secretion mobilization techniques are generally indicated for pulmonary conditions with more than 30 ml of secretions per day (e.g., cystic fibrosis, chronic bronchitis, bronchiectasis, and possibly asthma), aspirations, and atelectasis. Despite wide acceptance, there are no controlled studies that show that they shorten hospital stays, decrease the number of exacerbations, or reduce morbidity or mortality. They do not seem to be beneficial in treating pneumonia or viral bronchiolitis or as a routine postoperative measure. In acutely ill patients, they can cause hypoxemia and oxyhemoglobin desaturation.

1) Postural drainage involves the use of nine distinct gravity-assisted positions to improve the mobilization of secretions from individual lung lobes and segments. In general, the affected lung segment is positioned uppermost for drainage as well as for oxygenation. A commonly used position is the head-down (or Trendelenburg) posture with the patient either supine or prone and in varying degrees of trunk rotation or side-lying. The head-down angle of drainage is usually between 10 and 45 degrees (except when the upper lobes are drained, which is accomplished by having the patient sit up or lie flat). Studies show that COPD patients are able to tolerate up to a 25-degree head-down tilt. Precautions for the head-down position include circulatory problems (e.g., pulmonary edema, congestive heart failure, and hypertension), abdominal problems (e.g., obesity, abdominal distention, hiatal hernia, nausea, and recent food consumption), and dyspnea. For the sidelying position, precautions include axillofemoral bypass graft and musculoskeletal pain (e.g., recent rib fracture) that could be aggravated by the position. In postural drainage, care must be taken to ensure that drainage from the uppermost part of the diseased lung does not spill into and compromise the dependent "good" lung. Postural drainage is best done after awakening in the morning (due to secretion accumulation at night) and 1 to 2 hours after meals (to avoid gastroesophageal reflux).

2) **Percussion (clapping)** is applied throughout the entire respiratory cycle by rhythmically striking the thoracic cage with cupped hands or by using a mechanical percussor to loosen airway secretions from bronchial walls. It is delivered at a frequency of about 5 Hz for 1 to 5 minutes (or longer) over the chest area that is draining. In patients with sensitive skin (e.g., elderly patients), a thin towel may be draped over the percussed zone. Precautions of percussion include circulatory problems (e.g., coagulation disorders, a platelet count below 50,000, and anticoagulation therapy) and musculoskeletal problems (e.g., fractured ribs, flail chest, degenerative bone disease, severe osteoporosis, or other fragile bone disorders). Contraindications include cardiovascular instability or failure, hemoptysis, increased intracranial or intraocular pressure, or aortic aneurysm.

3) **Shaking** is the application of a downward pressure type of bouncing maneuver (at 2 Hz) to a specific area on the thorax (corresponding to the underlying involved lung segment) throughout the expiratory phase of breathing. It is commonly used following percussion. It has the same precautions and contraindications as percussion.

4) **Vibration** is a gentler modification of shaking applied manually to specific areas of the thorax during expiration. A vibrator may also be used with a frequency of 10 to 15 Hz and applied throughout the respiratory cycle. Because vibration uses little or no pressure to the thorax, it may be used when percussion and shaking are contraindicated. The use of expensive vibrating modalities (e.g., vibrating vests, air vibration under chest shells, or high-frequency oscillators) has not been shown to be significantly effective to justify their costs.

b. **Airway clearance techniques** depend on intact mucociliary clearance mechanisms and the generation of optimal peak cough expiratory flow rates (PCEF) of more than 5 to 6 L/sec. The mucociliary clearance mechanisms (i.e., ciliary and alveolar macrophage activities) are incapacitated by intubation and tracheostomy tubes as well as during infections, while PCEF is decreased in patients with pulmonary restrictive disease, ventilator assistance, oropharyngeal muscle weakness, abdominal muscle weakness, or intubation/tracheostomy tube (because of inability to close the glottis to generate expiratory pressures). Although airway suctioning can clear secretions from the upper airways, it does not help clear or mobilize the deeper secretions. Moreover, suction can cause potential complications (see below). Techniques to increase PCEF (i.e., cough maneuvers and their variations) are more effective than airway suctioning. In patients with COPD, the most effective mechanical aid for clearing the airway is the use of mechanical insufflator-exsufflators.

1) **Cough maneuvers** are the most common and easiest means of clearing the larger upper and central airways. They must be controlled to prevent dynamic airway collapse, bronchospasm, syncope, chest wall pain, and dyspnea. The sequence of cough include deep inspiration, glottic closure, thoracoabdominal pressure generation, and glottic opening and expulsion. The glottis closure and the increased intrathoracic pressure can collapse the small airways in some patients with COPD, thus trapping the air behind the closed airway and making the cough ineffective (in these patients, huffing techniques describe below are recommended).

a) **Controlled cough** is a timed, deliberate, coordinated forceful expiration used to mobilize the mucus without causing airway collapse. It is most effective when done in an upright or seated position in patients with a PCEF of at least 5 to 6 L/sec, maximum insufflation capacity (MIC) over 500 ml, and excessive airway secretion production (e.g., more than 30 ml/day). During cough, a transient expiratory air velocity as high as 200 to 250 m/sec can be created in central airways to provide a shearing force to expel mucus that adheres to airway walls. The upright patient inhales deeply, holds the breath for several seconds (to close the glottis), contracts the abdominal muscles (i.e., "bears down" to create an increased intrathoracic pressure of 50 to 200 mm Hg), then opens the glottis and forcefully and rapidly expels the air while contracting the abdominal muscles and leaning slightly forward. The cough is done 2 to 3 times with open mouth without taking another breath. The patient then takes a slow deep inhalation and repeats the whole procedure for 2 to 3 times, then rests and breaths normally for several minutes before repeating the controlled coughing.

b) **Tracheal cough stimulation** is used for patients who are unable to cough on command (e.g., after stroke or head trauma). A quick inward and downward pressure on the trachea (applied by placing the clinician's finger or thumb just above the suprasternal notch) is used to elicit the cough reflex.

c) **Active-assistive cough** is used in patients with ineffective cough (i.e., PCEF of less than 6L/sec) due to weak or paralyzed abdominal muscles (e.g., due to cervical tetraplegia). If the patient's vital capacity is below 1200 to 1500 ml, a deep mechanical insufflation may be provided, followed by active-assistive cough to provide a PCEF of 5 to 7 L/sec. Active-assistive cough may be inadequate during severe upper respiratory tract infections (URIs) or in patients with scoliosis or impaired function of the glottis (i.e., MIC of less than 500 ml). In these patients, the mechanical insufflator-exsuflator (described below) is recommended.

(1) **Manually assisted cough** involves the use of the clinician's (or assisting person's) arm or heel of the hand to apply forces at various sites of the trunk in synchrony with the patient's expiratory or coughing effort. The pressure may be applied at the navel pushing up against the diaphragm while the patient is side-lying (i.e., Heimlich-type assist or abdominal thrust

assist); the costophrenic angles of the rib cage with the patient assuming any position (i.e., costophrenic assist); the upper and lower anterior chest while the patient lies on one side or on three-quarter supine position (i.e., anterior chest compression assist); or in a counterrotational stretch direction of chest expansion applied to the patient's shoulder and pelvis during inspiration followed by reversing the pressure direction to compress the thorax on all planes to facilitate forceful expulsion (i.e., counterrotation assist).

(2) **Self-assisted cough** is more advanced and involves more active participation from the patient. The patient assumes or is physically assisted into one of the following positions: prone-on-elbows, long-sitting, short-sitting (e.g., on bedside), hands-and-knees, or standing. The patient is then taught to extend the head and trunk during maximal inspiration followed by flexion of the head and trunk during cough.

d) **Electrically stimulated cough** has been used for patients with paralyzed or weak abdominal muscles (e.g., SCI above the midthoracic level) by timing the stimulation of the abdominal muscles with expiration; however, this method needs further study.

2) **Huffing** is similar to controlled coughing except that the glottis remains open. The patient inhales deeply and immediately expels the air out by contracting the abdominal muscles and saying, ''Ha, ha, ha.'' Huffing does not increase the intrathoracic pressure (as in coughing), hence the collapsible airway walls (e.g., in COPD patients) are stabilized, thus making expiration and secretion removal more effective in these patients.

a) **Forced expiratory technique (FET)** is a form of huffing used for ''milking'' the secretions from the more peripheral airways that coughing may not affect. The patient is first taught to expand the lower chest (i.e., diaphragmatic breathing, with or without percussion and shaking), then to inhale a normal amount of air (resting tidal volume) followed by abdominal contractions to produce 1 to 2 forced exhalations starting at midlung volume and continuing to a low lung volume. This is followed by expectoration or a controlled cough at high lung volume to clear mucus from the central airways and then by a period of diaphragmatic breathing. The advantages for FET include less fatigue, less likelihood of bronchospasm, and less dynamic airway collapse (because of reduced transpulmonary pressures). The FET can be used in patients with COPD (including cystic fibrosis and asthma).

b) **Positive expiratory pressure (PEP) technique** may be used prior to huffing. The patient exhales down to the functional residual capacity (FRC) through a face mask or a mouthpiece (including a nose clip) with a one-way valve (to which variable expiratory resistance is applied) to achieve a PEP of 10 to 20 cm H_2O (as measured by a pressure manometer in midexhalation), for 5 to 15 breaths. This is followed by a few short, quick huffs and spontaneous cough as needed. The use of PEP can theoretically limit the dynamic expiratory airway closure while also increasing lung volume and directing air distal to and behind airway secretions so that these secretions can be more easily expelled.

3) Mechanical insufflation-exsufflation technique (e.g., Emerson Mechanical In-Exsufflator) is highly effective in removing airway secretions in patients with chronic restrictive pulmonary disease. It provides a deep inspiration (by positive-pressure insufflation) either through a mask or through the tracheal tube (tracheostomy or endotracheal) followed rapidly by a controlled suction (by negative-pressure exsufflation) of secretions into the mouth, mask, or tracheal tube where it can easily be suctioned. The sudden drop of insufflation pressure to exsufflation pressure (usually about 80 cm H_2O) occurs in less than 0.1 second and is sustained for 1.5 to 3 seconds to create a PCEF of 7 to 11 L/sec. The duration of negative-pressure exsufflation is significantly longer than those produced by all other forms of airway clearance. The technique is easy, comfortable, and has no reported complications. Because it effectively clears secretions and mucus plugs, it also increases pulmonary volumes and normalizes SaO_2. It is effective even in patients with severe URIs, scoliosis, impaired function of the glottis, or dysphagia. It also allows earlier ventilator weaning of intubated or tracheostomized patients, as well as continued ventilatory support without a tracheostomy.

4) Suctioning may be done through the mouth or nose but is facilitated by an endotracheal tube (ET) or tracheostomy tube (TT). When suctioning the TT (or ET) in the hospital setting, a sterile technique is mandatory; while for suctioning (of TT) outside the hospital, a clean technique (using clean reusable suction catheters) is usually employed. Suctioning should be done in conjunction with other airway clearance techniques or when the other techniques fail to remove secretions adequately. Suctioning must be done judiciously as it may lead to complications including hypoxemia, brady- or tachycardia, hypo- or hypertension, increased intracranial pressure, atelectasis, tracheal damage, and nosocomial infections. Suctioning can also irritate the airway membranes and exacerbate secretion problems as well as cause airway edema and wheezing.

2. Controlled-breathing techniques (CBTs) are generally used to improve PFT parameters, reduce dyspnea, reduce the work of breathing, and improve ventilatory muscle function. These techniques also facilitate relaxation (see Chapter 4.2, section VI) and are indicated in patients with obstructive or restrictive pulmonary problems. Patients are usually instructed to inspire nasally (to ensure a slow, even inspiration, and prevent mouth drying) and to exhale orally (to provide the least resistance to air flow). The CBT can be classified by the intended specific goals as follows:

a. A CBT to improve PFT parameters, i.e., to increase lung volume, redistribute ventilation, maintain or restore FRC, and improve gas exchange.

1) Diaphragmatic breathing involves retraining the patient to use the diaphragm while relaxing abdominal muscles during inspiration (i.e., the abdomen rises while the chest wall remains stationary). It is first taught to the patient in a semi-Fowler's (semireclined sitting) position, then progressed to sitting, standing, walking, stair climbing, and other activities. Theoretically, the use of the diaphragm (the principal and most efficient muscle of inspiration) can make breathing more efficient with decreased oxygen cost; however, clinical studies remain unclear on the long-term and short-term physiological benefits of diaphragmatic breathing. The possibility of a placebo effect has not been completely ruled out. Diaphragmatic breathing may be used in conjunction with a **biofeedback** machine to help confirm diaphragmatic use and to inhibit the use of accessory muscles. Its use with other relaxation techniques are described in Chapter 4.2, section VI.A.

2) **Segmental breathing** is aimed at hypoventilated segments of the lungs in patients with pleuritic pain and splinting (e.g., because of surgery or trauma) as well as segmental atelectasis. Prior to segmental breathing, any airway obstruction must be cleared (e.g., mucus plugs must be removed by secretion removal techniques described above; bronchogenic tumors must be resected). The patient is asked to inspire against the resistance of the clinician's hand(s) placed at the thorax over the area of hypoventilation. As the clinician feels the local expansion of the thorax, the hand resistance is released to allow full inhalation.

3) **Sustained maximal inspiration (or incentive spirometer technique)** involves slow inspiration through the nose or pursed lips. When maximal inspiration is reached, it is held for 3 seconds before passively exhaling the volume. It is used in acute situations for patients with posttraumatic pain, postoperative pain, or acute lobar collapse. An incentive spirometer may be used to provide visual feedback of the volume of inspired air.

4) **Glossopharyngeal breathing (GPB) or frog breathing,** which can technically be considered an IPPV, is a technique used by patients with chronic restrictive pulmonary disease in which the patient takes a deep (maximum) breath, and then uses the pistoning action of the tongue and pharyngeal muscle to project boluses of air past the glottis into the lungs. The lips, soft palate, and vocal cords open and close in rhythm during each pistoning stroke. In one breath, the patient usually performs 6 to 8 (or up to 65) boluses or gulps, with each gulp consisting of 30 to 150 (usually 60-100) ml of air. For GPB to be effective, the patient must have intact oropharyngeal muscle strength and should not be tracheostomized (even if the tracheostomy tube is plugged, gulped air can still leak around the tube and out of the tracheostomy site). Glossopharyngeal breathing enables the patient (even those with little or no vital capacity) to breathe without mechanical ventilation (up to 4 or more hours if the lungs are normal; otherwise, GPB may only be tolerated for minutes). This ventilator-free time is important when switching between different types of noninvasive aids and for security in case of ventilator failure. The GPB can also improve the volume of the voice (some patients may be able to shout for help), improve the flow and rhythm of speech, provide the deep breath needed for an effective assisted cough, help prevent microatelectasis, and improve or maintain pulmonary compliance. If during GPB, the SaO_2 falls to 85 to 90% or less, the patient typically complains of fatigue and requires mechanical ventilatory assistance.

b. **Controlled-breathing techniques to reduce dyspnea and the work of breathing**
   1) **Pursed lip breathing (PLB)** is used to reduce dyspnea and the work of breathing in patients with chronic airflow obstruction (e.g., COPD) by preventing air trapping caused by the collapse of small airways. The patient inhales through the nose for several seconds with the mouth closed, then exhales slowly for 4 to 6 seconds through pursed

lips (i.e., a whistling or kissing position). During PLB, there should be no expiratory airflow through the nose and the patient usually bends forward slightly. The abdominal muscles are usually relaxed but may be contracted judiciously to increase the exhaled volume (making sure not to increase intrathoracic pressure as this might produce airway collapse). To prolong the expiration phase, the clinician may apply gentle pressure on the patient's abdomen. Pursed lip breathing, together with diaphragmatic breathing, is used during and following an exercise or activity that can induce tachypnea leading to dyspnea. Additional effects of PLB include reduced respiratory rate, increased tidal volume, maintenance of minute ventilation while decreasing the work of breathing, improved gas mixing at rest, and facilitation of relaxation.

2) **Paced breathing** is a process in which the patient breaks down an activity (that might otherwise be unattainable because of dyspnea) into small attainable tasks, then uses PLB and rest periods to complete each task at a comfortable tempo until the whole activity is completed without dyspnea and fatigue. For example, to climb one flight of stairs, the patient inhales at rest, then on exhalation (using PLB) the patient ascends one or two steps at a time and stops to rest until full recovery. The patient repeats this process until the whole flight is ascended without dyspnea.

c. **Controlled breathing technique to improve ventilatory muscle functions** (i.e., to increase the strength, endurance, and efficiency of ventilatory muscles). The strength and endurance of the ventilatory skeletal muscles can be improved by general aerobic exercise alone as well as by using controlled breathing for ventilatory muscle training. Recent studies have shown that the exercise-induced improvement in ventilatory muscle function appears to be mode-specific, that is, endurance training improves the ability to increase sustained hyperpnea, whereas pure strength training improves inspiratory pressures. There is currently, however, no definitive data on the long-term benefits of ventilatory muscle training, the effect on functional activities, or criteria for patient selection or which ventilatory muscle training protocol to use.

1) **Inspiratory resistive loading** can be attained by using an inspiratory muscle trainer (IMT), which loads the inspiratory muscles by having the patient inhale through inspiratory orifices of progressively decreasing diameter (and to exhale without resistance). The initial aperture opening is determined by using 30 to 40% of the maximum inspiratory pressure (MIP) or by selecting the smallest aperture the patient can tolerate for a 10-minute exercise period. The training is done at a rate of 10 to 20 breaths/minute for 15 to 30 minutes, 1 to 2 times per day. After attaining a duration of 30 minutes, the exercise intensity is progressed by narrowing the aperture. For endurance training, use either a lower percent of MIP or the aperture opening that would allow a longer exercise duration. The IMTs are indicated in stable patients with chronic restrictive pulmonary disease (i.e., with decreased compliance, decreased intrathoracic volume, or decreased strength of the respiratory muscle caused by long-term ventilatory support) and COPD (i.e., with resistance to airflow or alteration in length-tension relationship of ventilatory muscles in a barrel chest).

The use of IMTs has been shown to improve strength, endurance, and functional capacity (i.e., ability to do ADLs).

2) **Inspiratory threshold loading** can be attained by using a threshold loading device that permits inspiration only after reaching a threshold mouth pressure (set by means of a weighted plunger or by adjusting the tension of a spring-loaded valve). Unlike IMTs, the threshold loading device produces inspiratory resistance without relying on inspiratory flow rates. Inspiratory threshold loading improves ventilatory strength and endurance but not functional capacity.

3) **Voluntary isocapnic hyperpnea** uses prolonged periods of hyperpnea to provide low tension and a high level of repetitive activity for the diaphragm and other inspiratory muscles, thus leading to improved endurance. The patient is asked to maintain as high a level of minute ventilation as possible (breathing frequency is usually between 30 and 60 breaths per minute) for periods of 10 to 15 minutes usually twice daily. Voluntary isocapnic hyperpnea has been shown to improve endurance but not functional capacity.

3. **Abdominal muscle exercise and support**
   a. **Abdominal strengthening exercises** may be performed to help improve airway clearance (e.g., by increasing coughing force). These include partial sit-up exercises and possibly the use of neuromuscular electrical stimulation in innervated muscles (see Chapter 4.1, section V.B.3).
   b. **Abdominal binders** may be used to enhance the expiratory phase of breathing in patients with weak abdominal muscles (e.g., high thoracic and cervical spinal cord injuries). They must not be too tight, however, to restrict inspiration. In COPD patients, abdominal binders should not be used as they impede breathing.

4. **Postural relief techniques** involve the use of appropriate positioning to reduce dyspnea by optimizing aeration, improving perfusion, and/or maximizing ventilation-perfusion ratios. Patients with COPD frequently lean forward at the waist (about 20-45 degrees from the vertical) and bear weight on the elbows for support with the arms and shoulders (usually elevated) in a locked position. If seated, the patient supports himself or herself by bracing the elbows or hands on the knees or on a table. When ambulating, a rolling walker or bilateral canes may be used to allow forward leaning. The forward-leaning position has been shown to decrease dyspnea and to increase exercise tolerance. The physiologic basis for dyspnea relief in the forward-leaning posture is probably due to the improved length-tension status of the diaphragm thus making it more efficient. In some COPD patients with low, flat, and overly shortened diaphragms, the head down (Trendelenberg) position at 10- to 20-degrees tilt may facilitate diaphragm movement thus decreasing dyspnea. In general, a flat, supine position is poorly tolerated by most pulmonary patients.

5. **General reconditioning exercises** are used to improve functional capacity. If possible, a graded-exercise tolerance test (see Chapter 2.7, section II.A), a PFT (see Chapter 2.6), and an ABG should be done prior to starting the exercise program. A 10% decrease in FEV_1 or $FEF_{25\%-75\%}$ indicates the need for preexercise bronchodilator therapy. Supplemental oxygen (see section IV.A.3) is needed if there is a decrease in PaO_2 of more than 20 mm Hg or if the PaO_2 is less than 55 mm Hg during exercise. All exercises must emphasize proper breathing techniques, proper body mechanics, and

must include adequate warm-up and cool-down periods. In patients with neuromuscular diseases, exercises should not be done to the point of fatigue. All patients must be given an appropriate home exercise program and instructed to keep a log of their exercise. Patients must be followed at a regular interval to ensure that they are doing the exercises properly and with appropriate progression. Patients must maintain a regular exercise regime, or they will lose any gains made from the exercise.

  a) Aerobic (cardiopulmonary) endurance exercises are described in Chapter 4.2, section III.A. Parameters obtained from the graded-exercise tolerance test are used to determine the mode, intensity, duration, and frequency of exercise. The prescribed aerobic exercises are low-to-moderate impact and may include walking (e.g., treadmill), stair climbing, calisthenics, stationary bicycle, arm ergometry, and pool activities.

  b) Range of motion (ROM) exercises are described in Chapter 4.2, section I. The use of ROM exercises of the upper limbs can be synchronized with diaphragmatic breathing for lung expansion (e.g., shoulder elevation on inspiration).

  c) Strengthening exercises (see Chapter 4.2, section II) are directed to limb muscle weakness (commonly seen in patients with chronic pulmonary problems). For the upper limbs, strengthening exercises are usually done with free weights.

 6. Relaxation techniques (see Chapter 4.2, section VI)

 7. Energy-conservation techniques can lower the energy expenditure and the oxygen consumption of an activity, thus allowing patients with pulmonary problems to perform essential ADLs (without dyspnea or fatigue) independently or with the least amount of assistance. Energy conservation techniques involve the use of assistive and adaptive devices (see Chapter 4.5, section I.B.3), activity planning and preparation (i.e., scheduling, organizing, and prioritizing of tasks or choosing the ''best breathing'' time), pacing (see section IV.B.2.b.2), efficient breathing techniques (see section IV.B.2 on breathing exercises for relaxation and reduction of the work of breathing). Specific energy conservation and work simplification techniques used in pulmonary rehabilitation are described by Rashbaum and Whyte (see bibliography).

 8. Psychological, social, and vocational measures may need to be recommended for appropriate patients to help them cope with their chronic pulmonary problems.

V. Invasive management is used only if noninvasive methods fails or are inadequate.

 A. Tracheal intubation can be attained by either using an ET or TT. The indication for tracheal intubation or tracheostomy is acute respiratory failure (PaO_2 below 55 mm Hg or $PaCO_2$ above 50 mm Hg) due to acute pulmonary disease, intrinsic lung disease, or obstructive or restrictive respiratory disease that necessitate

 • Supplemental oxygen for which noninvasive mechanical ventilation is inadequate or not possible because of poor access to oral or nasal routes (e.g., facial fractures, osteogenesis imperfecta, inadequate bite for mouthpiece entry, or presence of nasogastric tube; or upper airway obstruction) or due to other reasons (e.g., mental incompetence, obtundation, uncooperativeness, substance abuse, heavy sedative or narcotic use, uncontrollable seizures, or oropharyngeal muscle weakness)

 • Ongoing aggressive management of respiratory tract secretions (e.g., due to PCEF less than 3 L/sec or an MIC of less than 500 ml) for which a mechanical exsufflation device may be contraindicated or unavailable, and there is unreliable access to effective assisted coughing.

In the PM&R setting, most patients with CAH who require 24-hour/day ventilatory support do not need nor desire tracheal intubation (using ET or TT) because of the availability of effective, safer, more comfortable, and cheaper noninvasive mechanical ventilation methods (see section IV.A.4.a.2.b). Irrespective of the extent of the ventilatory failure, a tracheostomized (or intubated) patient receiving pulmonary rehabilitation should, as soon as medically indicated, be weaned off the TT (or ET) and, if needed, be considered for noninvasive mechanical ventilation.

The guidelines for ventilator setting and ventilator weaning of intubated or tracheostomized patients is the same as those used for patients on noninvasive mechanical ventilation (see sections IV.A.4.a.4.a and IV.A.4.a.5). Suctioning is described in section IV.B.1.b.5. In intubated or tracheostomized patients, cuff care is important to avoid tracheal ischemia. A high-volume, low-pressure cuff should be used to seal the airway with minimal pressure against the tracheal wall, that is, cuff pressure maintained below capillary filling pressure (below 25 mm Hg) as monitored every 8 hours with a manometer (e.g., a sphygmomanometer may be used with an adaptor). The use of periodic cuff deflation is not recommended as it is inadequate in reducing tracheal trauma.

1. **Endotracheal tube** is usually applied in an emergency setting via the direct laryngoscopic technique for orotracheal placement. The preferred ET size is no. 8 (i.e., with 8-mm lumen) or larger to reduce airway resistance and the work of breathing in acute respiratory failure as well as to facilitate suctioning. The ET may be extubated if the patient can tolerate unassisted spontaneous breathing for 30 to 90 minutes, for example, through a T tube or other continuous airflow circuit tube. Prolonged T tube breathing may cause fatigue, especially if the ET size is small.

2. **Tracheostomy tube** should be considered if the ET cannot be successfully extubated after 2 weeks (or earlier than 2 weeks if a prolonged intubation period is anticipated). If weaning from mechanical ventilation is imminent, however, TT may be postponed safely for up to 4 weeks. To use a TT, a tracheostomy must first be created via a tracheotomy (i.e., a surgical incision in the trachea). A new tracheostomy site usually takes at least 72 hours to mature. If the TT is dislodged during this period, the TT should not be reinserted blindly as this may lead to malposition of the TT in the pretracheal space or elsewhere outside the trachea. The responsible surgical service should, therefore, be consulted; however, if the TT is dislodged after the initial 72-hour period (i.e., when the tracheostomy site has most likely matured into a well-formed track from the skin to the trachea), the TT can easily be reinserted and, if needed, position confirmed through radiograph.

The early major complications of a tracheostomy include mediastinal or subcutaneous emphysema, postoperative bleeding, pneumomediastinum, pneumothorax, tube displacement, and aspiration, while the late major complications include nosocomial pneumonia, tracheal stenosis, tracheoinnominate fistula (i.e., between trachea and innominate artery), tracheomalacia (i.e., erosion or thinning of the tracheal wall), tracheoesophageal fistula, swallowing dysfunction (see Chapter 5.6, section VI.A for management of dysphagia in tracheostomized patients), and stomal infection. Tracheomalacia is highly suspected if the ratio of cuff size to tracheal size (C/T ratio) is more than 1.5. The C/T ratio (determined by radiogram) should ideally be less than or equal to 1. If the C/T ratio is above 1.5, the cuff should be inflated at a different site, that is, by using a TT with a different length (e.g., Portex extra-long TT) or by inflating the second cuff of a double-cuffed TT or using an ET and cutting it to a different length.

All TTs contain an outer cannula (or main shaft) and a neckplate (or neck flange), which rests on the neck between the clavicles. The neckplate contains small holes on the outer edge, which are used to secure tracheostomy ties. Unlike the ET, the tip of the TT is not beveled but is straight cut to maximize air flow and prevent occlusion of the tip by the tracheal wall. Most adult TTs contain an inner cannula, although some do not (e.g., Bivona Fome-cuff and some other Portex tubes). The inner cannula can be removed from the outer cannula (e.g., every 8 hours) for cleaning of crusted secretions that may occlude the airway (e.g., in patients who are not suctioned frequently); while the outer cannula is left in place (to keep the tracheostomy stoma open) and can be changed every 6 weeks or more frequently. The outer cannula on most tubes or the inner cannula in some tubes has a 15-mm adapter for direct connection to the ventilator unit or manual resuscitator (e.g., AMBU bag). Because the TT completely bypasses the upper airway, the inspired air must be warmed and humidified. The more effective water-reservoir-type humidifier (e.g., Bennett Cascade Humidifier) is preferred by patients with increased secretions over the heat-and-moisture exchange-type humidifier (e.g., Artificial Nose); however, the Artificial Nose is more portable.

a. **Size.** The length of a TT is usually 2 to 6 inches (5-15 cm), with the exception of the Portex TT, which is available in extra-long size. In general, the shorter the tube, the smaller the internal diameter (ID) unless the TT is customized by using an ET, which can be cut into any desired length. The ID of the TT ranges from 5 to 11 mm; while the outer diameter (OD) ranges from 7 to 15.3 mm. In most tubes, the ID is about 3 mm smaller than the OD. The ID size (usually printed on the TT neck flange) determines the TT size. The TT size for Jackson metal TT and Shiley double-cannula TT uses the Jackson equivalent number, that is, a #6 tube is equal to a 7.0 mm ID. This can be confusing, hence the ID size should be used instead of the TT size. If the TT size is used, it can be converted to OD size (in mm) by adding 4. The OD (in mm) size can then be multiplied by 3 to obtain the French size.

b. **Types**
  1) **Metal versus plastic TT**
      a) **Metal TTs** (e.g., Jackson, Hollinger) are cuffless, reusable tubes made of durable stainless steel or silver. Although a latex cuff can be placed, it is not recommended as it may slip. Compared to plastic TTs, metal TTs cause less local tissue reaction, may be left in place for longer periods, and may be less costly in prolonged use than most plastic tubes. They are used to keep the tracheostomy stoma patent in spontaneously breathing patients until the tracheostomy is no longer needed.
      b) **Plastic TTs** (e.g., Shiley, Portex, Bivona) are disposable tubes most of which are made of polyvinyl chloride (PVC), whereas some are made of nylon, silicone, or Teflon. The rigidity of the PVC

ranges from hard to soft, and it is available in either single or double cannulae, with or without a cuff.

2) Cuff-inflated versus uncuffed TT

a) Cuff-inflated TTs are used to provide an adequate seal to protect the lower airway from aspiration (e.g., patients who are unconscious or when eating or drinking especially in patients with dysphagia) and to ensure adequate ventilation to the lungs and prevent air leaking upward through the upper airway (e.g., when using CPAP or in patients with poor laryngeal control). Cuff inflation does not guarantee complete safety from aspiration (see discussion in Chapter 5.6, section III.C.1.a.2.b), and it does not allow the patient to speak. Most modern cuff-inflated TTs have high-volume/low-pressure balloon cuffs (see section V.A for monitoring guidelines) which evenly distribute the intracuff pressure on the tracheal mucosa, thus minimizing the complications of tracheal lesions. The lowest volume and pressure required for maintaining adequate cuff seal is used. The Bivona Fome-cuff TT uses self-inflating foam (instead of a balloon), which does not require cuff pressure monitoring; however, it may not seal well (e.g., in patients using PEEP) and may require more frequent tube changes.

b) Uncuffed TTs allow some patients to talk while receiving mechanical ventilation; however, to assure adequate ventilation, the exhaled tidal volume and ABGs should be checked regularly. It may be used right after a tracheostomy when there is loose fit of the TT on the stoma (thus allowing considerable leakage) or to prevent subcutaneous emphysema. An uncuffed TT should not be used in patients known to aspirate.

3) Fenestrated versus nonfenestrated TT

a) Fenestrated TTs have a straw-sized hole cut into the outer cannula of a cuffed or cuffless TT (e.g., Portex or Shiley cuffed TT with precut fenestration), thus allowing increased flow to the upper airway so the patient can speak (as well as breath and cough) while the TT is uncuffed, the inner cannula is removed, and the TT plugged and disconnected from the mechanical ventilation. If the patient needs mechanical ventilation, the inner cannula (which has no fenestration) is reinserted to occlude the fenestration of the outer cannula. The fenestrations should lie within the lumen of the trachea (this can be checked by direct vision with a flashlight) and should not touch the tracheal wall (otherwise granulation tissue can form into and around the holes, thus causing obstruction or bleeding, i.e., when the TT is pulled out). The fenestrated TT should only be used if the patient can breath spontaneously for 2 hours or more without the need of mechanical ventilation and be able to swallow without aspiration when the TT is uncuffed (aspiration can be evaluated by doing a swallowing test using a blue food coloring as described in Chapter 5.6, section III.C.1.a.2). It also allows the patient to breath through the mouth.

b) Nonfenestrated TTs are used if the patient needs continuous mechanical ventilation (i.e., is unable to have more than 2 hours of ventilator-free time) or is unable to protect the airway when swallowing. If the patient wants to talk, a one-way talking valve (e.g., Passy-Muir Speaking Valve; see next section) may be used or the TT size can be decreased or its cuff deflated to allow air leakage.

4) **Talking tubes versus speaking valves.** Both specialized tubes allow patient to speak. As discussed above, other nonspecialized tubes may be used for speaking by allowing air leakage into the larynx (e.g., un-cuffed tubes, cuff-deflated fenestrated or unfenestrated tubes, or use of smaller TT size). The use of tracheal buttons or plugs (see below) may also divert air to the larynx for speaking. For nonspeaking communication options, see Chapter 5.5, section IV.B.2.

a) **Talking tracheostomy tubes (pneumatic speaking tubes)** are indicated for alert and motivated patients who need an inflated cuff for ventilation and who have intact vocal cord and the ability to mouth words. They are specialized TTs capable of supplying pressurized gas mixtures (at a flow rate of 1.5-10 L/min) through a cannula that travels through the wall of the talking tube then enters the trachea through small holes above the inflated tube cuff so the patient can use the larynx to speak while the cuff is inflated (thus leaving mechanical ventilation undisturbed). The quality of speech is altered (e.g., lower pitch, coarser, or whisper-like) and patients need to speak in short sentences (because constant flow through the vocal cords can cause the voice to fade away). Also, the patient needs a fair amount of manual dexterity and minimal strength to occlude the external port to initiate flow of gas through the vocal cord. Talking TTs should not be used within the first 5 to 7 days after tracheostomy because the pressurized gas may flow retrograde through the tracheostoma around the tube and cause subcutaneous emphysema. Talking TTs may not work if there are secretions or granulation tissue above the cuff, which may occlude the exit port for the gas. They are available as single-lumen cannula cuffed tubes (e.g., Portex ''Talk'' tube, Bivona Fome-cuff with sideport airway connector), which are easier for the patient to learn to use and less likely to get occluded or as a double-lumen cannula cuffed tube (e.g., Communi-trach; Pitt Trach Speaking Tube).

b) **One-way speaking valves** (e.g., Passy-Muir Speaking Valve [PMSV], Olympic Trach-talk) are made of plastic and can be fitted on any TT with a 15-mm adapter. The valve opens on inspiration, bypassing upper airway pathology, thus making it easier to in-spire; then on expiration, the valve closes and forces the air through the vocal cords, thus allowing vocalization (as well as helping to blow out any food residue in the trachea; see Chapter 5.6, section VI.A). They are used either in mechanically ventilated patients (with the cuff deflated) or in those who spontaneously breathe and are receiving nonmechanical forms but cannot tolerate tracheal plugs or buttons. The PMSV is most frequently used because of its simple-to-use one-piece design. In contrast, the multipiece Olympic Trach-talk has a spring loaded one-way valve attached to a T piece. Speaking valves should only be used when the patient is awake and medically stable, able to manage his or her secretions effectively and not aspirate, has no severe tracheal or laryngeal stenosis, and is able to tolerate cuff deflation.

5) Tracheal buttons versus plugs. Both are used to keep the tracheostomy stoma patent during tracheostomy weaning when there is some doubt about the success of the weaning (i.e., in case suction is needed or the patient needs to be reattached to the ventilator) or when a planned surgical procedure may require tracheostomy and mechanical ventilation. It can also be used to allow the patient to speak (but unlike speaking valves, it does not allow inspiration). There are other reasons for placement of these tubes, such as easy access for suctioning the lower airway, sleep apnea (leaving the plug open during sleep), vocal cord paralysis, and in neurologic disorders, such as myasthenia gravis.

  a) Tracheal buttons extend only to the inner surface of the anterior tracheal wall without encroaching on the lumen (and, therefore, do not cause tracheal lumen obstruction). To ensure that the tip does not extend into the trachea, spacers or rings are inserted on the outside of the button. The Olympic button is made of rigid plastic (Teflon), while the Kistner button is made of flexible plastic. Proper size must be used, because if the button is too short the tracheostomy tract may granulate and occlude ventilation; if too long, the button may occlude the trachea (thus limiting ventilation and removal of secretions); and if the button diameter is too small, it can be dislodged at night, thus inadvertently allowing the stoma to shrink.

  b) Tracheal plugs or decannulation cannulas are specially fitted short, closed-lumen cannula, inserted into the outer cannula for plugging. They can easily be removed for suctioning or for reconnection to the mechanical ventilator.

c. Guidelines for TT decannulation. In general, TT decannulation or removal is considered when the patient no longer needs mechanical ventilation (see section IV.A.4.a.5 for ventilator-weaning guidelines) and can adequately clear secretions from the airway. A cuffed TT is weaned to a cuffless TT by gradual cuff deflation. The patient should not have an increased propensity for pneumonia or aspiration (aspiration may be checked by a blue-food coloring test; see Chapter 5.6, section III.C.1.a.2), should be adequately ventilated with the cuff deflated, and should be able to cough secretions out of the TT. The cuffless TT is then downsized to the next smaller size and checked for the above parameters. Once the TT is downsized to about 8 mm outer diameter (e.g., Shiley or Portex #4) and the patient does not need excessive suctioning, then the TT can be discontinued or a tracheal button or plug may be used temporarily (see section V.A.2.b.5).

After decannulation, the tracheostomy stoma is covered with a dry dressing or a dressing with petrolatum-impregnated gauze (Vaseline or Xeroform gauze) taped in place. The patient's voice may be raspy or gravelly for several days until the stoma closes completely and spontaneously. During this time the stoma is assessed and cleaned and its dressing changed at least daily. Occassionally, the tracheostomy stoma does not heal and may require plastic surgery.

B. Diaphragmatic pacing (electrophrenic nerve pacing) is a highly sophisticated form of portable mechanical ventilation, which leaves the patient's face free for ADLs. It is indicated in patients who have central damage to the respiratory control centers or their pathways (in the brainstem and spinal cord); at least partially intact C3-C5 anterior horn cells, phrenic nerve, and diaphragm; and who are unable to use an OIPPV. Some of the common cases that can benefit from diaphragmatic pacing include idiopathic central hypoventilation syndrome (CHS) or Ondine's curse; acquired CHS; and high spinal cord injury (i.e., C1-C2). The diaphragmatic pacemaker, which can be implanted by a simple operation (with brief hospitalization), consists of an electrode (implanted cervically onto phrenic nerve fibers) and radio receivers (implanted on the anterior chest wall).

An external radio transmitter (whose batteries last up to 2-3 weeks) produces impulses, which are delivered via the external antenna loop taped to the skin over the implanted receiver site. The radio transmitter may be accessed via a telephone for remote assessment of stimulation effectiveness and diagnosis of technical problems. Simultaneous bilateral diaphragmatic pacing is more effective and is preferred. In some adults, unilateral pacing may be used, however it can lead to paradoxical diaphragm movement which results in marginal ventilation. Potential complications of diaphragmatic pacing include infection, sudden operational failure, and the need to retain a tracheostomy because of obstructive sleep apnea. Diaphragmatic pacing is relatively new and costly. Recent advances in technology have increased its reliability, and it has been used successfully by some patients for over 10 years.

C. **Other surgical treatments** include intercostal nerve-to-phrenic nerve anastomosis with implantation of a pacing electrode for the recently denervated diaphragm; bilateral carotid body resection (BCBR) for the relief of severe dyspnea; and lung-heart transplant for end-stage lung disease of various causes.

BIBLIOGRAPHY

Alba, AS: Concepts in pulmonary rehabilitation. In Braddom RL, editor: *Physical medicine and rehabilitation,* Philadelphia, 1996, WB Saunders, pp 671-685.

Bach JR: Pulmonary rehabilitation in neuromuscular disorders, *Seminars Resp Med* 14 (6):515-529, 1993.

Bach JR: Rehabilitation of the patient with respiratory dysfunction. In De Lisa JA, Gans BM, editors: *Rehabilitation medicine: principles and practice,* ed 2, Philadelphia, 1993, JB Lippincott, pp 952-972.

Bach JR, Alba AS, Garrison SJ: Pulmonary rehabilitation, *Arch Phys Med Rehabil* 71(suppl 4):s238-s243, 1990.

Brannon FJ, Foley MW, Starr JA, et al: *Cardiopulmonary rehabilitation: basic theory and application,* ed 2, Philadelphia, 1993, FA Davis.

Casaburi R: Principles of exercise training, *Chest* 101 (Suppl 5):263S–267S, 1992.

Casaburi R, Petty TL: *Principles and practice in pulmonary rehabilitation,* Philadelphia, 1993, WB Saunders.

Dettenmeier PA: *Pulmonary nursing care,* St. Louis, 1991, Mosby–Year Book.

Fishman AP, editor: *Pulmonary rehabilitation,* New York, 1996, Marcel Dekker.

Haas F, Axen K, editors: *Pulmonary therapy and rehabilitation. Principles and practice,* ed 2, Baltimore, 1991, Williams & Wilkins.

Hodgkin J, Connors GL, Bell CW, editors: *Pulmonary rehabilitation: guidelines to success,* ed 2, Philadelphia, 1993, JB Lippincott.

Hodgkin J, Farrell M, Gibson S, et al: Pulmonary rehabilitation: official American Thoracic Society statement, *Am Rev Respir Dis* 124:663-666, 1981.

Howder CL: *Cardiopulmonary pharmacology: a handbook for cardiopulmonary practitioners and other allied health personnel,* Baltimore, 1996, Williams & Wilkins.

Levenson C: Breathing exercises. In Zadai C, editor: *Clinics in physical therapy: pulmonary management in physical therapy,* New York, 1992, Churchill Livingstone.

Massery M: Manual breathing and coughing aids, *Phys Med Rehabil Clin North Am* 7(2):407-422, 1996.

O'Donohue WJ, Jr, editor: *Long-term oxygen therapy: scientific basis and clinical application,* New York, 1995, Marcel Dekker.

O'Donohue WJ, Giovannoni RM, Goldberg AF, et al: Long-term mechanical ventilation: guidelines for management in the home and alternate community site, *Chest* 90 (suppl):1S–37S, 1986.

Rashbaum I, Whyte N: Occupational therapy in pulmonary rehabilitation: energy conservation and work simplification techniques, *Phys Med Rehabil Clin North Am* 7(2):325-340, 1996.

Rogers RM, Donahoe M: Nutrition in pulmonary rehabilitation. In Fishman AP, editor: *Pulmonary rehabilitation,* New York, 1996, Marcel Dekker, pp 543-564.

Wilson DJ, Shepherd KE: Modern airway appliances and their long-term complications. In Roberts JT, editor: *Clinical management of the airway,* Philadelphia, 1994, WB Saunders.

Supplemental References

Eckert RC, Bartsch K, Dowell D, et al: *Being close,* Denver, 1984, National Jewish Hospital/National Asthma Center.

Hossler CJ, Cole SS: *Intimacy and chronic lung disease,* Ann Arbor, 1983, University of Michigan.

Kravetz HM: *A visit with Harry* (slide-tape program), Prescott AZ, 1982, HM Kravetz.

Kravetz HM: *A visit with Helen* (slide-tape program), Prescott AZ, 1982, HM Kravetz.

Kravetz HM, Weiss M, Meadows R: *Sexual counseling for the male pulmonary patient* (slide-tape program), Prescott AZ, 1980, HM Kravetz.

Selecky PA: *Sexuality and chronic breathing problems,* Santa Ana, CA, 1989, American Lung Association of Orange County.

CHAPTER 5.13

CARDIAC PROBLEMS

This chapter gives an overview of cardiac rehabilitation in patients with medical cardiac diagnoses (e.g., post–myocardial infarction, chronic stable angina, compensated congestive heart failure, increased risk for coronary heart disease [CHD], and cardiac arrhythmias) and surgical cardiac diagnoses (e.g., post–coronary arterial bypass graft surgery [post-CABG], post–coronary angioplasty, post–cardiac valvular surgery, and post–cardiac transplantation). The general goals of cardiac rehabilitation are to optimize the patient's physiologic, psychosocial, and vocational function, as well as to reduce the morbidity and mortality of cardiac diseases. The cardiac patient is given an educational program (e.g., lifestyle modification such as low-cholesterol diet, stress-reduction, and smoking cessation) to reduce the risk factors for heart disease, as well as reconditioning exercises to improve safety and tolerance of daily activities (e.g., vocational, recreational, and sexual activities). The approach to cardiac rehabilitation is usually interdisciplinary, involving physicians, nurses, physical therapists, occupational therapists, exercise physiologists, nutritionists, psychologists (or psychiatrists), social workers, and vocational counselors. Cardiac rehabilitation services must include comprehensive long-term programs involving medical evaluation, exercise prescription, modification of CHD risk factors, education, counseling, and vocational programs.

I. **Epidemiology.** Cardiovascular disease, which is responsible for 50% of all deaths, is the leading cause of morbidity and mortality in the adult population in the United States. In 1990, the estimated mortality cost of cardiovascular disease was over $70 billion, with an estimated 8.2 million lost in life-years. The major category of cardiovascular disease is CHD, which can clinically manifest as stable or unstable angina pectoris, myocardial infarction (MI), silent myocardial ischemia, or sudden death. Another category of cardiovascular disease is heart failure, which is increasing in prevalence and which ranks as the fourth most common discharge diagnosis for all hospitalized Americans. The death rate of CHD still remains high despite its decrease from 228.1 per 100,000 population (in 1970) to 102.6 per 100,000 (in 1990). This decline in mortality rate has been attributed to advances in medical treatment and technology, increase in exercise participation, and reductions in cigarette smoking and red meat consumption.

There are more than 13.5 million Americans with a history of MI or who have experienced angina pectoris. Every year, approximately 1.5 million Americans sustain an MI, of which nearly 500,000 are fatal. The majority of patients (over 50%) with acute MI are over age 65, whereas about 45% occur between age 40 and 65 and 5% under age 40. The MI survivors (approximately 1 million Americans per year) are potential candidates for cardiac rehabilitation as are those with stable angina pectoris (more than 7 million Americans per year), post-CABG (309,000 patients in 1993, 45% of whom are under age 65), and percutaneous transluminal coronary angioplasty (PTCA) and other transcatheter interventional procedures (362,000 in 1993, 54% of whom are under age 65). Among these potential candidates, only 11 to 38% participate in cardiac rehabilitation programs, despite studies showing that cardiac rehabilitation can reduce the mortality and morbidity of CHD.

II. Coronary heart disease risk factors

A. Modifiable CHD risk factors. Hypertension (blood pressure [BP] at least 140/90 mm Hg), cigarette smoking, obesity (over 30% ideal body weight, especially those with abdominal fat pattern), habitually sedentary lifestyle, hypercholesterolemia (over 5.20 mmol/L or over 200 mg/dl), high levels of low-density lipoprotein (LDL) cholesterol (over 3.4 mmol/L or over 130 mg/dl), low levels of high-density lipoprotein (HDL) cholesterol (less than 0.9 mmol/L or less than 35 mg/dl), hypertriglyceridemia (over 2.8 mmol/L or over 250 mg/dl), hyperinsulinemia, diabetes mellitus (DM), and "type A" behavior (controversial due to problems in measuring "type A" behavior).

B. Unmodifiable CHD risk factors. Advanced age (male at least 45; female at least 55 or prematurely menopausal without estrogen replacement therapy); male gender (rate of CHD is 3-4 times higher than women in the middle decades of life and roughly 2 times higher in the elderly); black race (due to higher rates of hypertension), family history of premature CHD (i.e., MI or sudden death before age 55 in a first-degree male relative or before age 65 in a first-degree female relative), past history of CHD, cardiac event, or abnormal ECG (e.g., left ventricular hypertrophy [LVH]); and a past history of occlusive peripheral vascular disease (PVD) or cerebrovascular disease.

III. Cardiac evaluation

A. History

1. **Chief complaint (CC)**

    a. **Chest pain,** that is typical anginal pain, which is described as tight, vise-like, aching, squeezing, burning, and pressing, is located at the substernal area but may also involve the left chest, arms, neck, or jaw; lasts 3 to 5 minutes or up to 15 minutes; is precipitated during exertion, emotional upset, cold weather, or exertion after meals; and is relieved within 3 to 5 minutes after rest or sublingual nitroglycerin.

    b. **Other CCs** are dyspnea (usually exertional), orthopnea (often with paroxysmal nocturnal dyspnea), palpitation, syncope, fatigue, edema, dizziness or lightheadedness, nausea or vomiting, cyanosis, and pallor.

2. **Past history,** such as past cardiac event (e.g., MI) or abnormal electrocardiogram (ECG) (e.g., LVH), cardiovascular (CV) surgery or procedure (e.g., CABG, PTCA, or cardiac pacemaker insertion), congestive heart failure (CHF), hypertension, DM, occlusive PVD, cerebrovascular disease, pulmonary embolism, bacterial endocarditis, rheumatic fever, ankylosing spondylitis (associated with aortic valve disease or conduction defects), Down syndrome (associated cardiac abnormalities), myasthenia or other neuromuscular disease (associated with cardiomyopathy or conduction disease), and congenital heart defects.

3. **Medication history,** such as antianginals (nitrates, β-adrenergic blockers, calcium channel blockers), antiarrhythmics (sodium channel blockers, β-adrenergic blockers, potassium channel blockers, calcium channel blockers), antihypertensives (diuretics, adrenergic blockers, angiotensin-converting-enzyme [ACE] inhibitors, calcium channel blockers), heart-failure treatment drugs (inotropics, diuretics, peripheral vasodilators), anticoagulants, antiplatelets, and antilipemic agents.

4. **Functional and occupational history,** such as the function and level of activity tolerance at present and prior to the cardiac event and level of activity required at home and at work.

5. **Personal history,** such as cigarette use, alcohol use, substance abuse, leisure activities, exercise history, diet history, personality type, and emotional adaptation to stress.

6. **Social history,** such as, home situation, support system, architectural barriers, and financial condition.

7. **Family history,** such as, premature MI or sudden death, hypercholesterolemia or hyperlipidemia, arrhythmias, hypertrophic cardiomyopathies, and Marfan's disease.

B. **Physical examination**

1. **General.** Weight, height, skinfold measurement, body habitus, skin (pallor, diaphoresis, xanthelasma; if post-surgery, check incisional drainage, wound healing, as well as tubes and drains that limit mobility), arcus cornealis, facial appearance, anxiety, and gait.

2. **Vital signs.** Temperature, blood pressure (resting hypertension, orthostatic and symptomatic hypotension), pulse and heart rate and rhythm, and respiratory rate and pattern.

3. **Cardiovascular**

   a. **Inspection.** Jugular venous pulse and waveform, and cyanosis (e.g., perioral).

   b. **Palpation.** Precordium (point of maximal impulse, thrills, systolic heave), major arterial pulses (carotid, brachial, radial, femoral, popliteal, posterior tibial, and dorsalis pedis pulses), and peripheral dependent edema.

   c. **Auscultation**

      1) **Heart sounds:** S1 (mitral and tricuspid valve closure; soft S1 is heard in mitral regurgitation, low-output states, and first-degree heart block; loud S1 is heard in mitral stenosis, high-output states, and short PR intervals), S2 (pulmonic and aortic valve closure), fixed S2 splitting with respiration (atrial septal defect), paradoxical S2 splitting during expiration (left bundle branch block, left ventricular failure, aortic stenosis), gallop sounds (S3 due to ventricular filling sounds, and S4 during atrial systole due to decreased ventricular compliance), ejection click (aortic or pulmonic valve opening), midsystolic click (mitral valve prolapse [MVP]), and opening snap (opening of mitral valve in mitral stenosis).

      2) **Heart murmurs.** Systolic ejection murmurs (functional or innocent flow murmurs, aortic stenosis, pulmonic stenosis, idiopathic hypertrophic subaortic stenosis, atypical mitral regurgitation), pansystolic or holosystolic murmurs (mitral regurgitation, tricuspid regurgitation, ventricular septal defects), late systolic murmurs (MVP), immediate diastolic decrescendo murmurs (aortic regurgitation, pulmonic regurgitation), delayed diastolic murmurs (mitral stenosis, tricuspid stenosis), and continuous systolic and diastolic murmurs (arteriovenous fistula, patent ductus arteriosus).

      3) **Pericardial rub** (pericarditis, acute MI).

4. **Pulmonary.** Breath sounds (decreased, crackles or rales, wheezes, ronchi).

5. **Neurologic and musculoskeletal.** Focal neurologic signs, altered mental status, joint range of motion, muscle strength, and endurance.

C. **Diagnostic tests** are needed to detect subclinical findings; however, they must be correlated with clinical findings, and, if needed, they must be done serially for follow-up.

1. **Chest radiograph** is used to detect cardiac and pulmonary pathologies (e.g., cardiac enlargement, aortic calcification, pulmonary congestion, and pneu-

monia). A systematic approach to reading chest radiographs includes (a) soft tissues, bones, and thorax, (b) pulmonary vasculature and lungs, (c) size and contour of the heart and individual chambers, (d) great vessels and mediastinal structures, (e) abnormal densities and lucencies, and (f) pleura and diaphragm.

2. **Cardiac tests**

   a. **Electrocardiography (ECG)** is commonly used to identify structural changes (e.g., ventricular or atrial enlargement), ischemic changes (e.g., ST-T segment displacement), infarction (e.g., Q-wave or non-Q wave), conduction abnormalities (e.g., bundle branch block and heart block), rhythm abnormalities (e.g., atrial fibrillation or flutter, premature atrial or ventricular contractions, and ventricular fibrillation), and metabolic abnormalities (e.g., hyperkalemia). It can also determine drug effects on the heart (e.g., digitalis or quinidine) and can be used to guide the exercise prescription. Table 5.13-1 shows a quick method of ECG interpretation.

   b. **Echocardiography** (or **cardiac ultrasound**; see Chapter 2.2, section III.B)

      1) **Transthoracic echocardiography** is used to evaluate known or suspected CHD or MI (e.g., global or segmental wall motion abnormalities; assessment of left ventricular ejection fraction; and detection of ventricular aneurysm, mural thrombus, or right ventricular infarction), valvular heart disease (e.g., functional murmur vs. organic valvular abnormality, aortic valve stenosis vs. hypertrophic cardiomyopathy, specific causes of mitral regurgitation murmurs, prosthetic valve abnormalities, valvular vegetations [e.g., endocarditis], and ventricular function in valvular heart disease), pericardial disease (e.g., pericarditis, pericardial effusion, and cardiac tamponade), cardiomyopathy, congenital heart disease, and cardiac tumors. It may also be used in cardiac stress testings (see below).

      2) **Transesophageal echocardiography (TEE)** is particularly useful in the diagnosis of atrial pathology (thrombus, tumor, atrial septal defect, patent foramen ovale), mitral valve dysfunction (endocarditis, regurgitation), aortic pathology (dissection, abscess, endocarditis), and pulmonary artery pathology (thrombus).

3. **Laboratory tests**

   a. **Blood tests** including complete blood count (hemoglobin and hematocrit); serum electrolytes; serum creatine kinase (CK), especially the CK-MB isoenzyme (increased within 4-8 hours after the onset of MI then peaks between 8 and 24 hours, and returns to normal by 48-72 hours); serum lactate dehydrogenase (LDH) especially LD_1 isoenzymes (elevated from 48-96 hours after the onset of MI); and serum drug levels (e.g., digoxin, procainamide, and quinidine).

   b. **Cardiac stress tests**

      1) **Cardiovascular exercise tolerance testing (CV-ETT)** uses a treadmill or cycle ergometry (bicycle or arm crank) for cardiac diagnostic, prognostic, and functional purposes. In the PM&R setting, it is used primarily as the basis for prescribing an individualized and safe exercise program. Chapter 2.7, section I describes fully CV-ETT.

      2) **Echocardiographic stress testing** is usually done in conjunction with a treadmill or bicycle ergometer (or occasionally with a pharmacologic stress test; see below) to detect cardiac ischemia (i.e., left ventricular dyssynergia, regional wall motion abnormalities, and wall motion

Table 5.13-1.   Quick method of electrocardiogram (ECG) interpretation

ECG PARAMETERS	NORMAL	COMMENTS
A. Measurement* 1. Heart rate†	50-90 bpm‡	• Measure atrial and ventricular rates, if different • <50 bpm = sinus bradycardia • >90 bpm = sinus tachycardia • Variable beat to beat rate = sinus arrhythmia
2. PR interval	0.12-0.20 sec	• <0.12 = ventricular preexcitation (e.g., Wolff-Parkinson-White syndrome); AV-junctional rhythm • >0.2 = 1st degree AV-block
3. QRS duration	0.06-0.10 sec	• >0.10 = BBB; nonspecific IVCD; ventricular tachycardia
4. QT interval	Depends on HR§	• Prolonged in: CHD; drug therapy (quinidine, procainamide, TCA); hypokalemia; stroke
5. QRS axis in frontal plane	+90° to −30°	• Deviated in: ventricular hypertrophy; fascicular blocks involving LBB

B. Rhythm and conduction analyses	Normal sinus rhythm	1. Abnormal-impulse (arrhythmia) analyses
		  a. Site of origin: atria, AV junction, ventricles
		  b. Rate of occurrence: normal, slow, fast
		  c. Response: regular, irregular
		  d. Onset: premature (active), escape (passive)
		2. Conduction-delay analyses
		  a. Site of delay: sinoatrial, intraatrial, AV junction, intraventricular (left or right BBB);
		  b. Direction of block: antegrade, retrograde
		  c. Degree of AV block: 1st degree, 2nd degree (type I [Wenckebach], type II [Mobitz]), 3rd degree

C. Waveform description
  1. P waves: RAE (tall, peaked P waves in II, III, aVF); LAE (wide, notched P wave in frontal plane; increased negativity of P wave in V_1).
  2. QRS complexes: RVH (increased R-wave voltage in V_{1-2}; increased S-wave voltage in V_{5-6}); LVH (increased R-wave voltage in V_{5-6}; increased S-wave voltage in V_{1-2}); MI (increased T wave amplitude and width; terminal position of T wave inverts as MI becomes evolved; ST-segment elevation [>2 mm]; ''pathologic'' Q wave (i.e., >0.04 sec wide; depth ~1/3 QRS amplitude).
  3. Nonspecific ST-T wave changes: myocardial ischemia or infarction; electrolyte abnormalities; drugs; ventricular hypertrophy; central nervous system disease.

bpm = beats per minute; AV = atrioventricular; BBB = bundle branch block; IVCD = intraventricular conduction disorder; CHD = coronary heart disease; TCA = tricyclic antidepressant; RAE or LAE = right or left atrial enlargement; RVH or LVH = right or left ventricular hypertrophy; LBB = left bundle branch.
* In measuring ECG tracings, one big box = 0.2 sec; one small box = 0.04 sec.
† For HR estimation (at a paper speed of 25 mm/sec), each successive big box (between successive P waves or between successive QRS complexes) corresponds to 300, 150, 100, 75, 60, 50 bpm
‡ The normal HR range of 50-90 bpm (based on actual data) is more clinically relevant than the traditional 60-100 bpm (See Spodick DH, Raju P, Bishop RL, et al: Operational definition of normal sinus heart rate, *Am J Cardiol* 69:1245-1246, 1992.)
§ QT interval is <0.40 sec at 70 bpm; for every 10 bpm increase in HR, the QT interval decreases by 0.02 sec, and vice versa.

changes). The use of bicycle ergometry allows for continuous monitoring and the detection of transient ischemic changes, while the use of treadmill testing is limited to scanning before and after exercise. Exercise echocardiography, which compares favorably with the results of ETT using ECG, is used when ECG-ETT is ambiguous or nondiagnostic, in women (due to a higher likelihood of a false-positive ECG tests), and in those with abnormalities on the resting ECG.

3) Radionuclide stress testing uses thallium-201 or technetium-99m perfusion scintigraphy to assess myocardial perfusion and to detect ischemia in CHD (and also to detect acute MI). The imaging can be performed in conjunction with a treadmill or a bicycle ergometer test or with pharmacologic stress testing (see below). Radionuclide scintigraphy can image all patients regardless of habitus and has been shown to be more accurate than stress echocardiography alone or ECG alone; however, it is invasive (injection of a radioactive agent with a long half-life) and is expensive.

4) Pharmacologic stress testing involves the injection of coronary artery vasodilators (e.g., dipyridamole and adenosine) or dobutamine (inotropic, chronotropic, and moderate coronary vasodilator) to induce cardiac stress for the diagnosis of CHD and for risk stratification. Coronary artery vasodilator causes a "cardiac steal" phenomenon in which normal arteries dilate (thus increasing blood flow), but diseased arteries (which are already dilated) are unable to further dilate (thus causing a relative "decrease" in blood flow). Pharmacologic stress testing is usually used in conjunction with ECG monitoring and either echocardiography or radionuclide perfusion scintigraphy. Although patients can be tested regardless of their ability to perform adequate levels of exercise, the usefulness of pharmacologic stress testing remains questionable for determining exercise prescription in cardiac rehabilitation.

5) Isometric hand-grip stress test is performed having the patient squeeze a hand dynamometer at 25 to 75% of maximum hand strength for as long as tolerable to provide exercise stress. This technique, however, does not provoke ischemia as effectively as ETT and other stress testings.

   c. Invasive CV diagnostic procedures, such as, cardiac catheterization (right and left side of the heart), coronary angiography, intracardiac electrophysiologic studies, and endomyocardial biopsy.

IV. Cardiac rehabilitation consists of four distinct, successive phases. Most clinicians, however, divide it into three phases by combining phases III and IV and calling it the "long-term" or "maintenance" cardiac rehabilitation phase. Each phase of cardiac rehabilitation has specific goals with educational or lifestyle modification component as well as activity or exercise component, but differs with respect to location (inpatient, outpatient, or community), duration of the phase, amount of supervision, and intensity of activity.

A. Phase I is the in-patient acute phase of cardiac rehabilitation (generally lasting from 3-6 days), which is designed primarily for those recovering from MI or CABGs. Other cardiac patients that may benefit from a phase I program include those with angioplasty (PTCA), valve surgery, cardiac transplantation, stable angina, and CHD risk factors. Phase I is started as soon as the patient's condition has stabilized, usually on the second to fourth day after MI or after surgery. It is considered the initial point and cornerstone for all other phases in preparing the patient for return to an active and productive lifestyle.

The goals of Phase I are as follows: (1) to prevent the sequelae of immobilization and assist the patient in tolerating self-care activities and household ambulation; (2) to prepare the patient (and family) for a healthy lifestyle (i.e., by identifying and modifying the risk factors of CHD); (3) to reduce psychologic and emotional disorders that accompany the cardiac diagnosis (anxiety and depression are the most common; they are usually self-limiting but may last more than 6 months in up to 30% of patients); (4) to facilitate adjustment to the acute event and to the hospital environment; and (5) to motivate the patient to make a long-term commitment to the cardiac rehabilitation program. By the end of phase I, the cardiac patient should be able to perform self-care, activities of daily living (ADLs), and household ambulation (except stair climbing); understand the benefits of exercise and be able to perform the prescribed exercises; understand and be able to take medications independently; adhere to the prescribed diet (e.g., low-fat diet); check the pulse rate; and identify cardiac symptoms. Phase I programs include:

1. **Education and risk-modification programs.** Patient education techniques are discussed in Chapter 5.10, section VI.A. Specific topics for the phase I educational program include orientation to cardiac rehabilitation, anatomy and physiology of the heart, disease and the healing process, recognition of angina and other cardiac symptoms, cardiovascular medications, pulse taking, benefits of physical activity and exercise, psychosocial adjustment to disability (for patient and family), and sexual counseling (see Table 5.13-2; see also Chapter 5.9). The patient is also taught to identify modifiable CHD risk factors and to take the following steps:

   a. **Hyperlipidemia control,** that is, lowering of cholesterol to desirable levels (below 200 mg/dl of total cholesterol; below 130 mg/dl of LDL) to reduce atherosclerotic cardiovascular disease. Based on the 1993 guidelines of the National Cholesterol Education Program (NCEP) Expert Panel on Detection, Evaluation, and Treatment of High Blood Cholesterol in Adults (see bibliography), treatment consists primarily of dietary modification (i.e., step I and step II diets) and exercise (see section IV.A.2.a). Both steps I and II diets consist of carbohydrate (50-60% of total calories), protein (15% of total calories), and fat (30% or less of total calories). In step I, the saturated fat is 8 to 10% or less of total calories and the cholesterol is less than 300 mg/day; whereas in step II, the saturated fat is further reduced to less than 7% of total calories, and the cholesterol to below 200 mg/day. The step I diet is instituted for 3 to 6 months and if the desired level of LDL or total cholesterol is not attained, then the patient is placed on step II diet (for 3-6 months). Low-fat diet program and recipes can be found in the books listed in the supplemental reference.

      If dietary modification fails (after a minimum of 6 months of intensive dietary counseling and therapy), the following drugs are considered: bile acid sequestrants or bile acids binding resins (cholestyramine [Questran, Cholybar], colestipol [Colestid]), nicotinic acid (niacin), HMG-CoA reductase inhibitors (lovastatin [Mevachol], pravastatin [Pravachol], simvastatin [Zocor]), fibric acid derivatives (gemfibrozil [Lopid], clofibrate [Atromid-S]), and antioxidants (probucol [Lorelco]). The use of Metamucil (see Chapter 5.8, section VI.B.3.a.1) in counteracting the constipating effects of bile acid sequestrants also helps lower

Table 5.13-2. **General sexual counseling for patients after a cardiac event (e.g., myocardial infarction or coronary artery bypass graft surgery)**

PARAMETER	GENERAL SEXUAL COUNSELING
MET requirement	• The maximal activity during sexual intercourse approximates 4.7-5.5 METS for <30 sec and ~3.5 METS during the pre- and postorgasmic periods.[a,b] • Noncoital activities (e.g., masturbation) have lower energy expenditures than coitus.[c]
Safe time of sexual resumption	• When patient is stable or asymptomatic; in general, if the patient can exercise at levels of 5-7 METS without symptoms, abnormal pulse rate, or changes in blood pressure or ECG.[a] • Time period is variable (usually within 3-6 weeks after cardiac event).
Tests for readiness to resume sexual activity	• Clinical test: two-flight stair-climbing test (i.e., 10 min of rapid walking at 120 paces/min or 3 mph, followed by climbing two flights of stairs [about 22 steps with 17 cm height] in 10 sec or at 2 steps/sec)[d] or • Laboratory test: Exercise tolerance test (see Chapter 2.7, section I) with maximum workload of at least 5-7 METS.
Benefits of exercise	• Exercise training can lessen the peak coital heart rate.[e]
Positions[f]	• Suggested positions: patient at the bottom; side-by-side; face-to-face, face-to-back; sitting on a chair with partner sitting on patient's lap. • Most patients do not make changes in patterns of foreplay or position adopted during coitus.
Precautions	• Avoid sexual activities in the following conditions (associated with sudden death during coitus)[g]: illicit sexual affairs; unfamiliar surroundings; after a large meal; or after high alcohol intake. • Also avoid sexual activities soon after physical or emotional stress.
Warning signs[f] that warrants a physician consultation	• Tachycardia and dyspnea/tachypnea that persist for 10-15 min after coitus; extreme fatigue persisting until the next day; arrhythmias; dizziness, lightheadedness or "blacking out"; chest pain during or after coitus; sexual dysfunction.

Data adapted from:

[a] Hellerstein HK, Friedman EH: Sexual activity and the postcoronary patient, *Arch Intern Med* 125:987-999, 1970.

[b] Douglas JE, Wilkes TD: Reconditioning cardiac patients, *Am Fam Physician* 11(1): 123-129, 1975.

[c] Bohlen JG, Held JP, Sanderson MO, et al: Heart rate, rate-pressure product, and oxygen uptake during four sexual activities, *Arch Intern Med* 144:1745-1748, 1984.

[d] Larson JL, McNaughton MW, Kennedy JW, et al: Heart rate and blood pressure responses to sexual activity and a stair-climbing test, *Heart Lung* 9:1025-1030, 1980.

[e] Stein RA: The effect of exercise training on heart rate during coitus in the post myocardial infarction patient, *Circulation* 55:738-740, 1977.

[f] Papadopoulos C: Education and counseling of the patient and family: sexual problems/interventions. In Wenger NK, Hellerstein HK, editors: *Rehabilitation of the coronary patient*, ed. 3, New York, 1992, Churchill Livingstone, pp 473-481.

[g] Massie E, Rose EF, Rupp JC, et al: Sudden death during coitus: fact or fiction? *Med Aspects Hum Sex* 3(6):22-26, 1969.

cholesterol. Other cholesterol-lowering agents under investigation include fish oils; vitamins A, C, and E; and estrogen replacement therapy.

b. Hypertension control, that is, lowering of BP to below 140/90, to reduce cardiovascular, renal, and central nervous system morbidity and mortality associated with long-standing hypertension. Based on the 1993 JNC-V (i.e., The Fifth Report of the Joint National Committee on Detection, Evaluation, and Treatment of High Blood Pressure), the following "stepped-care" approach is recommended:

- **Step 1.** Lifestyle modification, that is, weight reduction if overweight (refer to the article by the National Institute of Health Technology Assessment Conference Panel [see bibliography] for discussion about weight-loss programs, that is, dietary change, exercise, behavior modification, drug treatment, and combination therapies); moderation of alcohol intake (i.e., patients suspected of alcohol abuse as identified by a "yes" response on the CAGE questionnaire [see Table 1.1-1] should be referred to programs for the treatment of alcoholism; patients with no alcohol abuse problems should limit daily alcohol intake to no more than 1 oz of ethanol, 24 oz beer, 8 oz wine, or 2 oz 100-proof whiskey); restriction of daily sodium intake (i.e., less than 2.3 g sodium, which is approximately less than 6 g salt [sodium chloride] per day); smoking cessation (see section IV.A.1.c); aerobic exercise program (see section IV.A.2.a); reduction in saturated fat intake (see section IV.A.1.a); stress management (controversial; not recommended by the JNC-V due to lack of convincing data; see section IV.A.1.e).

- **Step 2.** Continue lifestyle modification; add first-line drugs (β-blockers or diuretics) or other effective alternatives (e.g., α₁-blockers, α-β-blockers; angiotensin-converting enzyme [ACE] inhibitors, calcium channel blockers).

- **Step 3.** Increase drug dose, substitute another drug, or add a second drug from a different class.

- **Step 4.** Add a second or third agent or diuretic (if not already prescribed).

c. Smoking cessation (see techniques in Chapter 5.12, section IV.A.1.a) to reduce the risk of CHD by 50 to 70% in the primary prevention of CHD and to reduce up to 50% the risk of sudden death and fatal reinfarction in patients with MI (i.e., tertiary prevention).

d. Diabetes mellitus control, that is, lowering of blood sugar to less than 140 mg/dl, to reduce the risk of cardiovascular disease (especially CHD), peripheral vascular disease, and cerebrovascular disease. Management includes nonpharmacologic (e.g., weight loss program if obese, dietary control, and exercise) and pharmacologic (e.g., oral hypoglycemics and insulin) treatment.

e. Stress management, that is, relaxation techniques (see Chapter 4.2, section VI), biofeedback (see Chapter 4.1, section VI), and psychological techniques on coping with stress have been reported to reduce coronary morbidity and mortality, especially in patients with "type A" behavior. These beneficial effects, however, are controversial because of the difficulty in diagnosing "type A" behaviors. Recent studies seem to indicate that impatience and free-floating hostility (rather than ambition and competitive drive) are the key elements of "type A" behavior pattern.

2. Exercise. The following cardiac patients may generally proceed with Phase

I exercises and activities: those with uncomplicated cardiac events, first-degree heart block, sinus bradycardia, and infrequent premature ventricular contractions (PVCs). Although significant improvement in cardiovascular fitness or other physical measurements are not expected during phase I, studies have shown that early physical activity reduces the complications of immobilization (i.e., by reducing venous thromboembolism, maintaining muscle tone, reducing orthostatic hypotension, and maintaining joint mobility).

Absolute contraindications for exercise in cardiac patients include unstable angina, heart failure (acute, uncompensated), uncontrolled arrhythmias, second- or third-degree AV block, resting ST-segment displacement over 3 mm, resting BP above 200/110 mm Hg, inappropriate asymptomatic postural or exertional BP responses, severe aortic stenosis (more than 50 mm Hg gradient), active pericarditis or myocarditis, recent embolism, acute or chronic thrombophlebitis, idiopathic hypertrophic subaortic stenosis, dissecting aneurysm, and acute systemic illness or fever (above 100°F).

Relative contraindications of exercise in cardiac patients include resting BP of over 180/100 mm Hg, hypotension, inappropriate rise in BP during exercise, sinus tachycardia at rest (more than 120 beats/min), resting ST-segment depression over 2 mm, moderate aortic stenosis, ventricular aneurysm, compensated heart failure, pericarditis associated with CABG, excessive incisional drainage after CABG, new ECG change suggestive of new infarction, poorly controlled DM, symptomatic anemia (hematocrit less than 30%), significant emotional stress or psychological disorders, or neuromuscular, musculoskeletal, or orthopedic problems that would prohibit exercise.

a. **Exercise programs** include low-metabolic demand exercises and activities that are performed for 5 to 10 minutes (progressed up to 20-30 minutes), 2 to 4 times daily. These activities require less than 4.0 METS (see Chapter 2.7, section I.A for discussion of METS or metabolic equivalents; see also Tables 4.2-2 and 4.2-3 for METS of different activities) and should generally not raise the patient's heart rate (HR) above 20 beats per minute over the resting heart rate. At the beginning of phase I, the exercises emphasize range of motion (ROM), which is advanced through a series of active exercises (and, if tolerated, mild resistance exercises) in the supine, sitting, and upright positions. If the patient is confined to bed, leg and feet exercises (e.g., ankle pumps) are encouraged to reduce venous stasis. Passive or active-assistive ROM exercises may be necessary for some patients (e.g., those with severe myocardial damage, status post–cardiac transplantation, or other compromising complications). Otherwise, due to the short duration of phase I, the patient is immediately advanced to active exercises and activities under close monitoring during and after the session (which may later be progressed to telemetric ECG-monitoring of activities).

Exercise parameters monitored include pulse or HR, BP, ECG, and activity-induced symptoms. In general, HR monitoring is preferred as it is easier to monitor during exercise than auscultatory BP. The exercise or activity should be stopped if the patient develops any of the following signs and symptoms: angina, light-headedness, nausea, dyspnea, fatigue, pallor, cyanosis, ataxia, hypoxia, altered mental status, peripheral circulatory insufficiency (e.g., leg claudication); inappropriate bradycardia (drop in HR of more than 10 beats per minute); activity-induced BP changes (e.g., a greater than 20 mm Hg drop in systolic blood pressure [SBP]; SBP over 220 mm Hg or diastolic BP [DBP] above 110 mm Hg); activity-induced ECG-changes (e.g., ST displacement over 2-3 mm from rest, ventricular tachycardia, symptomatic supraventricular tachycardia, new-onset left bundle branch block, new-onset second- or third-degree AV block, R on T PVCs, and frequent multifocal PVCs [i.e., more than 30% of PVCs]).

As soon as tolerable, the patient is progressed to independent self-care and short distance ambulation (in the corridor or on a treadmill) or bicycle ergometry). In general, the energy cost of almost all ADLs is less than 4 METS. Unless the patient is able to tolerate 5 to 7 METS (e.g., from exercise tolerance testing described in Chapter 2.7, section I.A), he or she should not do stair climbing, which generally requires 5 to 7 METS. Patients who have CABG and PTCA have little or no permanent damage to the myocardium, hence can generally be exercised more aggressively than those who have sustained an MI. For patients who are status post–cardiac transplantation, passive ROM exercises are initiated at extubation and performed twice a day. Borg's rating of perceived exertion (RPE) scale at an intensity of 11 to 13 in the original Borg's RPE scale (see Table 4.2-4; see also discussion of Borg's RPE scale in Chapter 4.2, section III.A.3) is recommended in cardiac transplant patients because cardiac denervation decreases the reliability of other parameters such as HR (i.e., HR does not increase until circulating catecholamines rise after 3-5 minutes of exercise and does not reach maximum levels predicted for the donor age).

b. **Exercise testing.** At the end of phase I or prior to starting phase II (i.e., from 3 days to 3 weeks after a cardiac event), a low-level exercise tolerance test (see Chapter 2.7, section I) is generally ordered. Endpoints for ETT are shown in Table 2.7-2. Other endpoints that may be used in low-level exercise tolerance testing include attaining the following: increase in HR of 20 to 30 beats above resting HR; maximal heart rate of 120 to 140 beats/min; 70 to 75% age-estimated maximal HR; 4 to 6 METS, or, in patients on β-blockers, a Borg's RPE scale of "hard" (see Table 4.2-4). The ETT is used to stratify patients based on prognostic risks (see Table 5.13-3). Its specific goals are (a) to assess the patient's progress, adequacy of the current medical regimen, and need for coronary revascularization, and (b) to help determine the extent of ECG-monitoring needed during exercise and the appropriateness of progression to supervised phase II or to a home exercise program. Based on ETT, the prognoses of patients with MI are (see Theroux et al, Fioretti et al; Weld et al; and Krone et al)

- Patients with at least 1 mm of ST-segment depression, or who cannot achieve a peak workload of 4 METS, or cannot increase their SBP at least 30 mm Hg (or at least to 110 mm Hg) during the ETT are at increased risk for coronary mortality within the first year after MI. The abnormal BP response is probably a more sensitive predictor of mortality at 1 year than the maximal workload achieved or ischemic ST-segment changes.
- Patients with exercise-induced ST-segment depressions within 10 to 21 days after MI have 2 to 20 times greater risk of having a subsequent coronary event than do patients without this ECG finding.
- Patients unable to achieve a peak workload of 4 METS during ETT by 3 weeks after MI are at significantly higher risk for recurrent MI,

Table 5.13-3.   Minimal guidelines for risk stratification of cardiac patients

RISK LEVELS AND CHARACTERISTICS

Low risk*
- No significant left ventricular dysfunction (i.e., EF ≥50%)
- No resting or exercise-induced myocardial ischemia manifested as angina and/or ST-segment displacement
- No resting or exercise-induced complex arrhythmias
- Uncomplicated myocardial infarction (MI), coronary artery bypass graft surgery, percutaneous transluminal coronary angioplasty, or atherectomy
- Functional capacity ≥6 METS on graded exercise test ≥3 weeks after clinical event

Intermediate risk†
- Mild to moderately depressed left ventricular function (EF = 31 to 49%)
- Exercise-induced myocardial ischemia (1-2 mm ST-segment depression) or reversible ischemic defects (echocardiography or nuclear radiography)
- Failure to comply with exercise intensity prescription
- Functional capacity <5-6 METs on graded exercise test ≥3 weeks after clinical event

High risk‡
- Severely depressed left ventricular function (EF ≤30%)
- Complex ventricular arrhythmias at rest or appearing or increasing with exercise
- Decrease in systolic blood pressure (SBP) of >15 mm Hg during exercise or failure to rise with increasing exercise workloads
- Survivor of sudden cardiac death
- MI complicated by congestive heart failure, cardiogenic shock, and/or complex ventricular arrhythmias
- Severe coronary artery disease and marked exercise-induced myocardial ischemia (>2 mm ST-segment depression)

Reprinted by permission from American Association of Cardiovascular and Pulmonary Rehabilitation (AACVPR). *Guidelines for cardiac rehabilitation programs*, Champaign, IL, 1995, Human Kinetics publishers, p. 34.
1 MET (metabolic equivalent) = 3.5 ml O_2/kg/min; EF = ejection fraction.
* May be recommended moderate level exercise intensity with ECG monitoring only as indicated.
† May be recommended low-to-moderate level exercise intensity with intermittent ECG monitoring.
‡ May be recommended low-level exercise intensity with continuous or intermittent ECG monitoring.

coronary death, cardiac arrest, or necessity for CABG at a 2-year follow-up than those capable of performing at least 4 METS of peak workload.

B. Phase II is a continuation of phase I and is usually conducted in an outpatient setting or towards the end of hospitalization. If the patient is discharged from the hospital, phase II should generally start within 2 weeks and last 8 to 12 weeks. Indications and contraindications to phase II are essentially the same as those for phase I. The goals of phase II are (1) to enhance cardiovascular function and physical work capacity (i.e., strength, endurance, and flexibility), (2) to detect ECG changes (e.g., arrhythmias) during exercise, (3) to teach the patient proper techniques of exercise and provide him or her with guidelines for long-term exercise, (4) to establish healthy lifestyles in the patient and family; and (5) to enhance the patient's psychologic function and prepare him or her for a return to work and resumption of normal familial and social roles. By the end of phase II, the cardiac patient should be able to perform the daily self-administered exercise program safely, have adequate knowledge of his or her disease and symptoms to pursue vocational, recreational, and sexual activities safely; sustain healthy habits (e.g., low-fat diet) to reduce CHD risks; and comply with medications and medical follow-up. Phase II programs include

1. **Education and risk-modification programs.** These programs are a continuation and reinforcement of programs learned in phase I (see section IV.A.1) and are designed to help patients maintain a healthy lifestyle. Prepared education programs may be used (e.g., *An Active Partnership for the Health of Your Heart,* American Heart Association, 7272 Greenville Avenue, Dallas, TX 75231-4596, tel. (214) 706-1347).

2. **Exercise.** Depending on the ETT (see section IV.2.b) and the patient's risk stratification (see Table 5.13-3), the patient is given an individualized prescription of intensity, duration, frequency, and mode of activity. The exercise is supervised with either continuous or intermittent ECG monitoring (telemetry or hard-wired ECG). Phase II activities emphasize physical reconditioning and begin with dynamic-rhythmic or aerobic exercises (see Chapter 4.2, section III.A for discussion of aerobic exercises) at a level of 5 METS. The exercise involves both the upper- and lower-limb muscle groups because there is little crossover of adaptation between arm and leg exercises. Equipment used generally includes treadmills, bicycle ergometers, arm ergometers, wall pulleys, steps, rowing machines, vertical climbing devices, cross-county ski simulators, and light weights. The patient performs 5 to 10 minutes of exercise at each station with approximately 1 minute of rest between bouts. Each exercise session generally lasts 1 hour (including warm-up and cool-down periods) and is performed 3 times per week. The goal is to exercise within the target heart rate (described in Chapter 4.2, section III.A.1) for at least 20 to 30 minutes for training adaptation to occur. The exercise intensity is increased on a weekly basis as the patient's symptoms and physical conditioning permit, ultimately progressing to 8 METS before starting phase III.

3. **Return-to-work (RTW) program** (see also Chapter 5.11, section IV). Patients are prepared to return to their original job (or to a modified duty initially) or, in some cases, to an alternative job. In general, patients who can perform more than 7 METS of workload without any abnormal responses should be able to return to most jobs except heavy industrial work (see Table 5.11-1 for correlation of MET levels with the U.S. Department of Labor classification of work). Studies show that in the United States, more than two-thirds (70-75%) of patients with MI return to work (usually within 2-3 months); however, only 30% of cardiac patients from low socioeconomic levels or with low educational achievement are able to return to work. Among those cardiac patients who initially return to work, about 20% drop out within 1 year.

C. **Phases III and IV** are considered the maintenance (long-term) phase of cardiac rehabilitation. The maintenance phase is important because if it is neglected, the benefits gained during the training phases (i.e., I and II) are lost within a few weeks. Low-risk patients who did not participate in phases I or II may participate in the maintenance phase. Phase III usually lasts from 6 to 24 months and generally includes clinical supervision and intermittent ECG monitoring (e.g., through real-time ECG transmission over the telephone for home-based exercise). Exercises may initially be performed in an out-patient setting, then progressed to a community or home setting. The goals of phase

III are similar to those of phase II. Phase III is designed to provide a smooth transition from the structured, closely supervised, and monitored phase II program to one that is less monitored, supervised, and structured.

Phase IV, which is an extension of phase III, is a lifelong program, which generally does not include clinical supervision or ECG monitoring. The goals of phase IV are to continue in improving and maintaining fitness and a healthy lifestyle (to minimize cardiac disease morbidity and mortality). Other noncardiac patients (including healthy adults interested in enhancing physical fitness) may enter the phase IV program (even without going through phase III). A minimum of 2 weeks is generally needed to assess the patient's readiness for unsupervised and nonmonitored activities. The unsupervised patients may periodically need supervised exercise and ECG-monitored classes at the rehabilitation center to assess the patient's progress, to update the exercise program, and to evaluate the patient's clinical status. Phase III and IV programs include

1. **Education and risk-modification programs.** These programs consist of review and reinforcement of topics learned in phases I and II (see sections IV.A.1 and IV.B.1) for patients who underwent the training phases. For patients who are directly entering phase III or IV, the education and risk-modification programs (discussed in phases I and II) are initiated.

2. **Exercise.** As with phase II, the results from the ETT are used to determine the intensity of phase III training. The exercises selected involve the muscle groups trained in phase II and should fit within the interests and lifestyle of the individual patient. Due to training specificity, upper-limb exercises should also be prescribed in addition to the lower-limb exercises. The minimum requirement is to exercise at least 3 times per week for 30 to 60 minutes (with a regimen of 5-10 minutes warm-up, 20-30 minutes aerobic training, and 5-10 minutes cooldown). For those who have completed phase II, a target heart rate range (THRR) of 80% of maximum heart rate (MHR) is usually used, and the patient progresses gradually until 85% MHR when training adaptation is normal. However, for low-risk cardiac patients or healthy subjects who did not participate in phase II, a more conservative intensity is initially used (e.g., THRR at 70% of MHR attained in an ETT), which may progress at a more rapid rate (especially in healthy individuals depending on such factors as physical condition, age, musculoskeletal limitations) to 85 to 90% MHR (for healthy individuals and other select patients). The types of exercise include

   a. **Aerobic exercises.** For full discussion of aerobic exercises, see Chapter 4.1, section III.A. To help ensure long-term compliance, fun games and recreational sports may be used, preceded by a program of general conditioning and clinical assessment, including ECG monitoring with telemetry during actual play.

   b. **Resistance training.** The use of resistance exercises has been shown to be safe and beneficial for cardiac patients. Contraindications and termination criteria for resistive exercises are similar to those described in section IV.A.2 and those shown in Table 2.7-2, respectively. A popular form of resistive exercise is circuit weight training (CWT) using resistive machines, which seem to be more beneficial than free weights. Specific benefits of CWT include improvement in strength, lean body mass, flexibility, and cardiovascular endurance, and perhaps increase in bone mineral content (thus reducing the possibility of osteoporosis with aging). Circuit weight training also reduces the potential for musculoskeletal discomfort, is generally safe, and provides added fun and satisfaction.

   Circuit weight training is usually done after the aerobic phase (to ensure adequate warm-up and to decrease the risk of musculoskeletal injury), on alternate days, 3 times per week. All major muscle groups are exercised starting from large muscles then progressing to small muscles. The level of resistance (i.e., low-to-moderate or 30-60% of 10 repetition maximum [RM]) should allow the exercise sets to be completed comfortably (without straining) with 8 to 20 (usually 10-15) repetitions per station. Depending on the patient's fitness level and time allotted for CWT, the number of sets varies from 1 to 3 and the number of stations varies from 5 to 18.

In the beginning, the patient should attempt one set of exercises then gradually build up to three sets. When the patient can easily complete 12 to 15 repetitions at a Borg's RPE of 12 to 13 (see Borg's RPE scale in Table 4.2-4), then resistance can be increased (depending upon the patient's time allotment for the session, fitness level, and fatigability). When lifting is involved, it must be done through the full arc (if possible) at the following speed: lift to a count of 2 and lower to a count of 4. Each CWT session should last from 20 to 30 minutes with rest intervals of 30 to 60 seconds between stations. In general, shorter rest intervals allow for greater improvement in cardiovascular endurance; while longer rest intervals provide for greater recovery of heart rate and blood pressure and less risk of cardiovascular complications.

c. **Aquatic-exercise programs.** Water exercises (including swimming) are safe and are less stressful on bones and joints than land-based weight-bearing activities. Moreover, they can be performed in a horizontal position, thus enhancing venous return and augmenting stroke volume by reducing the effects of gravity. The cooling effect of water can also decrease the risk of heat overload. The recommended water temperature for cardiac patients ranges from 26 to 33°C (80-92°F). Most patients find the warmer temperature range more comfortable (especially those with peripheral vascular disease as heat causes vasodilation); however, the cooler temperature range is better for dissipation of heat.

Aquatic activities with varying intensities include water walking (with and without use of the arms), swimnastics, water aerobics, aqua stepping or step aerobics, swimming that incorporates a variety of strokes, and water games (e.g., volleyball). The exercise intensity is individually prescribed based on the ETT (see Chapter 2.7, section I). Although bicycle ergometer or treadmill tests may be used, an arm ergometer test is preferred if the aquatic program consists mainly of upper body work (e.g., swimming). The exercise frequency (3 times per week) and intensity are similar to those for aerobic exercises (see Chapter 4.1, section III.A). However, the THRR is preferred for estimating intensity, because the Borg RPE scale may be less accurate with water exercise, and there is limited data on the actual energy cost (METS) of water activities in cardiac patients.

BIBLIOGRAPHY

American Association of Cardiovascular and Pulmonary Rehabilitation (AACVPR): *Guidelines for cardiac rehabilitation programs,* ed 2, Champaign, IL, 1995, Human Kinetics.

Expert Panel on Detection, Evaluation, and Treatment of High Blood Cholesterol in Adults: Summary of the second report of the National Cholesterol Education Program (NCEP) Expert Panel on Detection, Evaluation, and Treatment of High

Blood Cholesterol in Adults (Adult Treatment Panel II), *JAMA* 269:3015-3023, 1993.

Fardy PS, Yanowitz FG: *Cardiac rehabilitation, adult fitness, and exercise testing,* ed 3, Baltimore, 1995, Williams & Wilkins.

Fioretti P, Brower R, Simoons ML, et al: Prediction of mortality in hospital survivors of myocardial infarction: comparison of predischarge exercise testing and radionuclide ventriculography at rest, *Br Heart J* 52:592-598, 1984.

Flores AM, Zohman LR: Rehabilitation of the cardiac patient. In DeLisa JA, Gans BM, editors: *Rehabilitation medicine: principles and practice,* ed 2, Philadelphia, 1993, JB Lippincott, pp 934-951.

Halar EM, editor: Cardiac rehabilitation: Part 1, *Phys Med Rehabil Clin North Am* 6(1):1-223, 1995.

Joint National Committee on Detection, Evaluation, and Treatment of High Blood Pressure: The fifth report of the Joint National Committee on Detection, Evaluation, and Treatment of High Blood Pressure (JNC-V), *Arch Intern Med* 153: 154-183, 1993.

Krone RJ, Gillespie JA, Weld FM, et al: Low-level exercise testing after myocardial infarction: usefulness in enhancing clinical risk stratification; *Circulation* 71: 80-89, 1985.

Moldover JR, Bartels MN: Cardiac rehabilitation. In Braddom RL, editor: *Physical medicine and rehabilitation,* Philadelphia, 1996, WB Saunders, pp 649-670.

National Institute of Health Consensus Development Panel: Physical activity and cardiovascular health. *JAMA* 276(3):241-246, 1996.

National Institute of Health Technology Assessment Conference Panel: Methods for voluntary weight loss and control, *Arch Intern Med* 116:942-949, 1992.

Pashkow FJ, Dafoe WA, editors: *Clinical cardiac rehabilitation: a cardiologist's guide,* Baltimore, 1993, Williams & Wilkins.

Pollock ML, Wilmore JH: *Exercise in health and disease: evaluation and prescription for prevention of rehabilitation,* ed 2, Philadelphia, 1990, WB Saunders.

Theroux P, Waters DD, Halphen C et al: Prognostic value of exercise testing soon after myocardial infarction, *N Engl J Med* 301(7):341-345, 1976.

Weld FM, King-Lee C, Bigger JT, et al: Risk stratification with low-level exercise testing 2 weeks after acute myocardial infarction, *Circulation* 64:306-314, 1981.

Wenger NK, Froelicher ES, Smith LK, et al: *Cardiac rehabilitation: clinical practice guideline No. 17.* AHCPR Publication No. 96-0672, Rockville, MD, October 1995, Agency for Health Care Policy and Research and the National Heart, Lung, and Blood Institute, U.S. Department of Health and Human Services.

Wenger NK, Hellerstein HK, editors: *Rehabilitation of the coronary patient,* ed 3, New York, 1992, Churchill Livingstone.

Supplemental References

Connor SL, Connor WE: *The new American diet,* New York, 1986, Simon & Schuster.

Grundy SM, Winston M, editors: *American Heart Association: Low-fat, low-cholesterol cookbook.* New York, 1989, Times-Books.

National Cholesterol Education Program (NCEP): *The second report of the Expert Panel on Detection, Evaluation, and Treatment of High Blood Cholesterol in Adults (Adult Treatment Panel II).* NIH publication no. 93-3095, Bethesda, MD, September 1993, National Institute of Health, and National Heart, Lung, and Blood Institute.

Ornish D: *Dr. Dean Ornish's program for reversing heart disease,* New York, 1996, Ivy (Ballantine) Books.

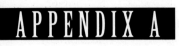

APPENDIX A

Appendix A-1. Average ranges of motion for the cervical spine and upper limbs

JOINT	MOTION	AAOS	AMA
Cervical spine	Flexion	0 to 130–150°*	0–60°
	Extension	0 to 130–150°*	0–75°
	Lateral flexion	0 to 80–100°*	0–45°
	Rotation	0 to 155–180°*	0–80°
Shoulder	Flexion	0–180°	0–180°
	Hyperextension	0–60°	0–50°
	Abduction	0–180°	0–180°
	Adduction	Not measured	0–50°
	Medial rotation	0–70°, or thumb tip reaches T6-T10	0–90°
	Lateral rotation	0–90°	0–90°
Elbow	Flexion	0–150°	0–140°
Forearm	Pronation	0–75°	0–80°
	Supination	0–80°	0–80°
Wrist	Flexion	0–80°	0–60°
	Extension	0–60°	0–60°
	Radial deviation	0–20°	0–20°
	Ulnar deviation	0–30°	0–30°
Thumb			
Carpometacarpal	Palmar abduction	0–70°	Not measured
	Radial abduction	0–80°	0–50°
	Adduction (radial)	Not measured	0–8 cm†
	Opposition	Thumb tip to 5th base	0–8 cm‡
Metacarpophalangeal	Flexion	0–50°	0–60°
	Hyperextension	Not measured	0–40°
Interphalangeal	Flexion	0–80°	0–80°
	Hyperextension	Not measured	0–30°
Fingers			
Metacarpophalangeal	Flexion	0 to 86–105°	0–90°
	Hyperextension	0 to 18–23°	0–20°
Proximal interphalangeal	Flexion	0 to 102–108°	0–100°
	Hyperextension	0 to 6–9°	0–30°
Distal interphalangeal	Flexion	0 to 63–72°	0–70°
	Hyperextension	0–8°	0–30°

Data adapted from Greene WB, Heckman JD, editors: *American Academy of Orthopaedic Surgeons (AAOS): The clinical measurement of joint motion.* Rosemont, IL, 1993, AAOS; and Engelberg AL, editor: *American Medical Association (AMA): Guides to the evaluation of permanent impairment,* ed 3, Chicago, 1988, AMA.

* Represents *total* values of passive cervical range of motion (i.e., right + left rotation or lateral flexion; flexion + extension); also age-dependent.

† Smallest possible distance from flexor crease of thumb interphalangeal joint to distal palmar crease of fifth metacarpophalangeal joint.

‡ Largest possible span from flexor crease of thumb IP joint to distal palmar crease of third metacarpal.

Appendix A-2. Average ranges of motion for the thoracolumbosacral spine and lower limbs.

JOINT	MOTION	AAOS	AMA
Thoracic spine	Flexion*	Not specified	0–50°
	Rotation*	0–30°	0–30°
Lumbar or lumbosacral spine	Flexion*	0 to 45–65°	0 to ≥60°
	Extension*	0–27°	0–25°
	Lateral flexion*	0 to 19–38°	0–25°
	Rotation*	0–21°	Not measured
Hip	Flexion	0–120°	0–100°
	Hyperextension	0–20°	0–30°
	Abduction	0–40°	0–40°
	Adduction	0–30°	0–20°
	Medial rotation	0–45°	0–40°
	Lateral rotation	0–45°	0–50°
Knee	Flexion	0–140°	0–150°
Ankle and foot	Dorsiflexion	0–20°	0–20°
	Plantarflexion	0 50°	0–40°
	Inversion	0 to 28–37°	0–30°
	Eversion	0 to 21–28°	0–20°
Toes			
1st metatarsophalangeal (MTP)	Flexion	Not measured	0–30°
	Extension	Not measured	0–50°
1st interphalangeal (IP)	Flexion	Not measured	0–30°
	Extension	0°	0°
2nd MTP	Flexion	Not measured	0–30°
	Extension	Not measured	0–40°
3rd MTP	Flexion	Not measured	0–20°
	Extension	Not measured	0–30°
4th MTP	Flexion	Not measured	0–10°
	Extension	Not measured	0–20°
5th MTP	Flexion	Not measured	0–10°
	Extension	Not measured	0–10°
2nd–5th proximal and distal IP	Flexion/extension	Not measured	Not measured

Data adapted from: Greene WB, Heckman JD, editors: *American Academy of Orthopaedic Surgeons (AAOS): The clinical measurement of joint motion.* Rosemont, IL, 1993, AAOS; and Engelberg AL, editor: *American Medical Association (AMA): Guides to the evaluation of permanent impairment,* ed 3, Chicago, 1988, AMA.
* Measured by double inclinometer technique.

Table A-3. Laboratory reference values (used at New York University Medical Center)

COMMON LABORATORY TESTS	NORMAL VALUES (ADULT)
Biochemistry, blood	
Acid phosphatase	0.1–0.8 IU/L
Alanine aminotransferase	3–36 U/L
Albumin	4.0–5.0 g/dl
Aldolase	<6 U/L
Alkaline phosphatase	39–117 U/L
Alpha-1-antitrypsin	85–313 mg/dl
Ammonia	11.0–35.0 Umol/L
Amylase	20–220 U/L
Anion gap at K^+	9–18 mEq/L
Aspartate aminotransferase	7–37 U/L
B-12	200–900 pg/ml
Bilirubin, direct	0–0.6 mg/dl
Bilirubin, indirect	0.2–0.7 mg/dl
Bilirubin, total	0.2–1.0 mg/dl
Blood urea nitrogen	10–20 mg/dl
Calcium	8.4–10.2 mg/dl
Carbon dioxide	21–29 mEq/L
Chloride	100–112 mEq/L
Cholesterol	
High-density lipoprotein	Male (M): 35–55 mg/dl; Female (F): 45–65 mg/dl
Low-density lipoprotein	65–175 mg/dl (calculated value)
Total cholesterol	120–240 mg/dl
Creatine kinase	25–225 U/L
Creatinine	0.6–1.6 mg/dl
Folic acid (folate)	5–15 mg/ml
Gamma glutamyl transpeptidase	7.0–60.0 IU/L
Glucose (fasting and nonfasting)	70–110 mg/dl
Iron group	
Iron	42–135 mcg/dl
Total iron binding capacity	280–400 mcg/dl
Saturation	11–46%
Lactic dehydrogenase	100–250 U/L
Magnesium	1.6–2.3 mg/dl
Osmolality	280–295 mosm/kg

Table A-3.—cont'd

COMMON LABORATORY TESTS	NORMAL VALUES (ADULT)
Phosphorus, inorganic	2.7–4.5 mg/dl
Potassium	3.5–5.3 mEq/L
Prealbumin	17–42 mg/dl
Protein, total	6.0–8.0 g/dl
Sodium	136–148 mEq/L
Triglyceride*	30–160 mg/dl (30–50 years old); 30–190 mg/dl (>50 years old)
Uric acid	2.5–7.0 mg/dl
Endocrine, blood	
Free thyroxine index	1.8 4.3
Thyroxine (T4)	4.5–11.5 mcg/dl
Triiodothyronine (T3)	90–185 ng/dl
T3 resin uptake	35–45%
Thyroglobulin RIA	≤25.0 ng/ml
Thyroid binding globulin	11–36 mcg/ml
Thyroid stimulating hormone	0.2–4.8 μU/ml
Hematologic	
Complete blood count	
White blood cell	$4.0–12.0 \times 10^9$/L
Red blood cell	M: $4.4–6.1 \times 10^{12}$/L F: $4.2–5.5 \times 10^{12}$/L
Hemoglobin	M: 14–18 g/dl F: 12–16 g/dl
Hematocrit	M: 41–51% F: 37–47%
Reticulocyte count	0.5–1.5%
Mean corpuscular volume	82–92 FL
Mean corpuscular hemoglobin	27–31 PG
MCH concentration	32–36 g/dl
Red-cell distribution width	11.5–14.5%
Platelets	$130–400 \times 10^9$/L
Erythrocyte sedimentation rate	M: 0–10 mm/hr F: 0–20 mm/hr
Glycosylated hemoglobin	5.5–9.5%
Coagulation	
Activated partial thromboplastin time	27–37 sec
Prothrombin time†	10.5–13.0 sec
Fibrinogen	150–380 mg%

Table A-3.—cont'd

COMMON LABORATORY TESTS	NORMAL VALUES (ADULT)
Immunologic, blood	
Total hemolytic complement (CH_{50})	150–250 units/ml
Complement components	
Clq	11–22 mg/dl
C3	55–120 mg/dl
C4	20–50 mg/dl
Urinalysis	
pH	5.0–7.0
Specific gravity	1.001–1.030
Color, appearance	Yellow, clear
White blood cell	0–2
Red blood cell	0–2
Urobilinogen	0.2–1.0 eu/dl
Casts, bilirubin, blood	Negative
Protein, glucose, ketones	Negative
Nitrate, yeasts, bacteria	Negative
Crystals, epithelial cells	Variable

* See also Chapter 5.13, sections II.A and IV.A.1.a, for undesirable and desirable levels, respectively.
† See Chapters 4.8 (VII.A.1) and 5.3 (IV.B.1.a and V.A.2) for therapeutic international normalized ratio (INR) levels.

Table A-4. Reference values for motor nerve conduction studies (these values are to be used as guidelines as every laboratory should ideally collect its own set of reference values; also, the patient's unaffected limb may be used as a "normal" reference)

MOTOR NERVE	DISTAL MOTOR LATENCY		MOTOR CONDUCTION VELOCITY	
	SEGMENT (DISTANCE FROM STIMULATING → PICK-UP ELECTRODE)	ONSET LATENCY MEAN ± 1 SD (RANGE)	SEGMENT (STIMULATING → PICK-UP ELECTRODE; USING TAPE MEASURE)	MEAN ± 1 SD (RANGE)
Median[a]	Wrist mid-crease → APB (8 cm along nerve course)	3.7 ± 0.3 msec (3.2–4.2 msec)	Above elbow → wrist	56.7 ± 3.8 m/sec (50.0–67.3 m/sec)
Ulnar[b,c]	Wrist → ADQ (6.5–8 cm)	3.0 ± 0.4 msec (2.2–3.8 msec)	Above elbow → wrist (elbow flexed ~70°)	62.7 ± 5.5 m/sec (52–74 m/sec)
Radial (PIN)[d,e]	Forearm → EIP[i] (8 cm)	2.4 ± 0.5 msec	Above elbow → EIP[i]	61.6 ± 5.9 m/sec (48–75 m/sec)
Deep peroneal[f,g]	Ankle → EDB (8 cm)	3.8 ± 0.7 msec (2.3–5.9 msec)	Fibular head → ankle	49.9 ± 5.9 m/sec (41.6–64.6 m/sec)
			Popliteal area → ankle	51.1 ± 6.3 m/sec (41.6–62.7 m/sec)
Tibial[h]	Ankle → AH[i] (8 cm)	3.4 ± 0.5 msec	Popliteal area → ankle	54.9 ± 7.6 m/sec

Data adapted from

[a] Melvin JL, Schuchmann JA, Lanese RR: Diagnostic specificity of motor and sensory nerve conduction variables in the carpal tunnel syndrome, *Arch Phys Med Rehabil* 54:69–74, 1973.

[b] Eisen A: Early diagnosis of ulnar nerve palsy, *Neurology* 24:256–262, 1974.

[c] Checkles NS, RussakovAD, Piero DL: Ulnar nerve conduction velocity: effect of elbow position on measurement, *Arch Phys Med Rehabil* 52:362–365, 1971.

[d] Trojaborg W, Sindrup EH: Motor and sensory conduction in different segments of the radial nerve in normal subjects, *J Neurol Neurosurg Psychiatry* 32:354–359, 1969.

[e] Jebsen RH: Motor conduction velocity in proximal and distal segments of the radial nerve, *Arch Phys Med Rehabil* 47:597–602, 1966.

[f] Jimenez J, Easton JKM, Redford JB: Conduction studies of the anterior and posterior tibial nerves, *Arch Phys Med Rehabil* 51:164–169, 1970.

[g] Checkles NS, Bailey JA, Johnson EW: Tape and caliper surface measurements in determination of peroneal nerve conduction velocity, *Arch Phys Med Rehabil* 50:217–218, 1969.

[h] Fu R, DeLisa JA, Kraft GH: Motor nerve latencies through the tarsal tunnel in normal adult subjects: standard determinations corrected for temperature and distance, *Arch Phys Med Rehabil* 61: 243–248, 1980.

[i] Needle recording electrode is inserted at the EIP.

[j] Ankle → AH segment specifically tests distal motor latency of medial plantar branch of tibial nerve.

SD = standard deviation; cm = centimeter; msec = millisecond; m/sec = meters per second; PIN = posterior interosseous nerve branch of radial nerve; APB = abductor pollicis brevis; ADQ = abductor digiti quinti; EIP = extensor indices propius; EDB = extensor digitorum brevis; AH = abductor hallucis.

Appendix A-5. Reference values for sensory nerve conduction studies (these values are to be used as guidelines as every laboratory should ideally collect its own set of reference values; also, the patient's unaffected limb may be used as a "normal" reference)

| SENSORY NERVE | DISTAL SEGMENT | | DISTAL LATENCY | | AMPLITUDE |
	ANTIDROMIC TECHNIQUE (STIMULATING → RECORDING ELECTRODE)	DISTANCE (CM)	ONSET LATENCY MEAN ± 1 SD	PEAK LATENCY MEAN ± 1 SD (RANGE)	MEAN ± 1 SD (RANGE)
Median[a,b]	Distal crease of wrist → 2nd or 3rd digit	14	2.4 ± 0.3 msec	3.0 ± 0.3 msec	41.6 ± 25 µV (10–90 µV)
Ulnar[a,c]	Wrist → 5th digit	14	2.4 ± 0.3 msec	3.0 ± 0.3 msec	(15–50 µV)
Superficial radial[d]	Forearm → 1st web space	10	1.8 ± 0.3 msec	2.3 ± 0.4 msec	31 ± 20 µV (13–60 µV)
		12	2.1 ± 0.3 msec	2.6 ± 0.4 msec	
		14	2.4 ± 0.3 msec	2.9 ± 0.4 msec	
Superficial peroneal[e]	Anterolateral leg → anteromedial area of lateral malleolus[g]	12		2.9 ± 0.3 msec	20.5 ± 6.1 µV
Sural[f]	Lower calf → area behind lateral malleolus[h]	14		3.5 ± 0.2 msec (3.0–4.0 msec)	(5–30 µV)

Data adapted from

[a] Cohn TG, Wertsch JJ, Pasupuleti DV, et al: Nerve conduction studies: orthodromic vs. antidromic latencies, Arch Phys Med Rehabil 71:579–582, 1990.
[b] Melvin JL, Schuchmann JA, Lanese RR: Diagnostic specificity of motor and sensory nerve conduction variables in the carpal tunnel syndrome, Arch Phys Med Rehabil 54:69–74, 1973.
[c] Johnson EW, Melvin JL: Sensory conduction studies of median and ulnar nerves, Arch Phys Med Rehabil 48:25–30, 1967.
[d] Mackenzie K, DeLisa JA: Distal latency measurement of the superficial radial nerve in normal adult subjects; Arch Phys Med Rehabil 62:31–34, 1981.
[e] Jabre JF: The superficial peroneal sensory nerve revisited, Arch Neurol 38:666–667, 1981.
[f] Schuchmann JA: Sural nerve conduction: a standardized technique, Arch Phys Med Rehabil 58:166–168, 1977.
[g] Normal sensory conduction velocity of superficial peroneal nerve (specifically intermediate dorsal cutaneous branch) = 65.7 ± 3.7 m/sec.
[h] Normal sensory conduction velocity of sural nerve for 0–14 cm = 40.1 m/sec.
cm = centimeter; SD = standard deviation; msec = millisecond; µV = microvolt; m/sec = meters per second.

Appendix A-6.   Reference values for F-wave studies (these values are to be used as guidelines as every laboratory should ideally collect its own set of reference values; also, the patient's unaffected limb may be used as a "normal" reference)

MOTOR NERVE	PICK-UP SITE	F-LATENCY[d] MEAN ± 1 SD	M-LATENCY MEAN ± 1 SD	F-WAVE CONDUCTION VELOCITY[e] (TO AND FROM SC) MEAN ± 1 SD	F-RATIO[f] MEAN ± 1 SD
Median[a,b]	APB	Wr = 29.1 ± 2.3 msec El = 24.8 ± 2.0 msec Ax = 21.7 ± 2.8 msec	Wr = 3.5 ± 0.5 msec El = 7.8 ± 0.8 msec Ax = 11.3 ± 1.0 msec	Wr = 59.2 ± 3.9 m/sec El = 62.2 ± 5.2 m/sec Ax = 64.3 ± 6.4 m/sec	El = 1.04 ± 0.09
Ulnar[a,b]	ADQ	Wr = 30.5 ± 3.0 msec bEl = 26.0 ± 2.0 msec aEl = 23.5 ± 2.0 msec Ax = 21.9 ± 1.9 msec	Wr = 2.9 ± 0.5 msec bEl = 6.7 ± 0.7 msec aEl = 9.2 ± 0.9 msec Ax = 11.2 ± 1.0 msec	Wr = 56.7 ± 2.9 m/sec bEl = 58.2 ± 2.9 m/sec aEl = 61.1 ± 5.4 m/sec Ax = 63.1 ± 5.9 m/sec	bEl = 1.40 ± 0.11
Peroneal[b,c]	EDB	An = 51.3 ± 4.7 msec Kn = 42.7 ± 4.0 msec	An = 4.5 ± 0.9 msec Kn = 12.9 ± 1.4 msec	An = 53.3 ± 3.8 m/sec Kn = 56.3 ± 4.9 m/sec	Kn = 1.11 ± 0.09
Tibial[b,c]	AH	An = 52.3 ± 4.3 msec Kn = 43.5 ± 3.4 msec	An = 4.1 ± 0.6 msec Kn = 12.9 ± 1.3 msec	An = 51.3 ± 2.9 m/sec Kn = 54.4 ± 3.6 m/sec	Kn = 1.17 ± 0.10

Data adapted from

[a] Kimura J: F-wave velocity in the central segment of the median and ulnar nerves: a study in normal subjects and in patients with Charcot-Marie-Tooth disease, *Neurology* 24:539–546, 1974.

[b] Kimura J: F-wave determinations in nerve conduction studies. In Desmedt JE, editor: Motor control mechanisms in health and disease, New York, 1983, Raven Press, pp 961–975.

[c] Kimura J, Bosch P, Linday GM: F-wave conduction velocity in the central segment of the peroneal and tibial nerves, *Arch Phys Med Rehabil* 56:492–497, 1975.

[d] The F latency is the shortest onset latency after 10–20 F-wave stimulations.

[e] F-wave conduction velocity (m/sec) = (nerve distance in mm × 2)/(F latency in msec − M latency in msec − 1), where nerve distance is measured using a tape measure as follows: (a) for the median or ulnar nerve, measure from the stimulus site along the course of the nerve to the axilla (with arm abducted 90°), then around the back of the shoulder (posteriorly) to the C7 spinous process; (b) for the peroneal or tibial nerve, measure from the stimulus site along the course of the nerve to the greater trochanter of the femur then posteriorly to the lower border of the T12 spinous process.

[f] The F ratio refers to the ratio between proximal and distal segments of the nerve, with cathode stimulation at the volar crease of the elbow (for median nerve); 3 cm above the medial epicondyle (for ulnar nerve), just above the fibular head (for peroneal nerve), and in the popliteal fossa (for tibial nerve). The F-ratio formula is (F latency in msec − M latency in msec − 1)/(M latency in msec × 2). By using the F ratio, there is theoretically less potential for errors as it circumvents the need for measuring nerve length. However, F ratio assumes that various limbs of different length have the same proportion for the proximal and distal segments (bisected at either the elbow or knee).

SD = standard deviation; msec = millisecond; m/sec = meters per second; Wr = wrist; El = elbow; bEl = below elbow; aEl = above elbow; Ax = axilla; An = ankle; Kn = knee; APB = abductor pollicis brevis; ADQ = abductor digiti quinti; EDB = extensor digitorum brevis; AH = abductor hallucis.

EMG FINDINGS

EMG Steps / LESION	NORMAL	NEUROGENIC LESION		MYOGENIC LESION		
		Lower Motor	Upper Motor	Myopathy	Myotonia	Polymyositis
1 Insertional Activity	Normal	Increased	Normal	Normal	Myotonic Discharge	Increased
2 Spontaneous Activity	—	Fibrillation Positive Wave		—	—	Fibrillation Positive Wave
3 Motor Unit Potential	0.5-1.0 mv 5-10msec	Large Unit Limited Recruitment	Normal	Small Unit Early Recruitment	Myotonic Discharge	Small Unit Early Recruitment
4 Interference Pattern	Full	Reduced Fast Firing Rate	Reduced Slow Firing Rate	Full Low Amplitude	Full Low Amplitude	Full Low Amplitude

Appendix A-7

Summary of typical findings of needle electromyography in normal muscle and in neurogenic and myogenic lesions. From: Kimura, J: *Electrodiagnosis in diseases of nerve and muscle: Principles and practice*, ed 2, Philadelphia, 1989, F.A. Davis, p. 252, with permission).

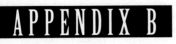

APPENDIX B

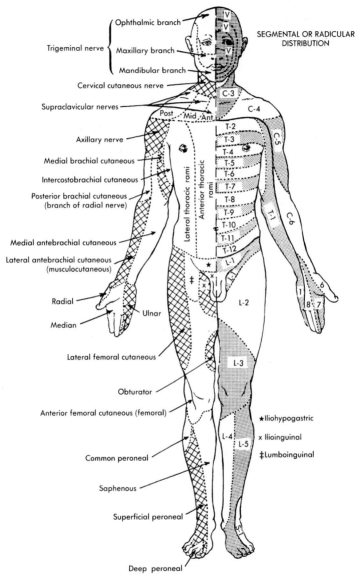

PERIPHERAL DISTRIBUTION

SEGMENTAL OR RADICULAR DISTRIBUTION

Trigeminal nerve — Ophthalmic branch
Maxillary branch
Mandibular branch

Cervical cutaneous nerve

Supraclavicular nerves

Axillary nerve

Medial brachial cutaneous

Intercostobrachial cutaneous

Posterior brachial cutaneous (branch of radial nerve)

Medial antebrachial cutaneous

Lateral antebrachial cutaneous (musculocutaneous)

Radial

Median   Ulnar

Lateral femoral cutaneous

Obturator

Anterior femoral cutaneous (femoral)

Common peroneal

Saphenous

Superficial peroneal

Deep peroneal

Lateral thoracic rami   Anterior thoracic rami

Post   Mid   Ant

★ Iliohypogastric
x Ilioinguinal
‡ Lumboinguinal

Appendix B-1

Sensory distribution of major peripheral nerves and dermatomes corresponding to spinal cord segments, anterior view. (From: Chusid JG: *Correlative neuroanatomy and functional neurology*, ed, 19, Los Altos, CA, 1985, Lange Medical Publications, p. 233, Copyright © 1985 Appleton & Lange, with permission).

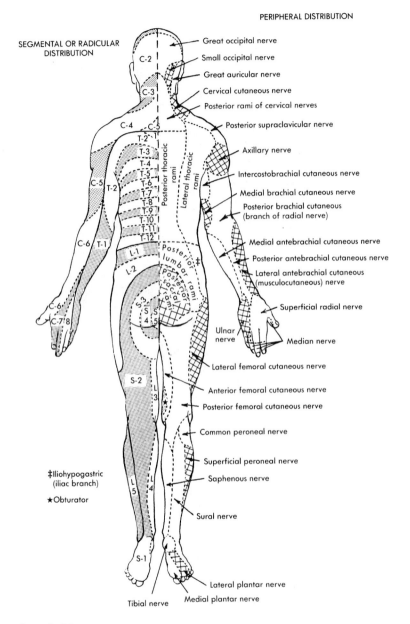

Appendix B-2
Sensory distribution of major peripheral nerves and dermatomes corresponding to spinal cord segments, posterior view. (From: Chusid JG: *Correlative neuroanatomy and functional neurology*, ed. 19, Los Altos, CA, 1985, Lange Medical Publications, p. 233, Copyright © 1985 Appleton & Lange, with permission.)

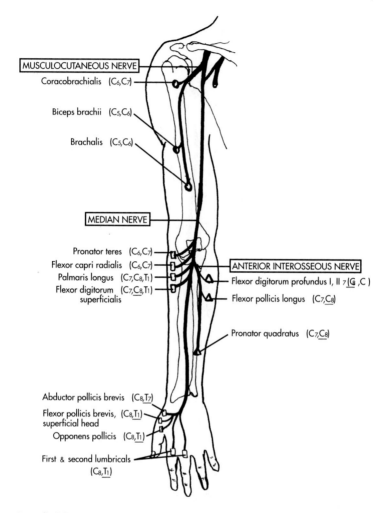

Diagram showing:

MUSCULOCUTANEOUS NERVE
Coracobrachialis (C_6, C_7)
Biceps brachii (C_5, C_6)
Brachialis (C_5, C_6)

MEDIAN NERVE

Pronator teres (C_6, C_7)
Flexor capri radialis (C_6, C_7)
Palmaris longus (C_7, C_8, T_1)
Flexor digitorum ($C_7, \underline{C_8}, T_1$)
superficialis

ANTERIOR INTEROSSEOUS NERVE
Flexor digitorum profundus I, II $_7$ ($\underline{C}$, C)
Flexor pollicis longus ($C_7, \underline{C_8}$)
Pronator quadratus ($C_7, \underline{C_8}$)

Abductor pollicis brevis (C_8, T_7)
Flexor pollicis brevis, ($C_8, \underline{T_1}$)
superficial head
Opponens pollicis ($C_8, \underline{T_1}$)
First & second lumbricals
($C_8, \underline{T_1}$)

Appendix B-3a
Diagram of motor innervation of the upper limb showing the branches of the musculocutaneous and median nerves. The predominant root supply is underlined. (Adapted from: The Guarantors of Brain: *Aids to the examination of the peripheral nervous system,* East Sussex, England, 1986, Balliere Tindall).

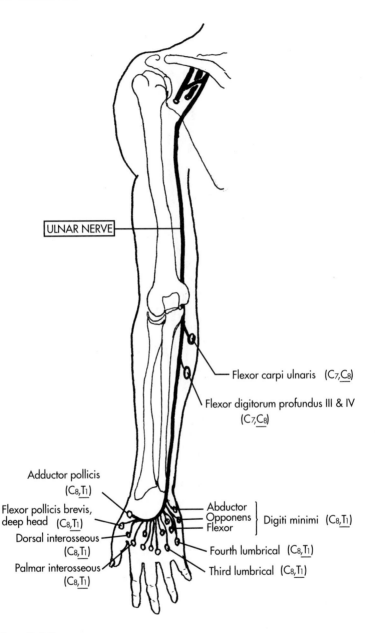

ULNAR NERVE

Flexor carpi ulnaris (C₇,C₈)

Flexor digitorum profundus III & IV
(C₇,C₈)

Adductor pollicis
(C₈,T₁)

Flexor pollicis brevis,
deep head (C₈,T₁)

Dorsal interosseous
(C₈,T₁)

Palmar interosseous
(C₈,T₁)

Abductor
Opponens } Digiti minimi (C₈,T₁)
Flexor

Fourth lumbrical (C₈,T₁)

Third lumbrical (C₈,T₁)

Appendix B-3b
Diagram of motor innervation of the upper limb showing the branches of the ulnar
nerve. The predominant root supply in underlined. (Adapted from: The Guarantors
of Brain: *Aids to the examination of the peripheral nervous system*, East Sussex,
England, 1986, Balliere Tindall).

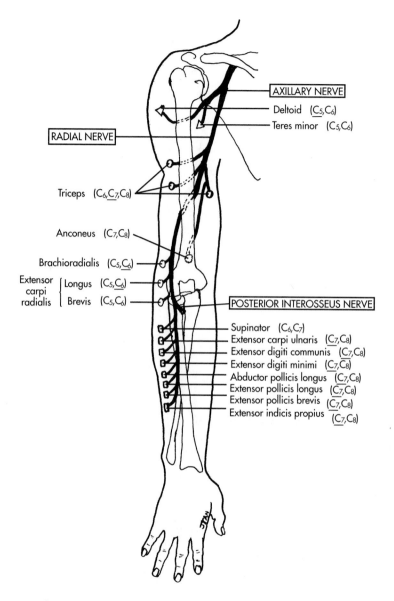

Appendix B-3c

Diagram of motor innervation of the upper limb showing the branches of the axillary and radial nerves. The predominant root supply is underlined. (Adapted from: The Guarantors of Brain: *Aids to the examination of the peripheral nervous system,* East Sussex, England, 1986, Balliere Tindall).

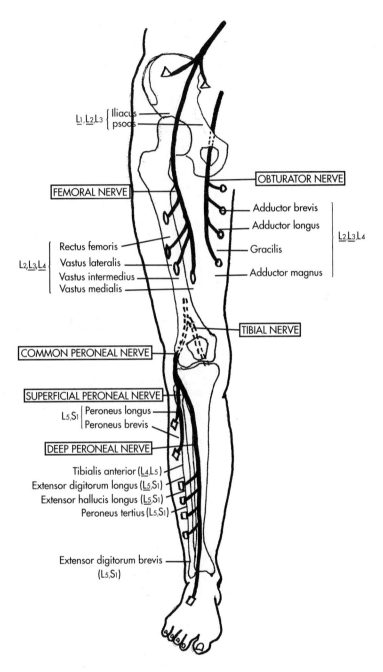

L1,L2L3 { Iliacus
          psoas

FEMORAL NERVE

OBTURATOR NERVE

Adductor brevis

Adductor longus

L2L3,L4 { Rectus femoris
          Vastus lateralis
          Vastus intermedius
          Vastus medialis

Gracilis

Adductor magnus

L2L3,L4

TIBIAL NERVE

COMMON PERONEAL NERVE

SUPERFICIAL PERONEAL NERVE

L5,S1 { Peroneus longus
         Peroneus brevis

DEEP PERONEAL NERVE

Tibialis anterior (L4,L5)
Extensor digitorum longus (L5,S1)
Extensor hallucis longus (L5,S1)
Peroneus tertius (L5,S1)

Extensor digitorum brevis
(L5,S1)

Appendix B-4a

Diagram of motor innervation of the lower limb showing the branches of the femoral, obturator and common peroneal nerves. The predominant root supply is underlined. (Adapted from: The Guarantors of Brain: *Aids to the examination of the peripheral nervous system*, East Sussex, England, 1986, Balliere Tindall).

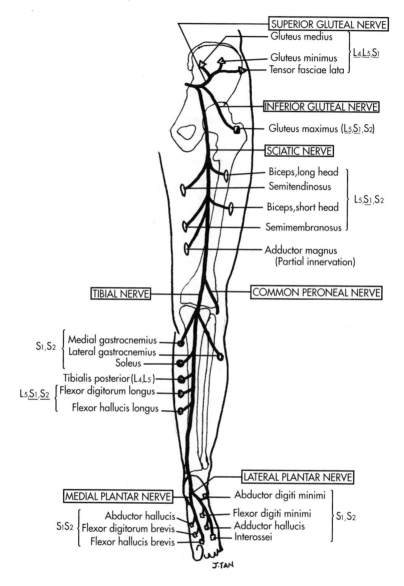

Appendix B-4b

Diagram of motor innervation of the lower limb showing the branches of the gluteal, sciatic, and tibial nerves. The predominant root supply is underlined. (Adapted from: The Guarantors of Brain: *Aids to the examination of the peripheral nervous system*, East Sussex, England, 1986, Balliere Tindall).

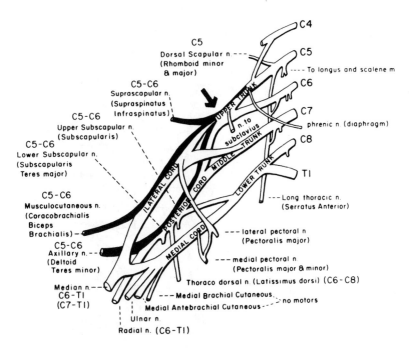

Appendix B-5

Diagram of the brachial plexus. The arrow indicates the Erb's point. Posterior nerves are shaded. (From: Torg JS, Shephard RJ. *Current therapy in sports medicine*, ed 3, St. Louis, 1995, Mosby, p. 62; with permission).

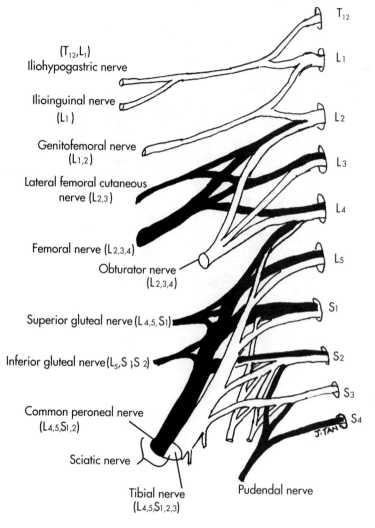

T_{12}

L_1

(T_{12}, L_1)
Iliohypogastric nerve

L_2

Ilioinguinal nerve
(L_1)

Genitofemoral nerve
$(L_{1,2})$

L_3

Lateral femoral cutaneous
nerve $(L_{2,3})$

L_4

Femoral nerve $(L_{2,3,4})$

L_5

Obturator nerve
$(L_{2,3,4})$

S_1

Superior gluteal nerve $(L_{4,5}, S_1)$

S_2

Inferior gluteal nerve $(L_5, S_1 S_2)$

S_3

Common peroneal nerve
$(L_{4,5}, S_{1,2})$

S_4

J.TAN

Sciatic nerve

Tibial nerve
$(L_{4,5}, S_{1,2,3})$

Pudendal nerve

Appendix B-6
Diagram of the Lumbosacral plexus. Posterior nerves are shaded.

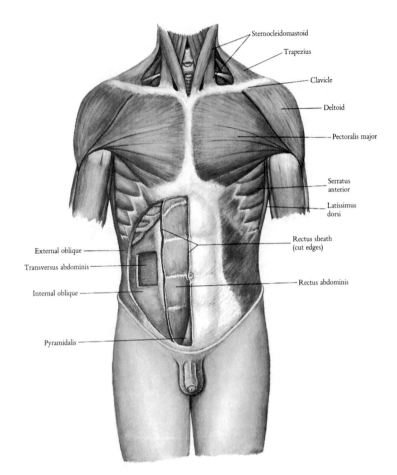

Appendix B-7
Superficial muscles of the trunk, anterior view. (From Seidel HM, Ball JW, Dains JE, et al: Mosby's guide to physical examination, ed 3, St. Louis, 1995, Mosby, p. 650, with permission).

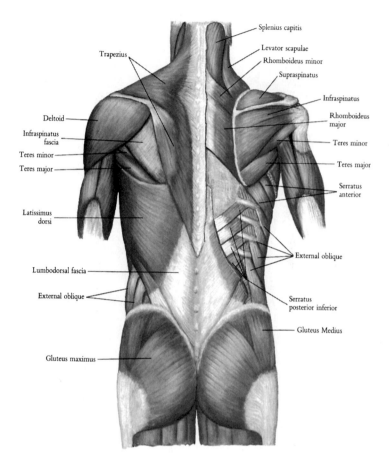

Splenius capitis

Levator scapulae

Rhomboideus minor

Supraspinatus

Trapezius

Infraspinatus

Deltoid

Rhomboideus major

Infraspinatus fascia

Teres minor

Teres minor

Teres major

Teres major

Serratus anterior

Latissimus dorsi

Lumbodorsal fascia

External oblique

External oblique

Serratus posterior inferior

Gluteus Medius

Gluteus maximus

Appendix B-8
Superficial muscles of the trunk, posterior view. (From Seidel HM, Ball JW, Dains JE, et al: Mosby's guide to physical examination, ed 3, St. Louis, 1995, Mosby, p. 651, with permission).

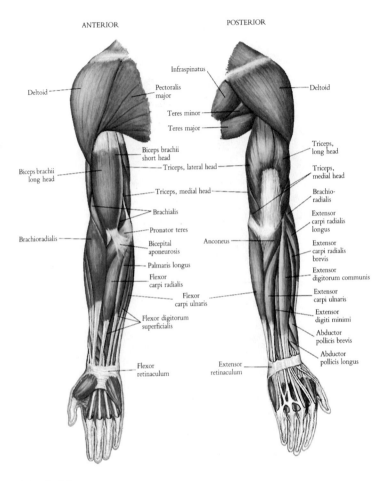

ANTERIOR

POSTERIOR

Deltoid

Pectoralis
major

Infraspinatus

Deltoid

Teres minor

Teres major

Biceps brachii
short head

Triceps, lateral head

Triceps,
long head

Triceps,
medial head

Biceps brachii
long head

Triceps, medial head

Brachialis

Brachio-
radialis

Brachioradialis

Pronator teres

Bicepital
aponeurosis

Palmaris longus

Flexor
carpi radialis

Flexor
carpi ulnaris

Flexor digitorum
superficialis

Flexor
retinaculum

Anconeus

Extensor
carpi radialis
longus

Extensor
carpi radialis
brevis

Extensor
digitorum communis

Extensor
carpi ulnaris

Extensor
digiti minimi

Abductor
pollicis brevis

Abductor
pollicis longus

Extensor
retinaculum

Appendix B-9
Muscles of the upper limbs. (From Seidel HM, Ball JW, Dains JE, et al: Mosby's guide to physical examination, ed 3, St. Louis, 1995, Mosby, p. 646, with permission).

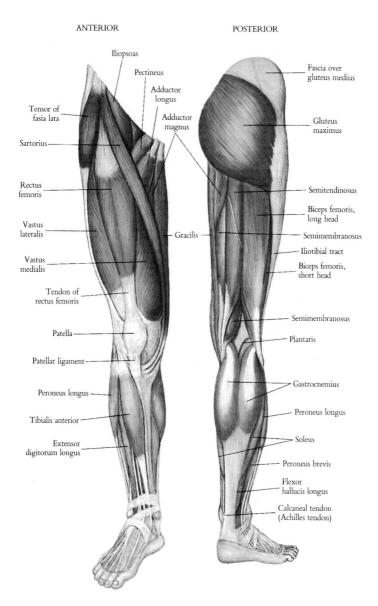

ANTERIOR

POSTERIOR

Iliopsoas

Pectineus

Adductor longus

Adductor magnus

Tensor of fasia lata

Sartorius

Rectus femoris

Vastus lateralis

Vastus medialis

Tendon of rectus femoris

Patella

Patellar ligament

Peroneus longus

Tibialis anterior

Extensor digitorum longus

Gracilis

Fascia over gluteus medius

Gluteus maximus

Semitendinosus

Biceps femoris, long head

Semimembranosus

Iliotibial tract

Biceps femoris, short head

Semimembranosus

Plantaris

Gastrocnemius

Peroneus longus

Soleus

Peroneus brevis

Flexor hallucis longus

Calcaneal tendon (Achilles tendon)

Appendix B-10
Muscles of the lower limbs. (From Seidel HM, Ball JW, Dains JE, et al: Mosby's guide to physical examination, ed 3, St. Louis, 1995, Mosby, p. 647, with permission).

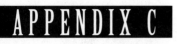

APPENDIX C

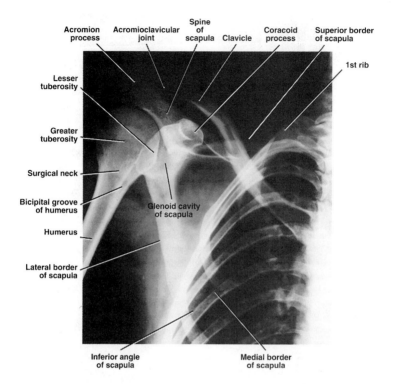

Appendix C-1

Anteroposterior radiograph of the shoulder joint with the humerus medially rotated. (From Snell R, Smith M: *Clinical anatomy for emergency medicine*, St. Louis, 1993, Mosby, p. 590, with permission).

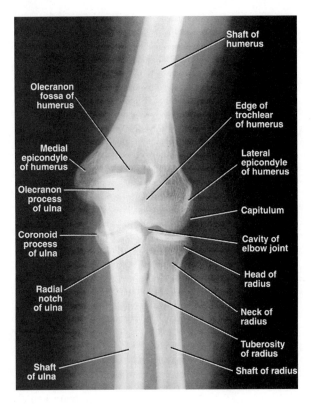

Appendix C-2

Anteroposterior radiograph of the elbow joint. (From Snell R, Smith M: *Clinical anatomy for emergency medicine*, St. Louis, 1993, Mosby, p. 592, with permission).

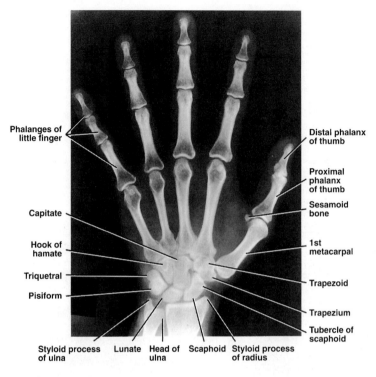

Phalanges of
little finger

Capitate

Hook of
hamate

Triquetral

Pisiform

Distal phalanx
of thumb

Proximal
phalanx
of thumb

Sesamoid
bone

1st
metacarpal

Trapezoid

Trapezium

Tubercle of
scaphoid

Styloid process   Lunate   Head of   Scaphoid   Styloid process
of ulna   ulna   of radius

Appendix C-3
Posteroanterior radiograph of the wrist and hand with the forearm pronated. (From
Snell R, Smith M: *Clinical anatomy for emergency medicine*, St. Louis, 1993,
Mosby, p. 650, with permission).

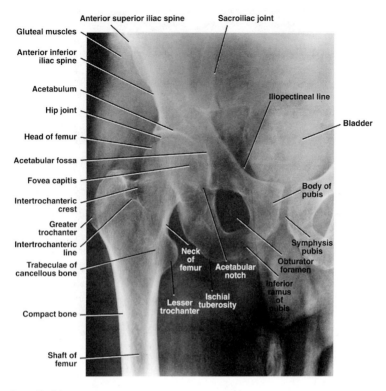

Appendix C-4
Anteroposterior radiograph of the hip joint and pelvis. (From Snell R, Smith M: *Clinical anatomy for emergency medicine*, St. Louis, 1993, Mosby, p. 703, with permission).

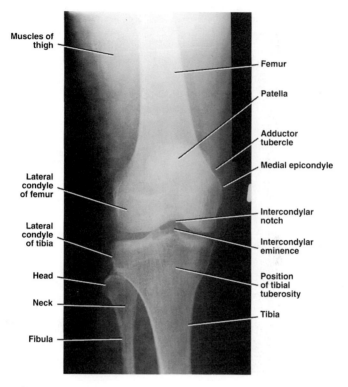

Muscles of thigh

Femur

Patella

Adductor tubercle

Medial epicondyle

Lateral condyle of femur

Intercondylar notch

Lateral condyle of tibia

Intercondylar eminence

Head

Position of tibial tuberosity

Neck

Tibia

Fibula

Appendix C-5
Anteroposterior radiograph of the knee joint. (From Snell R, Smith M: *Clinical anatomy for emergency medicine*, St. Louis, 1993, Mosby, p. 707, with permission).

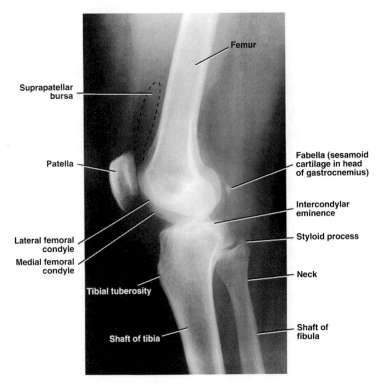

Appendix C-6
Lateral radiograph of the knee joint. (From Snell R, Smith M: *Clinical anatomy for emergency medicine*, St. Louis, 1993, Mosby, p. 708, with permission).

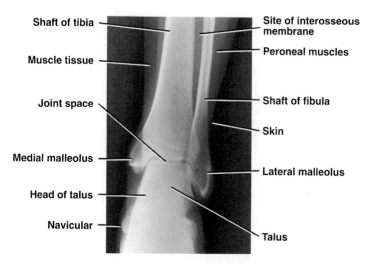

Shaft of tibia

Muscle tissue

Joint space

Medial malleolus

Head of talus

Navicular

Site of interosseous membrane

Peroneal muscles

Shaft of fibula

Skin

Lateral malleolus

Talus

Appendix C-7
Anteroposterior radiograph of the ankle joint. (From Snell R, Smith M: *Clinical anatomy for emergency medicine*, St. Louis, 1993, Mosby, p. 711, with permission).

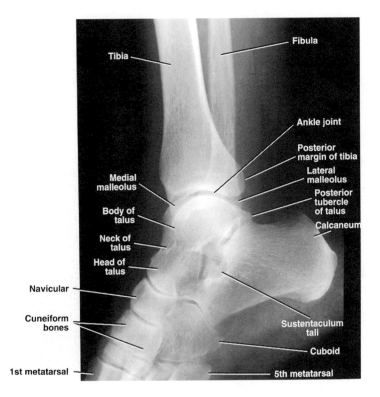

Appendix C-8
Lateral radiograph of the ankle joint. (From Snell R, Smith M: *Clinical anatomy for emergency medicine*, St. Louis, 1993, Mosby, p. 711, with permission).

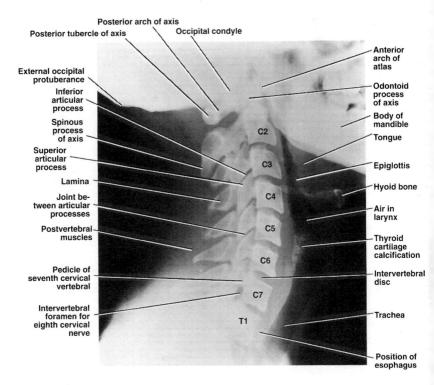

Appendix C-9

Lateral radiograph of the cervical spine. (From Snell R, Smith M: *Clinical anatomy for emergency medicine*, St. Louis, 1993, Mosby, p. 186, with permission).

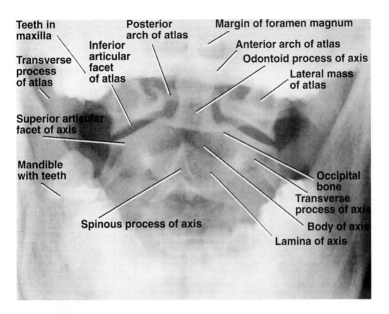

Teeth in maxilla

Posterior arch of atlas

Margin of foramen magnum

Inferior articular facet of atlas

Anterior arch of atlas

Transverse process of atlas

Odontoid process of axis

Lateral mass of atlas

Superior articular facet of axis

Mandible with teeth

Occipital bone

Transverse process of axis

Spinous process of axis

Body of axis

Lamina of axis

Appendix C-10
Anteroposterior radiograph of the upper cervical spine with the patient's mouth open to show the odontoid process. (From Snell R, Smith M: *Clinical anatomy for emergency medicine*, St. Louis, 1993, Mosby, p. 360, with permission).

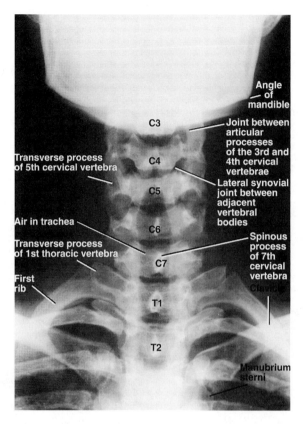

Appendix C-11
Anteroposterior radiograph of the cervical spine. (From Snell R, Smith M: *Clinical anatomy for emergency medicine*, St. Louis, 1993, Mosby, p. 360, with permission).

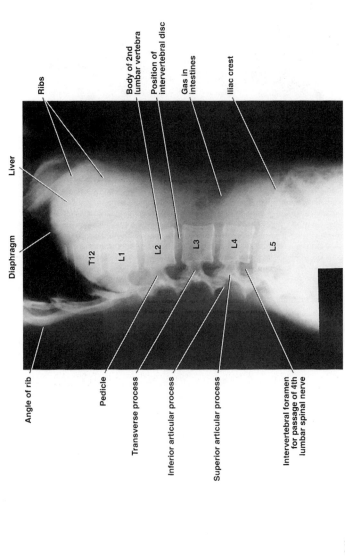

Appendix C-12

Lateral radiograph of the lumbar spine. (From Snell R, Smith M: *Clinical anatomy for emergency medicine,* St. Louis, 1993, Mosby, p. 365, with permission).

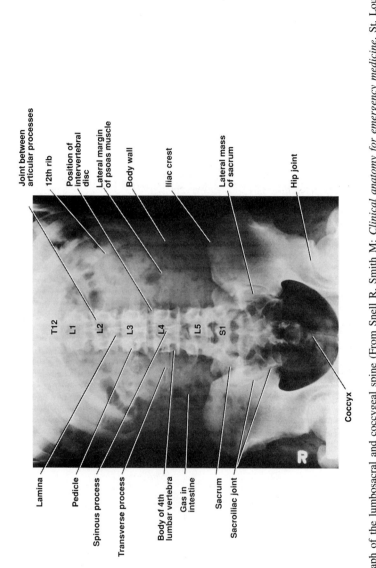

Appendix C-13

Anteroposterior radiograph of the lumbosacral and coccygeal spine (From Snell R, Smith M: *Clinical anatomy for emergency medicine,* St. Louis, 1993, Mosby, p. 364, with permission).

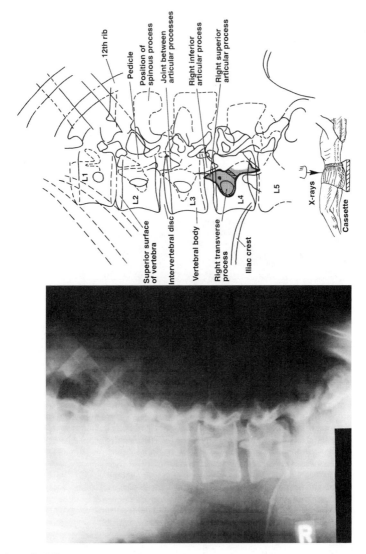

Appendix C-14

Oblique radiograph of the lumbar spine. The stippled "scotty dog" appearance is seen on the fourth lumbar vertebra. The ear of the dog is the superior articular process, the nose is the ipsilateral pedicle, the front leg is the inferior articular process, the body is the contralateral pedicle, the neck is the pars interarticularis (i.e., the area where the pedicle, lamina, and articular processes all converge), and the presence of a "collar" on the dog's neck indicates a defective area of ossification or a traumatic break in the pars interarticularis, called spondylolysis. (From Snell R, Smith M: *Clinical anatomy for emergency medicine*, St. Louis, 1993, Mosby, p. 366–367, with permission).

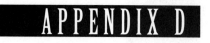

APPENDIX D

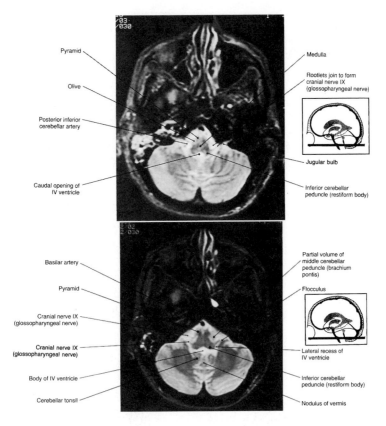

Appendix D

Normal brain MRI, axial view: The following are consecutive T$_2$-weighted magnetic resonance images (with repetition time/echo time [TR/TE] of 2000/80 msec) of the adult brain in axial sections. (Reprinted from Hayman LA, Pfleger MJ, Pagani JJ, et al: Atlas of the adult brain. In Hayman LA, Hinck VC, eds.: *Clinical brain imaging: Normal structure and functional anatomy*, St. Louis, 1992, Mosby, pp. 79–97, with permission).

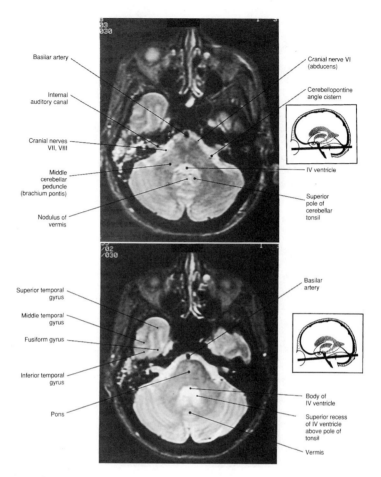

Basilar artery

Internal
auditory canal

Cranial nerves
VII, VIII

Middle
cerebellar
peduncle
(brachium pontis)

Nodulus of
vermis

Cranial nerve VI
(abducens)

Cerebellopontine
angle cistern

IV ventricle

Superior
pole of
cerebellar
tonsil

Superior temporal
gyrus

Middle temporal
gyrus

Fusiform gyrus

Inferior temporal
gyrus

Pons

Basilar
artery

Body of
IV ventricle

Superior recess
of IV ventricle
above pole of
tonsil

Vermis

Appendix D, cont'd
For legend see page 764.

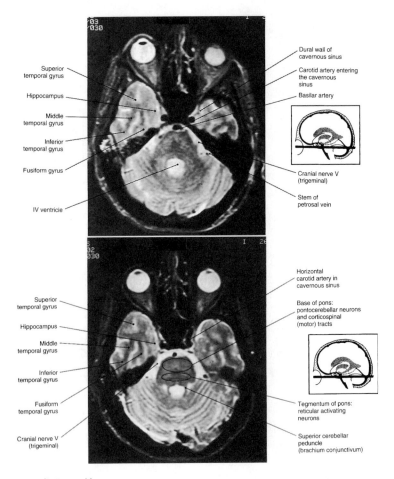

Superior temporal gyrus

Hippocampus

Middle temporal gyrus

Inferior temporal gyrus

Fusiform gyrus

IV ventricle

Dural wall of cavernous sinus

Carotid artery entering the cavernous sinus

Basilar artery

Cranial nerve V (trigeminal)

Stem of petrosal vein

Superior temporal gyrus

Hippocampus

Middle temporal gyrus

Inferior temporal gyrus

Fusiform temporal gyrus

Cranial nerve V (trigeminal)

Horizontal carotid artery in cavernous sinus

Base of pons: pontocerebellar neurons and corticospinal (motor) tracts

Tegmentum of pons: reticular activating neurons

Superior cerebellar peduncle (brachium conjunctivum)

Appendix D, cont'd
For legend see page 764.

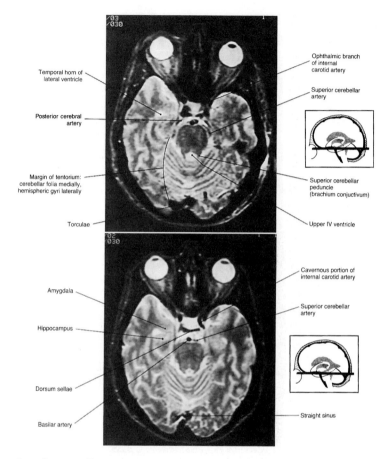

Ophthalmic branch
of internal
carotid artery

Superior cerebellar
artery

Temporal horn of
lateral ventricle

Posterior cerebral
artery

Margin of tentorium:
cerebellar folia medially,
hemispheric gyri laterally

Superior cerebellar
peduncle
(brachium conjuctivum)

Torculae

Upper IV ventricle

Cavernous portion of
internal carotid artery

Amygdala

Superior cerebellar
artery

Hippocampus

Dorsum sellae

Basilar artery

Straight sinus

Appendix D, cont'd
For legend see page 764.

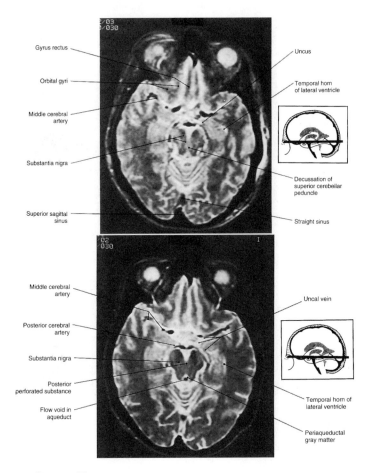

Appendix D, cont'd
For legend see page 764.

Appendix D **769**

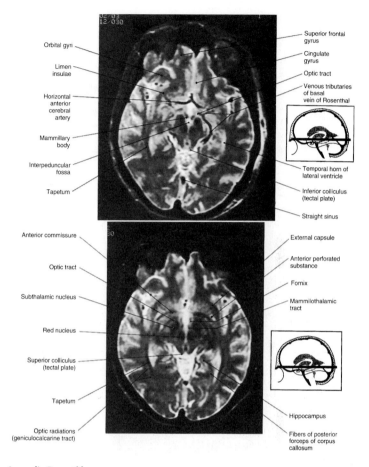

Appendix D, cont'd
For legend see page 764.

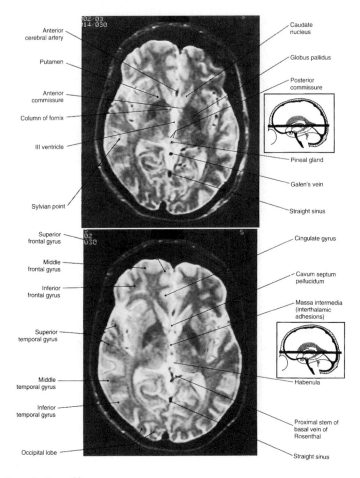

Appendix D, cont'd
For legend see page 764.

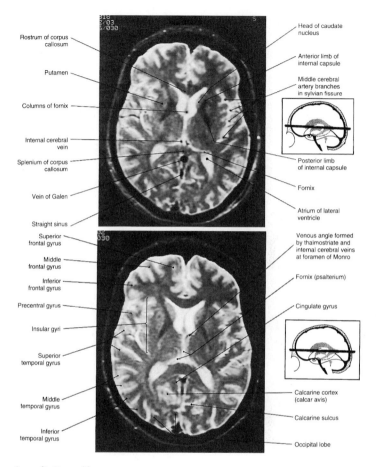

Appendix D, cont'd
For legend see page 764.

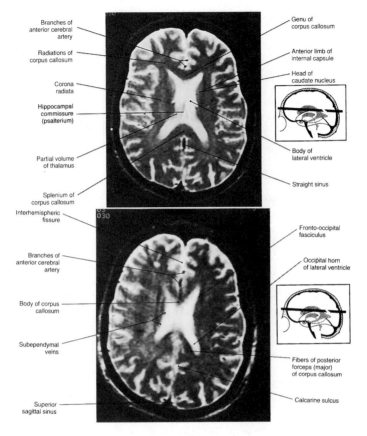

Appendix D, cont'd
For legend see page 764.

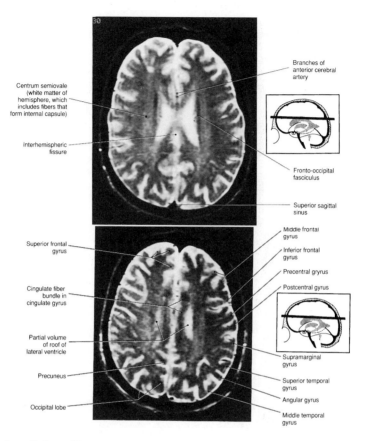

Appendix D, cont'd
For legend see page 764.

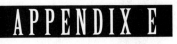

APPENDIX E

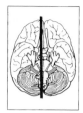

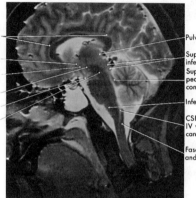

Cingulate gyrus with the fiber tract of the cingulum above

Anterior commissure

Anterior column of fornix

Mammillothalamic tract

Red nucleus

Mammillary body

Pulvinar of thalamus

Superior and inferior colliculi

Superior cerebellar peduncle (brachium conjunctivum)

Inferior olivary nucleus

CSF connection between IV ventricle and central canal of spinal cord

Fasciculi cuneatus and gracile (sensory)

Appendix E

Normal brain MRI (sagittal view). The following are consecutive T_2-weighted magnetic resonance images (with repetition time/echo time [TR/TE] of 2000/80 msec) of the adult brain in sagittal sections. (Reprinted with permission from Hayman LA, Pfleger MJ, Pagani JJ, et al.: Atlas of the adult brain. In Hayman LA, Hinck VC, eds.: *Clinical brain imaging: Normal structure and functional anatomy*, St. Louis, 1992, Mosby, pp. 99–111, with permission).

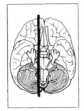

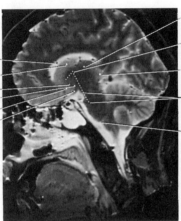

Thalamus

Genu of internal capsule extends ventrally as anterior limb and dorsally as posterior limb

Pulvinar of thalamus

Posterior limb of internal capsule continues inferiorly through cerebral peduncle (crus cerebri) as pyramidal (corticospinal) tract

Foramen caecum separates base of pons from olive of medulla

Frontal horn of the lateral ventricle

Head of the caudate

Anterior commissure

Putamen

Globus pallidus

Optic tract

Appendix E, cont'd
For legend see page 775.

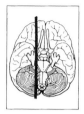

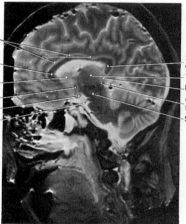

Cortex of the cingulate gyrus with overlying fiber tract (cingulum)

Genu of the corpus callosum

Head of the caudate nucleus

Anterior commissure

Optic tract

III cranial nerve

Splenium of the corpus callosum

Thalamus

Pulvinar of thalamus

Medial geniculate body

Subthalamic nucleus

Appendix E, cont'd
For legend see page 775.

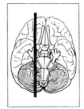

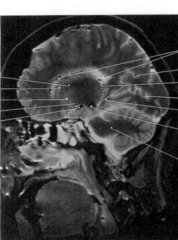

Anterior commissure

Caudate

Putamen

Anterior commissure

Optic tract

Central sulcus (Rolando)

Air and CSF in
the lateral ventricle

Parieto-occipital fissure

Wing of ambient cistern
joins choroidal fissure

Calcarine fissure

Isthmus of cingulate gyrus

Genu of internal capsule
becomes cerebral peduncle
(crus cerebri)

Middle cerebellar peduncle
(brachium pontis)

Appendix E, cont'd
For legend see page 775.

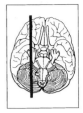

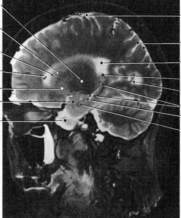

Posterior limb of internal capsule

Head of the caudate nucleus

Gliotic residual of germinal matrix

Frontal horn of the lateral ventricle

Putamen

Amygdala

Tip of the temporal lobe

Central fissure (Rolando)

Parieto-occipital fissure

Choroid glomus in the atrium (trigone) of the lateral ventricle

Fimbria of fornix

Occipital horn of the lateral ventricle

Subiculum

Dentate gyrus

Hippocampus

Appendix E, cont'd
For legend see page 775.

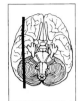

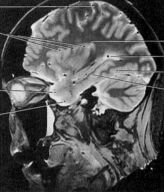

Central fissure (Rolando)

Insular cortex

Corona radiata

Atrium (trigone) of the lateral ventricle

Medial occipito-temporal gyrus

Superior temporal gyrus

Parahippocampal gyrus

Fusiform (lateral occipitotemporal) gyrus

Pathway of short association fibers that interconnect adjacent cerebral gyri throughout the brain

Transverse temporal gyrus of Heschl

Long gyri

Short gyri

Auditory radiations

Limen insulare

Optic radiations (Meyer's loop)

Appendix E, cont'd
For legend see page 775.

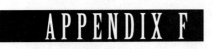

APPENDIX F

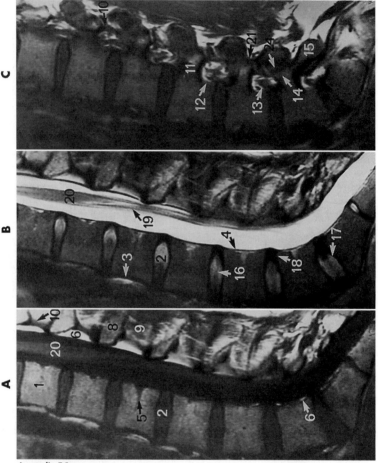

Appendix F-1

High resolution MR imaging of the sagittal section of the lumbar spine. A (T₁-weighted) and B (T₂-weighted) demonstrate normal midline anatomy. C is a T₁-weighted sagittal scan through the neural foramen showing the relationship of the soft tissues to the surrounding bone and intervertebral disk. 1, vertebral body. 2, intervertebral disk (nucleus pulposus). 3, anterior longitudinal ligament. 4, posterior longitudinal ligament. 5, basivertebral venous plexus. 6, epidural fat. 8, spinous processes. 9, interspinous ligament. 10, ligamentum flavum. 11, pedicle, 12, neural foramen with epidural fat and veins. 13, dorsal root ganglion. 14, superior articular facet. 15, inferior articular facet. 16, intranuclear cleft. 17, inner annular fibers of disk. 18, outer annular fibers of disk. 19, cauda equina. 20, conus medullaris. 21, pars interarticularis. 24, facet joint. (From Osborne AG: *Diagnostic neuroradiology,* vol 1, St. Louis, 1994, Mosby, p. 789, with permission).

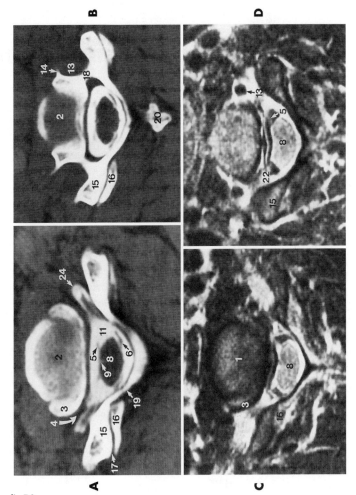

Appendix F-2

Multimodality imaging studies showing the axial anatomy of the spine. Axial CT scans (A and B) with intrathecal contrast are shown at the level of the uncovertebral joint and neural foramina (A) and the pedicles (B). C and D are axial T_2-weighted MR scans which depict normal cervical spinal cord and soft tissue anatomy. Prominent areas of high velocity signal loss from pulsatile CSF flow are present. 1, vertebral body. 2, intervertebral disk (nucleus pulposus). 3, uncinate process. 4, neural foramen. 5, anterior roots. 6, posterior roots. 8, cervical spinal cord. 9, ventral medial fissure. 11, subarachnoid space. 13, vertebral artery in foramen transversarium. 14, transverse process. 15, superior articular facet. 16, inferior articular facet. 17, facet joint. 18, pedicle. 19, lamina. 20, spinous process. 22, epidural fat. 24, root sleeve. (From Osborne AG: *Diagnostic neuroradiology,* vol 1, St. Louis, 1994, Mosby, p. 796, with permission).

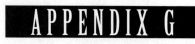

APPENDIX G

RESOURCES

G-1. **Accessibility (Home and Community) for the Disabled**

Access Board, 1331 F St. N.W., Ste. 1000, Washington DC 20004-1111, Tel (202) 272-5434; (202) 272-5449; (800) USA-ABLE

Access Equals Opportunity (Guidebook), Council of Better Business Bureau Foundation, 4200 Wilson Blvd., Ste. 800, Arlington, VA 22203, Tel. (703) 247-3656; Fax: (703) 525-8277

Access House *(Barrier-free regulations),* 1109 E. 139th Ave., Tampa, FL 33613, Tel. (813) 972-2289

Access for All *(Information book),* Hospital Audiences, Inc, 220 West 42nd St., New York, NY 10036, Tel. (212) 575-7660; Fax: (212) 575-7673

Accessibility Standards Illustrated *(Guidebook),* 401 South Spring St., Springfield, IL 62706

An Accessible Home of Your Own *(Guidebook),* Accent Books & Products, P.O. Box 700, Bloomington, IL 61702, Tel. (309) 378-2961; (800) 787-8444; Fax: (309) 378-4420

Accessible Housing Design File *(Book),* Van Nostrand Reinhold, 7625 Empire Drive, Florence, KY 41042, Tel. (606) 525-6600; (800) 942-3636

Adaptable Housing (Guidebook), Rehabilitation Institute of Chicago, 345 E. Superior St., Chicago, IL 60611

Adaptable Housing: A Technical Manual for Implementing Adaptable Dwelling *(Book),* HUD USER (Distributor), P.O. Box 6091, Rockville, MD 20850, Tel. (301) 251-5154; (800) 245-2691

Adaptive Environments Center, 374 Congress St., Ste. 301, Boston, MA 02210, Tel. (617) 695-1225; Fax: (617) 482-8099

Adaptive Environments Center Home Assessment Form, Massachusetts College of Art, 621 Huntington Ave., Boston, MA 02115

American National Standards Institute (ANSI), 1430 Broadway, New York, NY 10018, Tel. (212) 642-4900

An Approach to Barrier Free Design Magazine *(Guidebook),* A Positive Approach, P.O. Box 910, Millville, NJ 08332, Tel. (609) 451-4777; Fax: (609) 451-6678

Architectural & Transportation Barriers Compliance Board: Resource Guide *(Book),* see Access Board

Arts and 504: A 504 Handbook for Accessible Arts Programming, Office for Special Constituencies (Distributor), 1100 Pennsylvania Ave. NW, Washington, DC 20506, Tel. (202) 682-5531

AutoBOOK: ADA Disability Law Software and Subscription Service, ABA/Commission on Mental & Physical Disability Law, 1800 M St. N.W., Washington, DC 20036, Tel. (202) 331-2240; Fax: (202) 331-2220

Barrier Free Environments (BFE), P.O. Box 30634, Water Garden, Highway 70 West Raleigh, NC 27622

Center for Universal Design, North Carolina State University, P.O. Box 8613, Raleigh, NC 27695, Tel. (919) 515-3082; (800) 647-6777; TDD: (919) 737-3032

Directory of Accessible Building Products *(Book),* NAHB Research Center, 400 Prince George's Blvd., Upper Marlboro, MD 20774, Tel. (301) 249-4000; (800) 638-8556

Easy Street, Guynes Design, 1201 East Jefferson St., Ste. B125, Phoenix, AZ 85034

E.C.H.O. Housing: Recommended Construction and Installation Standards *(Book),* American Association of Retired Persons, 601 East St. N.W., Washington, DC 20049, Tel. (202) 434-2277

Electronic House: Journal of Home Automation *(Journal),* Electronic House, Inc., 205 W. 7th Ave., Ste. 202, Stillwater, OK 74074, Tel. (800) 375-8015

Fair Housing Design Guide for Accessibility *(Guidebook),* National Council on Multifamily Housing Industry, 15th & M St. N.W., Washington, DC 20005, Tel. (202) 822-0200

A Guide to Accessibility of Terminals (Access Travel: Airports), Airports Council International–North America, Consumer Information Center, Department 575A, Pueblo, CO 81009, Tel. (202) 501-1794

Handi-Lift, Inc. *(Stairway Lifts),* 436 W. Main St., Wykoff, NJ 07481, Tel. (201) 891-8097; (800) 432-LIFT

Ideas for Making Your Home Accessible *(Book),* Accent Books & Products, P.O. Box 700, Bloomington, IL 61702, Tel. (309) 378-2961; (800) 787-8444; Fax: (309) 378-4420

Inclinator Co. of America *(Residential Elevator),* 2200 Paxton St., P.O. Box 1557, Harrisburg, PA 17105, Tel. (717) 234-8065; Fax: (717) 234-0941

Institute for Law and Policy Planning, P.O. Box 5137, Berkeley, CA 94705, Tel. (415) 486-3352

Lifease, Inc., 2550 University Ave. W, Ste. 317 North St., Saint Paul, MN 55114

Medical Liability Advisory Service *(Newsletter),* Business Publishers, Inc., 951 Pershing Drive, Silver Spring, MD 20910, Tel. (301) 587-6300; (800) 274-6737; Fax: (301) 585-9075

National Health Law Program (NHeLP), 2639 South La Cienega Blvd., Los Angeles, CA 90034, Tel. (310) 204-6010; Fax: (310) 204-0891

National Legal Center for the Medically Dependent and Disabled, Inc., 50 South Meridian, Ste. 605, Indianapolis, IN 46204, Tel. (317) 632-6245; Fax: (317) 632-6542

North Carolina State Building Code, Volume I-C *(Book),* North Carolina Department of Insurance, P.O. Box 26387, Raleigh, NC 27611, Tel. (919) 733-3901

Planner's Guide to Barrier Free Meetings *(Book),* Barrier Free Environments, Inc., P.O. Box 30634, Raleigh, NC 27622, Tel. (919) 782-7823

Smart Kitchen/How to Design a Comfortable, Safe & Friendly Workplace *(Book),* Ceres Press, P.O. Box 87, Woodstock, NY 12498, Tel. (914) 679-5573

Sweet's Accessible Building Products File *(Book),* Sweet's Group–McGraw-Hill, 1221 Ave. of the Americas, New York, NY 10020, Tel. (800) 442-2258

UFAS Retrofit Guide: Accessibility Modifications for Existing Building *(Book),* Van Nostrand Reinhold (Distributor), 7625

Empire Dr., Florence, KY 41042, Tel. (606) 525-6600; (800)
842-3636

United States Architectural and Transportation Barriers Compliance Board, see Access Board

G-2. Adaptive Driving Suppliers and Associations

Adaptive Driving Conversions, Inc., 156 E. Commodore Blvd.,
Jackson, NJ 08527, Tel. (908) 928-2089; (800) 866-1529; Fax:
(908) 928-2449

Adaptive Mobility Services, 2201A E. Michigan St., Orlando, FL
32856-0996, (407) 897-7074

Aeroquip Wheelchair Securement System, 300 S. East Ave., Jackson, MI 49203, Tel (517) 787-8121

Ahnafield Corp., 3219 West Washington, Indianapolis, IN 46222,
Tel. (317) 636-8061

American Automobile Association, 1000 AAA Dr., Heathrow, FL
32746-5063, (407) 444-7962

American Driver and Traffic Safety Education Association, IUP
Highway Safety Center, Indiana, PA 15705-1092, (412) 357-
4051

Arcola Mobility, 51 Kero Road, Calstadt, NJ 07072, Tel. (201) 507-
8500; (800) ARCOLA-1

Association of Drivers Educators for the Disabled, P.O. Box 49,
Edgerton, WI 53534, (608) 884-8833

Auto-Mate (KG Engineering), 115 Front St., Woonsocket, RI
02895, Tel. (401) 765-0130; (800) 556-7355

Automotion, P.O. Box 6070, 731 Ulster Ave., Kingston, NY 12401,
Tel. (914) 331-2008

Braun Mobility Products, 1014 South Monticello, P.O. Box 310,
Winamac, IN 44996, Tel. (219) 946-6153; (800) THE-LIFT; Fax:
(219) 946-4670

The Chrysler Motors Physically Challenged Resource Center,
P.O. Box 159, Detroit, MI 48288-0159, (800) 255-9877

Commuter, 3353 West Osborn Road, Phoenix, AZ 85017, Tel. (602)
274-1432; (800) 288-8267

Contact Technologies, 11600 Western Ave., Stanton, CA 90680,
Tel. (714) 898-9263

The Department of Transportation, 400 Seventh St., SW, Washington, DC 20591, (202) 366-4000 or (800) 424-9153, TDD:
(202) 755-8919 or (800) 424-9153

Division Transportation, Inc., 9151 Hampton Overlook, Capital
Heights, MD 20743, Tel. (301) 499-1000; Fax: (301) 499-5529

Drive Master Co., Inc., 9 Spielman Rd., Fairfield, NJ 07004, Tel.
(201) 808-9709; Fax: (201) 808-9713

DW Auto and Home Mobility Specialties, 1208 N. Garth Ave.,
Columbia, MO 65203, Tel. (573) 449-3859; (800) 568-2271; Fax
(573) 449-4187

Explorer Van Co., P.O. Box 527, Warsaw, IN 46580, Tel. (219)
267-7666

EZ Wheelchair Rak Co., 1541 E. La Palma A3, Anaheim, CA
92805, Tel. (800) 248-9130

The Freedom Carrier, 3466 Great Neck St., Port Charlotte, FL 33952, Tel. (813) 624-6346

General Motors Mobility Program, P. O. Box 9011, Detroit, MI 48202, Tel. (313) 556-5445; (800) 323-9935; TDD: (800) 833-9935; Fax: (313) 974-4383

Gresham Driving Aids, P.O. Box 405, Wixom, WI 48096, Tel. (313) 624-1533; (800) 521-8930

Hand Control Systems (Wrightway, Inc.), P.O. Box 460907, Garland, TX 75046, Tel. (214) 240-8839; (800) 241-8839

Hand Drive, 311 Orchard St., Golden, CO 80401, Tel. (303) 271-3868; (800) 224-8156; Fax: (303) 271-3878

Handicapped Driving Aids of Michigan, 4020–30 Second St., Wayne, MI 48184, Tel. (313) 595-4400

Handicaps, Inc., 4335 S. Santa Fe Drive, Englewood, CO 80110, Tel. (303) 781-2062

Institute for Driver Rehabilitation, Inc., 156 E. Commodore Blvd., Jackson, NJ 08527, Tel. (908) 928-2088; (800) 866-1529; Fax: (908) 928-2449

Kneelkar Mednet, 555 Industrial Park Drive, Battle Creek, MI 49015, Tel. (616) 962-3800; Fax: (616) 962-8841

Kroepke Kontrols, 104 Hawkins City Island, Bronx, NY 10464, Tel. (212) 885-1100; Fax: (212) 885-1110

Mac's Lift Gate Corp., 2801 South St., Long Beach, CA 90805, Tel. (213) 634-5962

Mobility Plus Corp., 10 Birch St., Lisbon Falls, ME 04252, Tel. (207) 353-5503

Monarch Hand Controls, 7948 Ronson Rd, San Diego, CA 92111, Tel. (619) 292-1423

Monmouth Vans, Access, and Mobility, 5105 Routes 33/34, Farmingdale, NJ 07727, Tel. (908) 919-1444; (800) 221-0034; Fax: (908) 919-0256

National Mobility Equipment Dealers Association, 914 E. Skagway Ave., Tampa, FL 33604, (813) 932-8566

New Era Transportations, Inc., 810 Moe Drive, Akron, OH 44310, Tel. (330) 633-1118; (800) 638-8267; Fax: (330) 633-0330

R-D Butler and Co., Inc., 65 Ryan Drive F-1, Reynham, MA 02767, Tel. (508) 823-7799

RESNA (Society for the Advancement of Rehabilitation & Assistive Technology), 1700 North Moore St., Ste. 1540, Arlington, VA 22209-1903, (703) 524-6630

Ricon, 12450 Montague St., Pacoima, CA 91331, Tel. (818) 899-7588; (800) 322-2884; Fax: (818) 890-3354

Tim's Trim Inc., 30 Bermar Park, Rochester, NY 14624, Tel. (716) 429-6270

Vantage Mini Vans, 114 S. River Drive, #101, Tempe, AZ 85281, Tel. (602) 968-7011

Worldwide Engineering, Inc., 3240 North Delaware St., Chandler, AZ 85225, Tel. (602) 545-0033; (800) 848-3433; (800) 678-3433

G-3. Adaptive Equipment and Disability-Related Products (Major Catalog)

Abbey Home Healthcare, 3560 Hyland Ave., Costa Mesa, CA 92626, Tel. (800) 233-0098

Abbey Medical Equipment, 17390 Brookhurst St., Ste. 200, Fountain Valley, CA 92708, Tel. (714) 962-4477

AbleNet, Inc., 1081 10th Ave. SE, Minneapolis, MN 55414, Tel. (612) 379-0956; (800) 322-0956; Fax (612) 379-9143

Ableware (Maddak, Inc.), 6 Industrial Road, Pequannock, NJ 07440, Tel. (201) 628-7600; Fax. (201) 305-0841

Accent Buyer's Guide, P.O. Box 700, Bloomington, IL 61702, Tel. (309) 378-2961; (800) 787-8444; Fax (309) 378-4420

American Discount Medical, 2650 Jamaica Road #147-218, El Cajon, CA 92019, Tel. (619) 660-9100; (800) 877-9100

American Walker, Inc., 900 Market St., Oregon, WI 53575, Tel. (608) 835-9255; (800) 828-6808; Fax: (608) 835-5234

Arista Surgical Supply Co., 67 Lexington Ave., New York, NY 10010, Tel. (212) 679-3694; (800) 223-1984

Armstrong Medical, 575 Knightsbridge Parkway, Lincolnshire, IL 60069, Tel. (800) 323-4220; Fax: (708) 913-0138

Assistive Technology Sourcebook, 1482 East Valley Road #A-121, Santa Barbara, CA 93108, Tel. (800) 333-6867

At Home with Medical Equipment Distributors, 3223 S. Loop 289, Ste. 150, Lubbock, TX 79423, Tel. (806) 793-8421; (800) 253-4134

Bailey, 118 Lee St., P.O. Box 130, Lodi, OH 44254, Tel. (216) 948-1080; (800) 321-8372; Fax: (216) 948-4439

Best 25 Catalog Resources for Making Life Easier, 933 Chapel Hill Road, Madison, WI 53711, Tel. (608) 274-4380; Fax: (608) 274-6993

Bruno Independent Living Aids, Inc., 1780 Executive Dr., P.O. Box 84, Oconomowoe, WI 53066, Tel. (414) 567-4990; (800) 882-8183; Fax: (414) 567-4341

Card-Zine Therapy Products, 8912 Ewing Ave., Evanston, IL 60203, Tel. (708) 933-0406

CLEO of New York, Inc., South Buckout St., Trent Bldg., Irvington, NY 10533, Tel. (914) 251-1422; (800) 321-0595

Consumer Buyer's Guide for Independent Living, American Occupational Therapy Association, 4720 Montgomery Lane, Bethesda, MD 20824, Tel. (301) 652-AOTA; (800) OT-HELP-4-U

Danmar Products, Inc., 321 Jackson Industrial Drive, Ann Arbor, MI 48103, Tel. (313) 761-1990; (800) 783-1998; Fax: (313) 761-8977

Dayspring Associates, Inc., 2111 Foley Road, Havre De Grace, MD 21078, Tel. (301) 939-5900

Disability Bookshop Catalog, P.O. Box 129, Vancouver, WA 98666, Tel. (206) 694-2462; (800) 637-2256

Enrichments for Better Living, 145 Tower Drive, P.O. Box 579, Hinsdale, IL 60521, Tel. (800) 323-5547

Equipnet, Inc., 200 E. Del Mar Blvd., Pasadena, CA 91105, Tel. (800) 366-0232

Flaghouse Rehab Catalog, 150 North MacQuesten Parkway, Mount Vernon, NY 10550, Tel. (800) 221-5185

G.E. Miller, Inc., Sawmill River Road, Yonkers, NY 10701, Tel. (914) 969-4036; (800) 431-2924

Greatest of Ease Co. Catalog, 2443 Filmore #345, San Francisco, CA 94115, Tel. (415) 441-6649

Harris Communications, 6541 City West Parkway, Eden Prairie, MN 55344, Tel. (612) 946-0921; (800) 825-6758; TDD: (612) 946-0922

Health and Rehabilitation Products (Luminaud, Inc.), 8688 Atyler Blvd., Mentor, OH 44060, Tel. (216) 255-9082; (800) 255-3408; Fax: (216) 255-2250

Home Therapy Products, P.O. Box 7310, Jacksonville, FL 32238-7310, Tel. (904) 779-5605; Fax: (904) 771-0558

Maxi-Aids, 42 Executive Blvd., Farmingdale, NY 11735, Tel. (800) 522-6294

New Abilities Now, Inc., P.O. Box 208, Excelsior, MN 55331, Tel. (612) 930-5216; (800) 876-2300

New Breakthroughs, P.O. Box 25228, Eugene, OR 97402, Tel. (503) 741-5070; Fax: (505) 896-0123

Nightingale Medical Equipment Services (Rehabilitation Department), 6161 Stewart Rd, Cincinnati, OH 45227, Tel. (513) 527-3780; Fax: (513) 527-3686

North Coast Medical ADL Catalog, 187 Stauffer Boulevard, San Jose, CA 95125-1042, Tel. (800) 821-9319

Nottingham Rehab Health Care Catalog, 1307 West 22nd Place, Tulsa, OK, Tel. (800) 523-2729

Raymo Products, Inc., 212 S. Blake, P.O. Box 248, Olathe, KS 66051, Tel. (913) 782-1515

Rehabco Technology Guide, 1513 Olmstead Ave, Bronx, NY 10462, Tel. (718) 829-3800

Sammons-Preston Catalog, P.O. Box 5071, Bolingbrook, IL 60440-5071, Tel. (800) 323-5547; TDD: (800) 325-1745; Fax: (800) 547-4333

Walgreens Home Medical Center, 7173 W. Cermak, Berwyn, IL 60402, Tel. (708) 795-1295; (800) 323-2828; Fax: (708) 795-1308

Walton Way Medical, 948 Walton Way, Augusta, GA 30901, Tel. (800) 241-4636

Weitbrecht Communications, 2656 29th St., Ste. 205, Santa Monica, CA 90405, Tel. (310) 452-5460, (800) 233-9130; Fax: (310) 450-9918

G-4. Disability-Related Association and Professional Organizations

Agency for Health Care Policy and Research (AHCPR), Executive Office Center, Ste. 501, 2101 East Jefferson St., Rockville, MD 20852, Tel. (301) 227-6173

Alexander Graham Bell Association for the Deaf, 3417 Volta Pl. NW, Washington, DC 20007, Tel. (202) 337-5220

Academy of Dentistry for Persons with Disabilities, 211 East Chicago Ave., Ste. 948, Chicago, IL 60611, Tel. (312) 440-2661

American Academy of Orthotists and Prosthetists (see Orthotic and Prosthetic Association)

American Academy of Physical Medicine and Rehabilitation,

One IBM Plaza, Ste. 2500, Chicago, IL 60611, Tel. (312) 464-9700; Fax: (312) 464-0227

American Amputee Foundation, Inc., P.O. Box 250218, Hillcrest Station, Little Rock, AR 72225, Tel. (501) 666-2523; Fax: (501) 666-8367

American Art Therapy Association (AATA), 1202 Allanson Road, Mundelein, IL 60060

American Association for Music Therapy (AAMT), P.O. Box 80012, Valley Forge, PA 19484

American Association of Spinal Cord Injury Nurses (AASCIN), see American Paraplegia Society

American Association of Retired Persons (AARP), 601 East St., N.W., Washington, DC 20049, Tel. (202) 434-2277

American Association of Spinal Cord Injury Psychologists and Social Workers, see American Paraplegia Society

American Association of University Affiliated Programs for Persons with Developmental Disability, 8630 Fenton St., Ste. 410, Silver Spring, MD 20910, Tel. (301) 588-8252; Fax: (301) 588-2842

American Back Society, St. Joseph's Professional Center, 2647 East 14th St., Ste. 401, Oakland, CA 94601, Tel. (415) 536-9929

American Burn Association, New York Hospital Cornell Medical Center, 525 East 68th St., Room L-706, New York, NY 10021, Tel. (212) 746-5454

American Cancer Society, Inc. 1599 Clifton Road NE, Atlanta, GA 30329, Tel. (404) 320-3333; (800) ACS-2345; Fax: (404) 325-2217

American College of Sports Medicine, 401 W. Michigan St., Indianapolis, IN 46202, Tel. (317) 637-9200

American Congress of Rehabilitation Medicine, 4700 W. Lake Ave., Glenview, IL 60025-1485, Tel. (708) 375-4725; Fax: (708) 375-4777

American Council of the Blind, 1155 15th St. N.W., Ste. 720, Washington, DC 20005, Tel. (202) 467-5081; (800) 424-8666; Fax: (202) 467-5085

American Counseling Association, 5999 Stevenson Ave., Alexandria, VA 22304, Tel. (703) 823-9800

American Dance Therapy Association (ADTA), 2000 Century Plaza, Ste. 108, Columbia, MD 21044, Tel. (301) 997-4040

American Deafness and Rehabilitation Association (ADARA), P.O. Box 251554, Little Rock, AR 72225, Tel. (501) 663-7074

American Diabetes Association, National Service Center, 1660 Duke St., Alexandria, VA 22314, Tel. (703) 549-1500; (800) 232-3472; Fax: (703) 836-7439

American Dietetic Association, 216 W. Jackson Blvd., Chicago, IL 60606-6995, Tel. (312) 899-0040

American Foundation for the Blind, 11 Pennsylvania Plaza, Ste. 300, New York, NY 10001, Tel. (212) 502-7600; (800) 232-5463

American Geriatrics Society, 770 Lexington Ave., Ste. 300, New York, NY 10021, Tel. (212) 308-1414

American Group Pscyhotherapy Association, 25 E. 21st St., 6th Floor, New York, NY 10010, Tel. (212) 477-2677

American Hearing Research Foundation, 55 East Washington St., Ste. 2022, Chicago, IL 60602, Tel. (312) 726-9670

American Heart Association (AHA), 7272 Greenville Ave., Dallas, TX 75231, Tel. (800) 553-6321; (214) 748-7212; Fax: (214) 696-5211

American Lung Association, 1740 Broadway, New York, NY 10019, Tel. (212) 315-8700; (800) LUNG-USA

The American Lupus Society (TALS), 3914 Del Amo Boulevard, Ste. 922, Torrance, CA 90503

American Medical Association (AMA), 515 North State St., Chicago, IL 60610, Tel. (312) 464-4818; Fax: (312) 464-5835

American Occupational Therapy Association (AOTA), 4720 Montgomery Lane, Bethesda, MD 20824, Tel. (301) 652-AOTA; (800) 755-8550; (800) 729-AOTA; (800) OT-HELP-4-U

American Orthotics & Prosthetic Association (see Orthotic and Prosthetic Association)

American Osteopathic Association (AOA), 142 E. Ontario St., Chicago, IL, Tel. (312) 280-5800; (800) 621-1773

American Osteopathic College of Rehabilitation Medicine, 2214 Elmira Ave., Des Plaines, IL 60018, Tel. (708) 699-0048

American Pain Society (APS), 4700 W. Lake Ave., Glenview, IL 60025, Tel. (847) 375-4715; Fax: (847) 375-4777

American Paralysis Association, 500 Morris Ave., Springfield, NJ 07081, Tel. (201) 379-2690; (800) 225-0292; Fax: (201) 912-9433

American Paraplegia Society, 75-20 Astoria Boulevard, Jackson, Heights, NY 11370, Tel. (718) 803-3782; Fax: (718) 803-0414

American Parkinson Disease Association, 1250 Hylan Blvd., Staten Island, NY 10305, Tel. (718) 981-8001; (800) 223-2732; Fax: (718) 981-4399

American Printing House for the Blind, 1835 Frankfort Ave., P.O. Box 6085, Frankfort, KY 40206, Tel. (502) 895-2405

American Physical Therapy Association (APTA), 1111 North Fairfax St., Alexandria, VA 22314, Tel. (800) 999-APTA; Fax: (703) 706-3169

American Rehabilitation Association, 1910 Association Dr., Ste. 200, Reston, VA 20191, Tel. (703) 648-9300; (800) 368-3513; Fax: (703) 648-0346

American Rehabilitation Counseling Association (see American Counseling Association)

American Self-Help Clearinghouse, Northwest Covenant Medical Center, Denville, NJ 07834, Tel. (201) 325-7101; (800) 367-6274

American Speech-Language-Hearing Association (ASHA), 10801 Rockville Pike, Rockville, MD 20852, Tel. (301) 897-5700; Fax: (301) 571-0457

American Spinal Injury Association (ASIA), 250 E. Superior St., Room 619, Chicago, IL 60611, Tel. (312) 908-3425; ASIA Publications, 2020 Peachtree Road NW, Atlanta, GA 30309, Tel. (404) 355-9772; Fax: (404) 355-1826

American Trauma Society (ATS), 8903 Presidential Parkway, Ste. 512, Upper Marlboro, MD 20772-2656

Amyotrophic Lateral Sclerosis Association (ALSA), 21021 Ventura Blvd, Ste. 321, Woodland Hills, CA 91364, Tel. (818) 340-7500

Ankylosing Spondylitis Association, 511 North La Cienega, Box 216, Los Angeles, CA 90048, Tel. (800) 777-8189

Apple Computer, Inc., Worldwide Disability Solutions Group Mail Stop, 38DS 1 Infinite Loop, Cupertino, CA 95014

Arthritis Foundation, 1314 Spring St. N.W., Atlanta, GA 30309, Tel. (404) 872-7100; (800) 283-7800

The Arthritis Society, 250 Bloor Street East, Ste. 401, Toronto, Ontario M4W 3P2, Canada, Tel. (416) 967-1414

Associated Services for the Blind, 919 Walnut St., Philadelphia, PA 19107, Tel. (215) 627-0600

Association of Rehabilitatiion Nurses (ARN), 4700 W. Lake Ave., Glenview, IL 60025, Tel. (847) 679-8474

Association for the Retarded Citizens of the United States (ARC), 2501 Ave. J, P.O. Box 6109, Arlington, TX 76005-6109, Tel. (817) 640-0204

AT&T National Special Needs Center, 2001 Route 46, Ste. 310, Parsippany, NJ 07054, Tel. (800) 233-1222; TDD: (800) 833-3232

Behavior Therapy and Research Society, Temple University Medical School, Philadelphia, PA 19129, Tel. (215) 221-2000

Brain Injury Association, Inc., 1776 Massachusetts Ave., NW, Ste. 100, Washington, DC 20036, Tel. (800) 444-6443; (202) 296-6443; Fax: (202) 296-8850

Cancer Care, Inc., and the National Cancer Foundation, Inc. 1180 Ave. of the Americas, New York, NY 10036, Tel. (212) 221-3300

Cancer Connection, 4410 Main St., Kansas City, MO 64111, Tel. (816) 932-8453

Center for Rehabilitation Technology (CRT), 490-10th St. N.W., Atlanta, GA 30332-0156

Charcot-Marie-Tooth Association (CMTA), 601 Upland Ave., Upland, PA 19015, Tel. (610) 499-7486

Commission on Accreditation of Rehabilitation Facilities (CARF), 101 N. Wilmot, Ste. 500, Tucson, AZ 85711, Tel. (602) 748-1212

Committee for the Handicapped-People-to-People, P.O. Box 18131, Washington, DC 20036, Tel. (301) 774-7446

Council of Citizens with Low Vision International (CCLVI), 5707 Brockton Drive, Suite 302, Indianapolis, IN 46220-5481, Tel. (317) 254-1155; (317) 252-1185; (800) 733-2258

Council of State Administrators of Vocational Rehabilitation (CSAVR), 1055 Thomas Jefferson St. N.W., P.O. Box 3776, Ste. 401, Washington, DC 20007

Courage Center, 3910 Golden Valley Rd., Golden Valley, MN 55422, Tel. (612) 588-0811

The Deafness Research Foundation, 15 W. 39th St., New York, NY 10018, Tel. (212) 768-1181

Direct Link for the Disabled, P.O. Box 1036, Solvang, CA 93464, Tel. (805) 688-1603; (800) 686-5286; Fax: (805) 688-1603

Dysautonomia Foundation, Inc., 20 E. 46 St., Room 302, New York, NY 10017, Tel. (212) 949-6644

Dystonia Medical Research Foundation, One East Wacker Dr., Ste. 2430, Chicago, IL 60601-2098, Tel. (312) 755-0198; (312) 803-0138

Epilepsy Foundation of America, 4351 Garden City Drive, Landover, MD 20785, Tel. (301) 459-3700; (800) 332-1000; Fax: (301) 577-2684

Estate Planning for Persons with Disabilities, 3100 Arapahoe Ave., #112, Boulder, CO 80303, Tel. (303) 449-4103; (800) 448-1071; Fax: (303) 449-6003

Foundation For Dignity, 37 South 20th St., Ste. 601, Philadelphia, PA 19103, Tel. (215) 567-2828

Foundation for Hospice and Homecare, 513 C St., N.E., Stanton Park, Washington, DC 20002

Gazette International Networking Institute, 4207 Lindell Blvd., #110, St. Louis, MO 63108, Tel. (314) 534-0475; Fax: (314) 534-5070

Goodwill Industries International, 9200 Wisconsin Ave., Bethesda, MD 20814, Tel. (301) 530-6500; Fax: (301) 530-1516

Guide Dog Foundation for the Blind, Inc., 371 East Jericho Turnpike, Smithtown, NY 11787

Hearing Information Center, Swarthmore Medical Center, 300 South Chester Road, Swarthmore, PA 19081

Helen Keller International, 90 Washington St., 15th Floor, New York, NY 10006, Tel. (212) 943-0890

Huntington's Disease Society of America (HDSA), 140 W. 22nd St., 6th Floor, New York, NY 10011, Tel. (212) 242-1968; (800) 345-HDSA; Fax: (212) 243-2443

The Institute for Rehabilitation and Research, 1333 Moursund St., Houston, TX 77030, Tel. (713) 797-5945

International Association of Machinists, Placement Program for Persons with Disabilities, 3830 South Meridian, Wichita, KS 67217, Tel. (316) 522-1591

International Association of Psychosocial Rehabilitation Services (IAPSRS), 10025 Governor Warfield Pkwy, #301, Columbia, MD 21044

International Association for the Study of Pain (IASP), 909 NE 43rd St., Ste. 306, Seattle, WA 98105-6020, Tel. (206) 547-6409; Fax: (206) 547-1703

International Center for the Disabled (ICD), 340 East 24th St., New York, NY 10010, Tel. (212) 679-0100

International Federation of Physical Medicine and Rehabilitation (IFPMR), 600 University Ave., Ste. 1160, Toronto, Ontario M5G 1X5

International Hearing Society, 20361 Middlebelt Road, Livonia, MI 48152

International Pain Foundation, see International Association for the Study of Pain

International Polio Network (IPN), see Gazette International Networking Institute

International Rehabilitation Medicine Association (IRMA), 1333

Moursund Ave., A-221, Houston, TX 77030, Tel. (713) 799-5086

International Society for Augmentative and Alternative Communication (ISAAC), 428 East Preston St., Baltimore, MD 21202-3993

International Tremor Foundation, 833 W. Washington Blvd., Chicago, IL 60607, Tel. (312) 733-1893

International Ventilator Users Network (I.V.U.N.), see Gazette International Networking Institute

Juvenile Diabetes Foundation, 381 Park Ave. S, New York, NY 10010, Tel. (800) 533-8590

Juvenile Diabetes Foundation International, 120 Wall St., New York, NY 10005, Tel. (212) 785-9500; (800) JDF-CURE

The Lighthouse, Inc., 111 East 59th St., New York, NY 10022, Tel. (212) 821-9200; (800) 334-5497; (800) 829-0500

Lupus Foundation of America, Inc. 4 Research Place, Ste. 180, Rockville, MD 20850-3226, Tel. (800) 558-0121

Multiple Sclerosis Association of America, 601–603 White Horse Pike, P.O. Box 187, Oaklyn, NJ 08107, Tel. (800) 833-4MSA; (609) 858-3211

Multiple Sclerosis Foundation Inc., 6350 N. Andrews Ave., Fort Lauderdale, FL 33309, Tel. (954) 776-6805; (800) 441-7055; Fax: (954) 938-8708

Muscular Dystrophy Association, 3300 E. Sunrise Dr., Tucson, AZ 85718, Tel. (520) 529-2000

Myasthenia Gravis Foundation (MGF), 222 South Riverside Plaza, Ste. 1540, Chicago, IL 60606-6001, Tel. (312) 258-0522; (800) 541-5454; Fax: (312) 258-0461

Myoclonus Families United, 155 E. 35th St., Brooklyn, NY 11234, Tel. (718) 252-2133

Myoclonus Research Foundation, 200 Old Palisade Rd., Ste. 17D, Fort Lee, NJ 07024, Tel. (201) 585-0770; Fax: (201) 585-8114

National Academy of Certified Clinical Mental Health Counselors, 5999 Stevenson Ave., Alexandria, VA 22304, Tel. (703) 823-9800

National Amputation Foundation, 73 Church St., Malverne, NY 11565, Tel. (516) 887-3600

National Arthritis and Musculoskeletal and Skin Diseases Information Clearinghouse, 9000 Rockville Pike, Box AMS, Bethesda, MD 20892, Tel. (301) 495-4484

National Association of the Deaf, 814 Thayer Ave., Silver Spring, MD 20910, Tel. (310) 587-1788; TDD: (310) 587-1789

National Association for Hearing and Speech Action (NAHSA), 10801 Rockville Pike, Rockville, MD 20852

National Association for Music Therapy (NAMT), 8455 Colesville Road, Ste. 930, Silver Spring, MD 20910

National Association of Protection and Advocacy Systems, Inc., 900 Second St., N.E., Ste. 211, Washington, DC 20002, Tel. (202) 408-9514; Fax: (202) 408-9520

National Association of State Directors of Developmental Disabilities Services, 113 Oronoco St., Alexandria, VA 22314, Tel. (703) 683-4202

National Association for the Visually Handicapped, 22 W. 21st St., New York, NY 10010, Tel. (212) 889-3141

National Ataxia Foundation, 15500 Wayzata Blvd., #750, Wayzata, MN 55391, Tel. (312) 473-7666; Fax: (612) 473-9289

National Brain Tumor Foundation, 785 Market St., Ste. 1600, San Francisco, CA 94103

National Cancer Institute (NCI), National Institutes of Health, U.S. Department of Health and Human Services, 9000 Rockville Pike, Bethesda, MD 20892, Tel. (301) 496-5583

National Center for Medical Rehabilitation Research (NCMRR), 6100 Executive Boulevard, Room 2AO3, Rockville, MD 20852

National Center for Youth with Disabilities, University of Minnesota, P.O. Box 721, 420 Delaware St. S.E., Minneapolis, MN 55455, Tel. (612) 626-2825

National Clearinghouse for Alcohol and Drug Abuse, P.O. Box 2345, Rockville, MD 20857

National Clearinghouse of Rehabilitation Training Materials, Oklahoma State University, 816 West 6th Ave., Stillwater, OK 74078, Tel. (800) 223-5219; (405) 624-7650

National Clearinghouse on Technology and Aging, University Center on Aging, University of Massachusetts Medical Center, 55 Lake Ave. N., Worcester, MA 01655, Tel. (508) 856-3662

National Clearinghouse on Women and Girls with Disabilities, Educational Equity Concepts, Inc., 114 E. 32nd St., Ste. 701, New York, NY 10016, Tel. (212) 725-1803; Fax: (212) 725-0947

National Chronic Pain Outreach Association, 7979 Old Georgetown Rd., #100, Bethesda, MD 20814, Tel. (301) 652-4948; Fax: (301) 907-0745

National Council on Communicative Disorders (NCCD), 10801 Rockville Pike, Rockville, MD 20852

National Council on Disability, 1331 F St., N.W., Ste. 1050, Washington, DC 20004-1107

National Council on Independent Living (NCIL), 2111 Wilson Boulevard, Ste. 405, Arlington, VA 22201

National Council on the Aging, Inc. (NCOA), 409 3rd St. S.W., Washington, DC 20024

National Council on Spinal Cord Injury, 151 Tremont St., Boston, MA 02111, Tel. (617) 338-7777; Fax: (617) 338-4266

National Data Bank for Disability Support Services, Room 0126, Shoemaker Building, University of Maryland, College Park, MD 20742

National Diabetes Information Clearinghouse, 1 Information Way, Bethesda, MD 20892, Tel. (301) 654-3327

National Easter Seal Society, 230 West Monroe St., Chicago, IL 60606, Tel. (312) 726-6200; TDD: (312) 726-4258; (800) 221-6827

National Federation of the Blind (NFB), 1800 Johnson St., Baltimore, MD 21230, Tel. (410) 659-9314

National Heart, Lung, and Blood Institute (NHLBI), Information Center, P.O. Box 30105, Bethesda, MD 20824-0105, Tel. (301) 251-1222; Fax: (301) 251-1223

National Hospice Organization (NHO), 1901 North Moore St., Ste. 901, Arlington, VA 22209

National Institute of Art and Disabilities (NIAD), 551 23rd St., Richmond, CA 94804

National Institute on Deafness and Other Communication Disorders (NIDCD), National Information Clearinghouse, Program Planning and Health Reports Branch, Building 31, Room 3C 35, 9000 Rockville Pike, Bethesda, MD 20892, Tel. (301) 496-7243

National Institute on Disability and Rehabilitation Research, U.S. Department of Education, 330 C St., Washington, DC 20202; Mailing address: 600 Independence Ave. SW, Washington, DC 20202, Tel. (202) 205-8134; Fax: (202) 205-8997

National Institute of Neurological Disorders and Stroke (NINDS), National Institutes of Health, U.S. Department of Health and Human Services, Building 31, Room 8A 06, 9000 Rockville Pike, Bethesda, MD 20892, Tel. (800) 352-9424

National Library Service for the Blind and Physically Handicapped (NLS), Library of Congress, 1291 Taylor St. N.W., Washington, DC 20542, Tel. (800) 424-8567

National Neurofibromatosis Foundation (NNFF), 120 Wall St., New York, NY 10005, Tel. (212) 344-6633; Fax: (212) 747-0004

National Multiple Sclerosis Society, 733 3rd Ave., New York, NY 10017, Tel. (212) 986-3240, (800) 344-4867; Fax: (212) 986-7981

National Organization on Disability (NOD), 910 16th St. N.W., Ste. 600, Washington, DC 20006, Tel. (202) 293-5960; TDD: (202) 293-5968; Fax: (202) 293-7999

National Osteoporosis Foundation (NOF), 1150 17th St. N.W., Ste. 500, Washington, DC 20036-4603, Tel. (202) 223-2226

National Parent Network on Disabilities (NPND), 1600 Prince St., Ste. 115, Alexandria, VA 22314

National Parkinson's Foundation, 1501 N.W. 9th Ave., Miami, FL 33136, Tel. (800) 327-4545; (800) 433-7022 (in FL), (305) 547-6666; Fax: (305) 548-4403

National Pressure Ulcer Advisory Panel, State University of New York Buffalo, Beck Hall, 3435 Main St., Buffalo, NY 14214, Tel. (716) 881-3558

National Rehabilitation Association (NRA), 633 South Washington St., Alexandria, VA 22314-4193, (703) 836-0850

National Rehabilitation Information Center (NARIC), 8455 Colesville Road, Ste. 935, Silver Spring, MD 20910-3319, Tel. (301) 588-9284; Directory of National Information Sources on Disabilities (800) 346-2742

National Rehabilitation Hospital International Polio Institute, 102 Irving St. N.W., Washington, DC 20010

The National Scoliosis Foundation, 5 Cabot Place, Stoughton, MA 02072, Tel. (617) 341-6333; (800) 673-6922; Fax: (617) 341-8333

National Spasmodic Torticollis Association, P.O. Box 424, Mukwonago, WI 53149-0424, Tel. (800) HURTFUL; (414) 662-9886; Fax: (414) 662-9887

National Spinal Cord Injury Association, Information and Resource Center, 600 W. Cummings Park, Ste. 2000, Woburn, MA 01801, Tel. (800) 962-9629

National Spinal Cord Injury Hotline, 2200 Kernan Dr., Baltimore, MD 21207, Tel. (410) 448-6623; (800) 526-3456 (Outside MD)

National Stroke Association (NSA), 8480 E. Orchard Road, Ste. 1000, Englewood, CO 80111-5015, Tel. (303) 771-1700; (800) STROKES; Fax: (303) 771-1887

National Stuttering Project (NSP), 4601 Irving St., San Francisco, CA 94122

National Technical Information Service (NTIS), U.S. Department of Commerce, 5285 Port Royal Road, Springfield, VA 22161

Neurofibromatosis, Inc. (NF, Inc.), 8855 Annapolis Road, Ste. 110, Lanham, MD 20706-2924

Orthotic and Prosthetic Association (American Orthotic and Prosthetic Association; American Academy of Orthotists and Prosthetists), 1650 King St., Ste. 500, Alexandria, VA 22314, Tel. (703) 836-7116; Fax: (703) 836-0838

Paralyzed Veterans of America, Access Information Bulletin, 801 18th St. N.W., Washington, DC 20006, Tel. (202) 872-1300; (800) 424-8200

Parkinson's Disease-American-Information and Resource Center, Hospital for Joint Diseases, 301 E. 17th St., New York, NY 10003, Tel. (212) 598-6300

Parkinson's Disease Foundation, Inc. (PDF), Columbia-Presbyterian Medical Center, 710 West 168th St., 3rd Floor, New York, NY 10032, Tel. (212) 923-4700; (800) 457-6676; Fax: (212) 923-4778

Partners of the Americas PATH (Partners Appropriate Technology for the Handicapped) Americas Program, 1424 K St. N.W., Ste. 700, Washington, DC 20005

PRIDE Foundation (Promote Real Independence for the Disabled and Elderly), 391 Long Hill Road, Box 1293, Groton, CT 06340-1293

Rancho Los Amigos Research and Education Institute, Rancho Los Amigos Medical Center, 7601 East Imperial Highway, Downey, CA 90242, Tel. (562) 401-7111

Rehabilitation International, 25 East 21st St., New York, NY 10010, Tel. (212) 420-1500; Fax: (212) 505-0871

Rehabilitation Research and Training Center on Aging with Spinal Cord Injury, Craig Hospital, University of Colorado Health Science Center, Research Department, 3425 South Clarkson, Englewood, CO 80110

Rehabilitation Research and Training Center on Traumatic Brain Injury (TBI INFO), State University of New York (SUNY)/Buffalo, 194 Farber Hall, 3435 Main St., Buffalo, NY 14214

Rehabilitation Services Administration (RSA), Office of Special Education and Rehabilitative Services (OSERS), U.S. Department of Education, Switzer Building, Room 3028, 330 C St., S.W., Washington, DC 20202-2531, Tel. (202) 732-1362; Fax: (202) 732-1372

Rehabilitation Engineering and Assistive Technology Society of North America (RESNA), 1700 North Moore St., Ste. 1540,

Arlington, VA 22209-1903, Tel. (703) 524-6686; Fax: (703) 524-6630

Resources for Rehabilitation, 33 Bedford St., Ste. 19A, Lexington, MA 02173, Tel. (617) 862-6455; Fax: (617) 861-7517

Rusk Institute of Rehabilitation Medicine, New York University Medical Center, 400 East 34th St., Ste. 600, New York, New York 10016, Tel. (212) 263-7300

Scleroderma Federation, Peabody Office Building, One Newbury St., Peabody, MA 01960, Tel. (508) 535-6600; Fax: (508) 535-6696

Self Help for Hard of Hearing People (SHHH), 7910 Woodmont Ave., Ste. 1200, Bethesda, MD 20814

Sensory Aids Foundation, 385 Sherman Ave., Ste. 2, Palo Alto, CA 94306, Tel. (415) 329-0430

Sjogren's Syndrome Foundation, Inc., 333 N. Broadway, Jericho, NY 11050, Tel. (516) 933-6365

Society for Cognitive Rehabilitation, Inc. (SCR), P.O. Box 53067, Albuquerque, NM 87153-3067

Society for Muscular Dystrophy Information International (SMDI International), P.O. Box 479, Bridgewater, Nova Scotia, Canada, B4V 2X6

Spina Bifida Association of America (SBAA), 4590 MacArthur Boulevard NW, Ste. 250, Washington, DC 20007-4226, Tel. (202) 944-3285

Spinal Cord Injury Network International (SCINI), 3911 Princeton Drive, Santa Rosa, CA 95405-7013

Spinal Cord Society (SCS), Route 5, Wendell Road, Fergus Falls, MN 56537

Stroke Club International, 805 12th St., Galveston, TX 77550, Tel. (409) 762-1022

Stuttering Foundation of America (SFA), 3100 Walnut Grove Road, #603, P.O. Box 11749, Memphis, TN 38111-0749

Tardive Dyskinesia/Tardive Dystonia National Association, 4244 University Way NE, P.O. Box 45732, Seattle, WA 98145-0732, Tel. (206) 522-3166

Telecommunications for the Deaf, Inc. (TDI), 8719 Colesville Road, Ste. 300, Silver Spring, MD 20910

Technical Aids and Assistance for the Disabled, 1950 W. Roosevelt Rd., Chicago, IL 60608, Tel. (313) 421-3373, (800) 346-2959

Typewriting Institute for the Handicapped, 3102 W. Augusta Ave., Phoenix, AZ 85051, Tel. (602) 939-5344

Trace Research and Development Center on Communication, Control and Computer Access for Handicapped Individuals, University of Wisconsin, S-151, Waisman Center, 1500 Highland Ave., Madison, WI 53705, Tel. (608) 262-6966

Uniform Data System for Medical Rehabilitation, Research and Training Center on Functional Assessment and Evaluation of Rehabilitation Outcomes, State University of New York (SUNY/Buffalo), Department of Rehabilitation Medicine, 232 Parker Hall, SUNY South Campus, 3435 Main St., Buffalo, NY 14214-3007, Tel. (716) 829-2076; Fax: (716) 829-2080

United Cerebral Palsy Association, 1522 K St., N.W., Ste. 1112, Washington, DC 20005, Tel. (202) 842-1266, (800) 872-5827

United Parkinson Foundation, 933 W. Washington Blvd., Chicago, IL 60607, Tel. (312) 733-1893

United Scleroderma Foundation, Inc., P.O. Box 399, Watsonville, CA 95077-0399, Tel. (800) 722-HOPE; Fax: (408) 728-3328.

United States Government TDD Directory, Consumer Information Center, Department 575A, Pueblo, CO 81009, Tel. (202) 501-1794

Vermont Rehabilitation Engineering Research Center for Low Back Pain, 1 South Prospect St., Burlington, VT 05401, Tel. (802) 656-4582; (800) 527-7320

Visiting Nurse Associations of America (VNAA), 3801 East Florida Ave., Ste. 900, Denver, CO 80210

Vocational Evaluation and Work Adjustment Association (VEWAA), 202 East Cheyenne Mountain Boulevard, Colorado Springs, CO 80906

Worldwide Education and Awareness for Movement Disorders (WE MOVE), Mount Sinai Medical Center, One Gustave L. Levy Place, Box 1052, New York, NY 10029-6574, Tel. (800) 437-MOV2; (212) 241-8567; Fax: (212) 987-7363

World Institute on Disability, 510 16th St., Ste. 100, Oakland, CA 94612, Tel. (510) 764-4100; Fax: (510) 763-4109

G-5. Electronic Resources and Bulletin Boards for the Disabled

ABLE-DATA, see National Rehabilitation Information Center

AppleLink, Apple Computer, Inc., Office of Special Education and Rehabilitation, 20525 Mariani Ave., MS 43S, Cupertino, CA 95014, Tel. (408) 974-7910

CompuServe, CompuServe Information Service, 500 Arlinton Centre Blvd., Columbus, OH 43220, Tel. (800) 848-8199

Deaftech, USA, International Communications Limited, P.O. Box 81, Fayville, MA 01745, Tel. (508) 620-1777

4-Sights Network, Greater Detroit Society for the Blind, 16625 Grand River, Detroit, MI 48227, Tel. (313) 272-3900

HyperABLEDATA, TRACE Research & Development Center, 1500 Highland Ave., Waisman Center, Madison, WI 53705-2280, Tel. (608) 262-6966

Project Enable, Rehabilitation Technology Associates, West Virginia Research & Training Center, One Dunbar Plaza, Ste. E, Dunbar, WV 25064-3098

National Rehabilitation Information Center (NARIC), 8455 Colesville Road, Ste. 935, Silver Spring MD 20910-3319, (301) 588-9284; Directory of National Information Sources on Disabilities (800) 346-2742; **ABLE-DATA,** Tel (800) 227-0216; (301) 608-8998

Scan-GTE Education Services, GTE Place, West Airfield Dr., P.O. Box 619810, DFW Airport, TX 75261-9810, Tel. (800) 927-3000

G-6. Leisure and Sports Associations and Organizations for the Disabled

Access America, Northern Cartography, 4050 Williston Road, #131, S. Burlington, VT 05403, Tel. (802) 860-2886

Access to Sailing, 19744 Beach Blvd., Ste. 340, Huntington Beach, CA 92648, Tel. (714) 722-5371

Access Yosemite National Park, Special Needs Project, 1482 East Valley Road, #A-121, Santa Barbara, CA 93108, Tel. (800) 333-6867

Achilles Track Club, 9 East 89th St., New York, NY 10128, Tel. (212) 967-9300

American Athletic Association of the Deaf (AAAD), 3607 Washington Boulevard, Ogden, UT 84403-1731

American Blind Bowling Association, 411 Sheiff, Mencer, PA 16137, Tel. (412) 662-5748

American Blind Skiing Association, 610 South William St., Mt. Prospect, IL 60056, Tel. (708) 225-1739

American Camping Association, 5000 State Road 67 North, Martinsville, IN 46151-7902, Tel. (765) 342-8456; (800) 428-2267

American Canoe Association, Committee for Disabled Paddlers, 8580 Cinderbed Rd., Suite 1900, P.O. Box 1900, Newington, VA 22122-1190, Tel. (703) 550-7495

American Hearing Impaired Hockey Association, Inc., 1141 West Lake St., Chicago, IL 60607, Tel. (312) 829-2250

American Therapeutic Recreation Association, Inc., 3417A Sapula Rd., Box 377, Sand Springs, OK 74063, Tel. (904) 644-6014

American Wheelchair Archers (AWA), 5318 Northport Drive, Brooklyn Center, MN 55429

American Wheelchair Bowling Association, N54W 15858 Larkspur Lane, Menomonee Falls, WI 53051, (414) 781-6876

American Wheelchair Pilots Association, 1621 East Second Ave., Mesa, AZ 85204

American Wheelchair Table Tennis Association (AWTTA), 23 Parker St., Port Chester, NY 10573, Tel. (203) 629-6283

Amputee Sports Association, 11705 Mercy Blvd., Savannah, GA 31419, Tel. (912) 927-5406

Blind Outdoor Leisure Development (BOLD), 533 East Main St., Aspen, CO 81611, (303) 923-3811

Boating for the Handicapped: Guidelines for the Physically Disabled *(Book by E. Hedley),* Products Manager, Human Resources Center, 1 U Willets Road, Albertson, NY 11507

Canadian Wheelchair Sports Association, 1600 James Naismith Drive, Gloucester, Ontario, Canada K1B5N4, Tel. (613) 748-5685; Fax: (613) 748-5722

Diabetic Traveler, P.O. Box 8223 RW, Stamford, CT 06905, Tel. (203) 327-5832

Directory for Disabled Travelers (Travelin' Talk), P.O. Box 3534, Clarksville, TN 37043, Tel. (615) 552-6670

Directory of Travel Agencies for the Disabled, Twin Peaks Press, P.O. Box 129, Vancouver, WA 98666, Tel. (206) 694-2462; (800) 637-2256

Fun Vacations, Accent Books & Products, P.O. Box 700, Bloomington, IL 61702, Tel. (309) 378-2961; (800) 787-8444; Fax: (309) 378-4420

Handicapped Boaters' Association, P.O. Box 1134, Ansonia Station, NY 10023

Handicapped Scuba Association, 1104 E. Prado, San Clemente, CA 92672, Tel. (714) 498-6128; Fax: (714) 498-6128

Handicapped Travel Newsletter, P.O. Box 269, Athens TX 75751, Tel. (903) 677-1260

International Wheelchair Aviators, 1117 Rising Hill, Escondido, CA 92029, Tel. (619) 746-5018

International Foundation of Wheelchair Tennis, 3857 Birch St., Box 111, Newport Beach, CA 92660, Tel. (714) 851-1707

International Wheelchair Road Racers Club, Inc., 30 Myamo Lane, Stamford, CT 06902, Tel. (203) 967-2231

International Wheelchair Tennis Federation, 940 Calle Amenecer, Ste. 8, San Clemente, CA 92672, Tel. (714) 361-6811

National Amputee Golf Association (NAGA), P.O. Box 1228, Amhearst, NH 03031-1228, Tel. (800) 633-NAGA

National Amputee Summer Sports Association, 215 West 92nd St., New York, NY 10025, Tel. (212) 874-4138

National Association for Disabled Athletes, 33 Leonard Ave., Tenafly, NJ 07670

National Association of Handicapped Outdoor Sportsmen, Inc., RR 6, Box 25, Centralia, IL 62801, Tel. (618) 532-4565

National Association of Sports for Cerebral Palsy, 66 East 34th St., New York, NY 10016

National Council for Therapy and Rehabilitation Through Horticulture, 9041 Comprint, Ste. 103, Gaithersburg, MD 20877, Tel. (301) 948-3010

National Deaf Bowling Association, 9244 East Mansfield Ave., Denver, CO 80237, Tel. (303) 771-9018

National Foundation of Wheelchair Tennis, 4000 MacArthur Boulevard, Newport Beach, CA 92660

National Foundation of Wheelchair Tennis, 940 Calle Amanecer, Ste. B, San Clemente, CA 92673

National Handicap Motorcyclist Association, 35–34 84th St., #F8, Jackson Heights, NY 11372, Tel. (718) 565-1243

National Handicapped Sports, 451 Hungerford Drive, Ste. 100, Rockville, MD 20850, Tel. (301) 217-0960; Fax: (301) 217-0968

National Handicapped Sports and Recreation Association, Capitol Hill Station, P.O. Box 18664, Denver, CO 80218

National Inconvenienced Sportsmen's Association (NISA), 3738 Walnut Ave., Carmichael, CA 95608

National Ocean Access Project, 410 Severn Ave., Ste. 107, Annapolis, MD 21403, Tel. (301) 280-0464

National Skeet Shooting Association, 5931 Roft Road, San Antonio, TX 78253, Tel. (800) 877-5338

National Sports Center for the Disabled (NSCD), 2107 Templerton Gap Rd., Ste. C, Colorado Springs, CO 80907, (303) 632-0698

National Therapeutic Recreation Society (NTRS), National Recreation and Park Association, 2775 South Quincy St., Ste. 300, Alexandria, VA 22206

National Wheelchair Athletic Association, 40–24 62nd St., Woodside, NY 11377

National Wheelchair Basketball Association, 110 Seaton Building, Lexington, KY 40506, Tel. (606) 257-1623

National Wheelchair Raquetball Association, 65 Quaker Hills Road, Lancaster, PA 17603, Tel. (717) 394-2111

National Wheelchair Softball Association (NWSA), 1616 Todd Court, Hastings, MN 55033, Tel. (612) 437-1792

New England Handicapped Sportmen's Association, 26 McFarlin Road, Chelmsford, MA 01824

North American Riding for the Handicapped Association (NARHA), Box 33150, Denver, CO 80233, Tel. (303) 452-1212

North American Wheelchair Athletic Association, P.O. Box 26, Riverdale, NY 10471, Tel. (212) 796-5084

One-Arm Dove Hunt Association, P.O. Box 582, Olney, TX 76374, Tel. (817) 564-2102

Physically Challenged Swimmers of America, 22 William St., #225, South Glastonbury, CT 06073, Tel. (203) 548-4500

Project Magic, P.O. Box 100, Inglewood, CA 90306

Riding for Rehabilitation: A Guide for Handicapped Riders and Their Instructors *(Book by J. Bauer),* Can Ride, 209 Deloraine Ave., Toronto, Ontario, M5M 2B2 Canada

Seat-A-Robics, Inc., P.O. Box 630064, Little Neck, NY 11363, Tel. (800) 484-7046; (718) 631-4007

Senior Olympics, 5670 Wilshire Boulevard, Los Angeles, CA 90036

The Sierra Club Guide for the Disabled (for easy access to national parks), Sierra Club Books, 100 Bush St., Ste. 1300, San Francisco, CA 94104, Tel. (415) 291-1600

Skating Association for the Blind and Handicapped (SABAH), 1255 Niagara Falls Boulevard, Buffalo, NY 14226

Society for the Advancement of Travel for the Handicapped (SATH), 26 Court St., Ste. 1110, Brooklyn, NY 11242

Society for the Advancement of Travel for the Handicapped (SATH), 347 Fifth Ave., Ste. 610, New York, NY 10016

Special Olympics, 1350 New York Ave., NW, Ste. 500, Washington, DC 20005, Tel. (202) 628-3630

Special Recreations, Inc. 362 Koser Ave., Iowa City, IA 52246, Tel. (319) 337-7578

Therapeutic Horsemanship, Inc., c/o Sandy Rafferty, Director, Route 1, Valley Road, Pacific, MO 63069

United States Amputee Athletic Association, P.O. Box 560686, Charlotte, NC 28256, Tel. (704) 598-0407

United States Association of Blind Athletes (USABA), 33 North Institute St., Colorado Springs, CO 80903

United States Association for Blind Athletes, 55 West California Ave., Beach Haven Park, NJ 08008

United States Blind Golfers Association, 3094 Shamrock St. N, Tallahassee, FL 32308

United States Cerebral Palsy Athletic Association, 3810 W. Northwest Highway, Ste. 205, Dallas, TX 75220

United States Deaf Skiers Association, Inc. (USDSA), 0400 SW Palatine Hill Road, Portland, OR 97219-6551

United States Disabled Ski Team, P.O. Box 100, Park City, UT 84060

United States Hang Gliding Association, 559 East Pikes Peak Ave., Colorado Springs, CO 80903, Tel. (719) 632-8300

United States Racquet-Sports Association, 1 Devasage St., Jeannette, PA 15644, Tel. (412) 744-3320

United States Rowing Association, Adaptive Rowing Committee, 11 Hall Place, Exeter, NH 03833, Tel. (603) 778-0315

United States Wheelchair Swimming, 229 Miller St., Middleboro, MA 02346

United States Wheelchair Weightlifting Federation, 39 Michael Place, Levittown, PA 19057, Tel. (215) 945-1964

Wheelchair Bowling Association, Inc., N54 W 15858 Larkspur Lane, Menomonee Falls, WI 53051, Tel. (414) 781-6876

Wheelchair Motorcycle Association (WMA), 101 Terrey St., Brockton, MA 02401, Tel. (508) 583-8614

Wheelchair Sports, U.S.A., 3595 East Fountain Boulevard, Ste. L1, Colorado Springs, CO 80910

Wheelchair Tennis Players Association, 940 Calle Amanecer, Ste. B, San Clemente, CA 92672, Tel. (714) 361-6811

Winter Park Recreational Association, P.O. Box 36, Winterpark, CO 80482, Tel. (303) 726-5514

World Recreation Association of the Deaf/USA (WRAD), P.O. Box 3211, Quartz Hill, CA 93586

G-7. Musculoskeletal and Work-Related Testing Devices

ARCON, 309 McLaws Circle, Ste. F, Williamsburg, VA 23185

Baltimore Therapeutic Equipment (BTE), 7456-L New Ridge Road, Hanover, MD 21076

Biodex Medical Corp., P.O. Box S, Shirley, NY 11967, (800) 622-0460; (516) 924-9300

Blankenship, P.O. Box 5084, Macon, GA 31208

Chattanooga Corp., P.O. Box 4287, Chattanooga, TN 37405, (615) 8709-2281; (800) 729-5436

Computerized Motion Diagnostic Imaging (CMDI), Motion Diagnostic Laboratories, Inc., 2001 Marcus Ave., Ste. S90, Lake Success, NY 11042, (516) 352-2700

Cybex, A Division of Lumex, 2100 Smithtown Ave., Ronkonkoma, NY 11779, (800) 645-5392 or 222-3245; (516) 585-9000

Employment and Rehab Institute of California, P.O. Box 80864, Rancho Santa Margarita, CA 92688

ERGASYS, 25532 Terreno, Mission Viejo, CA 92691

Fred Sammons, 145 Tower Drive, Burr Ridge, IL 60521

Isernhagen Work Systems, 2202 Water St., Duluth, MN 55812

Key Functional Assessments, 1010 Park Ave., Minneapolis, MN 55404

Lafayette Instruments, P.O. Box 5729, Lafayette, IN 47903

Med-X Corp, 1155 NE 77th St., Ocala, FL 32670, (352) 622-2112

Motion Analysis Corp., 3650 N. Laughlin Rd, Santa Rosa, CA 95403

Smith and Nephew Rolyan, N93 W14475 Whittaker Way, P.O. Box 555, Menomonee Falls, WI 53051

Valpar International, 2450 W. Ruthrauff Road, Tucson, AZ 87505

Work Evaluation Systems Technology (WEST), P.O. Box 2477, Fort Bragg, CA 95437

Work Recovery System, 2341 S. Friebus, Ste. 14, Tucson, AZ 85713

G-8. Scooters

Amigo Mobility International, Inc. *(Amigo Centra),* 6693 Dixie Highway, Bridgeport, MI 48722, Tel. (517) 777-0910

Bruno Independent Living Aids, Inc. *(Regal Scooters),* 1780 Executive Dr., P.O. Box 84, Oconomowoc, WI 53066, Tel. (414) 567-4990; (800) 882-8183; Fax: (414) 567-4341

Burke, Inc. *(Super Scout 3-Wheeler),* 1800 Meriam Lane, Kansas City, KS 66106, Tel. (913) 722-5658; (800) 255-4147

Electric Mobility *(Electric Mobility Sparky 4-Wheeler; Rascal 3-Wheeler; Rascal Convertible),* Mobility Plaza, Sewell, NJ 08080, Tel. (800) 662-4548

Everest & Jennings, *(New E&J Scooter),* 3233 E. Mission Oaks Blvd., Camarillo, CA 93010, Tel. (905) 987-6911

Golden Technologies *(Scoota Bug; Sterling),* 4 Conyngham Ave., Wilkes-Barre, PA 18702, Tel. (717) 829-4119; Fax: (800) 628-5165

Gopher Research and Development *(GopherII),* P.O. Box 2199, Fullerton, CA 92663, Tel. (714) 879-0681

Invacare Fulfillment Center, 561 Ternes Ave., Elyria, OH 44035, Tel. (216) 329-6456; (800) 828-6282; Fax: (216) 365-7330

Jubilee Scooter, Inc. *(California Comfort; Jubilee 3-Wheel Scooter),* 324 Lakeside Drive, Foster City, CA 94404, Tel. (415) 571-5323

Leisure-Lift *(Pace Saver Plus II),* 1800 Merrimam Lane, Kansas City, KS 66106, Tel. (913) 722-5658

Mobilelectrics Co. *(Shuttle; Sidekick Scooter),* 4311 Woodgate Lane, Louisville, KY 40220

Motovator *(Motovator Three-Wheel Scooter),* 1732 Border Ave., Torrance, CA 90501, Tel. (310) 320-5941

Ortho-Kinetics, Inc. *(Bravo! + Three-Wheel Scooter; Explorer + 4-Wheel Scooter; MVP + 3-Wheel Scooter; Triumph Scooter),* P.O. Box 1647, Waukesha, WI 53187, Tel. (414) 542-6060; (800) 824-1068; Fax: (414) 542-3990

Palmer Industries *(Outdoor Independence; Palmer Independence; Palmer Twosome),* Box 707, Endicott, NY 13760, Tel. (607) 754-1954

Wheels For Freedom, Inc. *(Freedom Wheel Rover),* 2266 S. Dobson Road #207, Mesa, AZ 85202, Tel. (602) 730-5533

G-9. Wheelchair (Manual and Powered) Manufacturers and Suppliers

Active Aid, One Active Aid Road, P.O. Box 259, Redwood Falls, MN 56203-0359

Arista Surgical Supply Co., *(Vista WC),* Lexington Ave., New York, NY 10010, Tel. (212) 679-3694; (800) 223-1984

Artec, Inc., *(WC Rocker),* P.O. Box 25103-A, Greenville, SC 29616, Tel. (800) 445-0234

Convaid Products, Inc. *(Compax 12),* P.O. Box 2458, Rancho Palos Verdes, CA 90274, Tel. (213) 539-6814

Damaco, Inc. *(Damaco portable power unit for WC),* 20542 Plummer St., Chatsworth, CA 91311, Tel. (818) 709-4534; (800) 432-2434; (818) 709-5282

Eagle Sportschairs, 2351 Parkwood Place, Snellville, GA 60278, Tel. (404) 972-0763; (800) 932-9380; Fax: (404) 985-4885

ETAC-USA, Inc. *(Cross WC; Edge WC; Elite WCs; Swede Sting),* 2325 Parklawn Drive, Ste. J, Waukesha, WI 53186, Tel. (414) 796-4600; (800) 678-3822; Fax: (414) 796-4605

Everest & Jennings *(Formula Series Active WC; Power WCs),* 3233 E. Mission Oaks Blvd., Camarillo, CA 93010, Tel. (905) 987-6911

Fortress *(Custom WC; Freestyle II; Liberty; Sports WCs; Power WCs),* 827 Jefferson Ave., Clovis, CA 93612, Tel. (209) 323-0292; Fax: (209) 323-0299

Fortress Scientific, 61 Miami St., Buffalo, NY 14204

Gadabout Wheelchairs *(Gadabout Portable WC),* 1165 Portland Ave., Rochester, NY 14621, Tel. (716) 544-9060; (800) 828-4242

Garaventa Canada Ltd. *(Emergency Evacuation Chair),* P.O. Box L-1, Blaine, WA 98230, Tel. (800) 663-6556

Gaymar Industries *(HiRider WC),* 10 Centre Drive, Orchard Park, NY 14127, Tel. (716) 662-2551; (800) 828-7341

Gendron, Inc. *(WC for obese patients; Sport Lite),* Lugbill Road, Archbold, OH 43502, Tel. (800) 537-2521

Gunnell, Inc., 221 North Water St., Vassar, MI 48768

Invacare Corp., *(Rolls 2000; YM 9000 Ride-Lite),* 899 Cleveland St., Elyria, OH 44036, Tel. (216) 329-6000; (800) 333-6900

Iron Horse Productions, Inc. *(Iron Horse WC),* 2624 Conner St., Port Huron, MI 48060, Tel. (810) 987-6700; (800) 426-0354

K-Chair Corp. *(K-Chair),* 105 W. Dakota, #114, Clovis, CA 93612

Kareco International *(Klassic-Plus WC),* Colony Road, Jersey, NJ 07305, Tel. (201) 434-8301

Kuschall of America, *(Champion; Rigid WC),* 753 Calle Plano, Camrillo, CA 93010, Tel. (805) 484-3595; (800) 654-4768; Fax: (805) 987-9844

LDC Corp. of America, Inc. *(Stand-up WC),* 780-B2 Primos Ave., Folcroft, PA 19032, Tel. (610) 586-0986; (800) 782-6324; Fax: (610) 586-0847

Magic in Motion, Inc. *(Shadow Rigid WC; Rigid Sports WC),* 239 W. Stewart, Puyallup, WA 98371, Tel. (206) 848-6845

Motion Designs, Inc. *(Breezy; Quickie),* 2842 Business Park Ave., Fresno, CA 93727, Tel. (209) 292-2171

Permobil of America, Inc. *(Power WCs),* 30 Ray Ave., Burlington, MA 01803, Tel. (617) 229-9748; Fax: (617) 229-9841

Redman Wheelchairs *(Apache WC; Crow WC; Power WCs),* 3840 South Palo Verde, Tucson, AZ 85714, Tel. (800) 727-6684

Roleez Wheel System *(Sports WCs)*, 5717 Sellger Drive, Norfolk, VA 23502, Tel. (804) 461-1122; (800) 369-1390; Fax: (804) 461-0383

RX-Rocker *(RX-Rocker WC)*, 2495 Teller Road, Newbury Park, CA 91320, Tel. (805) 499-0696

Sportaid *(Sports WCs and parts)*, 2462 Centerville-Rosebud Road, Loganville, GA 30249, Tel. (404) 979-5185; (800) 743-7203; Fax: (404) 979-7203

Steven Motor Chair Co. *(Power WCs)*, 120 N. Gunter St., Siloam Springs, AR 72761, Tel. (501) 524-8448

Sunrise Medical *(Breezy; Quickie)*, 2842 Business Park Ave., Fresno, CA 93727, Tel. (209) 292-2171

21st Century Scientific, Inc., *(Power WCs)* 4915 Industrial Way, Coeur d'Alene, ID 83814, Tel. (208) 667-8800; (800) 448-3680; Fax: (208) 667-6600

Top End by Action *(Sports WCs)*, 4501 63 Circle North, Pinellas Park, FL 34665, Tel. (812) 522-8677; (800) 532-8677; Fax: (813) 522-1007

Wheelchair Institute of Kansas *(Wizzard WC)*, P.O. Box 777, La Crosse, KS 67548, Tel. (800) 537-6454

X-L Manufacturing Co., Inc., 4950-D Cohasset Stage Road, Chiro, CA 45926

G-10. Wheelchair and Scooter Accessories

Accent Books & Products *(Wheelchair Batteries)*, P.O. Box 700, Bloomington, IL 61702, Tel. (309) 378-2961; (800) 787-8444; Fax: (309) 378-4420

Ahnafield Corp. *(Latchloc Automatic Wheelchair Tiedown)*, 3219 West Washington, Indianapolis, IN 46222, Tel. (317) 636-8061

Air Lift Unlimited, Inc. *(Air Lift: Wheelchair Walker Oxygen Carry)*, 1212 Kerr Gulch, Evergreen, CO 80439, Tel. (303) 526-0132

APT Technology, Inc. *(Recline Control)*, 8765 Twp. Road 513, Shreve, OH 44676, Tel. (216) 567-2001

Bailey Manufacturing Co. *(Wheelchair Work Table)*, 118 Lee St., Lodi, OH 44254, Tel. (216) 948-1080

Cleo of New York, Inc. *(Lift and Carry Wheelchair Caddy; Transfer Board)*, South Buckout St., Trent Bldg, Irvington, NY 10533, Tel. (914) 251-1422; (800) 321-0595

Curtis Instruments, Inc. *(Scooter and WC battery fuel gauges and motor speed controller)*, 200 Kisco Ave., Mt. Kisco, NY 10549, Tel. (914) 666-2971; Fax: (914) 666-2188

D.A. Schulman, Inc. *(Battery Operated Cushion)*, 7701 Newton Ave., North, Brooklyn Park, MN 55444, Tel. (612) 561-2908

Dow Medical *(Electric Scooter Covers)*, 4230 Clipper Drive, Manitownc, WI 54220, Tel. (414) 682-7796

East Penn Manufacturing Co. *(Deka Dominator Batteries)*, Box 147, Lyon Station, PA 19536, Tel. (610) 682-6361

Falcon Rehabilitation Products, Inc. *(Power Recline System)*, 4404 East 60th Ave., Commerce City, CO 80022

Featherspring *(Foot Suport)*, 712 North 34th St., Seattle, WA 98103, Tel. (206) 545-8585

George H. Snyder Enterprises *(WC attachments)*, 5809 NE 21st Ave., Fort Lauderdale, FL 33308, Tel. (954) 491-2886

Graham-Field, Inc. *(Wheelchair Aide)*, 400 Rabro Drive, East Hauppauge, NY 11788, Tel. (516) 582-5900

Grandmar, Inc. *(Torso Support)*, 5675 C. Landregan St., Emery-ville, CA 94608, Tel. (415) 428-0441

LaBac Systems, Inc. *(Power Recline System)*, 8955 South Ridgeline Boulevard, Highlands Ranch, CO 80126

Laurel Designs *(Advantage Bags)*, 5 Laurel Ave., Beivedere, CA 94920, Tel. (415) 435-1891; Fax: (415) 435-1451

Lester Electrical, Inc. *(Lester Dual-Mode Battery Charger; Lestronic II Battery Charger)*, 625 West A St., Lincoln, NE 68522, Tel. (402) 477-8988

Med Covers, Inc. *(Wheelchair Back Pack and Tote Bag)*, 1639-D Green St., Raleigh, NC 27603, Tel. (919) 832-9711

MK Battery *(MK U-1 Gel Battery)*, 13752 Harbor Blvd., Garden Grove, CA 92643, Tel. (714) 554-9903

Osterguard Enterprises *(Camera Holder; Tilt-N-Table)*, 3228 West Olive, Fresno, CA 93722, Tel. (209) 275-4695

Pac-All Carriers, Inc. *(Pac-All Wheelchair Carrier)*, 2321 Carolton Road, Maitland, FL 32751, Tel. (407) 830-6604; Fax: (407) 339-2847

Skyway Machine, Inc., 4451 Caterpillar Road, Redding, CA 96003, Tel. (916) 243-5151; (800) 332-3357; Fax: (916) 243-5104

Thomas Hardware *(WC parts & fasteners)*, 1001 Rockland St., Reading, PA 19604, Tel. (215) 921-2723; (800) 634-4293; Fax: (800) 634-3099

G-11. Ventilator Manufacturers

Aequitron Medical Inc. *(Aequitron LP-6 and LP-10)*, 14800 28th Ave., N., Minneapolis, MN 55447-4834, Tel. (612) 557-9200; (800) 824-7103; Fax: (612) 557-8200

Bear Medical Systems, Inc. *(Intermed Bear 33)*, 2085 Rustin Ave., Riverside, CA 92507-2437, Tel. (714) 788-2460; (800) 232-7633; Fax: (714) 351-4609

Lifecare International Inc. *(Lifecare PLV-100 and 102)*, 655 Aspen Ridge Dr., Lafayette, CO 80026-9341, Tel. (303) 666-9234; (800) 669-9234; Fax: (303) 666-0415

Puritan-Bennett Corp. *(Puritan-Bennett Companion 2800 or 2801)*, Portable Ventilator Division, 4865 Sterling Dr., Boulder, CO 80301, Tel. (303) 443-3350; (800) 248-0890; Fax: (303) 443-4673

Respironics, Inc. *(Respironic BiPAP unit)*, 1001 Murry Ridge Drive, Murrysville, PA 15668-8550, Tel. (412) 733-0200; Fax: (412) 722-0299

G-12. Work-Related Organizations, Associations, and Government Agencies

American Board of Independent Medical Examiners, 55 West Seegers Rd, Arlington Heights, IL 60005, Tel. (800) 234-3940; Fax: (847) 228-1856

American College of Occupational and Environmental Medicine, 55 West Seegers Rd, Arlington Heights, IL 60005-3919, Tel. (847) 228-6850; Fax: (847) 228-6849

American Occupational Medicine Association, 2340 S. Arlington Heights Rd, Arlington Heights, Il 60005, Tel. (312) 228-6850

Barrier Free Environments (BFE), P.O. Box 30634, Water Garden, Highway 70, West Raleigh, NC 27622

Department of Transportation, 400 Seventh St., S.W., Washington, DC 20590, Tel. (202) 366-1656; TDD: (202) 366-4567

Equal Employment Opportunity Commission, 1801 L St. N.W., Washington, DC 20507, Tel. (800) 669-3362; TDD: (800) 800-3302

Federal Communications Commission, 1919 M St. N.W.,Washington, DC 20554, Tel. (202) 632-7260; TDD: (202) 632-6999

Federal Transit Administration (FTA), 400 7th St., S.W., Room 9400, Washington, DC 20590

Foundation on Employment and Disability, 3820 Del Amo Blvd., #201, Torrance, CA 90503, Tel. (213) 214-3430

Job Accommodation Network (JAN), President's Committee on Employment of People with Disabilities, West Virginia University, 918 Chestnut Ridge Road, Ste. 1, P.O. Box 6080, Morgantown, WV 26506-6080, Tel. (800) 526-7234; (800) 526-4698; (in WV); Fax: (800) 304-5407

National Institute for Occupational Safety and Health (NIOSH), 1095 Willowdale Rd, Morgantown, WV 26505-2888, Tel. (304) 285-5704

National Safety Council (NCS), P.O. Box 558, Itasca, IL 60143-0558, Tel. (800) 621-7619; Fax: (630) 285-0797

Occupational Safety and Health Administration (OSHA), Department of Public Affairs, 200 Constitution Ave. NW, Washington, DC 20210, Tel. (202) 219-8148

President's Committee on Employment of People with Disabilities (PCEPD), 1331 F St., N.W., 3rd floor, Washington, DC 2004-1107, Tel. (202) 376-6200; TDD: (202) 376-6205; Fax: (202) 376-6219

U.S. Architectural and Transportation Barriers Compliance Board ("Access Board"), 1331 F St. N.W., Ste. 1000, Washington, DC 20004-1111, Tel. (800) USA-ABLE

U.S. Department of Justice, Office on the American With Disabilities Act, Civil Rights Division, P.O. Box 66738, Washington, DC 20035, Tel. (202) 514-0301, (800) 514-0301; Fax: (800) 514-0383

U.S. Department of Labor, Employment Standard Administration, Office of Federal Contract Compliance Programs (OFCCP), 200 Constitution Ave. NW, Washington, DC 20210

INDEX

A

Absorptiometry, 38
Academic achievement tests, 100
Accessibility
  community, ADL adaptations for, 277
  external building, 277
  home
    ADL adaptations for, 272–276
    elevators for, 273
  internal building, 277
Acetaminophen, 321–322
  with caffeine, 332
Acetylsalicylic acid, 329
  with caffeine, 332
  with muscle relaxants, 332
Acid phosphatase, 23
Activities of daily living
  adaptations for, *see* ADL adaptations
  basic, 262–269
    mobility, 262
    positioning, 262
    transfers and, 262–264
  classification of, 262–281
  communication, 268–269
  community living skills, 276
  functional scales of, 16, *see also* ADL
      scales
  home management and, 270–276
  instrumental, 270–281
  occupational activities and, 281
  physiatric evaluation and, 3
  self-maintenance tasks, 264–268
  spasticity and, 462
Acupuncture, 153–154
Adapin, 357, 366
ADL, *see* Activities of daily living
ADL adaptations, 260–282
  for child care, 271
  for clothing care, 271
  for communication, 268–269
  community accessibility, 277
  for community living, 276
  community mobility, 278–280
  for cooking, 270

environmental, 269
  for home accessibility, 272–276
  for home management, 270–276
  household maintenance, 271
  for laundry, 271
  positioning, 262
  principles for, 260–262
    general, 260–261
    specific, 261
  for self-maintenance tasks, 264–268
  for sexual expression, 269
  for transfers, 262–264
ADL scales
  Functional Independence Measure, 16
  Katz index of independence in, 97
  Kenny self-care evaluation, 97
  Klein-Bell, 95
Adrenergic drugs, 382–383
Adverse drug reactions
  nonsteroidal antiinflammatory drugs,
      323–326
  opioid analgesics, 334–335
  to skeletal muscle relaxants, 344
Advil, 331
Aerobic-work capacity testing, 60
AFO, *see* Ankle-foot orthoses
Age-adjusted maximal heart formula,
      168
Airway clearance, 693–696
Airway obstruction, mechanical,
      dysphagia and, 536
Alendronate, 379
Alexander technique, 176
Alkanone NSAIDs, 332
Allergies, history of, 4
Aleve, 331
Alprazolam, 365
Ambien, 368
Americans with Disabilities Act of 1990,
      646
Amitriptyline, 357
  trigger point therapy and, 415
Amphetamines, 369
  administration guidelines, 370

adverse drug reactions, 369–370
contraindications/precautions to, 370
mechanism of action of, 369
Amyotrophic lateral sclerosis, muscle
  weakness and, 124
Anabolic steroids, 381
Anaerobic threshold, pulmonary ETT
  and, 92
Anafranil, 357
Anal continence studies, 561
Anal stretch voiding, 544
Analgesics, 321–343
  adjuvant, 343
  nonnarcotic, 321–332
  nonnarcotic combinations, 332
  nonopioid, 321–332
  opioid, 332–343
    administration guidelines, 336
    adverse drug reactions, 334–335
    contraindications/precautions for,
      336
    mechanism of action of, 333
    opioid classification and, 333
    physical dependence and, 335
    pure-agonist, 340–342
    semisynthetic pure-agonist, 340
    synthetic pure-agonist, 340–342
  pain management and, 636
Anaprox, 331
Androgens, 381
Anemia, treatment of, 439
Anesthetics
  local, 389
  pain management and, 635
Angiography, 40–41
Ankle, prostheses for, 232–242
Ankle pain, differential diagnoses of,
  119
Ankle-foot orthoses, 188–194
  with flange, 192
  guidelines for prescription of, 189
  hemispiral, 192
  hinged, 192
  metal, 192–194
  posterior leaf spring, 191
  solid, 191–192
  spiral, 192
  thermoplastic, 191–192
  tone-reducing
Anorectal catheter manometry, 560
Ansaid, 331

Antiaggression drugs, 371–372
Antiarrhythmic drugs, 384
Anti-bone-mineralization agents, 382
Anticoagulant therapy, 373–376
Anticonvulsants, 350–353
  administration guidelines, 350
  adverse drug reactions, 350
  contraindications/precautions, 350
  mechanism of action, 350
  pain management and, 634
Antidepressants, 353–360
  administration guidelines, 356–357
  adverse drug reactions, 356
  classification of, 353
  contraindications to, 356
  mechanism of action, 353
  tricyclic, 357
Antihistamines, 372–373
  adverse drug reactions, 372
  contraindications/precautions to, 372
  mechanism of action of, 372
Antihypertensive agents, pain
  management and, 638
Antiinflammatory drugs, nonsteroidal,
  323–332
  administration guidelines, 328–329
  adverse drug reactions, 323–326
  alkanone, 332
  arylpropionic acid, 331
  contraindications/precautions, 328
  enolic acid, 332
  fenamate, 332
  gastrointestinal toxicity, 326–328
  hepatic toxicity, 326
  heteroaryl acetic acid, 331–332
  indene acetic acid, 330
  indole, 330
  mechanism of action, 323
  nonsalicylate, 330–332
  opioids and, 342–343
  renal toxicity of, 326
  salicylate, 329–330
Antinuclear antibodies, 25
Antiplatelets, 376–377
Antispasticity agents, pain management
  and, 638
Antispasticity medications, 463–465
Anxiety, differential diagnoses of, 128
Anxiolytics, 361–366
  nonbenzodiazepines, 365–366
  pain management and, 637

Aphasia, 482–495
  assessment tools for, 486–489
  Broca's, 485
  classification of, 482–486
  comprehensive language tests,
    487–488
  conduction, 484–485
  fluent, 484
  functional communication tests,
    488–489
  global, 486
  major fluent, 484
  major nonfluent, 485
  minor fluent, 485
  minor nonfluent, 486
  mixed transcortical, 486
  nonfluent, 485
    anomic, 485
    transcortical sensory, 485
  prognosis for speech recovery,
    489–491
    medical variables, 489–490
    patient variables, 490
    speech/language variables, 490
  specialized tests for, 489
  transcortical motor, 486
  treatment for, 491–495
    interdisciplinary team approach,
      495
    speech therapy aids, 495
  Wernicke's, 484
Apraxia of speech, 503–505
  assessment of, 504
  retraining approaches, 504
  treatment of, 504
Aptitude tests, 101
Arm sling, 218
Arthrography, 42
Arthropathy
  crystal-associated, musculoskeletal
    pain and, 110
  degenerative, musculoskeletal pain
    and, 110
  inflammatory, musculoskeletal pain
    and, 110
Arylpropionic acid NSAIDs, 331
Ashworth Spasticity Scale, Modified,
  461
Aspirin, 377, *see* Acetylsalicylic acid
Atarax, 366, 372
Ataxia, differential diagnoses of, 126
Athletes, speed training and, 174

Ativan, 364
Atrophy, *see* Muscle atrophy
Attentional disorders, 501
Attitude tests, 101
Audiometry
  pure tone, 510
  speech, 510–511
Autotraction, 148
Axillary pain, differential diagnoses of,
  114

B

Back pain
  differential diagnoses of, 113
  low, *see* Low back pain
Baclofen, intrathecal, for spasticity,
  471–473
Bacterial infection, dysphagia and, 535
Balance, evaluation of, 15
Barbiturates, 369
Bartel Index, 95
Bathing, ADL adaptations for, 267–268
Beck Depression Inventory, 101
Bed mobility, 262
Behavioral management, voiding
  dysfunction and, 542–544
Benadryl, 369, 372
Bench-stepping test, 88
Benzodiazepines, 363–365, 367–369
  administration guidelines, 364
  adverse drug reactions, 363
  contraindications/precautions for, 364
  long-acting anxiolytic, 365
  mechanism of action of, 363
  physical dependence on, 363
  short-acting anxiolytic, 364
Bilateral Adductor Tone Score, 461
Biofeedback, 144–145
  dysphagia and, 534
  spasticity and, 463
  for voiding dysfunction, 544
Biopsy
  muscle, 28
  synovial, 28
Biphosphonates, 379–380
Bladder augmentation, 548
Bladder cancer, voiding dysfunction and,
  551
Bladder outlet procedures, 549–550
Bladder stimulation, 544

Bladder training, 542
Blink reflex/response, 50
Blocks, *see also* Nerve blocks; Spinal
        blocks
    brachial plexus, 408
    epidural, 402
    plexus, 408
    subarachnoid, 402
Blood gas
    measurement of, 76
    pulmonary ETT and, 91
Blood pressure, exercise tolerance
        testing and, 81
Bobath approach, 173
Bone mineral analyses, 38
Bone scanning, radionuclide, 38–39
Bone-formation agents, 381
Bone-metabolism regulators, 377–382
Borg's rate of perceived exertion scale,
        169–172
Borrelia burgdorferi, 27
Boston Diagnostic Aphasia Examination,
        487
Boston thoracolumbosacral orthosis, 223
Botox, for spasticity, 468–469
Bowel dysfunction, 553–579
    classification by causative factors,
        561–563
    complications of, 578–579
    diagnosis of, 558–561
    diagnostic tests for, 559–561
    epidemiology of, 557–558
    management of
        nonsurgical, 563–577
        surgical, 577–578
    neuroanatomy/neurophysiology of,
        553–554
Bowel evacuation, phases of, 555–557
Brace
    long leg, *see* Knee-ankle-foot orthoses
    short leg, *see* Ankle-foot orthoses
Braden scale, 434
Brain tumor, hemiplegia and, 126
Breast feeding, *see* Lactation
Breasts, review of systems and, 6
Breathing
    controlled, 175
        techniques for, 696–699
    diaphragmatic, 175, 696–697
    eye-movement technique for, 175
    "one" technique for, 175
    segmental, 697

Broca's aphasia, 485
Bronchodilators, 675
Brunnstrom approach, 173
Bulbar palsy, muscle weakness and, 124
Bupropion, 360
BuSpar, 365, 371
Buspirone, 365, 371
Buttock pain, differential diagnoses of,
        113
Butyrophenone, 361

C

Caffeine
    acetaminophen and, 332
    acetylsalicylic acid and, 332
Calcimar, 378–379
Calcitonin, 378–379
Calcium, 380
Calcium-channel blockers, 383–384
Camber, of manual wheelchairs, 297
Canadian Elbow Extensor Crutches, 288
Cancer, pain syndromes associated with,
        112–113
Canes, 288–289
    gait patterns with, 290
Carbamazepine, 352
Carbon Cop II foot, 235
Cardiac deconditioning, changes due to,
        427
Cardiac problems, 708–723
    diagnostic tests for, 710–711
    epidemiology of, 708–723
    evaluation for, 709–713
    laboratory tests for, 711
    physical examination for, 710
Cardiac rehabilitation, 713–722
Cardiac system and, review of systems
        and, 6
Cardiovascular drugs, 382–384
Carisoprodol, 344
Carpal tunnel syndrome, soft tissue
        injections and, 399
Carpometacarpal joint, pain, differential
        diagnoses of, 116
Carr and Shepherd approach, stroke
        patients and, 173–174
Carts, electric, 319–320
Casts, serial, spasticity and, 463
Cataflam, 331
Catapres, spasticity and, 464

Cellular immunity testing, for Lyme disease, 27
Central pain, 106
Centrally mediated pain, intravenous tests for, 403
Cerebrospinal fluid analysis, 24
Cervical orthoses, 220–223
Cervical traction, 146–147
Child care, ADL adaptations for, 271
Children, orthoses for, 206
Chloral hydrate, 368
Chlordiazepoxide, 365
Chlormezanone, 366
Chlorpromazine, 361
Chlorzoxazone, 344
Choline magnesium trisalicylate, 330
Chorea, 127
Circuit weight training, 164
Clinoril, 330
Clomipramine, 357
Clonazepam, 353
Clonidine, spasticity and, 464
Clorazepate, 365
Clothing care, ADL adaptations for, 271
Codeine, 340
    Tylenol with, 342
Cognition, evaluation of, 12
Cognitive-communication impairment, 495–500
    assessment of, 497
    classification of, 496
    cognitive deficits and, 496
    prognosis of, 497
    psychopharmacologic interventions, 499
    treatment of, 497–499
Cold, therapeutic, 136–137
Cold laser, low-power, 139–140
Communication, ADL adaptations for, 268–269
Communication Effectiveness Index, 488
Communication impairment, right hemisphere, 500–503
    assessment of, 501–502
    classification of, 500–501
    prognosis of, 502
    treatment of, 502–503
Communicative Abilities in Daily Living, 488
Compazine, 361, 366
Complement assay, 26

Comprehensive language tests
    Boston Diagnostic Aphasia Examination, 487
    Minnesota Test for Differential Diagnosis of Aphasia, 488
    Neurosensory Center Comprehensive Examination for Aphasia, 488
    Porch Index of Communicative Ability, 487
    Western Aphasia Battery, 487
Compression stockings, for venous thromboembolism, 451
Computer-assisted tomography, description of, 31
Conditioning, 165
Confusional states, differential diagnoses of, 128
Consciousness, level of, 10
Continent diversion, 549
Continuous passive movement machine, 159
Contraception methods, 599–603
Contrast bath, 138
Contrast imaging, 40–42
Cooking, ADL adaptations for, 270
Coordination
    approach for improving, 173–174
    evaluation of, 15
COPD, see Pulmonary disease, chronic obstructive
Cordectomy, for spasticity, 480
Cordotomy, for spasticity, 480
Coronary heart disease, risk factors for, 709
Corset, spinal, 227
Cortical disorders
    muscle weakness and, 124
    paraplegia and, 125
    tetraplegia and, 125
Corticosteroids, 345–350
    administrations guidelines, 346
    adverse drug reactions, 346
    alternate-day therapy guidelines, 347
    classification, 350
    contraindications/precautions, 346
    daily regimen guidelines, 347
    discontinuation guidelines, 347
    intraarticular, 386–389
    mechanism of action of, 346
    pain management and, 639
Cough preparations, 677

Cough reflex, dysphagia and, 517
Coumadin, 373
Cranial nerves, evaluation of, 13
Craniosacral therapy, 150
Crank ergometer, cardiovascular exercise
    tolerance testing and, 87–88
C-reactive protein, 24
Crede's maneuver, 544
Cricopharyngeal myotomy, for
    dysphagia, 535
Crutches, 286–288
  axillary, 287
  gait patterns with, 289–290
  Lofstrand, 287
Cryoglobulins, 25
CT, *see* Computer-assisted tomography
CTS, *see* Carpal tunnel syndrome
Cycle-ergometer, cardiovascular exercise
    tolerance testing and, 86–87
Cyclobenzaprine, 344
  trigger point therapy and, 415
Cylert, 370
Cystometrogram, voiding dysfunction
    and, 541
Cystoscopy, voiding dysfunction and,
    541

D

Dacron webbing hip rotation strap, 201
Dantrium, spasticity and, 464
Dantrolene sodium, spasticity and, 464
Daypro, 331
de Quervain's syndrome, tendon
    injections and, 398
Dead space volume, pulmonary ETT
    and, 92
Deconditioning, 425–430
  cardiac, changes due to, 427
  cardiovascular changes in, 427–428
  contractures and, 425
  dependent edema and, 428
  disuse osteoporosis and, 426–427
  endocrine changes, 429
  fluid balance changes in, 427–428
  gastrointestinal changes and, 428–429
  genitourinary changes and, 429
  metabolic changes, 429
  muscle weakness/atrophy and, 426
  musculoskeletal changes in, 425–427

  neurological changes in, 430
  nutritional changes, 429
  pressure ulcers and, 428
  respiratory changes in, 428
  skin changes in, 428
  subcutaneous bursitis and, 428
  venous thromboembolism and, 428
Defecography, 561
DeLorme technique, 163
Dementia, differential diagnoses of, 129
Demyelinating disease, hemiplegia and,
    126
Depakene, 352
Desoxyn, 370
Desyrel, 360, 369
Dexedrine, 370
Dexterity, poor, ADL adaptations for,
    261
Dextran-40 solution, 376–377
Dextroamphetamine, 370
Diaphragm, evaluation of, 7
Diaphragmatic breathing, 175, 696–697
Diarrhea, 561–562
Diathermy
  microwave, 136
  short wave, 135–136
Diazepam, 345, 365
  spasticity and, 464
Diclofenac, 331
Didronel, 380, 382
Differential diagnoses
  of nonpain problems, 124–130
  of pain, 105–124
Diflunisal, 330
Dilantin, 351
Diphenhydramine, 369, 372
Dipyridamole, 377
Disability, definition of, 3
Disalcid, 330
Disarticulation prostheses
  elbow, 256–259
  shoulder, 258
Discography, 42
Disequilibrium, differential diagnoses of,
    129
Dissociative visualization, 176
Distal interphalangeal joint, pain,
    differential diagnoses of, 116
Dizziness, ill-defined, differential
    diagnoses of, 129
Documentation, 3–20

Dolobid, 330
Doppler
  continuous-wave, 35
  pulsed-wave, 36
  vascular, 35
Doxepin, 357, 366
Dressing, ADL adaptations for, 265
Driving, ADL adaptations for, 278–279
Dual energy x-ray absorptiometry, 38
Dynamometry
  cervical, 57
  for limb muscle groups, 55–56
  physical examination and, 10
  of trunk, 56–57
  whole-body, 57
Dysarthria, 505–508
  assessment of, 506–507
  ataxic, 506
  classification of, 505–506
  flaccid, 505–506
  hyperkinetic, 506
  hypokinetic, 506
  spastic, 506
  treatment of, 507–508
Dyskinesia, 127
Dysphagia, 514–537
  biofeedback and, 534
  bolus modifications, 526–528
  classification by causative factors, 524
  complications of, 535–537
  cough reflex and, 517
  diagnostic tests for, 518–524
  epidemiology of, 515
  evaluation for, 515–524
  feeding modification for, 525
  gag reflex and, 517
  imaging studies for, 523
  management of
    nonsurgical, 525–534
    patient education, 525
    surgical, 534–535
  pathophysiology of, 514–515
  physical examination for, 516–517
  sensory stimulation for, 530–531
  strengthening exercise for, 532–533
  swallowing maneuvers for, 533
  swallowing reflex modulation, 531
  therapeutic exercises for, 531–532
Dysphasia, *see* Aphasia
Dysreflexia, autonomic, voiding
    dysfunction and, 551

Dystonia, involuntary movement
    disorders and, 126–127
Dystropin, 24

E

Echocardiography, 35
Effexor, 360
Ejaculation, chemical, 598
Elastic suspension belt, 247
Elavil, 357
Elbow
  differential diagnoses of pain, 114
  mobilization orthoses, 219
  orthoses for, 218
  prostheses for, 248–259
Electrocardiogram, 23
Electrocardiogram pattern, exercise
    tolerance testing and, 82
Electrodiagnostic testing, 44–50
Electroejaculation, 598
Electrogoniometer, 53
Electromyography, 46–48
Electrotherapy, 140–144
  TES classification
    by current type, 140–142
    by stimulation effect, 142–144
Elevators, 272
EMG, *see* Electromyography
Endep, 357
Endocrine system
  deconditioning and, 429
  review of systems and, 7
Endotracheal tube, 701
Endurance, low, ADL adaptations for,
  261
Endurance exercise/training
  aerobic, 166–168
    Borg's rate of perceived exertion
      scale, 169–172
  anaerobic, 172
    neurodevelopment technique of,
      173
    Rood approach, 173
    sensorimotor approach, 173
  cardiopulmonary, 165–172
  relaxation exercise, 174–176
  speed training and, 174
  total body, 165–172
Enolic acid NSAIDs, 332

Enoxaparin, 376
Enzyme-linked immunosorbent assay,
    for Lyme disease, 27
Epicondylar strap, 218
Erectile dysfunction, 588
Erythrocyte sedimentation rate, 24
Estrazolam, 367
Estrogen replacement, 377–378
    administration guidelines, 378
    adverse drug reactions to, 378
    contraindications/precautions, 378
    mechanism of action of, 378
Ethchlorvynol, 369
Etidronate, 380
Etidronate disodium, 382
Etodolac, 331
ETT, *see* Exercise tolerance testing
Evaluation, *see also* Physiatric
        evaluation
    clinical, 3–20
Evoked potential studies, 48–49
Exercise
    cardiopulmonary endurance, 165–172
    endurance, *see* Endurance exercise/
        training
    mobility, 158–161
    motor coordination, 172–173
    reciprocal unit for, 159
    therapeutic, *see* Therapeutic exercise
Exercise tolerance testing, 79–94
    cardiovascular, 79–89
        intermittent-load, 88
        interpretation guidelines, 83–84
        single-load, 88–89
        treadmill, 84
    pulmonary, 89–93
Expirogram, forced, 70
Expressive deficits, 500
Extralinguistic deficits, 500
Extremities, *see* Limbs

F

Facet injections, diagnostic, 404
Facial pain, differential diagnoses of,
    111, 113
Fatigue, chronic, differential diagnoses
    of, 128
Fecal impaction, 578

Fecal incontinence, 561–562
    biofeedback and, 144
Feeding, ADL adaptations for, 264
Feeding tube insertion, for dysphagia,
    535
Feldenkrais method, 176
Femoral fracture, orthosis for, 205
Fenamate NSAIDs, 332
Fenoprofen, 331
Fertility, male, 597–599
Fever, nosocomial, differential diagnoses
    of, 128
FIM, *see* Functional independence
        measures
Finger
    differential diagnoses of pain, 116
    ladder device for, 159
    orthoses for, 207–219
Flecainide, 384
Flexeril, 344
Flex-foot, 235
Flexibility
    evaluation of, 15
    exercises for, 158–159
    measurements of, 51
Flexirule, 53
Flow-volume curve, 72
Fluency disorders, 509
Fluoride, 381
Fluphenazine, 361
Flurbiprofen, 331
Foot
    drop, differential diagnoses of, 126
    orthoses for, 186–188
        heel cup, 186
        University of California
            Biomechanics Laboratory
                insert, 186
    pain, differential diagnoses of,
        119–120
    partial prostheses for, 230
    pressure measurement, 64
    problems
        orthoses for, 179–186
        shoes for, 179–186
    prostheses for, 232–242
Forced expiratory flow rate, 74
Forearm pain, differential diagnoses of,
    114
Forefoot pain, differential diagnoses of,
    120
Fosamax, 379

Frenkel exercise, 172
Friction mechanisms, 242
Functional assessment, instruments for, 95–99
Functional capacity evaluation, 60
  return to work and, 650
Functional communication analyses, for aphasia, 488–489
Functional Communication Profile, 488
Functional community analyses, 64
Functional independence measure, 16, 95

G

Gag reflex, dysphagia and, 517
Gait
  abnormal, causes of, 65
  aids for, 283–292
  assessment techniques, 60–66
  disorders of, differential diagnoses of, 126
  evaluation of, 15
  patterns of, using gait aids, 289–291
  reciprocating orthoses, 202
  stride analyses, 66
  training programs, 290–291
Gallium 67 citrate scan, 39
Gastrointestinal tract
  deconditioning and, 428–429
  pharmacologic agents for, 384
  review of systems and, 6
Genitourinary system
  deconditioning and, 429
  evaluation of, 7
  review of systems and, 6
Gloves
  compression, 214
  shock absorbing, 214
Goniometric techniques, 51–53
Gravity traction, 148
Greenfield filter, for venous thromboembolism, 455
Grooming, ADL adaptations for, 266–267
Guillain-Barre syndrome, muscle weakness and, 124

H

Hair, evaluation of, 7
Halcion, 367

Haloperidol, 361
Halo-vest cervicothoracic orthosis, 222
Halstead-Reitan neuropsychological Battery, 101
Hand
  measurement of strength, 54–55
  orthoses for, 207–219
  pain, differential diagnoses of, 116
  prostheses for, 248–259
Handicap, definition of, 3
Harness, upper limb, 254–255
Headache, differential diagnoses of, 111–112, 113
Health, state of, 7
Health care, personal, ADL adaptations for, 276
Hearing aid, 511
Hearing impairment, 509–512
  assessment of, 510
  auditory tests for, 510
  classification of, 510
  treatment of, 511–512
Heart rate, exercise tolerance testing and, 82
Heat, therapeutic, 133–136
Heating agents
  deep, 134–136
  radiant, 134
  superficial, 133–134
HEENT
  evaluation of, 7
  review of systems and, 6
Hematologic system, review of systems and, 7
Hematological agents, 373–377
Hemiparesis, differential diagnosis of, 125–126
Hemiplegia, differential diagnosis of, 125–126
Hemorrhoids, 578–579
Heparin, 375
Hindfoot eversion, shoe modifications for, 183
Hindfoot pain, differential diagnoses of, 121
Hinges, elbow, 253
Hip, disarticulation prosthesis, 248
Hip joints, 201
Hip locks, 201
Hip orthoses, 204–206
Hip rotation, Dacron webbing strap for, 201

Hip-knee-ankle-foot orthoses, 201–202
History
  of allergies, 4
  chief complaint and, 4
  of cigarette smoking, 5
  current medications and, 4
  economic, 5
  family, 6
  information source and, 4
  lifestyle and habits, 5
  past, 4
  personal, 4
  of present illness, 4
  review of systems, 6
  social, 5
  vocational, 5
HKAFO, *see* Hip-knee-ankle-foot
  orthoses
Household maintenance, ADL
  adaptations for, 271
HPI, *see* History of present illness
Hubbard tanks, 138
Hydrocodone, 342
Hydrotherapy, 134, 137–138
Hydroxyzine, 366, 372
Hygiene, personal, ADL adaptations for,
  266–267
Hypotension
  orthostatic, 427
  postural, 427

I

Ibuprofen, 331
Ice massage, 136–137
Imaging studies
  invasive, 38–43
  noninvasive, 30–37
Imipramine, 357
Immobilization, 425
Immunofluorescent assay, for Lyme
  disease, 27
Impairment, definition of, 3
Inclinometer, 52
Incoordination, ADL adaptations for,
  261
Indene acetic acid, 330
Inderal, 366, 371
Indocin, 330
Indole, 330
Indomethacin, 330

Inserts
  longitudinal arch, 188
  metatarsal, 188
  sesamoid, 188
  University of California Biomechanics
    Laboratory insert, 186
Integument system, evaluation of, 7
Intellectual ability tests, 100
Intermittent catheterization, 545
Intrathecal medications, 471
Intravenous pyelography, 41
Isometric strengthening, 162
  regimens for, 162–163
Isotoner gloves, 214
Isotonic strength testing,
  nondynamometric, 54
Isotonic strengthening, equipment for,
  164
IVP, *see* Intravenous pyelography

J

Jacobson exercise, 176
Job analyses, 651
Jobst gloves, 214
Joint
  contracture, 425–426
  counterstrain, 151
  dysfunction, differential diagnoses of,
    105–106
  injections, 386–410
    supplies for, 386–389
    techniques for, 389–397
  mobilization/manipulation, 161
  pain
    acute generalized, differential
      diagnoses of, 121
    differential diagnoses of, 105–106
    monoarticular, differential
      diagnoses of, 121–122
    polyarticular, differential diagnoses
      of, 133
  stability, evaluation of, 10
Jones technique, 150

K

Kabat and Voss approach, 172
KAFO, *see* Knee-ankle-foot orthoses

Karvonen formula, 168
Katz index of independence in ADLs, 97
Kegel exercises, 544
Kenny self-care evaluation, 97
Kenny Stick, 288
Ketoprofen, 331
Ketorolac, 332
Klein-Bell ADL scale, 95
Klonopin, 353
Knee
    disarticulation prosthesis, 247–248
    orthoses for, 198–201
    pain, differential diagnoses of,
        117–118
    prostheses for, 242–247
    stabilizer, three-way, 199
Knee-ankle-foot orthoses, 194–198
    plastic, 194–198
Knight technique, 163
KO, *see* Knee orthoses
Kymography, bowel dysfunction and,
    560

L

Labor, 603
Laboratory tests, 23–29
    biopsy, 28–29
    rheumatologic, 24–28
    for venous thromboembolism, 449
Lactation, 603–604
Language, *see also* Speech
    evaluation of, 12
Language impairments, 482–499
Laryngeal protection procedures, for
    dysphagia, 535
Laryngoscopy, 523
Lateral sclerosis, muscle weakness and,
    124
Laundry, ADL adaptations for, 271
Leg pain, differential diagnoses of,
    116–117, 118–119
Leukocyte antigen typing, human, 26
Leukocyte scans, 39
Levoprome, 361
Libido, 580
Libritabs, 365
Librium, 365
Lidocaine, 384
Lidocaine test, intravenous, 404

Lifting capacity testing, 57–60
Lifts, mechanical, 272
Light therapy, 138–140
Limber protocol, trigger point therapy
    and, 414
Limbs, *see also* Lower limbs; Upper
    limbs
    evaluation of, 7
    radiography of, 30
Lodine, 331
Lorazepam, 364
Lovenox, 376
Low back pain
    chronic, differential diagnoses of, 111
    differential diagnoses of, 111
Low back syndrome, failed, differential
    diagnoses of, 111
Lower limb
    orthoses for, 179–206
        special-purpose, 204–206
    pain, differential diagnoses of,
        116–121
    prostheses for, 229–248
Lubrication dysfunction, 593
Ludiomil, 360
Lumbar traction, 147–148
Lumbosacral orthoses, 224–225
Lung diffusion capacity, 75
Lung scan, radionuclide ventilation-
    perfusion, 39
Lung volume
    dynamic, 69
    static, 68
Luria-Nebraska Neuropsychological
    Battery, 101
Lyme disease, laboratory testing for, 27
Lyme serologic testing, 27
Lymph nodes, evaluation of, 7
Lymphatic system, review of systems
    and, 6

M

Magnetic resonance imaging, description
    of, 31
Malnutrition, dysphagia and, 536
Manipulation, 148–151
    spinal, 148–151
Manual muscle testing, 54
    physical examination and, 10

Maprotiline, 360
Massage, 151–153
Master's test, 88
McGill-Melzack Pain Questionnaire, 613
Meclofenamate, 332
Meclomen, 332
Medicine, physical, *see* Physical
    medicine and rehabilitation
Mefenamic acid, 332
Mendelsohn maneuver, 534
Mental status, evaluation of, 10
Meprobamate, 366
Metabolic disorders, painful
    polyneuropathy and, 108
Metabolic equivalent
    cardiovascular ETT and, 82
    pulmonary ETT and, 91
Metabolic imbalance, 127
Metabolic system, deconditioning and,
    429
Metacarpometacarpal joint, pain,
    differential diagnoses of, 116
Metaxalone, 345
Methamphetamine, 370
Methocarbamol, 345
Methotrimeprazine, 361
Methylmorphine, 340
Methylphenidate, 370
Methylxanthines, 676
Mexiletine, 384
Mexitil, 384
Miacalcin, 378–379
Millon Behavioral Health Inventory, 617
Millon Clinical Multiaxial Inventory II,
    99
Miltown, 366
Minnesota Multiphasic Personality
    Inventory, 99
Minnesota Test for Differential
    Diagnosis of Aphasia, 488
MMT, *see* Manual muscle testing
Mnemonics
    for admission orders, 16
    for discharge summary, 19
    for history of present illness, 4
    for progress notes, 19
    SOAP, 19
Mobilization, for venous
    thromboembolism, 451
Modalities, physical, *see* Physical
    modalities
Monoamine oxidase inhibitors, 359

Monoarthritis
    acute, 121–122
    chronic, 122
Mononeuropathy, painful, differential
    diagnoses of, 108
Mood assessment, 101
Morphine, 340
    intrathecal, for spasticity, 473
Morton's neuroma, soft tissue injections
    and, 400
Motion analysis system, gait assessment
    and, 64
Motor control
    approach for improving, 173–174
    dysphagia and, 518
    evaluation of, 15
Motor coordination, 172–173
Motor neuron disorders
    lower
        paraplegia and, 125
        tetraplegia and, 125
    muscle weakness and, 124
    upper
        paraplegia and, 125
        tetraplegia and, 125
Motor relearning program, 173–174
Motrin, 331
Movement disorders, involuntary
    differential diagnoses of, 126–127
    evaluation of, 15
Movement patterns, evaluation of, 15
Movement therapy, 173
MRI, *see* Magnetic resonance imaging
Munster supracondylar socket, 252
Muscle
    active inhibition of, 160–161
    biopsy of, 28
Muscle atrophy, deconditioning and, 426
Muscle enzymes, 23
Muscle relaxants
    acetylsalicylic acid and, 332
    skeletal, 343–345
        adverse drug reactions, 344
        contraindications/precautions for,
            344
        drug administration guidelines, 344
        mechanism of action of, 343–344
        single formulations of, 344–345
Muscle strength
    assessment of, 54–57
    evaluation of, 10, 15

Muscle strengthening exercises,
161–165
isometric, 162
equipment for, 162–163
regimens for, 162–163
isotonic, 164–165
equipment for, 164–165
manual, 162
mechanical, 162–165
Muscle tone, evaluation of, 15
Muscle weakness
ADL adaptations for, 261
deconditioning and, 426
differential diagnoses of, 124
Muscular atrophy, muscle weakness and,
124
Muscular dystrophy, muscle weakness
and, 124
Musculoskeletal changes, deconditioning
and, 425–427
Musculoskeletal disorders
joint/soft tissue injections, 386–410
work-related, 645–664
Musculoskeletal pain
acute generalized, differential
diagnoses of, 121
differential diagnoses of, 110–111
Musculoskeletal system
evaluation of, 7
review of systems and, 6–7
Musculoskeletal testing, 51–67
Myasthenia gravis, lower motor neuron
disorders and, 125
Myelography, 41
Myelotomy, for spasticity, 480
Myoclonus, 127
Myoglobinuria, muscle weakness and,
124
Myopathy
drug-induced, muscle weakness and,
124
metabolic, muscle weakness and, 125
toxin-induced, muscle weakness and,
124

N

Nails, evaluation of, 7
Nalfon, 331
Naprelan, 331

Naprosyn, 331
Naproxen, 331
Neck, evaluation of, 7
Neck pain, differential diagnoses of, 113
Nefazodone, 360
Nerve blocks, 401–410
chemical, for spasticity, 465–469
diagnostic, 401–404
peripheral, for spasticity, 469–471
preemptive, 404
prognostic, 404
somatic, 404–408
sympathetic, 408–409
therapeutic, 404–408
Nerve conduction studies, 44–46
Neurectomy, peripheral, for spasticity,
480
Neurodevelopment technique, of
endurance exercise, 173
Neurogenic communication disorders,
482–513
Neurogenic dysphagia, differential
diagnoses of, 127
Neuroleptic drugs, 360–361
adverse drug reactions, 360
contraindications to, 361
mechanism of action of, 360
pain management and, 633
Neurologic drugs, 384
Neurologic status, deconditioning and,
430
Neurologic system
evaluation of, 10–16
review of systems and, 7
Neuromuscular assessment, functional,
16
Neuromuscular electrical stimulator, 144
Neuromuscular junction studies, 49–50
Neuromusculoskeletal problems,
differential diagnoses of, 105–122
Neuropathic pain, differential diagnoses
of, 106
Neuropathy, peripheral, 127
Neuropsychologic battery tests, 100–101
Neurosensory Center Comprehensive
Examination for Aphasia, 488
Noctec, 368
Nonlinguistic deficits, 500
Norflex, 345
Norton scale, 434
NSAIDs, *see* Antiinflammatory drugs,
nonsteroidal

Nuclear medicine, 38–40
Nutrition, restoration of, 439
Nutritional needs, deconditioning and, 429
Nutritional therapy, pulmonary disorders and, 671
Nystagmus, differential diagnoses of, 130

O

Occupational activities, ADL adaptations for, 281
Opponens orthoses, 207–209
Orphenadrine, 345
Orthoses, 178–228
  above knee, *see* Knee-ankle-foot orthoses
  ankle-foot, *see* Ankle-foot orthoses
  below knee, *see* Ankle-foot orthoses
  construction of, 178
  fracture, 204
  hip-guidance, 202
  hip-knee-ankle-foot, *see* Hip-knee-ankle-foot orthoses
  knee, *see* Knee orthoses
  knee-ankle-foot, *see* Knee-ankle-foot orthoses
  lower limb, *see* Lower limb, orthoses for
  lumbosacral, 224–225
  mobilization, 214–219
  for pain management, 623
  patellar-tendon-bearing, 204
  pediatric, 206
  prehension, 210
  spasticity and, 463
  spinal, 219–227
  thoracolumbosacral, 223–224
  trunk-hip-knee-ankle-foot, *see* Trunk-hip-knee-ankle-foot orthoses
  upper limb, 207–219
  weight-bearing, 204
Orudis, 331
Oruvail, 331
Osteoporosis
  disuse, deconditioning and, 426
  immobilization, deconditioning and, 426
Oxaprozin, 331

Oxazepam, 364
Oxycodone, 342
Oxygen therapy, home, 679

P

Pain, *see also* specific types
  acute, 607–644, 617
  assessment of, 610–617
  behavioral assessment of, 616–617
  chronic, 607–644, 617
    biofeedback and, 144
  classification by duration, 617
  diagnostic tests for, 617
  differential diagnoses of, 105–124
  management of, 618–643
    nonpharmacologic, 622
    orthoses for, 623
    pharmacologic, 622
    physical modalities for, 623
    psychosocial techniques for, 641–642
    therapeutic exercises and, 623
  measurement tools, 611
  neuroanatomy/neurophysiology of, 607–608
  numerical rating scale, 612
  patient education and, 618
  physiologic effects of, 608–609
  psychosocial factors, 609–610
  scales of, 611–616
Pain patterns, location of, 416–422
Pain problems, nonneuromusculoskeletal, 122
Pamidronate, 380
Panwarfin, 373
Paraffin, 134
Parafon Forte, 344
Parallel bars, gait training programs and, 291
Paraplegia, differential diagnoses of, 125
Paresthesia, differential diagnoses of, 127
Patellar-tendon-bearing orthoses, 204
Patellofemoral disorder, knee orthoses for, 198–199
Patient history, *see* History
Patten-bottom orthosis, 204
Peak inspiratory flow rate, 73
Peak O_2 pulse, pulmonary ETT and, 91

Pediatrics, *see* Children
Pelvic band, 201
    belt suspension and, 247
Pelvic floor exercises, 544
Pemoline, 370
Penile prostheses, implantable, 592
Perception, evaluation of, 12
Percussion, 693
Peripheral joint
    counterstrain, 151
    manipulation/mobilization of,
        150–151
Peripheral neuromuscular facilitation,
    172
Peripheral vascular system
    evaluation of, 7
    review of systems and, 6
Persantine, 377
Personality tests, 99–100
Phantom pain, differential diagnoses of,
    107
Pharmacologic agents, 321–385
Phenothiazines, 361, 366
Phentolamine test, intravenous, 404
Phenytoin, 351
Phlebography, 40
    for venous thromboembolism, 448
Phleborrheography, 37
Photometric motion analysis system,
    53–64
Physiatric examination, 7–17
    history taking during, 4–7
Physiatric orders/referrals, 18
Physical medicine and rehabilitation,
    scope of, 3
Physical modalities, 133–155
    for pain management, 623
    spasticity and, 463
    trigger point therapy and, 415
Pindolol, 371
Placidyl, 369
Plethysmography, 36–37
    body, 75
    for venous thromboembolism, 448
PM&R, *see* Physical medicine and
    rehabilitation
Pneumonia, aspiration, dysphagia and,
    535
Pneumonitis, chemical, dysphagia and,
    535
PNF, *see* Peripheral neuromuscular
    facilitation

Polyarthritis
    acute, 122
    chronic, 122
Polyneuropathy, painful, differential
    diagnoses of, 108
Ponstel, 332
Pool therapy, 138
Porch Index of Communicative Ability,
    487
Postphlebitic syndrome, venous
    thromboembolism and, 458–459
Postural reactions, evaluation of, 15
Postvoid residual, voiding dysfunction
    and, 540
Preambulation programs, 290–291
Pregnancy, 603
Pressure ulcer, 431–444
    biochemical factors, 432
    biomechanical factors, 431–432
    classification of, 432
    conservative wound care for, 440–441
    diagnosis of, 432–434
    epidemiology of, 431
    evaluation of, 7
    medical factors, 432
    pathophysiology of, 431
    pressure-relieving devices for, 440
    prevention of, 434–438
    risk assessment scales, 434
    risk/etiologic factors, 431–432
    surgical treatment for, 441–444
        complications after, 444
        postoperative care, 443
        procedure selection, 443
    treatment of predisposing factors,
        439–444
Procaine, 384
Procan, 384
Prochlorperazine, 361, 366
Progressive resistance exercise, 163
Prolixin, 361
Propoxyphene, 342
Propranolol, 366, 371
ProSom, 367
Prostheses, 229–259
    above-elbow, 256–259
    above-knee, 242–247
    below-knee, 232–242
    disarticulation, 247–248
    elbow disarticulation, 256–259
    lower limb, 229–248
    partial-foot, 230

Syme, 231–232
transfemoral, 242–247
transhumeral, 256–259
transradial, 250–256
transtibial, 232–242
upper limb, 248–259
Proximal interphalangeal joint, pain, differential diagnoses of, 116
Proximal phalanx, pain, differential diagnoses of, 116
Psychiatric state, review of systems and, 7
Psychoimmunology, biofeedback and, 144
Psychologic tests, 99–102
Psychostimulants, 369
Psychotherapy, biofeedback and, 144
Psychotropic drugs, 353–372
Pubic pain, differential diagnoses of, 113
Pulleys, overhead, 159
Pulmonary disease/disorders
chronic, 665–707
epidemiology of, 665
etiologic classification, 668–670
evaluation of, 665–668
invasive management of, 700–706
noninvasive management of, 670–700
chronic obstructive, 668
chronic restrictive, 669–670
obstructive, 77
pharmacotherapy for, 674–679
rehabilitation modalities, 692–700
restrictive, 77–78
Pulmonary drugs, 384
Pulmonary embolism
diagnosis of, 457–458
pathophysiology of, 457
treatment of, 457–458
venous thromboembolism and, 457
Pulmonary function tests, 68–78
interpretation of, 76–78
Pulmonary mechanics, tests of, 75
PULSES profile, 95
Pyelogram, intravenous, 540
Pyelonephritis, voiding dysfunction and, 551

R

Radicular pain, differential diagnoses of, 106

Radiography
conventional, 30
plain, 23
Radionuclide bone scanning, 38–39
Ramps, 272
Range of motion
evaluation of, 10
exercises for, 158–159
limited, ADL adaptations for, 261
measurements of, 51
Rate-pressure product
cardiovascular ETT and, 82
pulmonary ETT and, 91
Raynaud's disease, biofeedback and, 144
Reading, ADL adaptations for, 268–269
Receptive deficits, 500
Reciprocal exercise unit, 159
Rectal bleeding, 579
Rectal prolapse, 579
Rectodynamics, bowel dysfunction and, 560
Reflex sympathetic dystrophy causalgia, 109–110
Reflexes
evaluation of, 15
pathologic, evaluation of, 15
segmental, evaluation of, 15
Rehabilitation, *see also* Physical medicine and rehabilitation
Relaxation exercise, 174–176
progressive muscle, 176
Relaxation strategies
autogenic, 176
cognitive, 176
controlled-breathing, 175–176
physiologic, 175–176
Renal scans, 40
Renal ultrasound, voiding dysfunction and, 540
Resistance training, 162
Respiratory quotient, pulmonary ETT and, 92
Respiratory system, review of systems and, 6
Restoril, 367
Review of systems, 6–7
Rheumatic problems, soft tissue, crystal-associated, 110–111
Rheumatoid factors, 24
Rheumatologic disorders
dysphagia and, 524
muscle weakness and, 124

Rhizotomy, spasticity and, 473–474
Ritalin, 370
Robaxin, 345
RSD, *see* Reflex sympathetic dystrophy

S

Salicylates, nonacetylated, 330
Salsalate, 330
Scapular pain, differential diagnoses of, 114
Scintiscanning, thyroid radioisotope, 40
Scooters, 319–320
Seattle foot, 234
Secretion removal techniques, 692
Sedative-hypnotics, 366–369
  nonbenzodiazepine, 368–369
Sedatives, pain management and, 637
Seizures, differential diagnoses of, 129
Sensation, decreased, ADL adaptations for, 261
Sensory evaluation, 14
Sepsis, differential diagnoses of, 128
Serax, 364
Serum protein electrophoresis, 23
Serzone, 360
Sexual dysfunction, 580
  classification of, 588–595
  diagnostic tests for, 586–588
  erectile dysfunction, 588
  laboratories tests for, 586
  management of, 588–595
  psychosocial, 594–595
  questionnaire assessments, 588
Sexual expression, ADL adaptations for, 269
Sexual rehabilitation counseling, 595–597
Sexual response
  assessment of, 583–586
  neurophysiology of, 581–583
Sexuality, problems in, 580–606
Shoes, 179–186
  heel modifications, 183–185
    internal, 186
  modifications to, 183–186
    internal, 186
  sole modifications, external, 185–186
Shopping, ADL adaptations for, 276
Shoulder, abduction stabilizer, 218

Shoulder pain, differential diagnoses of, 114
Shoulder sling, 218
Silesian belt, 201, 247
Sinequan, 357, 366
Single photon emission computed tomography, 40
Skelaxin, 345
Skin
  deconditioning and, 428
  evaluation of, 7
  review of systems and, 6
Skull, radiography of, 30–31
Smoking cessation, 670
Socket, transtibial, 236–238
Sockets, transfemoral, 243–244
Soft tissue injections, *see* Joint injections
Soma, 344
Spasm Frequency Score, 461
Spasticity, 460–481
  assessment scales for, 461
  care for, 462–480
  clinical evaluation of, 460
  cordectomy for, 480
  cordotomy for, 480
  exercise program for, 463
  functional evaluation of, 462
  myelotomy for, 480
  orthopedic surgery for, 474–480
  pathophysiology of, 460
  patient education for, 462
  peripheral neurectomy for, 480
  physical examination of, 460–461
  physical modalities for, 463
  positioning and handling and, 463
  qualitative/quantitative assessment of, 461
  rhizotomy and, 473–474
Speech, *see also* Language
  evaluation of, 12
Speech disorders, 503–508
  apraxia of speech, 503–505
Speech therapy, for aphasia, 495
Speed training, 174
Sphincterotomy, 550
Spinal blocks, 402–403
Spinal cord, disease of, 127
Spinal manipulation, 148–151
Spinal traction, 145–148
Spine
  corsets for, 227
  evaluation of, 7

orthoses for, 219–227
radiography of, 30
range of motion measurement of, 53
Spirometry, 68–75
indirect techniques for, 74–75
Splints, spasticity and, 463
Sports medicine, biofeedback and, 144
Stabilizers, mechanical, 242
Stairs, ADL adaptations for, 272
Stanford-Binet Intelligence Test, 100
Stelazine, 366
Stellate ganglion, sympathetic blocks, 408
Sterile needles, 389
Stiff-man syndrome, involuntary movement disorders and, 127
Stones, voiding dysfunction and, 551
Stored Energy foot, 234
Strengthening, *see* Muscle strengthening exercises
Strengthening exercise, for dysphagia, 532–533
Stretching, passive, 159–160
Stroke patients, motor relearning program and, 173–174
Strong Interest Inventory, 100
Strong Vocational Interest Blank, 100
Stuttering, 509
Sulindac, 330
Suspension, 159
Suspension mechanisms, transfemoral, 244–247
Suspensions, transtibial, 238–242
Swallowing studies, 518–523
Swanson postarthroplasty orthoses, 216
Swedish knee cage, 199
Syme prostheses, 231–232
Sympathetically maintained pain, differential diagnoses of, 107–109
Synovial fluid, 27
biopsy of, 28
Systems, review of, 6

T

Tai chi chuan, 176
Tape measures, 53
Task-oriented approach, motor control and, 174
Tegretol, 352

Temazepam, 367
Tendon injections, 397–399
Tendon reflexes, evaluation of, 15
TENS, *see* Transcutaneous electrical nerve stimulation
Terminal devices, 250–251
Tetraplegia, differential diagnoses of, 125
Therapeutic exercise, 156–177
active inhibition, 160–161
continuous passive movement machine and, 159
for dysphagia, 531–532
for pain management, 623
passive stretching and, 159–160
spasticity and, 463
strengthening, 161–165, *see also* Muscle strengthening exercises
trigger point therapy and, 414
Thermography, 37
Thigh pain, differential diagnoses of, 116–117
Thiopental test, intravenous, 403
Thoracolumbosacral orthoses, 223–224
Thorax, evaluation of, 7
Thorazine, 361
Thumb pain, differential diagnoses of, 116
Thyroid function testing, 23
Tibial fracture, orthosis for, 204
Ticlid, 377
Ticlopidine, 377
Tidal volume, pulmonary ETT and, 92
Timed walking test, 93
Tizanidine, spasticity and, 465
Tocalnamide, 384
Toe pain, differential diagnoses of, 120
Tofranil, 357
Toileting, ADL adaptations for, 268
Tolectin, 332
Tolmetin, 332
Tonocard, 384
Tone-reduction orthoses, 213
Toradol, 332
Tracheal intubation, 700
Tracheostomy, for dysphagia, 534
Tracheostomy tube, 701
Trager psychophysical integration, 176
Tramadol, 321–322
Trancopal, 366
Transcutaneous electrical nerve stimulation, 142–144

Transfemoral socket, 243–244
Transfers
    ADL adaptations for, 262–264
    depression, 263
    lift, 263
    sliding board, 263
    stand-pivot, 263
Transtibial socket, 236
Tranxene, 365
Trazodone, 360, 369
Treadmill, cardiovascular exercise
    tolerance testing and, 84–86
Tremor, 127
Triazolam, 367
Trifluoperazine, 366
Trigger point therapy, 411–422
    injections and, 412
        postinjection care, 414
        techniques for, 412–413
    noninjection, 414–415
Trigger points, location of, 416–422
Trigger thumb, tendon injections and,
    399
Trilisate, 330
Trunk-hip-knee-ankle-foot orthoses,
    202–204
Tubigrip gloves, 214
Tumbocor, 384
Tumescence constriction therapy, 589
Tylenol, with codeine, 342
Typing, ADL adaptations for, 268–269

U

Ulcer, pressure, *see* Pressure ulcer
Ultram, *see* Tramadol
Ultrasonography, diagnostic, 33–36
Ultrasound, 134–135
Ultraviolet radiation, 138–139
Upper extremity pain, differential
    diagnoses of, 114
Upper limb, orthoses for, 206–219
Upper limb prosthesis, 248–259
Uric acid serum, 27
Urinalysis, voiding dysfunction and, 540
Urinary incontinence, biofeedback and,
    144
Urinary tract infection
    spasticity and, 462
    voiding dysfunction and, 550–551

Urine collection devices, 544–545
Urodynamics, voiding dysfunction and,
    541
Urography, excretory, 41
Urologic history, 539
US, *see* Ultrasonography
Utensil holders, 210
Utensils, ADL adaptations for, 264

V

Valium, 345, 365
    spasticity and, 464
Valproic acid, 352
Valsalva's maneuver, 544
Vapocoolant spray, trigger point therapy
    and, 414
Venlafaxine, 360
Venography
    radionuclide, 40
    for venous thromboembolism, 448
Venous duplex scanning, for venous
    thromboembolism, 447
Venous thromboembolism, 445–459
    anticoagulation therapy for, 455
    clinical evaluation of, 446–447
    complications of, 457–458
    deconditioning and, 428
    diagnosis of, 446–449
    diagnostic tests for, 447–449
    epidemiology of, 446
    Greenfield filter for, 455
    inferior vena caval filter for, 455
    laboratory work-up for, 449
    management of, 455
    pathophysiology of, 445
    pharmacologic agents for, 452–455
    postphlebitic syndrome and, 458–459
    prophylaxis for, 449–455
    recurrence of, 458
    surveillance of, 455
    thrombolytic therapy for, 456
Ventilation
    mechanical, 682
    tests of, 68–75
Ventilatory equivalent, pulmonary ETT
    and, 92
Vertigo, differential diagnoses of, 130
Vesicoureteral reflux, voiding
    dysfunction and, 551

Vibroejaculation, 598
Vision, limited, ADL adaptations for, 261
Visken, 371
Vistaril, 366, 372
Visual analog scale, 461
    pain and, 611
Visualization, dissociative, 176
Vital signs, physical examination and, 7
Vitamin D, 380, 381
Vocational training, 663
Voice disorders, 508–509
    assessment of, 508
    speaking options, 509
Voiding, neuroanatomy/neurophysiology of, 538–539
Voiding cystourethrography, voiding dysfunction and, 540
Voiding dysfunction, 538–552
    classification of, 542
    complications of, 550–552
    diagnostic tests for, 540–542
    evaluation of, 539–542
    invasive procedures for, 548–550
    pharmacologic agents for, 545–548
    physical examination for, 539
    treatment of, 542–550
        behavioral management, 542–544
        bladder training, 542
Voltaren, 331
Voluntary ventilation, maximum, 74

W

Walkers, 283–286
    gait patterns with, 289
Warfarin, 373
Wechsler Adult Intelligence Scale, revised, 100
Weight training, circuit, 164
Wellbutrin, 360
Western Aphasia Battery, 487
Western blotting, for Lyme disease, 27
Wheelchairs
    attendant-propelled, 315–316
    manual, 293–315
        camber, 297
        checkout and training, 294
        classification by user needs, 312–315
        complications of, 293

contraindications to, 293
downhill-turning tendency, 296
dynamic stability of, 296
frames for, 297–300
head and neck support, 307
lower limb support, 310–311
maneuverability, 296
parts and subtypes of, 297–312
pitch-axis control, 296
proper seating and positioning goals, 294
propulsion efficiency, 296
propulsion of, 300–304
rolling resistance and, 296
safety components, 311–312
seating prescriptions for, 293–294
seating systems in, 304–307
side-slope effect, 296
static stability of, 297
trunk support systems, 307–308
upper limb support, 308–310
weight/portability, 297
yaw-axis control, 296
    mechanical lifts for, 272
    powered, 316–320
        battery systems for, 318–319
        contraindications to, 316–317
        control systems for, 318
        electric carts and, 319–320
        indications for, 316
        potential benefits of, 316
        potential disadvantages of, 316
        power-drive systems for, 317–318
        prescription guidelines for, 317
        user requirements for, 316
Whirlpools, 137–138
Wide-range Achievement Test, revised, 100
Woodcock-Johnson Psycho-educational Battery-revised, 100
Word discrimination test, 510
Work assessment, 60
Work rehabilitation, 656–664
Workload, exercise tolerance testing and, 82
Work-related musculoskeletal problems, 645–664
    Americans with Disabilities Act of 1990 and, 645–646
    costs of, 645–646
    epidemiology of, 645
    return to work issues, 646
    work assessment and, 648

Work-related testing, 51–67
Worksite evaluations, 651
Wrist
  orthoses for, 207–219
  prostheses for, 248–259
Wrist pain, differential diagnoses of, 115
Writing, ADL adaptations for, 268–269

X

Xanax, 365
Xylocaine, 384

Y

Yale cervicothoracic orthosis, 222
Yoga, 176

Z

Zanaflex, spasticity and, 465
Zinovieff's Oxford technique, 163
Zolpidem, 368
Zung Self-rating Depression Scale, 101